Edition 3

Functional Performance in Older Adults

Bette R. Bonder,
PhD, OTR/L, FAOTA
Professor, Depts. of Health Sciences and Psychology
Dean, College of Science
Cleveland State University

Vanina Dal Bello-Haas,
PhD, MEd, BSc(PT)
Associate Professor
School of Physical Therapy
University of Saskatchewan

 F A Davis Company • Philadelphia

F. A. Davis Company
1915 Arch Street
Philadelphia, PA 19103
www.fadavis.com

Printed in the United States of America

Last digit indicates print number: 10 9 8 7 6 5 4 3 2

Senior Acquisitions Editor: Christa Fratantoro
Manager of Content Development: George W. Lang
Developmental Editor: Peg Waltner
Art and Design Manager: Carolyn O'Brien

As new scientific information becomes available through basic and clinical research, recommended treatments and drug therapies undergo changes. The author(s) and publisher have done everything possible to make this book accurate, up to date, and in accord with accepted standards at the time of publication. The author(s), editors, and publisher are not responsible for errors or omissions or for consequences from application of the book, and make no warranty, expressed or implied, in regard to the contents of the book. Any practice described in this book should be applied by the reader in accordance with professional standards of care used in regard to the unique circumstances that may apply in each situation. The reader is advised always to check product information (package inserts) for changes and new information regarding dose and contraindications before administering any drug. Caution is especially urged when using new or infrequently ordered drugs.

Library of Congress Cataloging-in-Publication Data

Functional performance in older adults/[edited by] Bette R. Bonder, Vanina Dal Bello-Haas.—3rd ed.
   p. ; cm.
Includes bibliographical references and index.
ISBN-13: 978-0-8036-1688-2
ISBN-10: 0-8036-1688-0
1. Older people—Rehabilitation. 2. Aging. I. Bonder, Bette. II. Dal Bello-Haas, Vanina.
[DNLM: 1. Aging—physiology. 2. Aged. 3. Health Promotion. 4. Health Services for the Aged. 5. Mental Disorders. WT 104 F9789 2009]
RC953.5.F86 2009
612.6'7—dc22

                                                                                    2008034206

In loving memory of our friend and colleague,
Marilyn (Lynne) B. Wagner

B.R.B. and V.D.B.H.

FOREWORD

Question: How do health professionals help older adults live long past the "usual date of disintegration" so that they can retain the activities and roles that support their interests, curiosity, and happiness?

Answer: By understanding the process of aging, the theories that guide our interventions, how disease and injury can threaten the daily experiences of life, how to support the activities that make participation possible, how to build services, and context that supports the older individuals as they seek to live lives with meaning, purpose, and growth.

In the 3rd Edition of *Functional Performance in Older Adults,* Drs. Bonder and Dal Bello-Haas have authored and edited a volume that will provide the health professional with the concepts, theories, knowledge, and tools to use best practices and evidence as they design and provide services for our nations aging population. Congratulations to them for gaining the commitment for this project from people who are leaders in the field of aging. Each chapter is an elegant essay that offers a contemporary review of the literature and engages the reader in a greater understanding of the importance of employing this knowledge to address the needs of individuals, communities, and society.

The chapters reviewing the impact of normal aging give context to our increased understanding of the intrinsic determinants (cardiovascular, pulmonary, sensory, neuro-musculoskeletal, and mental function) that must be considered in determining the capabilities of the older adult. The major issues that threaten performance (falls, dementia, and depression) are covered in essays that call our attention to critical points requiring prevention. The activities central to self maintenance and plasticity (self-care, leisure, work and retirement, community mobility, interactions and relationships, and sexuality) are carefully put into a contemporary context. The section on service delivery stresses evaluation, wellness and health promotion, and community-based as well as home health, rehabilitation, and long-term care; all written to foster care to maximize the performance and the experiences of older adults who need services. The last section gives context that can be enabling (culture and aging, and products and technology), that can help practitioners recognize and manage an issue that requires our attention (elder abuse), and that highlights a very important aspect to our care and the needs of people and their families—end-of-life care. Each of these chapters has been written by scientists and clinicians that dedicate their work to enabling participation in the elderly. They are superbly written, conceptually linked, and strongly referenced, which makes this an excellent book to use with students who will be providing care to the largest population of older adults in the history of the world.

Our nations' elderly deserve care from knowledgeable practitioners. The body of knowledge exists to support excellence in the delivery of services. It is our individual and collective responsibility to shape the care that our elderly will receive. Policy makers and a dministrators of health and community services are looking for ways to meet the needs of a growing population of older adults. Let's help them design the services and systems. This wonderful book gives us the tools.

Carolyn Baum, PhD, OTR/L, FAOTA
St. Louis, Missouri
June, 2007

For age is opportunity no less
Than youth itself, though in another dress,
And as the evening twilight fades away
The sky is filled with stars, invisible by day.
—Henry Wadsworth Longfellow

This book considers what it means to grow old. Specifically, it examines what it is that older individuals want to do, need to do, what facilitates accomplishment of those tasks, and what interferes. These are not simple matters. Philosophers, scientists, novelists, and religious leaders have examined them for generations and debate continues to this day about what constitutes a satisfying later life.

Perhaps a reason for the continuing discussion is the fact that aging is such a complex phenomenon. Personal experience and characteristics, biological factors, culture, historical events, and context all influence later life for a particular individual. Theory and research have typically focused on describing groups, an approach that explains a great deal about aging in general but little about the experience for a particular person. Recent advances in our understanding of individuals' unique development in later life can be attributed to the growing interest in qualitative research that emphasizes description of perceptions and experiences in depth and detail.

While researchers struggle to find the best strategies for explaining later life, health-care providers are concerned primarily with individuals; thus, they focus on research that can guide their practice and describe the best possible intervention strategies. Although there is increasing attention being paid to population-based interventions such as careful community planning, and to public policy that affects older adults and their families, for most care professionals, the focus is on maximizing well-being for each client.

Of course, well-being is also a complex phenomenon. Rowe and Kahn (1998) popularized the concept of **successful aging,** which they distinguish from usual (or typical) and unsuccessful aging. They suggested that avoiding disease, maintaining health, and engaging in meaningful activities are the three main elements of successful aging. However, as will be seen in the pages of this volume, critics contend that the factors Rowe and Kahn identified as the main elements for successful aging are incomplete or even inaccurate. After all, while there are strategies that elders can pursue to avoid disease, most will at some point develop one or more chronic or acute diseases. And clearly many elders who have various health or functional problems find ways to pursue the meaningful occupations that promote positive quality of life. Occupational therapists would argue that regardless of physical status, the ability to pursue these occupations would be a measure of success at any stage of life.

Every health profession that provides care to elders has its own focus in the broader context of promoting successful aging and quality of life. Some, medical professionals, for example, emphasize preventing or treating biological disease; others, like physical therapists, emphasize enhancing physical capacity. Occupational therapists focus on promoting engagement in meaningful occupation. For all these professions, adequate care for the individual requires an understanding of the societal and physical environment in which care is provided, and the characteristics and needs of the service recipient from a historical, cultural, biological, and social perspective. In addition, health-care providers must understand the unique combination of these factors that make up the individual person.

This book is designed to provide both foundational information about aging and concrete strategies for supporting successful aging. It describes optimal aging, the normal aging process, and the factors that can interfere with normal aging. The material is presented from the perspective of functional performance of everyday activities, taking the stance that it is accomplishment of these activities that defines well-being and life satisfaction for older adults, and that "we who are interested in reducing the risk to elders of unproductive aging need to concentrate our attention and our efforts on enhancing the opportunities for older persons" (Grams & Albee, 1995, p. 13). It is inevitable that every older adult will experience some degree of physical or cognitive decline, but it is not a given that this will lead to a commensurate decline in function. Further, if function does decline in a particular area, substitution of new occupations may serve to ensure satisfaction of personal meanings and values in life.

The book is divided into five main parts. The first provides a demographic, historical, and theoretical context for understanding the aging process. In doing so, it reviews biological theories as well as psychosocial theories of aging, and emphasizes understanding of the importance of occupational engagement in later life.

Part 2 focuses on normal aging and interruptions in normal aging that can impede engagement in occupation. The chapters are organized based on the American Occupational Therapy Association's *Practice Framework* (2002), a model that is based on a hierarchy of factors contributing to occupational performance. Section 1, Chapters 4 through 7, focuses on normal age-related change in body functions and body structures. These changes occur to some degree for every elder, although as these chapters make clear, there is considerable individual variation. In spite of these individual differences, the aging process does have a somewhat predictable sequence, with some decrements in function more likely to occur earlier than others and some functions more likely to remain intact, or even to improve over time. These chapters also consider the ways in which the aging process can, at some point almost certainly will, lead to some deterioration of function. Most elders experience periodic abrupt or severe personal, social, or environmental losses.

There are some predictable factors that can lead to sudden major performance decrements. Loss of a spouse can precipitate a debilitating depression that might interfere with accomplishment or even identification of desired activities. Ice on the sidewalk can cause a fall that might have devastating effects for an older adult. Section 2, Chapters 8 through 10, describes common kinds of dysfunction that may signal the beginning of a downward spiral of functional loss. These three chapters are not meant to be an exhaustive survey of medical conditions; rather, they have been chosen to typify common musculoskeletal (falls/fractures), psychosocial (depression), and cognitive (dementia) problems that interfere with function. It is important to recognize that elders are affected by all the diseases and disabilities that affect younger individuals, and that they may also have to deal with the long-term consequences of such disorders as diabetes that may have emerged in earlier life. These issues are addressed in subsequent chapters.

Part 3, Chapters 11 through 16, considers activities and participation, with an emphasis on how typical elders engage in various kinds of occupations and the normal developmental challenges occupations can present as people age. There is also discussion about what health-care providers, particularly occupational therapists, can do to prevent or minimize dysfunction. It reviews theoretical issues related to aging, the meaning of activity, and our current understanding of the biological and psychosocial processes that influence various aspects of participation.

Part 4, Chapters 17 through 22, focuses on provision of care from the perspective of various health-care systems. Because most health care in the United States is paid by third-parties, therapists must understand the systems in which they work to ensure they provide the best possible care in the specific environment, and work to change systems that are unfair or inadequate. In these chapters, information is presented about the kinds of functional problems most often seen in each setting, strategies for assessing functional abilities and deficits, and for intervening to maximize older adults' ability to engage in the occupations that matter most to them.

The last part of the book, Chapters 23 through 26, presents several special issues. These include the interaction of culture with individual and community experiences of later life; the impact of emerging technologies on functional performance for older adults; and the issue, all too common in the United States, of elder abuse. Finally, the unavoidable issue of loss is addressed. Occupational therapists and other health professionals are increasingly involved in supporting elders and their families at the very end of life. Effective intervention can assist individuals as they cope with this final life task.

More and more individuals are spending longer and longer periods in the later stages of life. Quality of life and functional ability are crucial considerations. It is in everyone's best interests to understand the process and develop effective mechanisms for maximizing well-being. Our ability to accomplish this is, of course, a "work in progress." As the elderly population increases, more attention is being paid to its circumstances. New information emerges daily that increases our ability to provide high-quality service. It is our hope that this volume will generate new questions, the answers to which may further enhance our ability to assist older adults in leading meaningful and satisfying lives.

References

American Occupational Therapy Association (AOTA) (2002). Occupational therapy practice framework: Domain and process. *American Journal of Occupational Therapy, 56,* 609–639.

Grams, A., & Albee, G. W. (1995). Primary prevention in the service of aging (pp. 5–33). In L. A. Bond, S. J. Cutler, & A. Grams (Eds.), *Promoting successful and productive aging.* Thousand Oaks, CA: Sage.

Rowe, J. W., & Kahn, R. L. (1998). *Successful aging.* New York: Random House.

ACKNOWLEDGMENTS

A project like this one is complex and challenging and requires help from a vast array of individuals. We would like to thank the many older adults and their families who have shared their lives and their stories with us. We also thank the many professionals from whom we have learned about strategies for improving quality of life for elders.

Many of the chapter authors in this book have been with us from the beginning, and we greatly appreciate their contributions. Thank you to the authors who are new to this edition. The reviewers have provided invaluable insight and advice as this book was developed. We appreciate their thoughtfulness and thoroughness.

A large team was assembled at F.A. Davis. Christa Fratantoro served as senior acquisitions editor, ably aided by Elizabeth Zygarewicz. Peg Waltner, developmental editor, spent many hours getting the chapters formatted and making sure the materials were user-friendly. The production team included: David Orzechowski, managing editor, Bob Butler, production manager, Carolyn O'Brien, art and design manager, and Linda Kern at PPA.

Special thanks to our "on the scene" assistants: Tasha Thornhill, School of Physical Therapy (Class of 2008), University of Saskatchewan.

And last, but certainly not least, we thank our families. Tom Haas and Pat, Aaron, and Jordan Bray were patient when we weren't available for other tasks, and were supportive during the lengthy writing and editing process.

CONTRIBUTORS

Georgia J. Anetzberger, PhD, ACSW
Assistant Professor
Health Care Administration Program
Cleveland State University
Cleveland, OH

Ben Atchison, PhD, OTR, FAOTA
Professor
Department of Occupational Therapy
Western Michigan University
Kalamazoo, MI

Patrick Baker, MSHS, CDRS, OTR/L
Clinical Specialist
The Cleveland Clinic
Cleveland, OH

Vern Bengtson, PhD
Chair and Professor
University of Southern California
Davis School of Gerontology
Ethel Percy Andrus Gerontology Center
Los Angeles, CA

Anita Bundy, ScD, OTR, FAOTA
Professor and Chair of Occupational Therapy
Faculty of Health Sciences
The University of Sydney
Lidcombe, Australia

Rosalind Bye, PhD, MAppSc(OT), BAppSc(OT)
Senior Lecturer in Occupational Therapy
School of Biomedical and Health Sciences
College of Health and Science
University of Western Sydney
Penrith South, Australia

Cameron Camp
Director of Research and Product Development
Hearthstone Alzheimer Care
Woburn, MA

Boin Chang, M.A.
Doctoral Candidate
Industrial/Organizational Psychology
The University of Akron
Akron, OH

Charles Christiansen, EdD/L
College of Health Sciences
University of Texas Medical Branch
Galveston, TX

Lindy M. Clemson, PhD
Sesquicentenary Senior Research Fellow
and Senior Lecturer
Faculty of Health Sciences
The University of Sydney
Lidcombe, Australia

Elizabeth Dean, PhD, PT
Professor
Department of Physical Therapy
Faculty of Medicine
University of British Columbia
Vancouver, Canada

Armele D. De Andrade
Universidad Federal de Pernambuco
Recife, PE, Brazil

Vanina Dal Bello-Haas, PhD, PT
Associate Professor
School of Physical Therapy
University of Saskatchewan
Saskatoon, Canada

Karl Christl, BAppSc(PT), LLB(Hons)
Consultant Aged Care Physiotherapist
Company Director
Christl, Bye & Associates Pty Ltd
Aged Care Physiotherapy Services

Susan E. Doble, PhD, OTReg (NS)
Associate Professor
School of Occupational Therapy
Dalhousie University
Halifax, Nova Scotia, Canada

Beth A. Ekelman, JD, OTR/L
Director and Associate Professor
Department of Health Sciences
Cleveland State University
Cleveland, OH

Kristine Haertl, PhD, OTR/L
Associate Professor
Occupational Science and Occupational Therapy
College of St. Catherine
St. Paul, MN

Eric Hicks, MS, OTR/L
Doctoral Candidate and Research Assistant
Department of Occupational Therapy
Public Health & Health Professions
University of Florida
Gainesville, FL

Celia R. Hooper, PhD
Professor and Dean
School of Health and Human Performance
University of North Carolina Greensboro
Greensboro, NC

Greta A. Lax, M.S.
Doctoral Candidate
Industrial/Organizational Psychology
The University of Akron
Akron, OH

Lori Letts, PhD
Associate Professor
McMaster University
School of Rehabilitation Science
Hamilton, Ontario, Canada

**Gwynnyth Llewellyn, PhD, Med, BA,
Grad Dip ContEd, Dip OT**
Professor and Dean
Faculty of Health Sciences
University of Sydney
Lidcombe, Australia

William C. Mann, OTR, PhD
Distinguished Professor and Chair
Department of Occupational Therapy & PhD
Program in Rehabilitation Science
University of Florida
Gainesville, FL

**Andrew Miracle, PhD (deceased) and
Tina Miracle**
Fort Worth, TX

Steven Mitchell, OTR/L, ATP
SCI Occupational Therapy Supervisor
Louis Stokes Cleveland Department of
Veterans Affairs Medical Center
Cleveland, OH

Pam O'Dell-Rossi, MPA, OT
Coordinator
Occupational Therapy Education
The Cleveland Clinic
Cleveland, OH

Ruth E. Plautz, OTR/L, MHS
Director of Rehabilitation
Menorah Park Center for Senior Living
Beachwood, OH

Julie Richardson, PhD
Associate Professor
McMaster University
School of Rehabilitation Science
Institute of Applied Health Sciences
Hamilton, Ontario, Canada

Kathryn Perez Riley, PhD
Associate Professor
Department of Preventive Medicine
School of Public Health
University of Kentucky
Lexington, KY

Lauren Robinson
University of Texas Medical Branch
Galveston, TX

Marjorie E. Scaffa, PhD, OTR/L, FAOTA
Professor
Department of Occupational Therapy
University of South Alabama
Mobile, AL

Wendy Stav, PhD, OTR/L, SCDCM
Assistant Professor
Towson University
Towson, MD

Harvey Sterns, PhD
Professor of Psychology
Director and Senior Fellow
Institute of Life-Span Development and
Gerontology
The University of Akron
Research Professor of Gerontology
Northeastern Ohio Universities College of
Medicine and Pharmacy
Akron, OH

Rein Tideiksaar, PhD
President
FallPrevent, LLC
Blackwood, NJ

**Joyce Tryssenaar, PhD, BScOT, OT
Reg (Ont.)**
Associate Professor
School of Rehabilitation Science
McMaster University
Hamilton, Ontario, Canada

Seanne Wilkins, PhD
Associate Professor
McMaster University
School of Rehabilitation Science
Institute of Applied Health Sciences
Hamilton, Ontario, Canada

REVIEWERS

Jane Painter, EdD, OTR/L
Associate Professor
Occupational Therapy
East Carolina University
Greenville, NC

Lois J. Ricci, RN, GNP, EdD
Education Coordinator
Geriatric Medicine
Emory University
Atlanta, GA

Rhonda K. Stanley, PT, PhD
Associate Professor
Physical Therapy
Univerity of Texas
El Paso, TX

Sharon Stoffel, MA, OTR/L, FAOTA
Associate Professor
Occupational Therapy & Occupational Science
College of St. Catherine
St, Paul, MN

Ronald G. Stone, MS, OTR/L
Associate Professor
Occupational Therapy
University of Puget Sound
Tacoma, WA

Pamela E. Toto, MS, OTR/L, BCG, FAOTA
Occupational Therapist, Adjunct Faculty
Occupational Therapy
University of Pittsburgh
Pittsburgh, PA

Manon Tremblay
Director
Occupational Therapy
University of Ottawa
Ottawa, Canada

Stephanie J. D. Wong, MS, PT, OTR
Assistant Professor
Occupational Therapy
Touro College
Bay Shore, NY

CONTENTS

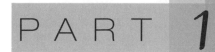

PART 1

Introduction

T he data about the aging population are reported in some detail in the pages of this volume. Life expectancy increased dramatically in the United States and elsewhere during the twentieth century (United Nations Secretariat, 1998). This increase is associated with reductions in deaths from infectious diseases like polio and measles (Riley, 2001), as well as improved health promotion habits including healthful eating, smoking cessation, and the use of seat belts. However, as we enter the 21st century, some populations face a decrease in life expectancy as a result of poor health habits associated with increases in chronic diseases like diabetes. Projecting demographic trends is tricky, although there is growing evidence for both increased longevity and compression of morbidity and mortality—that is, increased **active life expectancy** (Mor, 2005; Velkoff, He, Sengupta, & DeBarros, 2006)

The vast majority of older adults live in the community and adapt well to the changes that are an inevitable part of the aging process. Individuals find ways to compensate for the typical graduate decrements in physical and cognitive skills that accompany aging. Many older adults are adaptive, and when necessary, creative in finding ways to continue meaningful occupations. Furthermore, changes are not all negative. Individuals may have to adjust to reduced vision or hearing, but they also have increased life experience and knowledge that can help them cope. For example, as noted in this book, although older adults may learn differently than younger people, they are still quite capable of acquiring new skills and abilities, and may offer valuable insights and observations to younger people as well.

Part I of this book provides an overview of the aging experience and an introduction to biological and psychosocial theories of aging. In addition, it explores the meanings of occupation in later life. These chapters offer a context in which the experience of growing old can be understood. To ensure the best care, providers must understand the individual, including his or her history, needs, and wishes. It is essential to think of the individual in context, not as separate from life experiences and community. This section of the book is designed to provide an understanding of the context in which aging occurs, and the experiences of individuals and populations as they age.

Mor, V. (2005). The compression of morbidity hypothesis: A review of research and prospects for the future. *Journal of the American Geriatrics Society, 53*, S308–S309.

Riley, J. S. (2001). *Rising life expectancy: A global history*. New York: Cambridge University Press.

United Nations Secretariat: Department of Economic and Social Affairs. (1998). *World population prospects, the 1998 revision, Volume II: Sex and Age*. New York: Author.

Velkoff, V. A., He, W., Sengupta, M., & DeBarros, K. A. (2006). *65+ in the United States: 2005*. Washington, DC: U.S. Census Bureau.

CHAPTER 1

Growing Old in Today's World

Bette R. Bonder

"*The great thing about getting older is that you don't lose all the other ages you've been*"

Madeleine L'Engle

OBJECTIVES

By the end of this chapter, readers will be able to:

1. Discuss the problems in defining old age and provide a current definition.
2. Describe historical definitions of aging and identify reasons for increased longevity in modern times.
3. Identify demographic characteristics, including age, education, gender, and ethnicity, of older adults in the United States and globally.
4. Discuss how these demographic characteristics affect the experience of aging.
5. Analyze the effect of place of residence on the experience of aging.
6. Identify the impact of cohort effects and individual differences on the experience of aging.
7. Describe the interaction of public policy with the experience of aging.
8. Define successful aging and list its three components.
9. Discuss the importance of these factors to the health-care provider working with older adults.

Methuselah lived 969 years (Genesis 5:27). So goes the story in the Old Testament. Even though everyone would agree that 969 is old, this is one of the few certainties in discussions of old age. In some cultures, and at some times in history, individuals who survived to age 40 were considered old. More recently, longevity has increased so that the age at which one is viewed as "elderly" is considerably later in life (although no one in recent times has made it to 969).

Understanding what happens in later life has become increasingly important because of the rapid change in demographics worldwide. "Our global population is aging, and aging at an unprecedented rate" (Kinsella & Velkoff, 2001, p. 8). This demographic trend is the result of such factors as reductions in infant mortality and death due to infectious disease, as well as improved health care throughout the life span. And while this aging of the population is

4 PART 1 Introduction

typically associated with developed countries, it holds true in most of the developing world as well (*World Population Prospects*, 2003).

This rapid change has uncertain consequences for both individuals and societies. It may be that older adults are functional and healthy for a longer period, with compression of morbidity and mortality, or it may be that there is an expanding period of dysfunction as life is extended (Olshansky & Carnes, 2001). Although it remains to be established categorically, current research suggests that the former is accurate (Waidmann & Liu, 2000). However, in 1997, more than half of elders reported at least one disability that interfered with function; a third reported that they had at least one serious disability (Administration on Aging, 2004). And by age 80, three-quarters reported at least one disability. Fifty percent reported a serious disability.

Social circumstances are also uncertain; the costs associated with an aging population, for example in terms of retirement funding, availability of skilled workers, and health-care costs late in life have received considerable attention in the literature. However, there is less than absolute consensus about how these issues will develop over time. For example, a recent report from the U.S. Census Bureau (Velkoff, He, Sengupta, & DeBarros, 2006) suggests that individuals in the United States turning 60 in 2005 were healthier, better educated, and more financially stable than the previous cohort. Thus, they are expected to age more successfully than previous generations. This suggests that even though the demography of the developed world will be dramatically affected by the aging of the "baby boom" generation that will begin to turn 65 in 2011 (Weiss, 2003), some of the concerns may be overstated. Pessimistic projections suggest that the large population of elders will place an undue financial and social burden on younger individuals. More optimistic projections suggest that elders will be a source of significant support for younger individuals and that they will continue to contribute to society in meaningful ways. The one certainty is that around the world there will be more older individuals in the next several decades, both in absolute numbers and as a percentage of the population (*World Population Prospects*, 2003).

Changing definitions of aging and differing perceptions of the aging process contribute to confusion about appropriate performance or expected roles and activities of older adults. The concept of **successful aging** (Rowe & Kahn, 1998) has received increasing attention as demographic trends place more pressure on social and health-care agencies. The evolution of the United States from a primarily agricultural society to a primarily industrial society and now to a technological society has changed the experience of aging. Retirement is a recent development; in earlier times, people rarely lived long enough to retire, and those who lived to old age often had ongoing responsibilities. A historical and cultural context for understanding the aging process is important because, as Achenbaum and Sterns (1978) noted, "We cannot discuss old age without some sense of trend, of where we are coming from and where we are heading" (p. 307).

Factors such as gender, economic situation, and societal perceptions affect the health-care providers' beliefs and actions in working with elders, as well as those of the client. There is evidence that stereotypes of aging contribute to relatively pervasive, if increasingly subtle, ageism (Palmore, 2005). This extends to the views care providers hold about older adults' abilities to benefit from care (c.f. Harrington, Collier, & Burdin, 2005; Shipp, 2005), meaning that providers must understand their own beliefs about aging and about the clients being served to ensure that personal biases do not negatively impact care for the client.

This chapter provides an overview of some of the many factors that affect an individual's experience of growing old. The first section focuses on historical perspectives on aging. A current definition of aging is provided. Then the effects of gender, place of residence, socioeconomic status, cohort, and individual history are considered. The interrelationships among perceptions of aging, public policy, and experience of aging are examined, as are concepts of successful, usual, and pathological aging. Finally, the implications of these interrelated factors for care provider are discussed. Box 1-1 lists these factors.

BOX 1-1 Factors Affecting the Experience of Aging

- Gender
- Roles
- Cohort effects
- Cultural factors
- Place of residence
- Social attitudes
- Individual characteristics and experiences
- Socioeconomic factors
- Public policy

History of Aging

What do we mean by old age? Who is elderly? The definition of old age has not been static over time. First, there is the basic issue of longevity. In very early civilizations, the average life expectancy was 25.6 years (Hendricks & Hendricks, 1977). This is somewhat misleading because mortality was extremely high during the first year of life. Those who survived that year might hope to reach 30 or so. As time went on, life expectancy soared to 40. This figure remained stable until about 6000 B.C.E. In ancient Greece, Rome, and Egypt, men who reached the age of 25 could expect to live to 48 or so. In the Middle Ages, life expectancy was roughly 33 to 35 years, although those in the upper classes might survive to age 50. By the end of the Renaissance, it was increasingly common to find individuals living as long as 70 years, as promised by the biblical reference to three score and ten. During Shakespearean times, old age was said to begin at 40 (Sherman, 1997). This may be misleading, however, because many people did not know their actual ages (Covey, 1989).

Throughout this time, as is true in modern days, efforts to prolong life were evident (Gruman, 1966/2003). These efforts were recorded not only in the Old Testament, but in Greek, Indian, and Celtic myths. Long life was something to be sought, although the search for the Fountain of Youth suggests that although long life was valued, old age was not.

Life expectancy soared in the 20th century, primarily as a result of advances in public health, such as reductions in infant mortality and improved treatment of communicable disease (Riley, 2001). At the beginning of the 20th century, average life expectancy was between 45 and 49 years (Olshansky & Carnes, 2001), although as has been true throughout history, some individuals far outlived this age. In contrast, for those born in the United States in 2001, life expectancy was 80.2 years for white women, 75.5 years for African American women, 75 years for white men, and 68.6 years for African American men (Federal Interagency Forum on Aging Related Statistics [FIFARS], 2004). White men and women who were 65 years of age in 2001 could expect to live on average another 18.2 years; African Americans aged 65 in 2001 could expect another 16.4 years of life on average. According to the United Nations Department of Economic and Social Affairs, this increased longevity holds true worldwide to some extent (*World Population Prospects,* 2003).

Impact of Economic Circumstances and Gender

Historically, economic circumstances had an effect on longevity, with nobles surviving longer than their peasant counterparts. The factors contributing to this difference may be similar to those that persist to this day: access to adequate diet, health care, and information. Wealth also affected general perceptions about older adults. Men of wealth were more likely than poor men to be thought of as wise. In societies in which they retained their property and the right to dispose of that property as they wished, they were most likely to be accorded respect. Those who were impoverished worked until they could no longer do so and were then perceived as burdensome (Haber, 1997).

Gender has also been related to longevity throughout history. Whereas women generally were thought to reach old age well before men (Achenbaum & Sterns, 1978), they also lived longer. Thus, at least in terms of perception, women have traditionally spent a much greater proportion of their lives being old than have men (Moody, 1986). As is true for men, though, their specific circumstances depended in part on their wealth. Because in many societies widows lost all of their property, they were likely to live miserably from the time of the husband's death. In some places, they received a small "widow's share" of their deceased husbands' property, enough to live in genteel poverty. In a few societies, they were able to retain considerable resources. In these cases, though, they were generally treated with suspicion (Haber, 1997). In general, gender differences have been substantial throughout history (Achenbaum, 1995). When pensions were introduced as a benefit of employment, they often stopped at the husband's (probably earlier) death. To this day, older women are far more likely than older men to live in poverty. Although this may change as more women who have held paying jobs reach old age, the economic situation continues to be bleak for many older women. In the United States, anticipated problems funding Social Security and Medicare may make it more likely that elderly women will be impoverished. Much of the early writing about aging simply subsumed women under the description of men, or ignored women completely (Cole, 1992), so the lives of elderly women are less well documented.

Until recently, old age for women was defined by loss of procreative ability, and for men, by loss of the work role (Sterns, 1980). As a precursor of modern circumstances during later life, women had greater difficulty with old age because they were poorly prepared and did not have adequate support, either financial or societal. Older men seemed to retain some prestige through their moral leadership, but women enjoyed no such advantage.

There are also ways in which women have aged more satisfactorily than men, primarily because of ongoing responsibility for households and for grandparenting activities. These defined roles were a continuation of those women filled earlier in life, minimizing the transition to old age. It may also have been more comfortable, or at least more socially acceptable, for women to accept dependency. The woman pictured in Figure 1-1 has found an acceptable role that does not rely on family relationships.

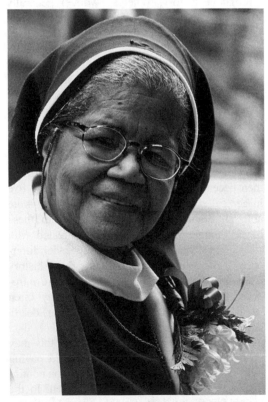

FIGURE 1-1 Gender and religion affect the experience of aging. (Photo from Jeffrey M. Levine, MD, Copyright 2007.)

Another largely economic issue is that of retirement. Until relatively recently, the gerontology literature suggested that retirement was an innovation of the mid-20th century, when social policy established a variety of pension strategies such as Social Security (in the United States) and other forms of financial support in late life (in other developed countries). However, recent authors indicate that, in fact, retirement has existed as an option for centuries, at least for some individuals (Achenbaum, 2002; Vinovskis, 2005). Shahar (1997) notes that during medieval times, landlords might well provide support for those peasants they wished to remove from farming activities. Vinovskis (2005) describes the pension system that emerged following the American Civil War, when soldiers were provided with pensions as were their surviving spouses. Hayward (2005) indicates that similar trends can be seen in the histories of European countries.

Attitudes About Aging From a Historical Perspective

Ambiguity of attitudes about aging is not new (Achenbaum & Sterns, 1978; Shahar, 1997). "Perceptions of the aged's worth, as well as their demographic and socioeconomic status, have varied enormously according to historical time and societal context" (Achenbaum & Sterns, 1978, p. 307). On the whole, Old Testament descriptions of age and aging are positive (Hays, Hays, & Hays, 2005). However, other historical sources suggest ambivalence or even disparagement of aging.

Older men are described in some sources as foolish and burdensome, in others, as respected, wise, and revered (Sherman, 1997). Women have sometimes been portrayed as wise, although more commonly as irrational and childish (Covey, 1989). The Old Testament suggests that older adults should be revered for their wisdom, and the ancient Hebrews believed that a long life was accorded to good people. The Greeks, in contrast, believed that aging was unpleasant, as did the Romans. Historically, individuals who might now be considered middle class seem to have had the best experience both in terms of resources and respect. During colonial times in the United States, there was a Calvinist ideal of veneration for older adults, who at that time represented 4 to 7% of the population. Throughout history, aging has been associated with wisdom (Edmonson, 2005), but reality was somewhat different, with older adults often shunted aside (Covey, 1989).

Attitudes have shifted over time, as well. Note, for example, that the word "hag" derives from a Greek word meaning "holy one" (Sokolovsky, 1997). It retained that positive meaning until the 13th century, when the Catholic church felt threatened by independent older women. At that time, "hag" became associated with evil and ugliness, a connotation that persists to current times. Similarly, "crone" had positive meanings when originally applied to women. It is noteworthy that there are many more such negative terms for women than for men.

As early as the mid-1800s, because of recognition that aging could have quite different courses in different individuals, advice was provided to assist older adults in sustaining health and self-reliance, while avoiding decay (Cole, 1992). One strategy suggested for accomplishing this was to stay engaged in meaningful activity for as long as possible.

Historical Roles of Older Adults

Expectations about appropriate or expected functions for older people have varied over time (Cole, 1992). In ancient and medieval society, contemplation was considered the appropriate use of old age (Covey, 1989). It was thought of as a time to review life and seek spiritual insights. Other activities, including work, sex, and military activities, were not considered appropriate. Particularly for women, marriage was unacceptable in later life.

For years, conventional wisdom has suggested that older adults did well in agrarian societies, where their supportive efforts were a vital part of the culture (Achenbaum & Sterns, 1978). More recently, this assumption has been questioned. Although some elderly individuals did have clearly defined roles, such as care of grandchildren, there was a perception of elders as being too weak or frail to contribute adequately to society. In addition, even in agrarian cultures, individuals who did not live on farms or with extended families were denied clear roles (Hagestad, 1986). Likewise, older adults in industrial settings have been denigrated throughout history (Achenbaum & Sterns, 1978). However, in some specific areas, including politics, religion, and academe, elderly

people, that is, elderly men, have been valued for their experience and wisdom.

Aging has been described as a mystery, presenting spiritual and philosophical dilemmas. It has also been described as a problem (Easterlin, 1996). For centuries, writers have struggled to understand aging, resulting in confusion about the meaning of this stage of life. Throughout history, however, writers have linked the value of the individual and the acceptability of the aging experience to ability to engage in useful activity (Achenbaum & Sterns, 1978).

Cohort Effects

Historical events exercise an effect on current elders. Individuals age in particular generations or cohorts that experience particular historical events that affect their behavior and values. For example, today's **cohort** of elders in the United States lived through the Great Depression of the 1930s. These individuals tend to watch their expenditures closely, having survived those economic hard times. Likewise, they experienced World War II, an event that inspired great patriotism that may have contributed to their likelihood to vote in large numbers today. Cohort effects influence personal behavior and the experience of aging. Alwin and McCammon (2001) found cohort differences in verbal ability, a finding they speculate may be due to differences in educational level among generational groups. Likewise, disease and disability prevalence differ by cohort (Reynolds, Crimmins, & Saito, 1998). The current cohort of elders includes long-term survivors of polio who are now experiencing renewed disability attributed to "post-polio syndrome" (National Institute of Neurological Disorders and Stroke, 2006). Members of the Baby Boom generation following them were the recipients of the first polio vaccine that has now all but eliminated polio around the world. Cohort experiences influence attitudes toward such issues as Social Security benefits and other policy considerations (Silverstein, Angelelli, & Parrott, 2001). It remains to be seen how cohort experiences of the Baby Boom generation, including such events as the Vietnam War, the women's liberation movement, and Watergate, will affect the coming group of elders. Table 1-1 shows the characteristics attributed to some of the

TABLE 1-1 **Characteristics of Cohorts in the United States**

Generation	Born	Characteristics	Personality
Silent generation	1925–1942	Dedication Sacrifice Hard work Duty before pleasure	Conformist Conservative spender Past-oriented
Baby boomers	1946–1964	Optimism Teamwork Personal gratification/growth	Driven Soul-searchers Love–hate relationship with authority
Generation X	1965–1981	Diversity Balance Self-reliance Pragmatism	Risk-takers Skeptical Family-oriented Job focused
Generation Y	1982–?	Confidence Civic duty Achievement Morality	Optimistic Collectivistic Tenacious

Data from AIA Practice Management Digest.

generations currently alive in the United States. Groups in other countries will have different experiences that affect cohort values and behaviors. And, of course, individuals within a given cohort may vary significantly from these stereotypes.

Current Definitions

Current definitions of old age are influenced by both public policy and by the rapid increase in life expectancy. According to the 2000 U.S. Census, there were 35.9 million people aged 65 or over (Administration on Aging, 2004). The elderly population continues to grow, both in absolute numbers and as a percentage of the population, both in the United States and elsewhere in the world (U.S. Census Bureau, 2001). The most rapid growth is in the group that is over 85 years.

Neugarten (1976, 1978) identified two groups of older adults, the "young-old," those from 55 to 75 years, and "old-old," those 76 and older. She noted that these chronological definitions are only rough categories, an imperfect reflection of individual circumstances and abilities. In today's world, the "young-old" may have more in common with individuals in their middle years than with the very old, those over 85 years (Velkoff, et al., 2006). Some definitions go further to describe a group of **oldest-old** who are 85 years or older, and add a group of

middle-old individuals aged 76 to 84. It is worth noting, however, that to some extent, chronological definitions are not relevant because they predict functional capacity so poorly; extreme individual variability characterizes later life (McMullin, 2000; Snowdon, 2001).

Definitions of old age must differentiate the old person (an individual) from old people (a group) (Settersten, 2005). And it is important to distinguish old age (a period of life) from aging (which occurs throughout life). The experiences of a single older person may vary substantially from that of old people in general, and old age implies a definite start point, whereas aging is a continuous process.

For purposes of this book, old age will be considered in the context of function, rather than absolute chronological age. Uhlenberg (2000) among others notes that this is perhaps a more profitable mechanism for examining human development in later life. However, it is important to keep in mind that, particularly in terms of public policy, old age most often refers to those individuals 65 years or older. This definition is based largely on legislative decisions such as, for example, eligibility for Medicare and Social Security in the United States, and public pensions in other developed countries. Even in policy, the definition of old age is a moving target. For example, in an effort to reduce Social Security outlays as the Baby Boom generation reaches old age, the United States instituted a gradual change in age of eligibility. By the time the last of the Baby Boomers reach old age in 2030, the year to attain eligibility will have increased from 65 to 67.

Current Attitudes

The best word to describe current attitudes about aging is *ambivalent*. Stereotypes of aging compete with the various realities, leading to considerable confusion of views (Biggs, 2005). At one end of the spectrum are extremely negative perspectives, leading Butler (1975) to ask "Why survive?" A survey of television images of older adults in 1988 (Dail) revealed that most portrayals were quite negative, showing individuals who were infirm, querulous, and difficult. Although there has been some positive progress in terms of media portrayals of elders, considerable bias remains (Hilt & Lipschultz, 2005).

Some experts present relatively unpleasant (and arguably inaccurate) descriptions of older adults (Harris, 2005). There is a perception that elders should not participate in a variety of kinds of activities, and they may find themselves dismissed with the comment: "You are too old for that" (Harris, 2005, p. 15). Such images have contributed to somewhat pervasive ageism (Palmore, 2001; Ragan & Bowen, 2001) that is evident in both "high-tech" and "low-tech" societies (Sokolovsky, 1997).

More recently, however, a number of researchers have begun to study what they label successful aging (Litwin, 2005; Rowe & Kahn, 1998). They have also begun to publicize their findings widely in the popular press as a means of reversing negative stereotypes (Lichtenstein et al., 2001) and encouraging the kinds of behaviors that support satisfying later life. This research suggests that the majority of older adults make significant contributions to society and enjoy life as well. There is some danger that the idea of successful aging will lead to a different kind of ageism, one that marginalizes elders who are disabled or "simply old and not well preserved" (Minkler & Holstein, 2005, p. 308). However, the image of the successfully aging elder is becoming more accepted, particularly as the Baby-Boom generation approaches old age.

It may be that some of the difference in perspectives is the result of experience with elders of different ages. There is no question that the picture is somewhat more grim (although by no means automatically bleak) for the oldest-old,

those older than 85 (FIFARS, 2004). These individuals are likely to have some degree of dependence and infirmity. However, as we shall see throughout this volume, this does not necessarily limit the individual's ability to enjoy a meaningful life. And there are more and more examples like the 92-year-old woman who appeared on television's Regis and Kathy Show (1998) to demonstrate traditional cooking and who also demonstrated physical energy and wit beyond that of many younger individuals.

Attitudes toward older adults can be changed through systematic efforts at education (Lichtenstein et al., 2001). Individual experiences with older adults whose behavior and appearance contrast with personal stereotypes can also challenge negative beliefs and lead to reexamination. Elders seem to find strategies for resisting negative stereotypes (Biggs, 2005; Zebrowitz, 2003) and, in many instances, for maintaining continuity of identity.

Cultural Factors

Historical and demographic trends are important to understand, but they are not the same for all cultures. To understand the experience of aging, cultural factors must also be examined. "Age is a social construction and the experience of growing old is culturally mitigated" (Fry, 1996, p. 123).

Demographic trends are a good indicator of some important cultural and societal differences. In the developed world (Canada, the United States, Europe, Australia, and Russia), 13% or more of the population was aged 65 years or over in 2000 (U.S. Census Bureau, 2001). In the developing world, the current percentage of the population over 65 years is less than 8% (and less than 3% in central Africa, where AIDS has taken a toll). But an increase in the proportion of the population that is older is growing worldwide. Fifty-nine percent of the world's elderly population now live in Africa, Asia, Latin America, the Caribbean, and Oceania. By 2050, two important population trends, already evident, will be far more pronounced:

1. The absolute number and percentage of elders worldwide
2. The change in demographic structure from a pyramid to a more rectangular shape (*World Population Prospects,* 2003)

As shown in Figure 1-2, this latter trend means that there will be fewer young adults to help support elders.

China provides an intriguing example of the influences of cultural and societal trends on the experience of aging. As a way to reduce its extremely rapid population growth, China instituted a "one-child" policy for families (Hesketh, Lu, & Xing, 2005). Cultural preference for male children resulted in selective abortion and other strategies for ensuring that the sole child would be male. These two factors resulted in both a reduction in the available young adults to support elders, and a lack of marriageable young women to produce the next generation. China has the world's largest population of older adults, nearly 88 million in 2000. The percentage of elders in the Chinese population mirrors that of developed countries, over 13%. However, because of efforts at population control, the country faces serious challenges in providing an acceptable quality of life for its elders. This will have an enormous impact on public policy and on services.

Culture may affect individuals' expectations about what old age will be like, their plans and goals for this period of their lives, their values and attitudes about being older and about health care, and their motivations for engaging in or withdrawing from activity. To understand the individual, an observer must set aside beliefs based on a view from without, possibly the view held by the health-care practitioner, and take the time to really understand the perspective from within—that is, the experience of the specific individual in the context of his or her culture.

Cultural factors affect societal beliefs about the aging process, social and economic supports for elders, self-identity of older adults, expected and accepted roles and activities, and health status. In the United States, one reason for increasing interest in cultural factors is the growing recognition of significant health disparities (Kahn & Fazio, 2005; Smedley, Stith, & Nelson, 2003). Over the past decade, many researchers have found that racial and ethnic differences are associated with rates of disease, views on health care, access to care, and outcomes of care. For elders, an accumulation of disadvantage throughout the life course may intensify these disparities. The reasons for the differences are not clearly understood, with hypotheses ranging from genetic differences to

socioeconomic factors to systematic discrimination. Researchers have adopted multiple strategies for trying to explain health disparities. Cultural factors will be discussed in greater detail in Chapter 23.

Place of Residence

Another important factor in understanding the experience of an aging individual is the geographic location in which he or she resides and the quality of housing in that location. As Rowles (1991) noted, place is of crucial importance to older adults. There is evidence of a strong link between housing and health (Cagney, Browning, & Wen, 2005), perhaps because of differences in support systems and service use among elderly individuals living in rural, suburban, and urban settings (Auchincloss, Van Nostrand, & Ronsaville, 2001). Golant (2003) suggested that environments have the potential to either facilitate or impede activities as well as health.

In rural environments, older adults form strong informal support networks (McCulloch, 1995). The grocery store, post office, bank, and so on are important sources of socialization and support, and informal networks are effective for both maintaining health and providing care for those who are ill. A clear set of social norms and social supports appears to emerge over time (Rowles, 1991). These supports are essential to positive quality of life, whether they are provided by family or by others (McCulloch, 1995).

Although there is good social support in small towns, older adults who live at a distance from town may have more difficulty obtaining needed assistance. Rural populations are quite diverse, and distance can be a problem (Sokolovsky, 1997). In addition, rural elders face challenges from the collapse of some rural economies and the resultant out-migration of younger individuals.

Elders provide benefits to rural locations in spite of their need for a greater number of support services than younger residents (Stallmann, Deller, & Shields, 1999). Among other factors, on average they introduce more money into the local economy than they require in services. Further, there is considerable evidence that elders provide reciprocal services as well, often looking after grandchildren or

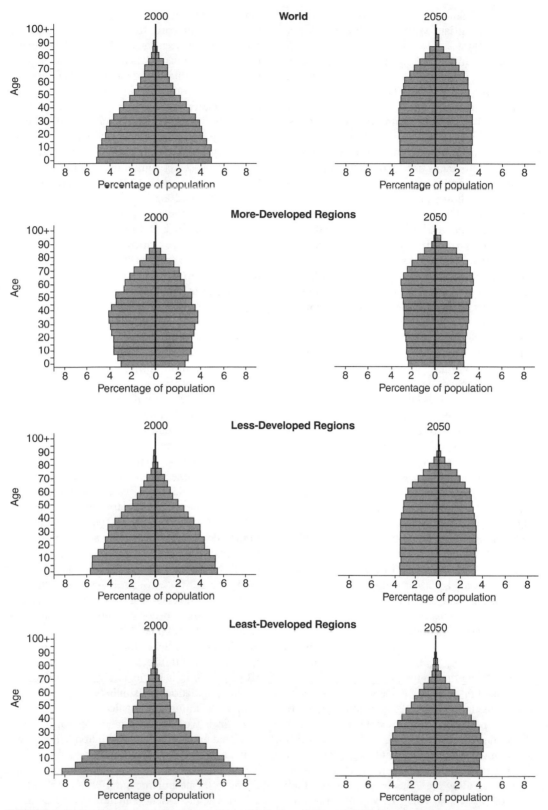

FIGURE 1-2   Population pyramids: Age and sex distribution, 2000 and 2050. (From *The Sex and Age Distribution of the World Populations: 1998* Revision, Vol. II, United Nations Publications, Department of Public Information, New York, New York.)

providing financial support to their adult children (Siegrist, von dem Knesebeck, & Pollack, 2004).

For suburban elderly individuals, transportation is frequently a problem (Logan & Spitze, 1988). They tend to have the greatest financial resources but fewer community resources. The lack of community resources is, in part, the result of an assumption by service providers that they are more affluent and that income shields them from problems confronted by those with fewer economic resources. Activity patterns, however, are often dictated by access to facilities. Some older adults, particularly those who are more affluent, deal with the dilemmas of suburban life by moving to communities designed specifically for them (McHugh & Larson-Keagy, 2005). Although this change may address some of the instrumental problems they may experience, such communities can be experienced as isolating.

The experience of the urban elderly population is unique in some respects from that of their rural and suburban counterparts. Urban elders may have greatest geographic access to transportation and services but have less access to the economic capacity to take advantage of those services. There also tends to be greater ethnic diversity among urban older adults, requiring that the aging process be understood in the context of both cultural and environmental factors.

The impact of rural versus urban residence is an issue in many developed countries (Mollenkopf et al., 2004). This study of five European countries found that rural elders were more likely to own their homes but had less access to services and amenities. Life satisfaction was similar in rural and urban settings, assuming that there was adequate access to leisure activities.

Regardless of place of residence, most elders express a wish to age in place—that is, to remain in their own homes. This wish is shared by their families (Gitlin, 2003). According to Gitlin, "living at home promotes a sense of personhood or normalcy in view of discontinuity and disjunction experienced as a consequence of multiple personal losses associated with age-related declines and chronic illness" (p. 629). Remaining at home allows elders to draw upon well-learned habits for self-care and other activities, allowing them to focus their energies on other roles they find fulfilling. Remaining at home, assuming that younger

family members are nearby, also allows elders to draw upon care from those individuals as needed. As will be seen in Chapter 15, living near family also allows elders to provide care supportive of their adult children and grandchildren.

Type of housing, in addition to location, can correlate with relative well-being of elders. Those living in more affluent neighborhoods, regardless of whether they are located in the inner city, a suburb, or a small town, tend to age more successfully than those in poor neighborhoods (Cagney, et al., 2005; Evans, Kantrowitz, & Eshelman, 2002). A particular example of problematic housing is residence in mobile homes (George & Bylund, 2002). Residence in such dwellings is associated with distance from family support networks. In addition, mobile homes tend to depreciate in value, while elders who live in homes they own can anticipate some appreciation in value and thus some added financial resources as they age. Both mobile homes and dilapidated inner-city residences may lack the environmental supports that can enhance function (Gitlin, 2003).

Migration has consequences for elders (Wolf & Longino, 2005) in all its various forms. First, some individuals choose to move permanently following retirement. They may move to a warmer climate, or they may attempt to identify prosperous communities, making the assumption that such communities would have greater availability of needed services (Serow, 2001). Second, some individuals develop a pattern labeled "snowbirding," in which they maintain two households: one in their community of long-standing and one in a warmer climate where they live during the winter (Wolf & Longino, 2005). Third, some elders who have moved to a warmer location ultimately decide on "reverse migration" to be closer to family as they become more frail (Stoller & Longino, 2001). Finally, attention is warranted to the ultimate migration, that of elderly immigrants from their countries of origin to the United States (Becker, 2002). It seems likely that the dilemmas of this population are similar in many countries with large immigrant populations. Some of these individuals wish to die in their homelands, a wish mediated by the presence of strong family supports in their new place of residence.

An added, often overlooked, issue is that of homelessness (Cohen, 1999; Crane et al., 2005). The number of homeless individuals in the United States has increased over time. Estimates about the percentage of these individuals who are elders range from 2.5% to 27% (Cohen, 1999). There are a variety of reasons for this phenomenon, among them the deinstitutionalization of individuals who are chronically mentally ill. Older adults are found among the homeless, although their exact numbers are difficult to measure. Clearly, homelessness presents an array of problems to the individual. Survival is, of necessity, a primary focus of activity, leaving little time for concern about "successful" aging.

Contrary to popular opinion, few older adults are institutionalized. In 1997, 4% of the population over age 65 lived in nursing homes (FIFARS, 2004). In 1999, 11 individuals per 1000 aged 65 to 74 years resided in nursing homes, as did 43 per 1000 of those 75 to 84 years of age, and 183 per 1000 of those 85 years and older. The oldest-old, women, and individuals without family support are disproportionately represented in this group. These women are most likely to become permanent residents of nursing homes. A wide array of alternative supported living arrangements is emerging, including assisted living facilities and other community housing with support services. It is possible that alternative supportive housing arrangements will play a role in reducing institutionalization further.

Although considerable recent attention has been paid to residence options that support successful aging, much remains to be learned. For example, evidence that religious faith can reduce stress of elders living in deteriorated neighborhoods (Krause, 1998) deserves further study. Findings that shortly after migration, elders experience increased dysfunction in activities of daily living (ADL) and instrumental activities of daily living, but that these are short-lived changes (Chen & Wilmoth, 2004) contravene the conventional wisdom that **aging in place** is more supportive of function. Such research could offer insight into the environmental factors that support good-quality later life and guide care providers in constructing optimal situations and helping elders make effective decisions about their residential situations.

Gender

The experiences of older women and older men diverge in significant ways. Demographics

alone dictate that their circumstances will differ. On average, women outlive men by 7 years. Because of this, women are much more likely than men to live alone in later life. This means women may experience greater isolation and loneliness and lower life satisfaction in later life (Inglehart, 2002). They may face financial difficulties because, for the current cohort of older women, any work history might have been interrupted by the demands of families, leaving them with lower pensions (Hardy & Shuey, 2000). If this results in reliance on spousal pensions, loss of a spouse may increase financial difficulties (Herd, 2005; Johnson, Sambamoorthi, & Crystal, 1999; Rupp, Strand, & Davies, 2003). These financial effects are found not only in the United States but also in other countries, including both Germany (Hungerford, 2001) and Hong Kong (Lee, 2001), where social welfare policies have been enacted to avoid such problems.

Widowhood, for both men and women, brings significant challenges, although the consequences are complex and different for the two genders. Older men who are alone face social isolation whether their status derives from widowhood or divorce (Davidson, 2004). They are more likely to have relied on their wives to establish and maintain the social support network, and to have difficulty reestablishing ties when they lose a spouse. In fact, research shows that men experience a greater decline in life satisfaction than women following death of a spouse (Chipperfield & Havens, 2001). However, for those whose marital status remains stable, women's life satisfaction declines over time while men's remains stable. Further, men who gain a spouse in later life have an increase in life satisfaction while women do not. As shown in Figure 1-3, men can acquire important family roles in later life that bring them closer to family.

Another issue of importance is that of financial resources. As already noted, older women, especially those who are widowed, experience poverty at substantially higher rates than men. Estimates suggest that there are twice as many older women than older men living in poverty (Rupp et al., 2003). The current cohort of older women tended not to work outside the home and, therefore, may have few financial resources of their own. Widowed women, in particular, are vulnerable to decreases in financial assets (Zick & Holden, 2000). Social

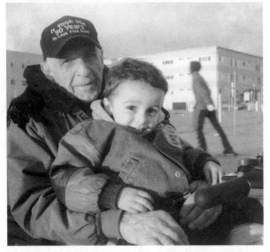

FIGURE 1-3 This man enjoys a close relationship with his grandson. Grandparenting often allows men closer ties with young people than they may have had with their children. (Photo from Jeffrey M. Levine, MD, Copyright, 2007.)

Security provides only a very modest livelihood and was never intended to be the sole source of support for older adults. However, for a significant subset of older women, it is their primary, or only, income.

The fact that women live so much longer also means that they will experience greater disability later in life (Denton & Walters, 1999; Wray & Blaum, 2001). They are more likely to develop Alzheimer's disease, to experience bone fractures, and to have other compromising health conditions. These problems influence quality of life and ability to function. There are particular challenges for older women who have completed rehabilitation and must return to homes where they live alone (Lysack, MacNeill, Neufeld, & Lichtenberg, 2002). There is less understanding of health conditions among older women because so much research has been done using primarily male study groups (Cattell, 1996). The National Institutes of Health in the United States now requires researchers to include women as research participants, but it will take time for research reports to fully reflect that requirement. At the same time, men have been largely ignored in the research on osteoporosis and breast cancer, even though small but identifiable groups of men have to deal with these conditions, and prostate cancer, which is even more common among men than breast cancer is for women, has not received adequate research attention.

Individual Experiences and Characteristics

The factors discussed so far in this chapter relate to the environment and history. However, the experience of aging is unique to each individual even in the context of the broader society. Individual personality characteristics and personal experience throughout the lifespan are central to a person's later life circumstances, behaviors, and attitudes. Later life is characterized by tremendous variability (Gatz, 1995), making it essential to understand the circumstances of the individual. As Hooker and McAdams (2003) noted, earlier theorists "have written persuasively about the necessity of taking this 'N-of-one-at-a-time' approach for understanding how intraindividual change is the mechanism for producing individual differences over time" (pp. P297–P298).

Genetic factors are the first individual difference to consider. As human genetic structure is better understood, it is clear that differences in DNA among individuals (and among species) is very small, but that those differences can have profound implications for development of the person (Johnson & Krueger, 2005; Ryff & Singer, 2005). Genetic explanations have been proposed for a variety of disorders commonly seen in later life. These include (among many others) Alzheimer's disease, osteoporosis, diabetes, and heart disease (National Center for Health Statistics Data Warehouse, 2006). However, there is also compelling evidence that a variety of environmental and social factors can mediate the expression of genes. As Johnson and Krueger (2005) indicate, "genetic expression may be buffered in some environmental circumstances but manifested in others" (p. 50). Snowdon (2001), for example, found that some nuns whose cognition remained intact in later life showed significant anatomical signs of Alzheimer's disease on autopsy. He suggests that some protective factors either in behavior or the environment, or both, served to reduce the signs of the disorder even in the presence of the biological characteristic.

One factor proposed as serving to buffer genetic characteristics is individual personality. Researchers examining such characteristics as neuroticism and extraversion have found that elders vary widely on such traits (Mroczek & Spiro, 2003). Personality traits are very stable across the life course (Small, Herzog, Hultsch, & Dixon, 2003) and across cultures (Labouvie-Vief, Diehl, Tarnowski, & Shen, 2000), and they influence both outlook and behavior. So, for example, extraversion is associated with positive aging (Lang, Staudinger, & Carstensen, 1998). It may be that extraverts are likely to establish and maintain the broad social networks that are known to support successful aging.

Among the effects of personal experience is the cumulative advantage or disadvantage that results from differences in socioeconomic status and education that can influence health status and outlook in later life (Dannefer, 2003). Stress has a significant influence on well-being in later life (Martin, Gruendahl, & Martin, 2001), as does self-identity (Franks, Herzog, Holmberg, & Markus, 2003). Early life events such as parental loss among African Americans are associated with poor integration into family life and friendships and fewer social resources very late in life (Johnson & Barer, 2002).

Personal skills and abilities like skill at constructing a social network can also affect the experience of aging either for good or ill. Individuals who are effective problem solvers are able to draw upon resources to address problems (Collins, Luszcz, Lawson, & Keeves, 1997). Individual resources include the ability to establish a social network (Steverink, Westerhof, Bode, & Dittmann-Kohli, 2001). Some research has found that it is the act of helping others that is important, as opposed to simply receiving help from a social network (Brown, Consedine, & Magai, 2005).

Attitudes have significant impact. Positive self-esteem (Bailis & Chipperfield, 2002), and optimistic expectations about what later life will be like may influence decisions to seek help when difficulties arise (Sarkisian, Steers, Hays, & Mangione, 2005). In fact, positive outlook is consistently associated with well-being in later life (Chipperfield, Perry, & Weiner, 2003; Isaacowitz & Smith, 2003), as is feeling younger than one's actual age (Westerhof & Barrett, 2005). Considerable research has found that perceived circumstances (e.g., having acquired self-perceived wisdom) are more important than objective reality (Ardelt, 1997).

Some older adults seem to age with grace and to identify old age as a time of special fulfillment. Others seem pessimistic and dour. It is likely that individual factors persist in old age, possibly diminishing or increasing somewhat, but rarely altering entirely. Identifying and drawing upon individual strengths is an important strategy in providing interventions that are helpful in enhancing later life for elders. These factors will be discussed in greater detail in later chapters.

Socioeconomic Status

As can be seen from the discussion to this point, socioeconomic (SES) factors play a significant role in aging. In particular, education, occupation, and income level influence the experience of aging as well as morbidity and mortality. As health disparities continue to be center stage in the health-care literature, the consequences of long-standing socioeconomic disadvantage have received particular attention (Hatch, 2005). This is true not only in the United States, but also in countries that provide universal health care, such as Canada (Buckley, Denton, Robb, & Spencer, 2004a, 2004b; Luo & Waite, 2005)

At its most basic, the influence of socioeconomic status can be summarized to suggest that better education and higher income are associated with a longer and healthier life. A growing body of literature establishes a causal relationship, with the direction being from SES to health (Chandola, Bartley, Sacker, Jenkinson, & Marmot, 2003). Further, there is increasing evidence that the impact of adverse SES is cumulative over the lifespan (George, 2005; Hatch, 2005).

SES affects many aspects of the experience of aging. Individuals who are wealthy and well educated are less likely to experience cognitive decline in later life (Cagney & Lauderdale, 2002; Turrell et al., 2002). Individuals from higher SES groups are more likely to feel they have access to caregivers (Talamantes, Cornell, Espino, Lichtenstein, & Hazuda, 1996). They experience more positive self-identities (Barrett, 2003) and greater subjective well-being (Pinquart & Sorensen, 2000).

Lower SES is associated with increased risky health behaviors (Wray, Alwin, & McCammon, 2005), poor health literacy (Baker, Gazmararian, Sudano, & Patterson, 2000), and poorer follow-through with health promotion and screening behaviors (Fox et al., 2004). Socioeconomic factors such as self-perceived adequacy of income and housing tenure are associated with risk for onset of disability (Matthews, Smith, Hancock, Jagger, & Spiers, 2005).

For a variety of reasons, the financial circumstances of elders tend to deteriorate as they live longer (Lee, 2004). There are a number of possible explanations for this, including increased health-care costs, need for support services, and outliving savings. However, individuals whose educational levels and previous SES are higher do not experience these decrements in financial resources in as detrimental a fashion as those who experienced lifelong poverty and low educational and occupational attainment.

An area that is not well understood is the potential for protective resources that ameliorate the negative consequences of low SES (Hatch, 2005). Some elders who have been impoverished all their lives tend to age very well while others struggle. There are complex interactions among all the factors discussed in this chapter that undoubtedly contribute to differential outcomes of aging experienced by different individuals (George, 2005). One potential explanation, which will be considered in Chapter 3, is the differential occupational patterns in which elders engage.

Public Policy and Aging

Socioeconomic factors associated with later life are inextricably linked to public policy. Retirement income and health-care coverage are among the issues closely tied to legislation. Policies about pensions, investments, and health care can greatly influence the extent to which elders are sufficiently secure financially in later life (Bergstrom & Holmes, 2004). Policy can also support or impede successful aging as it supports or impedes individual function (Lee & Frongillo, 2001).

An array of policies directly affect the health and well-being of older adults. One such U.S. law is the Older Americans Act (OAA) (PL89-73) (Hudson, 1996). Originally passed in 1965, the Act is now awaiting reauthorization by the federal legislature after years of disagreement about its provisions (Hudson, 2005). Its original purpose was to provide support and restorative services, both institutional and community based. The holdup regarding its reauthorization may relate to concerns about the increase in numbers of elders and rapidly escalating costs for their care. Increasing diversity among elders makes it more difficult to establish effective policy, because what works well for one group may have unintended (or even predictable) negative impact on another group. There is a veritable alphabet soup of legislation in the United States that affects elders, including the Americans with Disabilities Act (ADA, 1990), the Age Discrimination in Employment Act of 1967 (Neumark, 2006), and many others. Other countries also enact policies that affect the experience of growing old. For example, the United Kingdom provides universal health care, but only recently enacted legislation to forbid age discrimination in employment (*Statutory Instrument no. 1031, 2006*).

In the United States, pensions from employers are rapidly disappearing, after roughly 60 years as a major source of financial support for elders (Westerman & Sundali, 2005). Many developed countries, including Great Britain and Germany, also face changes in pension structure as a result of the rapid growth in the proportion of older adults in their populations (Asghar, Frick, & Buchel, 2005). The future of pensions has received considerable recent attention as evidence emerges that the demographic changes described earlier in this chapter, coupled with policies that have allowed employers to under-fund pension plans, has resulted in a serious shortfall in available resources.

Another historical source of financial support in the United States, Social Security, has gone a long way toward reducing (although not eliminating) poverty among older adults (Kingston & Herd, 2004). Recent concern about Social Security focuses on the fact that the population of the United States has an increasing proportion of elders relative to the population of working age individuals (typically defined as 22 to 65 years of age). This **"dependency ratio"**—that is, the ratio of those in the workforce to those (children and retired elders) depending on the taxes workers pay to provide their financial support—is difficult to calculate (Gratton, 1997). This is particularly true as elders increasingly remain at work (by choice) beyond the policy-determined retirement age, previously 65 and now being gradually increased to 67 in the United States (*The Economist,* 2005a). The United States is not the only country dealing with this issue, with many developed countries examining their financial supports for elders and age of eligibility (*The Economist,* 2005b). Changes in the age for eligibility for retirement benefits do influence choice to retire (Fronstin, 1999) but are far from the only factor affecting the decision.

Public and private sources of payment for health care are also issues largely determined through public policy. Because health-care expenditures go up toward the end of life (Yang, Norton, & Stearns, 2003), elders are more directly affected by the nature of these policies. For the past decade or more in the United States, there has been a trend toward increasing individual and family responsibility to cover health-care costs (Cohen, 1998; Crystal, Johnson, Harman, Sambamoorthi, & Kumar, 2000). This creates a significant problem for elders at the lower end of the socioeconomic scale (Lima & Allen, 2001). Ironically, but not surprisingly, individuals who can afford supplemental health insurance are less likely to develop disability than those who cannot (Landerman et al., 1998). This is almost certainly due to the fact that elders with more resources have better access to care throughout life and maintain better health habits as a result of better information.

Changes in family structure can exacerbate this problem, because so much care is provided by family members, particularly daughters and daughters-in-law (Levine, 2004). Such "informal" care has tremendous economic value, and also has influence on the growth of health-care spending for elders. When informal care is available, it continues even when formal care is provided (Li, 2005). However, as adult women are increasingly likely to work and the number of adult children per family decreases, informal care is less available for some elders, putting increasing upward pressure on health-care costs.

Not only does policy affect the extent to which health care is available, it often influences the location for such service. One example is the impact of the Balanced Budget Act (BBA) of 1997 (Spector, Cohen, & Pesis-Katz, 2004) which changed the rules about access to therapy in home health settings. The BBA was enacted in an effort to control the rapidly escalating costs associated with Medicare. At the same time, it shifted costs to individual states through Medicaid and Medicare waivers that allowed states to try various kinds of home health care beyond those traditionally covered by the federal government (Leutz, 1999).

As with pensions, problems of paying for health care for elders are not confined to the United States. Britain, with its universal health insurance system, has begun to shift toward privatization (Filinson, 1997). Bermuda, which has a system not unlike the combination payment program in the United States (including both employer- and government-provided insurance) has found that these structural features, as well as individual behavior, affect health-care utilization (Chappell & Penning, 1996). Chappell and Penning noted that "In Bermuda, health factors are important to the use of both physician and other health services. We also see, however, that economic factors, indirectly through health, may influence the utilization of physician services, as does education" (pp. 68–69). Some Asian countries have legislated family responsibility to provide care, building on traditional norms for family behavior (Ofstedal et al., 2002). So, for example, the Philippine Constitution states: "the family has the duty to care for its elderly members but the State may also do so" (p. 66).

There is widespread belief that there is intergenerational conflict in the United States about these policies (Cornman & Kingson, 1996; Greene & Marty, 1999). The reality is that considerable intergenerational exchange of financial and emotional support occurs in all directions (Keyes, 2002). The notion that younger adults resent support provided for elders is not borne out by the research (Greene & Marty, 1999). Likewise, there is a widespread belief that elders "hide" resources through formation of trusts that shift savings to their adult children to make themselves eligible for Medicaid coverage of nursing home care (Taylor, Sloan, & Norton, 1999). This is not borne out by the research either.

Elders tend to be politically active (Binstock & Day, 1996). Because they are somewhat conservative about social issues, they are inclined to support changes that occur gradually. Wholesale changes in Social Security would not meet with approval among this group. In addition, every policy enacted has both intended and unintended consequences. Effective in January 2006, Medicare has provided coverage for prescription medications required by seniors. Its enactment was the result of pressure from politically active elders and their lobbying groups, AARP most notably, and recognition that for some elders the cost of prescription medications was unaffordable. However, the legislation ultimately enacted was far from satisfactory, resulting in a confusing array of choices for elders and, according to some, unwarranted protections for pharmaceutical companies. At the writing of this chapter, elders and pharmacies are struggling to make sense of this convoluted plan.

A new concern with regard to public policy and aging emerged at the 2005 White House Conference on Aging (www.whcoa.gov). The administration in office at the time clearly pushed an agenda of "individual responsibility." Even though many would agree that elders bear the responsibility for preparing adequately for later life, it is also the case that in all sectors of society, there are times when social and economic supports may be needed. The decreases in pension plans, the complexities of saving, and the uncertainties of health may, in some instances, be beyond the control of the individual. For example, some retirees have had the experience of losing both pension and health insurance coverage after their retirement when the company for which they worked declared bankruptcy. In such instances, individual responsibility cannot remedy the resulting problems. Many European and other developed countries have policies in place to ensure that elders can manage during their later years. It will be important to monitor policies that result from the White House Conference to ensure that older adults do not suffer unduly.

There is a complex maze of legislative initiatives intended to address the needs of elders while at the same time attempting to constrain costs. Care providers working with older adults also must negotiate a confusing and ever-changing set of rules and regulations that determine where care will be provided—in the community, a hospital, a nursing home—and what kinds of care will be reimbursed. In this context, care providers must stay focused on their primary goal, which is to support successful aging. The idea of successful aging was well described by Rowe and Kahn (1998) who found that it involved three interrelated objectives.

Successful Aging

Having considered some of the many factors that affect the experience of aging for individuals and for populations, we now turn our attention to the role of health-care providers, and occupational therapists specifically, in working with older adults. Both physical and psychosocial change is inevitable with age; thus the idea that health care should be directed toward ensuring perfect health leads to unrealistic expectations. As a way to describe the realistic but also optimistic expectations for later life, Rowe and Kahn (1998) identified components of successful aging. Their initial description of this state of being suggested that elders could, by pursuing three main goals, live their lives with a sense of satisfaction and well-being. The three goals they identify are as follows:

1. Avoiding disease and disability
2. Maintaining high cognitive and physical functioning
3. Staying involved with life and living

The third of these recommendations has been explicitly identified as the domain of occupational therapy (American Occupational Therapy Association [AOTA], 2002). Furthermore, an emphasis on "assisting people to engage in daily life activities that they find meaningful and purposeful" (p. 610) is interwoven with strategies to maintain cognitive and physical function, which thereby minimizes disease and disability. "Occupational therapists' and occupational therapy assistants' expertise lies in their knowledge of occupation and how engaging in occupations can be used to affect human performance and the effects of disease and disability" (AOTA, 2002). The Canadian Association of Occupational Therapists endorses this view as well, embracing the Canadian Model of Occupational Performance, noting that "occupational performance refers to the ability to choose, organize, and satisfactorily perform meaningful occupations that are culturally defined and age appropriate for looking after one's self, enjoying life, and contributing to the social and economic fabric of a community" (CAOT, 2002, p. 30). Indeed, around the globe, and regardless of the age of the clients, occupational therapists recognize that their main role is to enable individuals to stay involved with meaningful occupations.

Clearly, successful aging is complex, and many of the factors discussed in this chapter are associated with individuals' perceptions, as well as professional evaluations, that they are aging successfully. As will be discussed in the next two chapters, an important starting point for considering the appropriate roles of professionals is the identification of theories that can help guide interventions focused on supporting successful aging and facilitate thoughtful evaluation of outcomes.

■ Summary

What does all this mean for health-care professionals? First, there is no unitary description of old age that adequately conveys the roles and circumstances of all older adults. Individual and cultural differences are great. Further, roles and circumstances change over time. What is true today may not be true tomorrow, and predictions based on current situations may or may not turn out to be accurate. For example, in Chapter 14, Sterns and his colleagues describe current trends in retirement in the United States, primarily in terms of earlier departure from the workforce, followed by reentry into part-time jobs. If labor shortages emerge in this country, public policy would shift to encourage employees to remain in the workforce longer, as has happened with recent changes in Social Security to increase age of eligibility from 65 to 67. If unemployment rises, incentives to retire might increase as a way to open jobs for younger individuals.

Changes in cognitive, physical, sensory, and psychosocial performance occur to some degree in all elderly individuals, as is discussed in the chapters that follow. Individual differences exist within the broad parameters of these predictable changes. Social and environmental events are also at least somewhat predictable. For example, whether married, single, or divorced, whether from a large or small family, older individuals experience loss of significant others.

We know that functional limitations increase as individuals age and are found with increased frequency in the oldest-old age group.

However, statistics reflect averages and do not provide definitive information about a given individual. The challenge for occupational therapists and other health-care providers is to understand not only the general patterns but also the factors that mold individual experience of growing older. Every client must be regarded as a unique individual with special interests, abilities, and needs. This is as true for elderly individuals as for those who are younger. However, the common realities of the aging process must also be understood, to help the individual prepare for probable changes.

Health care for older adults is often provided in settings other than traditional hospitals and clinics. Relationships among professionals may be affected by this, as in the case of a home health situation in which not all services can be provided. In these situations, it is essential for all health providers to understand the complexity of the situation and the range of possible interventions that may be employed and to make informed referrals when necessary.

Situations that influence the performance of the older adult are highly complex, including all the factors described in this chapter as well as the normal biological, social, and psychological changes that accompany aging, and the likelihood that a person will have two to three chronic conditions. All health-care providers must be sensitive to the myriad of interacting considerations that affect function.

Attitudes toward older adults, regardless of historical or cultural context, have always been somewhat ambivalent (Kastenbaum, & Ross, 1975). Even in those cultures where elders are revered, some ambivalence toward aging is evident. As Glascock and Feinman (1980) note, the ability to function is critical for elderly people in all cultures. "Nowhere is decrepitude valued" (Nydegger, 1983, p. 26).

Interventions risk being irrelevant to the client if they are planned without attention to the nature of the culture, family structure, and place and types of residences; demographic factors; the demands of life both in terms of physical and social environment and cultural institutions; work and leisure roles and the value placed on each; the degree of choice of activity available to the individual; and the unique characteristics of the individual.

For example, plans to return an individual to his or her home, with an assumption that adult children will provide support services, work only when there is a cultural expectation that adult children will do so and an adequate family network. Expecting individuals to shift interests from productive to leisure activities will work only when cultural values encourage (or at least do not discourage) this shift. Hendricks and Hendricks (1977) indicate that "it is only when mankind is not preoccupied with the necessities of survival that a humane treatment of nonproductive members can be realized" (p. 139). In the United States, most older adults are at that point, although some continue to be primarily preoccupied with survival. In determining what constitutes humane treatment, it is important to note that there is no single group that can be called "the old." In addition, the productivity that characterizes much of this population must be better described and acknowledged. As with other segments of the population, diversity is great. An individual must be considered in the context of personal history, ethnic background, and environment. Without adequate attention to each of these factors, generalizations will fail to reflect personal realities.

Increasingly, occupational therapists and other health-care providers are being called upon to intervene at the level of the community. Ideas of occupational justice (Townsend, 1999; Whiteford, 2000) suggest that therapists have an obligation to help structure environments and policies that enable all individuals, regardless of age or background, to have access to meaningful occupations. To achieve this goal, it may be necessary to work toward policy changes (Kam, 2002; Starkloff, 2001). Doing this requires that therapists stay informed about the evidence related to effective interventions and environmental structures and that they are able to translate this information for policy makers (Feldman, Nadash, & Gursen, 2001).

As health-care professionals, we must focus on well-being rather than on physical health alone. As John F. Kennedy (1963) said, "Our senior citizens present this Nation with increasing opportunity to draw upon their skill and sagacity and the opportunity to provide the respect and recognition they have earned. It is not enough for a great nation merely to have added new years to life—our objective must also be to add new life to those years" (p. 10).

Case Study

Mr. Smith is a 70-year-old Native American. His wife died 2 years ago following a lengthy period of disability. A year before his wife's death, Mr. Smith moved with her away from the state in which he had a job as a machinist to his original home on the Reservation. He lives alone in a rented house next door to his sister. His three children live out of town; he sees two of them on a monthly basis. He has always been careful about his health. He was a jogger until his hip recently "gave out," and he now bikes almost daily. He has minor back problems and mild arthritis that causes him difficulty particularly when he tries to lift something heavy. He is thankful for his good health. He is relatively well-off because his industrial job has provided him with a good pension. Although he can cook simple meals, he prefers to eat out, having breakfast at a local fast food restaurant, and lunch at a local diner. He tries to eat foods that are healthy, such as fruit, vegetables, and whole grains. He eats twice weekly with his sister, but otherwise his social encounters focus mostly on his restaurant meals. Mr. Smith describes himself as a Christian, and he prays daily. He also values his Native American spiritual origins and tries to adopt the outlook on life that characterizes his nation (adapted from McDonald, Quandt, Arcury, Bell, & Vitolins, 2000).

Questions

1. What do you see in this description of Mr. Smith that might contribute to successful aging?

   Mr. Smith's background as a Native American may imbue him with a sense of comfort with the natural order of things. If he subscribes to this cultural value, the prospect of death at some later point may be less anxiety provoking than for those less accepting of this natural order. His children appear to provide some social support, and his meals out provide additional social interaction. He has had a number of good health habits, including regular exercise and good eating habits, and he has strong spiritual beliefs that give him comfort.

2. What do you note as factors discussed in this chapter that might affect his experience of growing older?

   Mr. Smith's gender, his socioeconomic status, his cultural beliefs, his personality, and his personal experiences all influence the nature of his later life. The loss of a spouse is a significant stressor for individuals, regardless of the quality of the relationship. In this case, Mr. Smith left his familiar surroundings to provide her with added support; however, this may have limited his own social networks. The rural nature of the reservation may further complicate access to support networks.

3. Do you see any particular risk factors in this description of Mr. Smith?

   Living alone can be problematic. This is particularly true if the Reservation is one on which homes are distant from each other and roads are limited and hard to travel. The absence of such services as public transportation may eventually make it very difficult for Mr. Smith to grocery shop or manage other tasks of daily life. Further, it is possible that at some later point Mr. Smith would need assistance that would make it impossible for him to live by himself. Mr. Smith's health is good now, but his hip problem, arthritis, and back problems can become worse with age. It is difficult to tell from the description above, but it is also possible that Mr. Smith lacks the kind of meaningful occupations that would enhance successful aging.

Review Questions

1. In what ways have attitudes toward aging changed over time? How can they best be described in the United States now?
2. What societal and biological factors have altered definitions of old age?
3. How do socioeconomic status and culture affect the experience of aging?
4. In what ways is the experience of aging different for women and for men? For people in rural, suburban, and urban areas? Why might these differences exist?
5. How does public policy in the United States affect the lives of older adults? How might changes in demographic factors alter policy?
6. What is meant by successful aging?

For helpful information about the experience of aging, visit:

www.csis.org/gai, **Center for Strategic and International Studies,** date connected 3/10/07. This site describes the Global Aging Initiative, established in 1999. The site includes many links to information about specific countries and their experiences with changing demographics.

www.aginginstride.org, **Aging in Stride,** date connected, 3/10/07. This site includes a great deal of information that is useful in working directly with clients. It provides consumer-friendly advice about physical safety, aging in place, senior living options, health issues, choosing a nursing home, financial concerns, death and dying, and social networks.

www.cdc.gov/nchs/fastats/olderramericans.htm, **National Center for Health Statistics,** date connected 3/10/07. Provides excellent data regarding life expectancy, disability, and other important statistics about older adults. Includes many links to other sites as well.

REFERENCES

Achenbaum, W. A. (1995). Images of old age in America, 1790–1970. In M. Featherstone & A. Wernick (Eds.), *Images of Aging: Cultural Representations of Later Life* (pp. 19–28). London: Routledge.

Achenbaum, W. A. (2002). Shades of gray, revisited. *Hallym International Journal of Aging, 4*(1), 1–14.

Achenbaum, W. A., & Sterns, P. N. (1978). Essay: Old age and modernization. *Gerontologist, 18,* 307–312.

Administration on Aging. (2004). A profile of older Americans: 2004. Washington, DC: U.S. Department of Health & Human Services. www.aoa.dhhs.gov/prof/ Statistics/profile/2004/2.asp. Accessed March 30, 2006.

Alwin, D. F., & McCammon, R. J. (2001). Aging, cohorts, and verbal ability. *Journal of Gerontology: Social Sciences, 56B,* S151–S161.

American Occupational Therapy Association. (2002). Occupational Therapy Practice Framework: Domain and Process. *American Journal of Occupational Therapy, 56,* 609–639.

Americans with Disabilities Act of 1990, Public Law 101-336, 104 Stat. 327.

Ardelt, M. (1997). Wiedom and life satisfaction in old age. *Journal of Gerontology: Psychological Sciences, 52B,* P15–P27.

Asghar, Z., Frick, J., & Buchel, F. (2005). Income mobility in old age in Britain and Germany. *Ageing and Society, 4,* 543–565.

Auchincloss, A. H., Van Nostrand, J. F., & Ronsaville, D. (2001). Access to health care for older persons in the United States: Personal, structural, and neighborhood characteristics. *Journal of Aging and Health, 13,* 329–354.

Bailis, D. S., & Chipperfield, J. G. (2002). Compensating for losses in perceived personal control over health: A role for collective self-esteem in health aging. *Journal of Gerontology: Psychological Sciences, 57B,* P531–P539.

Baker, D. W., Gazmararian, J. A., Sudano, J., & Patterson, M. (2000). The association between age and health literacy among elderly persons. *Journal of Gerontology: Social Sciences, 55B,* S368–S374.

Barrett, A. E. (2003). Socioeconomic status and age identity: The role of dimensions of health in the subjective construction of age. *Journal of Gerontology: Social Sciences, 58B,* S101–S109.

Becker, G. (2002). Dying away from home: Quandaries of migration for elders in two ethnic groups. *Journal of Gerontology: Social Sciences, 57B,* S79–S95.

Bergstrom, M. J., & Holmes, M. E. (2004). Organizational communication and aging: Age-related processes in organizations. In M. J. Bergstrom & M. E. Holmes (Eds.), *Handbook of communication and aging research* (2nd ed., pp. 305–327). Mahwah, NJ: Lawrence Erlbaum Associates.

Biggs, S. (2005). Beyond appearances: Perspectives on identity in later life and some implications for method. *Journal of Gerontology: Social Sciences, 60B,* S118–S128.

Binstock, R. H., & Day, C. L. (1996). Aging and politics. In R. H. Binstock & L. K. George (Eds.), *Handbook of aging and the social sciences* (4th ed., pp. 362–387). San Diego: Academic Press.

Brown, W. M., Consedine, N. S., & Magar, C. (2005). Altruism relates to health in an ethnically diverse sample of older adults. *Journal of Gerontology: Psychological Sciences, 60B,* P143–P152.

Buckley, N. J., Denton, F. T., Robb, L. A., & Spencer, B. G. (2004a). Healthy aging at older ages: Are income and education important? *Canadian Journal on Aging, 23* (Suppl1), S155–S169.

Buckley, N. J., Denton, F. T., Robb, L. A., & Spencer, B. G. (2004b). The transition from good to poor health: An econometric study of the older population. *Journal of Health Economics, 23,* 1013–1034.

Butler, R. N. (1975). *Why survive? Being old in America.* New York: Harper & Row.

Cagney, K. A., Browning, C. F., & Wen, M. (2005). Racial disparities in self-rated health at older ages: What difference does the neighborhood make? *Journal of Gerontology: Social Sciences, 60B,* S181–S190.

Cagney, K. A., & Lauderdale, D. S. (2002). Education, wealth, and cognitive function in later life. *Journal of Gerontology: Psychological Sciences, 57B,* P163–P172.

Canadian Association of Occupational Therapists. (2002). *Enabling occupation: An occupational therapy perspective* (Revised ed.). Ottawa, Ontario: Author.

Cattell, M. G. (1996). Gender, aging, and health: A comparative approach. In C. F. Sargent & C. B. Brettell (Eds.), *Gender and health: An international perspective* (pp. 87–122). Upper Saddle River, NJ: Prentice Hall.

Chandola, T., Bartley, M., Sacker, A., Jenkinson, C., & Marmot, M. (2003). Health selection in the Whitehall II study, UK. *Social Science and Medicine, 57,* 1631–1641.

Chappell, N. L., & Penning, M. J. (1996). Employer-based health insurance and seniors: The case of Bermuda. *Gerontologist, 36,* 63–69.

Chen, P., & Wilmoth, J. M. (2004). The effects of residential mobility on ADL and IADL limitations among the very old living in the community. *Journal of Gerontology: Social Sciences, 59B,* S164–S172.

Chipperfield, J. G., & Havens, B. (2001). Gender differences in the relationship between marital status transitions and life satisfaction in later life. *Journal of Gerontology: Psychological Sciences, 56B,* P176–P186.

Chipperfield, J. G., Perry, R. P., & Weiner, B. (2003). Discrete emotions in later life. *Journal of Gerontology: Psychological Sciences, 43,* P23–P34.

Cohen, C. I. (1999). Aging and homelessness. *The Gerontologist, 39,* 5–14.

Cohen, M. A. (1998). Emerging trends in the finance and delivery of long-term care: Public and private opportunities and challenges. *The Gerontologist, 38,* 80–89.

Cole, T. R. (1992). *The journey of life: A cultural history of aging in America.* Cambridge: Press Syndicate of the University of Cambridge.

Collins, K., Luszcz, M., Lawson, M., & Keeves, J. (1997). Everyday problem solving in elderly women: Contributions of residence, perceived control, and age. *Gerontologist, 37,* 293–302.

Cornman, J. M., & Kingston, E. R. (1996). Trends, issues, perspectives, and values for the aging of the baby boom cohorts. *Gerontologist, 36,* 15–26.

Covey, H. C. (1989). Old age portrayed by the ages-of-life models from the middle ages to the 16th century. *Gerontologist, 29,* 692–698.

Crane, M., Byrne, K., Fu, R., Lipmann, B., Mirabelli, F., Rota-Bartelink, A., Ryan, M., Shea, R., Watt, H., & Warnes, A. M. (2005). The causes of homelessness in later life: Findings from a 3-nation study. *Journal of Gerontology. Social Sciences, 60B,* S152–S159.

Crystal, S., Johnson, R. W., Harman, J., Sambamoorthi, U., & Kumar, R. (2000). Out-of-pocket health care costs among older Americans. *Journal of Gerontology: Social Sciences, 55B,* 551–562.

Dail, P. W. (1988). Prime-time television portrayals of older adults in the context of family life. *Gerontologist, 28,* 700–706.

Dannefer, D. (2003). Cumulative advantage/disadvantage and the life course: Cross-fertilizing age and social science theory. *Journal of Gerontology: Social Sciences, 58B,* S327–S337.

Davidson, K., (2004). "Why can't a man be more like a woman?" Marital status and social networking of older men. *Journal of Men's Studies, 13,* 25–43.

Denton, M., & Walters, V. (1999). Gender differences in structural and behavioral determinants of health: An analysis of the social production of health. *Social Science & Medicine, 48,* 1221–1235.

Easterlin, R. A. (1996). Economic and social implications of demographic patterns. In R. H. Binstock & L. K. George (Eds.), *Handbook of aging and the social sciences* (4th ed., pp. 73–93). San Diego: Academic Press.

The Economist. (November 26, 2005a). Retirement age: 65 not out (2005). 16.

The Economist. (November 26, 2005b). Aging population must try harder. 72.

Edmondson, R. (2005). Wisdom in later life: Ethnographic approaches. *Aging & Society, 25,* 339–356.

Evans, G. W., Kantrowitz, E., & Eshelman, P. (2002). Housing quality and psychological well-being among the elderly population. *Journal of Gerontology: Psychological Sciences, 57B,* P381–P383.

Federal Interagency Forum on Aging Related Statistics (FIFARS). (2004). *Older Americans 2004: Key indicators of well-being.* FIFARS. Washington, DC: U.S. Government Printing Office.

Feldman, P. H., Nadash, P., & Gursen, M. (2001). Improving communication between researchers and policy makers in long-term care: Or, researchers are from Mars; Policy makers are from Venus. *Gerontologist, 41,* 312–321.

Filinson, R. (1997). Legislating community care: The British experience, with U.S. comparisons. *Gerontologist, 37,* 333–340.

Fox, P., Arnsberger, P., Owens, D., Nussey, B., Zhang, X., Golding, J. M., Tabnak, F., & Otero-Sabogal, R. (2004). Patient and clinical site factors associated with rescreening behavior among older multiethnic, low-income women. *Gerontologist, 44,* 76–84.

Franks, M. M., Herzog, A. R., Holmberg, D., & Markus, H. R. (2003). Self-complexity: Linking age and education with self-rated health and depression. *Hallym International Journal of Aging, 5*(2), 91–110.

Fronstin, P. (1999). Retirement patterns and employee benefits: Do benefits matter? *Gerontologist, 39,* 37–47.

Fry, C. (1996). Age, aging, and culture. In R. H. Binstock & L. K. George (Eds.), *Handbook of aging and the social sciences* (4th ed., pp. 117–136). San Diego: Academic Press.

Gatz, M. (1995). Questions that aging puts to preventionists. In L. A. Bond, S. J. Cutler, & A. Grams (Eds.), *Promoting successful and productive aging* (pp. 36–68). Thousand Oaks, CA: Sage.

George, L. K. (2005). Socioeconomic status and health across the life course: Progress and prospects. *Journal of Gerontology: Series B, 60B* (Special Issue II), 135–139.

George, L. K., & Bylund, R. (2002). Rural Midwestern seniors and mobile homes: Characteristics and issues. *Rural Research Report, 13*(4), 1–8.

Gitlin, L. N. (2003). Conducting research on home environments: Lessons learned and new directions. *Gerontologist, 43,* 628–637.

Glascock, T., & Feinman, S. (1980). A holocultural analysis of old age. *Comparative Social Research, 3,* 311–332.

Golant, S. (2003). Conceptualizing time and behavior in environmental gerontology: A pair of old issues deserving new thought. *Gerontologist, 43,* 638–648.

Gratton, B. (1997). The politics of dependency estimates: Social Security Board statistics, 1935–1939. *Journal of Gerontology: Social Sciences, 52B,* S117–S124.

Greene, V. L., & Marty, K. (1999). Editorial essay: Generational investment and social insurance for the elderly: Balancing the accounts. *Gerontologist, 39,* 645–647.

Gruman, G. J. (1966/2003). *A history of ideas about the prolongation of life.* New York: Springer.

Haber, C. (1997). Witches, widows, wives, and workers: The historiography of elderly women in America. In J. M. Coyle (Ed.), *Handbook on women and aging* (pp. 29–51). Westport, CT: Greenwood Press.

Hagestad, G. O. (1986). The aging society as a context for family life. *Daedalus, 115,* 119–139.

Hardy, M. A., & Shuey, K. (2000). Pension decisions in a changing economy: Gender, structure, and choice. *Journal of Gerontology: Social Sciences, 55B,* S271–S277.

Harrington, C., Collier, E., & Burdin, A. (2005). Nursing. In E. B. Palmore, L. Branch, & D. K. Harris (Eds.), *Encyclopedia of ageism* (pp. 233–236). Binghamton, NY: Haworth Press.

Harris, D. K. (2005). Age norms. In E. B. Palmore, L. Branch, & D. K. Harris (Eds.), *Encyclopedia of ageism* (pp. 14–15). Binghamton, NY: Hayworth Press.

Hatch, S. L. (2005). Conceptualizing and identifying cumulative adversity and protective resources: Implications for understanding health inequalities. *Journals of Gerontology: Series B, 60B* (Special Issue), 130–134.

Hayward, M. D. (2005). Commentary: What happened to America's elderly population? In K. W. Schaie & G. Elder (Eds.), *Historical influences on lives and aging* (pp. 35–42). New York: Springer.

Hays, J. C. D., Hays, R. B., & Hays, C. B. (2005). Ageism in the Bible. In E. B. Palmore, L. Branch, & D. K. Harris (Eds.), *Encyclopedia of ageism* (pp. 20–25). New York: Haworth Press.

Hendricks, J., & Hendricks, C. D. (1977). The age old question of old age: Was it really so much better back when? *Journal of Aging and Human Development, 8,* 139–154.

Herd, P. (2005). Ensuring a minimum: Social Security reform and women. *Gerontologist, 45,* 12–25.

Hesketh, T., Lu, L., & Xing, Z. W. (2005). The effect of China's one-child family policy after 25 years. *New England Journal of Medicine, 353*(11), 1171–1177.

Hilt, M., & Lipschultz, J. H. (2005). *Mass media, an aging population, and the baby boomers.* Mahwah, NJ: Lawrence Erlbaum Associates.

Hooker, K., & McAdams, D. P. (2003). Personality reconsidered: A new agenda for aging research. *Journal of Gerontology: Psychological Sciences, 58B,* P296–P304.

Hudson, R. B. (1996). Social protection and services. In R. H. Binstock & L. K. George (Eds.), *Handbook of aging and the social sciences* (4th ed., pp. 446–466). San Diego, CA: Academic Press.

Hudson, R. B. (Ed.). (2005). *The new politics of old age policy.* Baltimore, MD: Johns Hopkins Press.

Hungerford, T. L. (2001). The economic consequences of widowhood on elderly women in the United States and Germany. *Gerontologist, 41,* 103–110.

Inglehart, R. (2002). Gender, aging, and subjective well-being. *International Journal of Comparative Sociology, 43*(3–5), 391–402.

Isaacowitz, D. M., & Smith, J. (2003). Positive and negative affect in very old age. *Journal of Gerontology: Psychological Sciences, 58B,* P143–P152.

Johnson, C. L., & Barer, B. M. (2002). Life course effects of early parental loss among very old African Americans. *Journal of Gerontology: Social Sciences, 57B,* S108–S116.

Johnson, R. W., Sambamoorthi, U., & Crystal, S. (1999). Gender differences in pension wealth: Estimates using provider data. *Gerontologist, 39,* 320–333.

Johnson, W., & Krueger, R. F. (2005). Predictors of physical health: Toward an integrated model of genetic and environmental antecedents. *Journals of Gerontology: Series B, 60B* (Special Issue I), 42–52.

Kahn, J. R., & Fazio, E. M. (2005). Economic status over the life course and racial disparities in health. *Journals of Gerontology: Series B, 60B* (Special Issue II), 76–84.

Kam, P. (2002). From disempowering to empowering: Changing the practice of social service professionals with older people. *Hallym International Journal of Aging, 4,* 161–183.

Kastenbaum, R., & Ross, B. (1975). Historical perspectives on care. In J. G. Howells (Ed.), *Modern Perspectives in the Psychiatry of Old Age* (pp. 421–449). New York: Brunner/Mazel.

Kennedy, J. F. (1963). Elderly Citizens of Our Nation, 88th congress, 1st session, House of Representatives. In Document No. 72. Washington, DC: Government Printing Office, p. 10.

Keyes, C. L. M. (2002). The exchange of emotional support with age and its relationship with emotional well-being by age. *Journal of Gerontology: Psychological Sciences, 57B,* P518–P525.

Kingston, E., & Herd, P. (2005). Reframing Social Security: Cures worse than the disease. In R. B. Hudson (Ed.), *The new politics of old age policy* (pp. 183–204). Baltimore, MD: Johns Hopkins Press.

Kinsella, K., & Velkoff, V. A. (2001). *An aging world: 2001.* Washington, DC: U.S. Census Bureau publication P95/01-1.

Krause, N. (1998). Neighborhood deterioration, religious coping, and changes in health during late life. *Gerontologist, 38,* 653–664.

Labouvie-Vief, G., Diehl, M., Tarnowski, A., & Shen, J. (2000). Age differences in adult personality: Findings from the United States and China. *Journal of Gerontology: Psychological Sciences, 55B,* P4–P17.

Landerman, L. R., Fillenbaum, G. G., Pieper, C. F., Maddox, G. L., Gold, D. T., & Guralnik, J. M. (1998). Private health insurance coverage and disability among older Americans. *Journal of Gerontology: Social Sciences, 53B,* S258–S266.

Lang, F. R., Staudinger, U. M., & Carstensen, L. L. (1998). Perspectives on socioemotional selectivity in late life: How personality and social context do (and do not) make a difference. *Journal of Gerontology: Psychological Sciences, 53B,* P21–P30.

Lee, J. S., & Frongillo, E. A. (2001). Factors associated with food insecurity among U.S. elderly persons: Importance of functional impairments. *Journal of Gerontology: Social Sciences, 56B,* S94–S99.

Lee, W. K. M. (2001). The feminization of poverty among the elderly population of Hong Kong. *Asian Journal of Women's Studies, 7*(3), 31–54.

Lee, Y. G. (2004). Financial status of older Americans aged 70 and above: A comparison of successive age cohorts. *Hallym International Journal of Aging, 6*(1), 37–55.

Leutz, W. (1999). Policy choices for Medicaid and Medicare waivers. *Gerontologist, 39,* 86–93.

Levine, C. (Ed.) (2004). *Always on call: When illness turns families into caregivers.* Nashville, TN: Vanderbilt University Press.

Li, L. W. (2005). Longitudinal changes in the amount of informal care among publicly paid home care recipients. *Gerontologist, 45,* 465–473.

Lichtenstein, M. J., Pruski, L. A., Marshall, C. E., Blalock, C. L., Murphy, D. L, Plaetke, R., & Lee, S. (2001). The *Positively Aging®* teaching materials improve middle school students' images of older people. *Gerontologist, 47,* 322–332.

Lima, J. C., & Allen, S. M. (2001). Targeting risk for unmet need: Not enough help versus no help at all. *Journal of Gerontology: Social Sciences, 56B,* S302–S310.

Litwin, H. (2005). Correlates of successful aging: Are they universal? *International Journal of Aging and Human Development, 61,* 313–333.

Logan, J. R., & Spitze, G. F. (1988). Suburbanization and public services for the aging. *Gerontologist, 28,* 644–647.

Luo, Y., & Waite, L. J. (2005). The impact of childhood and adult SES on physical, mental, and cognitive well-being in later life. *Journal of Gerontology: Social Sciences, 60B,* S93–S101.

Lysack, C. L., MacNeill, S. E., Neufeld, S. W., & Lichtenberg, P. A. (2002). Elderly inner city women who return home to live alone. *OTJR: Occupation, Participation, and Health, 22*(2), 59–69.

Martin, M., Grunendahl, M., & Martin, P. (2001). Age differences in stress, social resources, and well-being in middle and older age. *Journal of Gerontology: Psychological Sciences, 56B,* P214–P222.

Matthews, R. J., Smith, L. K., Hancock, R. M., Jagger, C., & Spiers, N. A. (2005). Socioeconomic factors associated with the onset of disability in older age: A longitudinal study of people aged 75 years and over. *Social Science & Medicine, 61,* 1567–1575.

McCulloch, B. J. (1995). The relationship of family proximity and social support to the mental health of older rural adults: The Appalachian context. *Journal of Aging Studies, 9,* 65–81.

McDonald, J., Quandt, S. A., Arcury, T. A., Bell, R. A., & Vitolins, M. Z. (2000). On their own: Nutritional self-management strategies of rural widowers. *Gerontologist, 40,* 480–491.

McHugh, K. E., & Larson-Keagy, E. M. (2005). These white walls: The dialectic of retirement communities. *Journal of Aging Studies, 12*(2), 241–256.

McMullin, J. A. (2000). Diversity and the state of sociological aging theory, *Gerontologist, 40,* 517–530.

Minkler, M., & Holstein, M. (2005). Successful aging. In E. B. Palmore, L. Branch, & D. K. Harris (Eds.), *Encyclopedia of ageism* (pp. 306–309). Binghamton, NY: Hayworth Press.

Mollenkopf, H., Kaspar, R., Mracellini, F., Ruoppila, I., Szeman, Z., Tacken, M., & Wahl, H. (2004). Quality of life in urban and rural areas of five European countries: Similarities and differences. *Hallym International Journal of Aging, 6*(1), 1–36.

Moody, H. (1986). The meaning of life and the meaning of old age. In T. R. Cole & S. Gadow (Eds.), *What does it mean to grow old?* (pp. 9–40). Durham: Duke University Press.

Mroczek, D. K., & Spiro, A. (2003). Modeling intraindividual change in personality traits: Findings from the normative aging study. *Journal of Gerontology: Psychological Sciences, 58B,* P153–P165.

National Center for Health Statistics, Data Warehouse on Trends in Health and Aging (2006). www.cdc.gov/nchs/agingact.htm. Accessed March 20, 2006.

National Institute of Neurological Disorders and Stroke. (2006). *Post-polio syndrome fact sheet.* www.ninds.nih.gov/disorders/post_polio/detail_post_polio.htm. Accessed February 6, 2006.

Neugarten, B. (1976). Adaptation and the life cycle. *Counseling Psychologist, 6,* 16–20.

Neugarten, B. (1978). The rise of the young-old. In R. Gross, B. Gross, & S. Seidman (Eds.), *The new old: Struggling for a decent aging* (pp. 47–63). Garden City, NJ: Doubleday Anchor.

Neumark, D. (2006). Age discrimination legislation in the United States. http://ideas.repec.org/a/oup/coecpo/v21y 2003i3p297-317.html Accessed February 22, 2008.

Nydegger, C. N. (1983). Family ties of the aged in cross-cultural perspective. *Gerontologist, 23,* 26–32.

Ofstedal, M. B., Chan, A., Chayovan, N., Chuang, Y., Perez, A., Mehta, K., & Hermalin, A. I. (2002). Policies and programs in place and under development. In A. I. Hermalin (Ed.), *The well-being of the elderly in Asia: A four country comparative study* (pp. 65–97). Ann Arbor: University of Michigan Press.

Olshansky, S. J., & Carnes, B. A. (2001). *The quest for immortality: Science at the frontiers of aging.* New York: Norton Press.

Palmore, E. (2001). The ageism survey: First findings. *Gerontologist, 41,* 572–575.

Palmore, E. B. (2005). Biological definitions of aging. In E. B. Palmore, L. Branch, & D. K. Harris (Eds.), *Encyclopedia of ageism* (pp. 50–52). New York: Haworth Press.

Pinquart, M., & Sorensen, S. (2000). Influences of socioeconomic status, social network, and competency on subjective well-being in later life: A meta-analysis. *Psychology and Aging, 15,* 187–224.

Ragan, A. M., & Bowen, A. M. (2001). Improving attitudes regarding the elderly population: The effects of information and reinforcement for change. *Gerontologist, 41,* 511–515.

Reynolds, S. L., Crimmins, E. M., & Saito, Y. (1998). Cohort differences in disability and disease presence. *Gerontologist, 38,* 578–590.

Riley, J. C. (2001). *Rising life expectancy: A global history.* New York: Cambridge University Press.

Rowe, J., & Kahn, R. (1998). *Successful aging: The MacArthur Foundation study.* New York: Pantheon.

Rowles, G. D. (1991). Beyond performance: Being in place as a component of occupational therapy. *American Journal of Occupational Therapy, 45,* 265–271.

Rupp, K., Strand, A., & Davies, P. S. (2003). Poverty among elderly women: Assessing SSI options to strengthen Social Security reform. *Journal of Gerontology: Social Sciences, 58B,* S359–S368.

Ryff, C. D., & Singer, B. H. (2005). Social environments and the genetics of aging: Advancing knowledge of protective health mechanisms. *Journals of Gerontology: Series B, 60B* (Special Issue I), 12–23.

Sarkisian, C. A., Steers, W. N., Hays, R. D., & Mangione, C. M. (2005). Development of the 12-item Expectations Regarding Aging survey. *Gerontologist, 45,* 240–248.

Serow, W. J. (2001). Retirement migration counties in the Southeastern United States: Geographic, demographic, and economic correlates. *Gerontologist, 41,* 220–227.

Settersten, R. A. (2005). Linking the two ends of life: What gerontology can learn from childhood studies. *Journal of Gerontology: Social Sciences, 60B,* S173–S180.

Shahar, S. (1997). *Growing old in the middle ages: "Winter clothes us in shadow and pain."* New York: Routledge.

Sherman, S. R. (1997). Images of middle-aged and older women: Historical, cultural, and personal. In J. M. Coyle (Ed.), *Handbook on women and aging* (pp. 14–52). Westport, CT: Greenwood Press.

Shipp, K. M. (2005). Physical therapy. In E. B. Palmore, L. Branch, & D. K. Harris (Eds.), *Encyclopedia of ageism* (pp. 248–249). Binghamton, NY: Haworth Press.

Siegrist, J., von dem Knesebeck, O., & Pollack, C. E. (2004). Social productivity and well-being of older people: A sociological exploration. *Social Theory and Health, 2,* 1–17.

Silverstein, M., Angelelli, J. J., & Parrott, T. M. (2001). Changing attitudes toward aging policy in the United States during the 1980s and 1990s: A cohort analysis. *Journal of Gerontology: Social Sciences, 56B,* S36–S43.

Small, B. J., Hertzog, C., Hultsch, D. F., & Dixon, R. A. (2003). Stability and change in adult personality over 6 years: Findings from the Victoria longitudinal study. *Journal of Gerontology: Psychological Sciences, 58B,* P166–P176.

Smedley, B. D., Stith, A. Y., & Nelson, A. R. (2003). *Unequal treatment: Confronting racial and ethnic disparities in healthcare.* Washington, DC: National Academies Press.

Snowdon, D. (2001). *Aging with grace: Leading longer, healthier, and more meaningful lives.* New York: Bantam Books.

Sokolovsky, J. (1997). Culture, aging and context. In J. Sokolovsky (Ed.), *The cultural context of aging: Worldwide perspectives* (2nd ed., pp. 1–15). Westport, CT: Bergin & Garvey.

Spector, W. D., Cohen, J. W., & Pesis-Katz, I. (2004). Home care before and after the Balanced Budget Act of 1997: Shifts in financing and services. *Gerontologist, 44,* 39–47.

Stallmann, J. I., Deller, S. C., & Shields, M. (1999). The economic and fiscal impact of aging retirees on a small rural region. *Gerontologist, 39,* 599–610.

Starkloff, C. (2001). A consumer's perspective on aging: Challenges for independent living. *Rehabilitation Education, 15,* 439–444.

Statutory Instrument 2006 No. 1031 (2006). The Employment Equality (Age) Regulations 2006. http://www. opsi.gov.uk/si/si2006/20061031.htm#3. Accessed February 22, 2008.

Sterns, P. N. (1980). Old women: Some historical observations. *Journal of Family History 5,* 44–57.

Steverink, N., Westerhof, G. J., Bode, C., & Dittmann-Kohli, F. (2001). The personal experience of aging, individual resources, and subjective well-being. *Journal of Gerontology: Psychological Sciences, 56B,* P364–P373.

Stoller, E. P., & Longino, C. F. (2001). "Going home" or "leaving home"? The impact of person and place ties on anticipated counterstream migration. *Gerontologist, 41,* 96–102.

Talamantes, M. A., Cornell, J., Espino, D. V., Lichtenstein, M. J., & Hazuda, H. P. (1996). SES and ethnic differences in perceived caregiver availability among young-old Mexican Americans and non-Hispanic whites. *Gerontologist, 36,* 88–99.

Taylor, D. H., Sloan, F. A., & Norton, E. C. (1999). Formation of trusts and spend down to Medicaid. *Journal of Gerontology: Social Sciences, 54B,* S194–S201.

Townsend, E. (1999). Enabling occupation in the 21st century: Making good intentions a reality. *Australian Occupational Therapy Journal, 46,* 147–159.

Turrell, G., Lynch, J. W., Kaplan, G. A., Everson, S. A., Helkala, E., Kauhanen, J., & Salonen, J. T. (2002). Socioeconomic positions across the lifecourse and cognitive function in late middle age. *Journal of Gerontology: Social Sciences, 57B,* S43–S51.

Uhlenberg, P. (2000). Essays on age integration: Introduction: Why study age integration? *Gerontologist, 40,* 261–308.

U.S. Census Bureau. (2001). Introduction. In *An aging world: 2001* (pp. i–iv). Washington, DC: Author.

Velkoff, V. A., He, W., Sengupta, M., & DeBarros, K. A. (2006). *65+ in the United States: 2005.* Washington, DC: U.S. Census Bureau.

Vinovskis, M. A. (2005). Historical changes and the American life course. In K. W. Schaie & G. Elder (Eds.), *Historical influences on lives and aging* (pp. 1–21). New York: Springer.

Waidman, T. A., & Liu, K. (2000). Disability trends among elderly persons and implications for the future. *Journal of Gerontology: Social Sciences, 55B,* S298–S307.

Weiss, M. J. (May 1, 2003). GREAT expectations—Baby Boomer wealth forecasts wilt. LookSmart. www.findarticles.com/p/articles/mi_m4021/is_4_25/ ai_100751507/print. Accessed January 17, 2006.

Westerhof, G. J., & Barrett, A. E. (2005). Age identity and subjective well-being: A comparison of the United States and Germany. *Journal of Gerontology: Social Sciences, 60B,* S129–S136.

Westerman, J. W., & Sundali, J. (2005). The transformation of employee pensions in the United States: Through the looking glass of organizational behavior. *Journal of Organizational Behavior, 26,* 99–103.

White House Conference on Aging. (2005). *The booming dynamics of aging: From awareness to action.* www.whcoa.gov/press/05_Report_1.pdf. Accessed September 29, 2006.

Whiteford, G. (2000). Occupational deprivation: Global challenge in the new millennium. *British Journal of Occupational Therapy, 63,* 200–204.

Wolf, D. A., & Longino, C. F. (2005). Our "increasingly mobile society"? The curious persistence of a false belief. *Gerontologist, 45,* 5–11.

World Population Prospects, The 1998 Revision, Volume II: Sex and Age (2003). The Population Division, Department of Economic and Social Affairs. United Nations Secretariat. www.un.org/esa/.socdev/ageing/ageing/agewpop1.htm. Accessed February 22, 2008.

Wray, L. A., Alwin, D. F., & McCammon, R. J. (2005). Social status and risky health behaviors: Results from the Health and Retirement Study. *Journals of Gerontology: Series B, 60B* (Special Issue II), 85–92.

Wray, L. A., & Blaum, C. S. (2001). Explaining the role of sex on disability: A population-based study. *Gerontologist, 41,* 499–510.

Yang, Z., Norton, E. C., & Stearns, S. C. (2003). Longevity and health care expenditures: The real reasons older people spend more. *Journal of Gerontology: Social Sciences, 58B,* S2–S10.

Zebrowitz, L. A. (2003). Aging stereotypes—internalization or inoculation? A commentary. *Journal of Gerontology, Psychological Sciences, 58B,* P214–P215.

Zick, C. D., & Holden, K. (2000). An assessment of the wealth holdings of recent widows. *Journal of Gerontology: Social Sciences, 55B,* S90–S97.

CHAPTER 2

Theories of Aging: A Multidisciplinary Review for Occupational and Physical Therapists

Vern L. Bengtson • Bette R. Bonder

"It is better to know some of the questions than all of the answers."

James Thurber

OBJECTIVES

By the end of this chapter, readers will be able to:

1. Discuss the importance of understanding various theories of aging.
2. Describe the various biological theories of aging.
3. Describe psychological theories of aging.
4. Describe sociological theories of aging.
5. Discuss the impact of these theories on approaches to intervention with older adults.

Mrs. Arthur is a 73-year-old widow who has the appearance of a wizened 90-year-old. Her hair is pure white, and her skin is wrinkled. She walks slowly with feet wide apart. She spends most of her time in her apartment alone, and she complains to family and her few surviving friends about how her life is not worth living.

Mr. Morales is a 76-year-old married man who appears much younger than his age. His hair retains some of its original dark color, and his skin has a relatively youthful look. He provides care for his infirm wife and helps his adult son as

well. He enjoys the company of many friends and is busy much of the time playing pool, going to dominoes tournaments, and driving friends to the Hispanic Senior Center. He loves to dance, and he expresses enthusiasm for life.

What makes these two stories so different? Why do some people seem to age well, while others spend their later years infirm and unhappy? These questions raise more fundamental issues about the life course. Why do we age? What is the nature of senescence, and can its process be altered? How can we live healthier and more fulfilling lives? How can we better address the needs of elderly people and unleash their potentialities? Why do some people age successfully, and others don't? Why do some 80-year-olds look like 60-year-olds while some 60-year-olds look like they're 80?

These are important questions, and to answer them, scientific theory is required. *Theory* is an attempt to explain what we observe in empirical research or practice. *Theories of aging* are attempts to go beyond the *what* of symptoms or disabilities associated with aging to examine the *why* and *how* of changes related to age. The need for theory is most obvious in biomedical fields, where therapies represent the end of a sequence of laboratory research about causes and effects. But theory is equally important in psychology, sociology, and public policy. At the societal level, the rapid aging of populations presents researchers and policy makers with new and difficult questions. In all countries of the world, population aging is altering dependency ratios and dramatically increasing the number of elders who will need care. Gerontologists—whether as scientists, practitioners, or policy makers—concern themselves with these questions.

What Do We Want to Explain?

Gerontologists focus on three sets of issues as they attempt to analyze and understand the phenomena of aging.

The first set concerns *the aged*: the population of those who can be categorized as elderly in terms of their length of life lived or expected life span. Most gerontological research in recent decades has focused on the functional problems of aged populations, seen in human terms as medical disability or barriers to independent living.

A second set of issues focuses on *aging* as a developmental process. Here the principal interest is in the situations and problems that accumulate during the life span and cannot be understood separate from developmental experiences and processes across a lifetime. Gerontologists examine the biological, psychological, and social aspects of the aging process as including variable rates and consequences.

A third set of issues involves the study of *age* as a dimension of structure and behavior within species. Social gerontologists are interested in how social organizations are created and changed in response to age-related patterns of birth, socialization, role transitions, and retirement or death. The phenomena to be explained relate to how institutions such as labor markets, retirement and pension systems, health care organizations, and political institutions take into account or deal with "age." The study of age is also a concern of zoologists, primate anthropologists, and evolutionary biologists who note its importance as an organizing principle in many species, behaviors, and survival (Wachter & Finch, 1997). Although these three emphases are quite different in focus and inquiry, they are nonetheless interrelated in gerontological research and practice. Theoretical engagement helps to distinguish among these basic categories of interest.

The New Problem of Societal Aging

Rapid population aging and higher dependency ratios as described in Chapter 1 will create major challenges for states and economies over the next half century. Less obvious but equally important is the profound effect that population aging will have on social institutions such as families. Who will care for the growing numbers of very old members of human societies? Will it be state governments? The aged themselves? Their families? Private care providers? These challenges are the result of four remarkable sociodemographic changes that have occurred since the start of the 20th century and particularly during the past three decades.

Extension of the Life Course
Over this period, there has been a remarkable increase in life expectancy and an astonishing change in the typical, expected life course of individuals, especially in industrialized societies. Remarkably, an entire generation has been added to the average span of life over the past century.

Changes in the Age Structures of Nations
This increase in longevity has also added a generation to the social structure of societies. In many economically developed nations, those aged 80 and over are the fastest-growing portion of the total population. At the same time, total fertility rates in developed nations have plummeted. Several countries in Europe (notably

Germany) as well as Japan are beginning to show declining population numbers. Most nations today have many more elders, and many fewer children, than they did 50 years ago.

Changes in Family Structures and Relationships

Families look different today than they did 50 years ago. We have added a whole generation to the structure of many families. Some of these differences are the consequence of the expanding life course. Others are the result of trends in family structure, notably higher divorce rates and the higher incidence of single parents raising children. Still others are outcomes of changes in values and political expectations regarding the role of the state in the lives of individuals and families.

Changes in Governmental Expectations and Responsibilities

For most of the 20th century, governmental states in the industrialized world increasingly assumed more responsibility for their citizens' welfare and well-being. In the last decade, however, this trend appears to have slowed or reversed as states make efforts to reduce welfare expenditures. The economic and social implications of aging and the aged for societies are vast.

The Current State of Theory in Gerontology

Gerontology in the United States emerged as a distinct field of study following World War II when a number of U.S. scientists from biology, psychology, and human development founded the Gerontology Society of America. Since its beginnings, gerontology's scholarly and scientific interests were broadly defined because old age was considered "a problem" that was unprecedented in scope (Achenbaum, 1987). Indeed, aging has become one of the most complex subjects facing modern science (Birren, 1999). To understand and explain the multifaceted phenomena and processes of aging required the scientific insights of biology and biomedicine, psychology, and the social sciences. Over time, the field expanded beyond these core disciplines to include anthropology, demography, economics, epidemiology, history, the humanities and arts, political science, and

social work, as well as the many professions that serve older persons.

Over the past several decades, gerontology has endeavored to build better scientific theories (Achenbaum, 1995; Troen, 2003). Scientific theories are premised on the idea that the natural universe has fundamental properties and processes that explain phenomena in specific contexts, that knowledge can be value free, that it can explain the actual workings of the empirical world, and that it can be revised by a better theory as a result of careful observations of empirical events (Turner, 2003).

The process of building theory involves observations and abstractions. Scientists most often start with definitions of general concepts and put forward a number of logically ordered propositions about the relationships among concepts. Concepts are linked to empirical phenomena through operational definitions, from which hypotheses are derived and then tested against empirical observations. A general theory allows investigators to deduce logically a number of specific statements, or explanations, about the nature and behavior of a large class of phenomena (Turner, 2003; Wallace & Wolf, 1991). Because such theories are useful in predicting and hence manipulating our environments, they are considered essential for the design of programs aimed at ameliorating problems associated with aging, especially by the government.

Biological Theories of Aging

Biological theories address aging processes at the organism, molecular, and cellular levels. Instead of a defining theory of biological aging, there are a multitude of smaller theories, no doubt reflecting the fact that there is no single cause, mechanism, or basis for senescence. Biological theories of aging might explain why one individual remains flexible, as is true for the woman in Figure 2-1, while others lose physical function. Most of these biological theories fall into one of two general classes: **stochastic theories,** and **programmed (developmental-genetic) theories** (Cristofalo, Tresini, Francis, & Volker, 1999; Troen, 2003). In the past decade, however, evolutionary senescence theory has gained prominence as an explanation of why and how aging occurs. These theories focus on body systems and body function as classified in the International Classification of Function (ICF; WHO, 2001) or as

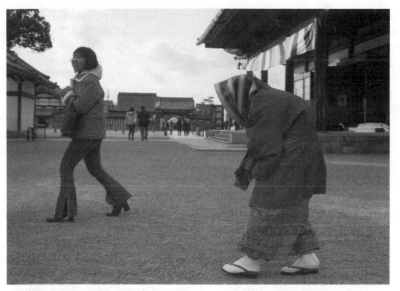

FIGURE 2-1 Cultural factors influence how elders dress and what they do. (Copyright © 2007 Jeffrey M. Levine.)

described in the Occupational Therapy Practice Framework (AOTA, 2002) as performance skills and client factors. Table 2-1 summarizes biological theories of aging.

Stochastic Theories

This class of theories explains aging as resulting from the accumulation of "insults" from the environment, which eventually reach a level incompatible with life. The best known is the *somatic mutation theory,* which came to prominence after World War II as a result of research on radiation exposure and damage. The theory states that mutations (genetic damage) will produce functional failure eventually resulting in death. Cristofalo (1996) notes, however, that an explanation of a shortened life span as a consequence

---

TABLE 2-1 **Biological Theories of Aging**

Stochastic ("insults")	Somatic mutation	Genetic damage leads to functional failure and death
	Error catastrophe	Defect in protein synthesis mechanism leads to errors in proteins
Developmental-genetic	Neuroendocrine	Functional decrements in neurons and hormones
	Immunological	Functional decrements in immune system
	Free radical	Damage from highly chemically reactive agents
	Caloric restriction	Excess calories damage tissues
Cellular aging	Cell–cell hybridization	All these theories posit cellular level changes affecting organismal changes
	Growth factor signal transduction	
	DNA replication	
Evolutionary	Mutation accumulation	Genetic errors/accidents over time lead to aging
	Antagonistic pleiotropy	Late-acting deleterious genes accumulate if they have any benefit in early life
	Disposable soma	Soma cells have limited durability because they have a short expected duration of use
Neuropsychological	Normal age-related change	Cognitive change is an inevitable part of aging
	Neurodegenerative change	Cognitive change is the result of damage and degeneration

of gene-altering exposure is not at all the same as explaining the normal processes of aging. In general, experiments have not supported somatic mutation theory. Another stochastic explanation, *error catastrophe theory,* proposes that a defect in the mechanism used for protein synthesis could lead to the production of error-containing proteins, resulting in the dysregulation of numerous cellular processes which eventually results in the death of the individual. Although appealing, there is no convincing evidence for error catastrophe (Cristofalo et al., 1999).

Developmental-Genetic Theories

This class of biological theories of aging proposes that the process of aging is continuous with and probably operating through the same mechanisms as development and, hence, is genetically controlled and programmed. Three categories of developmental-genetic theories have received empirical support (Cristofalo et al., 1999; Troen, 2003). First are the *neuroendocrine theories* that posit functional decrements in neurons and their associated hormones as central to the aging process. One such theory proposes that the hypothalamic/pituitary/adrenal axis is the primary regulator of the aging process, and that functional changes in this system are accompanied by or regulate functional decrements throughout the organism (Finch & Seeman, 1999). There is considerable evidence relating aging of the organism to loss of responsiveness of the neuroendocrine tissue to various signals. A second neuroendocrine explanation, the *immunological theory of aging* (Walford, 1969), is based on the observation that the functional capacity and fidelity of the immune system declines with age, as indicated by the strong age-associated increase in autoimmune disease.

A third neuroendocrine explanation, *free radical theory,* initially proposed by Harman (1956), suggests that most aging changes are due to the production of free radicals during cellular respiration (Frisard & Ravussin, 2006; Wolkow & Iser, 2006). Free radicals are highly chemically reactive agents that are generated in single electron transfer reactions to metabolism. This theory is among those currently attracting the greatest research attention, as it appears that oxidative stress is clearly at the center of cell damage and death. Comparative studies show that long-lived species have low levels of oxidative damage in the mitochondria (Sanz, Pamplona, & Barja, 2006). This would reduce mutations or the accumulation of "junk" that might be the source of cell death (Lenaz, Baracca, Fato, Genova, & Solaini, 2006; Terman & Brunk, 2006).

Some of the support for free radical theory comes from evidence about adaptive mechanisms that reduce oxidative stress and seem, thereby, to increase longevity (Yu & Chung, 2006). Estrogen, for example, has a protective role in reducing free radical production. Exercise also has protective effects, perhaps by suppressing inflammatory response in cells.

Even though free radical theory has gained widespread acceptance, it is not without its critics. Howes (2006) notes that extensive study has failed to conclusively demonstrate its value, and he further suggests that use of antioxidants that might be expected to reduce oxidative damage has not lived up to its early promise. Linnane and Eastwood (2006) present data to suggest that oxygen-free radical formation is not a direct cause of aging and is, in fact, essential for biological function.

Another explanation that relates differential rates of metabolism and life span expectancy is that of *caloric restriction* (Cristofalo et al., 1999; Ruggiero & Ferrucci, 2006; Sanz et al., 2006). This theory suggests that caloric restriction might slow metabolism and reduce oxidative damage. This theory, of course, gives one hope that simply by eating less, one might not only extend life, but also extend healthy life. Unfortunately, the evidence suggests that the needed caloric restriction would be draconian—something most individuals would be unwilling or unable to sustain. Further, caloric restriction theories do not explain why such restriction might extend life (Ruggiero & Ferrucci, 2006). They also do not clearly delineate whether it is total calories or calories of certain types that may produce the desired effect, for example, whether reducing protein might be as effective as reducing total calories.

Thus, even though theories of aging may give clues about how one ages, these theories do not promise Ponce de Leon's much sought after fountain of youth. Further, as can be seen in this discussion, in spite of extensive research, none has been conclusively demonstrated to be the primary cause of aging.

Theories of Cellular Aging

Although most well-known theories deal with the organism and its integrative functioning, the idea of aging as a cell-based phenomenon is relatively recent (Cristofalo, 1996). Three cellular-level research directions have emerged. The first focuses on a genetic analysis of senescence primarily based on cell–cell hybridization. A second strand relates to analyzing steps in the growth factor signal transduction. More recently, a third area of cellular-level research focuses on DNA replication and telomere shortening as a mechanism, which eventually curtails replication.

Evolutionary Theories

Martin (2003) argues that the single most important shift in biology of aging paradigmatic thinking in the past 20 years has been the widespread acceptance of evolutionary senescence theory as an explanation for why aging happens. Challenging the developmental-genetic approach is the idea of the 'selection' of aging mechanisms through evolution. This has been accompanied by growing skepticism that the diverse scenarios and trajectories of aging can be controlled by a process whose mechanisms regulate the precise processes of development (Cristofalo, 1996). Evolutionary theories attempt to explain the origin of aging as well as the divergence of species' life spans (Harman, 2006; Kirkwood, 2001). Evolutionary explanations of aging are based on three major theories. First is the *mutation accumulation theory* (Medawar, 1952) that states that aging is an inevitable result of the declining force of natural selection with age (that is, deleterious genes associated with senescence may be delayed until the postreproductive period). Mutation accumulation theory supposes the accumulation of heritable, late-acting deleterious constitutional mutations, as distinct from the accumulation of somatic mutations. The second evolutionary theory of aging, *antagonistic pleiotropy theory* (Williams, 1957), states further that late-acting deleterious genes might even be favored by selection and actively accumulated if they have any beneficial effects early in life. Simply put, the theory posits there are genes that have good effects early in life and bad effects later in life. The third evolutionary theory is *disposable soma theory* (Kirkwood, 2001). This refers to a process whereby there is limited investment in soma cell durability because such cells have a short expected duration of use. Soma are those parts of the body which are distinct from the "germ-line" that produces the reproductive cells. From this perspective, an increased rate of aging occurs through optimizing the investment in reproductive function as opposed to somatic maintenance functions.

Neuropsychological Theories of Aging

Drawing from the fields of neurology, physiology, and psychology, the neuropsychology of aging is a relatively new discipline that scientifically investigates, clinically assesses, and develops treatments for age-related and neurodegenerative changes in brain function and behavior. Theorizing proceeds induc-tively from empirical observations to models and theoretical explanations—a "bottom-up" approach. In a sense, the diagnosis is the theory (Woodruff-Pak & Papka, 1999). Contemporary theories of neuropsychology and aging differentiate between typical age-related changes in brain function, and neurodegenerative changes.

Theories of Typical Age-Related Change

There are two major configurations of change in cognitive functioning related to aging: (1) change in the prefrontal cortex and (2) change in the ability to form declarative memory. The prefrontal cortex is involved in executive function, attention, and working memory (Woodruff-Pak & Papka, 1999). Based on the principle that neural structures and related abilities laid down last should be the most vulnerable to processes of aging, evidence indicates that the frontal lobes (the last structure to develop) are the part of the brain affected earliest by normal aging. Declarative memory, which is dependent on circuitry in the medial temporal lobe or mammillary body, is involved in the manipulation and organization of memory (for example, "trying to learn" a task as opposed to performing a task) (Woodruff-Pak & Papka, 1999). Even though memory resides in a constellation of interacting brain areas, the medial temporal lobe circuitry for declarative memory appears to be most affected by processes of both normal and neuropathological aging.

Theories of Neurodegenerative Change

There are several age-linked neuropathological changes of the brain which produce observable degenerative deficits in cognitive functioning (the most prominent being Alzheimer's, but also Lewy body, Parkinson's, Huntington's, epilepsy, and Creutzfeldt-Jakob disease). Theories of Alzheimer's Disease relate to its neuropathological mechanisms (amyloid plaques and tangles associated with neuronal death); its genetic predisposition (presence of e4 allele within the ApoE genotypes and other factors modulating its expression) (Woodruff-Pak & Papka, 1999); and various existing and potentially new biochemical therapies (theories)—manipulating the cholinergic system (acetylcholine), manipulating brain excitation or signaling (blocking glutamate's ability to activate N-methyl-D-aspartate (NMDA) receptors, controlling the effect of calcium on NMDA receptors), blocking the formation of beta-amyloid (secretase inhibitors), and reducing brain inflammation (nonsteroidal anti-inflammatory drugs [NSAIDs], statins) (Walsh, 2004).

There are emerging hints that current neuropsychological theories of aging may be too pessimistic. There is increasing evidence that older adults can engage in a variety of lifestyle choices, including exercise, challenging cognitive activities (Sudoku and crossword puzzles are frequently mentioned in the popular press), and eating fruits and vegetables to stave off neuropsychological decline, or at least to slow it significantly. It is also clear that although much research has been done to explore the various biological theories of aging, much remains to be done. No one theory adequately explains observed phenomena. It seems increasingly likely that aging is the result of complex phenomena that incorporate elements of many of the theories presented here, and others yet to be identified (Troen, 2003). As is true of much research, it will be years before findings can be confirmed, refined, or refuted through replication of research longitudinal study.

Psychological Theories of Aging

The psychology of aging is a complex field with several subfields (cognitive development, personality development, social development) and topic areas (memory, learning, sensation and perception, psycholinguistics, social psychology, motor skills, psychometrics, and developmental psychology). (See Baltes, Freund, & Li, 2005.) Disciplinary boundaries can be amorphous. Schroots (1996) observes that sometimes psychological theories of aging are labeled as psychosocial; at other times they are conceived as biobehavioral, behavioral genetic, or neuropsychological. Theories in the psychology of aging seek to explain the multiple changes in individual behavior, across these domains, in the middle and later years of the life span. As with biological and sociological theories of aging, there is no defining psychology of aging theory. Psychological theories of aging focus largely on activity as described in the ICF (WHO, 2001), and on client factors, performance skills, and performance patterns as discussed in the Practice Framework (AOTA, 2002). See Table 2-2 for a summary of psychological theories of aging.

Life-Span Development Theory

One of the most widely cited explanatory frameworks in the psychology of aging, life-span development theory conceptualizes ontogenetic development as biologically and socially constituted and as manifesting both developmental universals (homogeneity) and interindividual variability (for example, differences in genetics and in social class). This perspective also proposes that the second half of life is characterized by significant individual differentiation, multidirectionality, and intraindividual plasticity. Using the life-span development perspective, Baltes and Smith (1999) identify three principles regulating the dynamics between biology and culture across the ontogenetic life span: (1) evolutionary selection benefits decrease with age, (2) the need for culture increases with age, and (3) the efficacy of culture decreases with age. Their focus is on how these dynamics contribute to the optimal expression of human development and the production of outcomes of adaptive fitness. Drawing from evolutionary theory and ontogenetic theories of learning, Baltes and Smith (1999) also postulate that a condition of loss, limitation, or deficit could play a catalytic role for positive change.

TABLE 2-2 Psychological Theories of Aging

Life span		The second half of life is characterized by significant individual differentiation, multidirectionality, and intraindividual plasticity
Selective optimization with compensation		A model of psychological and behavior adaptation identifying three fundamental mechanisms for managing adaptive development in later life
Socioemotional selectivity		Describes individual choices in interaction, based on self-interested need for emotional closeness that leads to selective interactions
Cognition and aging	Distal determinant	Factors that affect cognition reside outside the individual, for example, in the social and cultural environment
	Proximal determinant	Specific individual differences are the cause of cognitive change
Personality and aging		Theories that focus on the extent and nature of personality stability and change over time

Selective Optimization with Compensation Theory

Life-span development theory has produced one overall theory to explain how individuals manage adaptive (successful) development in later life (Baltes & Smith, 1999). The theory identifies three fundamental mechanisms or strategies: selection, optimization, and compensation (Baltes & Carstensen, 1996, 1999). This is a model of psychological and behavior adaptation where the central focus is on managing the dynamics between gains and losses as one ages. Selection refers to the increasing restriction of an individual's life to fewer domains of functioning because of age-related loss in the range of adaptive potential. Optimization reflects the idea that people engage in behaviors that augment or enrich their general reserves and maximize their chosen life courses. Like selection, compensation results from restriction of the range of adaptive potential and becomes operative when specific behavioral capacities are lost or are reduced below a standard required for adequate functioning. This life-long process of selective optimization with compensation enables people to age successfully (Schroots, 1996).

Socioemotional Selectivity Theory

In this theory, Carstensen (1992) combines insights from developmental psychology—particularly the selective optimization with compensation model developed by Baltes and Baltes (1990)—with social exchange theory to explain why the social exchange and interaction networks of older persons are reduced over time (a phenomenon that disengagement theory tried to explain). Through mechanisms of socioemotional selectivity, individuals reduce interactions with some people as they age and increase emotional closeness with significant others, such as an adult child or an aging sibling. Carstensen's (1992) theory provides a concise development-behavioral explanation for selective interaction in old age. This theory explains the change in social contact by the self-interested need for emotional closeness with significant others, which leads to increasingly selective interactions with others in advancing age. Such chosen interactions reflect the levels of reward these exchanges of emotional support achieve for older persons.

Cognition and Aging Theories

Researchers of cognition differentiate between types of cognitive abilities: *fluid* intelligence, reflecting genetic-biological determinants; and *crystallized* abilities, representing social-cultural influences on general world knowledge. The primary phenomenon to be explained by a theory of cognition is the age-related decline in *fluid* cognitive performance (the efficiency or effectiveness of performing tasks of learning, memory, reasoning, and spatial abilities) (Salthouse, 1999). Fluid abilities have been shown to decline with age, but crystallized abilities are more stable across the life span and may even display some growth with age.

Salthouse (1999) suggests there are apparently no theoretical accounts of the stability of crystallized cognition.

Most theories of fluid cognition and aging can be categorized by whether the primary determinants are distal or proximal in nature (Salthouse, 1999). *Distal determinant explanations* postulate factors that exert their influence over time and are responsible for age-related differences evident in the level of cognitive performance. One type of distal explanation emphasizes changes in the social and cultural environment as opposed to changes within the individual. For example, changes in educational patterns may explain age-related declines in cognitive functioning (although these differences in education probably account for only a small proportion of age-related differences in cognitive functioning). Another distal explanation is the disuse or "use it or lose it" perspective. Although popular among the public and some researchers, this perspective has had little empirical support (Salthouse, 1999).

Proximal determinant explanations of age-related differences in fluid cognition tend to incorporate specific mechanisms linking theoretical constructs to cognitive performance. They are as follows:

- Strategy-based explanations, of which there are two types:
  - a production deficiency version that posits that older people have similar capacities as younger people but use less than optimal strategies, and
  - a processing deficiency version that posits that differences in strategy are less important than differences in more fundamental abilities; empirical results tend to support the processing deficiency explanation (Salthouse, 1999).
- Specific-deficit explanations postulate age-related differences in the efficiency of "particular" information-processing stages or components.
- Reduced processing resource explanations postulate there are age-related declines in the efficiency or effectiveness of "elementary" cognitive operations or processing resources.

These theories hold that aging leads to a reduction in the quantity of one or more processing resources, such as attentional capacity, working memory capacity, or speed of processing. Experimental studies have shown processing speed to be a fundamental construct in human cognition, linked to explicit changes in neural structure and functioning as well as to higher-order cognitive processes like reasoning and abstraction (Salthouse, 1991). Because the key constructs of reduced processing resources theory are broader than in the specific deficit model and presumably affect a wide variety of tasks, this theoretical approach has proven to be more useful and found wide support (Salthouse, 1999; Schroots, 1996). Cognitive change in later life is discussed in greater detail in Chapter 7.

Personality and Aging Theories

Theories of personality and aging focus on the extent and nature of personality stability and change over the life span. There are two categories of explanation of age-related changes in personality. First are the *developmental explanations* as represented by Erikson's (1950) stages of development (in adulthood and old age, the stages of generativity versus stagnation and integration versus despair), and Levinson's (1978) stage theory of personality development. "Stage" theories of personality have fallen out of favor in recent years. Second are the *personality trait explanations,* based on the "big five" factors of personality (neuroticism, extroversion, openness to experience, agreeableness, and conscientiousness). These personality theories postulate that people show a high degree of stability in basic dispositions and personality, particularly during the latter half of their life course. There is growing consensus that personality traits tend to be stable with age, whereas key aspects of self, such as goals, values, coping styles, and control beliefs, are more amenable to change (Baltes & Smith, 1999). In research on the self and personality in old age, the current emphasis is on understanding the mechanisms that promote the maintenance of personal integrity and well-being in the face of social loss and health constraints (Baltes & Baltes, 1990; Baltes & Smith, 1999).

Sociological Theories of Aging

Sociological theories of aging consider the context in which aging occurs. That is, they focus on participation (WHO, 2001) and on the context in which occupation occurs and the demands of the activities and the environment (AOTA, 2002). As you will see, several of these theories focus specifically on activity. These will be discussed in greater detail in Chapter 3. These theories are summarized in Table 2-3. There are several important theoretical traditions that should be exploited in developing explanations and understandings of empirical phenomena.

Historical Foundations of Explanations in Social Gerontology

Scholars in gerontology have invested much intellectual effort in theory building. Early researchers on aging, such as Hall (1922), Cowdry (1939), Linton (1942), Parsons (1942), and Havighurst (1943), integrated empirical findings into theoretical insights and established the foundations of gerontology. Out of these pioneering efforts grew four theories, representing a first generation of social gerontology theories (Bengtson, Burgess, & Parrott, 1997): *disengagement theory* (Cumming & Henry, 1961); *activity theory* (Lemon, Bengtson, & Peterson, 1972); *modernization theory* (Cowgill & Holmes, 1974); and *subculture theory* (Rose, 1964). The most explicitly developed of these, disengagement theory (Cumming & Henry, 1961), attempted to explain human aging as an inevitable process of individuals and social structures mutually disengaging and adaptively withdrawing from each other in anticipation of the person's inevitable death. Drawn from structural-functionalism, this general theory of aging was elegant, multidisci-

plinary, parsimonious, and intuitively provocative (Achenbaum & Bengtson, 1994). However, its ambitious propositions were roundly criticized (Hochschild, 1975). The theory had attempted to explain both macro- and micro-level changes with one "grand theory," but when tested against the cited data, its validity and generalizability claims could not be supported. Even though many older people do appear to be "disengaging" or withdrawing from their social connections and activities, many do not.

In a second period of theoretical development, from about 1970 to 1985, several new theoretical perspectives emerged: *continuity theory* (Atchley, 1993), *social breakdown/ competence theory* (Kuypers & Bengtson, 1973), *exchange theory* (Dowd, 1975), the *age stratification perspective* (Riley, Johnston, & Foner, 1972), and the *political economy of aging perspective* (Estes, Gerard, Jones, & Swan, 1984). Since the late 1980s, many of these theories have been refined and reformulated, and new theoretical perspectives have emerged. Following is an overview of contemporary theoretical perspectives in social gerontology.

The Life Course Perspective

This perspective is perhaps the most widely cited theoretical framework in social gerontology today. Its proponents argue that to understand the present circumstances of older people, we must take into account the major social and psychological forces that have operated throughout the course of their lives (George, 1996). Although there is debate as

---

TABLE 2-3 Sociological Theories of Aging

Life course	Focuses on expected and normal changes in life over its entire span
Social exchange	Individuals, including elders, make rational choices about interactions with others, based on their needs and on norms of reciprocity
Social constructionist	Focuses on individual agency and social behavior within the larger structures of society, and on subjective meanings of age and the aging experience
Feminist	Give priority to gender as an organizing principle for social life across the life span
Political economy of aging	Focus on the interaction of economic and political forces in explaining how the treatment and status of older adults can be understood
Critical perspectives of aging	Focuses either on humanistic dimensions of aging or on structural components in attempting to create positive models emphasizing strengths and diversity of age

to whether the life course is a "theory" or an orienting perspective, it represents a convergence of thinking in sociology and psychology about processes at both macro- and micro-social levels of analysis and for both populations and individuals over time. Researchers using this perspective are attempting to explain the following:

1. The dynamic, contextual, and processual nature of aging
2. Age-related transitions and life trajectories
3. How aging is related to and shaped by social contexts, cultural meanings, and social structural location
4. How time, period, and cohort shape the aging process for individuals as well as for social groups (Bengtson & Allen, 1993; Elder, 1992; Elder & Johnson, 2002)

This approach is multidisciplinary, drawing content and methods from sociology, psychology, anthropology, and history, and emphasizing the kinds of social and cultural factors that might influence the experience of growing old for individuals from many cultures, like the woman in Figure 2-1. The life course approach is also explicitly dynamic, focusing on the life cycle in its entirety while allowing for deviations in trajectories (Dannefer & Sell, 1988). Although studies so far have not incorporated all four of these life course perspective dimensions in their empirical analyses, new methodological advances suggest such a multilevel, cross-time model in the future (Alwin & Campbell, 2001).

Social Exchange Theory

This micro-level theory has been useful in many recent studies in the sociology of aging, particularly those focusing on intergenerational social support and transfers. Developed and extended by Dowd (1975), the social exchange theory of aging draws from sociological formulations by Homans (1961) and Blau (1964) and work in economics that assumes a *rational choice* model of decision-making behavior. Applied to aging, this perspective attempts to account for exchange behavior between individuals of different ages as a result of the shift in roles, skills, and resources that accompany advancing age (Hendricks, 1995). It explicitly incorporates the concept of power differentials. A central

assumption is that the various actors (such as parent and child or elder and youth) each bring resources to the interaction or exchange, and that resources need not be material and will most likely be unequal. A second assumption is that the actors will only continue to engage in the exchanges for as long as the benefits are greater than the costs and while there are no better alternatives. This theoretical approach also assumes that exchanges are governed by norms of reciprocity; that when we give something, we trust that something of equal value will be reciprocated.

Social Constructionist Perspectives

Social constructionist theories draw from a long tradition of micro-level analysis in the social sciences: *symbolic interactionism* (Mead, 1934), *phenomenology* (Berger & Luckmann, 1966), and *ethnomethodology* (Garfinkel, 1967). Using hermeneutic or interpretive methods, social constructivism focuses on individual agency and social behavior within larger structures of society, and particularly on the subjective meanings of age and the aging experience. Researchers working in this tradition emphasize their interest in understanding, if not explaining, individual processes of aging as influenced by social definitions and social structures. Examples include Gubrium's (1993) study of the subjective meanings of quality of care and quality of life for residents of nursing homes, and how each resident constructs meanings from her or his own experiences. These meanings emerge from analyses of life narratives but cannot be measured by predefined measurement scales, such as those used by most survey researchers.

Feminist Theories of Aging

Feminist gerontology gives priority to gender as an organizing principle for social life across the life span that significantly alters the experience of aging, often in inequitable ways (Calasanti, 1999; McMullen, 1995). This theoretical perspective also challenges what counts as knowledge and how it functions in the lives of older women and men. Current theories and models of aging are regarded as insufficient, because they fail to address gender relations, the experience of women in the context of aging and caregiving demands, or issues of race, ethnicity, or class (Blieszner, 1993; Calasanti, 1999; Ray, 1996). At the macro-level of analyses, feminist theories of aging combine with political economy and critical perspectives to examine differential access to key material, health, and caring resources which substantially alters the experience of aging for women and men (Arber & Ginn, 1991). For example, feminist researchers seek to explain the comparatively high rates of poverty among older women and to propose changes in the ideologies and institutions that perpetuate it. From a feminist perspective, family caregiving can be understood as an experience of obligation, structured by the gender-based division of domestic labor and the devaluing of unpaid work (Stroller, 1993). At the micro-level, feminist perspectives hold that gender should be examined in the context of social meanings, reflecting the influence of the social constructivist approach.

Political Economy of Aging Perspective

These theories, which draw originally from Marxism (Marx, 1967/1867), conflict theory (Simmel, 1904/1966), and critical theory (Habermas, 1971), attempt to explain how the interaction of economic and political forces determines how social resources are allocated, and how variations in the treatment and status of the elderly can be understood by examining public policies, economic trends, and social structural factors (Estes, 2001). Political economy perspectives applied to aging maintain that socioeconomic and political constraints shape the experience of aging, resulting in the loss of power, autonomy, and influence of older persons. Life experiences are seen as being patterned not only by age, but also by class, gender, and race and ethnicity. These structural factors, often institutionalized or reinforced by economic and public policy, constrain opportunities, choices, and experiences of later life. Another focus of the political economy of aging perspective is how ageism is constructed and reproduced through social practices and policies, and how it negatively affects the well-being of older people (Bytheway, 2005).

Critical Perspectives of Aging

Critical perspectives are reflected in several theoretical trends in contemporary social gerontology, including the political economy of aging, feminist theories, theories of diversity, and humanistic gerontology. Coming primarily out of the Frankfort School of Critical Theory (Habermas, 1971; Horkheimer & Adorno, 1944) and post-structuralism (Foucault, 1975), these perspectives share a common focus on criticizing "the process of power" (Baars, 1991) as well as traditional positivistic approaches to knowledge. Critical gerontology has developed two distinct patterns, one that focuses on humanistic dimensions of aging, and the other on structural components. Moody (1993) postulates four goals of the humanistic strand of critical theory: (1) to theorize subjective and interpretive dimensions of aging, (2) to focus on praxis (involvement in practical change) instead of technical advancement, (3) to link academics and practitioners through praxis, and (4) to produce "emancipatory knowledge." A second strand emphasizes that critical gerontology should create positive models of aging focusing on the strengths and diversity of age, in addition to critiquing positivist knowledge (Bengtson, Burgess, & Parrott, 1997). To reach the goals of critical gerontology, researchers focus on the key concepts of power, social action, and social meanings in examining the social aspects of age and aging. Social constructionism, feminist theories, and critical perspectives have gained prominence in social gerontology theorizing, mirroring recent theoretical developments in sociology and the humanities. Not uncommonly, gerontologists will combine insights from all three perspectives to guide their research and interpret findings. At the same time, these theoretical perspectives pose a challenge to the scientific assumptions that have traditionally guided gerontological research.

■ Summary

Our goal in this chapter was, first, to examine the state of theory and knowledge building in the field of gerontology and gauge its prospects for future development; and second, to present an overview of the major theories in each of its core disciplines: the biology of aging, the psychology of aging, and the sociology of aging.

In the quest to understand the diverse phenomena of aging, gerontologists focus on three sets of issues: biological and social processes of aging, the aged themselves, and age as a dimension of structure and social organization. Societal aging poses new problems for gerontologists. We suggested that developing knowledge that informs policies that can effectively deal with the challenges posed by growing numbers of older persons will be crucial in the coming decades. There are good practical reasons for theory development in the field of gerontology.

Yet theory development is difficult. There are several reasons: the difficulty of integrating theory-based knowledge across topic areas and disciplines; the strong problem-solving focus of gerontology that detracts from theorizing, which has played such an important role in the advancement of basic research; and the excessive focus on individuals and micro settings while ignoring wider social contexts.

Researchers need to make explicit their assumptions and theoretical orientations when presenting their results and interpretations. Second, there has been a proliferation of single aspect research findings—too frequently generated by overly narrow research inquiries—that lack theoretical grounding and explanation. There is a need to raise these "empirical generalizations" to an explanatory level and integrate explanations and understandings with previous knowledge and explanations. Third, there is the need to cross disciplinary boundaries and develop multidisciplinary and interdisciplinary causal explanations of broader theoretical scope. Fourth, researchers need to be more sensitive to the social dimensions of scholarly research and values that imbue paradigmatic frameworks, affecting the kinds of questions asked, the analytic approaches and methods chosen, and the interpretations put forth.

Yet there is a way that these seemingly incommensurate epistemological positions can be accommodated. Explanation and understanding in the complex field of gerontology should draw from a range of theories and theoretical perspectives developed by its constitutive disciplines. It builds knowledge not only through the methods of formal theory development that characterize science, but also from the understandings developed by interpretavists and critical theorists. This diversity of theoretical perspectives can offer complementary insights. But in order for this to happen, it is important that researchers pay more attention to the accumulated knowledge of the field and to be explicit in their theoretical perspectives and insights.

From the perspective of occupational therapy, there is an added consideration. Given the profession's focus on what people need and want to do, the theories presented here must be integrated with specific emphasis on performance skills, performance patterns, client factors, and other issues related to satisfactory and satisfying occupational performance (AOTA, 2002). Chapter 3 addresses these concerns, revisiting some of the theories presented here and adding others, all of which are directly relevant to occupation.

Future Trends in Social Gerontological Thinking

- In this review of theoretical development in the gerontology, it is obvious that positivism is still with us. Yet changes are on the horizon. Perhaps in response to political economy and critical theorists' critiques, there appears to be increasing concern over the "microfication" of theories of social gerontology (Hagestad & Dannefer, 2001). This refers to the overemphasis on micro-level analysis, agency, and the individual subject.

- In future theorizing, we expect to see greater emphasis being placed on macro-level phenomena and the structural contexts of aging. This is because there is increased awareness of structures as having effects on processes of aging independent of individual actions, and the recognition that structures and institutions are not socially constructed but have a certain facticity (Turner, 2003). This shift in awareness may promote renewed interest in theory building and in social gerontology's development as a science.

- Theory development in social gerontology may be promoted by trends within sociology. The epistemological wars in sociological theorizing continue.

- Shifting the emphasis from theories *of* aging to theories *in* aging opens up a novel strategy for developing cross-disciplinary explanations and understanding in gerontology (Turner, 2003). The process starts with the collective identification of the major problems in aging research by practitioners of various disciplines and theoretical perspectives.

The process then inquires what discipline-specific theoretical knowledge can be brought to bear on illuminating and resolving these problems. Engaging in such a process holds the potential for forging a cross-disciplinary fertilization of ideas and possibly new approaches. Such a process tests the usefulness of theories in gerontology in a very practical way. It also becomes possible to evaluate whether theoretical integration across disciplines is needed.

Case Study

At the beginning of this chapter, you met Mr. Morales. To learn more about him, visit: http://academic.csuohio.edu/Aging/case_1/index.html.

At this website you will learn a great deal about Mr. Morales' performance skills and patterns, and the context in which he pursues his occupations. Overall, he is a healthy (except for the diabetes he has learned to manage well), active, and upbeat individual who describes his life as very satisfying. Both casual and well-informed observers would assert that Mr. Morales has a zest for life.

Review Questions

1. How might the various biological theories contribute to an understanding of the ways in which Mr. Morales has aged well?
   Mr. Morales may well be the beneficiary of a good genetic heritage. Perhaps his diet may have helped him avoid an excess of free radicals that some theorize contribute to age-related change. Or perhaps his activities have played a role in maintaining his physical vigor, given his active physical and cognitive life.
2. What psychosocial theories might explain Mr. Morales' positive aging trajectory?
   Mr. Morales maintains an active life. He has an upbeat, optimistic outlook. So, for example, while he must care for his wife, he perceives this in a positive way, finding personal satisfaction in what others might perceive as a situation that imposes a burden.
3. What sociological theories do you think help explain Mr. Morales' current status?
   Note that Mr. Morales has a rich social life. While he must care for his wife, he clearly loves her and values the relationship.

Web-Based Resources

www.prolongyouth.com/theories.html, date connected May 23, 2007. A summary of theories with an emphasis on implications for actions individuals might take to maintain wellness. Prolongyouth.com is the listed organization that developed this summary.

www.worldhealth.net/p/90,4863.html, **American Academy of Anti-Aging Medicine,** date connected May 23, 2007. A broad listing of theories with brief summaries and links to other resources.

www.healthandage.com/html/min/afar/content/other2_2.htm, **American Federation for Aging Research,** date connected May 23, 2007. Focused primarily on biological theories of aging.

REFERENCES

Achenbaum, W. A. (1987). Can gerontology be a science? *Journal of Aging Studies, 1*(1), 3–18.

Achenbaum, W. A. (1995). *Crossing frontiers: Gerontology as a science.* New York: Cambridge University Press.

Achenbaum, W. A., & Bengtson, V. L. (1994). Re-engaging the disengagement theory of aging: On the history and assessment of theory development in gerontology. *The Gerontologist, 34,* 756–763.

Alwin, D., & Campbell, R. T. (2001). Quantitative approaches. In R. H. Binstock & L. K. George (Eds.), *Handbook of aging and the social sciences* (5th ed., pp. 22–43). San Diego, CA: Academic Press.

American Occupational Therapy Association. (2002). Occupational Therapy Practice Framework: Domain and Process. *American Journal of Occupational Therapy, 56,* 609–639.

Arber, S., & Ginn, J. (1995). *Connecting gender and aging: A sociological approach.* Philadelphia: Open University Press.

Atchley, R. C. (1993). Critical perspectives on retirement. In T. R. Cole, W. A. Achenbaum, P. L. Jakobi, & R. Kastenbaum (Eds.), *Voices and visions: Toward a critical gerontology* (pp. 3–19). New York: Springer.

Baars, J. (1991). The challenge of critical theory: The problem of social construction. *The Journal of Aging Studies, 5,* 219–243.

Baltes, P. B., & Baltes, M. M. (1990). Psychological perspectives on successful aging. The model of selective optimization with compensation. In P. B. Baltes & M. M. Baltes (Eds.), *Successful aging: Perspectives from the behavioral science* (pp. 1–34). New York: Cambridge University Press.

Baltes, M. M., & Carstensen, L. L. (1996). The process of successful ageing. *Ageing and Society, 16,* 397–422.

Baltes, M. M., & Carstensen, L. L. (1999). Social-psychological theories and their applications to aging: From individual to collective. In V. L. Bengtson & K. W. Schaie (Eds.), *Handbook of theories of aging* (pp. 209–226). New York: Springer.

Baltes, P. B., Freund, A. M., & Li, S. -C. (2005). The psychological science of human aging . In *The Cambridge handbook of age and aging* (pp. 47–71). Cambridge: Cambridge University Press.

Baltes, P. B., & Smith, J. (1999). Multilevel and systemic analyses of old age: Theoretical and empirical evidence for a fourth age. In V. L. Bengtson & K. W. Schaie (Eds.), *Handbook of theories of aging* (pp. 153–173). New York: Springer.

Bengtson, V. L., & Allen, K. R. (1993). The life course perspective applied to families over time. In P. Boss, W. Doherty, R. La Rossa, W. Schumm, & S. Steinmetz (Eds.), *Sourcebook of family theories and methods: A contextual approach* (pp. 469–498). New York: Plenum.

Bengtson, V. L., Burgess, E. O., & Parrott, T. M. (1997). Theory, explanation, and a third generation of theoretical development in social gerontology. *Journal of Gerontology, 52B,* S72–S88.

Berger, P. L., & Luckmann, T. (1966). *The social construction of reality.* New York: Doubleday.

Birren, J. E. (1999). Theories of aging: A personal perspective. In V. L. Bengtson & K. W. Schaie (Eds.), *Handbook of theories of aging* (pp. 459–471). New York: Springer.

Blau, P. M. (1964). *Exchange and power in social life.* New York: Wiley.

Blieszner, R. (1993). A socialist-feminist perspective on widowhood. *Journal of Aging Studies, 17,* 171–182.

Bytheway, B. (2005). Ageism and age categorization. *Journal of Social Issues, 61,* 361–374.

Calasanti, T. M. (1999). Feminism and gerontology: Not just for women. *Hallym International Journal of Aging, 1,* 44–55.

Carstensen, L. (1992). Social and emotional patterns in adulthood: Support for socioemotional selectivity theory. *Psychology and Aging, 7,* 331–338.

Cowdry, E. V. (Ed.). 1939. *Problems of aging.* Baltimore, MD: Williams and Wilkins.

Cowgill, D. A., & Holmes, L. D. (1974). Aging and modernization. A revision of theory. In J. Gubrium (Ed.), *Laterlife: Community and environmental policies* (pp. 305–323). New York: Basic Books.

Cristofalo, V. J. (1996). Ten years later: What have we learned about human aging from studies of cell cultures? *The Gerontologist, 36,* 737–741.

Cristofalo, V. J., Tresini, J., Francis, M. K., & Volker, C. (1999). Biological theories of senescence. In V. L. Bengtson & K. W. Schaie (Eds.), *Handbook of theories of aging* (pp. 98–112). New York: Springer.

Cumming, E., & Henry, W. (1961). *Growing old: The process of disengagement.* New York: Basic Books.

Dannefer, W. D., & Sell, R. R. (1988). Age structure, the life course and aged heterogeneity: Prospects for research and theory. *Comprehensive Gerontology, 2,* 1–10.

Dowd, J. J. (1975). Aging as exchange: A preface to theory. *Journal of Gerontology, 30,* 584–594.

Elder, G. H., Jr. (1992). Models of the life course. *Contemporary Sociology: A Journal of Reviews, 21,* 632–635.

Elder, G. H., Jr., & Johnson, M. K. (2002). The life course and aging: Challenges, lessons, and new directions. In R. A. Settersten, J. (Ed.), *Invitation to the life course: Toward new understandings of later life* (pp. 49–81). Amityville, NY: Baywood.

Erikson, E. H. (1950). *Childhood and society.* New York: W. W. Norton.

Estes, C. L. (2001). Political economy of aging: A theoretical framework. In C. L. Estes & Associates. *Social policy and aging: A critical perspective* (pp. 1–22). Thousand Oaks, CA: Sage.

Estes, C. L., Gerard, L. E., Jones, J. S., & Swan, J. H. (1984). *Political economy, health, and aging* (pp. 1–22). Boston, MA: Little, Brown.

Finch, C. E., & Seeman, T. E. (1999). Stress theories of aging. In V. L. Bengtson & K. W. Schaie (Eds.), *Handbook of theories of aging* (pp. 81–97). New York: Springer.

Foucault, M. (1975). *Discipline and punish: The birth of a prison.* Trans. A. Sheridan. New York: Vintage/Random House.

Frisard, M., & Ravussin, E. (2006). Energy metabolism and oxidative stress: Impact on the metabolic syndrome and the aging process. *Endocrine, 29,* 27–32.

Garfinkel, H. (1967). *Studies in ethnomethodology.* Englewood Cliffs, NJ: Prentice Hall.

George, L. K. (1996). Missing links: The case for a social psychology of the life course. *The Gerontologist, 36,* 248–255.

Gubrium, J. F. (1993). *Speaking of life: Horizons of meaning for nursing home residents.* New York: Aldine de Gruyter.

Habermas, J. (1971). *Knowledge and human interests.* Trans. J. J. Shapiro. Boston: Beacon Press.

Hagestad, G. O., & Dannefer, D. (2001). Concepts and theories of aging: Beyond microfication in social science approaches. In R. H. Binstock & L. K. George (Eds.), *Handbook of aging and the social sciences* (5th ed., pp. 3–21). San Diego, CA: Academic Press.

Hall, G. S. (1922). *Senescence.* New York: Appleton.

Harman, D. (1956). Aging: A theory based on free radical and radiation chemistry. *Journal of Gerontology, 11,* 298–300.

Harman, D. (2006). Free radical theory of aging: An update: Increasing the functional life span. *Annals of the New York Academy of Sciences, 1067,* 10–21.

Havighurst, R. J. (1943). *Human development and education.* New York: Longman.

Hendricks, J. (1995). Exchange theory in aging. In G. Maddox (Ed.), *The Encyclopedia of aging* (2nd ed. p. 274). New York: Springer.

Hochschild, A. R. (1975). Disengagement theory: A critique and a proposal. *American Sociological Review, 40,* 553–569.

Homans, G. C. (1961). *Social behavior: Its elementary forms.* New York: Harcourt Brace Jovanovich.

Horkheimer, M., & Adorno, T. W. (1944). The cultural industry: Enlightenment as mass deception. In M. Horkheimer and T. W. Adorno (Eds.), *Dialectic of enlightenment.* Trans. J. Cumming. New York: Continuum.

Howes, R. M. (2006). The free radical fantasy: A panoply of paradoxes. *Annals of the New York Academy of Sciences, 1067,* 22–26.

Kirkwood, T. B. L. (2001). Why does aging occur? In V. J. Cristofalo, R. Adelman, and K. W. Schaie (Eds.), *Annual review of gerontology and geriatrics, Volume 21* (pp. 41–55). New York: Springer.

Kuypers, J. A., & Bengtson, V. L (1973). Social breakdown and competence: A model of normal aging. *Human Development, 16,* 181–201.

Lemon, B. W., Bengtson, V. L., & Peterson, J. A. (1972). An exploration of the activity theory of aging. *Journal of Gerontology, 27,* 511–523.

Lenaz, G., Baracca, A., Fato, R., Genova, M. L., & Solaini, G. (2006). New insights into structure and function of mitochondria and their role in aging and disease. *Antioxidants & Redox Signaling, 8,* 417–437.

Levinson, D. J. (1978). *The seasons of a man's life.* New York: Knopf.

Linnane, A. W., & Eastwood, H. (2006). Cellular redox regulation and prooxidant signaling systems: A new perspective on the free radical theory of aging. *Annals of the New York Academy of Sciences, 1067,* 47–55.

Linton, R. (1942). Age and sex categories. *American Sociological Review, 7,* 589–603.

Martin, G. M. (2003). Biology of aging: The state of the art. *The Gerontologist, 43,* 272–274.

Marx, K. (1967[1867–1895]). *Capital: A critique of political economy.* New York: International Publishers.

McMullen, J. (1995). Theorizing age and gender relations. In S. Arber & J. Ginn (Eds.), *Connecting gender and aging: A sociological approach.* Philadelphia: Open University Press.

Mead, G. H. (1934). *Mind, self, and society.* Chicago: University of Chicago Press.

Medawar, P. B. (1952). *An unsolved problem of biology.* London: H. K. Lewis.

Moody, H. R. (1993). Overview: What is critical gerontology and why is it important? In T. R. Cole, W. A. Achenbaum, P. L. Jakobi, & R. Kastenbaum (Eds.), *Voices and visions: Toward a critical gerontology* (pp. xv–xviii). New York: Springer.

Parsons, T. (1942). Age and sex in the social structure of the United States. *American Sociological Review, 7,* 604–616.

Ray, R. E. (1996). A postmodern perspective on feminist gerontology. *The Gerontologist, 36,* 674–680.

Riley, M. W., Johnson, M., & Foner, A. (1972). *Aging and society. Vol III: A sociology of age stratification.* New York: Russell Sage Foundation.

Rose, A. (1964). A current theoretical issue in social gerontology. *The Gerontologist, 4,* 46–50.

Ruggiero, C., & Ferrucci, L. (2006). The endeavor of high maintenance homeostasis: Resting metabolic rate and the legacy of longevity. *Journals of Gerontology: Medical Sciences, 61A,* M466–M471.

Salthouse, T. A. (1991). *Theoretical perspectives on cognitive aging.* Hillsdale, NY: Lawrence Erlbaum Associates.

Salthouse, T. A. (1999). Theories of cognition. In V. L. Bengtson & K. W. Schaie (Eds.), *Handbook of theories of aging* (pp. 196–208). New York: Springer.

Sanz, A., Pamplona, R., & Barja, G. (2006). Is the mitochondrial free radical theory of aging intact? *Antioxidants & Redox Signaling, 8,* 582–599.

Schroots, J. J. F. (1996). Theoretical developments in the psychology of aging. *The Gerontologist, 36,* 742–748.

Simmel, G. (1904/1966). *Conflict.* Trans. K.H. Wolff. Glencoe, IL: Free Press.

Stroller, E. P. (1993). Gender and the organization of lay health care: A socialist-feminist perspective. *Journal of Aging Studies, 7,* 151–170.

Terman, A., & Brunk, U. T. (2006). Oxidative stress, accumulation of biological "garbage," and aging. *Antioxidants & Redox Signaling, 8,* 197–204.

Troen, B. R. (2003). The biology of aging. *Mount Sinai Journal of Medicine, 70,* 3–22.

Turner, J. H. (2003). *The structure of sociological theory.* Belmont, CA: Wadsworth/Thomson Learning.

Wachter, K. W., & Finch, C. E. (Eds.). (1997). *Between Zeus and the salmon: The biodemography of longevity.* Washington, DC: National Academy Press.

Walford, R. (1969). *The immunologic theory of aging.* Copenhagen: Munksgaard.

Wallace, R. A., & Wolf, A. (1991). *Contemporary sociological theory: Continuing the classical tradition* (3rd ed.). Englewood Cliffs, NJ: Prentice Hall.

Walsh, J. P. (2004). Drug therapy in Alzheimer's Disease. Andrus Gerontology Center's Research Roundtables presentation, University of Southern California, December.

Williams, G. C. (1957). Pleiotropy, natural selection and the evolution of senescence. *Evolution, 11,* 398–411.

Wolkow, C. A., & Iser, W. B. (2006). Uncoupling protein homologs may provide a link between mitochondria, metabolism and lifespan. *Ageing Research Reviews, 5,* 196–208.

Woodruff-Pak, D. S., & Papka, M. (1999). Theories of neuropsychology and aging. In V. L. Bengtson & K. W. Schaie (Eds.), *Handbook of theories of aging* (pp. 113–132). New York: Springer.

World Health Organization. (2001). International Classification of Function. Geneva: author. Retrieved February 26, 2006, from www3.who.int/icf.

Yu, B. P., & Chung, H. Y. (2006, Feb. 21) Adaptive mechanisms to oxidative stress during aging. *Mechanics of Aging Development.*

CHAPTER 3

Meaningful Occupation in Later Life

Bette R. Bonder

"What I enjoy most is talking to men who are really old. It seems right to inquire of them, as if they have traversed a long journey which we perhaps will have to traverse, to ask what the journey is like, rough and difficult or easygoing and smooth."

Socrates, cited in *Plato,* 1956, p. 126

OBJECTIVES

By the end of the chapter, readers will be able to:

1. Discuss the role of occupation in the lives of older adults.
2. Discuss occupational therapy theories regarding occupation and well-being.
3. Discuss the ways in which occupation in later life affects subjective well-being, self-efficacy, and life satisfaction.
4. Discuss the ways in which elders engage in various types of activities.
5. Describe the interrelationship between occupation and health, and between poor health and loss of meaningful occupations.
6. Describe strategies for assessing occupations and their meanings for elders.
7. Discuss the evidence regarding outcomes of occupational therapy focused on promoting meaningful occupations.

Every stage of life presents unique occupational challenges. Infants must learn to interact with and manipulate their environments. Adolescents must learn to choose the work and relationships that will shape their adult lives. Adults engage in work and family occupations. In later life, the occupational challenges focus on finding meaning in the absence of clearly defined roles. Engagement in meaningful occupations in later life is associated with better physical and emotional health (Chipperfield & Greenslade, 1999; Krause, 2004), greater life satisfaction and subjective well-being (George, 2006; Hilleras, Jorm, Herlitz, & Winblad, 2001), and continued hope and optimism (Rowe & Kahn, 1998).

All individuals strive to find meaning in their lives (Baumeister, 1991; Crabtree, 1998; Hasselkus, 2002). They ascribe meaning to the objects around them, to their social relationships, and to what they do with their time. For older adults, the process of finding meaning is the culmination of a life of choice—of occupation, friends, and environment (Thompson, 1993). Occupation is central to the process of making meaning in life (Peloquin, 1997). "When we build our identities through occupations, we provide ourselves with the contexts necessary for creating meaningful lives, and life meaning helps us to be well" (Christiansen, 1999, p. 547). Aristotle noted that "all human happiness or misery takes the form of action, the end for which we live is a certain kind of activity, not a quality" (cited in Lind, 1957, p. xviii).

In their summary of successful aging, Rowe and Kahn (1998) indicate that active engagement with life (that is "happy activities" [p. 45]) is one of three key factors, along with avoidance of disease and maintaining function. Other researchers have criticized Rowe and Kahn, noting that individuals who have not successfully avoided disease and disability still have meaningful lives if they are able to sustain occupations that are meaningful to them (George, 2006; Wong, 2000). In fact, Wong suggested that "personal meaning is the hidden dimension of successful aging, because having a positive meaning and purpose in life will not only add years to one's life but also add life to one's years" (p. 23).

This latter view is certainly consistent with the fundamental principles of occupational science (Yerxa, 1998). "The human spirit for activity is actualized, in a health way, through engagement in occupation: self-initiated, self-directed activity that is productive for the person (even if the product is fun) and contributes to others" (Yerxa, p. 412).

Later life is characterized by a reduction in prescribed roles and activities. The notion of retirement commonly found in developed countries allows, even encourages, withdrawal from paid employment. Children have been raised and are creating their own lives. Thus, elders have the option of withdrawing from two of the most significant occupations of middle age. At least hypothetically, this offers a greater degree of personal choice. Perhaps because of the diversity introduced by this greater choice, there is little clarity about activity patterns among older adults, or the personal meanings of the activities that they undertake.

Because U.S. society provides less guidance about expected occupations for older individuals than for younger individuals, "we have not, as a nation, channeled equal energy into defining the nature of those added years or creating positive roles or meaningful institutions through which they may be enjoyed" (Kaufman, 1986, p. 4). Thus, for older adults, the search for meaning is highly individual and begins with few reference points. At the same time, however, Baumeister (1991) has suggested an alternative way of thinking about meaning. He noted that "actual modern human lives are full of meaning, contrary to the misconceptions about existentialist theories. In a sense, the modern affliction is to have too much meaning, rather than not enough" (Baumeister, p. 5).

Many disciplines have explored the importance of occupation in later life (Yerxa, 1998). In particular, psychologists have begun to explore "positive psychology" focused on understanding what makes life worth living (Seligman & Csikszentmihalyi, 2000). Csikszentmihalyi (1990) described optimal experience as "flow," the intense and consuming engagement in occupations that promote a sense of well-being and happiness. Optimal experiences as he describes them are characterized by concentration, attention, and creative use of personal skills.

In what ways does occupation contribute to well-being? Among the outcomes reported among elders are enhanced self-efficacy (McAuley et al., 1999; Seeman, Unger, McAvay, & Leon, 1999), perceived usefulness and competence (Ranzijn, Keeves, Luszcz, & Feather, 1998), perceived control (Kunzmann, Little, & Smith, 2002; Menec & Chipperfield, 1997; Mirowsky, 1997; Smith, Kohn, Savage-Stevens, Finch, Ingate, & Lim, 2000; Wolinsky, Wyrwich, Babu, Kroenke, & Tierney, 2003), and mastery (Jang, Borenstein-Graves, Haley, Small, & Mortimer, 2003). Each of these constructs is a contributing factor in subjective well-being for older adults (Salmela-Aro & Schoon, 2005). Thus, there is a direct link between engagement in meaningful occupation and well-being in later life, as is true in other developmental phases.

The relation of occupation to meaning is central to understanding quality of life for older adults. However, the creation of personal meaning is not a one-time event, but a process (Thompson, 1993). In later life, individuals engage in "a constant struggle to maintain cherished life-styles against the threatening impact of both external events and internal changes, in which different styles of life will prove to have different kinds of resilience" (Thompson, p. 686). In this chapter, some types of meaning that have particular relevance in the lives of elders and the relationship of those meanings to the occupations in which they engage will be discussed. Also discussed are some important therapeutic considerations in helping elders create and maintain meaningful occupational patterns.

Occupation of Meaning

There is general agreement that occupation is an essential component of meaning in later life (Christiansen, 1999; Lawton, Moss, Hoffman, Grant, Have, & Kleban, 1999; Rudman, Cook, & Polatajko, 1997; Wilcock, 2001). At the same time, occupational scientists and occupational therapists "have debated how occupational engagement is associated with the development and maintenance of people's occupational identity, and how life meaning and self-esteem are linked to this concept" (Howie, Coulter, & Feldman, 2004, p. 446). Occupation plays a central role in identity throughout the life span, and factors that interfere with occupation, such as chronic illness, can interfere with identity (Charmaz, 2002).

Although most researchers and care providers recognize that activity or occupation is an essential component of quality of life in later life, there is a certain lack of clarity about the essential components of meaningful occupations for elders. One of the many ways in which the aging process complicates maintenance of meaningful performance patterns is the inevitable change in performance skills and client factors that characterize later life. Davidson (1997), describing the experiences of her husband in adjusting to Alzheimer's disease, indicates "it was hard to let go . . . but it's part of life. The challenge is to let go with pride and *find new things to do*" (p. 60) (emphasis added).

Although living a meaningful life is central to life satisfaction, difficulties abound in describing precisely what that means. Part of the problem is the establishment of a satisfactory definition of meaning. The literature presents an array of possible choices. Csikszentmihalyi (1990) provided a three-part definition:

meaning includes achieving purpose, expressing intentionality, and creating internal harmony. Baumeister (1991) suggested that meaning represents a coherent worldview, identified by each individual's choices among the culturally and societally available options. Thus, he noted that "life-meanings do not originate from some mysterious well deep inside the individual. Meaning itself is acquired socially, from other people and from the culture at large" (Baumeister, p. 6). Although occupations have socially constructed meanings, those meanings are filtered through the screen of personal interpretation to create what we will call personal meaning. Alternative views suggest that "personal meaning is defined as having a purpose in life, having a sense of direction, a sense of order and a reason for existence" (Reker, 1997, p. 710).

Themes of Meaning

The literature includes a number of models for conceptualizing the meanings of occupation. These, of course, begin with some of those developed by the theorists described in Chapter 2. So, for example, Erikson (1963) suggested that the major tasks of later life are generativity (productivity and creativity) versus stagnation, and ego integrity versus despair. Neugarten (1975) identified acceptance of imminent death, coping with increasing infirmity, dealing with care decisions, and maintaining social ties as the important developmental tasks of later life. Levinson (1986) described two stages for older adults. The first is a transition stage, during which tasks involve coping with physical decline and moving from formal authority to a more informal life structure. The second, in late adulthood, is characterized by decreasing concern with formal authority, status, and formal rewards, forming a broader life perspective and greater inner resources, and contributing to the wisdom of others. In each of these theories, there is an implicit or explicit assumption that in accomplishing these tasks, elders will find later life meaningful and satisfying.

A problem with the life-span theories is that they were developed before it became clear that later life would extend substantially in duration. It is unlikely that in 1963 Erikson anticipated that later life might last two or more decades. Thus, it seems probable that the struggles between generativity and stagnation and between ego integrity and despair have become more complex, and that there may well be other important tasks associated with meaning in later life.

Baumeister (1991) found that individuals seek meaning in their efforts to meet four fundamental needs: purpose, efficacy, value, and self-worth. He suggested that even though every individual strives to create his or her own personal meaning, it is difficult to do so, because meaning is socially and culturally structured. Rather, he believed, "at most, the person chooses among the meanings offered by culture and society" (Baumeister, p. 6). The cross-cultural literature on meaning supports this belief. Much of that research has explored subjective well-being across cultures (George, 2006), study that has resulted in the concept of "**happy life expectancy (HLE)**" (p. 331). HLE is highest in Europe and lowest in Africa and seems correlated not only with affluence, but also with individualism and human rights protections. A study exploring the factors contributing to a sense of well-being among Thai elders (Ingersoll-Dayton, Saengtienchai, Kespichayawattana, & Aungsuroch, 2004) found that, in direct contrast to Western components of well-being, these individuals identified acceptance, interdependence, and harmonious relationships as primary factors.

Then what are the socially and culturally mediated meanings found in later life occupations in the United States? A qualitative exploration of elders' perspectives on activity (Rudman et al., 1997) found that elders perceived activity as contributing to well-being, as a means to express and manage identity, as an organizer of time, and as a connector to the past, present, and future. Crabtree (1998) suggested that occupation organizes performance to meet the demands of self-maintenance and identity. Christiansen (1999) confirms that creation of identity is an important meaning of occupation. "When we build our identities through occupations, we provide ourselves with the context necessary for creating meaningful lives" (Christiansen, p. 547). Further, reasons for engaging in occupations are more important than simply the number of occupations (Everard, 1999).

Based on these suggestions, meanings will be clustered in this discussion into four main themes: instrumental meanings, existential meanings, emotional meanings, and sustaining self-identity. Even though there are undoubtedly many other ways to organize themes of meaning, the literature about aging seems to suggest that these are particularly salient in later life. As you will see, these themes overlap to some extent. Instrumental meanings are not completely separate from self-identity or evaluative meanings. But because ability to complete instrumental activities is much more central in the lives of elders than in younger individuals, it is an important theme to consider.

Instrumental Meanings

Instrumental meanings are those typically associated with occupations that support daily life. For younger individuals, accomplishing daily tasks is habitual. As performance skills diminish with age, those habits may be disrupted. Elders may need to focus much greater attention on bathing, dressing, and taking nourishment than do their younger counterparts. And these activities become imbued with important meanings, particularly in terms of the individual's perceptions about independence and dependence. Having proactive goals in later life is strongly associated with well-being and life satisfaction (Holahan & Chapman, 2002), and maintaining independence is often a valued proactive goal (Zirkel & Cantor, 1990). One possible reason that instrumental tasks structure meaning in later life is that they provide everyday routines (Gallimore & Lopez, 2002). "**Everyday competence,**" a person's ability to perform the activities that are central to independence," contributes to both physical and psychological well-being (Diehl, 1998, p. 422).

It is not just actual functional ability that matters, it is also perceived ability (Bernard, Kincade, Konrad, Arcury, Rabiner, Woomert et al., 1997). Both subjective usefulness and self-rated functional ability correlate with mortality, suggesting that elders who perceive themselves as capable are likely to live longer than others (Bernard et al., 1997; Okamata & Tanaka, 2004). Indeed, function is one of the factors identified in an exploration of valuation of life that contributes to elders' wish to live (Lawton et al., 1999). Valuation of life is "the extent to which the person is attached to his or her present life, for reasons related to a sense not only of enjoyment and the absence of distress, but also hope, futurity, purpose, meaningfulness, persistence, and self-efficacy" (Lawton et al., p. 407).

Adaptation to changing circumstances is one factor frequently addressed in considering the contributions of instrumental tasks to meaning in life (Anderson, James, Miller, Worley, & Longino, 1998; Jonsson, Moller, & Grimby, 1999; Ludwig, 1998). As the chapters that follow will demonstrate, aging is associated with both some degree of decline in performance skills and change in contexts like family and social networks. Elders who are able to reorganize their routines (Ludwig, 1998) and to maintain a sense of control (Wolinsky et al., 2003) are more likely to find life meaningful and gratifying.

Evaluative Meanings

For most of us, occupations contribute to our evaluation of well-being and happiness. Life-span theories suggest that this evaluation is a central concern of later life, and research confirms that for older adults, occupation has a central role in subjective assessments about satisfaction with life. A number of interrelated constructs are used in the research examining this issue: **happiness, life satisfaction, subjective well-being (SWB),** and **quality of life.** There are subtle distinctions among these constructs. Happiness refers to a sense of pleasure or a positive effect in the present, and life satisfaction refers to an overall life evaluation with which one is content. Well-being reflects a feeling that current circumstances are, in general, positive. Quality of life is perhaps the most inclusive of these evaluative terms, because it conveys satisfaction with circumstances and health, and also reflects external, concrete markers of well-being, such as income, type of housing, and education.

There is a great deal of research literature suggesting that these positive evaluations of life are associated with occupation. Some of the literature examines specific performance areas such as leisure (Lennartsson & Silverstein, 2001), work (Altschuler, 2004), and social participation (Bukov, Maas, & Lampert, 2002). Other literature examines more global aspects of the association between occupation and well-being (Salmela-Aro & Schoon, 2005). Although there are differences among nations in reported SWB, work and social occupations are associated with SWB around the world. Research examining the opposite side of the same coin finds that decreased activity is associated with decreased happiness (Menec, 2003). And stressors that affect highly valued roles erode meaning (Krause, 2004). "Engagement in meaningful activities contributes to good health, satisfaction with life, and longevity, as well as providing a potentially effective means of reducing costs of physical and emotional illness in later life" (Butler, 2002, p. S323).

Of course, there is somewhat less clarity about what constitutes optimal engagement; to a large extent, the purpose of the occupational therapy process in later life is to ascertain this for each individual and to facilitate the ability of the individual to sustain or regain those occupations. A third option is to substitute new occupations that convey similar meanings. Freund and Baltes (2002) referred to these three options as composing a process of substitution, optimization, and compensation (SOC). Because meaningful occupation is so closely tied to successful aging (Knight & Ricciardelli, 2003), elders who are able to satisfactorily manage this SOC are more likely to perceive life as worth living.

Existential Meanings

Of course, the question about whether or not life is worth living defines the existential challenge of living, a challenge that certainly becomes more critical as death nears. When describing tasks associated with various stages during the life course, early life course theorists discussed age as a time to address the tension between ego integrity and despair (Erikson, 1963). One of the major ways in which elders maintain ego integrity and avoid despair is through engagement in meaningful occupations. These are the occupations through which elders address important philosophical questions about their lives: Has my life been worth living? Have I made a contribution to the world around me? Bauman (1992) suggested that for elders, a good life in later life is one that can answer these existential questions in the affirmative. Elders must draw on "human strengths that act as buffers against mental illness: courage, future mindedness, optimism, interpersonal skill, faith, work ethic, hope, honesty, perseverance, and the capacity for flow and insight" (Seligman & Csikszentmihalyi, 2000). Meaningful occupations allow elders to sustain these attributes in the face of the challenges of later life. People need to engage in purposeful activity to provide meaning for existence (Howard & Howard, 1997).

Spirituality, identified as a contextual factor in the *AOTA Practice Framework* (2002), is an occupation whose central purpose is to address existential meanings. The gerontology literature is replete with studies of participation in religious or spiritual occupations. Religious occupations are those undertaken in association with formally constituted religious organizations, such as churches, mosques, or synagogues. "**Religion** consists of socially shared patterns of behavior and belief that seek to relate humans to the superhuman" (Howard & Howard, 1997, pp. 181–182). Spiritual occupations are those that individuals identify as connecting them to a higher power. "**Spirituality** stresses the person's subjective perception and experience of something or someone greater than himself or herself" (Howard & Howard, p. 181). These occupations may not have an obvious association with organized religion, so that, for example, someone who enjoys hiking and canoeing might report that being close to the natural world has a spiritual component.

Both religion and spirituality are associated with positive outcomes in later life. Individuals who participate in religious activities report higher levels of life satisfaction, self-esteem, and optimism, a finding that is particularly pronounced among African Americans in the United States as compared with whites (Krause, 2003). Similar findings are reported for participation in spiritual occupations (Kirby, Coleman, & Daley, 2004). Religious or spiritual occupations are associated with other positive outcomes as well. Religious grandparents are more involved with grandchildren than those who are not (King & Elder, 1999). Religious and spiritual activities are associated with lower levels of chronic illness and higher levels of activity (Benjamins, Musick, Gold, & George, 2003) and with lower mortality (Hill, Angel, Ellison, & Angel, 2005; Pandya, 2005). Religion and spirituality help individuals cope with chronic pain (Rippentropp, 2005). Religion can reduce the stress associated with the transition from independent living to residential care (Lewis, Edwards, Roe, Jewell, Jackson, & Tidmarsh, 2005). Caregivers who had religious or spiritual coping strategies reported lower stress levels than those who did not (Chang, Noonan, & Tennstedt, 1998).

Individuals who scored high on religiousness expressed less fear of death and dying than those who were less religious (Wink & Scott, 2005). It is important to note here, however, that low religiousness was also related to less fear of death and dying. Individuals who demonstrated inconsistency between religious beliefs and practices had the greatest fear of dying. This may be explained by the finding that religious doubt is associated with the highest levels of distress in later life (Krause, Ingersoll-Dayton, Ellison, & Wulff, 1999).

Spiritual and religious occupations clearly address existential meanings. But they are not the only occupations to do so. Leaving a legacy (Hunter & Rowles, 2005) or otherwise connecting with past, present, and future (Rudman et al., 1997) also allows elders to resolve existential questions. Elders feel a need "to be remembered positively, to pass along beliefs, values andideals they felt made them strong and contributed to positive aspects of their identity" (Hunter & Rowles, p. 344). The woman shown in Figure 3-1 derived great satisfaction by combining her love of music with her need to remember her heritage

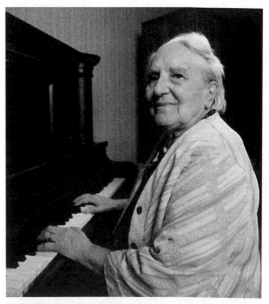

FIGURE 3-1 Playing traditional songs on the piano helps this woman maintain emotional ties with her ethnic heritage. (Courtesy of Menorah Park Nursing Home, Cleveland, Ohio, with permission.)

and was, therefore, eager to seek opportunities to enjoy playing the piano. By teaching a grandchild to play, she might pass along some of that heritage, and by playing at family gatherings, she might provide her family with positive memories of her. Other individuals become more interested in family history and genealogy as a way to leave information for families, or they may keep journals to pass their own stories along to children and grandchildren. Reminiscence has long been identified as an occupation that is important to elders (Fry, 1991), one that also allows elders to convey a legacy. These occupations all reflect the fact that "we want to leave something positive behind and exhibit an optimism that allows us to find something positive even in the darkest of situations" (Hunter & Rowles, p. 344).

What individuals choose to leave varies among individuals, just as spiritual expression varies among individuals (Wilding, May, & Muir-Cochrane, 2005). There can be no doubt, though, that a large number of older adults find comfort and optimism in the opportunity to engage in occupations with religious or spiritual significance, or that enable them to leave a legacy for others. These occupations provide comforting answers to questions about the meaning of life.

Meaning and Identity

To a great extent, we are what we do. Thus, a third meaning of occupations in later life is the maintenance of a sense of identity (Howie et al., 2004). Occupations allow elders to explore possible selves (Freund & Smith, 1999; Smith & Fruend, 2002). This is particularly important as the self changes with age. Discovering through occupation that it is possible to experience positive personal growth and to continue to make a contribution to the world enables elders to sustain a sense of hope both in the present and the future (Howie et al.).

For elders, later life occupations allow a continued sense of mastery (Jang et al., 2003) and control in the face of significant physical and social change (Kunzmann et al., 2002; Mirowsky, 1997). **Self-efficacy,** context-specific control, is strongly associated with occupation (McAuley et al., 2005; Seeman et al., 1999). Elders who retain a sense of personal agency and control sustain function later into life than those who do not (Smith et al., 2000), while individuals

who perceive control as resting largely with others tend to have higher rates of depression and general dissatisfaction with life than those who continue to feel they are in control (Kunzmann et al., 2002). Perhaps for these reasons, individuals who experience stressful life events tend to become more committed to valued roles, rather than to abandon them (Krause, 1999).

Several personal factors seem salient in supporting perceived control for elders. One of these is a sense of optimism (Leung, Moneta, & McBride-Chang, 2005; Reker, 1997). Another is a belief in the possibility of continued personal growth (Mack, Salmoni, Viverais-Dressler, Porter, & Garg, 1997). Positive self-perceptions have long-term benefits for functional health (Levy, Slade, & Kasl, 2002), and in all probability, function has long-term consequences for self-perceptions.

What, then, are the essential elements of occupations that provide for a sense of control? Among the factors that seem most important are perceived usefulness and competence (Ranzijn et al., 1998), maintaining personal control (Holahan & Chapman, 2002), and ability to sustain physical activity (McAuley et al., 2005). Individuals who are able to provide social support for others, as well as to receive it, typically experience a greater sense of mastery (Schieman & Meersman, 2004). Individuals who are able to sustain everyday routines feel a greater sense of agency (Gallimore & Lopez, 2002).

Consider the example of volunteering, a late-life occupation in which many elders participate (Hendricks & Cutler, 2004). Volunteering is a socially recognized contribution to others, one that enhances a sense of purpose and competence. It has clear meaning beyond simply keeping busy (Shmotkin, Blumstein, & Modan, 2003). It has thus been identified as an occupation that has major implications for well-being for older adults as a way to maintain identity (Greenfield & Marks, 2004; Morrow Howell, Hinterlong, Rozario, & Tang, 2003).

Supporting Meaning in Occupational Therapy Interventions

Throughout this volume, you will read about particular aspects of occupational performance and the performance skills necessary to enable them. You will also read about the contexts in which occupational performance occurs. As you do so, it will be important to remember that it is **meaningful** occupation that is critical later in life. Having personal goals (Riediger, Freund, & Baltes, 2005) is a critical component of successful aging. Strategies for selecting the most salient occupations, optimizing the ability to engage in those occupations, and compensating for those that must be abandoned can greatly enhance life satisfaction and subjective well-being (Duke, Leventhal, Brownlee, & Leventhal, 2002; Lang, Rieckmann, & Baltes, 2002). SOC is certainly not the only model for considering the occupations of elders.

The *Occupational Therapy Practice Framework* (AOTA, 2002) identifies the steps in occupational therapy intervention. These include evaluation, composed of completion of an occupational profile and an analysis of occupational performance; intervention, composed of establishing an intervention plan, implementing it, and reviewing its effectiveness; and outcomes defined in terms of engagement in an occupation to support participation as described in the International Classification of Function (ICF) (WHO, 2001). At every step in this process, having a model or framework that organizes the kinds of questions and forms of intervention can help ensure that the therapist works with the client to establish a helpful, comprehensive, and meaningful plan.

Early theories about occupation focused on efforts to provide a global description of elders' activity patterns as they aged. Perhaps the first of these was Disengagement Theory (Cummings & Henry, 1961). This theory suggested that as people age, they gradually withdraw from occupations that had been important to them. According to the theory, this occurs in terms of both actual participation and psychological participation. In other words, older adults do less and become less invested in activities. Relatively soon, this theory was called into question. Social scientists and care providers felt that it presented an unnecessarily pessimistic view of elders and that it ran counter to their observations about what older adults appeared to do. And, it was noted that disengagement theory was based on research with recent retirees who would be expected to report disengaging from activity because they had just

stopped activity that is recognized as central to identity. (See Chapter 13 for further discussion of work and retirement.) More recently, though, some researchers (Achenbaum & Bengtson, 1994: Ekerdt, 1986) suggested that it is appropriate for elders to withdraw from some activity, and that it may not make sense to assume that every older adult should or wants to continue occupation at levels that were desired in middle age. Ekerdt (1986) called this belief the "busy ethic" and noted that many theorists believe that reflection is an important part of later life that is too often overshadowed.

In the 1920s and 1930s, Russian psychologists proposed a theory of human activity that holds that the need to meet a goal is the primary human motivation for activity (cf. Vygotsky, 1978). Activity theory (Havighurst, 1963) was later applied to the experience of aging and emerged as a counterpoint to disengagement theory. Activity theory proposed that greater activity leads to greater life satisfaction in aging individuals, making activity an end in itself. It suggested that older adults live longer and have more satisfactory adjustment to old age when they maintain the activity levels that characterized their middle years and add new activities to substitute for any lost. Even though both disengagement and ongoing activity can be seen in certain individuals in their later years, neither of these seemed to describe the majority of elders. Atchley (1989) suggested that perhaps what was actually seen was continuity. Continuity theory proposed that activity patterns in older adults are similar to those they had when they were younger. Individuals who were relatively inactive in their younger years would continue to be so, and those who were more active would find ways to continue this pattern as well. Realizing that abilities change as individuals age, Atchley suggested that "in making adaptive choices, middle-aged and older adults attempt to preserve and maintain existing internal and external structures and . . . they prefer to accomplish this objective by using continuity" (p. 183).

The Model of Human Occupation (MOHO) (Kielhofner, 2004) is a well-known occupational-based model of behavior. Based on early philosophical work by Meyer (1922/1977) and Slagle (1933) and later work by Reilly (1974), this model views activity in terms of systems theory. The individual is conceptualized as an open, and therefore changing, system, with a number of subsystems that are directly relevant to activity. These subsystems include volition, habituation, and mind–brain–body performance.

The volition subsystem encompasses personal causation, values, and interests (Kielhofner, 2004). According to Kielhofner, an important early discovery in life is the connection between personal intention, action, and consequences. The individual must identify those actions that are important and that he or she wishes to pursue.

The desire to act is insufficient to ensure the ability to act, however. Roles must be identified and habits developed. These processes constitute the habituation subsystem. In many ways, roles dictate activity patterns. For example, the role of mother may involve such activities as dressing children, cooking, and talking with teachers. Roles alone, however, are not sufficient to fully explain activity. Mothers differ greatly in the specific types of activities they undertake in that role, selecting from the many activities that make up the role. One mother might take her children to see her office, whereas another might sew elaborate Halloween costumes.

Even when values, goals, and roles have been identified, the ability to perform affects activity. Skills must be developed that permit the mother to cook, to talk with her children, and so on. Skills include the ability to perceive and respond, to process information, and to communicate.

In determining what activity means to older adults in this framework, each of the subsystems must be considered (Kielhofner, 2004). A problem that becomes immediately obvious is the absence of prescribed roles for older adults, other than "retiree" (if indeed the person has retired) and grandparent (if indeed the person has grandchildren). In addition, elders vary greatly with regard to values, habits, and, to some extent, even skills.

Another model that can guide intervention in occupational therapy is Occupational Adaptation (OA) (Schkade & Schultz, 1992; Schultz & Schkade, 1992). OA suggests that throughout life, individuals are presented with new situations that require acquisition of new occupations and adaptation of existing occupations. It suggests that dysfunction is the result of ineffective adaptive responses and focuses on enhancing occupational adaptation as change in circumstances occurs.

Lawton's Ecological Model of Aging (Lawton, 1983) focuses on the fit between individuals and environments. It proposes that when the demands of the environment, which Lawton called **environmental press,** match the skills of the individual, function will be enhanced. Cvitkovich and Wister (2002) note that the environment can be considered in the context of three domains: structural resources, social support, and service support. Occupational therapists have added occupation to the mix, proposing the model of person–environment–occupation (PEO) (Christiansen & Baum, 1997). PEO describes "what people do in their daily lives, what motivates them, and how their personal characteristics combine with the situations in which occupations are undertaken to influence successful occupational performance" (p. 48) (Table 3-1).

Both the SOC and PEO models have particular applicability to occupations in late life. SOC (Freund & Baltes, 2002) suggests ways in which elders and their caregivers can ensure good fit among the person, the environment, and the occupation. What follows is consideration of the occupational therapy process through the lens of SOC. Although some therapists might find other models preferable, selection of a model is essential to effective intervention, as it ensures that assessment and intervention are coherent and comprehensive.

There is growing evidence with regard to the importance of meaningful occupation in later life. Research by Vaillant and colleagues (Vaillant, 2002; Vaillant, DiRago, & Mukamal, 2006) has demonstrated the importance of sense of purpose and meaningful activity in later life. Atchley (1999) documented the importance of maintaining activities and roles to adapt to change as one ages. Therapists can assist in helping to modify occupations to allow for continuation, as is seen in Figure 3-2.

Assessing meaningfulness in occupations and identifying strategies for selection, optimization, and compensation can be challenging. Certainly, it is easier to determine whether a client can dress independently than it is to discern whether this occupation has meaning for the individual, or whether he or she would rather get help with this and invest energy in other occupations. One recommended strategy is the use of a "personal projects" approach (Christiansen, Little, & Backman, 1998). To accomplish this, the

TABLE 3-1 **Summary of Theories of Activity of Older Adults**

Theory	Theorists	Constructs
Disengagement	Cummings & Henry (1961)	Elders typically withdraw from previous activities in preparation for death
Activity Theory	Havighurst (1963)	Elders maintain activity and do best when they are active and engaged
Continuity Theory	Atchley (1989)	Individuals in later life sustain previous beliefs, values, and characteristics
		Elders strive to retain previous activities
		When previous activities cannot be sustained, elders strive to replace those with activities that carry the same meanings
Life span	Neugarten (1975)	Old age is a continuation of the developmental process, representing a new development stage
	Erikson (1963)	Tasks specific to the stage can be identified
		Successful aging results from accomplishing tasks
Model of Human Occupation	Kielhofner (2004)	Individual is open system
		Subsystems are volition, habituation, performance
		Effectiveness of development of each subsystem reflects successful performance
Occupational Adaptation	Schultz & Schkade (1992)	Occupations change across the life span
	Schkade & Schultz (1992)	Individuals need to adapt to occupational change
Person–Environment– Occupation Selection, Optimization, Compensation	Christiansen & Baum (1997)	Individual, occupations, and environments interact Interaction can be effective or problematic
	Freund & Baltes (2002)	Elders adapt through these three mechanisms to change in functional ability

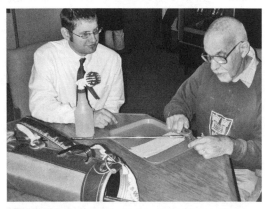

FIGURE 3-2 Sometimes the occupation must be changed significantly to enable the individual to continue some aspect of it, as is the case with this man, who has been a lifelong golfer.

therapist first asks the individual to list important projects and then to rate these along the dimensions that matter in the assessment process. The client might be asked to rate each project for importance, for impact on stress management, on meanings, or on other variables that help prioritize the projects in terms of centrality for the intervention process.

In addition to this kind of qualitative assessment, there are a number of instruments that can assess particular aspects of occupational meaning. The Spirituality Index of Well-Being (SIWB) (Frey, Daaleman, & Peyton, 2005) is one such instrument that explores self-efficacy and life scheme as related to spirituality. The Spiritual History Scale in Four Dimensions (SHS-4) (Hays, Meador, Branch, & George, 2001) measures factors labeled "God helped," "family history of religiousness," "lifetime religious social support," and "cost of religiousness." Other quantitative measures designed for elders capture different elements of life satisfaction or well-being. These include the Life Satisfaction Index (Havighurst, Neugarten, & Tobin, 1968) and the Satisfaction with Life Scale (SWLS) (Pavot & Diener, 1993). The SWLS, in particular, is quick and easy to administer and can provide a global view of the elder's well-being, and it has been adequately tested for reliability and validity. The Life Satisfaction Inventory has questionable validity and is particularly problematic when used with individuals from cultures with different values (Bonder, 2001). In administering this instrument to Maya elders in Guatemala, it was clear that the constructs did not translate conceptually, in spite of the careful linguistic translation that had been done. Because it is based, to some extent, on comparing current circumstances with the past, and with other individuals, it did not fit Mayan values, as Mayans view comparison as promoting jealousy or dissatisfaction.

One instrument that incorporates both qualitative and quantitative methods is the Canadian Occupational Performance Measure (COPM) (Law, Baptiste, Carswell, McColl, Polatajko, & Pollock, 2005). Like the personal project assessment, this instrument asks the individual first to identify important occupations. These are then rated numerically in terms of satisfaction with ability to perform it and its importance in the individual's life. These numbers can be tracked throughout the intervention process to determine whether progress is being made toward enabling those important occupations.

The kinds of occupations most likely to support meaning in later life are those that help the individual sustain a sense of hope (Spencer, Davidson, & White, 1997). Likewise, those that encourage expression and management of identity and those that connect the elder to the past, present, and future (Rudman et al., 1997) can enhance the individual's sense of meaning and purpose in later life. Once meaningful occupations have been identified and their characteristics explored, intervention can focus on what the *Practice Framework* (AOTA, 2002) calls "Create, promote; Establish, restore; Maintain; Modify; Prevent" (p. 627).

There has been a tremendous growth of attention in occupational therapy to the importance of interventions that emphasize spirituality (Belcham, 2004; Collins, Paul, & West-Frasier, 2001; Engquist, Short-DeGraff, Gliner, & Oltjenbruns, 1997; Howard & Howard, 1997; Schulz, 2004; Taylor, Mitchell, Kenan, & Tacker, 2000; Townsend, 1997;

Udell & Chandler, 2000). Certainly, the growing awareness of the centrality of religion in some cultural groups has increased awareness in occupational therapy of the relevance of interventions that facilitate the ability to attend church or otherwise participate in faith-based occupations, and to express spirituality through creative expression.

Evidence suggests that occupational therapy interventions emphasizing wellness and meaningful occupation promote mental health, social functioning, functional status, and physical functioning (Clark et al., 2001; Matuska, Giles-Heinz, Flinn, Neighbor, & Bass-Haugen, 2003). It is noteworthy that some of this research (Clark et al.) has compared occupational therapy intervention to a nonintervention control group and a generalized group activity group. The occupational therapy intervention, perhaps because of its emphasis on meaningful occupation, was superior to the two other conditions, in one of the few well-controlled studies of occupational therapy interventions with elders.

Among other occupations, reminiscence is particularly valued by elders (Cully, LaVoie, & Gfeller, 2001). This is an occupation that relates directly both to leaving a legacy and to the importance of connections with the past, present, and future. It seems to be an activity that translates well across cultures (Backerman, 1998). Likewise, creative writing offers opportunities for self-reflection, for connection with others, and with meaning-making generally (Wolf, 2005).

How does this process translate into an individual life? Mrs. A was a 72-year-old widow who had been working full time for the past 30 years. However, her hearing had worsened, making it difficult to continue her job as a social worker. Her daughter was recently divorced and was a single parent with two young children. An occupational therapist and Mrs. A reviewed her occupational profile and occupational performance, as well as performance patterns, skills, contexts, and client factors. Applying the SOC model, Mrs. A and the therapist considered a careful selection of meaningful occupations, and strategies for optimizing her performance and satisfaction in those occupations. In addition, they considered ways to substitute new occupations for those she could no longer perform. Based on this evaluation, Mrs. A decided to retire and to assume a substantial role in the care of her grandchildren. The specific constellation of activities that constituted the roles of "retiree" and "grandparent," in Mrs. A's view, included spending days with her grandchildren, arriving early enough that her daughter could get to work on time, taking them to school, or on days when they had no school, engaging in "enriching activities" like touring the art museum and baking cookies.

Unfortunately, as much as she loved her grandchildren, Mrs. A did not like baking cookies and felt personally unfulfilled in the new roles she had identified. She was frustrated by what she perceived as a lack of productivity. Thus, the outcomes of this first plan were unsatisfactory, so the therapist and Mrs. A revisited her occupational profile and reconsidered her decisions. This led to a new set of choices. One possibility was to redefine "retiree" and "grandparent" to reflect more adequately her personal values and beliefs. This included substituting some activities that Mrs. A perceived as productive, because this is an important value for her. She decided to volunteer at a hospital while her grandchildren were in school and to give guest lectures at the local school of social work. She optimized her involvement with her grandchildren by engaging with them in more "productive" kinds of activities as well, including homework and visits to museums to enhance their education. She also considered whether her volunteer and grandparenting roles compensated for the worker role she had relinquished, along with the possibility of returning to work, and alternatives such as part-time employment. If she decided to do so, and felt that she was abandoning her daughter, providing financial assistance might resolve the dilemma. Concerns about her decreasing ability to work effectively could be assuaged by identifying a job in which she could function in spite of any decline in abilities.

In this kind of intervention planning and implementation, it is essential to recognize the unique ways in which different individuals enact important occupations. In studying occupations of older women, it became clear that broad categories of occupation, religious participation, for example, led to very different activities (Bonder & Martin, 2000). Two women identified themselves as very religious. One went regularly to church, rarely missing a Sunday, and participated in a number of church committees and activities. The other never went to church services but instead choreographed intergenerational dance at the church.

These women were actively engaged in an array of other occupations as well. Within a given category or role, variability in the occupations that were undertaken and the meanings participants assigned to them were so great as to make the role label almost meaningless. For example, one woman enacted her role of grandmother as one of having fun with her new granddaughter through such activities as Halloween trick-or-treating. She looked forward to providing child care as a way to get to know her granddaughter. The other enacted grandparenting through child care provided on days when school was closed and during the summer. She experienced these activities as somewhat burdensome but expected. Reducing activity patterns through simple categorization on a single dimension may mask issues of vital importance to the individual—in particular, the unique contribution of each occupation to meaning and quality of life.

It is important to note that these issues of meaning are not unique to the developed world. Even in cultures where subsistence is the first order of business, and elders are expected to pitch in to contribute to efforts to secure food and shelter, they are concerned with how they are perceived, and how well they are able to manage expectations (Draper & Harpending, 1994). Even though older adults in developed nations may have greater time to focus on existential questions, they are not absent in other environments.

Throughout this book, evidence will be presented with regard to the importance of various occupations in the lives of older adults, and the outcomes of interventions focused on enabling occupational performance. This evidence clearly indicates that occupation contributes to sustained health, function, and even to survival (Avlund et al., 2004; Bukov et al., 2002; Everard, Lach, Fisher, & Baum, 2000; Krause, 2002; Lennartsson & Silverstein, 2001; Lovden, Ghisletta, & Lindenberger, 2005). There is also a growing body of evidence that occupational therapy intervention is central to enhanced outcomes of care (Arling, Williams, & Kopp, 2000; Carlson, Fanchiang, Zemke, & Clark, 1996; Clark et al., 1997). Therapists interested in fostering successful aging can look to this literature for guidance about how best to proceed. They can also use these findings to support efforts to improve the context in which aging occurs, through interventions focused on policy change and on access to care for older adults.

■ Summary

The ultimate goal of occupational therapy services is well-being, not health. This presents dilemmas for care providers who design programming or individual interventions for older adults. Public policy emphasizes self-care as the sole desired outcome of care and provides reimbursement according to guidelines that reflect this emphasis. Although this focus is understandable, given the lack of clarity about what occupations contribute to life satisfaction in later life, it may well be misguided, because it is clear that "there is more to life than putting on your pants" (Radomski, 1995, p. 487). As will be seen in subsequent chapters, occupational therapists must consider strategies other than direct care in hospital settings, and community-based and population-based care has grown considerably.

Pursuing an evaluation that incorporates all aspects of occupational performance is challenging, as is designing meaningful intervention plans. Further, intervention is not complete until reevaluation has occurred and outcomes are carefully examined. Mrs. A was not as satisfied as she once had been with her worker role because of changes in her abilities. However, she felt strongly about the importance of working, and the alternatives she first attempted did not have the same meaning for her.

As is clear in the example of Mrs. A, intervention is not straightforward. Simply developing a list of occupations is inadequate, because the nature of the occupation, the context in which it occurs, and individual skills, performance, and patterns are essential considerations. Because roles can be expressed in many ways, the job of the health care team, and the occupational therapist in particular, is to help the individual examine not only the occupation but also the activities that constitute the occupation for the individual. The next step is to facilitate the substitution, optimization, and compensation process through which the individual establishes new occupational performance patterns that are meaningful. A number of methods for accomplishing these goals are presented in the chapters that follow. It is clearly crucial that both evaluation and intervention must be undertaken with recognition of meanings that are important to the client.

Successful aging has become the focus of considerable research interest. Comprehensive review supports the idea that individuals who have lives with purpose are most likely to be among successful (as opposed to usual, or even unsuccessful) agers. As Swensen (1983) noted, "People live as long as they have something to do that needs to be done" (p. 331). Health care providers, policy planners, and older adults must develop a clear understanding of what it means, both to the individual and to society, to have something that needs to be done.

Case Study

Emma[1] was a patient in an in-patient mental health facility. She "was an 83-year-old woman with major depression who had lost her husband about 6 months before admission. Because she had become increasingly unable to cope with her daily activities, she moved in with her son who anticipated that Emma would be permanently unable to live independently. At the time of admission, she had stopped doing all daily activities, was experiencing difficulty with intentionality, and

was struggling to find meaning in her daily life" (Spencer, Davidson, & White, 1997, p. 194).

The therapist completed both an occupational profile and an analysis of occupational performance. Emma did not appear to have any physical limitations, but had poor memory and was experiencing a sense of hopelessness. The therapist and Emma worked on goal setting, initially identifying only a few goals to avoid leaving Emma feeling

continued on page 58

overwhelmed. One goal Emma identified was increased participation in leisure activities. She indicated she wanted to be able to participate in at least one or two activities per week in her son's home. The therapist provided the initial energy for this task, providing cues and "goal-focused expectations." At discharge, Emma was able to return to her son's home and participate in one or two leisure activities each week, the goal she had originally specified. This gave her the hope to continue to set goals with regard to leisure, self-care, and productive activities. In particular, she had added such activities as

visiting the sick. Among the many positive consequences of this improvement, Emma perceived a renewed sense of spirituality.

1. In what ways did Emma demonstrate a lack of meaningful engagement in occupation?
2. Initially, Emma was reported to have stopped self-care activities. Why might the therapist have focused on leisure activities?
3. What role did the son play in this situation?

Review Questions

1. How is occupation associated with meaning in later life?
2. Discuss the importance of environment and context to meaning.
3. Describe the characteristics of the theories of disengagement, activity, continuity, life span, human occupation, occupational adaptation, person–environment–occupation, and substitution, optimization, and compensation.
4. What is meant by instrumental meanings? Evaluative meanings? Existential meanings?
5. How can occupational therapy interventions support meaning?

Web-Based Resources

www.ppc.sas.upenn.edu/lifesatisfactionscale.pdf, **University of Pennsylvania,** date connected March 10, 2007. This site contains the questions for the Satisfaction with Life Scale. Diener has other sites providing analysis of psychometric properties, including www.psych.uiuc.edu/~ediener/hottopic/hottopic.html, **University of Illinois at Chicago,** date connected March 10, 2007. For information about the Life Satisfaction Index, go to www.gesher.org/Myers-Briggs/life_satis_index.html, **Winer Foundation** (for the actual instrument) and www.atsqol.org/sections/instruments/ko/pages/isia.html, **American Thoracic Society** (for an analysis), date connected March 10, 2007.

www.upa.pdx.edu/IOA/newsorn/gsaquant/wallace.ppt, **Gerontological Society of America Contact,** date connected March 10, 2007. The actual questions can be found at www.gesher.org/Myers-Briggs/life_satis_index.html, **Winer Foundation** (for the actual instrument, listed above).

REFERENCES

Achenbaum, W. A., & Bengtson, V. L. (1994). Re-engaging the disengagement theory of aging: On the history and assessment of theory development in gerontology. *The Gerontologist, 34,* 756–762.

Atchley, R. C. (1989). Continuity theory of normal aging. *Gerontologist, 29,* 183–190.

Altschuler, J. (2004). Beyond money and survival: The meaning of paid work among older women. *International Journal of Aging and Human Development, 58,* 223–239.

American Occupational Therapy Association. (2002). Occupational therapy practice framework: Domain and process. *American Journal of Occupational Therapy, 56,* 609–639.

Anderson, R. T., James, M. K., Miller, M. E., Worley, A. S., & Longino, C. F. (1998). The timing of change: Patterns in transitions in functional status among elderly persons. *Journal of Gerontology: Social Sciences, 53B,* S17–S27.

Arling, G., Williams, A. R., & Kopp, D. (2000). Therapy use and discharge outcomes for elderly nursing home residents. *The Gerontologist, 40,* 587–595.

Atchley, R. C. (1989). Continuity theory of normal aging. *The Gerontologist, 29,* 183–190.

Atchley, R. C. (1999). *Continuity and adaptation in aging: Creating positive experiences.* Baltimore, MD: Johns Hopkins University Press.

Avlund, K., Lund, R., Holstein, B. E., Due, P., Sakari-Rantala, R., & Heikkinen, R. (2004). The impact of structural and functional characteristics of social relations as determinants of functional decline. *Journal of Gerontology: Social Sciences, 59B,* S44–S51.

Backerman, G. H. (1998). Reminiscence in the elder: An exploration of identity and meaning making. *Dissertation Abstracts International: Section B: The Sciences and Engineering. 58*(10-B), 5668.

Bauman, Z. (1992). *Mortality, immortality, and other life strategies.* Cambridge, UK: Polity Press.

Baumeister, R. F. (1991). *Meanings of life.* New York: Guilford Press.

Belcham, C. (2004). Spirituality in occupational therapy: Theory in practice? *British Journal of Occupational Therapy, 67*(1), 39–46.

Benjamins, M. R., Musick, M. A., Gold, D. T., & George, L. K. (2003). Age-related declines in activity level: The relationship between chronic illness and religious activity. *Journal of Gerontology: Social Sciences, 58B,* S377–S385.

Bernard, S. L., Kincade, J. E., Konrad, T. R., Arcury, T. A., Rabiner, D. J., Woomert, A., et al. (1997). Predicting mortality from community surveys of older adults: The importance of self-rated functional ability. *Journal of Gerontology: Social Sciences, 52B,* S155–S163.

Bonder, B. R. (2001). Culture and occupation: A comparison of weaving in two traditions. *Canadian Journal of Occupational Therapy, 65,* 310–319.

Bonder, B. R., & Martin, L. (2000). Personal meanings of occupation for women in later life: Two women compared. *Women and Aging, 12,* 177–193.

Bukov, A., Maas, I., & Lampert, T. (2002). Social participation in very old age: Cross-sectional and longitudinal findings from BASE. *Journal of Gerontology: Psychological Sciences, 57B,* P510–P517.

Butler, R. N. (2002). Guest editorial: The study of productive aging. *Journal of Gerontology: Social Sciences, 57B,* S323.

Carlson, M., Fanchiang, S., Zemke, R., & Clark, F. (1996). A meta-analysis of the effectiveness of occupational therapy for older persons. *American Journal of Occupational Therapy, 50,* 89–98.

Chang, B., Noonan, A. E., & Tennstedt, S. L. (1998). The role of religion/spirituality in coping with caregiving for disabled elders. *The Gerontologist, 38,* 463–469.

Charmaz, K. (2002). The self as habit: The reconstruction of self in chronic illness. *Occupational Therapy Journal of Research, 53,* 547–558.

Chipperfield, J. G., & Greenslade, L. (1999). Perceived control as a buffer in the use of health care services. *Journal of Gerontology Series B: Psychological Sciences & Social Sciences, 54,* 146–154.

Christiansen, C. H. (1999). Defining lives: Occupation as identity: An essay on competence, coherence, and the creation of meaning. *American Journal of Occupational Therapy, 53,* 547–558.

Christiansen, C., & Baum, C. (1997). Person-environment occupational performance: A conceptual model for practice. In C. Christiansen & C. Baum (Eds.), *Occupational therapy: Enabling function and well-being* (2nd ed., pp. 46–70). Thorofare, NJ: Slack.

Christiansen, C. H., Little, B. R., & Backman, C. (1998). Personal projects: A useful approach to the study of occupation. *American Journal of Occupational Therapy, 52,* 439–446.

Clark, F., Azen, S. P., Carlson, M., Mandel, D., LaBree, L., Hay, J., Zemke, R., Jackson, J., & Lipson, L. (2001). Embedding health-promoting changes into the daily lives of independent-living older adults: Long-term follow-up of occupational therapy intervention. *Journal of Gerontology: Psychological Sciences, 56B,* P60–P63.

Clark, F., Azen, S. P., Zemke, R., Jackson, J., Carlson, M., Mandel, D., et al. (1997). Occupational therapy for independent-living older adults: A randomized controlled trial. *Journal of the American Medical Association, 278,* 1321–1326.

Collins, J. S. D., Paul, S., & West-Frasier, J. (2001). The utilization of spirituality in occupational therapy: Beliefs, practices, and perceived barriers. *Occupational Therapy in Health Care, 14*(3/4), 73–92.

Crabtree, J. L. (1998). The end of occupational therapy. *American Journal of Occupational Therapy, 52,* 205–214.

Csikszentmihalyi, M. (1990). *Flow: The psychology of optimal experience.* Grand Rapids, MI: Harper & Row.

Cully, J. A., LaVoie, D., & Gfeller, J. D. (2001). Reminiscence, personality, and psychological functioning in older adults. *The Gerontologist, 41,* 89–95.

Cummings, E. M., & Henry, W. E. (1961). *Growing old: The process of disengagement.* New York: Basic Books.

Cvitkovich, Y., & Wister, A. (2002). Bringing in the life course: A modification to Lawton's Ecological Model of Aging. *Hallym International Journal of Aging, 4*(1), 15–29.

Davidson, A. (1997). *Alzheimer's: A love story. One year in my husband's journey.* Secaucus, NJ: Birch Lane Press.

Diehl, M. (1998). Everyday competence in later life: Current status and future directions. *The Gerontologist, 38,* 422–433.

Draper, P., & Harpending, H. (1994). Cultural considerations in the experience of aging: Two African cultures. In B. R. Bonder & M. B. Wagner (Eds.), *Functional Performance in Older Adults* (pp. 15–27). Philadelphia: F.A. Davis.

Duke, J., Leventhal, H., Brownlee, S., & Leventhal, E. A. (2002). Giving up and replacing activities in response to illness. *Journal of Gerontology: Psychological Sciences, 57B,* P367–P376.

Ekerdt, D. J. (1986). The busy ethic: Moral continuity between work and retirement. *The Gerontologist, 26,* 239–244.

Engquist, D. E., Short-DeGraff, M., Gliner, J., & Oitjenbruns, K. (1997). Occupational therapists' beliefs and practices with regard to spirituality and therapy. *American Journal of Occupational Therapy, 51,* 173–180.

Erikson, E. H. (1963). *Childhood and society.* New York: W. W. Norton.

Everard, K. M. (1999). The relationship between reasons for activity and older adult well-being. *Journal of Applied Gerontology, 18,* 325–340.

Everard, K. M., Lach, H. W., Fisher, E. B., & Baum, M. C. (2000). Relationship of activity and social support to the functional health of older adults. *Journal of Gerontology: Social Sciences, 55B,* S208–S212.

Freund, A. M., & Baltes, P. B. (2002). Life-management strategies of selection, optimization, and compensation: Measurement by self-report and construct validity. *Journal of Personality and Social Psychology, 82,* 642–662.

Freund, A. M., & Smith, J. (1999). Content and function of the self-definition in old and very old age. *Journal of Gerontology: Psychological Sciences, 54B,* P55–P67.

Frey, B. B., Daaleman, T. P., & Peyton, V. (2005). Measuring dimension of spirituality for health research: Validity of the Spirituality Index of Well-Being. *Research on Aging, 27,* 556–577.

Fry, P. S. (1991). Individual differences in reminiscence among older adults: Predictors of frequency and pleasantness ratings of reminiscence activity. *International Journal of Aging and Human Development, 33,* 311–326.

Gallimore, R., & Lopez, E. M. (2002). Everyday routines, human agency, and ecocultural context: Construction and maintenance of individual habits. *Occupational Therapy Journal of Research, 22*(suppl.), 70S–77S.

George, L. K. (2006). Perceived quality of life. In R. H. Binstock & L. K. George (Eds.), *Handbook of aging and the social sciences* (6th ed., pp. 320–335). Burlington, MA: Academic Press.

Greenfield, E. A., & Marks, N. F. (2004). Formal volunteering as a protective factor for older adults' psychological well-being. *Journal of Gerontology: Social Sciences, 59B,* S258–S264.

Hasselkus, B. R. (2002). *The meaning of everyday occupation.* Thorofare, NJ: Slack.

Havighurst, R. J. (1963). Successful aging. In R. H. Williams, C. Tibbetts, & W. Donahue (Eds.), *Processes of Aging, Vol. I* (pp. 299–320). New York: Atherton.

Havighurst, R. J., Neugarten, B. L., & Tobin, S. S. (1968). Life Satisfaction Index. In R. A. Kane & R. L. Kane, *Assessing the Elderly: A Practical Guide to Measurement* (pp. 174–189). Lexington, MA: Lexington Books.

Hays, J. C., Meador, K. G., Branch, P. S., & George, L. K. (2001). The Spiritual History Scale in Four Dimensions (SHS-4): Validity and reliability. *The Gerontologist, 41,* 239–249.

Hendricks, J., & Cutler, S. D. J. (2004). Volunteerism and socioemotional selectivity in later life. *Journal of Gerontology: Social Sciences, 59B,* S251–S257.

Hill, T. D., Angel, J. L., Ellison, C. G., & Angel, R. J. (2005). Religious attendance and mortality: An 8-year follow-up of older Mexican Americans. *Journal of Gerontology: Social Sciences, 60B,* S102–S109.

Hilleras, P. K., Jorm, A. F., Herlitz, A., & Winblad, B. (2001). Life satisfaction among the very old: A survey on a cognitively intact sample aged 90 years or above. *International Journal of Aging and Human Development, 52*(1), 71–90.

Holahan, C. K., & Chapman, J. R. (2002). Longitudinal predictors of proactive goals and activity participation at age 80. *Journal of Gerontology: Psychological Sciences, 57B,* P418–P425.

Howard, B. S., & Howard, J. R. (1997). Occupation as spiritual activity. *American Journal of Occupational Therapy, 51,* 181–185.

Howie, L., Coulter, M., & Feldman, S. (2004). Crafting the self: Older persons' narratives of occupational identity. *American Journal of Occupational Therapy, 58,* 446–454.

Hunter, E. G., & Rowles, G. D. (2005). Leaving a legacy: Toward a typology. *Journal of Aging Studies, 19,* 327–347.

Ingersoll-Dayton, B., Saengtienchai, C., Kespichayawattana, J., & Aungsuroch, Y. (2004). Measuring psychological well-being: Insights from Thai elders. *The Gerontologist, 44,* 596–604.

Jang, Y., Borenstein-Graves, A., Haley, W. E., Small, B. J., & Mortimer, J. A. (2003). Determinants of a sense of mastery in African American and white older adults. *Journal of Gerontology: Social Sciences, 58B,* S221–S224.

Jonsson, A. T., Moller, A., & Grimby, G. (1999). Managing occupations in everyday life to achieve adaptation. *American Journal of Occupational Therapy, 53,* 353–362.

Kaufman, S. R. (1986). *The ageless self: Sources of meaning in later life.* Madison, WI: University of Wisconsin Press.

Kielhofner, G. (2004). *Conceptual foundation of occupational therapy* (3rd ed.). Philadelphia: F.A. Davis.

King, V., & Elder, G. H. (1999). Are religious grandparents more involved grandparents? *Journal of Gerontology: Social Sciences, 54B,* S317–S328.

Kirby, S. E., Coleman, P. G., & Daley, D. (2004). Spirituality and well-being in frail and nonfrail older adults. *Journal of Gerontology: Psychological Sciences, 59B,* P123–P129.

Knight, T., & Ricciardelli, L. A. (2003). Successful aging: Perceptions of adults between 70 and 101 years. *International Journal of Aging and Human Development, 56,* 223–245.

Krause, N. (1999). Stress and the devaluation of highly salient roles in late life. *Journal of Gerontology: Social Sciences, 54B,* S99–S108.

Krause, N. (2002). Church-based social support and health in old age: Exploring variations by race. *Journal of Gerontology: Social Sciences, 57B,* S332–S347.

Krause, N. (2003). Religious meaning and subjective well-being in late life. *Journal of Gerontology: Social Sciences, 58B,* S160–S170.

Krause, N. (2004). Stressors arising in highly valued roles, meaning in life, and the physical health status of older adults. *Journal of Gerontology: Social Sciences, 59B,* S287–S297.

Krause, N., Ingersoll Dayton, B., Ellison, C. G., & Wulff, K. M. (1999). Aging, religious doubt, and psychological well-being. *The Gerontologist, 39,* 525–553.

Kunzmann, U., Little, T., & Smith, J. (2002). Perceiving control: A double-edged sword in old age. *Journal of Gerontology: Psychological Sciences, 57B,* P484–P491.

Lang, F. R., Rieckmann, N., & Baltes, M. M. (2002). Adapting to aging losses: Do resources facilitate strategies of selection, compensation, and optimization in everyday functioning? *Journal of Gerontology: Psychological Sciences, 57B,* P501–P509.

Law, M., Baptiste, S., Carswell, A., McColl, M. A., Polatajko, H., & Pollock, N. (2005). *Canadian Occupational Performance Measure.* Toronto: Canadian Association for Occupational Therapy.

Lawton, M. P. (1983). Environment and other determinants of well-being in older people. *The Gerontologist, 23,* 349–357.

Lawton, M. P., Moss, M., Hoffman, C., Grant, R., Have, T. T., & Kleban, M. H. (1999). Health, valuation of life and the wish to live. *The Gerontologist, 39,* 406–416.

Lennartsson, C., & Silverstein, M. (2001). Does engagement with life enhance survival of elderly people in Sweden? The role of social and leisure activities. *Journal of Gerontology: Social Sciences, 56B,* S335–S342.

Leung, B. W., Moneta, G. B., & McBride-Chang, C. (2005). Think positively and feel positively: Optimism and life satisfaction in late life. *International Journal of Aging and Human Development, 61,* 335–365.

Levinson, D. J. (1986). A conception of adult development. *American Psychologist, 49,* 3–13.

Levy, B. R., Slade, M. D., & Kasl, S. V. (2002). Longitudinal benefit of positive self perceptions of aging on functional health. *Journal of Gerontology: Psychological Sciences, 57B,* P409–P417.

Lind, L. R. (1957). *Ten Greek plays in contemporary translations.* Boston: Houghton Mifflin.

Lovden, M., Ghisletta, P., & Lindenberger, U. (2005). Social participation attenuates decline in perceptual speed in old and very old age. *Psychology and Aging, 20,* 423–434.

Lowis, M. J., Edwards, A. C., Roe, C. A., Jewell, A. J., Jackson, M. I., & Tidmarsh, W. M. (2005). The role of religion in mediating the transition to residential care. *Journal of Aging Studies, 19,* 349–362.

Ludwig, F. M. (1998). The unpackaging of routine in older women. *American Journal of Occupational Therapy, 52,* 168–178.

Mack, R., Salmoni, A., Viverais-Dressler, G., Porter, E., & Garg, R. (1997). Perceived risks to independent living: The views of older, community-dwelling adults. *The Gerontologist, 37,* 729–736.

Matuska, K., Giles-Heinz, A., Flinn, N., Neighbor, M., & Bass-Haugen, J. (2003). Outcomes of a pilot occupational therapy wellness program for older adults. *American Journal of Occupational Therapy, 57,* 220–224.

McAuley, E., Elavsky, S., Motl, R. W., Konopack, J. F., Hu, L., & Marquez, D. X. (2005). Physical activity, self-efficacy, and self-esteem: Longitudinal relationship in older adults. *Journal of Gerontology: Psychological Sciences, 60B,* P268–P275.

McAuley, E., Katula, J., Mihalko, S., Blissmer, B., Duncan, T., Pena, M., et al. (1999). Mode of physical activity differentially influences self-efficacy in older adults: A latent growth curve analysis. *Journal of Gerontology: Psychological Sciences, 54B,* P283–P292.

Menec, V. H. (2003). The relation between everyday activities and successful aging: A 6-year longitudinal study. *Journal of Gerontology: Social Sciences, 58B,* S74–S82.

Menec, V. H., & Chipperfield, J. G. (1997). Remaining active in later life: The role of health locus of control in seniors' activity level, health, and life satisfaction. *Journal of Aging and Health, 9,* 105–125.

Meyer, A. (1922/1977). The philosophy of occupational therapy. *American Journal of Occupational Therapy, 31,* 639–642.

Mirowsky, J. (1997). Age, subjective life expectancy, and the sense of control: The horizon hypothesis. *Journal of Gerontology: Social Sciences, 52B,* S125–S134.

Morrow-Howell, N., Hinterlong, J., Rozario, P. A., & Tang, F. (2003). Effects of volunteering on the well-being of older adults. *Journal of Gerontology: Social Sciences, 58B,* S137–S145.

Neugarten, B. L. (1975). *Middle age and aging.* Chicago, IL: University of Chicago Press.

Okamata, K., & Tanaka, Y. (2004). Subjective usefulness and 6-year mortality risks among elderly persons in Japan. *Journal of Gerontology: Psychological Sciences, 59B,* P246–P249.

Pandya, L. (2005). Spirituality, religion and health. *Geriatric Medicine, 35*(5), 19–20, 22.

Pavot, W., & Diener, E. (1993). Review of the Satisfaction with Life Scale. *Psychological Assessment, 5,* 164–172.

Peloquin, S. M. (1997). Nationally speaking: The spiritual depth of occupation: Making worlds and making lives. *American Journal of Occupational Therapy, 51,* 167–168.

Radomski, M. V. (1995). There is more to life than putting on your pants. *American Journal of Occupational Therapy, 49,* 487–490.

Ranzijn, R., Keeves, J., Luszcz, M., & Feather, N. T. (1998). The role of self-perceived usefulness and competence in the self-esteem of elderly adults: Confirmatory factor analyses of the Bachman Revision of Rosenberg's Self-Esteem Scale. *Journal of Gerontology: Psychological Sciences, 53B,* P96–P104.

Reilly, M. (1974). *Play as exploratory learning*. Beverly Hills, CA: Sage.

Reker, G. T. (1997). Personal meaning, optimism, and choice: Existential predictors of depression in community and institutional elderly. *The Gerontologist, 37,* 709–716.

Riediger, M., Freund, A. M., & Baltes, P. B. (2005). Managing life through personal goals: Intergoal facilitation and intensity of goal pursuit in younger and older adulthood. *Journal of Gerontology: Psychological Sciences, 60B,* P84–P91.

Rippentrop, A. E. (2005). A review of the role of religion and spirituality in chronic pain populations. *Rehabilitation Psychology, 50,* 278–284.

Rowe, J., & Kahn, R. (1998). *Successful aging: The MacArthur Foundation study*. New York: Pantheon.

Rudman, D. L., Cook, J. V., & Polatajko, H. (1997). Understanding the potential of occupation: A qualitative exploration of seniors' perspectives on activity. *American Journal of Occupational Therapy, 51,* 640–650.

Salmela-Aro, K., & Schoon, I. (2005). Introduction to the special section: Human development and well-being. *European Psychologist, 10,* 259–263.

Schieman, S., & Meersman, S. C. (2004). Neighborhood problems and health among older adults: Received and donated social support and the sense of mastery as effect modifiers. *Journal of Gerontology: Social Sciences, 59B,* S89–S97.

Schkade, J. K., & Schultz, S. (1992). Occupational adaptation: Toward a holistic approach for contemporary practice, part 1. *American Journal of Occupational Therapy, 46,* 829–838.

Schulz, E. K. (2004). Spirituality and disability: An analysis of select themes. *Occupational Therapy in Health Care, 18*(4), 57–83.

Schultz, S., & Schkade, J. K. (1992). Occupational adaptation: Toward a holistic approach for contemporary practice, part 2. *American Journal of Occupational Therapy, 46,* 917–926.

Seeman, T. E., Unger, J. B., McAvay, G., & Mendes de Leon, C. F. (1999). Self-efficacy beliefs and perceived declines in functional ability: MacArthur studies of successful aging. *Journal of Gerontology: Psychological Sciences, 54B,* P214–P222.

Seligman, M. E. P., & Csikszentmihalyi, M. (2000). Positive psychology: An introduction. *American Psychologist, 55,* 5–14.

Shmotkin, D., Blumstein, T., & Modan, B. (2003). Beyond keeping active: Concomitants of being a volunteer in old-old age. *Psychology and Aging, 18,* 602–607.

Slagle, E. C. (1933). *Habit training. Syllabus for training of nurses in Occupational Therapy* (2nd ed.). Utica, NY: State Hospital Press.

Smith, G. C., Kohn, S. J., Savage-Stevens, S. E., Finch, J. J., Ingate, R., & Lim, Y. (2000). The effects of interpersonal and personal agency on perceived control and psychological well-being in adulthood. *The Gerontologist, 40,* 458–468.

Smith, J., & Freund, A. M. (2002). The dynamics of possible selves in old age. *Journal of Gerontology: Psychological Sciences, 57B,* P492–P500.

Spencer, J., Davidson, H., & White, V. (1997). Helping clients develop hopes for the future. *American Journal of Occupational Therapy, 51,* 191–198.

Swensen, C. H. (1983). A respectable old age. *American Psychologist, 9,* 327–334.

Taylor, E., Mitchell, J. E., Kenan, S., & Tacker, R. (2000). Attitudes of occupational therapists toward spirituality in practice. *American Journal of Occupational Therapy, 54,* 421–426.

Thompson, P. (1993). Comment: "I don't feel old": The significance of the search for meaning in later life. *International Journal of Geriatrics and Psychiatry, 8,* 685–692.

Townsend, E. (1997). Inclusiveness: A community dimension of spirituality. *Canadian Journal of Occupational Therapy, 64,* 146–155.

Udell, L., & Chandler, C. (2000). The role of the occupational therapist in addressing the spiritual needs of clients. *British Journal of Occupational Therapy, 63,* 489–494.

Vaillant, G. (2002). *Ageing well*. Melbourne: Scribe.

Vaillant, G. E., DiRago, A. C., & Mukamal, K. (2006). Natural history of male psychological health, XV: Retirement satisfaction. *American Journal of Psychiatry, 163,* 682–688.

Vygotsky, L. S. (1978). *Mind in society. The development of higher psychological processes*. Cambridge, MA: Harvard University Press.

Wilcock, A. A. (2001). Occupation for health: Re-activating the regimen sanitatis. *Journal of Occupational Science, 8*(3), 20–24.

Wilding, C., May, E., & Muir-Cochrane, E. (2005). Experience of spirituality, mental illness and occupation: A life-sustaining phenomenon. *Australian Occupational Therapy Journal, 52*(1), 2–9.

Wink, P., & Scott, J. (2005). Does religiousness buffer against the fear of death and dying in late adulthood? Findings from a longitudinal study. *Journal of Gerontology: Psychological Sciences, 60B,* P207–P214.

Wolf, M. A. (2005). Writers have no age, creative writing for older adults. *Educational Gerontology, 31,* 657–658.

Wolinsky, F. D., Wyrwich, K. W., Babu, A. N., Kroenke, K., & Tierney, W. M. (2003). Age, aging, and the sense of control among older adults: A longitudinal reconsideration. *Journal of Gerontology: Social Sciences, 58B,* S212–S220.

Wong, P. T. P. (2000). Meaning of life and meaning of death in successful aging. In A. Tomer (Ed.), *Death attitudes and the older adult* (pp. 23–35). New York: Brunner/Mazel.

World Health Organization. (2001). *International classification of functioning, disability, and health (ICF)*. Geneva, Switzerland: author.

Yerxa, E. J. (1998). Health and the human spirit for occupation. *American Journal of Occupational Therapy, 52,* 412–418.

Zirkel, S., & Cantor, N. (1990). Personal construal of life tasks: Those who struggle for independence. *Journal of Personality and Social Psychology, 58,* 172–185.

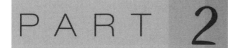

PART 2

Impact of Normal Aging, and Interruptions in Function

*A*lthough context is important, occupational therapists and other health-care providers are most often presented with an individual or a family confronting particular life challenges. Chapters 4 through 7 emphasize the normal aging process as it affects body systems and body functions. These are the capacities that support activities and participation, and, as is true throughout life, they are not stable and unchanging. As has been emphasized already, even though it is likely that body systems and functions will decline with age, such decline is not the same for everyone, and decline does not mean inevitable deterioration in participation.

Chapters 8 through 10 discuss examples of cognitive, musculoskeletal, and psychological disorders that can have major consequences for older adults. These are by no means the only interruptions encountered by older adults, but they demonstrate some of the special factors of performance interruption in older individuals.

Other common conditions such as cerebrovascular accident (CVA or stroke), cardiovascular diseases, arthritis, cancer, and, increasingly, diabetes, can similarly affect functional ability. While rates of CVA and heart disease are decreasing, diabetes incidence is increasing rapidly (Federal Interagency Forum on Aging Related Statistics [FIFARS], 2004). Thus, practitioners of the future may anticipate dealing with more individuals with diabetes-related vision loss and amputations than are currently encountered, while dealing with fewer clients with stroke. It will be interesting to see how these data change as the Baby Boom generation ages. Early reports suggest that they are entering old age healthier and more functional than those who preceded them (Velkoff, He, Sengupta, & DeBarros, 2006), although it may also be that there is a bimodal distribution based on education, socioeconomic status, and access to health care.

Federal Interagency Forum on Aging-Related Statistics (FIFARS). (2004). *Older Americans 2004: Key indicators of well-being.* Washington, DC: U.S. Government Printing Office.

Velkoff, V. A., He, W., Sengupta, M., & DeBarros, K. A. (2006). *65+ in the United States: 2005.* Washington, DC: U.S. Census Bureau.

Impact of Normal Aging

CHAPTER 4

Cardiovascular and Pulmonary Function

Elizabeth Dean, PhD, PT, • Armele Dornelas De Andrade, PhD, PT

T he weakest and oldest among us can become some kind of athlete, but only the strongest can survive as spectators, only the hardiest can withstand the perils of inertia, inactivity, and immobility.

J. H. Bland and S. M. Cooper,
Musculoskeletal system. In Leon Sokolof (Ed.),
The Musculoskeletal System. Baltimore: Williams & Wilkins, 1975.

OBJECTIVES

By the end of this chapter, the reader will be able to:

1. Understand health and the interrelationships among limitation of structure and function, activity, and social participation (World Health Organization International Classification of Functioning, Disability, and Health), and explain why these components are not consistently related.
2. Describe the age-related changes that are expected in cardiopulmonary and cardiovascular function.
3. Describe the impact of disease on any changes in cardiopulmonary and cardiovascular function secondary to primary or secondary disease.
4. Describe the impact of inactivity on any changes in cardiopulmonary and cardiovascular function secondary to recumbency and inactivity.

continued on page 66

5. Describe changes in cardiopulmonary and cardiovascular function secondary to extrinsic factors, such as to medical interventions and medications.
6. Describe changes in cardiopulmonary and cardiovascular function secondary to intrinsic factors, such as the individual's characteristics, culture and lifestyle, nutritional status, regular physical activity, long-term occupation, and coexistent morbidity.
7. Based on the changes identified in objectives 3 through 6, prioritize the goals of treatment and provide the rationale.
8. Based on the changes identified in objectives 3 through 6, outline the focus of the assessment and the measures that would be most relevant to record.
9. Based on the changes identified in objectives 3 through 6, outline the treatment plan vis-à-vis prescribing training for functional performance—that is, activities of daily living (ADLs), functional capacity, or both.
10. Describe the precautions that are necessary when assessing and prescribing ADLs, or exercise, or both.
11. Given that a maximum exercise test is not feasible, (a) outline the rationale for the short-term and long-term responses expected for the treatment plan, and (b) describe adverse responses the individual could exhibit in response to the treatment plan.

Human beings are designed to be bipedal, upright, and moving in a gravitational field, but they tend to spend less time upright and moving against gravity as they progress over the life cycle. This factor, combined with physiologic decline, contributes to overall losses in functional performance, ability to accomplish activities of daily living (ADLs), and functional capacity (i.e., aerobic capacity). As a result, an older person is more susceptible to debility and illness; even minor infections and afflictions can be a threat to life in an older recumbent, inactive person.

The primary goal of rehabilitation for older persons is to maximize function. The capacities of the cardiopulmonary and cardiovascular systems are significant determinants of an individual's functional abilities. Two components of function need to be addressed during rehabilitation. The first is to maximize the person's physiologic capacity to adapt to the upright position and move against gravity, which are central components of functional performance. Second, an older person's cardiopulmonary and cardiovascular reserve capacity must be maximized to exceed his or her critical functional performance threshold.

A person's ability to perform functional activities is primarily dependent on the integrity of the cardiopulmonary and cardiovascular systems and their combined ability to effect oxygen transport and tissue oxygenation. Functional performance reflects the integrated action of multiple systems. (See Chapters 5, 6, and 7.)

Over the life cycle, the changes in the cardiopulmonary and cardiovascular systems have important functional consequences (Tables 4-1 and 4-2). These effects are compounded by several other factors in older populations including the effects of cardiopulmonary and cardiovascular disease, the effects of **recumbency** and restricted mobility, extrinsic factors related to medical care the person may be receiving, and intrinsic factors related to his or her unique characteristics, lifestyle, physical activity level, nutritional status, and coexistent morbidity. Psychosocial factors are also important. (See Chapters 9, 10, 12, 13, 15, and 23.) An essential clinical consideration in contemporary rehabilitation is the translation of improvement of impairment to the improvement of capacity for physical activity and functional performance and, in turn, improvement in quality of life. The translation of these changes needs to be addressed clinically and not assumed.

The purposes of this chapter are to

• Understand the construct of health as it relates to older individuals.

TABLE 4-1 Age-Related Changes in the Cardiopulmonary System and Its Function

Morphological and Structural Changes	Functional Significance
THORAX	
Calcification of bronchial and costal cartilage ↑ Stiffness of costovertebral joints ↑ Anteroposterior diameter ↑ Wasting of respiratory muscles	↑ Resistance to deformation of chest wall ↑ Effective use of accessory respiratory muscles ↓ Tidal volume ↑ Exercise-induced hyperpnea ↓ Maximal voluntary ventilation ↓ Force of cough ↑ Risk of aspiration or choking
LUNG	
↑ Size of alveolar ducts ↓ Supporting duct framework ↑ Size of alveoli ↑ Mucous glands ↑ Alveolar compliance	↓ Surface area for gas exchange ↑ Physiologic dead space ↓ Elastic recoil ↓ Vital capacity ↓ Inspiratory reserve volume ↑ Expiratory reserve volume ↑ Functional residual volume and residual volume ↓ Ventilatory flow rates ↓ Distribution of ventilation ↑ Closure of dependent airways ↑ Arterial desaturation ↑ Resistance to airflow in small airways ↓ Pulmonary capillary network ↓ Distribution of perfusion ↑ Impaired diffusion capacity ↑ Fibrosis of pulmonary capillary intima ↓ Ventilation to perfusion matching

Data from Bates (1989) and West (2005).

- Examine the interrelationships among structure and function, activity, and social participation in relation to the International Classification of Functioning, Disability, and Health (ICF) (WHO, 2002).
- Describe age-related changes in the cardiopulmonary and cardiovascular systems and their function.
- Characterize other age-related factors that affect cardiopulmonary and cardiovascular function in the older adult.
- Analyze the functional consequences of age-related changes in the cardiopulmonary and cardiovascular systems.
- Describe the implications of age-related changes for care of older persons with respect to maintaining or improving functional performance.

- Examine means of optimizing an older person's ability to perform functional activities.

Health

Health is not merely the absence of disease. Based on the definition of the World Health Organization (WHO), health is psychosocial and physical well-being (WHO, 2006). Health is maximized with good nutrition, optimal body weight, regular physical activity and exercise, the absence of smoking and inhalation of other pollutants, stress reduction, and optimal rest (see review Dean, 2006a). Commonly today, rehabilitation professionals see people with considerable comorbidity. To design and plan appropriate programs, their risk factors and

TABLE 4-2 Age-Related Changes in the Cardiovascular System and Its Function

Morphological and Structural Changes	Functional Significance
HEART	
↑ Fat constituents	↓ Excitability
↑ Fibrous constituents	↓ Cardiac output
↑ Mass and volume	↓ Venous return
↑ Lipofuscin (by-product of glycogen metabolism)	↑ Cardiac dysrhythmias
↑ Amyloid content	
↓ Specialized nerve conduction tissue	
↓ Intrinsic and extrinsic innervation	
↑ Connective tissue and elastin	
↑ Calcification	
BLOOD VESSELS	
↑ Loss of normal proportion of smooth muscle to connective tissue and elastin constituents	↓ Blood flow to oxygenate tissues
↑ Rigidity of large arteries	↓ Blood flow and risk of clots in venous circulation
↑ Atheroma arterial circulation	↓ Cardiac output
↑ Calcification	↓ Venous return
↑ Dilation and tortuosity of veins	

Data from Campbell, Caird, and Jackson (1974); Higginbotham, Morris, Williams, Coleman, and Cobb (1986); Kantrowitz et al. (1986).

comorbidity need to be assessed. Such an assessment provides the optimal baseline for developing programs and establishing long-term goals. Rehabilitation professionals today need to understand basic health behaviors related to nutrition and physical activity, as these provide the backdrop for the functional consequences of other conditions for which the individual may be seeing the rehabilitation professional. Basic nutritional recommendations are included given that the rehabilitation profession typically makes physical demands of patients. To meet these demands and benefit from their cumulative effect, nutrition and body weight both need to be optimal. Generally, the food pyramid (Figure 4-1) (United States Department of Agriculture, 2006a) provides physiologically defensible nutritional guidelines, and if followed appropriately across the life cycle such that caloric intake meets metabolic demand, body weight should be normalized. A pedometer can be useful in objectifying an individual's general activity level. Ten thousand steps a day is consistent with a generally active lifestyle (Tudor-Locke & Bassett, 2004). The components

of different levels of exercise on a daily or weekly basis are illustrated in the physical activity pyramid (Figure 4-2) (United States Department of Agriculture, 2006b), which like the food pyramid provides a good teaching tool. Both of these can be discussed at the same time. Regular low–moderate aerobic-type exercise in the form of walking is needed daily, and this can be augmented with strength training a couple of times a week. Aerobic training at 70% to 85% of one's age-predicted maximal heart rate (i.e., 220 – age [years]) is a guide for generally healthy people. This intensity, however, needs to be modified based on an individual's specific functional capacity test (see the Assessing Functional Capacity section of this chapter), if morbidity exists. Sedentary activities including television watching and prolonged periods working at a computer should constitute a small proportion of time for optimal health in older as well as younger people. Smoking is the major cause of preventable death in adults (Mokdad, Marks, Stroup, & Gerberding, 2004); thus, smokers need to be identified, and smoking cessation resources and programs need to be

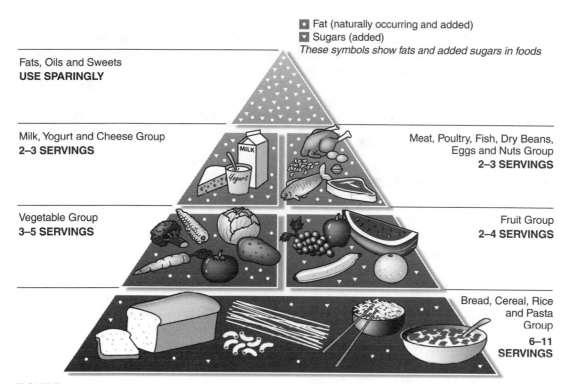

FIGURE 4-1 The nutrition food pyramid. (Source: United States Department of Agriculture (2006a).)

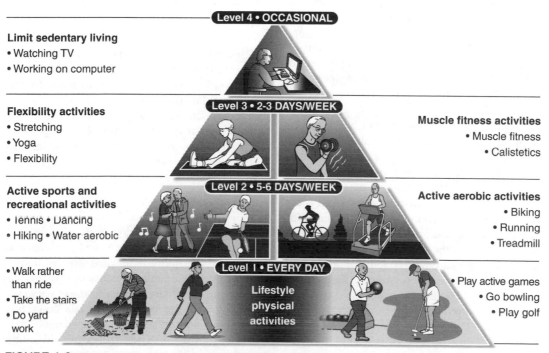

FIGURE 4-2 The physical activity and exercise pyramid. (Source: United States Department of Agriculture (2006b).)

made available. Smoking cessation needs to be a component of management in rehabilitation programs for older people to maximize functional and long-term health outcomes.

Interrelationships Among Structure and Function, Activity, and Social Participation with Reference to Cardiovascular and Cardiopulmonary Function

Based on the WHO's definition of health, the International Classification of Functioning, Disability, and Health (WHO, 2002) has become an important framework and basis for diagnosis in the rehabilitation professions and definition of outcomes of intervention. Each individual is viewed as a whole such that his or her social participation and quality of life are viewed distinctly, as well as interdependently with the capacity to perform activities and the integrity of anatomic structure and physiologic function. Specifically, activity includes ADLs and those activities associated with social participation and engagement in living. In turn, the framework includes the role of limitations in anatomical structure and physiology function on activity the individual can perform, and social participation.

Unlike the biomedical model in which remediation of limitations of structure and function are the primary focus of management, the ICF focuses on the components of an individual's life that are meaningful to him or her in addition to limitations of structure and function.

The ICF framework has particular relevance in health care today. First, this framework is consistent with a model of health care versus illness care. Second, it is consistent with contemporary health care priorities—namely, the diseases of civilization (i.e., ischemic heart disease, cancer, smoking-related conditions, hypertension and stroke, diabetes, and osteoporosis). The WHO has decreed that these conditions and their associated social and economic burdens are largely preventable (World Health Organization, 1999–2003). These conditions have achieved epidemic proportions. Further, people are developing comorbidities earlier in their lives than in the last century because of injurious lifestyles. Because the biomedical model can maintain people's lives when threatened, people today can

expect to experience long periods of morbidity, and particularly end-of-life morbidity. Prolonged morbidity is not associated with high rates of social participation or quality of life.

With the increased predominance of the diseases of civilization in high-income countries, and the increasing predominance in low- and middle-income countries, a reflection of their economic growth, and the chronicity of these diseases, there has been growing interest in quality of life issues. Two broad classifications of scales to assess quality of life have emerged: generic and condition specific. Generic scales include the Short-Form 36 and 12 (Stewart, Hays, & Ware, 1988) and the Sickness Impact Profile (SIP) (Gilson, Gilson, Bergner, Bobbit, Kressel, & Pollard, 1975). Condition-specific scales related to cardiopulmonary and cardiovascular conditions include the Outcome Institute Angina Type Specification (Rogers, Johnstone, Yusuf, Weiner, Galagher, & Bittner, 1994) and the Chronic Respiratory Disease Questionnaire (Guyatt, Berman, Townsend, Pugsley, & Chambers, 1987).

Age-Related Anatomic Changes in the Cardiopulmonary System and its Function

Aging has a direct effect on each component of the cardiopulmonary system including the airways, lung parenchyma and its interface with the circulation (the alveolar capillary membrane), chest wall, and respiratory muscles. Ventilation of the alveoli and oxygenation of venous blood depends on the anatomic and physiologic integrity of these components (Berne & Levy, 2000; West, 2005).

Airways

As in other systems, aging leads to a decrease in the amount of elastic tissue and an increase in fibrous tissue. Because the large airways are predominantly rigid connective tissue, few changes with aging are reported. Because the medium and small airways are composed of less connective tissue and more smooth muscle, a decrease in the elasticity of these structures occurs with aging, resulting in reduced structural integrity of the tissue and increased **compliance.**

Lung Parenchyma

The lung **parenchyma** is composed of spongy alveolar tissue that is designed to be ventilated and provide an interface with the pulmonary blood through the alveolar capillary membrane, which has a large surface area to promote the oxygenation of blood. Age-related increases in connective tissue and elastin disintegration reduce elastic recoil, the principal mechanism of normal expiration. The loss of normal recoil contributes to uneven distribution of ventilation, airway closure, air trapping, and impaired gas exchange. The net result of these changes is a decrease in alveolar surface area.

Alveolar Capillary Membrane

The alveolar capillary membrane is uniquely designed to optimize the diffusion of gases between the alveolar air and the pulmonary circulation. The **diffusing capacity**—that is, the ability of oxygen to diffuse from the alveolar airspaces into the pulmonary capillary— progressively declines with age and has been attributed to reduced alveolar surface area, alveolar volume, and pulmonary capillary bed.

Chest Wall

The chest wall is composed of the structures separating the thorax from the head and neck, the diaphragm separating the thorax from the abdomen, the rib cage, the intercostal muscles, and the spinal column. With age, the joints of the thorax become more rigid, and cartilage becomes calcified; hence, the chest wall becomes less compliant. The chest wall becomes barrel shaped, the anteroposterior diameter increases, and the normal three-dimensional motion of the chest wall during the respiratory cycle is diminished.

Respiratory Muscles

The diaphragm, the principal muscle of respiration, tends to flatten with age-related hyperinflation of the chest wall, reduced lung compliance, and air trapping in the lungs, and is possibly secondary to reduced muscle mass. Loss of respiratory muscle mass parallels the age-related reduction in skeletal muscle mass in general. Loss of abdominal muscle strength reduces the force of coughing, which can contribute to aspiration.

Net Effect of Age-Related Cardiopulmonary Changes

These anatomic changes give rise to predictable physiologic or functional changes in pulmonary function after the pulmonary system has matured (see Table 4-1). Respiratory mechanics that largely reflect the resistance to airflow and the compliance of the chest wall and lung parenchyma are altered. Specifically, both airflow resistance and lung compliance increase. With respect to pulmonary function, forced expiratory volumes and flows and inspiratory and expiratory pressures are reduced. **Functional residual capacity** and **residual volume** are increased. These effects are further accentuated in recumbent positions. Arterial oxygen tension and saturation are also reduced linearly with age. Thus, progressively over the life cycle, the lung becomes a less efficient gas exchanger.

Age-Related Changes in the Cardiovascular System and its Function

The cardiovascular system is composed of the heart and vasculature. Loss of efficiency of the cardiovascular system occurs with age.

Heart

Electrical Behavior

With aging, the heart's conduction system changes such that the frequency and regularity of cardiac impulses may become abnormal secondary to fibrotic changes in the specialized nerve conduction system of the heart and musculature. In cases in which the electrical activity of the heart cannot be stabilized or regulated with medications, artificial pacemakers are often implanted. Electrocardiographic irregularities, such as **premature ventricular contractions, atrial fibrillation,** and **heart blocks,** are common in persons older than 65 years of age.

Mechanical Behavior

The heart pumps less effectively with age as a result of changes in the mechanical properties of the cardiac muscle, which alter the length–tension and force–velocity relationships. Additionally, changes with age in both the integrity of the valves—the atrioventricular valves, the pulmonic valve, and the aortic valve—and variations in the aging pulmonary and systemic circulations can result in less-efficient pumping action of the heart (Higginbotham et al., 1986). Histologically, the heart tissue becomes fattier, and both heart mass and volume increase. **Amyloidosis,** a histologic feature of aging observed in many organs including the heart and vasculature, is characterized by the progressive deposition of amyloid protein. This waxy protein infiltrates tissue, rendering it dysfunctional.

In general, the walls of the heart become more compliant with age. The myocardial fibers no longer contract at optimal points on the length–tension or force–velocity curves, which reduces the efficiency of myocardial contraction.

Blood Vessels

Blood vessels require varying degrees of distensibility or compliance depending on their specific function. The forward motion of blood on the arterial side of the circulation is a function of the elastic recoil of the vessel walls and the progressive loss of pressure energy down the vascular tree. The decrease in elasticity of the arterial vessels with aging may result in chronic or residual increases in vessel diameter and vessel wall rigidity, which impair the function of the vessel. The reservoir function of the venous circulation is dependent on its being highly compliant to accommodate the greatest proportion of the blood volume at rest. Although the mechanical characteristics of venous smooth muscle have been less well studied compared with arterial smooth muscle, the efficiency of its contractile behavior can be expected to be reduced with aging. Furthermore, its electrical excitability and responsiveness to neurohumoral transmitters tend to be less rapid and less pronounced.

Blood
A discussion of the effects of aging on the cardiopulmonary and cardiovascular systems would not be complete without reference to the blood—both its volume and its constituents—and the ability of the heart and vasculature to move blood. The ability of the vasculature to move blood through the vascular system and shift volumes of blood between vascular beds depending on need is diminished with aging. Also, the rapidity with which these changes can be effected is correspondingly reduced. The ability to effect these vascular adjustments in response to gravity and exercise are tantamount to effective physical functioning.

Net Effects of Age-Related Cardiovascular Changes

The age-related anatomical and physiological changes of the heart and blood vessels result in reduced capacity for oxygen transport at rest and, in particular, in response to situations imposing an increase in metabolic demand for oxygen (see Table 4-2) (Davies, 1972). Therefore, activities associated with a relatively low metabolic demand are perceived by older persons as physically demanding. Certain activities may no longer be able to be performed, whereas others may require rest periods in between. Fifty percent of older persons have been reported to have electrical conduction abnormalities at rest, which has considerable implications for the mechanical behavior of the heart and the regulation of cardiac output, particularly when stressed during activity and exercise (Campbell, Caird, & Jackson, 1974). A high proportion of conduction irregularities occur in the absence of clinical heart disease (Davies & Pomerance, 1972).

Other Factors that Affect Cardiopulmonary and Cardiovascular Function

Numerous factors contribute to impaired oxygen transport in older persons; these factors are summarized in Box 4-1. Establishing the relative contribution of these factors is central to defining treatment goals and treatment parameters (see Implications for the Management of Care of Older Persons later in this chapter).

Pathophysiology

Cardiopulmonary disease is prevalent in older age groups. Chronic airflow limitation is most frequently manifested as chronic bronchitis and

---

BOX 4-1   Factors Contributing to Cardiopulmonary and Cardiovascular Dysfunction and Impaired Oxygen Transport in Older People

I. AGE-RELATED CHANGES
  Cardiopulmonary system
  Cardiovascular system
  Hematologic factors
II. CARDIOPULMONARY AND
    CARDIOVASCULAR DISEASE
  Acute
  Chronic
  Acute and chronic
III. RESTRICTED MOBILITY AND
    RECUMBENCY
  Removal of gravitational stress
  Removal of exercise stress
IV. EXTRINSIC FACTORS (I.E., THOSE
    IMPOSED BY MEDICAL OR SURGICAL
    CARE)
  Hospitalization
  Fever
  Malaise
  Reduced arousal
  Surgery (e.g., type, positioning, type and depth
    of sedatives and anesthesia, incisions, duration,
    blood and fluid administration, use of bypass
    machine, intraoperative complications)
  Dressings and bindings
  Casts or splinting devices, traction
  Incisions
  Invasive lines, catheter, or chest tubes
  Monitoring equipment (invasive and noninvasive)
  Medications
  Portable equipment (e.g., IVs, O_2 tanks)
  Intubation

  Mechanical ventilation
  Suctioning
  Pain
  Multisystem complications
V. INTRINSIC FACTORS (I.E., THOSE
    IMPOSED BY THE INDIVIDUAL'S
    CHARACTERISTICS, LIFESTYLE, AND
    MEDICAL AND SURGICAL HISTORIES)
  Gender
  Ethnicity
  Sociocultural background
  Smoking history
  Occupation
  Environment (e.g., humidity, temperature,
    oxygen concentration, and air quality)
  Quantity and quality of sleep
  Obesity
  Nutritional deficits
  Stress, anxiety, and depression
  Deformity
  Congenital abnormalities
  Walking aids and devices
  Habitual activity and conditioning level
  Reaction to medications
  Adherence to medication schedules
  Adherence to recommendations from health
    care professionals
  Immunity
  Fluid and electrolyte balance
  Anemia or polycythemia
  Thyroid and other endocrine abnormalities
  Previous medical and surgical histories

Data from Dean & Ross (1992a); Dean & Ross (1992b)

---

emphysema. Asthma, characterized by hyperexcitability of bronchial smooth muscle, may occur on its own or as a component of chronic airflow limitation. Although less common, restrictive lung disease is also prevalent in older age groups and results from prolonged exposure to a variety of pulmonary irritants often over the course of one's life through occupational or environmental exposure (Table 4-3) (Chung & Dean, 1989). Depending on the severity of the disease, individuals may report shortness of breath on exertion or at rest. In chronic airflow limitation, the person presents with a barrel chest. Loss of the elastic recoil of the lungs results in hyperinflation of the chest wall,

flattening of the hemi-diaphragms, and air trapping. Although total lung capacity is unchanged, these changes impair the efficiency of respiratory mechanics, resulting in inefficient ventilation, impaired gas mixing, and impaired ventilation and perfusion matching (Dean, 2006b). These individuals tend to adopt a breathing pattern characterized by prolonged expiration to help promote gas exchange in the lungs. The metabolic cost of breathing is also increased. Individuals with restrictive lung disease tend to have fibrotic, stiff lungs that have reduced compliance and thus are more difficult to expand and ventilate with normal ventilatory efforts. The work of breathing needed to inflate

TABLE 4-3 **Pulmonary Diseases and Cardiovascular Abnormalities**

Type	Presenting Symptoms and Signs	Anatomical and Physiological Changes	Impairments
Chronic airflow limitation	Barrel chest May have shortness of breath on exertion or rest Breathing pattern: prolonged expiration	Hyperinflation of chest wall Flattening of hemi-diaphragms Air trapping Increased metabolic costs of breathing	Inefficient ventilation Impaired gas mixing Impaired ventilation
Restrictive lung disease	Breathing pattern: rapid, shallow	Fibrotic stiff lungs	Reduced compliance Increased effort to inflate lungs
Atherosclerosis	High blood pressure Ischemic chest pain Myocardial infarction	Fatty atheromatous plaques within blood vessel walls Vessel wall rigidity	Stenosed arteries Increased peripheral resistance
Diabetes	Hypoglycemia with activity or exercise	Similar to atherosclerosis	Similar to atherosclerosis

the lungs and counter the greater proportion of **dead space,** particularly during exercise, is disproportionate. To reduce the work of breathing, individuals with restrictive disease adopt rapid shallow breathing patterns. Both types of lung pathology, airflow limitation and restriction, can lead to impaired oxygen tension in the blood during exercise and in severe cases even at rest. The additional metabolic cost of breathing in individuals with moderate to severe disease of either type contributes significantly to the overall metabolic cost of a given activity or exercise. These individuals are in danger of significantly desaturating their blood during increased workloads; thus, monitoring vital signs, arterial saturation, and subjective response during prescribed activities or exercise is essential. Cardiovascular abnormalities are common in older age groups. Atherosclerosis, blood pressure abnormalities, and the vascular components from diabetes are common in the older adult. Atherosclerosis is a degenerative disease of the arterial vasculature, especially the large arteries. Atherosclerosis affecting the coronary arteries is termed coronary artery disease and is the major cause of morbidity and mortality in older persons in the Western industrialized countries. Hypertension is the blood pressure abnormality that occurs most frequently in the older adult (Khan et al., 2006). Because hypertension is not generally associated with unpleasant symptoms, the individual may be unaware of the condition and may not

seek medical attention or be inclined to take medication regularly. The consequences of high blood pressure, stroke and heart disease, are dire, and its control significantly reduces complications, cardiovascular death, congestive heart failure, and stroke (Khan et al., 2006). Alternatively, some older people are prone to hypotension, particularly during positional changes. A diminished responsiveness of autonomic adjustments may be responsible. Another common disease in the older adult that has serious vascular consequences is diabetes, usually of the adult-onset type. Hypermetabolism associated with activity and exercise places increased demand on energy stores and insulin requirements. Another vascular consequence of diabetes is that the rate of atherosclerosis is accelerated by a decade compared with the non-diabetic older population, and these individuals are at additional risk during activity and exercise.

Gravitational Stress and Exercise Stress

Oxygen transport and tissue oxygenation are dependent on the body's ability to provide an adequate cardiac output to the peripheral tissues commensurate with tissue demand. Physical factors that normally challenge the body's ability to maintain or increase cardiac output include position change, activity or exercise, and emotional stress. The older adult may be limited in ability to adjust to the gravitational and exercise stress caused by normal activities if a greater proportion of time has been spent recumbent or if activity has been limited. Reduction in gravitational stress and exercise stress contributes to physiological deterioration and susceptibility to illness.

Physiological Responses to Gravitational Stress

Orthostatism refers to the ability of the body to maintain normal cardiac output, in particular, cerebral perfusion, during assumption of the upright body position. On moving from the recumbent to the upright position, blood volume is displaced toward the abdominal cavity and the legs (Blomqvist & Stone, 1983). This blood volume displacement reduces venous return and, hence, cardiac output, resulting in a compensatory increase in heart rate and peripheral vascular resistance to increased blood pressure and cardiac output. If this neurological compensation is ineffective, cerebral perfusion is compromised, and a blackout or fainting may ensue.

During recumbency, this sequence of events is reversed. The blood volume is displaced centrally toward the heart and lungs. Venous return is increased, resulting in a compensatory decrease in heart rate and peripheral vascular resistance to maintain cardiac output. The increased central blood volume leads to a compensatory **diuresis** within hours of assuming the recumbent position. Thus, overall blood volume is reduced, and the person is prone to orthostatic intolerance on assuming the upright position (Sandler, 1986). The loss of fluid-volume–regulating mechanisms, rather than cardiovascular deconditioning, has been reported to be the primary factor responsible for bedrest deconditioning (Convertino, 1992; Winslow, 1985). The only means of preventing **orthostatic intolerance** following recumbency is to assume the upright position frequently. This adaptation is further augmented if it is coupled with movement; however, exercise in the absence of being upright fails to counter orthostatic intolerance (Chase, Grave, & Rowell, 1966). In addition to the primary beneficial adaptive responses that being upright and moving have on oxygen transport, virtually every other organ system benefits when an individual is upright and moving (Dean & Ross, 1992a).

Physiological Responses to Exercise Stress

Exercise increases the metabolic demand for oxygen and substrates. With aging, the oxygen transport system is less capable of responding to exercise stress as a consequence of the diminished efficiency of the various steps in the oxygen transport pathway including oxidative metabolism at the cellular level (Astrand & Rodahl, 1986; Lesnefsky & Hoppel, 2006). Despite the reported age-related changes, the considerable reserve capacity of the cardiopulmonary and cardiovascular systems tends to offset the potential functional consequences. The degree of this compensation, however, is highly variable among individual older persons. Although this variability reflects genetic factors to a considerable extent, fitness and lifestyle factors also have a significant role. That cardiopulmonary and cardiovascular reserve capacity is maximized with exercise irrespective of age has been known for several decades. Further, age is not a limiter for the capacity to exhibit as exercise response (Shephard, 1986).

Extrinsic Factors

Extrinsic factors that can affect cardiopulmonary and cardiovascular function in older persons include iatrogenic factors—that is, secondary effects from the medical care that an individual may be receiving (Dean & Ross, 1992b). In the context of function in the older medically stable adult, the effects of medication and routine medical procedures are likely to be the most important extrinsic factors. It is not uncommon for older persons to be taking one or more medications. Although a medication may have a specific and beneficial effect, it may have an untoward effect elsewhere. For example, beta blockers are highly effective in improving the mechanical efficiency of the heart; however, these drugs blunt the normal hemodynamic responses to exercise, and some patients report experiencing undue fatigue when taking these medications. Routine medical procedures adversely affect cardiopulmonary and cardiovascular function secondary to confinement to a body position (typically recumbent) for a prolonged period, restricted mobility, insertion of invasive lines and leads, and associated medications and hospitalization. The morbidity and mortality associated with these routine procedures are accentuated in older persons.

Intrinsic Factors

Intrinsic factors that affect cardiopulmonary and cardiovascular function are those that are imposed by the general history, background, and characteristics of the individual (Dean & Perme, 2007). For example, the effects of non-primary cardiopulmonary and cardiovascular disease—that is, manifestations of diseases of the renal, hepatic, neurological, endocrine, gastrointestinal, immune, hematological, and musculoskeletal systems—can have significant consequences on cardiopulmonary and cardiovascular function (Dean, 1997). In addition, connective tissue disorders can have significant cardiopulmonary and cardiovascular manifestations. Although the secondary manifestations of diseases of these systems can be more obscure than manifestations of primary disease of the heart and lungs, their diagnosis is more difficult and their prognosis tends to be poorer.

Like other dynamic functions of the human body, the function of the heart and lungs is dependent on adequate nutrition and hydration. The appropriate energy sources must be available to the metabolically active tissues. Older persons may be uninformed or negligent about their nutritional and fluid needs or incapable of meeting these needs either physically or economically. On the other extreme is the problem of obesity, which has been described as being a problem of epidemic proportions in North America. With reduced muscle mass and reduced cardiopulmonary and cardiovascular reserves associated with aging, being overweight constitutes a significant additional load that can further impair heart and lung function and musculoskeletal function, and hence threaten functional independence. In Western countries, there is a tendency to gain weight with advancing years; however, this trend reverses in the very old age groups.

Reduced cardiopulmonary and cardiovascular function can result from factors other than dysfunction of the primary organ systems that are directly responsible for effecting functional activity. For example, sleep deprivation, nutritional deficits, or impaired cognition have obvious ramifications on function and independence. Some older persons may experience stress, anxiety, and depression, which contribute to low energy, fatigue, withdrawal, and social isolation (Fry, 1986). Impaired cognitive ability or dementia may significantly restrict an older person's activity level because of the need for supervision (American Psychiatric Association, 1994). Cultural background can also be an important determinant of health and well-being, illness, and disability. Beliefs about health practices and lifestyle can influence well-being (Purnell & Paulanka, 2003a). Eastern cultures compared with Western cultures, for example, are characterized as being collectivistic versus individualistic, high versus low on the power distance scale, high versus low on the uncertainty avoidance scale, and tightly versus loosely structured (Purnell & Paulanka, 2003b). In addition to having an influence on health and well-being, and on illness and disability, these four primary dimensions of culture affect people's response to health care interventions, particularly those requiring adherence and active participation. Occupational therapy and physical therapy in the United States and Canada, for example, focus on an individual's independence and self-reliance which are highly valued in Western cultures. However, in Eastern cultures, the group versus the individual is valued, and interdependence and relationships with others are more highly valued. Western practitioners may have less-effective therapeutic outcomes with people from Eastern cultures without an awareness of that culture and creative modifications in the interventions prescribed (Suh, 2004).

Other intrinsic factors that affect cardiopulmonary and cardiovascular function include current and long-term lifestyle practices such as level of physical activity and exercise, nutritional status, smoking history, and effectiveness of stress management strategies. Regular exercise, in which the heart rate reflecting exercise intensity is within the training-sensitive heart rate zone, is essential for aerobic conditioning. Such conditioning ensures aerobic reserve capacity, which provides a cardiopulmonary protective effect if the person becomes ill or requires routine medical and surgical procedures. Also, years of active and passive smoking are well-known risk factors for chronic airflow limitation and cancer. Poor coping strategies contribute to excessive levels of circulating **catecholamines,** cardiac irregularities,

coronary vasospasm, and hypertension. Occupational environments over the long term can
have significant long-term consequences (e.g.,
the occurrence of interstitial lung disease in
workers exposed to toxic environmental agents
and in farmers).

Functional Consequences of Age-Related Cardiopulmonary and Cardiovascular Changes

Function can be categorized as ADLs, exercise,
or general activity. The focus of this chapter is
on ADLs and exercise. ADLs include self-care
activities, sexual activity, home and family
management, and work and leisure. Exercise is
fundamental to those activities that require some
degree of endurance, demanding the maintenance of increased oxygen transport and tissue
oxygenation. Although other types of activity,
such as card playing, require a greater metabolic
demand than is required when one is at rest, the
increased metabolic demand is not usually
sustained. In addition, this chapter distinguishes
between functional performance and functional
capacity. Functional performance pertains to
task completion that imposes stress on the
oxygen transport system above that imposed by
resting metabolic demand. Functional capacity
refers to the capacity of the cardiovascular
system to transport oxygen.

Different types of exercise tests are used to
assess functional performance and functional
capacity. In both cases, appropriate standards,
procedures, and monitoring are essential to
ensure the tests are valid and reliable and are
performed with maximal safety. Tests of ADL
assess functional performance, whereas conventional exercise tests are designed to measure
functional capacity. The results of both types of
tests yield important but different types of information about an individual's level of functioning.

The Functional Performance Threshold

The ability to perform ADLs to meet the
minimum criterion compatible with personal
care and independent living can be thought of as
a functional performance threshold (Young,
1986). Young people have considerable physiological capacity and reserve that enable them to
perform activities and exercise well in excess of
the metabolic and physical demands required by
routine daily activities. With aging, however,
changes to the various organ systems, particularly the lungs, heart, nervous system, endocrine
system, and musculature, reduce physiological
capacity and reserve. If physical decline results
in a functional capacity below the functional
performance threshold, that individual will be
unable to meet the minimum criterion for
self-care and independent living. Falling below
this threshold can be a result of progressive
age-related changes, or restricted mobility or
illness sufficient to lower an individual's already
minimal reserves.

The rate of decline in functional capacity
with age and the decline in functional
performance are qualitatively different. Although
functional capacity deteriorates linearly with
advancing age, the decrease in functional
performance declines in a curvilinear manner.
Thus, an individual can lose significant capacity
yet retain considerable function over the years.

A rational objective of rehabilitation for
older persons is to maintain physiological
capacity and reserve well above the functional
performance threshold. The basis for this
objective is threefold. First, the individual will
be able to perform self-care and be functionally
independent. Second, this level of physical
performance will avoid the negative consequences of restricted mobility and is consistent
with health promotion. Third, should the
individual be exposed to a period of relative
inactivity or become ill, a greater initial
functional capacity provides a greater margin of
safety. Detraining effects will be minimized,
and faster recovery will be likely. Research is
needed to determine precisely the level of
functional performance that is needed in older
persons to minimize morbidity and mortality,
and the optimal parameters of an exercise
prescription that would best achieve this result.

Metabolic Demand of Activities of Daily Living and Exercise

The metabolic demand of an activity can be
defined by the unit called the **metabolic
equivalent** (MET). One MET is equal to 3.5 mL
O_2/kg of body weight per minute, the normal

basal metabolic demand for oxygen (American College of Sports Medicine, Whaley, Brubaker, Otto, & Armstrong, 2006; Blair, Painter, Pate, Smith, & Taylor, 1988). By convention, the metabolic demands of different activities are expressed as multiples of the basal metabolic rate (Table 4-4) (Fox, 1972). Theoretically, the metabolic demand for a given activity does not vary. Even though an individual is deconditioned or older and perceives an activity as more physiologically demanding, the metabolic demand of activities does not change (Shephard, 1985). The effect of skill level and biomechanical efficiency on metabolic cost of common activities is generally small. Research is needed, however, to examine the effect of aging on metabolic cost of activity. The effect of changes in stature over the life cycle, altered center of gravity on the metabolic cost of physical activities, and gender differences need to be studied.

The metabolic costs of sexual activity and the capacity to work have been relatively neglected in the literature, particularly with respect to older persons. The American Heart Association (American Heart Association, Committee on Exercise, 1975) recommends that sexual activity can be tolerated if the individual can maintain steady-state exercise of 6 to 8 cal/ min on the treadmill or 600 kp/m on the cycle ergometer. If aerobically conditioned, an older person can perform physical activity such as sexual intercourse with reduced heart rate, blood pressure, and overall exertion (Stein, 1977). To minimize further the metabolic demand and exercise stress, sexual encounters can be timed with medications and with energy peaks during the day. Body positions during intercourse can be modified; upright positions will likely be better tolerated than recumbency.

Increased longevity and non-mandatory retirement has raised interest in vocational assessment for older persons. The ability to perform a certain type of work can be predicted on the basis of an exercise test. If a given occupation exceeds 40% of an individual's peak oxygen consumption in an exercise test, the American Thoracic Society has advocated that the individual would not be able to tolerate working at that occupation for prolonged periods (American Thoracic Society, 1986). Research is needed to refine and extend guidelines for older persons who are considering changing occupations or reentering the labor force.

Progressive changes in the cardiopulmonary and cardiovascular systems, in conjunction with changes in the capacity for oxygen and substrate utilization in the musculature, result in less-efficient oxygen transport in the older adult. With activity and exercise, the increased metabolic demand for oxygen and substrate requires a commensurate increase in ventilation and cardiac output. Both maximal ventilation and cardiac output decline linearly with age, and maximal oxygen consumption is correspondingly reduced. The extraction of oxygen at the tissue level, however, which is measured by the arteriovenous oxygen difference, does not change significantly with age.

The degree of endurance needed to perform ADLs varies depending on the task. Those ADLs that are primarily skill based, such as dressing, toileting, grooming, shaving, bathing, and feeding, are associated with low metabolic demand and generally require little endurance. Restriction of skill-based ADLs in older persons tends to reflect musculoskeletal or neuromuscular deficits rather than difficulties with oxygen transport or gas exchange. However, other ADLs, including ambulation, climbing stairs and hills, yard work, housework, shopping, gardening, sexual activity, volunteer work, gainful employment, managing transportation, and social activities outside the home are associated with higher metabolic demand, require greater endurance, and tend to reflect the status of the cardiopulmonary and cardiovascular systems.

Whether an active lifestyle contributes to or results from cardiopulmonary and cardiovascular conditioning warrants discussion. The question can best be addressed by examining the elements of aerobic conditioning. To elicit an aerobic training response, the stimulus must be of sufficient intensity, frequency, and duration and be carried out over a sufficiently long period of time. The critical parameters of the prescription needed to effect an aerobic training response are the performance of aerobic exercise for 20 to 30 minutes, at 60% to 70% of the maximum oxygen consumption that is associated with a heart rate between 70% and 80% of the maximum heart rate, for a minimum of 3 days a week for 3 to 6 months (American College of Sports Medicine, 2006). The physiological adaptations that result reflect an increased

TABLE 4-4 **Metabolic Demands of Activity and Exercise**

Intensity, 70-kg person	Endurance Promoting	Occupational	Recreational
1½–2 MET 4–7 mL/kg/min 2–2½ kcal/min	Too low in energy level	Desk work, driving auto, electric calculating, machine operation, light housework, polishing furniture, washing clothes	Standing, strolling (1 mi/h), flying, motorcycling, playing cards, sewing, knitting
2–3 MET 7–11 mL/kg/min 2½–4 kcal/min	Too low in energy level unless capacity is very low	Auto repair, radio and television repair, janitorial work, bartending, riding lawn mower, light woodworking	Level walking (2 mi/h), level bicycling (5 mi/h), billiards, bowling, skeet shooting, shuffleboard, powerboat driving, golfing with power cart, canoeing, horseback riding at a walk
3–4 MET 11–14 mL/kg/min 4–5 kcal/min	Yes, if continuous and if target heart rate is reached	Bricklaying, plastering, wheelbarrow (100-lb load), machine assembly, welding (moderate load), cleaning windows, mopping floors, vacuuming, pushing light power mower	Walking (3 mi/h), bicycling (6 mi/h), horseshoe pitching, volleyball (6-person, noncompetitive), golfing (pulling bag cart), archery, sailing (handling small boat), fly fishing (standing in waders), horseback riding (trotting), badminton (social doubles)
4–5 MET 14–18 mL/kg/min	Recreational activities promote endurance; occupational activities must be continuous, lasting longer than 2 min	Painting, masonry, paperhanging, light carpentry, scrubbing floors, raking leaves, hoeing	Walking (3½ mi/h), bicycling (8 mi/h), table tennis, golfing (carrying clubs), dancing (foxtrot), badminton (singles), tennis (doubles), many calisthenics, ballet
5–6 MET 18–21 mL/kg/min	Yes	Digging garden, shoveling light earth	Walking (4 mi/h), bicycling (10 mi/h), canoeing (4 mi/h), horseback riding (posting to trotting), stream fishing (walking in light current in waders), ice or roller skating (9 mi/h)
6–7 MET 21–25 mL/kg/min 7–8 kcal/min	Yes	Shoveling 10 times/min (4½ kg or 10 lb), splitting wood, snow shoveling, hand lawn mowing	Walking (5 mi/h), bicycling (11 mi/h), competitive badminton, tennis (singles), folk and square dancing, light downhill skiing, ski touring (2½ mi/h), water skiing, swimming (20 yard/min)

continued on page 80

TABLE 4-4 **Metabolic Demands of Activity and Exercise** (continued)

Intensity, 70-kg person	Endurance Promoting	Occupational	Recreational
7–8 MET 25–28 mL/kg/min 8–10 kcal/min	Yes	Digging ditches, carrying 36 kg or 80 lb, sawing hardwood	Jogging (5 mi/h), bicycling (12 mi/h), horseback riding (gallop), vigorous downhill skiing, basketball, mountain climbing, ice hockey, canoeing (5 mi/h), touch football, paddleball
8–9 MET 28–32 mL/kg/min 10–11 kcal/min	Yes	Shoveling 10 times/min ($5\frac{1}{2}$ kg or 14 lb)	Running ($5\frac{1}{2}$ mi/h), bicycling (13 mi/h), ski touring (4 mi/h), squash (social), handball (social), fencing, basketball (vigorous), swimming (30 yard/min), rope skipping
10+MET 32+mL/kg/min 11+kcal/min	Yes	Shoveling 10 times/min ($7\frac{1}{2}$ kg or 16 lb)	Running (6 mi/h = 10 MET, 7 mi/h = $11\frac{1}{2}$ MET, 8 mi/h = $13\frac{1}{2}$ MET, 9 mi/h = 15 MET, 10 mi/h = 17 MET), ski touring (5+ mi/h), handball (competitive), squash (competitive), swimming (greater than 40 yard/min)

Source: From Fox (1972), with permission

ability to transport oxygen and to use oxygen and metabolic substrates at the tissue level.

Depending on an individual's age, most ADLs and habitual activity are not performed at a sufficient intensity, duration, or frequency or over a sufficient time period to effect long-term aerobic adaptations. However, habitual activity does maintain sufficient physiological adaptation to perform tasks associated with low metabolic demand. Given that maximal heart rate and aerobic capacity diminish with age, even skill-based ADLs can become aerobically demanding. Routine walks down hospital corridors, for example, can be associated with an intensity of exercise that exceeds acceptable limits in some older individuals using walkers (Baruch & Mossberg, 1983). This scenario is one in which individuals are frequently not monitored. Thus, routine tasks and activities not considered to be metabolically demanding must be analyzed at two levels: their relative physiological demand on a given individual and the individual's capacity to meet that metabolic demand such that the adaptation that is elicited is both therapeutic and safe.

Assessing Functional Performance

The objective of the assessment of functional performance is to determine the individual's ability to perform ADLs. Functional performance reflects the capacity of the individual to perform work. Nutritional status and body weight are important components of the assessment of a person's capacity to perform work. The nutrition pyramid (see Figure 4-1) illustrates some fundamental principles of nutrition that need to be assessed and discussed as a basis for maximizing an individual's capacity for work, much in the same way as for athletes. When nutritional status is optimal, an individual will be better able to engage in regular physical activity and structured exercise programs (see Figure 4-2).

Numerous performance tests have been described previously in the literature (Carey & Posavic, 1988; Katz, Ford, Moskowitz, Jackson, & Jaffe, 1963; Kruiansky & Gurland, 1976; Linn & Linn, 1982; MacKenzie, Charlson, DiGioia, & Kelley, 1986; Mahoney & Barthel, 1965). Such tests must be performed according to standardized criteria to ensure their validity and reliability. A major liability of these tests, however, is that patient monitoring is seldom considered an integral component of the test. Although they are not associated with large metabolic demands, ADLs are often experienced as physically demanding by older persons. With cardiopulmonary dysfunction superimposed, monitoring an older person's responses to normal ADLs and exercise is critical to assessment (see Chapter 17). Without appropriate monitoring, the rehabilitation specialist may underestimate the physiological demand placed on the patient.

Although it is fundamental to normal function, movement constitutes a physiological stressor and, thus, is inherently risky, particularly in older persons. Adverse effects may include abnormal heart rate, blood pressure, and breathing frequency; cardiac dysrhythmias; altered intra-abdominal and thoracic pressures; and reduced venous return, stroke volume, and cardiac output. In turn, the work of breathing and of the heart may be excessive, which adds further to the overall metabolic cost of the activity.

Assessing the person's ability to perform an ADL should be viewed as a unique form of exercise test. Although motor control and performance may be the focus of ADL reeducation, important cardiovascular and pulmonary responses should be monitored at least initially. Baseline measures including heart rate and rhythm, breathing frequency, systolic and diastolic blood pressure, rate pressure product (the product of heart rate and systolic blood pressure, which is highly correlated with myocardial oxygen consumption and the work of the heart), and perceived exertion provide valuable information about an individual's ability to perform an activity. One of the most commonly used scales for rating perceived exertion is the Borg's scale, and this has been adapted to other symptoms such as pain and fatigue (Table 4-5).

The rehabilitation specialist needs a thorough understanding of the physiological demands of the activity or exercise that the person is performing so that the exercise response can be anticipated and is appropriate. For example, aerobic activities with incremental work rates, preferably involving the legs, will result in a commensurate increase in heart rate, blood pressure, breathing depth and rate, and increased perceived exertion (Wasserman & Whipp, 1975). Activities involving primarily the arms, such as hair combing or snow shoveling, result in a disproportionate increase in blood pressure and work of the heart compared with dynamic leg exercise. These activities should be monitored carefully in the older person.

TABLE 4-5 Subjective Scales of Exercise Responses

	Perceived Exertion	Breathlessness	Discomfort/Pain	Fatigue
0	Nothing at all	Nothing at all	Nothing at all	Nothing at all
0.5	Very, very weak	Very, very light	Very, very weak	Very, very light
1	Very weak	Very light	Very weak	Very light
2	Weak	Light	Weak	Light
3	Moderate	Moderate	Moderate	Moderate
4	Somewhat strong	Somewhat strong	Somewhat strong	Somewhat strong
5	Strong	Hard	Strong	Hard
6				
7	Very strong	Very heavy	Very strong	Very strong
8				
9				
10	Very, very strong/maximal	Very, very strong/maximal	Very, very strong/maximal	Very, very strong/maximal

Note: Based on the Borg rating of perceived exertion scale (Borg, 1982).

Many ADLs require a change in body position, such as getting out of bed, the tub, or a chair, or picking up something off the floor. Although these activities may not be metabolically demanding, they lead to significant fluid shifts secondary to the effect of gravity and have profound hemodynamic consequences. Because the fluid-volume–regulating mechanisms in older persons may be blunted, dizziness, blackouts, or fainting can result. Thus, the hemodynamic status of these individuals needs to be monitored until the rehabilitation specialist is sure that these activities can be safely performed.

Activities such as getting out of bed, the tub, or a chair, or getting off the toilet may appear comparable; however, the mechanisms of orthostatic intolerance—that is, postural hypotension—associated with each activity can differ. Getting out of bed in the morning may be accompanied by morning stiffness, imbalance, slowed vital signs, slowed autonomic responsiveness, and reduced muscle pump activity in the legs. Getting out of the tub is associated with significant peripheral vasodilation from having been in warm water for a period of time. Thus, adaptation of the normal fluid shifts will be poorer on assuming the standing position. In addition, there is enormous drag in lifting oneself out of water either in the tub or a swimming pool, and increased cardiac work is required secondary to the postural stabilization. Getting off the toilet may follow a period of autonomic changes and physical straining and, hence, may result in reduced venous return. Orthostatic intolerance associated with getting out of a chair may reflect fluid shifts and pooling of blood in the abdomen and legs during sitting. Finally, orthostatic intolerance associated with picking an item off the floor may reflect reduced cerebral blood flow secondary to the sudden movement to the erect position and the lack of the normal rapid compensatory response. Observing and monitoring each individual's objective and subjective responses to changes in body position enables the rehabilitation specialist to make specific recommendations aimed at reducing the risk of blackouts, fainting, and falling.

Another critical factor that may have significant effects on an older person's ability to perform an activity or exercise is impaired thermoregulation. Older people have a reduced capacity to thermoregulate. A significant proportion have hypothermia (Martyn, 1981), and others may have an impaired ability to lose exercise-induced body heat. The increase in peripheral blood flow to dissipate heat during activity, especially in a warm ambient environment, may compromise cardiac output and blood flow to the working muscles. Failure of blood-pressure–regulating mechanisms may be responsible. Activity in warm environments taxes the individual to an even greater extent and may exacerbate congestive heart failure and dehydration. The individual may show signs of lightheadedness, disorientation, instability, fainting, and heart irregularities. Some common submaximal tests of functional performance, whose validity, reliability, and safety have been established in older subjects, are summarized in Table 4-6 with respect to their specific purpose and procedures. These include the self-paced walking test (SPWT) (Bassey, Fentem, MacDonald, & Scriven, 1976; Cunningham, Rechnitzer, Pearce, & Donner, 1982), modified shuttle walking test (MSWT) (Singh, Morgan, Hardman, Rowe, & Bardsley, 1994; Singh, Morgan, Scott, Walters, & Hardman, 1992), bag-and-carry test (BCT) (Posner et al., 1995), timed up and go test (TUGT) (Mathias, Nayak, & Isaacs, 1986; Podsiadlo & Richardson, 1991), and the 6- and 12-minute walk test (6- and 12-MWT) (McGavin, Artvinli, Naoe, & McHardy, 1978; McGavin, Gupta, & McHardy, 1976).

Functional Capacity

Functional capacity refers to the capacity to respond to an exercise stimulus, maintain the physiological adjustments necessary to sustain aerobic exercise for a period of time (work), and then recover appropriately from that stimulus on cessation of exercise. Although this capacity declines with increasing age, individual differences among older people are considerably greater than among young people. The physical activity pyramid illustrates the general principles for various levels of physical activity for optimal health irrespective of age (see Figure 4-2). Formal exercise in the older adult accrues the same physiological benefits as in younger people with respect to enhanced oxygen transport. Older people, however, may increase their maximal cardiac output and stroke volume in response to training, in favor of peripheral adaptation (Spina, Rashid, Davila-Roman, & Ehsani, 2000; Thomas, Cunningham, Rechnitzer, Donner, & Howard, 1985).

TABLE 4-6 Common Submaximal Tests Used to Assess Functional Performance in Older Individuals

Test	Purpose	Procedure
Self-paced walking test (SPWT) (Bassey et al, 1976, Cunningham et al, 1982)	To assess functional performance in older individuals	Individual is instructed to walk a measured distance (e.g. 250 meters) at three different speeds with 5 min rests between each one: (a) a slow pace, (b) a normal pace, and (c) a fast pace, without overexerting yourself. At least one practice trial required. Outcomes: For each walking trial, speed, time to complete the distance, and stride frequency are calculated; also, average heart rate, stride length, and predicted VO_2 max can be determined.
Modified shuttle walking test (MSW1) (Singh et al, 1992, 1994)	1. To assess patients with a wide range of cardiac and respiratory disabilities 2. To prescribe an appropriate walking program	Set up includes a measured corridor 10 meters in length, with two pylons placed 0.5 meter from each end. The individual walks up and down a 10-meter course at a speed dictated by a prerecorded audio signal on a cassette deck. The individual is instructed to "Walk at a steady pace, aiming to turn around when you hear the signal. You should continue to walk until you feel that yo<None>u are unable to maintain the required speed without becoming unduly breathless." Outcome: The number of levels the patient can attain.
Bag-and-carry test (BCT) (Posner et al., 1995)	To evaluate functional performance including endurance, strength, and balance	Individual is instructed to walk 7.5 meters, climb four stairs, and return carrying 0.9 kg with both arms. On completion of each circuit, 0.9 kg is added to the package The individual continues until he or she can no longer complete the circuit carrying the package. At least one practice trial is required. Outcome: The heaviest weight the individual can carry is recorded.

continued on page 84

TABLE 4-6 **Common Submaximal Tests Used to Assess Functional Performance in Older Individuals** (continued)

Test	Purpose	Procedure
Timed up and go test (TUGT) (Podsiadlo, Richardson, 1991, Mathias et al., 1986)	To assess basic functional mobility in the elderly	Individual rises from a standard office arm chair, walks 3 meters, turns around a cone, and returns to the chair. At least one practice is required. Outcome: Time in seconds to complete the task.
6- and 12- minute walk test (6- and 12- MWT) (McGavin et al., 1976, 1978)	To assess functional performance in individuals with low functional capacity such as the elderly and those with chronic cardiac and respiratory disabilities	For the 12-MWT, the instructions are "to cover as much ground as possible in 12 minutes and to keep going continuously if possible but not to be concerned if you have to slow down or rest." At the end of the test, the subject should feel he or she could not have covered more ground in the time. For the 6-MWT, the instructions are "to walk from end to end, covering as much ground as possible in 6 minutes." Two practices are required for each test; encouragement is standardized. Outcome: Total distance covered in either 6 or 12 minutes.

Assessing Functional Capacity

Assessing functional capacity involves determining an individual's peak aerobic power or ability to sustain aerobic exercise over time. These assessments are typically based on the results of a peak exercise test or endurance test. Although exercise testing is a well-established practice for patients with cardiopulmonary and cardiovascular dysfunction, as well as for healthy people, exercise testing and training in older age groups is not as advanced. This may reflect the inherent challenges of dealing with older age groups related to the prevalence of multisystem complications such as arthritis, cardiopulmonary and cardiovascular dysfunction, hypertension, obesity, diabetes, thyroid problems, depression, and cognitive impairment. Although peak aerobic power may be of physiological interest in older people, endurance is likely to have greater practical value with respect to functional capacity overall.

To assess functional capacity in young people, maximum exercise testing is considered the gold standard. The results of a maximum exercise test provide a profile of the individual's capacity to transport oxygen during progressive increments in work rates and the upper limit of oxygen consumption for that individual.

Although maximum tests have a role in assessing older athletes, they are of less value in assessing older people in general. Maximum exercise tests are neither feasible nor safe for most nonathletic older people, and the criterion for defining the test as a true maximum test is unlikely to be achieved in this population. Instead, peak or submaximal exercise tests are used in older people because they provide practical information regarding an individual's functional capacity and endurance. In a maximum exercise test, the individual undergoes an incremental protocol until the maximum oxygen consumption is reached. Submaximal testing is associated with less risk, is more pleasant to perform, and can be readily administered by a knowledgeable rehabilitation specialist.

Principles for selecting and administering submaximal exercise tests have been described in detail in the literature previously (Noonan & Dean, 2000); the clinical decision-making process is summarized in Box 4-2. The goal of the test needs to be determined and a decision made as to whether a symptom or sign limited test, or both, or a steady-state exercise test is indicated. Endurance can be tested with either a continuous steady-state test or a test involving

an interrupted protocol for individuals with very low functional work capacity.

Considerable research is needed to maximize the validity and reliability of submaximal exercise testing procedures and thereby to increase the diagnostic and clinical value of performing these tests in populations in which maximum testing has fewer indications. Despite their limitations, if carefully administered and the procedures appropriately documented, submaximal exercise testing can provide a basis for prescribing activity and exercise that is both therapeutic and safe for older people (Shephard et al., 1968).

BOX 4-2   Clinical Decision-Making Process: Principles for Selecting and Administering Submaximal Exercise Tests

PRESESSION PATIENT CHECK
Appropriateness of time of day for activity or exercise for individual
Quality of night's sleep
Activity before the session (e.g., visitors, tests, agitation, or irritations)
Discomfort or pain
Competing demands
Timing with respect to medications
Types of changes in medications
Lability of vital signs or hemodynamic instability
General well-being
Interest and motivation

ESTIMATE FUNCTIONAL CAPACITY
Estimate based on history and assessment
Possible outcomes: high, intermediate, or low

IF THE ESTIMATED FUNCTIONAL CAPACITY IS HIGH*
Test Options
Peak exercise test
Continuous incremental protocol on treadmill or ergometer

Maximal Exercise Test
Continuous incremental protocol on treadmill or ergometer (*Note:* Depending on the individual's age, history, and assessment, either type of test may require a physician present.)
ADLs
High metabolic demand

Test End Points
Based on the history and assessment, determine relative and absolute end points that indicate the discontinuation of ADLs or exercise

IF THE ESTIMATED FUNCTIONAL CAPACITY IS INTERMEDIATE
Test Options
Submaximal exercise test
Continuous incremental or steady-state protocol on modality or 6- or 12-min walk test
ADLs
Intermediate metabolic demand

Test End Points
As above

IF THE ESTIMATED FUNCTIONAL CAPACITY IS LOW
Test Options
Submaximal exercise test
Interrupted protocol on modality or 3- or 6-min walk test
ADLs
Low metabolic demand either interrupted or uninterrupted

Test End Points
As above

MONITORING
Level of monitoring before, during, and after testing determined by history and assessment

Basic
Heart rate
Systolic and diastolic blood pressure
Rate pressure product (product of heart rate and systolic blood pressure provides an index of myocardial oxygen consumption and work of the heart)
Breathing frequency

continued on page 86

BOX 4-2 **Clinical Decision-Making Process: Principles for Selecting and Administering Submaximal Exercise Tests** (continued)

Chest or breathing discomfort	*Advanced*
Perceived exertion	EKG
Breathlessness	Arterial saturation (noninvasive pulse oximeter)
Fatigue	Respiratory gas analysis† (i.e., oxygen uptake,
General discomfort or pain	minute ventilation, tidal volume, etc.)
Other parameters: color, perspiration, orientation,	Cardiac output (can be determined noninvasively)
coordination, stability, facial expression, comfort,	Serum enzymes and lactate (require blood work)
and ability to talk	

*Estimated high functional work capacity: approximately equal to or greater than that of a healthy normal sedentary person.

†Oxygen consumption studies can provide detailed profile of respiratory, hemodynamic, and metabolic responses to incremental or steady-state exercise; this information is used to aid diagnosis of the mechanisms of exercise limitation and define the parameters of the exercise prescription.

Functional Consequences of Fitness in Older People

Deconditioning

The effects of deconditioning following restricted mobility have been well documented over the past 60 years and are multisystemic (Mascitelli & Pezzetta, 2004; Mackinnon, 2000). Other than reduced respiratory muscle strength and endurance, most of the effects of restricted mobility on the cardiopulmonary system have been those associated with recumbency—reduced lung volumes and capacities, with the exception of closing volume of the airways, which increases (Clauss, Scalabrini, Ray, & Reed, 1968; Craig, Wahba, Don, Couture, & Becklake, 1971; Ray et al., 1974; Svanberg, 1957). The alveolar-arterial oxygen difference and arterial oxygen tension are reduced. In the cardiovascular system, resting and submaximal heart rates and blood pressure increase (Deitrick, Whedon, & Shorr, 1948), and maximal oxygen consumption is reduced (Convertino, Goldwater, & Sandler, 1986). Total blood volume and plasma volume are reduced (Deitrick et al., 1948; Saltin, Blomqvist, Mitchell, Johnson, Wildenthal, & Chapman, 1968), and blood viscosity is increased, along with the risk of thromboembolism (Lentz, 1981; Sandler, Popp, & Harrison, 1988). The rate of deconditioning has been reported to exceed that of conditioning (Harper & Lyles, 1988; Sandler et al., 1988), which has particular consequences in the older individual with less physiological reserve. The effects of deconditioning are accentuated in older people.

Older men and women may decondition differently. Men and women residing in a long-term facility have been reported to differ in terms of physical fitness components and functional performance (Singh, Chin, Paw, Bosscher, & van Mechelen, 2006). Although functional performance was not different between the two genders, peripheral muscle strength and eye–hand coordination were reported to be better preserved in deconditioned men in the facility, whereas women were more flexible and had superior motor coordination. These findings have implications for rehabilitation assessments and potential interventions indicated.

Conditioning

Exercise training elicits the same physiological benefits in older persons with respect to oxygen transport and oxygen and substrate use as in younger people (Bijnen et al., 1998; De Vito, Hernandez, Gonzalez, Felici, & Figura, 1997; de Wild, Hoefnagels, Oeseburg, & Binkhorst, 1995; DiPietro, 1996; Evans, 1995; Lavie & Milani, 1995, 1997; Levine & Balady, 1993; Levy, Cerqueira, Abrass, Schwartz, & Stratton, 1993; Mazzeo, 1994; McCartney, Hicks, Martin, & Webber, 1995; Pollock, Graves, Swart, & Lowenthal, 1994; Rogers & Evans, 1993; Satoh, Sakurai, Miyagi, & Hohshaku, 1995; Shinkai, Konishi, & Shephard, 1997; Silman, O'Neill, Cooper, Kanis, & Felsenberg, 1997; Stratton, Levy, Cerqueira, Schwartz, & Abrass, 1994; Taaffe, Pruitt, Pyka, Guido, & Marcus, 1996; Tai, Gould, & Iliffe, 1997;

Vaitkcvicius et al., 1993; Vorhies & Riley, 1993; Warren et al., 1993), and these effects are still apparent in individuals with chronic diseases. Adaptation to exercise training in older people results in increases of 10% to 20% in aerobic power and strength, which is comparable to the magnitude of change observed in younger people (Shephard, 1986). Submaximal heart rates, blood pressure, and ventilatory rates are reduced. **Stroke volume** increases, and oxygen extraction at the tissue level is also increased. Comparable to young people, exercise can augment peripheral vasodilatation in older adults which supports the preservation of vascular plasticity in this population (Wray, Uberoi, Lawrenson, & Richardson, 2006). Further, aerobic fitness can improve the plasticity of the brain and, thus, may reduce cognitive as well as physical age-related changes (Colcombe et al., 2004). These improvements translate into increasing functional capacity over and above the critical functional performance threshold (Aniansson, Grimby, Rundgren, Svanborg, & Orlander, 1980; Clark, Wade, Massey, & Van Dyke, 1975; De Vries, 1970; Stamford, 1972; Thomas et al., 1985).

Even though the absolute metabolic cost is theoretically constant, older people experience a given activity as more physiologically demanding than younger people because of the reduced capacity of their oxygen transport systems and their musculature to respond to the physical demand. Decline in the economy of movement in older adults, however, may also contribute (Davies & Dalsky, 1997). Thus, even fit older people report that activities such as walking, climbing stairs, and carrying objects are demanding. With increasing age, these seemingly innocuous activities can be the equivalent of a maximal effort and may increase an older individual's heart rate, blood pressure, and oxygen consumption to maximal values.

The prescription parameters of an exercise program are based on the results of an exercise test. The clinical decision-making process involved in defining the parameters of an exercise program has been described in detail in the literature previously (Dean, 2006b) and is summarized in Box 4-3. However, there are two additional principles of exercise physiology that have particular relevance in prescribing therapeutic activity and exercise for older people—namely, the principles of training specificity and reversibility. The human body is extremely efficient in that physiological adaptation to exercise stress is unique to a specific activity or exercise. Thus, to improve an individual's ability to perform an activity, that activity should be the primary object of training. The lower the initial functional capacity, the more significant is the principle of specificity. Also, once training has been discontinued, the training effect does not carry over, and deconditioning begins immediately. Thus, to maintain a given level of activity or exercise, the training stimulus must be presented at the required intensity, duration, and frequency, and over the requisite period of time that is consistent with eliciting physiological adaptation (American College of Sports Medicine, 2006; Blair et al., 1988).

Implications for the Management of the Care of Older People

Goals

The primary goal of rehabilitation for older people is maximizing function and occupational performance, of which cardiopulmonary and cardiovascular capacity is a significant determinant. The two principal subgoals are as follows:

1. To maximize the cardiopulmonary and cardiovascular reserve capacity such that this capacity exceeds an individual's critical functional performance threshold with consideration of physical activity and exercise stimuli and nutritional status.
2. To maximize an individual's ability to perform ADLs. The ability to perform ADLs largely requires the physiological capacity to adapt to the upright position and to move against gravity; these are both central components of functional performance.

Whether the focus is directed toward functional performance, functional capacity, or both, rehabilitation is based on a detailed analysis of these factors that contribute to functional impairment of that individual which may reflect nutritional deficits (Figure 4-3). A nutritionist may need to be consulted; however, the occupational therapist needs to be familiar with basic nutritional requirements across the life span, *text continued on page 90*

BOX 4-3 **Clinical Decision-Making Process: Principles for Prescribing Activities of Daily Living and an Exercise Program**

PRESESSION PATIENT CHECK

Appropriateness of time of day for activity or exercise for individual

Quality of night's sleep

Activity prior to the session (e.g., visitors, tests, agitations, or irritations)

Discomfort or pain

Competing demands

Timing with respect to medications

Types or changes in medications

Lability of vital signs or hemodynamic instability

General well-being

Interest and motivation

PRESCRIPTION OF ACTIVITIES OF DAILY LIVING

Object

To maximize functional performance by promoting the appropriate physiological adaptation and task endurance, with maximum movement economy, comfort, and least risk

Parameters

Type

Based on individual's needs; prioritize

Intensity

Activity Phases: If feasible, tailor a specific ADL or sequential ADL into:

• Warm-up (up to 75% of the intensity for the steady state)
• Steady state (performed within target range based on predetermined levels of physiologic or subjective variables)
• Warm-down
• Recovery (monitored until within 10% of baseline values, and individual appears to have returned to baseline)
• Lower target limit: None other than pathologically low values for physiological variables (e.g., consistent with a hypotensive episode)
• Upper target limit: Physiological variables not to exceed a predetermined level of physiological variable (e.g., heart rate, blood pressure, exertion level, or subjective experience of exertion, breathlessness, discomfort or pain, fatigue, chest pain)

Duration

If recovery is less than 30 min, patient can likely tolerate an increase in duration.

If recovery is between 30 min and 3 h, duration is probably optimal.

If recovery is longer than 3 h, duration is likely too long. (This recovery excludes the anticipated cumulative fatigue over the course of the day.)

Frequency

If recovery is within 30 min, likely too infrequent

If recovery is between 30 min to 3 h, optimal frequency

If recovery is longer than 3 h, likely too frequent

Time Course

Based on adaptation to performance criterion, optimal movement economy, sufficient cardiopulmonary—cardiovascular conditioning, velocity, and safety

Progression

Reduce demands of activity if individual is consistently in the upper limit of the target range; individual can tolerate higher demand activities if the physiological responses are not consistently reaching the target therapeutic range.

If low functional work capacity, performance and adaptation are enhanced with lighter-intensity, shorter, more frequent sessions.

EXERCISE PRESCRIPTION

Object

To maximize functional capacity by promoting physiological adaptation to an exercise stimulus, with maximum movement economy, comfort, and safety, and thereby increase functional capacity reserve above the functional performance threshold commensurate with the individual's needs if the estimated functional capacity is high

Parameters

Type

Based on goals and results of the exercise test

Intensity

If normal exercise response and adaptation can be expected, then steady-state exercise at 70% to 85% of peak physiological parameters on peak test (e.g., heart rate, blood pressure, perceived exertion)

If abnormal aerobic responses and adaptation to exercise are expected (e.g., chronic airflow limitation, restrictive lung disease or heart disease), define target training range on the basis of breathlessness scale, exertion, or chest pain provided that physiological parameters remain within acceptable limits

continued on page 89

BOX 4-3   Clinical Decision-Making Process: Principles for Prescribing Activities of Daily Living and an Exercise Program (continued)

Duration
20 to 40 min per session

Frequency
3 to 5 times per week

Time Course
In health, 3 to 6 months; but in sedentary persons, change can be observed in 4 to 8 weeks

Progression
With adaptation, target range is no longer maintained (i.e., heart rate, blood pressure, and exertion levels consistently below selected range based on initial exercise test); progression based on a repeated exercise test to redefine exercise prescription parameters

IF ESTIMATED FUNCTIONAL CAPACITY IS INTERMEDIATE
Parameters
Set between those for high and low

Type
For example, treadmill, ergometer, walking, swimming, water exercises

Intensity
60% to 75% of peak work rate achieved on exercise test

Duration
20 min or less

Frequency
1 to 2 times per day

Time Course
With pathology, can expect prolonged course

Progression
Maintain exercise parameters: if exceeding values, cut back; if consistently below, can increase the duration or frequency

IF ESTIMATED FUNCTIONAL CAPACITY IS LOW
Parameters
Type
For example, walking, water exercise, and general light activity or exercise

Intensity
Based on heart rate: lower limit = resting heart rate + 0.60 (peak heart rate from the exercise test resting heart rate)
Upper limit = resting heart rate + 0.75 (peak heart rate from the exercise test—resting heart rate)
If heart rate inappropriate or invalid measure of exercise intensity, blood pressure, perceived exertion, or the talk test
Can be used to define the target training range

Duration
Maximize tolerance by maintaining power output constant and velocity changes to maintain perceived exertion constant
Emphasis on prolonging duration by using an interrupted regimen of alternating higher- and lower-demand work, or low-demand work with rest

Frequency
Several times daily guided by pre-exercise-session check

Time Course
If reduced functional capacity due to deconditioning, adaptation will be observed daily and weekly
If reduced functional capacity due to physical limitations, it is weeks to months for central or peripheral adaptation, or both, to occur

Progression
Exercise progressed as soon as the target training parameters are no longer consistently reached in the exercise session

MONITORING
Refer to guidelines in Box 4–2.
Essential to guide exercise prescription, training, and for general safety.
Note: Supplemental oxygen may be a component of the ADL or exercise training session.

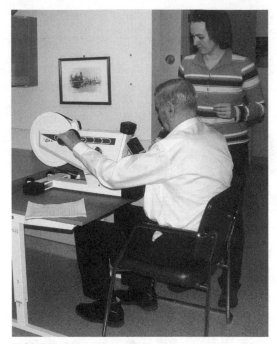

FIGURE 4-3 Although this man has difficulty walk-ing, he is able to work toward enhancing his functional capacity, using an arm ergometer to exercise. (Courtesy of the Geriatric Day Hospital, Specialized Geriatric Services, Saskatoon Health Region, Saskatoon, Saskatchewan, with permission.)

and assess nutritional adequacy at a basic level, making general recommendations related to nutrition, weight loss, or both.

The rationale for improving an individual's ability to perform ADLs and functional capacity appears inherently reasonable. However, the goal of enhancing functional capacity in an indi-vidual with cardiopulmonary or cardiovascular dysfunction may appear paradoxical and war-rants some discussion. Given that the purposes of the cardiopulmonary and cardiovascular sys-tems are oxygen transport and gas exchange and that these functions are effected through an inte-grated system of steps along the oxygen trans-port pathway, it becomes clear that augmenting the function and efficiency of the steps in the pathway can enhance oxygen transport overall. Although there may be weak links in the pathway because of disease, these links can be compensated for by improved efficiency of other steps in the pathway (Chung & Dean, 1989; Dean & Ross, 1992b; Wasserman & Whipp, 1975). The net result of improved efficiency of various steps in the pathway is improved maximum functional capacity.

Individuals with severe cardiopulmonary and cardiovascular dysfunction who cannot achieve an intensity of exercise that is sufficient to stimulate improved aerobic capacity can improve their functional capacity through other mechanisms, including desensitization to shortness of breath, increased motivation, and improved movement efficiency (Belman & Kendregan, 1981, 1982).

Endurance is a primary objective with respect to optimizing function in the older person. Although muscle strength, balance, and coordina-tion are also central to function, these features can frequently be optimized commensurate with endurance activities and exercise. The princi-ple of exercise specificity indicates that optimal adaptation results if the target activity serves as the training stimulus. Although it is commonly practiced, the precise relationship between strength training, for example, and functional activity and its efficacy in relation to function has not been studied in detail.

Assessment

To prescribe ADLs or exercises for older people, the mechanisms contributing to impaired function must be analyzed in detail. Prescribing activity and exercise for older people is as exacting as drug prescription, in that exercise is inherently risky, particularly in older age groups, and needs to be prescribed based on clear indications. Exer-cise can be associated with side effects and has some contraindications. Maximizing therapeutic gain and minimizing risk is the objective and may be achieved with the application of a six-point system of analysis of function (Box 4-4). Collec-tively, the contribution of these six factors is established so that the mechanisms of functional impairment are understood and ADLs and exer-cise can be prescribed appropriately by directing the intervention at specific causes of functional impairment and within an individual's capacity. The exercise or activity prescription can maxi-mize oxygen transport and hence function in the long term.

The object of the assessment is to deter-mine the individual's ability to meet the meta-bolic demands of the activities or exercise of interest. Common parameters that are meas-ured during exercise include heart rate, systolic and diastolic blood pressure, rate pressure product, and breathing frequency.

**BOX 4-4   Exercise Requirements for Analysis of Function
and Prescribing Activity in the Older Adult**

1. Know effects of normal aging on all organ systems.
2. Understand normal exercise responses and effects of position stress in combination with exercise stress.
3. Determine contribution of cardiopulmonary or cardiovascular dysfunction to functional impairment.
4. Establish impact of recumbency and restricted mobility to functional impairment.
5. Verify effect of extrinsic factors, such as medications or medical procedures, on function.
6. Consider intrinsic factors related to specific characteristics of individual and lifestyle.

Oxygen consumption can be measured using a metabolic measurement cart; however, this measure is not routinely performed. Rather, oxygen consumption is estimated based on tables, provided that the work rate or work performed can be accurately determined. Other responses that need to be monitored will depend on the specific individual and the particular factors that contribute to functional deficit. For example, cardiopulmonary disease would require continuous arterial saturation monitoring. Although the availability and sophistication of monitoring equipment has increased, the rehabilitation specialist needs to determine what measures are of particular interest, clinically relevant, and meet the requirements of being valid and reliable.

Because exercise testing is an exacting procedure and must be methodically executed to be meaningful, the rehabilitation specialist must standardize and appropriately record the pretest, testing, and posttest conditions of the exercise test. The details of the specific protocol must be established and the times of work rate changes and measurement recording clearly noted so that the test can be performed in precisely the same way on another occasion or by another person, if necessary. There is greater potential for variability in performing tests of ADLs than standardized exercise tests; thus, such tests need to be strictly standardized to maintain quality control, validity, and reproducibility.

Prescription of Activities of Daily Living and Exercise

The rehabilitation specialist must consider several factors when prescribing ADLs or exercise for a given individual. First, the object of the prescription needs to be defined in order to enhance functional performance, functional capacity, or both. If the object is to enhance functional performance of an ADL, then activity is the focus of training. The activity must be analyzed in terms of its cardiopulmonary and cardiovascular demands in addition to whether the individual is capable of performing the activity from a neuromuscular and musculoskeletal perspective. The body position assumed in performing an activity and the use of any assistive device can alter the metabolic demand. Although some degree of aerobic fitness is desirable in the older adult, maximal aerobic fitness is not needed to perform ADLs and live independently. Rather, activity performance, velocity, and safety are the primary considerations. Assessment of an individual's functional capacity should be based on the demands expected in the individual's living environment. For example, an individual who is to be ambulatory in the community will need to be able to walk 332 m at 50% normal velocity (greater than 40 m/min) and be able to negotiate three steps and a 3% ramp with rails and a curb (Cohen, 1987). An individual's ability to perform an ADL or exercise will also depend on such factors as the time of day, whether the individual has eaten recently, what medications the individual may be receiving, and general well-being on a given day. Also, how rested and energetic the individual feels will influence the ability to perform the activity or exercise. A low-demand activity that needs to be performed once is less demanding overall than the same or more demanding activity that has to be performed multiple times. High-demand activities can be effectively interspersed with rest periods. Even in healthy young people, this type of interval training can significantly increase the overall amount of work performed.

Two concepts applied nonspecifically in the clinic are energy conservation and pacing. Although conserving energy may be a goal, energy sparing needs to be balanced with energy expenditure to avoid the deleterious effects of inactivity and deconditioning. The pace of an activity or exercise affects the overall metabolic cost. Performing an activity too slowly as well as too fast can increase metabolic cost; therefore, the pace at which optimal efficiency is achieved needs to be included as a component of the prescription. Research is needed to examine the concepts of energy conservation and activity pacing so that these concepts can be prescribed on a rational basis and exploited therapeutically.

The assessment identifies ADL deficits and the type of exercise program that will improve function. The capacity of the individual to meet the metabolic demand, however, must also be evaluated. An exercise stimulus, whether prescribed to promote adaptation to ADLs or exercise, should involve no more than 60% to 70% of peak effort and be tolerated without undue fatigue or distress.

Metabolism for daily activities requires the interplay of anaerobic and aerobic metabolic processes. Sprint-type activities demand rapid release from sources of oxygen; thus, the anaerobic system of metabolism is stimulated. Light activities and activities demanding more prolonged submaximal endurance require aerobic metabolism. A physiological steady state is achieved during aerobic exercise and is more functional than anaerobic training. Aerobic adaptation can be achieved with a maximum training intensity of 40% of the **heart rate reserve** [heart rate reserve = resting heart rate + (maximum heart rate − resting heart rate)] in older persons, whereas in young people, a minimum training intensity of 60% of the maximum heart rate is required. Anaerobic activities or exercise are seldom indicated for older people because these can be excessively demanding physiologically and are associated with greater risk. In addition, high levels of anaerobic capacity are not as essential in daily living compared with aerobic capacity.

The parameters of activity or exercise prescription include a warm-up, a steady state, a warm-down, and a recovery period (American College of Sports Medicine, 2006). Even in prescribing ADLs, these components are essential if maximal benefit is to be derived with the least risk. The warm-up and warm-down are critical in priming the cardiopulmonary, cardiovascular, and musculoskeletal systems for work and recovery, respectively. An appropriate warm-up will improve the efficiency during the steady-state portion of the prescription. Monitoring during all portions of the prescription is important, including during the warm-down and recovery. These components are needed to ensure that the physiological adjustments needed to perform work have returned to baseline conditions (e.g., the degradation of lactate and circulating catecholamines). Also, adequate warm-down and recovery reduce late-onset fatigue and soreness.

Older people, particularly those with low functional capacities, can perform large amounts of work in an interval exercise program. Interval training, analogous to "fartlek" training in the athlete, involves alternating either relatively high and low metabolically demanding activity or low metabolically demanding activity and rest periods (Astrand and Rodahl, 1986; Sheffield & Roitman, 1977). Cumulatively, an individual can perform an overall amount of work that would not be achievable if it was attempted all at once. In addition, such a schedule is considerably safer and subjectively tolerated better. Rehabilitation specialists need to exploit interval training regimens in a systematic manner in therapeutic programs for older people.

A balance of activity and rest can also be incorporated over the course of a day to maximize function (Dean, 1991). Theoretically, judicious rest periods contribute to physiological restoration, enabling the individual to perform more work and activity over time. The prescription of rest periods warrants as much attention as the prescription of exercise, given that the negative effects of excessive rest as well as exercise are particularly hazardous in the older person. Rest needs to be viewed as a therapeutic intervention, and similarly, the appropriate parameters need to be selected to optimize function. Considerable research is needed to improve the prescription of rest in conjunction with activity and exercise so that its inclusion will maximize work output and minimize the deleterious effects of inactivity. The overall success of the prescription of ADLs and exercise reflects not only knowledge of exercise physiology but also consideration of psychosocial factors (see Chapters 9, 10, 12, 13, 15, 23). The attitudes, values, and beliefs of older persons and those of their families and peers toward them and their physical status also have a significant impact on the outcomes of the program.

Physical activity is essential to life. Physical decline related to aging has been associated with deconditioning. Thus, promoting active lifestyles in children is probably the most effective way to ensure an active adulthood. Studies related to motivating older adults to be physically active are limited. One recent study, however, examined this relationship in older Australians. In that culture, primary motivating factors to be physically active included keeping healthy, liking the activity, improving physical fitness, and maintaining joint mobility (Kolt, Driver, & Giles, 2004).

Special mention needs to be made of walking and strength training. Walking capacity and a certain level of strength are fundamental to many ADLs. Although walking may not be essential, it can often facilitate the performance of ADLs. Exercise can improve many domains of functional fitness even among very old, previously sedentary individuals, which may in turn facilitate the performance of ADLs (Simons & Andel, 2006).

Monitoring

Although they may appear to be performing activities associated with low metabolic demand, many individuals will be working at loads that would be unacceptable in young people or that alternatively are not within the therapeutic threshold to elicit the maximal benefit. Given that exercise constitutes a risk and that to be therapeutic its intensity needs to be gauged, objective as well as subjective monitoring should be a standard component of assessment and therapeutic interventions. All too often, however, stringent monitoring is neglected in medically stable older people.

The inherent risk of exercise is accentuated in older people for several reasons that add further to the need to monitor these individuals. There are many conditions associated with aging that require special attention. For example, individuals with a history of cardiopulmonary or cardiovascular disease should be monitored closely during activity or exercise. Some people may have no cardiac history but report ischemic leg pain at rest or during exercise. These individuals have a high probability of having cardiac involvement and require cardiac and blood pressure monitoring. Older people are prone to high blood pressure and, in general, are more apt to experience blood pressure irregularities during exercise than young people. Alternatively, some older people are prone to hypotensive episodes. Thus, judicious blood pressure monitoring is essential. Although many individuals are taking medications for heart disease and hypertension, monitoring hemodynamic status is still essential. Individuals with heart disease who are on drugs such as nitrates for coronary artery dilatation should not be treated unless monitoring devices are readily available. The rehabilitation specialist needs to be very familiar with how these and other medications will affect exercise response. Some medications interfere with normal hemodynamic responses to exercise, in which case other parameters need to be used. Special provision needs to be made for diabetic patients, and a sugar source must be available in the event of a hypoglycemic episode associated with increased activity or exercise.

Safety

Safety issues are a foremost concern when testing and prescribing ADLs and exercise (Shephard, 1991). An activity or exercise is prescribed within the anticipated upper limit of an individual's physiological capacity yet above the lower limit of the therapeutic threshold range, and appropriate monitoring is conducted to verify this. A thorough knowledge of signs and symptoms of distress during exercise is essential, and these signs need to be anticipated for each individual and taught to an older person when self-monitoring is appropriate. Rehabilitation specialists involved with prescribing activity or formal exercise for any population must have current certification in cardiopulmonary resuscitation. Rehabilitation departments and clinics should have facilities in the case of an emergency and a procedure outlined in the event of a respiratory or cardiac arrest. All members of the department need to be reacquainted with emergency procedures on a regular basis.

Customizing the Environment to Maximize Function

An astronaut living and working in space is not considered disabled. Modifications with respect to bathing, toileting, washing, exercising, and working have been made to enable the astronaut to survive and be functionally independent in space. Hence, an individual is only as restricted as the surrounding environment (either physically or psychosocially) is restrictive. The physical environment of older people requires constant surveillance to optimize this environment and to promote function and independence as the individual continues to age. Adaptive equipment, mobility aids, and assistive devices within and outside the home need to be reevaluated. In this way, independent living is promoted, the amount of time the individual is upright and moving is maximized, and the risk of morbidity, falls, and injury is reduced.

Cultural considerations are also important in that they provide the basis for each individual's lifestyle, nutrition, physical activity, and preferences related to these. The principles underlying the nutrition pyramid and the physical activity pyramid can be qualitatively modified to meet an individual's cultural preferences. Such sensitivity and attention to cultural issues will enable each individual to adhere to the rehabilitation specialist's recommendations related to health and function.

■ Summary

The principal goals of rehabilitation in the care of the older person are to maximize health, improve the ability to perform ADLs, and enhance functional capacity, the reserve of the cardiopulmonary and cardiovascular systems, and the efficiency of oxygen transport overall. Such an approach raises the individual's functional capacity above the critical functional performance threshold so that with progressive aging and in the event of illness or restricted mobility the individual has sufficient reserve to minimize functional deterioration and dependency. Most of what has been associated with lost function with aging can be attributed significantly to inactivity, disuse, and deconditioning.

The rehabilitation specialist must have a high level of expertise in the assessment and prescription of ADLs and exercise. Such expertise is based on a knowledge base encompassing the following areas:

• An understanding of the determinants of health including optimal nutrition and

physical activity, abstinence from smoking, and quality sleep and rest.
• Normal age-related changes in the cardiopulmonary and cardiovascular systems in addition to multiple other systems that work in an integrated manner to effect functional performance and enhance functional capacity with training.
• Primary and secondary pathophysiological changes resulting in cardiopulmonary and cardiovascular dysfunction and the implications of these changes on functional performance and capacity.
• Effects of nutritional status and weight on health and functional capacity.
• Effects of gravitational stress and acute and long-term exercise stress on the cardiopulmonary and cardiovascular systems.
• Effects of extrinsic factors related to the individual's medical care. For example, in the medically stable individual, these factors include medications and medical procedures.
• Effects of intrinsic factors related to the general history and characteristics of the individual, as well as the individual's nutritional status, regular physical activity, and occupations and lifestyle over the life cycle.
• Knowledge of exercise physiology in health and disease, the principles of adaptation to activity and exercise in older people, and the basis for activity–exercise prescription in this population where multiple factors (the first five listed here) contribute to functional deficits.

Rehabilitation specialists are in a unique position to maximize functional performance and functional capacity in the older adult based on the scientific literature and to identify areas that warrant further study. Moreover, based on a thorough knowledge of exercise physiology in health and disease, these specialists have a responsibility to advise other health care professionals in the promotion of activity and exercise in the older population from both a therapeutic and a lifestyle perspective.

Case Study

Ms. Beverly Hamel, a Muslim African American who is 85 years of age, underwent total hip replacement surgery 1 week ago. She had fallen in her two-story home 10 days ago after getting up in the night because she does not sleep well. She was found by a neighbor who helps with her bath and breakfast each day. On admission to the hospital, she was mildly dehydrated; her blood work indicated that she was moderately anemic. Ms. Hamel's height and weight were 154 cm and 40.5 kg, respectively. She lived and worked on a farm most of her life. She has a long history of bronchial asthma. She reports being frequently short of breath during the day, although she claims to use her inhaler faithfully every morning. She has never smoked. She is having difficulty praying.

Questions

1. Describe the impact of disease on any changes in cardiopulmonary and cardiovascular function secondary to primary or secondary conditions.
2. Describe the impact of recumbency and restricted activity on cardiopulmonary and cardiovascular function.
3. Describe any changes in cardiopulmonary and cardiovascular function secondary to extrinsic factors (i.e., to medical interventions and drugs).
4. Describe any changes in cardiopulmonary and cardiovascular function secondary to intrinsic factors (i.e., to the individual's characteristics, for example, age gender, ethnicity, culture and lifestyle, nutritional status, physical activity, long-term occupation, and coexistent morbidity).
5. Based on the changes identified in questions 1 through 4, prioritize the goals of treatment and provide the rationale.
6. Based on the changes identified in questions 1 through 4, describe the focus of the assessment and the measures and outcomes that would be most relevant to record.
7. Based on the changes identified in questions 1 through 4, describe the treatment plan vis-à-vis prescribing training for functional performance—that is, ADLs, functional capacity, or both.
8. Describe the precautions that you would take in assessing and prescribing ADLs or exercise, or both.
9. Given that a maximum exercise test was not feasible, (a) describe the rationale for the short-term and long-term responses that you would expect to include in your treatment plan and (b) describe what adverse responses this individual could exhibit in response to your treatment plan.

Review Questions

1. Describe the interrelationships among limitation of structure and function, activity, and social participation (World Health Organization International Classification of Function), and explain why these relationships are often limited in people.
2. Describe the age-related changes in cardiopulmonary and cardiovascular function that you would expect to see.
3. Describe the impact of primary or secondary disease on changes in cardiopulmonary and cardiovascular function.
4. Describe the impact of restricted activity and recumbency on any changes in cardiopulmonary and cardiovascular function.
5. Describe changes in cardiopulmonary and cardiovascular function secondary to extrinsic factors (i.e., to medical interventions and drugs).
6. Describe changes in cardiopulmonary and cardiovascular function secondary to intrinsic factors (i.e., to the individual's characteristics, for example, age gender, culture and lifestyle, nutritional status, physical activity, long-term occupation, and coexistent morbidity).

Web-Based Resources

www.mypyramid.gov/professionals/index.html, **United States Department of Agriculture,** date connected March 30, 2007. This website provides information specifically for health care professionals, but also has appropriate content for consumers about the *MyPyramid* food guidance system.

www.cdc.gov/nccdphp/dnpa/physical/health_professionals/index.htm, **Centers for Disease Control and Prevention,** date connected March 30, 2007. This website provides physical activity resources for health care professionals.

http://nutritionandaging.fiu.edu/index.asp, **National Resource Center on Nutrition, Aging and Physical Activity (Florida International University),** date connected March 30, 2007. This website provides numerous resources for health care professionals and older adults.

www.acsm-msse.org/pt/re/msse/positionstandards.htm, **American College of Sports Medicine (ACSM),** date connected March 30, 2007. This website has a collection of ACSM position stands, including exercise-related position stands that have been published in *Medicine & Science in Sports & Exercise®*.

www.hc-sc.gc.ca/hl-vs/seniors-aines/index_e.html, **Health Canada (Government of Canada),** date connected March 30, 2007. This website provides various healthy aging resources for older adults.

www.alcoa.ca, **Active Living Coalition for Older Adults,** Date connected March 30, 2007. This website provides educational materials related to the health benefits of active living for older adults.

REFERENCES

American College of Sports Medicine, Whaley, M. H., Brubaker, P. H., Otto, R. M., & Armstrong, L. E. (2006). *ACSM's guidelines for exercise testing and prescription* (7th ed.). Baltimore: Lippincott Williams & Wilkins.

American Heart Association, Committee on Exercise. (1975). Recommendations concerning sexual activity in post-coronary patients. *Exercise testing and training of individuals with heart disease or at high risk for its development: A handbook for physicians* (pp. 57–58). New York: American Heart Association.

American Psychiatric Association. (1994). *Diagnostic and statistical manual of mental disorders, ed 3 (DSM-IV R)* (4th ed.). Washington, DC: American Psychiatric Association.

American Thoracic Society. (1986). Evaluation of impairment/disability secondary to respiratory disorders. *American Review of Respiratory Disease, 133*(6), 1205–1209.

Aniansson, A., Grimby, G., Rundgren, A., Svanborg, A., & Orlander, J. (1980). Physical training in old men. *Age and Ageing, 9*(3), 186–187.

Astrand, P. O., & Rodahl, K. (1986). Body dimensions and muscular exercise. *Textbook of work physiology. Physiological bases of exercise* (pp. 391–411). New York: McGraw-Hill.

Baruch, I. M., & Mossberg, K. A. (1983). Heart-rate response of elderly women to nonweight-bearing ambulation with a walker. *Physical Therapy, 63*(11), 1782–1787.

Bassey, E. J., Fentem, P. H., MacDonald, I. C., & Scriven, P. M. (1976). Self-paced walking as a method for exercise testing in elderly and young men. *Clinical Science & Molecular Medicine—Supplement, 51*(6), 609–612.

Bates, D. V. (1989). Altered physiologic states and associated syndromes. *Respiratory function in disease* (3rd ed.) (pp. 81–105). Philadelphia: W.B. Saunders.

Belman, M. J., & Kendregan, B. A. (1981). Exercise training fails to increase skeletal muscle enzymes in patients with chronic obstructive pulmonary disease. *American Review of Respiratory Disease, 123*(3), 256–261.

Belman, M. J., & Kendregan, B. A. (1982). Physical training fails to improve ventilatory muscle endurance in patients with chronic obstructive pulmonary disease. *Chest, 81*(4), 440–443.

Berne, R. M., & Levy, M. N. (2000). *Cardiovascular physiology* (8th ed.). St. Louis: Mosby.

Bijnen, F. C., Caspersen, C. J., Feskens, E. J., Saris, W. H., Mosterd, W. L., & Kromhout, D. (1998). Physical activity and 10-year mortality from cardiovascular diseases and all causes: The zutphen elderly study. *Archives of Internal Medicine, 158*(14), 1499–1505.

Blair, S. N., Painter, P., Pate, R. R., Smith, L. K., & Taylor, C. B. (1988). *Resource manual for guidelines for exercise testing and prescription.* Philadelphia: Lea & Febiger.

Blomqvist, C. G., & Stone, H. L. (1983). Sec 2: Circulation: Cardiovascular adjustments to gravitational stress.

In J. T. Shepherd, & F. M. Abboud (Eds.), *Handbook of physiology* (Vol. 2, pp. 1025–1063). Bethesda, MD: American Physiological Society.

Borg, G. (1982). Psychophysical basis of perceived exertion. *Medicine and Science in Sports and Exercise, 14,* 377–381.

Campbell, A., Caird, F. L., & Jackson, T. F. (1974). Prevalence of abnormalities of electrocardiogram in old people. *British Heart Journal, 36*(10), 1005–1011.

Carey, R. G., & Posavic, E. J. (1988). Rehabilitation program evaluation using the revised level of rehabilitation scale (LORS-II). *Physical Medicine and Rehabilitation, 69,* 337–343.

Chase, G. A., Grave, C., & Rowell, L. B. (1966). Independence of changes in functional and performance capacities attending prolonged bed rest. *Aerospace Medicine, 37*(12), 1232–1238.

Chung, F., & Dean, E. (1989). Pathophysiology and cardiorespiratory consequences of interstitial lung disease—review and clinical implications: A special communication. *Physical Therapy, 69*(11), 956–966.

Clark, B. A., Wade, M. G., Massey, B. H., & Van Dyke, R. (1975). Response of institutionalized geriatric mental patients to a twelve-week program of regular physical activity. *Journal of Gerontology, 30*(5), 565–573.

Clauss, R. H., Scalabrini, B. Y., Ray, J. F., 3rd, & Reed, G. E. (1968). Effects of changing body position upon improved ventilation-perfusion relationships. *Circulation, 37*(4 Suppl), II214–II217.

Cohen, J. J. (1987). Establishing the criteria for community ambulation. *Topics in Geriatric Rehabilitation, 3,* 71–77.

Colcombe, S. J., Kramer, A. F., Erickson, K. I., Scalf, P., McAuley, E., Cohen, N. J., et al. (2004). Cardiovascular fitness, cortical plasticity, and aging. *Proceedings of the National Academy of Sciences of the United States of America, 101*(9), 3316–3321.

Convertino, V. A. (1992). Effects of exercise and inactivity on intravascular volume and cardiovascular control mechanisms. *Acta Astronaut, 27,* 123–129.

Convertino, V. A., Goldwater, D. J., & Sandler, H. (1986). Bedrest-induced peak VO_2 reduction associated with age, gender, and aerobic capacity. *Aviation Space & Environmental Medicine, 57*(1), 17–22.

Craig, D. B., Wahba, W. M., Don, H. F., Couture, J. G., & Becklake, M. R. (1971). "Closing volume" and its relationship to gas exchange in seated and supine positions. *Journal of Applied Physiology: Respiratory, Environmental and Exercise Physiology, 31*(5), 717–721.

Cunningham, D. A., Rechnitzer, P. A., Pearce, M. E., & Donner, A. P. (1982). Determinants of self-selected walking pace across ages 19 to 66. *Journal of Gerontology, 37*(5), 560–564.

Davies, C. T. (1972). The oxygen-transporting system in relation to age. *Clinical Science, 42*(1), 1–13.

Davies, M. J., & Dalsky, G. P. (1997). Economy of mobility in older adults. *Journal of Orthopaedic & Sports Physical Therapy, 26*(2), 69–72.

Davies, M. J., & Pomerance, A. (1972). Quantitative study of aging changes in the sinoatrial and internodal tracts. *British Heart Journal, 34,* 150–155.

De Vito, G., Hernandez, R., Gonzalez, V., Felici, F., & Figura, F. (1997). Low intensity physical training in older subjects. *Journal of Sports Medicine & Physical Fitness, 37*(1), 72–77.

De Vries, H. A. (1970). Physiological effects of an exercise training regimen upon men aged 52 to 88. *Journal of Gerontology, 25*(4), 325–336.

de Wild, G. M., Hoefnagels, W. H., Oeseburg, B., & Binkhorst, R. A. (1995). Maximal oxygen uptake in 153 elderly Dutch people (69–87 years) who participated in the 1993 Nijmegen 4-day march. *European Journal of Applied Physiology & Occupational Physiology, 72*(1–2), 134–143.

Dean, E. (1991). Clinical decision making in the management of the late sequaelae of poliomyelitis. *Physical Therapy, 71,* 752–761.

Dean, E. (1997). Oxygen transport deficits in systemic disease and implications for physical therapy. *Physical Therapy, 77,* 187–202.

Dean, E. (2006a). Epidemiology and the practice of physical therapy. In D. Frownfelter & E. Dean (Eds.), *Cardiovascular and pulmonary physical therapy: Evidence and practice* (4th ed.). St. Louis: Mosby Elsevier.

Dean, E. (2006b). Mobilization and exercise. In D. Frownfelter & E. Dean (Eds.), *Cardiovascular and pulmonary physical therapy: Evidence and practice* (4th ed.). St. Louis: Mosby Elsevier.

Dean, E., & Perme, C. (2008). Effects of positioning and mobilization. In J. A. Pryor & S. A. Prasad (Eds.), *Physiotherapy for respiratory and cardiac problems* (4th ed., pp. 115–133). Edinburgh: Churchill Livingstone.

Dean, E., & Ross, J. (1992a). Mobilization and body conditioning. In C. Zadai (Ed.), *Pulmonary management in physical therapy.* (pp. 157–191). New York: Churchill Livingstone.

Dean, E., & Ross, J. (1992b). Oxygen transport: The basis for contemporary cardiopulmonary physical therapy and its optimization with body positioning and mobilization. *Physical Therapy Practice, 4*(1), 34–44.

Deitrick, J. E., Whedon, G. D., & Shorr, E. (1948). Effects of immobilization upon various metabolic and physiologic functions of normal men. *American Journal of Medicine, 4,* 3–36.

DiPietro, L. (1996). The epidemiology of physical activity and physical function in older people. *Medicine & Science in Sports & Exercise, 28*(5), 596–600.

Evans, W. J. (1995). Exercise, nutrition, and aging. *Clinics in Geriatric Medicine, 11*(4), 725–734.

Fox, S. M. III, Naughton, J. P., & Gorman, P. A. (1972). Physical activity and cardiovascular health. III. The exercise prescription: Frequency and type of activity. *Modern Concepts of Cardiovascular Disease, 41,* 25–30.

Fry, P. S. (1986). Functional disorders in the elderly: Description, assessment, and management considerations. In P. S. Fry (Ed.), *Depression, stress, and adaptations in the elderly* (pp. 205–254). Rockville, MD: Aspen.

Gilson, B. S., Gilson, J. S., Bergner, M., Bobbit, R. A., Kressel, S., Pollard, W. E., et al. (1975). The sickness impact profile. Development of an outcome measure of health care. *American Journal of Public Health,* 65(12), 1304–1310.

Guyatt, G. H., Berman, L. B., Townsend, M., Pugsley, S. O., & Chambers, L. W. (1987). A measure of quality of life for clinical trials in chronic lung disease. *Thorax,* 42(10), 773–778.

Harper, C. M., & Lyles, Y. M. (1988). Physiology and complications of bed rest. [Review] [80 refs]. *Journal of the American Geriatrics Society,* 36(11), 1047–1054.

Higginbotham, M. B., Morris, K. G., Williams, R. S., Coleman, R. E., & Cobb, F. R. (1986). Physiologic basis for the age-related decline in aerobic work capacity. *American Journal of Cardiology,* 57(15), 1374–1379.

Kantrowitz, F. G., Munoz, G., Roberts, N., Schatten, S., & Stern, S. (1986). Rheumatology in geriatrics. In S. R. Gambert (Ed.), *Contemporary geriatric medicine* (Vol. 2, pp. 197–200). New York: Plenum Medical Books.

Katz, S., Ford, A. B., Moskowitz, R. W., Jackson, B. A., & Jaffe, M. W. (1963). Studies of illness. *JAMA, 185,* 914–919.

Khan, N. A., McAlister, F. A., Rabkin, S. W., Padwal, R., Feldman, R. D., Campbell, N. R., et al. (2006). Canadian Hypertension Education Program. The 2006 Canadian Hypertension Education Program recommendations for the management of hypertension: Part II—Therapy. *Canadian Journal of Cardiology,* 22(7), 583–593.

Kolt, G. S., Driver, R. P., & Giles, L. C. (2004). Why older Australians participate in exercise and sport. *Journal of Aging and Physical Activity,* 12(2), 185–198.

Kruiansky, J., & Gurland, B. (1976). The performance test of activities of daily living. *International Journal of Aging & Human Development,* 7(4), 343–352.

Lavie, C. J., & Milani, R. V. (1995). Effects of cardiac rehabilitation programs on exercise capacity, coronary risk factors, behavioral characteristics, and quality of life in a large elderly cohort. *American Journal of Cardiology,* 76(3), 177–179.

Lavie, C. J., & Milani, R. V. (1997). Benefits of cardiac rehabilitation and exercise training in elderly women. *American Journal of Cardiology,* 79(5), 664–666.

Lentz, M. (1981). Selected aspects of deconditioning secondary to immobilization. *Nursing Clinics of North America,* 16(4), 729–737.

Lesnefsky, E. J., & Hoppel, C. L. (2006). Oxidative phosphorylation and aging. *Ageing Research Reviews,* 5(4), 402–433.

Levine, G. N., & Balady, G. J. (1993). The benefits and risks of exercise training: The exercise prescription. *Advances in Internal Medicine, 38,* 57–79.

Levy, W. C., Cerqueira, M. D., Abrass, I. B., Schwartz, R. S., & Stratton, J. R. (1993). Endurance exercise training augments diastolic filling at rest and during exercise in healthy young and older men. *Circulation,* 88(1), 116–126.

Linn, M. W., & Linn, B. S. (1982). The rapid disability rating scale-2. *Journal of the American Geriatrics Society,* 30(6), 378–382.

MacKenzie, C. R., Charlson, M. E., DiGioia, D., & Kelley, K. (1986). A patient-specific measure of change in maximal function. *Archives of Internal Medicine, 146*(7), 1325–1329.

Mackinnon, L. T. (2000). Chronic exercise training effects on immune function. *Medicine and Science in Sports and Exercise, 32*(7 Suppl.), S369–S376.

Mahoney, F. I., & Barthel, D. W. (1965). Functional evaluation: The Barthel Index. *Maryland State Medical Journal, 14,* 61–65.

Martyn, J. W. (1981). Diagnosing and treating hypothermia. *Canadian Medical Association Journal, 125*(10), 1089–1096.

Mascitelli, L., & Pezzetta, F. (2004). Anti-inflammatory effect of physical activity. *Archives of Internal Medicine, 164*(4), 460.

Mathias, S., Nayak, U. S., & Isaacs, B. (1986). Balance in elderly patients: The "get-up and go" test. *Archives of Physical Medicine & Rehabilitation, 67*(6), 387–389.

Mazzeo, R. S. (1994). The influence of exercise and aging on immune function. *Medicine & Science in Sports & Exercise, 26*(5), 586–592.

McCartney, N., Hicks, A. L., Martin, J., & Webber, C. E. (1995). Long-term resistance training in the elderly: Effects on dynamic strength, exercise capacity, muscle, and bone. *Journals of Gerontology Series A-Biological Sciences & Medical Sciences, 50*(2), B97–B104.

McGavin, C. R., Artvinli, M., Naoe, H., & McHardy, G. J. R. (1978). Dyspnea, disability and distance walked: Comparison of estimates of exercise performance in respiratory disease. *British Medical Journal, 1,* 243–248.

McGavin, C. R., Gupta, S. P., & McHardy, G. J. (1976). Twelve-minute walking test for assessing disability in chronic bronchitis. *British Medical Journal, 1*(6013), 822–823.

Mokdad, A. H., Marks, J. S., Stroup, D. F., & Gerberding, J. L. (2004). Actual causes of death in the United States, 2000. *JAMA, 291*(10), 1238–1245.

Noonan, V., & Dean, E. (2000). Submaximal exercise testing: Clinical application and interpretation. *Physical Therapy, 80,* 782–807.

Podsiadlo, D., & Richardson, S. (1991). The timed "Up & Go": A test of basic functional mobility for frail elderly persons. *Journal of the American Geriatrics Society, 39,* 142–148.

Pollock, M. L., Graves, J. E., Swart, D. L., & Lowenthal, D. T. (1994). Exercise training and prescription for the elderly. *Southern Medical Journal, 87*(5), S88–S95.

Posner, J. D., McCully, K. K., Landsberg, L. A., Sands, L. P., Tycenski, P., Hofmann, M. T., et al. (1995). Physical determinants of independence in mature women. *Archives of Physical Medicine & Rehabilitation, 76*(4), 373–380.

Purnell, L. D., & Paulanka, B. J. (2003a). The Purnell model for cultural competence. *Transcultural health care: A culturally competent approach* (pp. 8–39). Philadelphia: F.A. Davis.

Purnell, L. D., & Paulanka, B. J. (2003b). Transcultural diversity and health care. In L. D. Purnell & B. J. Paulanka (Eds.), *Transcultural health care: A culturally competent approach* (2nd ed., pp. 1–7). Philadelphia: F.A. Davis.

Ray, J. F., 3rd, Yost, L., Moallem, S., Sanoudos, G. M., Villamena, P., Paredes, R. M., et al. (1974). Immobility, hypoxemia, and pulmonary arteriovenous shunting. *Archives of Surgery, 109*(4), 537–541.

Rogers, M. A., & Evans, W. J. (1993). Changes in skeletal muscle with aging: Effects of exercise training. *Exercise & Sport Sciences Reviews, 21,* 65–102.

Rogers, W. J., Johnstone, D. E., Yusuf, S., Weiner, D. H., Gallagher, P., Bittner, V. A., et al. (1994). Quality of life among 5,025 patients with left ventricular dysfunction randomized between placebo and enalapril: The studies of left ventricular dysfunction. The SOLVD investigators. *Journal of the American College of Cardiology, 23*(2), 393–400.

Saltin, B., Blomqvist, G., Mitchell, J. H., Johnson, R. L., Jr, Wildenthal, K., & Chapman, C. B. (1968). Response to exercise after bed rest and after training. *Circulation, 38*(5 Suppl.), 1–78.

Sandler, H. (1986). Cardiovascular effects of inactivity. In H. Sandler & J. Vernikos (Eds.), *Inactivity physiological effects* (pp. 11–47). New York: Academic Press.

Sandler, H., Popp, R. L., & Harrison, D. C. (1988). The hemodynamic effects of repeated bed rest exposure. *Aviation Space & Environmental Medicine, 59*(11 Pt. 1), 1047–1054.

Satoh, T., Sakurai, I., Miyagi, K., & Hohshaku, Y. (1995). Walking exercise and improved neuropsychological functioning in elderly patients with cardiac disease. *Journal of Internal Medicine, 238*(5), 423–428.

Sheffield, L. T., & Roitman, D. (1977). Stress testing methodology. In E. H. Sonnenblick & M. Lesch (Eds.), *Exercise and heart disease* (pp. 152–168). New York: Grune & Stratton.

Shephard, R. J. (1985). Limitations upon the rate of working. In R. J. Shephard (Ed.), *Physiology and biochemistry of exercise* (pp. 47–94). New York: Praeger.

Shephard, R. J. (1986). Physical training for the elderly. *Clinics in Sports Medicine, 5*(3), 515–533.

Shephard, R. J. (1991). Safety of exercise testing—the role of the paramedical exercise specialist. *Clinical Journal of Sport Medicine: Official Journal of the Canadian Academy of Sport Medicine, 1,* 8–11.

Shephard, R. J., Allen, C., Benade, A. J., Davies, C. T., Di Prampero, P. E., Hedman, R., et al. (1968). Standardization of submaximal exercise tests. *Bulletin of the World Health Organization, 38*(5), 765–775.

Shinkai, S., Konishi, M., & Shephard, R. J. (1997). Aging, exercise, training, and the immune system. *Exercise Immunology Review, 3,* 68–95.

Silman, A. J., O'Neill, T. W., Cooper, C., Kanis, J., & Felsenberg, D. (1997). Influence of physical activity on vertebral deformity in men and women: Results from the European vertebral osteoporosis study. *Journal of Bone & Mineral Research, 12*(5), 813–819.

Simons, R., & Andel, R. (2006). The effects of resistance training and walking on functional fitness in advanced old age. *Journal of Aging and Health, 18*(1), 91–105.

Singh, A. S., Chin, A., Paw, M. J., Bosscher, R. J., & van Mechelen, W. (2006). Cross-sectional relationship between physical fitness components and functional performance in older persons living in long-term care facilities. *BMC Geriatrics, 6,* 4–12.

Singh, S. J., Morgan, M. D., Hardman, A. E., Rowe, C., & Bardsley, P. A. (1994). Comparison of oxygen uptake during a conventional treadmill test and the shuttle walking test in chronic airflow limitation. *European Respiratory Journal, 7*(11), 2016–2020.

Singh, S. J., Morgan, M. D., Scott, S., Walters, D., & Hardman, A. E. (1992). Development of a shuttle walking test of disability in patients with chronic airways obstruction. *Thorax, 47*(12), 1019–1024.

Spina, R. J., Rashid, S., Davila-Roman, V. G., & Ehsani, A. A. (2000). Adaptations in beta-adrenergic cardiovascular responses to training in older women. *Journal of Applied Physiology, 89,* 2300–2305.

Stamford, B. A. (1972). Physiological effects of training upon institutionalized geriatric men. *Journal of Gerontology, 27*(4), 451–455.

Stein, R. A. (1977). The effect of exercise training on heart rate during coitus in the post-myocardial patient. *Circulation, 55,* 738–740.

Stewart, A. L., Hays, R. D., & Ware, J. E., Jr. (1988). The MOS short-form general health survey: Reliability and validity in a patient population. *Medical Care, 26*(7), 724–735.

Stratton, J. R., Levy, W. C., Cerqueira, M. D., Schwartz, R. S., & Abrass, I. B. (1994). Cardiovascular responses to exercise: Effects of aging and exercise training in healthy men. *Circulation, 89*(4), 1648–1655.

Suh, E. E. (2004). The model of cultural competence through an evolutionary concept analysis. *Journal of Transcultural Nursing: Official Journal of the Transcultural Nursing Society/Transcultural Nursing Society, 15*(2), 93–102.

Svanberg, L. (1957). Influence of posture on the lung volumes, ventilation and circulation in normals; a spirometric-bronchospirometric investigation. *Scandinavian Journal of Clinical and Laboratory Investigation, 9*(Suppl. 25), 1–195.

Taaffe, D. R., Pruitt, L., Pyka, G., Guido, D., & Marcus, R. (1996). Comparative effects of high- and low-intensity resistance training on thigh muscle strength, fiber area, and tissue composition in elderly women. *Clinical Physiology (Oxford, Oxfordshire), 16*(4), 381–392.

Tai, S. S., Gould, M., & Iliffe, S. (1997). Promoting healthy exercise among older people in general practice: Issues in designing and evaluating therapeutic interventions. *British Journal of General Practice, 47*(415), 119–122.

Thomas, S. G., Cunningham, D. A., Rechnitzer, P. A., Donner, A. P., & Howard, J. H. (1985). Determinants of the training response in elderly men. *Medicine & Science in Sports & Exercise, 17*(6), 667–672.

Tudor-Locke, C., & Bassett, D. R., Jr. (2004). How many steps/day are enough? Preliminary pedometer indices for public health. *Sports Medicine (Auckland, N.Z.), 34*(1), 1–8.

United States Department of Agriculture. (2006a). *Food pyramid.* Retrieved December 2006 from www.usda.gov.

United States Department of Agriculture. (2006b). *Physical activity and exercise pyramid.* Retrieved December 2006 from www.islandcounty.net/health/CHAB/phyactpyr.pdf.

Vaitkevicius, P. V., Fleg, J. L., Engel, J. H., O'Connor, F. C., Wright, J. G., Lakatta, L. E., et al. (1993). Effects of age and aerobic capacity on arterial stiffness in healthy adults. *Circulation, 88*(4 Pt. 1), 1456–1462.

Vorhies, D., & Riley, B. E. (1993). Deconditioning. *Clinics in Geriatric Medicine, 9*(4), 745–763.

Warren, B. J., Nieman, D. C., Dotson, R. G., Adkins, C. H., O'Donnell, K. A., Haddock, B. L., et al. (1993). Cardiorespiratory responses to exercise training in septuagenarian women. *International Journal of Sports Medicine, 14*(2), 60–65.

Wasserman, K., & Whipp, B. J. (1975). Exercise physiology in health and disease. *American Review of Respiratory Diseases, 112,* 219–249.

West, J. B. (2005). *Respiratory physiology: The essentials* (7th ed.). Philadelphia: Lippincott Williams & Wilkins.

Winslow E. H. (1985). Cardiovascular consequences of bed rest. *Heart Lung, 14,* 236–246.

World Health Organization. (1999–2003). *Annual health reports 1999–2003.* Geneva, Switzerland.

World Health Organization. (2002). *International Classification of Functioning, Disability and Health.* Retrieved December 2006 from www.sustainable-design.ie/arch/ICIDH-2PFDec-2000.pdf.

World Health Organization. (2006). *Definition of health.* Retrieved June 2006 from www.who.int.

Wray, D. W., Uberoi, A., Lawrenson, L., & Richardson, R. S. (2006). Evidence of preserved endothelial function and vascular plasticity with age. *American Journal of Physiology. Heart and Circulatory Physiology, 290*(3), H1271–H1277.

Young, A. (1986). Exercise physiology in geriatric practice. *Acta Medica Scandinavica - Supplementum, 711,* 227–232.

CHAPTER 5

Sensory Function

Celia Routh Hooper, PhD, CCC-SLP • Vanina Dal Bello-Haas, PT, PhD

The spiritual eyesight improves as the physical eyesight declines.

Plato (427–347 BCE)

It is a mistake to regard age as a downhill grade toward dissolution. The reverse is true. As one grows older, one climbs with surprising strides.

George Sand, French author (1804–1876)

OBJECTIVES

By the end of this chapter, the reader will be able to:

1. Explain the relationship between sensory changes that occur in older adults and resultant physical and behavioral compensation.
2. Discuss the age-related changes of the eye, its support structures, and the visual pathway of the nervous system.
3. Describe major ocular diseases that affect vision in older adults.
4. Describe the changes associated with aging in the auditory system, particularly as they relate to the reception of speech sounds.
5. Identify common age-related changes that occur in taste, smell, and touch.
6. Relate common sensory deficits of older adults to functional performance and lifestyle issues.
7. Relate common sensory deficits of older adults to functional performance and lifestyle issues.
8. Identify the recurrent themes regarding changes in the sensory systems.
9. Explore Internet resources for additional information.

Our bodies receive information about the physical world through generalized and specialized sensory receptors. These receptors begin functioning in most cases in utero, and beginning in early adulthood start a slow, progressive decline (Cech & Martin, 2002). The "senses" or systems of sensation provide information from the surrounding environment to the brain. The senses send information via a **modality,** or sensory channel, in the peripheral nervous system (PNS) to the central nervous system (CNS), where the information is comprehended. *Perception,* a higher sensory function and a middle ground between sensation and comprehension, enables the organism to receive and perceive that a stimulus has occurred, process the information, and attach meaning to the information. The exact anatomy and physiology of perception is not well understood, and it is unclear when or where reception ends and perception begins. Our perceptions are changed with experience as we learn the likely meaning of signals, and learned perceptions may aid us as our sensory receptors begin to decline. The parieto-temporal and parieto-occipital areas of the cerebral cortex, important sensory areas, are responsible for the

integration, or association, of information regarding sensory modalities. Sensory information does not travel through a direct route of **monosynaptic connections** from receptor cells to the CNS. Rather, somatosensory input and sensory fiber tracts travel through several relay stations, or integrating centers, in the brain stem reticular system and the thalamus (Lynch, 2006). Any neuronal degeneration in these sensory integrative and relay structures reduces the quality of information received at the CNS level. The information contained in this chapter should be viewed in the context of the many typical changes that take place in the aging nervous system, as sensory and sensory integrative changes are a reflection of those systemic changes.

Age-related changes in the sensory systems (summarized in Table 5-1) can have a major impact on the social, psychological, and physical function of the older person. This chapter describes common changes found in older adults that affect the senses, specifically,

- Vision
- Hearing
- Taste

TABLE 5-1 Summary of Effects of Age-Related Sensory Changes on Functional Activities

Sensory System	Primary Changes Related to Aging	Functional Results
Vision	Loss of subcutaneous fat around the eye	Decreased near vision
	Decreased tissue elasticity and tone	Poor eye coordination
	Decreased strength of the eye muscles	Distortion of images
	Decreased corneal transparency	Blurred vision
	Degeneration of sclera, pupil, and iris	Compromised night vision
	Increase in density and rigidity of lens	Loss of color sensitivity, especially green, blue, and violet shades
	Increased frequency of disease processes	Difficulty with recognition of moving objects,
	Slowing of CNS information processing	items with a complex figure, or items that appear in and out of light quickly
Hearing	Loss or damage to sensory hair cells of cochlea and the lower basal turn of the inner ear	Difficulty in hearing higher frequencies, tinnitus Diminished ability for pitch discrimination
	Nerve cell diminution of cochlear ganglia	Reduced speech recognition and reception
	Degeneration in central auditory pathways	Loss of speech discrimination
	Loss of neurotransmitters	
Taste	Decrease in taste buds	Higher thresholds for identification of
	Varicose enlargement	substances
Smell	Degeneration of sensory cells of nasal mucosa	Decline in suprathreshold sensitivity for odors
Superficial sensation	Slower nerve conduction velocities	Decreased response to tactile stimuli
		Alterations in perception of pain
		Adversely affected by thermal extremes

• Smell
• Somatic senses—touch, pain, and temperature

Vision and Functional Performance

Because of a number of structural and function changes in the eye, all older adults experience a decrease in visual ability as they age. Even though the older adult may not be acutely aware of the changes because they occur gradually, and the older adult can often adapt to these changes, visual problems are of great significance for many older adults. In 2002, more than 161 million people worldwide were reported to have visual impairments—124 million people had low vision and 37 million were blind. More than 82% of all people with visual impairments are 50 years of age and older (World Health Organization, 2005). As illustrated in Figure 5-1, the prevalence of visual impairments increases significantly with age. It has been estimated that direct and indirect care and vision services for older adults with vision loss are between $30 billion and $40 billion each year (Butler, Faye, Guazzo, & Kupfer, 1997). The relationship

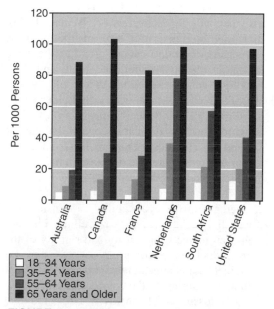

FIGURE 5-1 Prevalence of visual impairments in six countries. (Data from G. E. Hendershot & J. E. Crews. (2006). Toward international comparability of survey statistics on visual impairments. The DISTAB project. *Journal of Visual Impairment & Blindness, 100*(1), 11–25.)

between vision impairments and activity and participation limitations, as well as depression and psychological distress, has been well documented (Brody et al., 2001; Crews & Campbell, 2001; DiNuzzo, Black, Lichtenstein, & Markides, 2001; Ramrattan et al., 2001; West, Gildengorin, Haegerstrom-Portnoy, Schneck, Lott, & Brabyn, 2002; West et al., 1997).

The term **low vision** describes a serious visual loss that is uncorrectable by medical or surgical intervention or with eyeglasses (Faye, 1984). It is a term used to describe the person's problem, not the underlying pathology or etiology. The term low vision, along with *visually impaired, visually handicapped,* and *partially sighted,* implies that an individual has some vision remaining. In other words, a person with low vision has some usable vision, but the visual loss is significant enough that it affects work, recreation, and other activities of daily living. A separate term, **legally blind,** is typically used by governments to define a person whose degree of sight loss entitles them to special benefits. Legal blindness is defined as **visual acuity** of 20/200 or less in the better eye after best possible standard correction or visual field of no greater than 20 degrees (United States Social Security Administration, 1992). Visual acuity of 20/200 means that a person can see a letter or word at a distance of 20 feet that can be seen by a normally sighted person at a distance of 200 feet. It is important to note that legal blindness is not necessarily the same as total blindness. About 85% of those legally blind have low vision rather than total blindness (Faye, 1984).

Normal Age-Related Changes

Age-related changes occur in the support structures of the eye, the eye, and the visual pathway. See Figure 5-2 for an illustration of a healthy eye. Changes in the support structures include loss of subcutaneous fat and decreased tissue elasticity and tone, all of which may make the eyes appear sunken or may result in redundancy of the skin of the eyelids and eyelid malpositions (Kalina, 1997). Tear production may decrease, causing symptoms of foreign body sensation and burning and, for some, corneal ulceration (Mathers, Lane, & Zimmerman, 1996; Smith, 1998). Increased use of over-the-counter topical ophthalmic solutions by

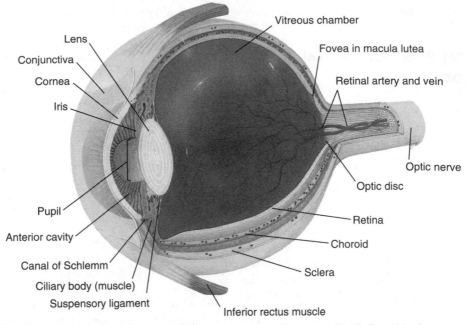

FIGURE 5-2 Internal anatomy of the eyeball. (From V. C. Scanlon & T. Sanders. (2007). *Essentials of anatomy and physiology,* 5th ed. Philadelphia: F.A. Davis, p. 205, with permission.)

older adults may mask symptoms of "dry eye" and may cause additional problems in those who have concomitant cardiac, respiratory, or neurological system pathology (Diamond, 1997). Additionally, the levator palpebrae superioris eye muscle becomes weak, causing problems with upward gaze and **convergence** (Sullivan, 1984), which in turn results in poor eye coordination and difficulty focusing.

Changes in the eye begin with the **cornea,** where light first enters. The cornea thickens, flattens, and becomes less smooth and more rigid after age 60 to 65 years, causing or increasing **astigmatism** and resulting in images that are distorted or blurred. These changes also affect the way in which light is reflected. A ring of opaqueness forms in the cornea of some individuals, and a deposit of pigment occurs in most corneas (Leslie, 1978). These changes result in a reduced corneal transparency that limits the amount of light reaching the retina and may reduce the visual field. In addition, decreased corneal sensitivity may cause older adults to be less aware of injury or infection.

The **sclera, pupil,** and **iris** undergo degenerative changes. The scleral tissue loses water and increases its fatty deposits, causing a yellow cast and decreased opacity (Sullivan,1984).

The pupil decreases in size and becomes more fixed. The iris decreases in dilation ability because of several processes, including an increase of connective tissue, sclerosis of the blood supply, and muscle weakness (Kasper, 1978; Schaefer & Weale, 1970). Because the maximum size of the pupil is decreased, the pupil cannot dilate to the same extent in response to reduced light, and thus, less light gets to the retina. As a result, there is a gradual loss of visual acuity, and older adults have more difficulty seeing clearly in low light situations. Every 10 years between the ages of 20 and 80, significant changes in visual acuity occur due to this gradual decrease in light available to the retina (Woodruff-Pak, 1997).

The **lens** also changes with age, resulting in a decrease in the eye's ability to transmit and focus light (Sullivan, 1984). Cellular changes cause an increase in density and rigidity of the lens, which may compromise near and far vision. These changes in the lens may also contribute to filtering of the color spectrum, resulting in a loss of color sensitivity across the total spectrum but especially for green, blue, and violet shades (Dye, 1983). Loss of color sensitivity results in reduced visual acuity for subtle differences in color shadings.

The central area of the retina, the **macula,** has a concentration of cone cells that allow for color vision and fine-detail discrimination and rod cells that are extremely sensitive to light and are responsible for peripheral vision and night vision. Conflicting results have been reported regarding the loss of cone cells with aging (Dorey, Wu, Ebenstein, Garsd, & Weiter, 1989; Gartner & Henkind, 1982). However, rod density has been found to decrease by 30% with advancing age (Curcio, Millican, Allen, & Kalina, 1993). As the retina ages, it gradually loses neurons, and the retinal nerve fiber layer has been found to thin by 20% to 30% with increased age (Lovasik, Kergoat, Justino, & Kergoat, 2003).

As a result of the above changes, older adults experience a narrower field of vision (deceased ability to see objects at the corner of their gaze), have problems with seeing clearly in low light settings, have problems with light and dark adaptation, and have increased sensitivity to glare. Older adults may need three times more lighting than younger people to see clearly (Hooyman & Kiyak, 2005). Because light and dark adaptation is compromised, more time is needed for an older adult to adjust his or her eyes when entering or leaving a dark room. This may predispose older adults to falls as they ambulate in rooms with varying light levels and may cause problems with reading signs at night. Glare from shiny objects, polished floors, headlights, and wet pavements is poorly tolerated for many people as they age, and older adults need more time to recover from glare situations. Avoidance of night driving is common due to glare and light and dark adaptation problems, which in turn affects participation in evening social activities.

All individuals begin to lose the ability to focus on near objectives around the age of 40 to 45, due to normal age-related changes in the lens, the structure responsible for properly focusing an image on the retina. As the lens ages, it loses elasticity, resulting in decreased ability of the lens to change shape or accommodate in response to the distance of the object being viewed. This difficulty focusing on near objects, **presbyopia,** makes it difficult to read print and perform close-vision tasks. In addition, the **accommodation** loss further reduces overall visual acuity in middle-age and older adults. Bifocals or reading glasses are often prescribed for presbyopia.

Evidence suggests that not all age-related visual problems result from changes in the eye but are also due to changes in the nervous system (Baltes & Lindenberger, 1997; Madden, 1990). Older adults are slower at processing visual stimuli and need to see stimuli longer before accurately identifying them. Some of these visual perception changes may occur because of degeneration along the optic pathway or in areas of the cortex responsible for processing visual information, and result in slowed information processing and increased perceptual inflexibility that affects image judgment (Bergman, 1980; Moscovitch, 1982; Walsh, 1982). This slowed processing translates into more difficulty with recognition of moving objects, items with a complex figure or ground, and items that appear in and out of light quickly. Personal care tasks as well as instrumental tasks (i.e., driving, housekeeping, and meal preparation) depend on such recognition.

Pathological Changes

In addition to the natural aging process changes, several specific and common visual conditions have a more profound effect on an older adult's functional abilities: cataracts, age-related macular degeneration, glaucoma, and diabetic retinopathy.

Cataracts

The lens may undergo protein degeneration and aggregation with advancing age. The resulting lenticular opacity, a **cataract,** reduces light transmission to the retina, and the lens of the eye will appear cloudy and yellowish. Individuals with cataracts will experience the following:

- Decreased acuity
- Hazy or blurred vision
- Altered color perception
- Increased sensitivity to glare
- Difficulty driving at night
- Difficulty seeing low-contrast objects
- Image distortion (straight lines appear wavy) (Valluri, 1999)

When the cataract interferes with vision to such an extent that functional activities are affected, cataract extraction and lens prosthesis implantation surgery is performed (Brodie, 2003).

Age-Related Macular Degeneration

Age-related macular degeneration (AMD) is a condition affecting people over the age of 50, and about 30% of the population between ages 75 and 81 (Leibowitz et al., 1980). Globally, AMD ranks third as a cause of irreversible visual loss and blindness, and it is the primary cause of visual impairment in industrialized countries (WHO, 2005). AMD is more common in whites and smokers, and those with a blue iris, hypertension, hypercholesteremia, and a family history of the disease. AMD is characterized by retinal atrophy and scarring and hemorrhages in the macula, and it results in a gradual loss of the central field of vision. There are two types of AMD:

1. Dry AMD (nonexudative). This type of AMD is characterized by yellow deposits of extracellular material in the macula (**drusen**). Areas of retinal atrophy may lead to vision loss over time. Dry AMD is the most common type of AMD.
2. Wet AMD (exudative). This type of AMD is more rapidly progressive and is characterized by a proliferation of abnormal blood vessels that leak blood and fluid into the macula.

Medical treatment options are very limited. Wet AMD can sometimes be treated in the early stages of the disease with laser surgery or photocoagulation, to cauterize the new blood vessels and stop their development (Brodie, 2003). However, no known treatment prevents macular degeneration or can reverse the visual loss. Central vision loss can have very negative psychological and social effects. As the macula is responsible for fine-detail vision, reading, needlework, writing, and recognizing faces become very difficult, and problems with distance and depth cues and color and contrast perception are evident. As a result, safe mobility may be affected because of problems with distance and depth cues, and reluctance to participate in social activities, and limitations with ADLs, work, and leisure are common (Watson, 2001). Because people with AMD cannot see items in their central visual field, they may compensate by rotating the head or trunk in such a way as to see the missing information. Training in *eccentric viewing,* the process of aligning the image into a new retinal viewing area, allows the older adult to place the target outside of the blind spot so it can be seen (Fletcher, Schuchard, Livingstone, Crane, & Hu, 1994).

Glaucoma

Glaucoma is a group of diseases characterized by progressive optic nerve damage. Glaucoma is more common in Blacks and Hispanics (Minassian, Reidy, Coffey, & Minassian, 2000), and is projected to affect 79.6 million people by 2020 (Quigley & Broman, 2006). Among blacks, glaucoma presents at a younger age with higher intraocular pressures, is more difficult to control, and is the main irreversible cause of blindness (Sommer et al., 1991). There are several types of glaucoma; however, the two most common in older adults include:

1. Primary open-angle glaucoma (POAG). POAG has a slow and insidious onset. The major risk factor for developing POAG is raised intraocular pressure (IOP). The increased IOP may cause permanent loss of peripheral vision before the individual notes a change in vision, and if left untreated, blindness occurs (Sheldrick, Ng, Austin, & Rosenthal, 1994).
2. Angle-closure glaucoma (ACG). ACG is an acute condition resulting from a sudden blockage of aqueous fluid outflow and acute elevation of IOP. Gradual increase in lens size with advancing age or because of cataracts predisposes the eye to ACG. Symptoms include severe pain, blurry vision, and halos around lights. ACG is a medical emergency (Brodie, 2003).

Glaucoma is treated medically or surgically depending on the type and stage of glaucoma. Medical treatment consists of either topical (eye drops) or systemic medications that will lower the intraocular pressure. If pressure is not relieved enough or if medications are not effective or tolerated, surgery (filtration surgery, laser trabeculectomy) is used to help remove the blockage and increase fluid drainage (Brodie, 2003).

The effect of loss of peripheral vision is great. The individual may not see objects in a path and may bump into objects in the periphery, making ambulation unsafe. Objects or people outside the person's peripheral field of view may suddenly appear, startling the person. In addition, reading and writing may be problematic, as only a small portion of the page can be seen at once (Watson, 2001). The adaptations used by persons with visual field loss resulting from glaucoma are similar to those used by individuals with AMD—the person must increase head or trunk rotation to gather missing sensory information. Regular eye examinations are essential, as early detection and treatment can prevent the visual loss that occurs if glaucoma is left untreated.

Diabetic Retinopathy

Although it can affect all ages, **diabetic retinopathy,** damage to the blood vessels of the retina as a result of diabetes, is a common cause of retina changes in the older adult. Because diabetic neuropathy is a complication of having diabetes, the incidence of diabetic neuropathy typically increases with the length of time a person has diabetes, and the degree and rate of progression of the retinopathy strongly correlate with the level and duration of elevated blood sugars. Thus, good control of blood sugars is essential to prevent diabetic retinopathy and delay its progression (The Diabetes Control and Complications Trial Research Group, 1993; UK Prospective Diabetes Study Group, 1998). Diabetic neuropathy occurs in stages. In the initial stage (nonproliferative stage), microaneurysms form but are reabsorbed by the retina. With time, the retinal capillaries begin to leak fluid into the surrounding tissue, causing retinal edema and producing exudate, which leads to decreased visual acuity. In the later stage (proliferative stage), new blood vessels grow in the retina. These blood vessels easily rupture and produced bleeding into the eye. **Scotomas** in the central vision field often occur (Brodie, 2003).

Symptoms of diabetic neuropathy include fluctuating and blurred vision, decreased contrast sensitivity, problems with driving at night, difficulty with color discrimination, "spotty" visual field losses, and complete blindness. The degree of activity and participation limitations resulting from diabetic retinopathy varies greatly and is dependent on time of diagnosis and severity of the disease. Medical management is dependent on the stage and may include laser to treat the microaneurysms or vitrectomy, a procedure used to remove blood and scar tissue from the vitreous (Brodie, 2003).

Functional and Behavioral Adaptations

What do these visual changes mean for functional performance of the older adult? Vision loss of any type is a significant event in the life of the older adult, not only to the individuals affected but also to their families, their communities, and the health care system. Horowitz (2004), in her review of the consequences of vision impairments in later life, found that vision impairments have one of the greatest impacts on functional ability in older adults, and relationships have been found between vision impairment, diminished overall function, and decreased quality of life (Lee, Spritzer, & Hays, 1997; Mangione, Lee, & Hays, 1996; Salive, Guralnik, Glynn, Christen, Wallace, & Ostfeld, 1994).

Whether acute or gradual in onset or partial or full loss, any vision changes can threaten the functional independence older adults strive to maintain. As mentioned previously, safe mobility is jeopardized because of visual problems. Aside from obvious acuity problems with reading, practical day-to-day tasks, such as housekeeping, shopping, and clothing selection, can be quite frustrating. Color discrimination of critical items, such as food and medication, can be challenging. Common leisure activities such as card playing, sports requiring eye–hand coordination, television viewing, and needlepoint can become extremely difficult for the older adult with age-related visual changes. Glare and sudden illumination contrasts can compromise vision because of slower adaptation. Night vision may be very poor, curtailing many activities, including driving. Dim lighting in restaurants and other public places may contribute to trips and falls. A number of researchers have documented the relationship between visual impairments and falls, and visual impairments and fear of falling, which may further limit social activities of older adults (Campbell, Crews, Moriarty, Zack, & Blackman, 1999; Ivers, Cumming, Mitchell, & Attebo, 1998; Ivers, Norton, Cumming, Butler, & Campbell, 2000).

Visual detail, distance, illumination, and facial acuity of a partner are all important factors for successful communication (Erber & Heine, 1996). Lip reading also plays a vital role in communication, as it provides visual cues to assist in the perception of speech (Erber & Osborn, 1994). Older adults with vision loss will have difficulty seeing their communication partner's face and will have problems picking up nonverbal cues, such as gestures, facial expressions, and body posture, and hearing loss cannot be compensated for by lip reading (Heine & Browning, 2002; Sullivan, 1984).

The older adult's psychological impact to loss of vision varies and is related to personal factors, such as personality characteristics and individual coping strategies; timing and degree of loss; and the use of compensatory strategies. Twenty-five percent of adults with vision impairments report symptoms of depression, compared to 10% of those without impairments (Center on an Aging Society, 2002). Older adults with vision loss may have to stop doing things they enjoy and may feel more isolated and vulnerable (Lambert, West, & Carlin, 1981; Stuen, 1990). It is important to note that the sensitivity of others as well as environmental modifications can assist the older adult in facing visual impairments without undue despair. Adaptation to age-related visual changes is positively affected by support received from one's social network, the use of coping strategies, and knowledge of and access to rehabilitation services (Brennan, 2002; Brennan, Horowitz, Reinhardt, Cimarolli, Benn, & Leonard, 2001).

There are many visual disability questionnaires that can be utilized to examine the impact of visual impairments on the older adult, including the Visual Activities Questionnaire (Sloane, Ball, Owsley, Bruni & Roenkar, 1992), the Activities of Daily Vision Scale questionnaire (Mangione et al., 1992), the VF-14 (Steinberg et al., 1994), the Visual Disability Assessment (VDA) (Pesudovs & Coster, 1998), the National-Eye Institute Visual Functioning Questionnaire-25 (VFQ-25) (Mangione, Lee, Gutierrez, Spritzer, Berry, & Hays, 2001), and the Catquest questionnaire (Lundström, Roos, Jensen, & Fregell, 1997). These questionnaires are widely used in different parts of the world. For example, the VF-14 and VFQ-25 are used in North America, the Catquest is widely used in Europe, and the VDA is used in Australia.

Low-vision rehabilitation is becoming a specialty area for occupational therapists (OTs). OTs working in conjunction with other professionals, including ophthalmologists, neuron-ophthalmologists, optometrists, nurses, social workers, orientation and mobility instructors, and psychologists, can assist older adults in managing and adjusting to their visual impairments through the use of optic devices (Table 5-2), compensation, and environmental

strategies (Box 5-1). The role of the OT in low-vision rehabilitation may be to

- Educate the older adult about low vision
- Teach the older adult how to use his or her prescribed optical and nonoptical devices in ADLs
- Teach the older adult how to function more effectively within the context of the vision loss
- Assist the older adult to develop appropriate adaptive techniques to expand their visual and physical capabilities
- Educate the older adult about vision substitution techniques
- Educate the older adult and the family about general compensation strategies and environmental modifications, such as management of lighting, contrast, and glare
- Address any psychosocial issues
- Refer the older adult to community resources (McCabe, Nason, Demers Turco, Friedman, & Seddon, 2007)

Environmental modifications are easier to implement with the availability of today's technology in older adults' homes or their adult children's homes and in libraries or resource centers. With the use of closed-circuit video units or computers (including laptop computers for those who cannot sit at a computer monitor), older adults can be quite creative in using any residual vision. A large computer screen can automatically increase word or picture size. Many documents available online can now be viewed in a variety of text sizes. It is unknown how many older adults have a personal computer or have access to one, but technology and aging experts report that the numbers are increasing each year (Fox, 2004). With the advent of sound files and personal digital accessories, text can be converted to sound for those with normal hearing.

Hearing and Functional Performance

About 30% of adults between the ages of 65 and 74 years and 50% of those between the ages of 75 and 79 years have some degree of hearing loss (U.S. Bureau of the Census, 1997), and European studies suggest a steady decline in hearing from the sixth to ninth decades (Jonsson & Rosenhall, 1998; Milne, 1977; Pedersen,

TABLE 5-2 Common Optic Devices Used for Older Adults with Vision Loss

Device	Description and Considerations
Strong prescription reading glasses	• Objects appear in focus only when held very close to the eyes • If older adults wear these glasses while walking, can lead to difficulty with mobility

Magnifiers	• Amount of magnification is determined by one's visual acuity
	• Different magnification strengths used for different uses
	• Enlarge objects held at a normal distance
	• Can be handheld (for spot reading), attached to a stand (for continuous reading), head-mounted, or attached to glasses (for hands-free work)
	• Advantages:
	  ◦ Can be used at a greater distance from the eye
	• Disadvantages:
	  ◦ Handheld devices require good hand control, and one hand is always in use

Telescopes	• Can be handheld or mounted onto a pair of glasses
	• Can be monocular or binocular
	• Used to view distant objects
	• Disadvantages:
	  ◦ Stronger telescopes allow only a small field of view—leads to the older adult getting "lost" trying to find the object of interest
	  ◦ Less acceptable cosmetically

Electronic magnification	• Can be achieved through closed-circuit television, video magnification, or computer software in which images are enlarged and contrast is enhanced
	• Advantages:
	  ◦ Provide very high magnification
	• Disadvantages:
	  ◦ Expensive and not very portable

Note that magnification devices can cause nausea and dizziness. Postural support and ergonomics are important aspects to consider.

Source: Data from Watson, G. R. (2001). Low vision in the geriatric population: Rehabilitation and management. *Journal of the American Geriatrics Society, 49,* 317–330.

BOX 5-1 Examples of Communication Strategies and Environmental Modifications for Older Persons with Low Vision

• Use voice or touch to get attention
• Face the older adult
• Ensure adequate lighting in the room (note: high levels of illumination my result in glare)
• Direct the light source from behind the older adult or on the side of the better-seeing eye for reading or writing to reduce glare
• Avoid fluorescent lighting
• Remove clutter and limit number of objects in the environment
• Avoid visual clutter in the environment (e.g., decrease number of prints, posters, or pictures on the walls; use solid colors for background surfaces)

• Enlarge educational/reading materials using a photocopier
• Provide written instructions on nonglossy paper; use high-contrast print and paper and at least 14 to 16 point font; may need even greater font size for people with very poor visual acuity
• Use a large black felt marker for written instructions
• Enhance contrast:
  ◦ Add strips of contrasting tape to the edge of steps
  ◦ Mark light switches with contrasting fluorescent tape

Rosenhall, & Moller, 1989). Vision and hearing along with speech contribute to human communication. Like the visual system, the auditory system likely undergoes many central changes and peripheral changes with age (Bergman, 1985). This fact becomes critical when we consider the importance of hearing for speech in the life of an older adult.

Discussions of hearing loss in old age are problematic because levels of "normal hearing" for the older adult have never been clearly defined (Gelfand & Silman, 1985). For younger people, normal hearing is reflected by a standard decibel level (*loudness*) at selected frequencies (*pitch*) based on published normative data. Normative data do not exist for the older adult. Instead, researchers and clinicians use either a comparison to published **audiograms** of older adults (Konkle, Beasley, & Bess, 1977; Newman & Spitzer, 1983) or some unspecified judgment of functional normalcy for age, such as subject report (Bosatra & Russolo, 1982; Rowe, 1978), to determine hearing problems. Having one's hearing termed "normal for your age" offers little consolation to the older person who cannot hear the water running or the speech sounds of grandchildren.

Since the 1940s and 1950s, there has been a growing body of data on **air conduction hearing,** or hearing tested with tones of various *pitches* (frequencies) through binaural headphones. Through World Fair screening, public health studies, and clinical screening records, age-associated hearing loss has been well documented, particularly higher-frequency loss (Glorig, Wheeler, Quiggle, Grings, & Summerfield, 1957; Montgomery, 1939). Whether hearing loss older adults experience is only **presbycusis,** age-related hearing loss, or hearing loss from and in combination with other causes, such as noise exposure (**sociocusis**), **ototoxic drugs,** or disease is difficult to determine. Environmental conditions can exacerbate age-related hearing loss. For example, deafness among long-term workers in heavy industry has been well documented (Sekuler & Blake, 1985). Studies of older, rural African tribal peoples have not demonstrated the hearing loss seen in older people of European descent (Jarvis & van Heerden, 1967; Rosen, Bergman, Plester, el-Mofty, & Satti, 1962), suggesting the contribution of factors other than age. A diet lacking in B_{12} can affect the rate of hearing loss

(Houston et al., 1999). It also appears that there is a genetic component to some types of hearing loss in later life (Gates, Couropmitree, & Myers, 1999). Regardless of additional factors that may affect hearing, the age effects are inclusive of slow, progressive changes throughout the auditory system (Katz, 2001).

Types of Hearing Loss

Audiologists, professionals who test hearing and treat hearing loss, usually divide hearing loss into conductive, sensorineural, and mixed loss (Figure 5-3).

Conductive hearing loss, or block of acoustic energy that prevents the conduction of sound to the inner ear, may occur because of problems in the external or middle ear (Figure 5-4). External ear infections or too much *cerumen* (wax) buildup in the external canal may cause blockage of sound. The middle ear may be filled with fluid from eustachian tube dysfunction or upper respiratory disease, preventing the three bones of the middle ear from conducting sound efficiently past the eardrum. Diseases of the middle ear that affect bone movement, such as tumors, also can affect the

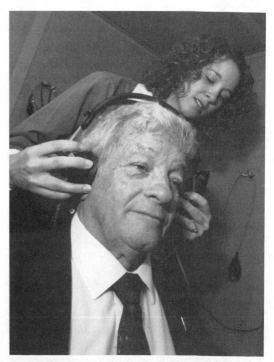

FIGURE 5-3 Audiologist assists client during tinnitus testing in a Tinnitus Clinic. (Photograph by Bert Vanderveen, with permission.)

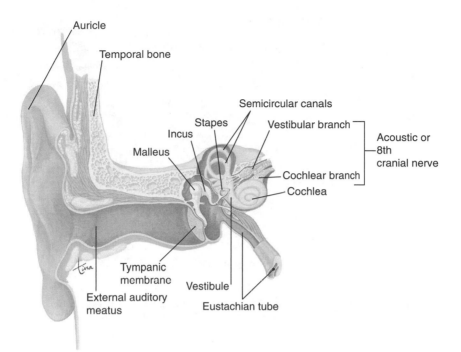

Auricle

Temporal bone

Semicircular canals

Stapes

Vestibular branch

Incus

Acoustic or
8th
cranial nerve

Malleus

Cochlear branch

Cochlea

Tympanic
membrane

Vestibule

External auditory
meatus

Eustachian tube

FIGURE 5-4 Outer, middle, and inner ear structures. (From Scanlon, V. C., & Sanders, T., *Essentials of anatomy and physiology,* 5th ed., F.A. Davis, Philadelphia, 2007, p. 211, with permission.)

mechanical transmission of energy (Davis, 1978; Glass, 1990). Interestingly, people with conductive hearing loss can hear better in noisy surroundings (Kanagala & Berkower, 2003). Conductive-related problems can often be corrected by cleaning of the ear, medication, or surgery. Unfortunately, conduction loss is not the primary cause of hearing loss in the elderly population.

Sensorineural hearing loss results from loss or damage to the sensory hair cells of the *cochlea,* a pea-sized snail-shaped organ of the inner ear (Figure 5-5), or to the nerve cells of the cochlear ganglion, brain stem tracts, or cortex, or a combination of any of these. Age-related changes (presbycusis), medications, noise, acoustic neuroma, and Meniere's disease can all cause sensorineural hearing loss. This type of hearing loss is characterized by better air conduction than bone conduction (Kanagala & Berkower, 2003). At the current time, sensorineural loss due to age-related changes is not correctable, but compensation with a hearing aid is possible.

Presbycusis results in progressive, bilateral high-frequency hearing loss, and four types have been distinguished:

- Sensory presbycusis—characterized by epithelial atrophy and degeneration of hair cells and supporting cells in the Organ of Corti
- Neural presbycusis—characterized by a gradual decrease in first-order neurons within the cochlea and neuron loss along the auditory pathway
- Strial presbycusis—characterized by atrophy and degeneration of the **stria vascularis**
- Cochlear conductive presbycusis—caused by a disorder in the motion mechanics of the cochlear duct (Schuknecht, 1974; Schuknecht & Gacek, 1993)

The hair cells of the cochlea are slowly lost and may be associated with the progressive high-frequency hearing loss of old age (Schuknecht, 1964). Damage to the hair cells can occur from exposure to a variety of drugs or noise. Although, technically, damage to the hair cells is not age related, as a person ages, there is increased opportunity for exposure to these noxious factors (Glass, 1990). Some investigators have found that the cochlear or spiral ganglion undergoes cell loss (Hawkins & Johnsson, 1985; Kirikae, Sato, & Shitara, 1964), but research has found that most sensorineural

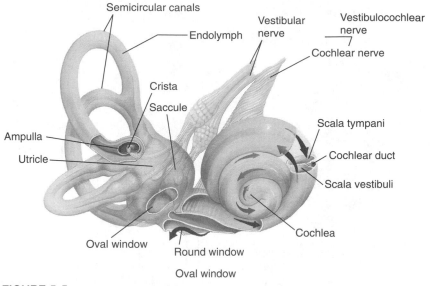

FIGURE 5-5 Inner ear structures. (From Scanlon, V. C., & Sanders, T., *Essentials of anatomy and physiology,* 5th ed., F.A. Davis, Philadelphia, 2007, p. 212, with permission.)

changes seem to occur in the hair cell loss of the lower basal turn of the inner ear (Hawkins & Johnsson, 1985). Investigation of the auditory system of aged monkeys, a system much like that of humans, has demonstrated minimal changes rather than broad nervous system otopathology. Degenerative changes in the *Organ of Corti,* the band containing hair cells, have been likened with those changes seen in AMD (Hawkins & Johnsson, 1985). Research into the role of the cochlea suggests that frequency processing within the cochlea is not affected by age alone and may interact with noise exposure over a lifetime (Bertoli & Probst, 1997; Miller, Dolan, Raphael, & Altschuler, 1998). There are likely age-related factors that may alter the stiffness of the basilar membrane (in the cochlea) or changes in the fluid of the cochlea. These changes can be considered mechanical cochlear changes that affect the hearing of an older adult (Ramotowski & Kimberley, 1998).

Age-related changes beyond the cochlea, those occurring in the brain stem tracts and cortical or central auditory pathways in the temporal lobe, have been very difficult to document from histological studies (Hansen & Reske-Neilsen, 1965; Kirikae et al., 1964; Konigsmark & Murphy, 1972). There may be loss of neurons in parts of the auditory pathway (Kirikae et al., 1964) or a decrease in the number of myelinated axons Konigsmark

& Murphy, 1970). Degeneration of white matter in the brain stem and hearing centers centrally has been reported (Hansen & Reske-Neilsen, 1965), and there appear to be bilateral cell loss in the temporal lobe (Hansen & Reske-Neilsen, 1965) and vascular and neurochemical changes throughout the aging auditory system (Caspary, Milbrandt, & Helfer, 1995; Corso, 1957). The confusing results from these studies of age-related changes in the central auditory pathway may be due to the small number of subjects studied and varied investigational methods (Corso, 1971; Ferraro & Minckler, 1977).

A relatively common, but often unrecognized, cause of hearing loss in the older adult is central auditory processing disorder. The typical pathology is either in the central neuronal connections or in the auditory cortex; however, the peripheral mechanisms are intact. This type of hearing loss is seen in people with neurodegenerative disorders, such as dementia (Kanagala & Berkower, 2003). An interesting and promising line of research in neural auditory problems is related to the study of neurotransmitter changes with aging. Similar to other parts of the CNS and PNS, the auditory nervous system appears to have synaptic areas that suffer from loss of specific neurotransmitters. For example, changes of glutamate and glutamate-related genes with age may be an important factor in the pathogenesis of presbycusis (Tadros, D'Souza, Zettel, Zhu, Waxmonsky, & Frisina, 2007).

An ever-increasing common problem in older adults is **tinnitus,** or the perception of sound in the absence of an acoustic stimulus. Tinnitus is unilateral in about 50% of the cases and is perceived as buzzing, whistling, or ringing in the ears. More than 35 million adults experience tinnitus, and 2 to 3 million are severely affected to the extent that quality of life is affected (Ahmad & Seidman, 2004). The prevalence of tinnitus increases with age and is correlated with both age-related hearing loss and noise-induced hearing loss. There do not appear to be gender differences, although preliminary data indicate there may be racial/ethnic differences (Tucker, Phillips, Ruth, Clayton, Royster, & Todd, 2005). Tinnitus can be caused by a number of factors, including medications and metabolic and vascular diseases, and is difficult to treat. Management can include cognitive therapy, counseling, ear or environment noise masking, and tinnitus retraining therapy (Fortune, Haynes, & Hall, 1999).

Effects of Age-Related Hearing Loss

The effects of conductive hearing loss are easy to understand. Sound is not conducted or is conducted through an obstruction (fluid or wax); thus, sound intensity is reduced. If sound is amplified loudly enough to reach the inner ear, it can then travel along the auditory pathway in a normal fashion—in other words, make it louder and the listener can hear you. Unfortunately, too many people, both young and old, have the misconception that all hearing loss is conductive loss. As stated previously, very few older adults have conductive hearing loss, primarily or at all. Rather, the majority have sensorineural hearing loss alone, or in combination with conductive hearing loss (mixed loss). The sensorineural component effects both hearing sensitivity and speech understanding in very complex ways.

Hearing sensitivity appears to change with age. Lebo and Reddell (1972) examined results from eight previous studies that attempted to specify typical threshold measures for individuals of increasing age (excluding noise-exposed subjects). Their results indicate that after about age 32 for men and age 37 for women, there is nearly always some increase in hearing level or poorer hearing. As age increases, hearing level increases, with the most dramatic difficulty being experienced in hearing the higher frequencies, such as those above 400 Hz. A big difference in hearing level for older men and women probably does not occur when the variable of noise exposure is controlled.

In addition to age-related changes in threshold sensitivity, there appear to be changes in pitch discrimination and auditory reaction time. The older adult's ability to detect small changes in pitch, a skill important for the understanding of both music and speech, may begin to diminish as early as the fourth decade (Koenig, 1957). Beyond age 55, the ability to detect small pitch changes decreases as a linear function of age and becomes more problematic in the higher frequencies. The mechanism or site of lesions for these changes is not known. Like pitch discrimination, auditory reaction time changes with age. Early studies of **dichotic listening,** or simultaneous presentation of different material to each ear, were intended to investigate short-term memory and aging (Ingles, 1962). Later researchers criticized these investigations and pointed out that they were more likely studies of reduced information input and changes in decision making for output responses (Clark & Knowles, 1973). Because older adults are more cautious in responding to auditory stimuli, several researchers have urged that both changes in pitch discrimination and auditory reaction time be evaluated as part of broader changes in perception and cognition that affect behavioral responses (Corso, 1957).

Understanding Speech and Aging

One of the most critical effects of hearing loss and aging is that of difficulties understanding speech. This very complex skill is related to several abilities: speech reception, speech discrimination, and speech understanding in stressful situations. Investigators are challenged to determine if changes in speech understanding are related to peripheral or central changes in the auditory nervous system or to a combination of changes throughout the auditory system. In any case, a reduction or inability to understand speech is the most common reported symptom among elderly hearing-impaired individuals presenting themselves to an audiology clinic.

Speech reception and recognition, typically measured as the intensity level required to produce 50% correct responses for a standard list of words, are reduced with age. This reduction often correlates with a decreased hearing sensitivity (Jerger, 1973). Pestalozza and Shore (1955) found that many older adults had poor speech recognition even with mild hearing loss. Gaeth (1948) described this concept as "phonemic regression"—as a person ages, he or she has less ability to understand **phonemes.** Many other investigators have reached the same conclusions when matching subjects for hearing sensitivity and not age (Jerger, 1971; Kasden, 1970; Luterman, Welsh, & Melrose, 1966).

A closely related auditory skill is speech discrimination. A common characteristic of age-related hearing loss is the decreased ability to hear high-frequency sounds, in particular, *th* and *f,* resulting in poor speech recognition or discrimination (Berry, Mascia, & Steinman, 2007). Speech discrimination is measured clinically by administering a test of phonetically balanced monosyllabic words. The loudness of the words is increased during the test. Corso (1957) and Feldman and Reger (1967) found that younger subjects were relatively stable in this skill; however, by age 80, there was some loss of discrimination. This poor discrimination acuity can affect speech understanding of older adults and can restrict their speech intelligibility input to a more narrow intensive range. This leads to the common complaint *"I can hear you but I can't understand you"* (Mascia, 1994). Speech may be difficult to understand or may not sound clear, and similar words may be confused— *"pat"* and *"bat"* or *"dinner"* and *"thinner"* (Berry et al., 2007).

Personal and Interpersonal Behavior and Hearing Loss

Hearing loss interferes with understanding people's words, detecting clues from the tone of voice, and quick recognition of who is talking (Luey, 1994). When working with older adults, it is important to be able to recognize behaviors that may indicate a hearing loss and the functional consequences that may occur because of the loss. These behaviors include the following:

- Making repeated requests for a person to speak louder or to repeat what was said
- Not responding to verbal questions or conversation

- Giving nonpertinent or inappropriate responses to questions
- Directing questions to spouse, family, or caregiver
- Leaning forward, tilting head to one side
- Showing distress or irritation; becoming disoriented or confused during conversations
- Withdrawing in social situations

Understanding speech during stressful listening conditions is probably the most common and most troublesome for the average older adult. Stressful listening conditions exist daily and everywhere, such as in the automobile, a room with background noise, or in a group speaking situation. Researchers have tried to duplicate these conditions experimentally by altering the acoustic signal, presenting competing noise, or altering the listening environment. Although speech understanding in the elderly population is markedly decreased in the presence of these stressful listening conditions, it should be noted that variability exists among elderly individuals. Each difficult listening condition does not result in the same degree of perceptual difficulty in every older person. Thus, it is difficult to translate speech perception research into a prognosis for any given older individual.

The cumulative consequences of these hearing problems have been shown to affect interpersonal behavior in the older adults. Safety may also be a concern if the older adults cannot hear alarms or if someone is moving toward them— this may increase feelings of vulnerability. At a basic level, older adults may no longer have access to familiar sounds in the environment— they may not hear birds chirping or footsteps approaching—which produces one more strain on the person already adjusting to changes. The embarrassment caused by misunderstanding others may lead to social withdrawal, and poor hearing raises the suspicion that others are mumbling. Thus, family relations may be strained, enjoyment of daily activities may be limited, social interactions may decrease, and isolation and paranoia may increase (Garstecki & Erler, 1998; Hyams, 1982). In people with existing mental health or behavioral problems, such as depression or Alzheimer's disease, a hearing loss may result in increased disability (Cohen, 1990). Investigators have noted that poor understanding of speech may appear to others as related to cognitive decline, when in fact it is likely a consequence of hearing loss (Schneider, Daneman, & Pichora-Fuller, 2002; Wahl & Heyl, 2003).

Beard (1969), in interviewing 270 centenarians, determined that hearing loss is much more gradual than loss of vision; however, the subjects reported more trouble adjusting to the changes in hearing. In more recent studies where both vision and hearing impairments were examined, vision impairments were found to consistently have the stronger effect on predicting negative mental health outcomes (Carabellese et al., 1993; Wallhagen, Strawbridge, Shema, Kurata, & Kaplan, 2001). However, older adults with concurrent impairments in both vision and hearing are most at risk of depression compared to those with a single impairment in either vision or hearing (Carabellese et al., 1993; Lupsakko, Mäntyjärvi, Kautiainen, & Sulkava, 2002).

Several attitude or perceptions scales exist for use with older adults with hearing loss, and these instruments are typically administered by an audiologist. One example, the Hearing Handicap Inventory for the Elderly (Figure 5-6), examines hearing difficulties and the impact on ADLs, such as time spent in conversation, reluctance to talk on the phone or in face-to-face conversations, and self and others' perceptions of the hearing loss (Ventry & Weinstein, 1982).

Treating the hearing loss can result in significant clinical improvement in the older person's functioning, particularly in an improved ability to attend to, understand, and respond to speech. It is particularly critical for older adults to be able to hear speech if they need the help of a mental health professional (Dunkle & Hooper, 1983; Hooper & Johnson, 1992). A variety of adaptation techniques, accommodations, and devices are available that can make communication easier. Box 5-2 outlines some communication strategies and environmental modifications that can be introduced to optimize communication and function in older adults with hearing loss.

An audiologist can introduce a hearing-impaired older adult to the many technologies that exist, which, coupled with "communication courtesy," will enhance aural functioning (Gates & Rees, 1997). Several kinds of hearing aids are available (Figure 5-7A, B, C): (1) behind the ear—fits behind the ear and has a small ear hook that extends over the top of the auricle into the ear canal; (2) in the canal—looks like a large earplug and fits in the ear canal; and (3) completely in the canal—is nearly invisible, because it is so small it almost completely inserts into the canal (Watson & Maino, 2007). The National Council on the Aging (1999) survey of 2300 hearing-impaired adults age 50 or older found that hearing loss in older persons can have a significant negative impact on quality of life. Those with untreated hearing loss were more likely to report depression, anxiety, and paranoia and less likely to participate in organized activities, compared to those who wore hearing aids. Unfortunately, most hearing aids work best in a quiet environment, because they amplify all sounds equally. As a result, communication with a hearing aid

BOX 5-2 Examples of Communication Strategies and Environmental Modifications for Older Persons with Hearing Loss

- Communication
  - Face the older adult directly
  - Get visual attention before speaking
  - Speak clearly using a low-tone voice and moderate rate of speech
  - Approach the older adult from the front to avoid startling
  - Reduce glare and ensure adequate lighting to enhance visual and nonverbal cues
  - Do not shout
  - Rephrase if the message is not understood
- Television, radio, music
  - Closed captioning, assisted listening devices, remote controls to select programming
  - Avoid having on constantly
- Background noise
  - Carpeting on floors, acoustical tiles on ceiling, drapes on windows, upholstered furniture rather than wood and metal furniture, and banners from high ceilings absorb sound
  - Older adult should sit away from distracting background noises, windows and plaster walls; should avoid crowded areas
- Safety
  - Alerting devices (e.g., flashing lights or vibro-tactile devices) or lower-pitched rings for smoke detectors, doorbells, and telephones
  - Volume controls for telephones
- Other
  - Amplified doorbells, voice and telephone ringers

Instructions:

The purpose of this scale is to identify the problems your hearing loss may be causing you. Answer YES, SOMETIMES, or NO for each question. Do not skip a question if you avoid a situation because of your hearing problem. If you use a hearing aid, please answer the way you hear without the aid.

	Yes (4)	SOMETIMES (2)	NO (0)
S-1. Does a hearing problem cause you to use the phone less often than you would like?	___	___	___
E-2. Does a hearing problem cause you to feel embarrassed when meeting new people?	___	___	___
S-3. Does a hearing problem cause you to avoid groups of people?	___	___	___
E-4. Does a hearing problem make you feel irritable?	___	___	___
E-5. Does a hearing problem cause you to feel frustrated when talking to members of your family?	___	___	___
S-6. Does a hearing problem cause you difficulty when attending a party?	___	___	___
E-7. Does a hearing problem cause you to feel "stupid" or "dumb"?	___	___	___
S-8. Do you have difficulty hearing when someone speaks in a whisper?	___	___	___
E-9. Do you feel handicapped by a hearing problem?	___	___	___
S-10. Does a hearing problem cause you difficulty when visiting friends, relatives, or neighbors?	___	___	___
S-11. Does a hearing problem cause you to attend religious services less often than you would like?	___	___	___
E-12. Does a hearing problem cause you to be nervous?	___	___	___
S-13. Does a hearing problem cause you to visit friends, relatives, or neighbors less often than you would like?	___	___	___
E-14. Does a hearing problem cause you to have arguments with your family members?	___	___	___
S-15. Does a hearing problem cause you difficulty when listening to TV or radio?	___	___	___
S-16. Does a hearing problem cause you to go shopping less often than you would like?	___	___	___
E-17. Does any problem or difficulty with your hearing upset you at all?	___	___	___
E-18. Does any problem cause you to want to be by yourself?	___	___	___
S-19. Does a hearing problem cause you to talk to family members less often than you would like?	___	___	___
E-20. Do you feel that any difficulty with your hearing limits or hampers your personal or social life?	___	___	___
S-21. Does a hearing problem cause you difficulty when in a restaurant with relatives or friends?	___	___	___
S-22. Does a hearing problem cause you to feel depressed?	___	___	___
S-23. Does a hearing problem cause you to listin to TV or radio less often than you would like?	___	___	___
E-24. Does a hearing problem cause you to feel uncomfortable when talking to friends?	___	___	___
E-25. Does a hearing problem cause you to feel left out when you are with a group of people?	___	___	___

FOR CLINICAN'S USE ONLY: Total Score: _____
Subtotal E: _____
Subtotal S: _____

This self-assessment tool is designed to assess the effects of hearing impairment on the emotional and social adjustment of elderly people. The inventory is comprised of 25 items and is divided into two subscales: the 13-item emotional subscale explores emotional consequences of hearing impairment; the 12-item social/situational subscale explores both social and situational effects. The scoring and response system of the Hearing Handicap Index for the Elderly (HHIE) is quite simple; a "yes" response is awarded 4 points, a "no" or *"nonapplicable"* response 0 points, and "sometimes" 2 points. Scores on the HHIE range from 0% suggesting no handicap to 100% suggesting total handicap.

FIGURE 5-6 Hearing Handicap Index for the Elderly. (From Ventry, I., & Weinstein, B. (1982). The Hearing Handicap Inventory for the elderly: A new tool. *Ear & Hearing, 3,*128–134.)

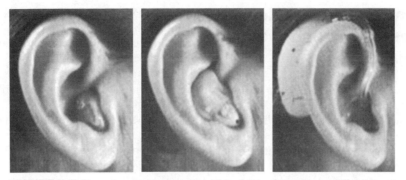

FIGURE 5-7 Three types of hearing aids (from left to right): (A) small in-the-ear, (B) larger in-the-ear, and (C) behind-the-ear aids. (Source: Celia Hooper's online course, CSD 250 Concepts in Communication Sciences, UNCG, Fall 2006, https:// blackboard.uncg.edu/webapps/portal/frameset.jsp?tab=courses&url=/bin/common/course. pl?course_id=_68452_1, with permission.)

can be frustrating because background noise is picked up. Although hearing aids can reduce depression, the remaining communication struggles can be depressing in themselves (The National Council on the Aging, 1999).

Assistive listening devices (ALDs), which consist of a headphone and a microphone, amplify the primary signal and not the competing noise (Figure 5-8A, B). Thus, ALDs are more advantageous when background noise exists (Watson & Maino, 2007). Telephone amplification, personal communication devices, and room amplification systems with individual receivers are examples of technologies that may be of benefit for older adults with hearing loss.

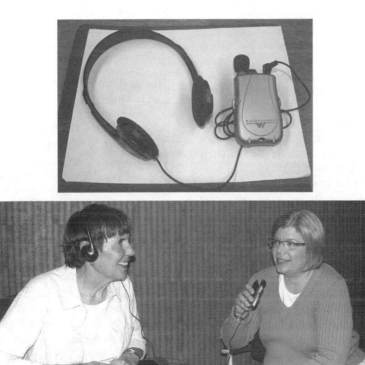

FIGURE 5-8 An assistive listening device, consisting of (A) a headphone and (B) a microphone, improves the ease of communication. (Courtesy of The Rural and Remote Memory Clinic, Saskatoon, Saskatchewan, Canada, with permission.)

Taste and Smell: Physical Changes and Functional Performance

Although taste and smell are quite different mechanisms anatomically, they are considered together because of their functional link to the flavor of food. Taste and smell change with age but are also very sensitive to environmental effects such as smoking. Both smell and taste complaints are common in older persons. Survey studies have found a large proportion of older individuals complain about the taste of food and of taste and smell problems (Murphy, 1993; Schiffman, 1983; Stevens & Lawless, 1981). Research indicates that taste changes relatively little with age in comparison to smell which undergoes more significant change; thus, chemosensory complaints and associated disturbances of older adults are more likely due to olfactory changes rather than alterations in taste (Deems et al., 1991; Stevens, Bartoshuk, & Cain, 1984).

The cause of taste changes in normal aging in the absence of disease and medications is not fully understood. Some have found decreased numbers of papillae or taste buds, but others have not found losses with normal aging. Poorer flavor discrimination (Cain, Reid, & Stevens, 1990; Stevens, Cain, Demarque, & Ruthruff, 1991) and a decreased ability to identify foods in the mouth (Murphy, 1985) have been reported in older adults. However, because food flavor arises largely from olfactory stimulation, it is possible these changes more likely reflect age-related declines in olfactory function. Changes in taste, or *gustation,* have been noted by researchers who have examined the basic tastes of sweet, salty, bitter, and sour substances— subjects are asked to sip a substance in a liquid and identify it or differentiate it from water. The ability to detect and discriminate between sweet, sour, salty, and bitter tastes deteriorates as one ages (Kaneda, Maeshima, & Goto, 2000), and the thresholds for salt and bitter tastes show age-related increases (Weiffenbach, Baum, & Burghauser, 1982). Some investigators have found that older subjects confuse tastes, which may be attributed to the presence of fungus in the mouth, the aspiration of oral contents, the wearing of dentures, or the commonly found changes in the mouth tissue of older adults (Shay & Ship, 1995). In addition, medications and medical conditions play a major role in taste losses and distortions. For example, clinical studies have implicated over 250 drugs in altered taste sensations (Schiffman, 1983; Schiffman, 1991).

As mentioned above, **olfaction** plays a major role in the sensory and pleasure experience of eating and provides early warning of dangers, such as fire, dangerous fumes, leaking gas, spoiled foods, and polluted environments. Thus, smell dysfunction can significantly diminish the quality of life and can even be life threatening (Doty, Shaman, & Dann, 1984). Changes in the olfactory tract and bulb are similar to overall CNS changes, typically generalized atrophy with a loss of neurons. Degeneration of the sensory cells of the nasal mucosa has been documented, such that by the ninth decade, the olfactory threshold increases by about 50%, contributing to poor smell recognition (Dharmarajan & Ugalino, 2000). Smell identification is impaired with increased age, even in generally healthy individuals. It appears that the ability to identify odors correctly increasingly deteriorates with greater age, especially in men (Ship, Pearson, Cruise, Brant, & Metter, 1996). Various aspects of age-related decline in olfactory function have been reported:

- Higher detection thresholds (Deems & Doty, 1987; Murphy, 1986; Stevens & Cain, 1987)
- A decline in suprathreshold sensitivity for odors (Murphy, 1983; Stevens & Cain, 1985, 1986; Stevens, Plantinga, & Cain, 1982)
- Impaired ability to identify and discriminate odors (Doty, Shaman, Applebaum, Giberson, Sikorski, & Rosenberg, 1984; Schemper, Voss, & Cain, 1981; Schiffman & Leffingwell, 1981; Schiffman & Warwick, 1991; Stevens & Cain, 1985, 1987; Stevens et al., 1982)

Taste and smell changes with age may be functionally important for the individual. For example, some older people report flavor changes, and that eating is less pleasurable (Rolls, 1999), a problem that may be compounded by the need to reduce salt intake in people with high blood pressure. Thus, older adults who need specific dietary regimens may not adhere to those regimens. Changes in taste and smell have a common factor in the neuronal degeneration of the lower part of the postcentral gyrus, where these sensations are "appreciated" (Purves et al., 2004). If this is the case, there would not be a sensory change per se but a change in sensory integration or sensory comprehension. Functionally, changes in these senses can reduce pleasure from eating and lead to decreased food intake or alterations in food choices. As a result, subsequent exacerbation of disease risk, weight loss, and nutritional and immune deficiencies can occur (Roberts & Rosenberg, 2006). In addition, some suggest that older adults with chemosensory decrements may be at greater risk for food poisoning or overexposure to environmentally hazardous chemicals that might otherwise be detected by taste and smell (Schiffman, 1997).

Somesthesis: Physical Changes and Functional Performance

Somesthesis includes the sensations that arise from light and deep touch of the skin and the viscera, vibration, pain, and temperature, as well as **kinesthesis,** the sensation and awareness of active or passive movement (see Chapter 6 for a discussion on age-related changes in vibration and proprioception). Similar to research of other sensory modalities, research in somesthesis demonstrates change with advancing age, but environmental effects cannot be ruled out; for example, neuropathies and structural changes in the skin (e.g., thinning) make age-related changes almost impossible to detect in the purest sense.

Touch and Pressure

The skin receptors responsible for the perception of pressure and light touch, **pacinian** and **Meissner's corpuscles,** undergo structural changes and decline in number (Gescheider, Beiles, Checkosky, Bolanowski, & Verrillo, 1994), such that by the ninth decade they are only one third of their original density (Bolton, Winkelmann, & Dyck, 1966). In addition, the sensory fibers innervating the peripheral receptors undergo changes and decline, and the speed, quantity, or quality of information processing may be affected (Woodward, 1993). Decreased response to tactile stimuli, higher touch thresholds (e.g., firmer stimulation of the skin is required before the stimulus is detected), and decreased ability to detect touch and pressure have been reported in some older adults (Desrosiers, Hebert, Bravo, & Dutil, 1996; Stevens & Choo, 1996;

Thornbury & Mistretta, 1981; Woodward, 1993). It is important to note that the degree of change is highly variable, in that the effects vary greatly in their magnitude across individuals. Donat and colleagues (2005) reported that although touch/pressure was decreased in individuals over 60, statistically significant differences were not found between age groups (60 to 69, 70 to 79, over 80), suggesting that age-related changes in touch/pressure may not be progressive in healthy older adults. Interestingly, a recent research study that had subjects train two-point discrimination tactile skills found tactile ability may be preserved and improved with therapeutic interventions (Dinse, Kleibel, Kalisch, Ragert, Wilimzig, & Tegenthoff, 2006).

Touch provides important information about one's environment, plays a role in communication, and is an important prerequisite for adequate performance of manual tasks (Carmeli, Patish, & Coleman, 2003; Francis & Spirduso, 2000). The extent to which age-related skin changes contribute to change of touch sensation has yet to be determined. Older adults who experience loss or a decrease in tactile acuity or sensitivity will have difficulty localizing and identifying stimuli. Response time may be decreased, as the speed and intensity in which the stimuli are perceived are reduced. An older person must take special care to avoid injury from prolonged pressure on the skin. Changes in tactile sensitivity will result in increased reliance on other sensory systems for information, a problem for older adults with contaminant changes in vision.

Pain

Age-related changes in the perception of pain have been a topic of interest for several years; however, the effects of aging on pain perception remain unclear. Although studies of experimental pain support the view that pain thresholds (e.g., the older adult can tolerate a more extreme stimulus without perceiving it to be painful) to short-duration noxious stimuli are increased in older adults, research has yielded inconsistent findings; for example, some researchers have reported increased thermal pain thresholds in older adults (Chakour, Gibson, Bradbeer, & Helme, 1996; Lautenbacher & Strian, 1991; Procacci, Bozza, & Buzelli, 1970; Sherman & Robillard, 1960), and an equal number of researchers have reported no age-related differences in heat pain thresholds (Edwards & Fillingim, 2001; Hardy, Wolff, & Goodell, 1943; Harkins, Price, & Martinelli, 1986; Heft, Cooper, O'Brien, Hemp, & O'Brien, 1996). It is likely that pain perception is decreased in later years, in particular, deep pain perception (Katzman & Terry, 1983). For example, a retrospective study of elderly people with peritonitis found that abdominal pain was absent in almost half of the cases (Wroblewski & Mikulowski, 1991), and myocardial infarction is often unrecognized in persons aged 75 to 79 years (Sigurdsson, Thorgeirsson, Sigvaldason, & Sigfusson, 1995).

How age affects the perception of pain, level of discomfort experienced, and suffering associated with pain is not certain. Psychological factors may alter pain experience in elderly people (Gibson & Helme, 1995), and older adults may be conservative in reporting pain and underreport pain intensity (Clark & Mehl, 1971; Yong, Gibson, Horne, & Helme, 2001). The nociceptive pathways of older adults undergo numerous and widespread changes in morphology, electrophysiology, neurochemistry, and function with aging (Box 5-3). Many of these changes could affect pain perception (Burchinsky, 1985), but more research is needed regarding the mechanisms involved in nociception in older adults, specific changes that are associated with pain perception and their related functional consequences.

Temperature

It is unclear how much of the thermoregulatory impairments seen in older adults are age related. Skin structure changes (e.g., thinning), decreased vascularization, chronic disease processes, personal health habits, such as smoking, and a sedentary lifestyle may all play a role (Lybarger & Kilbourne, 1985). Thermoreceptors, which are sensitive to the surrounding environment changes (external and internal), help to regulate and maintain a constant body temperature. Cold and heat receptors are found in the skin, spinal cord, and hypothalamus, and the skin receptors provide the hypothalamus with important information about the need to generate, converse, or dissipate heat (Hissa, 1990). Due to age-related changes, older adults are less able to sense changes in skin temperature and are more likely to experience thermoregulatory problems. Research on thermal extremes of hot and cold found that older adults have increased thresholds in the hand and foot compared to younger adults (Jamal, Hansen, Weir, & Ballantyne, 1985; Kenshalo, 1986). Stevens and Choo (1998) found thermal sensitivity declines with age, and that the greatest changes in sensitivity occurred in the extremities,

BOX 5-3 Structural and Biochemical Changes Affecting Pain Perception in Older Adults

- Decreased density of unmyelinated fibers by age 60 (Ochoa & Mair, 1969)
  - Selective loss of unmyelinated fibers 1.2–1.6 μm in diameter (Ochoa & Mair, 1969)
  - 50% loss in unmyelinated afferent fibers in persons aged 65–75 years (Verdu, Ceballos, Vilches, & Navarro, 2000)
- Decreased density of myelinated fibers
  - 35% loss in myelinated afferent fibers in persons 65–75 years (Verdu et al., 2000)
  - Decrease in large-diameter afferents and finely myelinated afferents (0.1–5.0 μm) (Jacobs & Love, 1985)
- Decreased peripheral nerve conduction velocity (Alder & Nacimiento, 1988)
- Marked reduction in **substance P** content—in aged human skin (Helme & McKernan, 1984), in thoracic and lumbar dorsal root ganglion cells (Khalil, Ralevic, Bassirat, Dusting, & Helme, 1994)

- Dorsal horn sensory neurons:
  - Marked loss of myelin; signs of damage (e.g., axonal involution especially in the medial lemniscal pathways); altered spinal neurochemistry (e.g., age-related loss of serotonergic and noradrenergic neurons in the dorsal horn (Ko, King, Gordon, & Crisp, 1997; Prineas & Spencer, 1975)
- Cortex, midbrain, brain stem:
  - Neuronal death, loss of dendritic arborization, neurofibrillary abnormalities (Pakkenberg & Gundersen, 1997)
  - Decreased synthesis, axonal transport, uptake, and receptor binding of neurotransmitters (Grachev, Fredrickson, & Apkarian, 2000; McGeer & McGeer, 1976; Rogers & Bloom, 1985; Wong et al., 1984)

especially the foot. Interestingly, they found that central regions of the body lost sensitivity more slowly compared to the extremities which showed the greatest and earliest change with age.

Part of the inability to cope with environmental temperature extremes is related to the decrease in perception of the thermal environment and changes in the ability to generate and conserve heat. In response to increased temperatures, older adults are not able to increase cutaneous blood flow as effectively as younger adults. Sweating is also impaired; and in response to a cold environment, the shivering response and the cutaneous vasoconstrictor response are less effective. The physiologic deficits could be compensated for by conscious behavioral responses (e.g., wearing appropriate clothing layers, moving to a cooler environment, decreasing activity level). However, because of the perception deficit, implementation of preventative measures may not be seen as necessary (Dharmarajan & Bullecer, 2003). Age-related changes may make it more difficult for the older adult to detect a difference between cool and cold or warm and hot, and decreased temperature sensitivity increases the risk of injuries, such as frostbite, hypothermia, and burns. Because older adults are more adversely affected by extremes of hot or cold, many social service agencies have special programs for the elderly population during the very hot or cold times of the year.

■ Summary

Although age-related changes in the sensory systems are numerous and may cause activity and participation limitations, many older adults can and do adapt to these changes. Sensation and perception in the sensory systems have some common themes:

1. Sensitivity may be decreased.
2. Perceptual changes may reflect general nervous system changes rather than specific changes of the sensory modality.
3. A reaction in an experimental condition may be conservative and more reflective of general slower CNS information processing, rather than a specific change to the sensory modality.
4. Perception over a lifetime may become learned and automatic, with a maintenance of functional skills even in the presence of sensory decline.

There are both positive and negative aspects to the learned sensory and perceptual patterns one adopts over a life span. On the one hand, the older adult can "fill in" missing information based on remembered events and learned contexts. On the other hand, life can be more challenging or even dangerous if sounds, sights, smells, tastes, and other sensory events are misperceived and erroneously interpreted—questions may be answered incorrectly, the struggle to communicate may result in withdrawal, unsafe situations may go undetected, something harmful may be touched, and enjoyment from previous pleasurable sensory events, such as movies, religious events, conversations, and music may be lost.

Some researchers have found that changes in sensory and perceptual information are reflective of overall nervous system deterioration and, in particular, cognitive function (Baltes & Smith, 1997). However, changes in cognition may affect adaptation to the physical environment, and research in age-related cognitive changes (see Chapter 9) may be biased by sensory and perceptual abilities of older subjects (Wahl & Heyl, 2003). Of course, there is much more to cognition, but the role of sensory sensitivity diminution must be taken into account. For example, a negative correlation between hearing sensitivity and scores on intelligence or memory tasks has been found (Kenshalo, 1977; Li & Lindenberger, 2002; Thomas, Hunt, Garry, Hood, Goodwin, & Goodwin, 1983).

There are two important facts about the sensory perceptual systems and their neural pathways that need to be considered: (1) they are integrated at a higher cortical level, the "association cortex"; and, (2) it is likely that sensory and perceptual losses share a common component of degeneration, such as neurotransmitter changes or basic cell action alterations. These common connections and associations may have functional effects. Just as the older adult "can't hear without my glasses on," he or she may find one sensory pathway aiding another as sensitivity decreases. Although, unlike a young adult who can compensate well if one sensory system is affected, the older adult may be compensating or adapting to sensory or perceptual losses with systems that are likewise impaired. Perhaps learned patterns and memory of sensory stimuli play a greater role than compensation for some events. This is an area that is yet to be examined.

Case Study

Mr. Elliott Fedricks is an 82-year-old man who lives in a condominium, with the support of a home health aide, Sally, who provides services for 3 hours a day, 3 days per week. Mr. Fedricks was diagnosed with mild cognitive impairment 2 years ago and has diabetes. Mr. Fedricks' only son, daughter-in-law, and three grandchildren live out of town. His son checks in every other day by telephone and visits every 2 months for the weekend. Mr. Fedricks had been very active with the social and recreational activities that are organized by the condominium's social club—he played bridge 3 days a week, he attended the weekly pot-luck social and movie night, he worked in the wood-working shop making toys for his grandchildren, and he participated in the daily water aerobics fitness class.

Sally tells you that Mr. Fedricks has been complaining of blurred vision on occasion, and she notices he has been having difficulty picking out his pills when she puts them on the placemat. Sally is also concerned that Mr. Fedricks' cognitive problems are getting worse—he seems to have difficulty understanding questions and frequently asks Sally to repeat what she has said or changes the subject when asked questions. In addition, Mr. Fedricks seems to be less interested in participating in his usual activities. He frequently tells Sally he is too tired to attend and often sleeps in the afternoon.

Questions

1. What might be contributing to Mr. Fedricks' recent visual complaints? What should you do?
2. What might be contributing to Mr. Fedricks' change in his participation in social and recreational activities?
3. What common assumption did Sally make regarding Mr. Fedricks' cognitive problems?
4. If Mr. Fedricks is experiencing both a visual loss and a hearing loss, what are the implications?

Review Questions

1. What general sensory changes occur with aging in all sensory organs or systems?
2. How might changes in sensory systems affect the older adult's behavior? Are any changes generally more devastating than others? Why or why not?
3. How might an older adult change his or her daily activities as a result of visual changes? Auditory changes?
4. How might social function change for an older adult who cannot understand speech sounds normally? Who has tinnitus?
5. What dangers might an older adult face because of changes in taste, smell, or superficial sensations? Based on known physiological changes, are any of these dangers more likely to occur than others in the vast majority of older adults?
6. Imagine that you are designing a retirement or life care center, or group home for well older adults. Taking the research about sensory system and sensory integrative changes into account, what are a few important steps you would take to ensure that sensory stimuli are received optimally by all residents of your facility? Think beyond local and federal legislation or regulations related to health and safety and (a) design the facility, taking into account financial constraints, and (b) design the ideal facility. Think sensory systems and technology!
7. Identify adaptations, strategies, and interventions commonly used for older adults to compensate for sensory deficits in vision, hearing, taste, touch, and smell. What suggestions might you, as an occupational therapist, be able to provide to an older adult experiencing sensory changes?

Web-Based Resources

www.lrc.rpi.edu/programs/lightHealth/AARP/index.asp, **Lighting Research Center,** date connected May 30, 2007. This page has guidelines for designing lighting for older adults. Three sets of guidelines are available in pdf format: (1) the general public, including older adults and their families; (2) designers and builders; and (3) health care professionals.

www.homemods.org/library/life%2Dspan/, **Stein Gerontological Institute** and the **American Association of Retired People** entitled *Life-Span Design of Residential Environments for an Aging Population,* date connected, May 30, 2007. The section on "Low-Tech Applications and Retrofit" has a subsection entitled *Sensory and Perceptual Considerations in Designing Environments for the Elderly* .

www.nei.nih.gov, **The National Eye Institute (NEI),** one of the **U.S.A.'s federal government's National Institutes of Health (NIH),** date connected, May 30, 2007. The website has numerous resources including educational information on eye diseases and disorders, eye care resources, photos images and videos, statistics and data on common eye disease, and information on eye health research.

www.asha.org/public/hearing/disorders/default.htm, **American Speech-Language Hearing Association,** date connected, May 30, 2007. This webpage contains information on the causes and effects hearing loss.

www.hear-it.org/page.dsp?page=2745, **Hear-it AISBL,** date connected, May 30, 2007. Hear-it AISBL is an international nonprofit and noncommercial organization whose objective is to collect, process, and circulate all and any up-to-date scientific (sociological, legal, medical, public, policy related) and other relevant information including personal stories pertaining to hearing impairments and their human and socioeconomic consequences. This particular weblink contains information related to hearing loss and the older adult. The site is also available in Español, Deutsch, and Francais.

www.healthinsite.gov.au/topics/Hearing_Impairments, **HealthInsite,** date connected, May 20, 2007. An Australian Government Initiative.

Many resources and weblinks related to hearing loss in older adults and other health-related topics are found on this site.

REFERENCES

Ahmad, N., & Seidman, M. (2004). Tinnitus in the older adult: Epidemiology, pathophysiology and treatment options. *Drugs & Aging, 21,* 297-305.

Alder, G., & Nacimiento, A. C. (1988). Age-dependent changes in short-latency somatosensory evoked potentials in healthy adults. *Applied Neurophysiology, 51,* 55-59.

Baltes, P. B., & Lindenberger, U. (1997). Emergence of a powerful connection between sensory and cognitive function across the adult lifespan: A new window to the study of cognitive aging? *Psychology and Aging, 12,* 12–21.

Baltes, P. B., & Smith, J. (1997). A systematic-wholistic view of psychological functioning in very old age. Introduction to a collection of articles from the Berlin Aging Study. *Psychology and Aging, 12,* 395–409.

Beard, B. B. (1969). Sensory decline in very old age. *Gerontologia Clinica, 11,* 149–158.

Bergman, M. (1980). *Aging and the perception of speech.* Baltimore, MD: University Park Press.

Bergman, M. (1985) Hearing and aging: An introduction and overview. In J. Roush (Ed), *Seminars in hearing: Aging and hearing impairment* (pp. 99–114). New York: Thieme-Stratton.

Berry, P., Mascia, J., & Steinman, B. A. (2007). Auditory impairment in the older adult. In A. A. Rosenbloom & M. W. Morgan (Eds.), *Vision and aging.* St. Louis, MO: Butterworth-Heinemann.

Bertoli, S., & Probst, R. (1997). The role of transient-evoked otoacoustic emission testing in the evaluation of elderly persons. *Ear & Hearing, 18,* 286–293.

Bolton, C. F., Winkelmann, R. K., & Dyck, P. J. (1966). A quantitative study of Meissner's corpuscles in man. *Neurology, 16,* 1–9.

Bosatra, A., & Russolo, M. (1982). Comparison between central tonal tests in elderly subjects. *Audiology, 21,* 334–341.

Brennan, M. (2002). Spirituality and psychosocial development in middle-age and older adults with vision loss. *Journal of Adult Development, 9* (1), 31–46.

Brennan, M., Horowitz, A., Reinhardt, J. P., Cimarolli, V., Benn, D. T., & Leonard, R. (2001). In their own words: Strategies developed by visually impaired elders to cope with vision loss. *Journal of Gerontological Social Work, 35* (1), 63–85.

Brodie, S. E. (2003). Aging and disorders of the eye. In R. C. Tallis & H. M. Fillit (Eds.), *Brocklehurst's textbook of geriatric medicine and gerontology* (6th ed., pp. 735–748). Philadelphia: Churchill Livingstone.

Brody, B. L., Gamst, A. C., Williams, R. A., Smith, A. M., Lau, P. W., Dolnak, D., et al. (2001). Depression, visual acuity, comorbidity, and disability associated with age-related macular degeneration. *Ophthalmology, 108* (10), 1893–1901.

Burchinsky, S. G. (1985). Changes in the functional interactions of neurotransmitter systems during aging: Neurochemical and clinical aspects: A review. *Journal of Clinical Experimental Gerontology, 7,* 1–30.

Butler, R., Faye, E., Guazzo, E., & Kupfer, C. (1997). Keeping an eye on vision: Primary care of age-related ocular disease. *Geriatrics, 52* (8), 30–38.

Cain, W. S., Reid, F., & Stevens, J. C. (1990). Missing ingredients: Aging and the discrimination of flavor. *Journal of Nutrition for the Elderly, 9,* 3–15.

Campbell, V. A., Crews, J. E., Moriatry, D. G., Zack, M. M., Blackman, D. K. (1999). Surveillance for sensory impairment, activity limitation, and health-related quality of life among older adults—United States 1993–1997. *Morbidity and Mortality Weekly Report, Centers for Disease Control and Prevention, 48,* 131–156.

Carabellese, C., Appollonio, I., Rozzini, R., Bianchetti, A., Frisoni, G. B., Frattola, L., et al. (1993). Sensory impairment and quality of life in a community elderly population. *Journal of the American Geriatrics Society, 41* (4), 401–407.

Carmeli, E., Patish, H., & Coleman, R. (2003). The aging hand. *Journal of Gerontology Series A: Biological Sciences and Medical Sciences, 58,* M146–M152.

Caspary, D. M., Milbrandt, J. C., & Helfer, R. H. (1995). Central auditory aging: GABA changes in the inferior colliculus. *Experimental Gerontology, 30,* 349–360.

Cech, D. J., & Martin, S. (2002). *Functional movement development across the lifespan* (2nd ed.). Philadelphia: W.B. Saunders.

Center on an Aging Society. (2002). *Visual impairment data profile, Number 3.* Retrieved May 13, 2007, from http://ihcrp.Georgetown.edu/agingsociety/pdfs/viual.pdf.

Chakour, M. C., Gibson, S. J., Bradbeer, M., & Helme, R. D. (1996). The effect of age on A-delta and C-fibre thermal pain perception. *Pain, 64,* 143–152.

Clark, L. E., & Knowles, J. B. (1973). Age differences in dichotic listening. *Journal of Gerontology, 28,* 173–178.

Clark, W. C., & Mehl, L. (1971). Thermal pain: A sensory decision theory analysis of the effect of age and sex on various response criteria, and 50 percent pain threshold. *Journal of Abnormal Psychology, 78,* 202–212.

Cohen, G. D. (1990). Psychology and mental health in the mature and elderly adult. In J. E. Birren & K. W. Schaie (Eds.), *Handbook of the psychology of aging,* (3rd ed., pp. 359–371). San Diego, CA: Academic Press.

Corso, J. F. (1957). Confirmation of normal discrimination loss for speech on CID Auditory Test W-22. *Laryngoscope, 67,* 365–370.

Corso, J. F. (1971). Sensory process and age effects in normal adults. *Journal of Gerontology, 26,* 90–105.

Crews, J. E., & Campbell, V. A. (2001). Health conditions, activity limitations and participation restrictions among older people with visual impairments. *Journal of Visual Impairment & Blindness, 95* (8), 458–467.

Curcio, C. A., Millican, C. L., Allen, K. A., & Kalina, R. E. (1993). Aging of the human photoreceptor mosaic: Evidence for selective vulnerability of rods in central retina. *Investigative Ophthalmology & Visual Science, 34,* 3278–3296.

Davis, H. (1978). Acoustics and psychoacoustics. In H. Davis & S. R. Silverman (Eds.), *Hearing and deafness* (pp. 8–45). New York: Holt, Rinehart and Winston.

Deems, D. A., & Doty, R. L. (1987). Age-related changes in the phenyl ethyl alcohol odor detection threshold. *Transactions—Pennsylvania Academy of Ophthalmology and Otolaryngology, 39,* 646–650.

Deems, D. A., Doty, R. L., Settle, R. G., Moore-Gillon, V., Shaman, P., Mester, A. F., et al. (1991). Smell and taste disorders, a study of 750 patients from the University of Pennsylvania smell and taste center. *Archives of Otolaryngology-Head and Neck Surgery, 117,* 519–528.

Desrosiers, J., Hébert, R., Bravo, G., & Dutil, E. (1996). Hand sensibility of healthy older people. *Journal of the American Geriatrics Society, 44* (8), 974–978.

Dharmarajan, T. S., & Bullecer, M. L. F. (2003). Thermoregulation and aging. In T. S. Dharmarajan, & R. A. Norman (Eds.), *Clinical geriatrics* (pp. 284–292). New York: The Parthenon Group.

Dharmarajan, T. S., & Ugalino, J. T. (2000). The aging process. In D. Dreger & B. Krumm (Eds.), *Hospital physician geriatric medicine board review manual* (Vol. 1, Part 1, pp. 1–12). Wayne, PA: Turner White Communications.

Diamond, J. P. (1997). Systemic adverse effects of topical ophthalmic agents: Implications for older patients. *Drugs Aging 11,* 252–260.

Dinse, H. R., Kleibel, N., Kalisch, T., Ragert, P., Wilimzig, C., & Tegenthoff, M. (2006). Tactile coactivation resets age-related decline of human tactile discrimination. *Annals of Neurology, 60,* 88–94.

DiNuzzo, A. R., Black, S. A., Lichtenstein, M. J., & Markides, K. S. (2001). Prevalence of functional blindness, visual impairment, and related functional deficits among elderly Mexican Americans. *Journal of Gerontology: Medical Sciences, 56* (9), M548–M551.

Donat, J., Özcan, A., Özdirenc, M., Aksakoğlu, G., & Aydinoğlu, S. (2005). Age-related changes in pressure pain threshold, grip strength and touch pressure threshold in upper extremities of older adults. *Aging: Clinical and Experimental Research, 17* (5), 380–384.

Dorey, C. K., Wu, G., Ebenstein, D., Garsd, A., & Weiter, J. J. (1989). Cell loss in the aging retina: Relationship to lipofuscin accumulation and macular degeneration. *Investigative Ophthalmology & Visual Science, 30,* 1691–1699.

Doty, R. L., Shaman, P., Applebaum, S. L., Giberson, R., Sikorski, L., & Rosenberg, L. (1984). Smell identification ability: Changes with age. *Science, 226,* 1441–1443.

Doty, R. L., Shaman, P., & Dann, M. S. (1984). Development of the University of Pennsylvania smell identification test: A standardized microencapsulated test of olfactory function. *Physical Behavior, 32,* 489–502.

Dunkle, R. E., & Hooper, C. R. (1983). Using language to help depressed elderly aphasic persons. *Social Casework, 64,* 539–545.

Dye, C. J. (1983). Sensory changes in aging. In N. S. Ernst & H. R. Glazer-Waldman (Eds.), *The aged patient* (pp. 142–157). Chicago, IL: Year Book Medical.

Edwards, R. R., & Fillingim, R. B. (2001). Age-associated differences in responses to noxious stimuli. *Journal of Gerontology A: Biological Sciences and Medical Sciences, 56,* M180–M185.

Erber, N. P., & Heine, C. (1996). Screening receptive communication of older adults in residential care. *American Journal of Audiology, 5,* 38–46.

Erber, N. P., & Osborn, R. R. (1994). Perception of facial cures by adults with low vision. *Journal of Vision Impairment and Blindness, 88,* 171–175.

Faye, E. (1984). *Clinical low vision* (2nd ed.). Boston: Little, Brown, and Company.

Feldman, R. M., & Reger, S. N. (1967). Relations among hearing, reaction time, and age. *Journal of Speech and Hearing Research, 10,* 479–495.

Ferraro, J. A., & Minckler, J. (1977). The human lateral lemniscus and its nuclei. *Brain and Language, 4,* 277–294.

Fletcher, D. C., Schuchard, R. A., Livingstone, C. L., Crane, W. G., & Hu, S. Y. (1994). Scanning laser ophthalmoscope macular perimetry and applications for low vision rehabilitation clinicians. *Ophthalmology Clinics of North America, 7*(2), 257–265.

Fortune, D. S., Haynes, D. S., & Hall, J. W. (1999). Tinnitus: Current evaluation and management. *Medical Clinics of North America, 83,* 153–162.

Fox, S. (2004). *Older Americans and the Internet,* Washington, DC: Pew Internet & American Life Project. Retrieved May 24, 2007, from www.pewinternet.org.

Francis, K. L., & Spirduso, W. W. (2000). Age differences in the expression of manual asymmetry. *Experimental Aging Research, 26,* 169–180.

Gaeth, J. (1948). A study of phonemic regression in relation to hearing loss. Unpublished doctoral dissertation. Northwestern University, Evanston, IL.

Garstecki, D. C., & Erler, S. F. (1998). Hearing and aging: Facilitating communication in the older person. *Topics in Geriatric Rehabilitation, 14*(2), 1–17.

Gartner, S., & Henkind, P. (1982). Aging and degeneration of the human macula. I. Outer nuclear layer and photoreceptors. *British Journal of Ophthalmology, 65,* 23–28.

Gates, G. A., Couropmitree, N. N., and Myers, R. H. (1999). Genetic associations in age-related hearing thresholds. *Archives of Otolaryngology, Head and Neck Surgery, 125,* 654–659.

Gates, G. A., & Rees, T. S. (1997). Hear ye—Hear ye—Successful auditory aging. *Western Journal of Medicine, 167,* 247–252.

Gelfand, S. A., & Silman, S. (1985). Future perspectives in hearing and aging: Clinical and research needs. In J. Roush (Ed.), *Seminars in hearing: Future perspective in hearing and aging: Clinical and research needs* (pp. 207–219). New York: Thieme-Stratton.

Gescheider, G. A., Beiles, E. J., Checkosky, C. M., Bolanowski, S. J., & Verrillo, R. T. (1994). The effects of aging on information-processing channels in the sense of touch: II. Temporal summation in the P channel. *Somotosensory and Motor Research, 11*(4), 359–365.

Gibson, S. J., & Helme, R. D. (1995). Age differences in pain perception and report: A review of physiological, psychological laboratory and clinical studies. *Pain Review, 2,* 111–137.

Glass, L. E. (1990) Hearing impairment in geriatrics. In B. Kemp, K. Brummel-Smith, J. W. Ramsdell (Eds.), *Geriatric rehabilitation* (pp. 235–251). Boston: College-Hill.

Glorig, A., Wheeler, D., Quiggle, R., Grings, W., & Summerfield, A. (1957). *1954 Wisconsin State Fair Hearing Survey.* New York: American Academy of Ophthalmology and Otolaryngology.

Grachev, I. D., Fredrickson, B. E., & Apkarian, A. V. (2000). Abnormal brain chemistry in chronic back pain: An in vivo proton magnetic resonance spectroscopy study. *Pain, 89,* 7–18.

Hansen, C. C., & Reske-Nielsen, E. (1965). Pathological studies in presbycusis. *Archives of Otolaryngology— Head & Neck Surgery, 82,* 115–132.

Hardy, J. D., Wolff, H. G., & Goodell, H. (1943). The pain threshold in man. *American Journal of Psychiatry, 99,* 744–751.

Harkins, S. W., Price, D. D., & Martinelli, M. (1986). Effects of age on pain perception: Thermonociception. *Journal of Gerontology, 41,* 58–63.

Hawkins, J. E., & Johnsson, L. (1985). Otopathological changes associated with presbycusis. In J. Roush (Ed.), *Seminars in hearing: Aging and hearing impairment* (pp. 115–133). New York: Thieme-Stratton.

Heft, M. W., Cooper, B. Y., O'Brien, K. K., Hemp, E., & O'Brien, R. (1996). Aging effects on the perception of noxious and non-noxious thermal stimuli applied to the face. *Aging: Clinical and Experimental Research, 8,* 35–41.

Heine, C., & Browning, C. J. (2002). Communication and psychosocial consequences of sensory loss in older adults: Overview and rehabilitation directions. *Disability and Rehabilitation, 24* (15), 763–773.

Helme, R. D., & McKernan, S. (1984). Flare responses in man following topical application of capsaicin. In L. A. Chahl, J. Szolcsanyi, & F. Lembeck (Eds.), *Antidromic vasodilatation and neurogenic inflammation* (pp. 303–315). Budapest: Akademiai Kiado.

Hissa, R. (1990). Central control of body temperature: A review. *Arctic Medical Research, 49*(1), 3–15.

Hooper, C. R., & Johnson, A. F. (1992). Assessment and intervention. In D. Ripich (Ed.), *Handbook of geriatric communication disorders* (pp. 307–332). Austin, TX: Pro-Ed.

Hooyman, N., & Kiyak, A. A. (2005). *Social gerontology: A multidisciplinary perspective.* Boston: Allyn & Bacon.

Horowitz, A. (2004). The prevalence and consequences of vision impairment in later life. *Topics in Geriatric Rehabilitation, 20,* 185–196.

Houston, D. K., Johnston, M. A., Nozza, R. J., Gunter, E. W., Shea, K. J., Cutler, G. M., et al. (1999). Age-related hearing loss, vitamin B-12 and folate in elderly women. *American Journal of Clinical Nutrition, 69,* 564–571.

Hyams, D. E. (1982). Psychological factors in rehabilitation of the elderly. *Gerontologica Clinica, 11,* 129–134.

Ingles, J. (1962). Effects of age on responses to dichotic stimulation. *Nature, 19,* 1101.

Ivers, R. Q., Cumming, R. G., Mitchell, P., & Attcbo, K. (1998). Visual impairment and falls in older adults. *Journal of the American Geriatrics Society, 46,* 58–64.

Ivers, R. Q., Norton, R., Cumming, R. G., Butler, M., & Campbell, A. J. (2000). Visual impairment and risk of hip fracture. *American Journal of Epidemiology, 152,* 633–639.

Jacobs, J. M., & Love, S. (1985). Qualitative and quantitative morphology of human sural nerve at different ages. *Brain, 108,* 897–924.

Jamal, G. A., Hansen, S., Weir, A. I., & Ballantyne, J. P. (1985) An improved automated method for the measurement of thermal thresholds. 1. Normal subjects. *Journal of Neurology, Neurosurgery, and Psychiatry, 48,* 354–360.

Jarvis, J. F., & van Heerden, H. G. (1967). The acuity of hearing in the Kalahari Bushman: A pilot study. *Journal of Laryngology and Otology, 81,* 63–68.

Jerger, J. (1971). *Audiological findings in aging.* Paper presented at the International Oto-Physiology Symposium, Ann Arbor, MI.

Jerger, J. (1973). Audiological findings in aging. *Advances in Oto-rhino-laryngology, 20,* 115–124.

Jonsson, R., & Rosenhall, U. (1998). Hearing in advanced age. A study of presbycusis in 85-, 88- and 90-year-old people. *Audiology, 37,* 207–218.

Kalina, R. E. (1997). Seeing into the future: Vision and aging. *Western Journal of Medicine, 167,* 253–257.

Kanagala, M., & Berkower, A. S. (2003). Disorders of the ear. In T. S. Dharmarajan & R. A. Norman (Eds.), *Clinical geriatrics* (pp. 381–390). New York: The Parthenon Group.

Kaneda, H., Maeshima, K., & Goto, N. (2000). Decline in taste and odor discrimination abilities with age, and relationship between gestation and olfaction. *Chemical Senses, 25,* 331–337.

Kasden, S. D. (1970). Speech discrimination in two age groups matched for hearing loss. *Journal of Auditory Research, 10,* 210–212.

Kasper, R. L. (1978). Eye problems of the aged. In W. Reichel (Ed.), *Clinical aspects of aging* (pp. 383–402). Baltimore: Williams & Wilkins.

Katz, J. (2001). *Handbook of clinical audiology* (5th ed.). Baltimore: Lippincott Williams & Wilkins.

Katzman, R., & Terry, R. D. (1983). *The neurology of aging.* Philadelphia: F.A. Davis.

Kenshalo, D. R., Sr. (1986). Somethetic sensitivity in young and elderly humans. *Journal of Gerontology, 41,* 732–742.

Kenshalo, D. R. (1977). Age changes in touch, vibration, temperature, kinesthesis and pain sensitivity. In J. E. Birren &

K. W. Schaie (Eds.), *Handbook of the psychology of aging* (pp. 562–579). New York: Van Nostrand Reinhold.

Khalil, Z., Ralevic, V., Bassirat, M., Dusting, G. J., & Helme, R. D. (1994). Effects of ageing on sensory nerve function in rat skin. *Brain Research, 641,* 265–272.

Kirikae, I., Sato, T., & Shitara, T. (1964). A study of hearing in advanced age. *Laryngoscope, 74,* 205–220.

Ko, M. L., King, M. A., Gordon, T. L., & Crisp, T. (1997). The effects of aging on spinal neurochemistry in the rat. *Brain Research Bulletin, 42,* 95–98.

Koenig, E. (1957). Pitch discrimination and age. *Acta Otolaryngologica, 48 ,* 475–489.

Konigsmark, B. W., & Murphy, E. A. (1972). Volume of ventral cochlear nucleus in man: Its relationship to neuronal population and age. *Journal of Neuropathology & Experimental Neurology, 31,* 304–316.

Konkle, D. F., Beasley, D. S., & Bess, F. H. (1977). Intelligibility of time-altered speech in relation to chronological age. *Journal of Speech and Hearing Research, 20,* 108–115.

Lambert, R. M., West, M., & Carlin, K. (1981). Psychology of adjustment to visual deficiency: A conceptual model. *Journal of Visual Impairment and Blindness, 75,* 193–196.

Lautenbacher, S., & Strian, F. (1991). Similarities in age differences in heat pain perception and thermal sensitivity. *Functional Neurology, 6,* 129–135.

Lebo, C. P., & Reddell, R. C. (1972). The presbycusis component in occupational hearing loss. *Laryngoscope, 82,* 1399–1409.

Lee, P. P., Spritzer, K., & Hays, R. D. (1997). The impact of blurred vision on functioning and well being. *Ophthalmology, 104,* 390–396.

Leibowitz, H. M., Krueger, D. E., Maunder, L. R., Milton, R. C., Kini, M. M., Kahn, H. A., et al. (1980). The Framingham eye study monograph: An ophthalmological and epidemiological study of cataract, glaucoma, diabetic retinopathy, macular degeneration, and visual acuity in a general population of 2631 adults, 1973–1975. *Survey of Ophthalmology, 24* (Suppl. 4), 335–610.

Leslie, W. J. (1978). Senescent changes of the cornea. *Journal of the American Optometric Association, 49,* 774–779.

Li, K. Z., & Lindenberger, U. (2002). Relations between aging sensory/sensorimotor and cognitive functions. *Neuroscience & Biobehavioral Reviews, 26,* 777–783.

Lovasik, J. V., Kergoat, M. J., Justino, L., & Kergoat, H. (2003). Neuroretinal basis of visual impairment in the very elderly. *Graefes Archives of Clinical and Experimental Ophthalmology, 241,* 48–55.

Luey, H. S. (1994). Understanding age-related hearing loss among older adults. In D. Watson, S. Boone, & M. Bagley (Eds.), *The challenge to independence: Vision and hearing loss among older adults* (pp. 159–172). Little Rock: University of Arkansas.

Lundström, M., Roos, P., Jensen, S., & Fregell, G. (1997). Catquest questionnaire for use in cataract surgery care: Description, validity, and reliability. *Journal of Cataract and Refractive Surgery, 23,* 1226–1236.

Lupsakko, T., Mäntyjärvi, M., Kautiainen, H., & Sulkava, R. (2002). Combined hearing and visual impairment and depression in a population aged 75 years and older. *International Journal of Geriatric Psychiatry, 17* (9), 808–813.

Luterman, D. M., Welsh, O. L., & Melrose, J. (1966). Responses of aged males to time-altered speech stimuli. *Journal of Speech and Hearing Research, 9,* 226–230.

Lybarger, J. A., & Kilbourne, E. M. (1985). Hyperthermia and hypothermia in the elderly: An epidemiology review. In B. B Davis & W. G. Wood (Eds.), *Homeostatic function and aging* (pp. 149–156). New York: Raven.

Lynch, J. C. (2006). The cerebral cortex. In Duane E. Haines (Ed.), *Fundamental neuroscience for basic and clinical applications* (pp. 511–526). Philadelphia: Churchill Livingstone.

Madden, D. J. (1990). Adult age differences in the time course of visual attention. *Journal of Gerontology, 45* (1), P9–P16.

Mangione, C. M., Lee, P. P., Gutierrez, P. R., Spritzer, K., Berry, S., & Hays, R. D. (2001). Development of the 25-item National Eye Institute Visual Function Questionnaire. *Archives of Ophthalmology, 119,* 1050–1058.

Mangione, C. M., Lee, P. P., & Hays, R. (1996). Measurement of visual functioning of health-related quality of life in eye disease and cataract surgery. In B. Spilker (Ed.), *Quality of life and pharmacoeconomics in clinical trials* (2nd ed., pp. 1045–1051). New York: Raven.

Mangione, C. M., Phillips, R. S., Seddon, J. M., Lawrence, M. G., Cook, E. F., Dailey, R., et al. (1992). Development of the "Activities of Daily Vision Scale." A measure of visual functional status. *Medical Care, 30,* 1111–1126.

Mascia, J. (1994). Understanding age-related hearing loss among older adults. In S. E. Boone, D. Watson, & M. Bagley (Eds.), *The challenge to independence: Vision and hearing loss among older adults* (pp. 93–98). Little Rock: University of Arkansas Rehabilitation Research and Training Center (RRTC) for Persons Who Are Deaf or Hard of Hearing.

Mathers, W. D., Lane, J. A., & Zimmerman, M. B. (1996). Tear film changes associated with normal aging. *Cornea, 15,* 229–234.

McCabe, P., Nason, F., Demers Turco, P., Friedman, D., & Seddon, J. M. (2007). Evaluating the effectiveness of a vision rehabilitation intervention using an objective and subjective measure of functional performance, *Ophthalmic Epidemiology, 7* (4), 259–270.

McGeer, E. G., & McGeer, P. L. (1976). Neurotransmitter metabolism in the ageing brain. In R. D. Terry & S. Gershon (Eds.), *Neurobiology of aging* (pp. 389–401). New York: Raven Press.

Miller, J. M., Dolan, D. F., Raphael, Y., & Altschuler, R. A. (1998). Interactive effects of aging with noise induced hearing loss. *Scandinavian Audiology, Supplementum 48,* 53–61.

Milne, J. (1977). A longitudinal study of hearing loss in older people. *British Journal of Audiology, 11,* 7–14.

Minassian, D. C., Reidy, A., Coffey, M., & Minassian, A. (2000). Utility of predictive equations for estimating the prevalence and incidence of primary open angle glaucoma in the UK. *British Journal of Ophthalmology, 84* (10), 1159–1161.

Montgomery, H. C. (1939). Analysis of World's Fairs' Hearing Tests. *Bell Laboratory Record, 18,* 98.

Moscovitch, M. (1982). A neuropsychological approach to memory and perception in normal and pathological aging. In F. I. M. Craik & S. Trehub (Eds.), *Aging and cognitive processes* (pp. 355–378). New York: Plenum.

Murphy, C. (1983). Age-related effects on the threshold, psychophysical function, and pleasantness of menthol. *Journals of Gerontology, 38,* 217–222.

Murphy, C. (1985). Cognitive and chemosensory influences on age-related changes in the ability to identify blended foods. *Journal of Gerontology, 40,* 47–52.

Murphy, C. (1986). Taste and smell in the elderly. In H. L. Meiselman & R. S. Rivlin (Eds.), *Clinical measurement of taste and smell* (pp. 343–371). New York: Macmillan.

Murphy, C. (1993). Nutrition and chemosensory perception in the elderly. *Critical Reviews in Food Science and Nutrition, 33,* 3–15.

Newman, C. W., & Spitzer, J. C. (1983). Prolonged auditory processing time in the elderly: Evidence from a backward recognition-masking paradigm. *Audiology, 22,* 241–252 .

Ochoa, J., & Mair, W. G. P. (1969). The normal sural nerve in man. II. Changes in the axon and Schwann cells due to ageing. *Acta Neuropathologica, 13* (3), 217–239.

Pakkenberg, B., & Gundersen, H. J. (1997). Neocortical neuron number in humans: Effect of sex and age. *Journal Comparative Neurology, 384,* 312–320.

Pedersen, K. E., Rosenhall, U., & Moller, M. B. (1989). Changes in pure-tone thresholds in individuals aged 70–81: Results from a longitudinal study. *Audiology, 28,* 194–204.

Pestalozza, G., & Shore, I. (1955). Clinical evaluation of presbycusis on basis of different tests of auditory function. *Laryngoscope, 65,* 1136–1163.

Pesudovs, K., & Coster, D. J. (1998). An instrument for assessment of subjective visual disability in cataract patients. *British Journal of Ophthalmology, 82,* 617–624.

Prineas, J. W., & Spencer, P. S. (1975). Pathology of the nerve cell body in disorders of the peripheral nervous system. In P. J. Dyck, P. K. Thomas, & E. H. Lambert (Eds.), *Peripheral neuropathy* (pp. 253–295). Philadelphia: W.B. Saunders.

Procacci, P., Bozza, G., & Buzelli, G. (1970). The cutaneous pricking pain threshold in old age. *Gerontologic Clinics, 12,* 213–218.

Purves, D., Augustine, G. J., Fitzpatrick, D., Hall, W. C., LaMantia, A., McNamara, J. O., et al. (Eds.). (2004). *Neuroscience* (3rd ed.). Sunderland, MA: Sinauer & Associates.

Quigley, H. A., & Broman, A. T. (2006). The number of people with glaucoma worldwide in 2010 and 2020. *British Journal of Ophthalmology, 90,* 262–267.

Ramotowski, D., & Kimberley, B. (1998). Age and the human cochlear traveling wave delay. *Ear & Hearing, 19,* 111–119.

Ramrattan, R. S., Wofs, R. C. W., Panda-Jones, S., Jonas, J. B., Bakker, D., Rols, H. A., et al. (2001). Prevalence and causes of visual field loss in the elderly and associations with impairment in daily functioning: The Rotterdam study. *Archives of Ophthalmology, 119* (12), 1788–1794.

Roberts, S. B., & Rosenberg, I. (2006). Nutrition and aging: Changes in the regulation of energy metabolism with aging. *Physiological Reviews, 86,* 651–667.

Rogers, J., & Bloom, F. E. (1985). Neurotransmitter metabolism and function in the aging nervous system. In C. E. Finch & E. L. Schnieder (Eds.), *Handbook of the biology of aging* (pp. 645–662). New York: Van Nostrand Reinhold.

Rolls, B. J. (1999). Do chemosensory changes influence food intake in the elderly? *Physiology and Behavior, 66* (2), 193–197.

Rosen, S., Bergman, M., Plester, D., el-Mofty, A., & Satti, M. H. (1962). Presbycusis study of a relatively noise-free population in the Sudan. *Annals of Otology, Rhinology, and Laryngology, 71,* 727–742.

Rowe, M. J. (1978). Normal variability of the brain-stem auditory evoked response in young and old subjects. *Electroencephalographic Clinical Neurophysiology, 4,* 459–470.

Salive, M. E., Guralnik, J., Glynn, R. J., Christen, W., Wallace, R. B., & Ostfeld, A. M. (1994). Association of visual impairment with mobility and physical function. *Journal of the American Geriatrics Society, 42,* 287–292.

Schaefer, W. D., & Weale, R. A (1970). The influence of age and retinal illumination on the pupillary near reflex. *Vision Research, 10,* 179–191.

Schemper, T., Voss, S., & Cain, W. S. (1981). Odor identification in young and elderly persons: Sensory and cognitive limitations. *Journal of Gerontology, 36,* 446–452.

Schiffman, S. S. (1983). Taste and smell in disease. *New England Journal of Medicine, 308* (22), 1337–1343.

Schiffman, S. S. (1991). Drugs influencing taste and smell perception. In T. V. Getchell, R. L. Doty, L. M. Bartoshuk, & J. B. Snow (Eds.), *Smell and taste in health and disease* (pp. 845–850). New York: Raven.

Schiffman, S. S. (1997). Taste and smell losses in normal aging and disease. *Journal of the American Medical Association, 278,* 1357–1362.

Schiffman, S. S., & Leffingwell, J. C. (1981). Perception of odors of simple pyrazines by young and elderly subjects: A multidimensional analysis. *Pharmacology, Biochemistry and Behavior, 14,* 787–798.

Schiffman, S. S., & Warwick, Z. S. (1991). Changes in taste and smell over the lifespan. In M. I. Friedman, M. G. Tordoff, & M. R. Kare (Eds.), *Chemical senses: Appetite and nutrition* (Vol. 4, pp. 341–365). New York: Marcel Dekker.

Schneider, B. A., Daneman, M., & Pichora-Fuller, M. K. (2002). Listening in aging adults: From discourse comprehension to psychoacoustics. *Canadian Journal of Experimental Psychology, 56,* 139–152.

Schuknecht, H. F. (1964). Further observations on the pathology of presbycusis. *Archives of Otolaryngology—Head & Neck Surgery, 80,* 369–382.

Schuknecht, H. F. (1974). *Pathology of the ear.* Cambridge, MA: Harvard University Press.

Schuknecht, H. F., & Gacek, M. R. (1993). Cochlear pathology in presbycusis. *Annals of Otolaryngology, Rhinology, and Laryngology, 102,* 1–16.

Sekuler, R., & Blake, R. (1985). *Perception.* New York: Random House.

Shay, K., & Ship, J. A. (1995). The importance of oral health in the older patient. *Journal of the American Geriatrics Society, 43,* 1414–1422.

Sheldrick, J. H., Ng, C., Austin, D. J., & Rosenthal, A. R. (1994). An analysis of referral routes and diagnostic accuracy in cases of suspected glaucoma. *Ophthalmic Epidemiology, 1,* 31–38.

Sherman, E. D., & Robillard, E. (1960). Sensitivity to pain in the aged. *Canadian Medical Association Journal, 83,* 944–947.

Ship, J. A., Pearson, J. D., Cruise, L. J., Brant, L. J., & Metter, E. J. (1996). Longitudinal changes in smell identification. *Journal of Gerontology, 51A,* (2), M86–M91.

Sigurdsson, E., Thorgeirsson, G., Sigvaldason, H., & Sigfusson, N. (1995). Unrecognized myocardial infarction: Epidemiology, clinical characteristics, and the prognostic role of angina pectoris. The Reykjavik study. *Annals of Internal Medicine, 122,* 96–102.

Sloane, M. E., Ball, K., Owsley, C., Bruni, S. R., & Roenkar, D. L. (1992). The visual activities questionnaire: Developing an instrument for assessing problems in everyday visual tasks. In *Everyday visual tasks. Technical digest of the noninvasive assessment of the visual system.* (Vol. 1, pp. 26–29). Washington, DC: Optical Society of America.

Smith, S. C. (1998). Aging, physiology, and vision. *Nurse Practitioner Forum, 9,* 19–22.

Sommer, A., Tielsch, J. M., Katz, J., Quigley, H. A., Gottsch, J. D., Javitt, J., et al. (1991). Relationship between intraocular pressure and primary open angle glaucoma among white and black Americans. *Archives of Ophthalmology, 109,* 1090–1095.

Steinberg, E. P., Tielsch, J. M., Schein, O. D., Javitt, J. C., Sharkey, P., Cassard, S. D., et al. (1994). The VF-14: An index of functional impairment in patients with cataract. *Archives of Ophthalmology, 112,* 630–638.

Stevens, D. A., & Lawless, H. T. (1981). Age-related changes in flavor perception. *Appetite, 2,* 127–136.

Stevens, J. C., Bartoshuk, L. M., & Cain, W. S. (1984). Chemical senses and aging: Taste versus smell. *Chemical Senses, 9,* 167–179.

Stevens, J. C., & Cain, W. S. (1985). Age-related deficiency in the perceived strength of six odorants. *Chemical Senses, 10,* 517–529.

Stevens, J. C., & Cain, W.S. (1986). Aging and the perception of nasal irritation. *Physiology and Behavior, 37,* 323–328.

Stevens, J. C., & Cain, W. S. (1987). Old-age deficits in the sense of smell as gauged by thresholds, magnitude matching, and odor identification. *Psychology of Aging, 2,* 36–42.

Stevens, J. C., Cain, W. S., Demarque, A., & Ruthruff, A. M. (1991). On the discrimination of missing ingredients: Aging and salt flavor. *Appetite, 16,* 129–140.

Stevens, J. C., & Choo, K. K. (1996). Spatial acuity of the body surface over the life span. *Somatosensory and Motor Research, 13,* 153–166.

Stevens, J. C., & Choo, K. K. (1998). Temperature sensitivity of the body surface over the life span. *Somatosensory & Motor Research, 15,* 13–28.

Stevens, J. C., Plantinga, A., & Cain, W. S. (1982). Reduction of odor and nasal pungency associated with aging. *Neurobiology of Aging, 3,* 125–132.

Stuen, C. (1990). Psychosocial consequences of vision loss among the elderly. In A. Johnston & M. Lawrence (Eds.), *Low vision ahead II: Proceedings of the International Conference on Low Vision* (pp. 149–153). Melbourne: Association for the Blind.

Sullivan, N. (1984). Vision in the elderly. In E. M. Stilwell (Ed.), *Handbook of patient care for gerontological nurses, Journal of Gerontological Nursing* (pp. 1–9). Thorofare, NJ: Slack.

Tadros, S. F., D'Souza, M., Zettel, M. L., Zhu, X., Waxmonsky, N. C., & Frisina, R. D. (2007). Glutamate-related gene expression changes with age in the mouse auditory midbrain. *Brain Research, 1127* (1), 1–9.

The Diabetes Control and Complications Trial Research Group. (1993). The effect of intensive treatment of diabetes on the development and progression of long term complications in insulin-dependent diabetes mellitus. *New England Journal of Medicine, 329,* 977–986.

The National Council on the Aging. (1999). *The consequences of untreated hearing loss in older persons.* Washington, DC: The National Council on the Aging Retrieved May 13, 2007, from www.ncoa.org/attachments/UntreatedHearingLossReport.pdf.

Thomas, P. D., Hunt, W. C., Garry, P. J., Hood, R. B., Goodwin, J. M., & Goodwin, J. S. (1983). Hearing acuity in healthy elderly population: Effects on emotional, cognitive and social status. *Journal of Gerontology, 38,* 321–325.

Thornbury, J. M., & Mistretta, C. M. (1981). Tactile sensitivity as a function of age. *Journal of Gerontology, 36,* 34–39.

Tucker, D. A., Phillips, S. L., Ruth, R. A., Clayton, W. A., Royster, E., & Todd, A. D. (2005). The effect of silence on tinnitus perception. *Otolaryngology-Head & Neck, 132,* 20–24.

UK Prospective Diabetes Study Group. (1998). Intensive blood-glucose control with sulphonylureas or insulin compared with conventional treatment and risk of complications in patients with type 2 diabetes: UKPDS 33. *Lancet, 352,* 837–853.

United States Social Security Administration. (1992). Code of Federal Regulations, Title 20, Ch. III, Pt. 404, Subpt. P, App. 1. List of Impairments. U.S. DHHS (SSA). Washington, DC.

U.S. Bureau of the Census. (1997). *Statistical abstract of the United States 1996,* Washington, DC: U.S. Government Printing Office.

Valluri, S. (1999). Gradual painless visual loss: Anterior segment causes. *Clinics in Geriatric Medicine, 15* (1), 87–93.

Ventry, I., & Weinstein, B. (1982). The hearing handicap inventory for the elderly: A new tool. *Ear & Hearing, 3,* 128–134.

Verdu, E., Ceballos, D., Vilches, J. J., & Navarro, X. (2000). Influence of aging on peripheral nerve function and regeneration. *Journal of the Peripheral Nervous System, 5,* 191–208.

Wahl, H. W., & Heyl, V. (2003). Connections between vision, hearing, and cognitive function in old age. *Generations, 27,* 39–44.

Wallhagen, M. I., Strawbridge, W. J., Shema, S. J., Kurata, J., & Kaplan, G. A. (2001). Comparative impact of hearing and vision impairment on subsequent functioning. *Journal of the American Geriatrics Society, 49* (8), 1086–1092.

Walsh, D. A. (1982). The development of visual information processes in adulthood and old age. In F. I. M. Craik & S. Trehub (Eds.). *Aging and cognitive processes* (pp. 99–125). New York: Plenum.

Watson, G. R. (2001). Low vision in the geriatric population: Rehabilitation and management. *Journal of the American Geriatrics Society, 49,* 317–330.

Watson, G., & Maino, J. H. (2007). Assistive technologies for the visually impaired older adult. In A. A. Rosenbloom, Jr. (Ed.), *Rosenbloom & Morgan's vision and aging* (pp. 285–298). St. Louis, MO: Butterworth-Heinemann.

Weiffenbach, J. M., Baum, B. J., & Burghauser, R. (1982). Taste thresholds: Quality specific variation with human aging. *Journal of Gerontology, 37* (3), 372–377.

West, S. K., Gildengorin, G., Haegerstrom-Portnoy, G., Schneck, M. E., Lott, L., & Brabyn, J. A. (2002). Is vision function related to physical function ability in older adults? *Journal of the American Geriatrics Society, 50* (1), 136–145.

West, S. K., Munoz, B., Rubin, G. S., Schein, O. D., Bandeen-Roche, S., Zeger, P. S., et al. (1997). Functional and visual impairment in a population-based study of older adults: The SEE project. *Investigative Ophthalmology & Visual Science, 38* (1), 72–82.

Wong, D. F., Wagner, H. N. J., Dannals, R. F., Links, J. M., Frost, J. J., Ravert, H. T., et al. (1984). Effects of age on dopamine and serotonin receptors measured by positron tomography in the living human brain. *Science, 226,* 1393–1396.

Woodruff-Pak, D. S. (1997). *Neuropsychology of aging.* Malden, MA: Blackwell.

Woodward, K. L. (1993). The relationship between skin compliance, age, gender and tactile discriminative thresholds in humans. *Somatosensory and Motor Research, 10,* 63–67.

World Health Organization. (2005). *Prevention of avoidable blindness and visual impairment.* Report by the Secretariat. Geneva: author (www.who.int/blindness/causes/priority/en/index8.html).

Wroblewski, M., & Mikulowski, P. (1991). Peritonitis in geriatric inpatients. *Age and Aging, 20,* 90–94.

Yong, H. H., Gibson, S. J., Horne, D., & Helme, R. D. (2001). Development of a pain attitudes questionnaire to assess stoicism and cautiousness for possible age differences. *The Journals of Gerontology Series B: Psychological Sciences and Social Sciences, 56,* 279–284.

ACKNOWLEDGMENT

The authors would like to acknowledge the assistance of UNCG graduate students Amy Sample and E. Thor Rasmussen, and the assistance of Tasha Thornhill, University of Saskatchewan Physical Therapy Student.

CHAPTER 6

Neuromusculoskeletal and Movement Function

Vanina Dal Bello-Haas, PhD, PT

Most old(er) people are young people in old bodies.

Bernard Isaacs, *The Challenge of Geriatric Medicine,* Oxford
Medical Publications, New York, 1992, p. 6

The life course is made up of change and transition
at least as much as periods of relative stability.

J. R. Kelly, *Peoria Winter: Styles and Resources in Later Life,*
Lexington Books, Lexington, MA, 1987, p. 52

OBJECTIVES

By the end of this chapter, readers will be able to:

1. Describe the International Classification of Functioning, Disability, and Health (ICF) framework in their own words.
2. Describe the typical age-related muscular, skeletal, and nervous system structural changes that may lead to impairments and affect functional abilities.
3. Discuss the effects of aging on muscle strength and power, joint range, posture, balance, coordination, and gait.
4. Explain assessment considerations for the older adult and the specific procedures used for assessing range of motion, strength, posture, coordination, and balance.
5. Describe the types of exercise programs that have been used to increase strength in the older adult.
6. Discuss the relationship between older adult function and muscle strength, muscle power, posture, balance, and coordination.
7. Identify interventions that may be used to prevent or lessen age-related neuromusculoskeletal changes in older adults.

A variety of tissues make up the neuromusculoskeletal system, including muscle, tendon, ligament, bone, cartilage, and nerves. As with the other body systems that were described in several chapters in this book (Chapters 4, 5, and 7), age-related body structure and function changes are also prevalent in the neuromusculoskeletal system. Because of these changes, older adults are at risk for common impairments, including decreased strength and decreased range of motion (ROM) and movement and function problems. As a result, older adults may experience a gradual decline in abilities and may have difficulty performing their daily activities and occupations. As with other systems the musculoskeletal and neurological aging process varies greatly from one person to another. However, for some individuals age-related changes may contribute to the development of several chronic conditions typically seen in older adults. In addition, changes secondary to disuse, other system pathologies, and personal factors, such as lifestyle and nutrition, may also contribute to or enhance the effects of aging. The purposes of this chapter are to

• Describe the typical age-related muscular, skeletal, and nervous system changes that may lead to impairments and affect functional abilities in the older adult.
• Discuss the effects of aging on muscle strength and power, joint range, posture, balance, coordination, and gait, and the resultant impact on the older adult's function.
• Explain the procedures used for range of motion, strength, posture, coordination, and balance assessments and the assessment considerations for the older adult.
• Identify interventions and specific exercise programs that may be used to prevent or lessen age-related neuromusculoskeletal changes in older adults.

The International Classification of Functioning, Disability, and Health and the Neuromusculoskeletal System

The World Health Organization (WHO) recently updated its framework to reflect an emerging understanding of health and how individuals live with their conditions. The International Classification of Functioning, Disability, and Health (ICF) was designed to serve diverse disciplines and sectors across different countries and various cultures in order to accomplish the following:

1. Provide a scientific basis for understanding and studying health and health-related states, issues, outcomes, and determinants.
2. Establish a common, international language for describing health and health-related states in order to improve communication between different users, such as health care professionals, researchers, health policy makers and managers, and the public.
3. Allow for comparison of data across countries, health care disciplines, and health services and sectors.
4. Provide a systematic coding scheme for health information systems.

The ICF framework is applicable to all people, regardless of their health condition, and places the emphasis on function rather than on condition or disease. Functioning and disability are viewed as a complex interaction between the health condition of the individual and the contextual factors of the environment, as well as personal factors. The ICF framework has three main domains—*Body, Activity,* and *Participation*—that can be used to classify the impact of health on an individual (WHO, 2001). The Body component includes classifications of body functions and body structures (i.e., functions of bones and joints, muscle functions). **Body functions** are defined as the physiological functions of body systems and also include psychological functions. **Body structures** are the anatomical parts of the body, such as organs, limbs, and their components. Abnormalities of function, as well as abnormalities of structure, are referred to as **impairments,** which are defined as a significant loss or deviation (e.g., deformity) of structures (e.g., joints) or functions (e.g., decreased range of motion [ROM] or muscle strength, pain, fatigue).

Activities and participation includes all aspects of functioning from both the individual and societal perspectives. **Activity** is the execution of a task or action by an individual and represents the individual perspective of functioning. **Participation** refers to the involvement of an individual in a life situation and represents the societal perspective of functioning. Difficulties at an activity level are referred to as *activity limitations,* and problems an individual may experience in his or her involvement in life situations are denoted as *participation restrictions* (e.g., restrictions in community life, recreation, and leisure).

The ICF describes the health of an individual according to how he or she is functioning within his or her environment. Within this context, *function* is an umbrella term for body structures, body functions, activities, and participation, and denotes the *positive* aspects of the interaction between an individual with a health condition and the contextual factors of the individual. *Disability* is an umbrella term for impairments, activity limitations, and participation restrictions, and denotes the *negative* aspects of the interaction between an individual with a health condition and the contextual factors of the individual. Because an individual's health includes his or her ability to carry out the full range of activities required to engage in all aspects of human life, the outcomes of interventions can be evaluated by recording performance in the individual's real-life environment.

The domains interact with each other, but not necessarily in a linear manner, are influenced by contextual factors (*environmental and personal factors*), and produce a visual of *the person in his or her world* through the combination of factors and domains (WHO, 2001). The contextual factors represent the complete background of an individual's life and living situation: (1) the *environmental* factors that make up the physical, social, and attitudinal environment in which an individual lives and conducts his or her life are external to the individual and can be facilitators (positive) or barriers (negative) for an individual; (2) *personal* factors, such as gender, age, race, fitness levels, lifestyle, habits, and social background, are the particular background of an individual's life and living situation (Figure 6-1a).

Typical age-related and abnormal biological alterations in the neuromusculoskeletal system (impairments) can lead to *activity restrictions* and *participation limitations* for many older adults. Figure 6-1b illustrates the ICF model and the dynamic interactions between the components for Mrs. Smithson, a 78-year-old female with osteoarthritis, whose history is described in Box 6-1. The ICF treats all dimensions as interactive and dynamic, rather than linear or static.

The interactions are in both directions, such that the presence of a disability may modify the health condition. Recent studies have linked

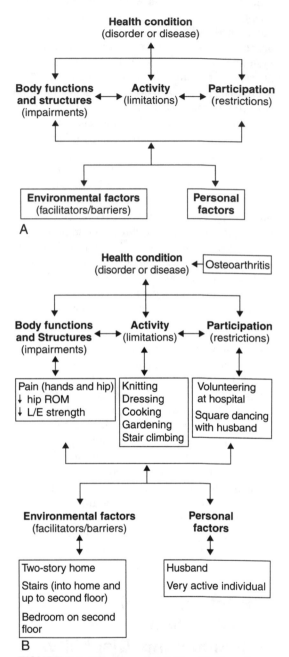

FIGURE 6-1 The International Classification of Functioning, Disability, and Health framework. (A) Interactions among dimensions are dynamic. (B) Interactions among the ICF dimensions for Mrs. Smithson, a 78-year-old female with osteoarthritis. (Adapted from World Health Organization. (2003). International Statistical Classification of Diseases and Related Health Problems, 10th Revision (ICD-10). Geneva, Switzerland: World Health Organization, with permission.)

BOX 6-1 **Mrs. Smithson**

Mrs. Smithson is a 78-year-old female who lives with her husband of 56 years in a two-story home. There are five steps up into the house with a railing on both sides of the steps. There are eight steps (no railing) from the main floor to the second floor, where Mr. and Mrs. Smithson's bedroom is located.

Mrs. Smithson has osteoarthritis of her hands diagnosed 10 years ago and experiences a great deal of pain. In addition, she has great difficulty with daily tasks such as dressing, especially buttons and clasps, and cooking, especially cutting food and juicing. Mrs. Smithson has started to notice pain in her right hip and has been having difficulty negotiating stairs. She must climb one step at a time and often has to hold onto her husband to negotiate the stairs, especially if there is no railing. She thinks she has less mobility of the hip and thinks her "legs are not as strong as they used to be." For example, she has difficulty bringing her legs up to put on her socks.

Mrs. Smithson has also been a very active woman. She volunteered at the local hospital visiting with patients twice a week. However, she is now only able to volunteer once every other week, as her hip is too sore to visit the hospital more frequently. The Smithson's enjoy square dancing and used to attend their local community center at least three times a week. Now Mr. and Mrs. Smithson attend square dancing only once a week, for the big community dance on Saturday evenings. Mrs. Smithson's hip is often too sore and she doesn't feel she has the strength or energy to attend more often.

Mrs. Smithson used to be an avid knitter, but her osteoarthritis has forced her to give up this activity. She is very disappointed she cannot continue with this activity, as she greatly enjoyed knitting socks, mittens, and sweaters for her 13 grandchildren.

Mrs. Smithson loves to garden and used to keep a small garden in her backyard and two flower boxes in front of her house. Due to the pain in her hip and hands, she is only able to keep the flower boxes in the front of her house.

outcome measures to the ICF domains to better reflect all aspects of health, body function, activity, and participation in musculoskeletal conditions (Cieza et al., 2002; Kjeken et al., 2005; Tremayne, Taylor, McBurney, & Baskus, 2002), and with the emergence of this broader model of health, clinical research has begun to focus on how the ICF might explain health outcomes across a spectrum of health conditions (Stucki, Ewert, & Cieza, 2003).

Neuromusculoskeletal and Movement Function in Older Adults

As described in Chapter 2, theories of aging abound. Aging has been conceptualized as an accumulation of microinsults that results in damage or changes in body tissues, and which eventually leads to the diminution of physiological systems (Johnson, 1985). These tissue and system changes affect older adults' function, mobility,

and ability to interact with the environment. Some of the most salient age-related changes in the neuromusculoskeletal system include

- Decreased muscle strength and power
- Marked loss of skeletal muscle mass
- Decreased number of functional motor units
- Decreased percentage of Type II fibers
- Changes in postural alignment
- Bone and cartilage changes
- Changes in balance and gait
- Decreased maximal speed of movement and initiation of responses to stimuli
- Increased threshold for vibration sensation and decreased proprioception

It is clear that alterations in the neuromuscular and skeletal systems occur with the passage of time. However, aging is a personal and unique experience, not only because older adults differ from one another with respect to their personal and environmental factors, but also because their physiological systems age at different rates. The rate of physiological change and resultant impact on function is highly individualized, and individual differences among older adults become strikingly more apparent with increasing age.

A continuum of function among older adults has been described by Spirduso, Francis, and MacRae (2005) (Figure 6-2). At the highest level of the hierarchy, *physically elite* older adults train on a daily basis, compete in sports competitions, or continue to work in a physically demanding occupation, such as firefighting or ski instruction. Although not many can continue working in these occupations into very old age, some do, and these individuals represent the maximum physical capabilities of older adults. *Physically fit* individuals may still work in their chosen occupation, may participate in activities with individuals younger than themselves, and continue to exercise on a regular basis for their health and well-being.

Physically independent older adults are those individuals whose physical function status allows them to participate in advanced activities of daily living (ADLs) and who continue to be active in hobbies and leisure and social activities. Although these individuals may have one or more chronic conditions, they are still able to function independently, although they engage in less physically demanding activities. *Physically frail* older adults can perform ADLs but may have a debilitating condition or disease that is physically challenging on a daily basis. They can live independently with human or environmental assistance but may be unable to engage in certain instrumental ADLs (IADLs). *Physically dependent* older adults cannot perform some or all basic ADLs (BADLs) as a result of acute or chronic conditions, cognitive problems, or personal factors, such as physical

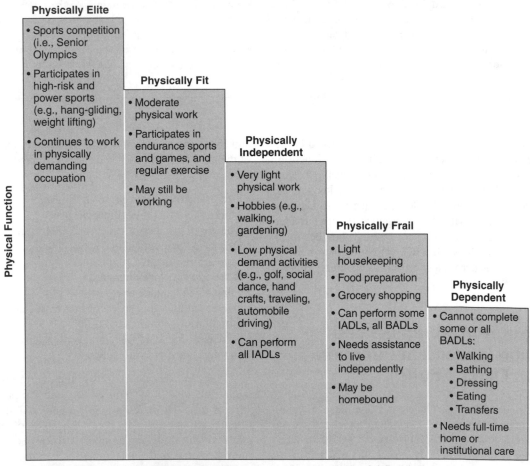

BADLs = basic activities of daily living; IADLs = instrumental activities of daily living.

FIGURE 6-2 The continuum of physical function for older adults. (Adapted from Spirduso & MacRae, 2005, with permission.)

inactivity, smoking, or increased weight. These individuals require institutional care or full-time assistance (Spirduso et al., 2005).

Considering the heterogeneity of aging and the continuum of physical functioning of older adults, it is important to remember that although age-related changes do occur, deterioration in physical abilities is not a guarantee for all older adults (Figure 6-3).

Age-Related Changes in Muscle Strength and Power

Muscle size and function change dramatically across the life span, with initial growth-related rapid increases and aged-related declines later on. Typically, it is believed that maximal muscle strength, the amount of force produced in a single maximum contraction of a muscle or muscle group, is achieved in the second or third decade and then declines. Different researchers have examined the effects of aging on muscle strength by investigating various factors, including type of strength loss (isometric, isotonic, or isokinetic), location of muscle strength loss, and physical activity and comorbidities of the individuals assessed. Thus, there have been some conflicting reports concerning the age at which the decline of muscle strength begins. For example, Larsson and associates (1979) reported that strength loss is moderate up to age 50 but then decreases at a rate of about 15% per decade to the age of 70 years, and between 70 and 80 years of age, the loss of strength accelerates and may be as great as 30% (Aniansson, Grimby, & Hedberg, 1992). Most agree that changes in absolute muscle strength are minor until about the sixth decade and then a steady decline becomes evident (McComas, 1996; Porter, Vandervoort, & Lexall, 1995).

Isometric strength has been found to change insignificantly until about the sixth decade but then decreases about 1% to 1.5% per year from 50 to 70 years of age and about 3% thereafter (Vandervoort, 2002). Upper extremity (U/E) isometric muscle strength tends to decline less than the lower extremities (L/E) (Lynch et al., 1999). Concentric strength decreases in a pattern similar to isometric strength, with the most dramatic losses occurring after 70 years of age, and the U/Es tending to decline less than the L/Es (Vandervoort, 2002). The total loss of concentric strength between 30 and 80 years of age has been reported to be 40% to 50% in the L/E and back muscles and 30% to 40% in the U/E (Frischknecht, 1998). Interestingly, eccentric strength declines are not as dramatic as concentric strength changes (Porter, Vandervoort, & Kramer, 1997; Vandervoort, 2002) (Figure 6-4).

Others have examined dynamic strength changes over time using an isokinetic dynamometer, which assesses **isokinetic strength,** the

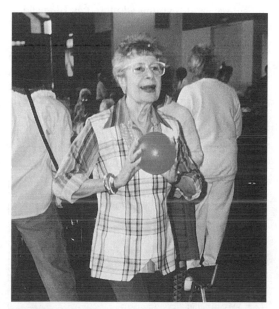

FIGURE 6-3 This woman continues to be vigorous and active, in spite of age-associated neuromusculoskeletal changes. (Courtesy of the Menorah Park Nursing Home, Cleveland, Ohio, with permission.)

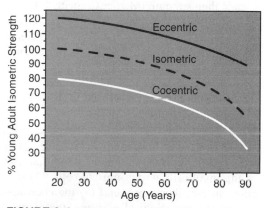

FIGURE 6-4 Effect of age on maximal strength throughout the human life span. The shape and height of the schematic curves depend on the type of strength being measured: isometric, concentric, or eccentric. (From Vandervoort, A. A. (2002). Aging of the human neuromuscular system. *Muscle and Nerve, 25,* 17–25, with permission).

maximum force that can be generated through full joint range of motion (ROM) at a preestablished velocity of limb movement. Isokinetic knee extension strength was found to decrease 25% to 35% over a 12-year period (Frontera et al., 2000), and Hughes and colleagues (2001) found a 14% decrease per decade in isokinetic knee extensor strength and a 16% decrease per decade in isokinetic knee flexor strength. The Hughes study examined both men and women and found that percent changes in knee extensor and flexor strength losses were similar in men and women. However, older women had only a 2% decline per decade in isokinetic elbow flexor and extensor strength, compared to a 12% decline in males, suggesting there is variability in the response to aging by different muscles groups, particularly in women. For more comprehensive reviews concerning muscle strength loss with aging, see Vandervoort (2002) or Porter, Vandervoort, and Lexall (1997).

Muscle power is the ability to generate force rapidly (calculated as the product of the muscle force generated multiplied by the velocity of movement). Thus, generating peak power requires timing and coordination. Strength and power are separate but related muscle attributes. Measuring muscle power requires more sophisticated and expensive instrumentation, and thus is used less frequently in clinical settings. Age-related decreases in muscle power are greater than declines in muscle strength. Although the onset of decline is similar for both, power has been found to decrease at a 10% greater rate per decade than strength (Metter, Conwitt, Tobin, & Fozard, 1997). Age-related absolute power and relative (scaled to body mass) power decrease about 6% to 11% and 6% to 8% per decade, respectively (Spirduso et al., 2005).

Sarcopenia and Age-Related Changes in Muscle Structure

Why do strength and power decrease with aging? Both muscle strength and muscle power are dependent on (1) the number and diameter of the myofibrils within muscle cells, (2) specific muscle fiber types, and (3) the coordination of the neurological elements that control muscle contraction.

A variety of changes in skeletal muscle structure occur with aging (Aniansson, Grimby, Hedberg, & Krotkiewski, 1981; Aniansson, Hedberg, Henning, & Grimby, 1986; Frolkis, Martynenko, & Zamostyan, 1976; Kirkendall & Garrett, 1998; Lexell, Henriksson-Larsen, Winblad, & Sjöström, 1983; Porter, Vandervoort, & Lexall, 1995), see Box 6-2. The loss of muscle mass associated with aging, **sarcopenia,** is one of the main determinants of musculoskeletal impairments and reduced function in older adults. The prevalence of clinically significant sarcopenia increases with age, and although sarcopenia is prevalent in both men and women, some have found sarcopenia to be more prevalent in older men. For example, Iannuzzi-Sucich, Prestwood, and Kenny (2002) found the prevalence of sarcopenia to be 22.6% in women and 26.8% in men. However, a subgroup analysis of those 80 years or older revealed prevalence rates of 31.0% in women and 52.9% in men.

Sarcopenia should not be confused with muscle atrophy that occurs with lack of physical activity, **disuse atrophy.** Sarcopenia is present in healthy, independent older adults and occurs even in master athletes who maintain very high levels of physical activity, suggesting that aging per se is the main cause of muscle mass loss (Roubenoff & Hughes, 2000). With sarcopenia, the size of the muscle mass that is able to contract decreases, and thus, there is a decrease in strength. This loss in muscle mass is clearly evident when comparing the cross-sectional muscle area of a young adult and an older adult (Figure 6-5) or muscles of a typical 60-year-old person with those of a 93-year-old person (Figures 6-6 and 6-7). Studies have found high correlations between muscle mass and strength in both longitudinal and cross-sectional studies (Frontera et al., 2000; Hughes et al., 2001;

BOX 6-2 Age-Related Changes in Muscle Morphology

- Decline of total muscle fiber number
- Atrophy of some fibers, hypertrophy of other fibers
- Loss of muscle mass
- Increased lipofusion
- Increased fatty and connective tissue
- Ringbinden found
- Cytoplasmic bodies found
- Myofibrillar degeneration
- Streaming of Z lines
- Denervation of muscle fibers

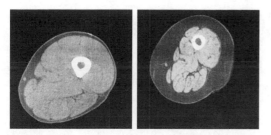

FIGURE 6-5 Magnetic resonance images through the mid-thigh of a healthy 25-year-old (left) and a healthy 75-year-old (right), illustrating sarcopenia. The older adult's image shows smaller muscle mass (light gray), more subcutaneous fat (dark gray), and increased intramuscular fat (dark gray lines). (From Roubenoff, R. (2003). Sarcopenia: Effects on body composition and function. *The Journals of Gerontology, 58A,* 1012–1017, with permission.)

Lynch et al., 1999). Decreases in muscle mass are consistent with respect to timing and magnitude of strength loss (Porter, Vandervoort, & Lexell, 1995) and directly or indirectly affect weakness (Frischknect, 1998). Although sarcopenia accounts for a large amount of strength loss in older adults, it does not fully explain the strength loss picture. The underlying cause of decreased muscle strength and function is multifactorial, and more than likely the extent of contributions and interactions of numerous factors varies among individual older adults (Figure 6-8). Additional factors that may contribute to age-related changes in muscle are briefly described below.

Muscle fibers are characterized as slow- or fast-twitch fibers. *Slow-twitch fibers* (type I) contract very slowly, are fatigue resistant, and are recruited when muscle contractions must be

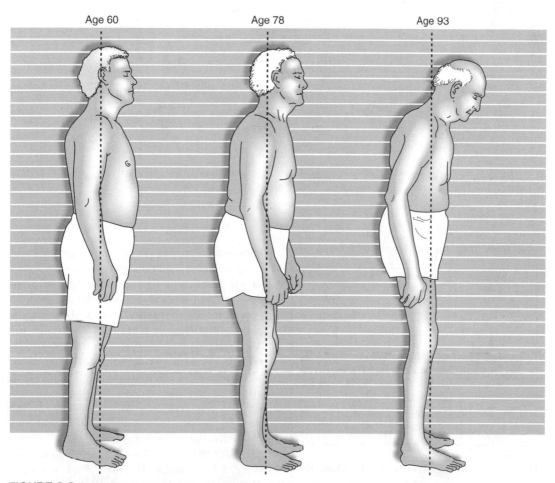

FIGURE 6-6 Lateral posture of (A) a 60-year-old man, (B) a 78-year-old man, and (C) a 93-year-old man. (From *Topics in geriatric rehabilitation,* Vol. 2, No. 4, Aspen, 1987, p. 16, with permission.)

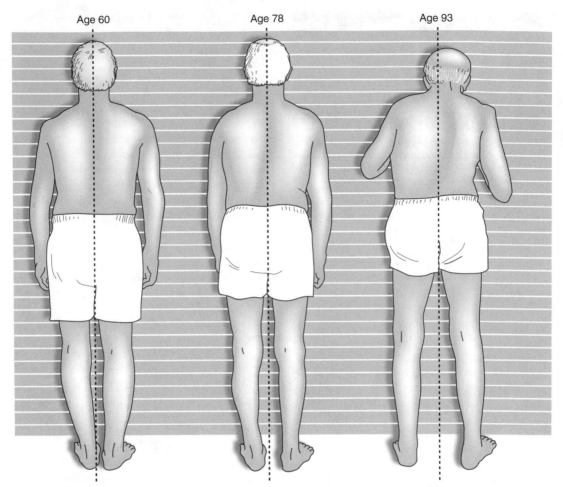

Age 60   Age 78   Age 93

FIGURE 6-7 Posterior posture of (A) a 60-year-old man, (B) a 78-year-old man, and (C) a 93-year-old man. (From *Topics in geriatric rehabilitation,* Vol. 2, No. 4, Aspen, 1987, p. 17, with permission.)

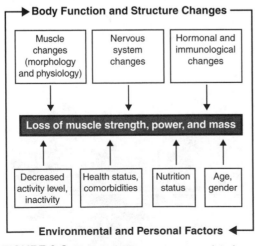

FIGURE 6-8 Multiple factors cause age-related changes in muscle strength and power.

maintained for long periods (e.g., during swimming or maintaining an upright position). *Fast-twitch fibers* (type II) contract very rapidly and develop high tension, although this tension can only be sustained for short periods. Type IIb (fast glycolytic) fibers are recruited for activities that require rapid and powerful contractions, whereas type IIa fibers (fast oxidative-glycolytic) contract at an intermediate speed. Studies of the aging effects on the microstructure of muscle, including fiber size, number, and arrangement of fibers have found that there is an overall loss of muscle fibers, both type I and type II, and a significant decrease in the average size and proportion of type II fibers (Essen-Gustavsson & Borges, 1986; Fiatarone Singh et. al, 1999; Hakkinen et al., 1998; Hikida et al., 2000; Larsson, Sjodin, &

Karlsson, 1978; Lexell, Taylor, & Sjöström, 1988). Anderson and colleagues (1999) suggest that in older adults there is a greater percentage of fibers that appear as a cross between type I and type II fibers (e.g., not distinguishable, neither strictly type I or type II).

Age-related muscle weakness may also be attributable to a decrease in muscle force, specifically the amount of force each muscle fiber can produce. Specific force has been reported to be decreased 20% in older adults, and this decrease is proposed to be attributable to changes in muscle architecture (Young, Stokes, & Crowe, 1985). An increase in fat and connective tissue has also been found in aging muscle, resulting in decreased muscle quality (Kent-Braun, Ng, & Young, 2000; Overend, Cunningham, Paterson, & Lefcoe, 1992). This replacement of muscle tissue is important because it may disrupt the normal orientation of the myofilaments. Loss of muscle tissue in combination with a decline in skeletal muscle fiber numbers reduces the tension a contracting muscle can generate. This is clinically manifested as weakness and possibly contributes to slowness and incoordination of muscle contractions.

Muscle fibers are innervated by a motor neuron, and the motor neuron, its axon, and all of the muscle fibers that it innervates make up the **motor unit.** Approximately 1% of the total number of motor neurons is lost per year, beginning in the third decade and increasing in rate after the age of 60 (Rice, 2000), and research suggests that age-related loss of motor neurons preferentially affects type II motor units (Carmeli & Reznick, 1994). This decrease results in an increase in size of the remaining motor units through collateral innervation. Age-related decreases in motor axon conduction velocity also occur (Doherty, Vandervoort, Taylor, & Brown, 1993; Wang, DePasqua, & Delwaide, 1999). These changes result in a decreased ability to generate muscle force in general and a decreased ability to generate force rapidly.

Skeletal muscle function relies on protein metabolism. Decreased rates of myofibrillar protein synthesis and increased protein turnover that occur with aging may be responsible for increased muscle fatigability and a decrease in type-II fibers, respectively (Rooyackers, Adey, Ades, & Nair, 1996; Short & Nair, 2001). Diets

low in protein have been shown to lead to decreased muscle mass and function in older individuals (Campbell, Trappe, Wolfe, & Evans, 2001; Iannuzzi-Sucich et al., 2002). Although decreased nutrition may be more prevalent in older adults in hospital or institutions, community-dwelling older adults may also have inadequate intakes of protein and energy requirements (Vellas et al., 2001) for a variety of reasons, including age-related changes in the digestive and sensory systems, depression, social isolation, and functional losses secondary to acute and chronic health problems.

Another factor that may affect age-related changes in muscle strength is a decrease in the number of capillaries per muscle fiber. The larger the number of capillaries per muscle fibers or the larger the number of capillaries that surround a muscle fiber, the greater is the capillarity and, thus, the better the oxygen exchange capacity. Last, hormonal and immunological alterations may contribute to sarcopenia. Aging is associated with a decrease in the growth hormone (GH), insulin-like growth factor-1 (IGF-1), and the sex hormones, testosterone and estrogen. These decreases may also contribute to age-related changes in muscle structure and strength.

Although disuse can contribute to sarcopenia, the etiology of sarcopenia is rather obscure. Simple disuse leads to reversible muscle atrophy but not to a loss of fiber number, whereas sarcopenia involves both (Lexell, 1995). Not all muscles demonstrate the same degree of decline with aging (Frolkis et al., 1976; Grimby, 1995; Kirkendall & Garrett, 1998; Potvin, 1980). Muscles of an older adult show different degrees of changes with respect to reduction in the numbers of fibers. Despite the inevitable changes with aging, a number of studies have demonstrated that older individuals who have higher levels of physical activities tend to preserve their muscle architecture and performance (Kiltgaard et al., 1990; Sipilä, Multanen, Kallinen, Era, & Suominen, 1996). For example, Smith and colleagues (2003) investigated the effects of 3 years of detraining following 2 years of resistance training in older adults with a mean age of 72 years. Subjects exercised for 2 years—high-intensity weight training (80% of a one repetition maximum [1RM]). Following 2 years of training, one group of subjects continued to train at a maintenance level (60% to 70% 1RM), and a second group stopped training. A third group (control) was monitored and refrained from any form of resistance training over the 5-year period. After 2 years of training, muscle strength increased, and the 3 years of training at the maintenance level maintained gains, with the authors reporting a ~44% increase in strength at the end of the 5 years compared with baseline measures. The nontrained control group demonstrated an 11.3% loss of muscle function over the 5 years. Although 3 years of detraining did result in some losses of strength, muscle strength was still 15.6% greater than pretraining baseline scores. Thus, older adults who remain physically active may have only moderate losses in skeletal muscle mass and function.

Age-Related Muscle Changes and Function

Physical function is dependent on muscle strength, muscle power, endurance, coordination, balance, and flexibility. The most obvious consequence of sarcopenia is a loss of muscle strength; however, the loss is much greater than that of muscle size. That is, there is a decrease in the intrinsic strength of skeletal muscle. Although neural factors, such as a decrease in neural drive, contribute to this phenomenon, muscle fibers are able to generate less force per unit size. Recent evidence suggests that this may be due to a decrease in myosin content as a result of aging, as well as inactivity (D'Antona et al., 2003).

Muscle strength is one of the main determinants of movement and performance of almost every ADL. Skeletal muscle weakness can lead to impaired mobility, loss of independence, and an increased risk of falls (Brown, Sinacore, & Host, 1995; Buchner, Beresford, Larson, La Croix, & Wagner, 1992; Whipple, Wolfson, & Amerman, 1987; Wolfson, Judge, Whipple, & King, 1995). Reductions in strength in older adults have been shown to decrease the ability to function normally:

- By reducing the maximum loads that can be lifted (Jette & Branch, 1981)
- By slowing walking speed and stride length (Bassey et al., 1992; Ferrucci et al., 1997; Fiatarone et al., 1990)
- By affecting the ability to stand up from a chair (Ferrucci et al., 1997; Fiatarone et al., 1990; Kauffman, 1982)

- By reducing the ability to balance in a position of decreased base of support, and to recover from postural perturbation (Ferrucci et al., 1997; Probst, 1989)
- By affecting the ability to get out of bed, cross a street, exit a car, and climb stairs (Bassey et al., 1992; Topp et al., 1998)

As a result of the lean body mass decreases and concomitant increase in fat mass associated with old age, displacement of the body, such as during walking, will place a greater metabolic load on muscle fibers, causing an increase in the energy cost of walking (Malatesta et al., 2003; Martin, Rothstein, & Larish, 1992). Hence, sarcopenia not only leads to muscle weakness and reduced function and mobility, but it is also associated with an increased metabolic cost of movement.

More recently, it has been noted that impairments in muscle power may be even more influential than strength on an older adult's function and mobility (Bean et al., 2002; Suzuki, Bean, & Fielding, 2001). Between the ages of 65 and 89 years, the rate of decrease in muscle power (3.5% per year) is greater than the rate of decrease of muscle strength (1% to 2% per year) (Skelton, Young, Greig, & Malbut, 1995). This is extremely relevant, as most ADLs, such as walking or rising from a chair, require the generation of power in addition to strength. A positive correlation between muscle power and ADLs has been described, especially if power is normalized for body weight (Bassey et al., 1992; Skelton, Greig, Davies, & Young, 1994). Lower extremity muscle power has been shown to be predictive of self-reported disability in community-dwelling older women (Foldvari et al., 2000) and has been found to correlate with gait speed, chair-rise time, and stair climb time (Bassey et al., 1992). Recent studies have determined that muscle power is more influential than muscle strength as a determinant of mobility and physical performance (Bean et al., 2002; Bean et al., 2003).

The link between impairments and the development of activity limitations and participation restrictions (disability) would seem obvious. Researchers have attempted to examine this link through longitudinal studies on aging. For example, data derived from community-dwelling healthy men (Honolulu Heart Study) have demonstrated that midlife hand grip strength is predictive of functional limitations and disability 25 years later (Rantanen et al., 1999a). Rantanen and colleagues (1999b) used cross-sectional data from baseline measurements of The Women's Health and Aging Study to examine the role of muscle strength in the decline of functional abilities in older adults. They concluded that hand grip strength and isometric strength of the knee extensor muscles had a mediating role between physical activity and disability in their sample. In other words, disability is associated with physical inactivity, inactivity leads to loss of muscle strength, and decreased muscle strength may be related to increased disability. In addition, impaired balance has been found to be a predictor of disability, and the risk increases when combined with muscle weakness (Jette et al., 1998; Rantanen, Guralnik, Ferrucci, Leveille, & Fried, 1999; Rantanen et al., 2001). Deficits in muscle power are closely associated with functional tasks (Bassey et al., 1992).

Data that allow for the prediction of function from strength values are not presently available, but studies that have investigated the relationship between functional activities and muscle strength and power suggest that there are important reasons to maintain or to increase muscle strength and power in older adults.

Age-Related Changes in the Skeletal System

The skeletal system functions to

- Provide mechanical support
- Protect soft tissues and organs
- Serve as a reservoir for calcium homeostasis and a site for red blood cell production
- Act as a lever system for muscle action

Changes in Bone

Adult bone undergoes continuous self-renewal (bone remodeling). **Bone remodeling** involves the coordinated activity of **osteoblasts,** cells responsible for bone formation, and **osteoclasts,** cells responsible for bone resorption. Maintenance of bone health throughout the life span is essential, because decreases in skeletal integrity increase the risk of skeletal conditions, such as fractures and osteoporosis. Factors affecting bone health include nonmodifiable factors such as

gender and ethnicity, and modifiable factors such as nutrition, exercise, body weight, and hormones.

Peak bone mass (PBM) is achieved in adulthood. Toward the end of the third decade the rate of osteoclast activity (resorption) exceeds the rate of osteoblast activity (bone formation), resulting in a bone remodeling imbalance. As a result of the bone remodeling imbalance, major changes occur in bone with aging. These include increased mineralization, increased porosity, and increased vulnerability to bone fatigue, resulting in microfractures. If there is an accumulation of microfractures, the integrity of the bone is compromised and a major fracture occurs.

Bone loss of about 0.7% to 1.0% a year occurs up until age 50 for men and women. However, women, particularly after menopause, have increased osteoclast activity, making them more susceptible to fractures. For example, bone loss in women increases to about 2% to 3% per year beginning after menopause and continues for 5 to 10 years, and lifetime risk of fractures in women is about three times that of men. Rate of bone loss after age 80 continues to increase similarly in both men and women (Spirduso et al., 2005). It is important to note that the balance between formation and resorption differs not only in different bones (weight-bearing and non-weight-bearing), but also in different bone tissue.

Changes in Cartilage, Joints, and Tendons

Age-related changes in cartilage, tendons, and joints are associated with alterations in collagen and elastin extensibility, and decreases in various proteins found in cartilage (Table 6-1). Connective tissue is found nearly everywhere in the body, and all types of connective tissue have similar features. Collagen is the basic protein component in fibrous connective tissue found in bone, tendon, ligaments, and cartilage. Collagen fibers are arranged in bundles that criss-cross (*cross-linkage*) to form structure in the body, and are strong and flexible in the younger years. As a person ages, there is increased cross-linkage of fibers resulting in more dense matrices. As these matrices become denser, the collagen structures become stiffer, and the cellular movement of nutrients and wastes becomes impaired. Elastin molecules also have a specific arrangement (*a lattice-type network*) that allows elastin to return to its original shape after being stretched.

TABLE 6-1 Normal Age-Related Changes that Affect Bone, Cartilage, Tendons, and Joints

	Description, Structure, and Function	Changes with Aging	Functional Implications
Collagen	The main protein of connective tissue and main component of cartilage, ligaments, tendons, and bone	Increased cross-linkage of fibers	Increased stiffness of tissues
		Increased shortening and distortion of collagen fibers	Decreased mobility of tissues
	Arranged in crisscross pattern to provide structure and tensile strength to connective tissue	Becomes more dense and stiff	Decreased hydration Decreased tensile strength
Elastin	A connective tissue protein	Progressive decrease in amount of elastin	Decreased elasticity of tissues
	Lattice-type network arrangement allows elastin to return to its original shape after being stretched		Decreased ease of movement of tissues
Hyaluronic acid	Secreted by connective tissue ribosomes, especially those in cartilage	Decrease in hyaluronic acid secretion	Decreased tensile strength
	Helps regulate viscosity of tissue	Decrease in hyaluronic acid molecule size	Tissue degradation
	Decreases amount of friction		
Glycoproteins	Small molecules of soluble protein	Decreased production and release of glycoproteins	Decreased hydration of tissues
	Produces osmotic force in ECM, which helps maintain fluid content of tissues		
Proteoglycans	Made up of a core protein to which chains of glycosaminoglycans are attached	Aggrecan (large proteoglycan found in articular cartilage) molecules become smaller and structurally altered	Decreased hydration of tissues
	Resist complete compression of cartilage during joint motion		

ECM, extracellular matrix.

With aging, the amount of elastin also decreases, further affecting the elasticity of tissues. Many of the cellular changes seen with aging are also seen in cases of inactivity or when the effects of weight-bearing are limited, such as bed rest. Thus, lack of exercise and activity can accentuate the normal effects of aging on connective tissue.

Synovial joints are typically found at the end of long bones of the U/E and L/E. The ends of the bones are covered with special articular cartilage, which acts as a shock absorber and decreases the amount of friction during movement. Cartilage is a unique connective tissue that has no direct blood supply. Rather, blood flow in adjacent bones and synovial fluid provide the nutrients to the chondroblasts. Chondroblasts secrete glycoproteins and hyaluranic acid and provide lubrication of the joint. The joint capsule that surrounds the joint is composed of a thick layer of dense connective tissue, and a synovial membrane lines most of the joint cavity. The membrane produces synovial fluid that fills the joint cavity and provides lubrication, nourishes the articular cartilage, and acts as a shock absorber when the joint is compressed. With aging, the cartilage that normally covers the joints thins and deteriorates, especially in the weight-bearing joints. Decreases in water content of the cartilage, decreased hydration of the joint, decreased elasticity of the joint capsule, and increased fibrous growth all contribute to increased joint stiffness. In addition to the muscle structure and characteristic changes described previously in this chapter, muscle tissue becomes less flexible and more rigid, secondary to a decrease in elastin and an increase in collagen. Tendons and ligaments also become less resilient to length changes.

Flexibility and range of motion (ROM) depend on the condition of the soft tissues of the joints, tendons, ligaments, and muscles, and are specific to each joint of the body. Inadequate range and inflexibility in older adults may affect functional tasks (e.g., putting on one's coat), ADLs (reaching into the cupboard to put away groceries), and general mobility (walking, bending, and stair climbing). Limited ROM and flexibility in the L/Es may also contribute to age-related gait changes and increase the risk of falls (Gehlsen & Whaley, 1990; Judge, Davis, & Ounpuu, 1996).

Maximum ROM is achieved in the mid- to late-twenties and gradually decreases with age, about 20% to 30% between the ages of 30 and 70. A gradual reduction in shoulder abduction ROM has been found with increasing age and is somewhat more pronounced in females. More than one-third of women aged 75 and older and more than one-fourth of men aged 75 and older had a shoulder abduction ROM below the functional threshold of 120 degrees, the ROM required to wash hair without difficulty (Skelton, Young, Walker, & Hoinville, 1999). Hamstring muscle and lower spine flexibility, as measured by a sit-and-reach test, has been shown to decline about 15% per decade (Golding & Lindsay, 1989), and Einkauf and colleagues (1987) found trunk extension ROM decreases the most with increased age, when compared to forward and side flexion. The ankle joint has also been shown to lose ROM with aging, with females losing 50% of their ROM between the ages of 55 and 85, and males losing 35% of ROM (Vandervoort et al., 1992). Loss of spinal flexibility and ankle ROM have important implications for older adults, as these impairments can lead to an increased risk of falls (see Chapter 8).

Changes in Postural Alignment

Posture is the biomechanical alignment of body parts in relation to one another and the orientation of the body as a whole to the environment. Posture is typically viewed as a static process, but gravity and neural control mechanisms constantly affect subtle shifts in weight and body alignment in order to counteract the effects of gravity, which necessitate a dynamic type of postural control. Posture is a key element to maintaining postural control, and the ability to control postural balance is a necessity for the safe performance of many daily tasks (Maki & McIlroy, 1996)

The aging process modifies normal postural alignment, and a flexed posture frequently predominates (see Figures 6-5 and 6-6). Thoracic kyphosis with a forward head position is typical, and many older adults develop an altered lordotic curve (flattened or exaggerated), rounded shoulders, and flexed hips and knees, as well (Kauffman, 1987). What causes this flexed posture is not clearly understood and is most likely multifactorial. Muscle weakness, decreased ROM, and loss of spinal flexibility can all be related to the postural changes seen frequently in older adults. For example, back extensor strength decreases with age and is associated with reduced levels of physical activity (Lexell, Henriksson-Larsen, Winblad, & Sjöström, 1983) and a decrease in bone mineral density (BMD) of the spine (Froklis et al., 1976; Frontera & Larsson, 1999).

A flexed or stooped posture can result in chronically stretched neck, trunk, and hip and knee extensor musculature, and may be associated with other changes in postural alignment, including a compensatory shift in the vertical displacement of the center of body mass back toward the heels. Kyphotic spinal changes may cause pain secondary to stretching of ligaments and muscles and a compensatory hyperlordosis in the lumbar spine can cause lower back pain. The more forward head position may cause impairments of anterior gaze, an important sensory modality for external world exploration and obstacle avoidance. In addition, the combination of abnormal postural alignment and decreased spinal mobility and flexibility interferes with the use of normal strategies for static and dynamic balance control.

Numerous changes have been described in the aging spine (Fielding, 1985; Sculco, 1985). The intervertebral disks undergo the most dramatic age-related changes of all connective tissue (Kauffman, 1987), causing kyphosis (Kendall, Kendall, Provance, Rodgers, & Romani, 1993; Kirkendall & Garrett, 1998). The forward head position alters load distribution on vertebral joint surfaces and can lead to spondylosis (Johnson, 1985) and deformities of vertebral bodies when bone structure is weakened by osteoporosis (Fiatarone et al., 1994). Cervical spondylosis has been reported in over 80% of persons over 55 years of age (Wyke, 1979). This problem has the effect of reducing postural stability and flexibility. Wyke (1979) postulated that age-related disequilibrium is influenced by progressive degeneration of mechanoreceptors of the spinal apophyseal joints and suggested that inflammatory degeneration or traumatic injury to the spine reduces the crucial afferent feedback to the central nervous system for postural stability.

In addition, changes in postural alignment may be a result of muscular impairments (e.g., weakness) or may result from compensating for other impairments secondary to neurologic (e.g., stroke) or musculoskeletal conditions (e.g., hip or knee arthritis).

The most common age-related changes in the axial skeleton are:

• Forward head position and rounded shoulders (Kaufman, 1987)
• Increased thoracic kyphotic curvature (O'Gorman & Jull, 1987)
• Decreased lumbar lordosis (Milne & Lauder, 1974)
• Increased knee flexion angle (Brocklehurst, Robertson, & James-Groom, 1982)
• A more posterior hip position (Woodhull-McNeal, 1992) (see Figures 6-5 and 6-6)

The head-forward position is often considered to be abnormal, but to some degree it may be a normal compensation necessitated by other postural changes, such as age-related flattening of the lumbar spine. Scoliotic curvatures occur in the older adult and may be due to spinal or appendicular changes (Kaufman, 1987). In the extremities, the most common postural variations in aged adults are rounded shoulders with protracted scapula and slightly flexed elbows, hips, and knees. In addition, changes in the articular surfaces and joint capsules often cause varus or valgus deformities at the hips, knees, or ankles. The normally obtuse angle between the neck and shaft of the femur may become more acute, which emphasizes the flexed posture.

As described above, the numerous changes that occur in the skeletal system with aging may diminish the maintenance of upright posture.

Postural variations have been shown to have a relationship to functional problems, such as falls (O'Brien, Culham, & Pickles, 1997), in the older adult. Additionally, changes in muscle, connective tissue, and skin alter postural alignment. Postural muscles, such as the quadriceps and soleus, have been noted to have more age-related atrophy than nonpostural muscles (Mahar, Kirby, & MacLeod, 1985). Trauma, lifestyle, or habits such as prolonged wearing of high heels also contribute to postural changes with aging.

Common Skeletal Pathology

Although the focus of this chapter is typical, normal aging, two conditions, *osteoporosis* and *osteoarthritis,* are so prevalent in older adults that they warrant a brief discussion.

Osteoporosis

Osteoporosis (OP) is a growing public health problem throughout the world, in part because of the increasing numbers of people living beyond the age of 65 years. Osteoporosis is defined as a skeletal disorder characterized by compromised bone strength predisposing a person to increased risk of fracture (NIH Consensus Development Panel on Osteoporosis Prevention, 2001). Low bone mass and microarchitectural deterioration in bone tissue lead to enhanced bone fragility and a consequent increase in fracture risk (NIH Consensus Development Panel on Osteoporosis Prevention, 2001).

Bone strength has two components: **bone mineral density** (BMD) and **bone quality.** Bone mineral density is determined by the amount of bone loss subtracted from the peak bone mass for a client, whereas bone quality considers bone architecture, bone mineralization, accumulated damage (e.g., microfractures), and bone turnover (NIH Consensus Development Panel on Osteoporosis Prevention, 2001). As described previously, bone is continuously turning over, with the bony skeleton acting as a reservoir for calcium, and a slow loss of bone mass beginning as a natural aspect of aging in about the mid-thirties to mid-forties. However, the process of osteoporosis is characterized by increased bone resorption over bone formation. Signs and symptoms in early disease are completely absent, whereas loss of height, pain, and kyphosis are common signs and symptoms of advanced osteoporosis. Skeletal fractures are the main clinical manifestation of the disease, and a history of atraumatic fracture has been included in the definition of osteoporosis (Kanis & the WHO Study Group, 1994). Older adults are the most severely affected by fractures, which cause substantial mortality, morbidity, and economic cost (van Balen et al., 2001).

Currently, there is no single measure for bone strength, and the diagnosis of OP is based on the bone mineral density. BMD has been used as the best measure of OP, because it accounts for approximately 70% of bone strength. Although BMD is the single best predictor of osteoporotic fracture, studies have shown that a major risk factor for osteoporotic fracture is a previous fracture, and clinically, osteoporosis is recognized by the occurrence of fractures (Woolf & Pfleger, 2003). Adults with a history of fracture, regardless of its location, have a 50% to 100% increased risk of subsequent fracture of a different type (Klotzbuecher et al., 2000; Wu et al., 2002). Hip fracture, forearm fracture, and vertebral fractures are the most common, and hip fracture is considered the most serious outcome of OP (Cummings & Melton, 2002). The number of hip fractures is increasing throughout the world, and the projected number for 2050 is 6.3 million worldwide (Cooper, Campion, & Melton, 1992). Although the majority of hip fractures occur in North America and Europe, demographic shifts over the next 50 years will lead to a relocation in the burden of disease from developed countries to the developing world. For example, 75% of hip fractures are expected to occur in the developing world by the year 2050 (Genant et al., 1999).

Nonpharmacologic interventions for osteoporosis mainly address nutritional management, fall prevention, and exercise, specifically weight-bearing and strengthening exercises, to improve bone health; whereas, pharmacologic interventions target bone loss through decreasing bone resorption, increasing bone formation, or a combination of both processes. Refer to the most recent osteoporosis guidelines for more information on osteoporosis management (www.cmaj.ca/cgi/content/full/167/10_suppl/s1).

Osteoarthritis

Osteoarthritis (OA) is the most common form of joint disease and one of the leading causes of disability in men and women aged 65 and older. More than 90% of adults over 40 years of age have radiographic changes consistent with OA in weight-bearing joints, and up to 30% of older adults report symptomatic pain and disability due to OA (Murray & Lopez, 1996). The significant prevalence of OA brings a high cost to society through the loss of self-care abilities and productivity, and major economic costs. For example, direct and indirect costs for hip and knee OA in the United States in 1994 were $12.9 billion (Yelin, 1998).

The precise cause of OA is unknown but is thought to be related to mechanical wear and tear. Risk factors for OA include nonmodifiable factors such as increased age and family history, and modifiable factors such as obesity, high physical workload occupations, and participation in contact sports. Osteoarthritis can occur in any joint but most often affects the hip, knee, spine, and hand and feet joints and is characterized by biochemical and biomechanical changes that cause the loss of articular cartilage, active bone remodeling, and deformities. With OA, the cartilage becomes thinner, tears, and disrupts the joint capsule. As the cartilage wears, ulceration (eburnation), spur formation (osteophytes), synovitis, and thickening of the capsule occur, resulting in less joint protection. Individuals with OA commonly report pain and stiffness, and frequent signs include joint pain and swelling, decreased ROM, and **crepitus** with movement. Pain is usually relieved by rest, and most individuals with OA report a period of morning stiffness.

Interventions are typically directed at multiple levels. One of the most important aspects of management is the reduction or modification of risk factors, especially obesity. Exercise to reduce pain and increase function, and joint protection education are also key elements to an overall management plan. Strength training and physical fitness exercise have been found to improve function, decrease pain and disability, increase endurance, and decrease risk of falls in older adults with OA (American Geriatrics Society Panel on Exercise and Osteoarthritis, 2001). Pharmacologic management consists of analgesics, nonsteroidal anti-inflammatory medications, topical agents, and glucosamine. Intra-articular injection of corticosteroids and arthroscopic surgery to remove loose cartilage or large osteophytes may be useful. For individuals with advanced disease, intractable pain, or severely compromised function, a joint replacement is performed. Surgery is the only effective intervention for advanced disease, and total hip replacement (THR) and total knee replacement (TKR) surgery have been shown to restore function and quality of life (Murray, 1998).

Age-Related Changes in the Nervous System

As it ages, the nervous system also undergoes numerous changes, resulting in alterations in sensory (see Chapter 5), reflex, and motor function. The changes that commonly occur in the nervous system of older adults are summarized in Box 6-3. Possible causes of these changes include the following:

- Biochemical and morphological changes in the neurons and receptors
- Loss of neurons
- Defects in neuronal transport mechanisms
- Decreases in myelin
- Gradual decreases in the conduction velocity of nerves
- Defects in protein synthesis
- Cumulative trauma
- Oxidative stress and vascular changes

Alterations in specific morphological and biochemical parameters have not always been directly correlated with functional changes. Additional research is needed to determine whether specific age-related changes occurring

---

BOX 6-3 Age-Related Changes of the Nervous System

- Cerebral atrophy
- Increased cerebrospinal fluid space
- Specific neuronal loss
- Reduced dendritic branching
- Increased lipofuscin granules
- Decreased effectiveness of neurotransmitter systems; selectively reduced activities in dopaminergic, cholinergic, and noradrenergic systems
- Reduced cerebral blood flow
- Diminished glucose utilization
- Alterations in electroencephalogram
- Loss of motor nerve fibers
- Decreased number and size of motor units
- Slowing of nerve conduction velocities
- Increased plaques and neurofibrillary tangles in selective brain regions

---

in the nervous system cause declines in functional performance.

The functional integrity of the nervous system in most healthy, older adults is maintained despite the reported structural, biochemical, and metabolic changes that have been reported to occur in the aging nervous system. However, disorders of the central nervous system (CNS), such as stroke, are the most common cause of disability in older adults. These disorders have been estimated to cause nearly half of the disability in adults older than 65 years of age and more than 90% of the cases of total dependency (Timiras, 1994).

Changes in the aging nervous system may contribute to postural instability, impaired sensation, muscle weakness, abnormal gait patterns, and falls. Each individual responds to changes in the neuromuscular system in a unique manner. For some older adults, profound structural changes can occur without inhibiting functional abilities, whereas in other older adults seemingly insignificant changes can cause serious functional impairments. For example, Sudarsky and Ronthal (1983) provide evidence that CNS changes are present in the brains of healthy, community-dwelling older adults, irregardless of functional limitations. Computerized tomography (CT) was used to study the brains of 50 adults with a mean age of 79.5 years with undiagnosed gait disorders. Although individuals with known neurological disorders were excluded from the study, pathological changes were found. Evidence of multiple cerebral infarcts was found in 16% of the sample. Four individuals had clear evidence of dementia, and hydrocephalus was found in two persons. Cerebellar atrophy, truncal ataxia, and peripheral neuropathy were found in four subjects, whereas another nine showed signs of multiple sensory disorders including decrements in visual, vestibular, or proprioceptive afferent responses. These nine individuals also had evidence of peripheral neuropathy. Seven persons had essential or idiopathic gait disorders and clinical findings of a wide-based gait with shortened strides and a tendency to be easily displaced in a posterior direction. However, none of the subjects had been diagnosed as having gait disorders, suggesting that they were able to accomplish the activities that were important to them irregardless of obvious clinical findings. These study findings typify "disabilities" or "problems" in the older adult—clinicians often identify deficits that at the time have no functional implications for the individual. Interestingly, autopsy findings of highly functional, cognitively intact older adults often show substantial cortical thinning and expansion of the ventricular spaces, which are consistent with findings in brains of individuals diagnosed with dementia.

Age-Related Changes in Balance, Coordination, Movement, and Function

The systems that control balance have an important role in the performance of functional activities. **Postural control,** the ability to control the body's position in space for the purposes of **postural orientation** and **postural stability** (balance), occurs through the complex interaction of many systems (Box 6-4). Thus, postural control is not regulated by a single system but instead by the integrated interaction of many systems (Shumway-Cook & Woollacott, 2007). Problems with balance may occur because of changes in one or more of the subsystems that contribute to postural control, rather than from an age-related decline in the nervous system alone. For a comprehensive discussion about postural control, the development of postural control, and the effects of aging on postural control, see Shumway-Cook and Woollacott (2007).

Age-related changes in the nervous system that may contribute to balance problems and functional decline in older adults have been identified (Tell, Lefkowitz, Kiehr, & Elster, 1998). These changes include visual and vestibular information (see Chapter 5), muscular atrophy, loss of proprioception and vibration sense, extrapyramidal dysfunction, and slowed reaction times (Richardson, 1999). In addition, decreases in muscle strength and power (discussed previously in this chapter) may also contribute to postural control and stability problems.

Both the visual and vestibular systems show a reduction of function in aging. The numerous changes in the eye described in Chapter 5 result in less light transmitted to the retina and an increase in visual threshold. Thus, older adults need more light to see an object. In addition, loss of visual field, decreases in visual acuity, and contrast sensitivity cause difficulties with depth perception. An intact vestibular system is important for balance, especially in older adults who have declines in other senses that provide orientation information to the CNS. Vestibular nerve and hair cells decrease by 40% by age 70 (Rosenhall & Rubin, 1975). Thus, a decrease in vestibular function with age would result in the nervous system having increased difficulty with resolving conflicting afferent information coming in from the visual and somatosensory systems (Shumway-Cooke & Woollacott, 2007).

The extrapyramidal system, which is used to refer to the basal ganglia and its connections, is reported to change with aging, resulting in the slowing of skilled motor movements and

---

BOX 6-4 **Postural Control for Stability and Orientation Requires a Complex Interaction of Many Components and Systems**

• Musculoskeletal system	Joint range of motion, spinal flexibility, muscle properties, biomechanical relationships among linked body segments
• Individual sensory systems	Visual, vestibular, somatosensory
• Sensory/perceptual processes	The organization and integration of individual sensory systems
• Neuromuscular synergies	Organization, coordination, and sequential activation of muscles and muscle groups
• Adaptive mechanisms	Sensory and motor system modifications in response to changing task and environmental demands
• Anticipatory mechanisms	Sensory and motor system pretuning based on previous experience and learning
• Higher-level neural processes	Cognitive influences essential for mapping sensation to action and for adaptive and anticipatory mechanisms; internal representations

Source: Data from Shumway-Cook & Woollacott, 2007.

alterations of gross movements (Clark & Siebens, 1998; Timiras, 1994). The basal ganglia and cerebellum play a major role in control of movement. Tics or tremors may become evident, and movement may be slowed (bradykinesia), altered or absent, leading to postural instability in the older adult (Timiras, 1994). Reaction time, the ability to respond to a stimulus, is often used as a measure of neuromuscular function in older adults because it requires afferent impulses, central processing, and efferent impulses to affect a response (Potvin, 1980; Sherwood & Selder, 1979; Spirduso, 1975).

Slowing of **simple reaction time** (SRT) is considered one of the most measurable and recognizable behavioral changes that occurs with aging (Spirduso et al., 2005). Studies of **choice reaction time** suggest that as the task difficulty increases, reaction times of older adults are significantly slower than the reaction times of those who are younger (Hale, Myerson, & Wagstaff, 1987; Hultsch, MacDonald, & Dixon, 2002). Very wide individual variations in reaction times at all ages have been reported, and as age increases, heterogeneity in reaction times increases (Hultsch et al., 2002; Spirduso et al., 2005). It has been suggested that slowed central processing is the primary factor leading to an increased reaction time, rather than declines in motor or sensory nerve conduction velocities or rate of muscle contraction (Katzman & Terry, 1992). Interestingly, older, physically inactive persons show the more typical age-related decline in speed of motor activities and slowing on tasks. Spirduso (1975) reported very little decline in reaction time tasks in older persons who were active in racket sports compared to young, physically active persons, and concluded that the decline in speed of movement reported in many older adults may relate more to the level of physical activity rather than being a function of age and neurological changes.

Coordination

The ability to perform coordinated movement requires the integration of multiple muscle groups (**muscle synergies**) and involves afferent as well as efferent pathways. Intact neuromusculoskeletal and sensory systems are necessary to produce movements that are smooth and accurate. Functional activities that require either gross- or fine-motor responses or a combination of both (e.g., walking,

getting out of bed, buttoning and zipping clothing) are dependent on coordinated movements, and timing and force of muscle contractions and joint motions are crucial for these controlled movements.

Coordination is the ability to execute smooth, accurate, controlled movements, which is dependent on an intact neuromusculoskeletal system, inputs from visual, somatosensory, and vestibular systems, and sensorimotor processing. Coordinated movements involve multiple joints and muscles, which need to be activated at the appropriate time and with the appropriate force, so the movement is accurate, smooth, and efficient (Shumway-Cook & Woollacott, 2007). Changes in the ability to execute smooth, accurate, and controlled motor responses occur with normal aging, and these changes may be accentuated further by impairments of the sensory systems.

Research has found that the following occurs with increasing age:

- Slowing of eye–hand coordination (Potvin, 1980)
- Poor inter-limb coordination (Serrien, Swinnen, & Stemach, 2000)
- Decreases in homolateral hand and foot movements (Capranica, Tessitore, Olivieri, Minganti, & Pesce, 2004)
- Decreases in motor coordination (Bornstein, 1986; Potvin, Syndulko, Tourtelotte, Lemmon, & Potvin, 1980; Verkek, Schouten, & Oosterhuis,1990)
- Decreases in manual dexterity (Kellor, Frost, Silberberg, Iversen, & Cummings, 1971; Laufer & Scheitz, 1968; Mathiowetz, Volland, Kashman, & Weber, 1985; Molbeck, 1976; Sperling,1980)

Proprioception and Vibration

As described in Chapter 5, virtually all sensory modalities decrease in acuity with age, and propriception and vibration are no exception. **Proprioception** is described as the awareness of body segments in relationship to each other and in relationship to the environment (orientation). Some research has found no major decline in small joint proprioception (e.g., finger and toes), but others have found joint position sense of the knee decreases with age (Skinner, Barrack, & Cook, 1984) and higher detection thresholds for angular displacement at the ankle (Thelen, Brockmiller, Ashton-Miller, Schultz, &

Alexander, 1998). In addition, older adults may have impaired integration of proprioceptive input at the spinal cord and higher centers (Hay, Bard, Fleury, & Teasdale, 1996). Decreased awareness of the body or limbs in space, combined with other sensory losses or cognitive changes (described in Chapters 5 and 9) may result in safety issues during daily activities, transfers, and ambulation.

A 97% decrease in vibration threshold has been reported in healthy men between the ages of 20 and 80 years, with the most profound differences in the L/E, specifically the toe and ankle (Potvin et al., 1980). In general, vibration thresholds increase more in the L/Es than the U/Es. For example, Stuart, Turman, Shaw, Walsh, and Nyugen (2003) confirmed decreased vibration sensitivity in older adults compared to young adults, but found a lack of significant difference in the fingers, and some have reported an inability to record vibratory responses at the ankle, because older adults were unable to perceive the sensation there at all (Whanger & Wang, 1974).

Changes in Gait

Balance control is a primary contributor to stable walking. Decreased postural stability is a major factor leading to a loss of ambulatory ability in the older adult (Shumway-Cooke & Woollacott, 2007). The gait of older adults and the manner in which they adjust their gait to accommodate obstacles have been found to differ from that of the younger or middle-aged adults. Various gait changes are predominant in the older adult and are the most common of all functional activities researched (Wolfson, Whipple, Amerman, Kaplan, & Kleinberg, 1985). The most typical gait changes with aging are:

- Decreased step length (Gabell & Nayak, 1984; Mbourou, Lajoie, & Teasdale, 2003)
- Decreased stride length (Hageman & Blanke, 1986; Kressig et al., 2004; Mbourou et al., 2003)
- Slower walking velocity (Hageman & Blanke, 1986; Kressig et al., 2004)
- Decreased cadence (Laufer, 2005; Mbourou et al., 2003)
- Decreased ankle range of motion (Hageman & Blanke, 1986)
- Decreased push-off with the toes (Winter, Patla, Frank, & Walt, 1990)

- Increased double-stance time (Kressig et al., 2004; Mbourou et al., 2003; Winter et al., 1990)
- Decreased vertical displacement of center of mass (Mbourou et al., 2003; Shkuratova, Morris, & Huxham, 2004)

It has been suggested that some of these gait changes occur because older adults try to improve their balance or adopt a more cautious walking pattern when confronted with obstacles (Chen, Ashton-Miller, Alexander, & Schultz, 1994). Gait changes have not been found in all healthy older adults (Blanke & Hageman, 1989). Active older adults tend to have greater gait speed than sedentary older individuals (Bendall, Bassey, & Pearson, 1989; Woo, Ho, Lau, Chan, & Yuek, 1995), and impairments are more predominant in persons with functional limitations or in those individuals who tend to fall (Wolfson et al., 1985).

Aging of the CNS has often been characterized as an irreversible loss of function and a decline in capabilities. This is probably an oversimplification of the real picture. In fact, the adult brain has the ability to compensate functionally for neuronal loss or atrophy (Timiras, 1994). The slowing in reaction time may not be a function of a decline in the nervous system, but rather may be related to the unique activity levels of older individuals. Many of the balance problems and gait disorders in the older adults are probably related to pathology, rather than a manifestation of a generalized aging process. Generally, the changes in the nervous system, although significant, do not usually become functionally important in terms of normal daily activities until after 75 years of age (Katzman & Terry, 1992).

Assessing the Neuromusculoskeletal System in Older Adults

Neuromusculoskeletal changes that occur normally with aging influence range of motion, flexibility, muscle strength, posture, coordination, balance, and ambulation. Age-related impairments can result in loss of independence and decreased ability to perform ADLs, and changes in lifestyle and decreases in activity levels may exacerbate these age-related changes. A comprehensive assessment provides the health care professional with the necessary information to design appropriate intervention and management programs. However, because the older adult may present with normal age-related changes in addition to changes related to chronic illnesses or comorbidities, assessment may be more challenging, and differentiating between what changes are due to normal aging versus pathology may not be straightforward. Chapter 17 provides extensive detail regarding the purposes of assessing the older adult, a philosophy of client-centered and contextually based assessment, assessment issues specific to the older adult, and methods used to assess older adults.

Range of Motion, Flexibility, and Strength Assessment

Range of Motion and Flexibility

Measurement of joint range of motion is commonly assessed using a standard goniometer or determined through observation of functional movement, and limits of movement are compared to the noninvolved limb or to norms expected for each joint. Comparison to standard norms may not be appropriate, as studies have found differences in ROM in older subjects compared to younger subjects and differences in older adults by age groups (Bassey, Morgan, Dallosso, & Ebrahim, 1989; Fitzgerald, Wynveen, Rheault, & Rothchild, 1983; James & Parker, 1989; Walker, Sue, Miles-Elkousy, Ford, & Trevelyan, 1984). These differences should be kept in mind in order to develop realistic management goals.

Flexibility is dependent on joint ROM, in addition to the extensibility of joint soft tissues, ligaments, tendons, and muscles. Lower and upper extremity flexibility can be measured by the "sit-and-reach test" (Nieman, 2003) and the "back-scratch test" (Rikli & Jones, 2001), respectively. With the sit-and-reach test, the individual completes a warm-up activity such as walking or cycling and then sits facing a flexibility box with shoes off, knees fully extended, and feet flat against the box. The individual is instructed to reach directly forward as far as possible along a measuring scale four times, and the distance point reached on the fourth trial is measured (Nieman, 2003). Rikli and Jones' (2001) "chair sit-and-reach test" is a modification of the sit-and-reach test, which allows the older adult

to remain seated in a chair for testing. The individual is instructed to reach toward his or her toes keeping the knee extended, and the distance beyond how far the person can reach beyond the toes is recorded. With the back-scratch test, the individual is asked to reach one hand over the shoulder and one up the middle of the back, and the distance between the extended middle fingers is recorded (Rikli & Jones, 2001).

Strength

Strength assessments are a very important aspect when providing care for the older adult. Baseline measurements of strength are necessary before the initiation of an exercise program to quantify the outcome of the intervention. In addition, measurement of strength can assist the clinician in targeting individuals who might receive the most benefit from an exercise intervention (Ferrucci et al., 1997). Muscle strength can be assessed in clinical settings using a variety of methods including manual techniques, instrumentation, and functional activities. It is important to note that with some older adults, it may be necessary to modify the methods that are commonly used when performing these procedures because of pain, joint deformities, or limitations in endurance and flexibility. These strength testing methods are summarized in Table 6-2.

One of the most commonly used assessments of strength is the manual muscle test (MMT). This test does not require sophisticated equipment and can be performed quickly in a clinical setting. Depending on the grading method used, manual muscle testing yields either an ordinal measurement from 0 to 5, or one of the following results: zero, trace, poor, fair, good, or normal. In one method of MMT, the evaluator applies an opposing force to the contracting muscle as the subject moves the extremity throughout the range of motion. An alternate method of strength assessment known as the break test may be necessary for older adults who have impaired flexibility or pain. This method can be used in a pain-free range or at the end range by asking the subject to resist or to hold against the evaluator's force. The strength is determined by the amount of force needed to overcome (i.e., to break) the subject's resistance. It is rated on the same ordinal scale of 0 to 5 and represents a maximal isometric contraction. With

text continued on page 152

TABLE 6-2 **Evaluating Muscle Strength in the Older Adult**

Assessment Method	Description	Scoring	Advantages	Disadvantages	Precautions for the Older Adult
Manual Muscle Test (MMT)	The examiner physically applies the matching force of the specific muscle being tested, either through arc of movement *(make test)* or in the client's pain-free ROM until the therapist overpowers the client *(break test)*	Ordinal scale from 0 to 5 or 0 to 10 Zero, trace, poor, fair, good, or normal	Does not require sophisticated equipment Can be performed quickly Safe Inexpensive	Lack of sensitivity to change Poor reliability Force application can be a source of variability Poor correlation with absolute muscle strength (especially in strong muscles) Grading scale represents ordinal data (may decrease statistical power)	Be careful not to apply too much pressure, especially if client has osteoporosis (bone may be susceptible to fracture) Ensure client avoids the Valsalva maneuver during testing
Handheld Dynamometer	The examiner uses a handheld device against the muscle that is strength tested, as described for MMT The device provides a force reading of the strength of the specific muscle being tested	Kilograms or pounds of muscle force generated	Easy to administer Portable May be muscle-group specific More sensitive to change than MMT Reliability has been demonstrated in older adults Norms for older adults available	Strength of tester must be greater than that of client Differing levels of reliability among instruments May be difficult to calibrate No standard design for point of force application or tester grasp Measures static force (not directly related to function)	Positioning of the dynamometer may cause temporary discomfort
Computerized Dynamometer • Isometric	Client is secured and stabilized and asked to exert a force against a strain gauge	Force generated during maximal contraction (measured in pounds or kilograms)	Performed in controlled conditions, so more easily reproducible Relatively safe Fatigue not typically induced in most clients	Measures static force (not directly related to function)	Precautions in the positions used to test the muscles (flexibility needed)

continued on page 152

TABLE 6-2 **Evaluating Muscle Strength in the Older Adult** (continued)

Assessment Method	Description	Scoring	Advantages	Disadvantages	Precautions for the Older Adult
Computerized Dynamometer • Isokinetic	An electromechanical device that monitors and changes resistance so that the movement velocity is held constant throughout ROM Body segment cannot accelerate beyond a pre-set angular velocity Assesses torque output with isolated joint movements	Provides measurement values for torque, muscle work, power, and endurance	Determine movement capability at different speeds Sensitive tool to quantify deficit Reliability demonstrated in older adults Norms available for older adults Correlates well with functional task May be more relevant because activities relate more to function and not absolute strength	Lack of extensive norms for older adults makes it difficult to interpret findings accurately Not transportable Expensive Constant velocity of joint motion may be difficult to control in some patients with weakness Not a standardized measure Subject to differences in rating among scorers	May cause an exaggerated blood pressure response May be fatiguing for some older adults May be unsafe for some older adults
Observation of performance of functional activities	Use of older adults' performance of functional activities to rate strength	Observation			

all strength assessments of older persons, the evaluator must be cautious when applying pressure. Because of the increased incidence of osteoporosis in older adults, the bone may be unable to withstand normal stresses and can be susceptible to a pathological fracture. Additionally, because cardiovascular problems commonly occur in older adults, the Valsalva maneuver should be avoided during the MMT by instructing the individual to breathe out during the test.

Dynamometers may be used to measure both static and dynamic muscle strength. Handheld dynamometers that are both portable and easy to administer may be used in conjunction with the MMT in order to quantify the tension that is generated. Cautious use of these instruments is necessary, because some are more reliable than others, and the strength of the tester must be greater than that of the subject. To improve the accuracy of the

isometric test, a belt anchored to a table leg or eye-hook can be used to stabilize the trunk or extremities.

The more sophisticated and expensive dynamometers that measure isokinetic torques also have their place in testing muscle force in older adults. One of the greatest advantages of isokinetic testing is that it can be used to determine movement capability at different speeds. Assessing dynamic strength is important in older adults, because common ADLs require individuals to move at speeds of about 300 degrees per second (Brown, 1993). Clinicians using isokinetic testing should be aware that even high velocities of 300 to 450 degrees per second are still significantly lower than many everyday movements (Hunter, White, & Thompson, 1998). The clinician should use caution, especially when testing the upper extremities of older, frail individuals, because testing the strength of these muscles isokinetically may cause an exaggerated blood pressure response. The use of isokinetic dynamometers is also limited because they are not transportable.

As an alternative to more standardized tests for muscle weakness, practitioners can use an older adult's performance of a functional activity to rate strength. Lower extremity strength can be assessed as an individual rises from a chair, climbs stairs, or walks. For example, a functional test might indicate that the individual is able to ascend six steps without assistance but needs minimal assistance to complete a total of 12 steps. The sit-to-stand test is a measurement of the time taken to complete a number of chair stands and examines L/E strength (Csuka & McCarty, 1985; MacRae, Lacourse, & Moldavon, 1992). For older adults, this kind of assessment may be the most relevant because function, rather than absolute strength, is the issue. It is not unusual for an older adult to be more functional than might be expected on the basis of MMT or dynamometer testing, because motivation and other factors work in combination with muscle strength to produce movement.

In addition, physical assessment measurement tools, such as the Physical Performance Test (Reuben & Sui, 1990) and the Continuous-Scale Physical Functional Performance Test (Cress, 1996), can be used in the clinical setting. Although they do not specifically measure muscle strength per se, the test items simulate activities of daily living and include components of fine or gross motor function and muscular endurance.

Static Posture Assessment

Standard assessment methods for postural alignment are appropriate for the older adult. Posture is visually assessed from the anterior, posterior, and lateral views, and using a plumb line may be of benefit as a reference point. The lateral view of normal postural alignment is represented by a straight line projecting through the ear, the acromion, the greater trochanter, the posterior patella, and the lateral malleolus (Kendall et al., 1993). When using a plumb line to assess posture in the older adult, **postural sway** may become more apparent to the evaluator and may increase the difficulty of the postural assessment. Postural sway, small oscillating movements of the body

over the feet during bipedal standing, can be assessed by observation or, more formally, through the use of a computer-assisted postural sway analyzer or force platforms in a laboratory setting.

Coordination and Balance Assessment

Coordination

The most common clinical approach to evaluating coordination in the older adult is to observe the performance functional movements and activities and the resultant movement characteristics. More formal clinical tests of coordination can be divided into tasks that require equilibrium, which generally reflect the coordination of multijoint movements required for postural control and ambulation (Box 6-6), and those that do not (nonequilibrium tests, Box 6-5) (Schmitz, 2007). When assessing coordination, the accurate ability to perform the task and the speed required to complete the task must be considered. Movement should be in the correct direction, and the movement trajectory should be smooth and fluid and well-timed throughout. In addition, problems with muscle tension and movement control achieved by groups of muscles working together (synergies) and difficulty initiating or stopping the movement should be noted. Body or extremity posture should be maintained during the movement, and movements should be easily reversed, even with changes in speed and direction of movement (Shumway-Cook & Woollacott, 2007).

Standardized assessments of arm–hand function and motor coordination, and eye–hand coordination for use in older adults are numerous and include the Purdue Pegboard Test (Desrosiers, Hebert, Bravo, & Dutil, 1995a; Tiffin, 1968), the Jebsen Hand Function Test (Jebsen, Taylor, Treischmann, Trotter, & Howard, 1969), the Timed Manual Performance (Williams, Gaylord, & McGaghie, 1990), and the Upper Extremity Performance Test for the Elderly (TEMPA) (Desrosiers, Hebert, Bravo, & Dutil, 1995b).

Balance

The ability to maintain balance is crucial for the successful performance of most ADLs. Assessment of balance in older adults

BOX 6-5 Nonequilibrium Coordination Tests*

• Finger to nose	The shoulder is abducted to 90 degrees with the elbow extended. The patient is asked to bring the tip of the index finger to the tip of the nose. Alterations may be made in the initial starting position to assess performance from different planes of motion.
• Finger to therapist's finger	The patient and therapist sit opposite each other. The therapist's index finger is held in front of the patient. The patient is asked to touch the tip of the index finger to the therapist's index finger. The position of the therapist's finger may be altered during testing to assess ability to change distance, direction, and force of movement.
• Finger to finger	Both shoulders are abducted to 90 degrees with the elbows extended. The patient is asked to bring both hands toward the midline and approximate the index fingers from opposing hands.
• Alternate nose to finger	The patient alternately touches the tip of the nose and the tip of the therapist's finger with the index finger. The position of the therapist's finger may be altered during testing to assess the patient's ability to change distance, direction, and force of movement.
• Finger opposition	The patient touches the tip of the thumb to the tip of each finger in sequence. Speed may be gradually increased.
• Mass grasp	An alternation is made between opening and closing fist (from finger flexion to full extension). Speed may be gradually increased.
• Pronation/supination	With elbows flexed to 90 degrees and held close to the body, the patient alternately turns the palms up and down. This test also may be performed with shoulders flexed to 90 degrees and elbows extended. Speed may be gradually increased. The ability to reverse movements between opposing muscle groups can be assessed at any joint. Examples include active alternation between flexion and extension of the knee, ankle, elbow, fingers, and so forth.
• Rebound test	The patient is positioned with the elbow flexed. The therapist applies sufficient manual resistance to produce an isometric contraction of biceps. Resistance is suddenly released. Normally, the opposing muscle group (triceps) will contract and "check" movement of the limb. Many other muscle groups can be tested for this phenomenon, such as the shoulder abductors or flexors, elbow extensors, and so forth.
• Tapping (hand)	With the elbow flexed and the forearm pronated, the patient is asked to "tap" the hand on the knee.
• Tapping (foot)	The patient is asked to "tap" the ball of one foot on the floor without raising the knee; heel maintains contact with floor.
• Pointing and past pointing	The patient and therapist are opposite each other, either sitting or standing. Both patient and therapist bring shoulders to a horizontal position of 90 degrees of flexion with elbows extended. Index fingers are touching or the patient's finger may rest lightly on the therapist's. The patient is asked to fully flex the shoulder (fingers will be pointing toward ceiling) and then return to the horizontal position such that index fingers will again approximate. Both arms should be tested, either separately or simultaneously. A normal response consists of an accurate return to the starting position. In an abnormal response, there is typically a "past pointing," or movement beyond the target. Several variations to this test include movements in other directions such as toward 90 degrees of shoulder abduction or toward 0 degrees of shoulder flexion (finger will point toward floor). Following each movement, the patient is asked to return to the initial horizontal starting position.
• Alternate heel to knee: heel to toe	From a supine position, the patient is asked to touch the knee and big toe alternately with the heel of the opposite extremity.

continued on page 155

BOX 6-5 **Nonequilibrium Coordination Tests*** (continued)

• Toe to examiner's finger	From a supine position, the patient is instructed to touch the great toe to the examiner's finger. The position of finger may be altered during testing to assess ability to change distance, direction, and force of movement.
• Heel on shin	From a supine position, the heel of one foot is slid up and down the shin of the opposite lower extremity.
• Drawing a circle	The patient draws an imaginary circle in the air with either upper or lower extremity (a table or the floor also may be used). This also may be done using a finger–eight pattern. This test may be performed in the supine position for lower extremity assessment.
• Fixation or position holding	Upper extremity: The patient holds arms horizontally in front. Lower extremity: The patient is asked to hold the knee in an extended position.

★Tests should be performed first with eyes open and then with eyes closed. Abnormal responses include a gradual deviation from the "holding" position and a diminished quality of response with vision occluded. Unless otherwise indicated, tests are performed with the patient in a sitting position.

Source: O'Sullivan, S. B., & Schmitz, T. J., *Physical rehabilitation*, 3rd ed. F.A. Davis, Philadelphia, 1994, p. 102, with permission.

BOX 6-6 **Equilibrium Coordination Tests**

- Standing in a normal, comfortable posture.
- Standing, feet together (narrow base of support).
- Standing, with one foot directly in front of the other (toe of one foot touching heel of opposite foot).
- Standing on one foot.
- Arm position may be altered in each of the above postures (i.e., arms at side, over head, hands on waist, and so forth).
- Displace balance unexpectedly (while carefully guarding patient).
- Standing, alternate between forward trunk flexion and return to neutral.
- Standing, laterally flex trunk to each side.
- Walking, placing the heel of one foot directly in front of the toe of the opposite foot.
- Walk along a straight line drawn or taped to the floor, or place feet on floor markers while walking.
- Walk sideways and backward.
- March in place.
- Alter speed of ambulatory activities (increased speed will exaggerate coordination deficits).
- Stop and start abruptly while walking.
- Walk in a circle, alternate directions.
- Walk on heels or toes.
- Normal standing posture. Observe patient both with patient's eyes open and with patient's eyes closed (or vision occluded). If patient is able to maintain balance with eyes open but not with vision occluded, it is indicative of a proprioceptive loss. This inability to maintain an upright posture without visual input is referred to as a *positive Romberg sign.*

Source: O'Sullivan, S. B., & Schmitz, T. J., *Physical rehabilitation,* 3rd ed., F.A. Davis, Philadelphia, 1994, p. 103, with permission.

can assist in defining movement capacity, and changes in balance scores are commonly used to judge improvement following therapeutic programs. As described above, because multiple systems contribute to postural stability, a comprehensive assessment of all systems that may contribute to balance problems is essential. Thus, an assessment of postural alignment, ROM, flexibility, muscle strength, sensation, and cognition, in addition to specific balance tests would compose the multiple evaluation components of balance.

Evaluation of balance in the laboratory setting typically includes (1) a force plate system that measures the changing pressures under the feet during the maintenance of static posture or during movement, (2) a computerized dynamic posturography system that assesses motor and sensory contributions to balance, and (3) electromyography and high-speed filming systems that evaluate the spatial and temporal components of muscle activation and inter-limb coordination during movement or balance perturbations. Balance in the older adult is assessed clinically using a variety of balance measures that evaluate the following areas:

1. Static balance—standing quietly
2. Limits of stability
3. Anticipatory postural control
4. Reactive postural control
5. Sensory strategies and integration
6. Functional balance skills
7. Effects of cognitive demand on balance
8. Self-report measures of balance activities

Several of the balance measures have well-established norms that can be used for comparisons, and many are used to identify older adults at risk for falls (Table 6-3). Because the older adult will be asked to perform a number of tasks that will cause instability, safety is essential, and the therapist should closely guard and protect the person at all times to prevent a fall.

Static Balance

To assess static balance, clinicians typically observe spontaneous postural sway during quiet stance. Altering the base of support by asking the older adult to bring his or her feet together, stand in tandem stance or on one leg, increases the difficulty of the initial static balance task. Differences in the amount of postural sway with eyes-open versus eyes-closed for each of the positions are also noted, and the amount of time the older adult can maintain each of the positions is recorded.

Postural sway increases with age (Sheldon, 1963) and is greater in older subjects with declining balance (Baloh, Corona, Jacobson, Enrietto, & Bell, 1998). The ability to perform one-legged stance in subjects from 20 to 80 years of age has been reported to decline 32% with eyes open and 100% with eyes closed (Potvin, 1980). Maintaining the ability to

balance with a reduced area of weight bearing is important when considering functional activities, because walking and stair climbing require the ability to stand on one leg.

Limits of Stability

The Functional Reach Test (FRT) is a single-item quick screening test to assess the capacity of an older adult to perform a voluntary movement while challenging balance. The older adult is asked to stand with feet shoulder distance apart, flex one arm to 90 degrees, and reach as far forward as he or she is able. The functional reach is recorded in inches as the greatest distance the person is able to reach forward beyond arm's length while maintaining a fixed base of support, and that can be compared to gender- and age-related norms. The FRT has been found to be predictive of falls among older adults. (Duncan, Weiner, Chandler, & Studenski, 1990).

The Multi-Directional Reach Test (MDRT), an expansion of the FRT, examines the older adult's limits of stability backward and laterally to the right and left, in addition to the forward direction (Newton, 2001). The distance the person can reach in each direction is recorded.

Anticipatory Postural Control

In the clinical setting, it is more difficult to quantitatively examine anticipatory postural control. This aspect of balance can be assessed by telling the older adult a nudge is going to be applied in advance of the action and he or she needs to resist it, or by asking the individual to negotiate an obstacle course. An older adult with good anticipatory postural control abilities will be able to quickly respond to the perturbation by stabilizing the body and negotiate the obstacles with little hesitation.

The Dynamic Gait Index is an eight-item measure of gait. Although considered a mobility test, several test items examine the older adult's ability to modify gait in response to changes in tasks, providing an indication of anticipatory postural control (e.g., "turn and stop," stepping over a shoe box, and going around a cone) (Shumway-Cook & Woollacott, 2001). Scores below 19 are associated with increased fall risk (Shumway-Cook, Gruber, Baldwin, & Liao, 1997).

Reactive Postural Control

The nudge test developed by Tinetti (1986) is one method of assessing reactive postural

TABLE 6-3 Norms and Other Scores for Common Balance Measures

Measure	Norms	Other Scores
Functional Reach Test (Duncan et al., 1990)	**Men (Mean reach, inches ± SD)** (Duncan et al., 1990) 20–40 yr 16.7 ± 1.9 41–69 yr 14.9 ± 2.2 70–87 yr 13.2 ± 1.6 **Women (Mean reach, inches ± SD)** (Duncan et al., 1990) 20–40 yr 14.6 ± 2.2 41–69 yr 13.8 ± 2.2 70–87 yr 10.5 ± 3.5	Reach ≤ 6 inches = high risk of falls (Duncan et al., 1992) Reach > 6 but < 10 inches = risk of falls (Duncan et al., 1992)
Multi-directional Reach Test (Newton, 2001)	**Men and Women (74.1 ± 7.9 yrs)** (Newton, 2001) FR (inches) 8.89 ± 3.4 BR (inches) 4.64 ± 3.1 RR (inches) 6.86 ± 3.0 LR (inches) 6.61 ± 2.9	**Below Average Scores** (Newton, 2001) FR < 5.6 inches BR < 1.6 inches RR < 3.8 inches LR < 3.8 inches **Above Average Scores** (Newton, 2001) FR > 12.2 inches BR > 7.6 inches RR > 9.4 inches LR > 9.4 inches
Timed Up and Go (Podsiadlo & Richardson, 1991)	**TUG (Mean seconds, 95% CI)** (Newton, 2001) 60–69 yr 8.1 s (7.1, 9.0) 70–79 yr 9.2 s (8.2, 10.2) 80–99 yr 11.3 s (10.0 – 12.7)	< 10 seconds = independent in balance and mobility skills (Podsiadlo & Richardson, 1991) < 20 seconds = mostly independently mobile (Podsiadlo & Richardson, 1991) > 30 = dependent in mobility and ADL (Podsiadlo & Richardson, 1991)
Berg Balance Scale (BBS) (Berg, Wood-Dauphinee, Williams, & Maki, 1989)		> 14 s = at risk for falls (Shumway-Cook, Brauer, & Woollacott, 2000) <45/56 = predictive of falls (Berg, Wood-Dauphinee, Williams, & Maki, 1989) <36/56 = fall risk close to 100% (Shumway-Cook, Baldwin, Polissar, & Gruber, 1997) Between 46/56 and 54/56 = a 1-point decrease in BBS: associated with a 6% to 8% increase in fall risk (Shumway-Cook, Baldwin, Polissar, & Gruber, 1997)
Tinetti Performance-Oriented Mobility Assessment (Tinetti, 1986)		< 19/28 = high risk for falls (Tinetti, 1986) 19 – 24 = moderate risk for falls (Tinetti, 1986)

FR = forward reach; BR = leaning backwards; RR = reaching sideways to right; LR = reaching sideways to left; ADL = activities of daily living control. An unexpected nudge is lightly applied against the older adult's sternum three times and the response is graded using a three-point scale. A more sophisticated test that has been developed to test reactive postural control clinically is the Postural Stress Test (Wolfson, Whipple, Derby, Amerman, & Kleinberg, 1986). The PST unexpectedly perturbs the older adult in a backward direction using a weighted pulley system connected to a belt worn around the pelvis. Weights representing 1.5%, 3.0%, and 4.5% of total body weight are used to simulate small, medium, and large perturbations.

Sensory Strategies and Integration

The Clinical Test of Sensory Interaction in Balance (CTSIB) assesses balance in six sensory conditions (Shumway-Cook & Horak, 1986). The CTSIB is based on postural stability research and the interaction of the somatosensory, visual, and sensory systems and is the clinical equivalent to more expensive laboratory-based assessments of sensory strategies and integration. The older adult individual is tested under the following six conditions, and the time balance that can be maintained in each of the conditions is recorded:

1. Without visual restrictions
2. With a blindfold
3. With a visual conflict dome
4. Without visual restrictions, but standing on foam to control proprioceptive sensory input
5. With a blindfold and standing on foam to control proprioceptive sensory input
6. With a visual conflict dome and standing on foam to control proprioceptive sensory output

The six-condition test has been modified to a four-condition version (the Modified-CTSIB), which eliminates the visual conflict dome (Rose, 2003). The CTSIB provides useful information about the individual's ability to use and integrate sensory information to maintain postural stability.

Functional Balance Skills

When the concern is centered on the functional performance of an older adult, the ability of the individual to respond appropriately while performing everyday activities and skills may provide meaningful information. There are numerous measures that examine functional balance skills. It is important to note that functional balance tests have limitations:

1. Tests typically do not examine all aspects of postural control.
2. Most do not provide insight into quality of movement used to accomplish the task. It may be difficult to determine the specific subsystem responsible for the performance problem.
3. The older adult's performance is examined under a limited environmental condition; thus, results may not be able to predict actual performance in more complex environments (Shumway-Cook & Woollacott, 2007).

The timed Get-Up-and-Go tests are used to measure an individual's functional dynamic balance. The Get-Up-and-Go test was originally described by Mathias, Nayak, and Isaacs (1986) and later modified by Podsiadlo and Richardson (1991). The Timed Up and Go test, a commonly used screening test, measures the time it takes a person to rise to standing from a standard armchair, walk a distance of 3 meters, turn, walk back to a chair, and sit down.

The Berg Balance Scale, and the balance portion of The Tinetti Performance-Oriented Mobility Assessment (POMA) are commonly used clinically to screen for balance impairments and to assess components of functional performance. The POMA, consisting of both a balance and gait section, was developed as a falls risk index and examines postural stability and mobility skills (Tinetti, 1986). The balance portion includes assessments of static sitting and standing balance, anticipatory and reactive balance, and the ability to use somatosensory inputs. The Berg Balance Scale (BBS) consists of 14 balance items common to many functional tasks, such as reaching, bending forward, transferring, standing, and getting up from a chair. The BBS includes items that examine static balance (including positions of reduced base of support), dynamic balance, anticipatory balance, the ability to use somatosensory inputs, and forward limits of stability (Berg, Wood-Dauphinee, Williams, & Maki, 1989). Both the POMA and the BBS have cut-off scores for increased falls risk.

The more recently developed Fullerton Advanced Balance (FAB) scale (Rose, 2003) is intended for use in higher-functioning older adults, as the majority of items are considerably more challenging than the POMA or BBS. No cut-off scores for falls risk are available for the FAB; however, more balance dimensions are examined, including the ability to use somatosensory and vestibular inputs, forward limits of stability, anticipatory and reactive postural control, and static and dynamic balance in a position of reduced base of support.

Effects of Cognitive Demand on Balance

Balance requires attentional resources (Lajoie, Teasdale, Bard, & Fleury, 1993; Teasdale, Bard, LaRue, & Fleury, 1993), and the effect of cognitive demand and attentional capacities on balance abilities has been the focus of recent research. The dual-task TUG (TUG$_{DT}$) was developed to examine whether adding a secondary task to the TUG would increase the specificity and sensitivity of the TUG as a fall risk measure (Shumway-Cook, Brauer, & Woollacott, 2000). The TUG$_{DT \ cognitive}$ asks the older adult to complete the TUG while counting backwards by threes, and the TUG$_{DT\_manual}$ asks the older adult to complete the TUG while carrying a cup of water. Although the TUG alone was found to be a sensitive and specific indicator of fall risk, the time to complete the TUG$_{DT}$ was significantly longer in the dual-task conditions. This finding indicates that adding a secondary task may provide insight into how an older adult can maintain balance under multitask conditions (Shumway-Cook et al., 2000).

Self-Report Measures of Balance Ability

An essential component of balance assessment is finding out from the older adult the circumstances that lead to a loss of balance and his or her perceptions about how balance abilities affect daily activities. Self-report measures that examine balance ability include the Activities-specific Balance Confidence (ABC) scale (Powell & Meyers, 1995) and the Modified Falls Efficacy Scale (MFES) (Hill, Schwarz, Kalogeropolous, & Gibson, 1996). The ABC is a 16-item questionnaire that examines how confident the older adult feels about performing various activities without losing his or her balance on a scale from 0% (no confidence) to 100% (complete confidence) (Powell & Meyers, 1995). The MFES, a 14-item questionnaire, asks the client to rate on a 10-point visual analogue scale how confidently he or she can do an activity without falling (0 = not confident/not sure at all; 5 = fairly

confident/fairly sure; 10 = completely confident/completely sure) (Hill et al., 1996). Gathering this type of information is useful in determining which aspects of postural control may be impaired and assists the clinician in structuring the examination, generating hypotheses, and developing an intervention plan (Shumway-Cooke & Woollacott, 2007).

Gait Assessment

In the clinical setting, visual observation is the most common method for assessing gait, but this method has poor inter-rater and retest reliability and poor criterion validity against **kinematic** (i.e., characteristics of movement) analysis (Eastlack, Arvidson, Snyder-Mackler, Danoff, & McGarvey, 1991; Goodkin & Diller, 1973; Krebs, Edelstein, & Fishman, 1985). Timed measures of gait using a stopwatch have moderate to high reliability but are limited to collecting data on gait **velocity, stride length,** and **cadence** (Morris, Morris, & Iansek, 2001; Wall & Scarbrough, 1997; Youndas & Atwood, 2000) and may require an individual to perform several repeat trials to collect the necessary information. Regardless, measuring gait velocity is simple and quick, and velocity is considered a composite measure of distance and temporal gait variables. Gait velocity has been demonstrated to be a sensitive test for detecting mobility impairments and a strong predictor of adverse events, even for highly functional older adults (Cesari et al., 2005; Montero-Odasso et al., 2005). Although there is no consensus regarding optimal testing distance for determining gait velocity, a common method is to calculate gait velocity over a longer distance, such as 10 meters, to accommodate the acceleration phase of walking (Bendall et al., 1989). Comfortable gait speeds for men in their fifties, sixties, and seventies are 83.6 meters/minute, 81.5 meters/minute, and 79.8 meters/minute, respectively. For women in their fifties, sixties, and seventies, comfortable gait speeds are 83.7 meters/minute, 77.8 meters/minute, and 76.3 meters/minute, respectively (Bohannon, 1997).

Clinicians may also use standardized gait assessment forms, such as the Gait Assessment Rating Scale (GARS; Wolfson, Whipple, Amerman, & Tobin, 1990) or the modified version of the GARS (VanSwearingen, Paschal, Bonino, & Yang, 1996), and the Dynamic Gait Index (DGI; Shumway-Cook & Woollacott,

1995). These measures have been tested in healthy adults and older adults with a history of falls, are reliable, are sensitive indicators of gait function changes, and have been found to distinguish older adults with or without a history of recurrent falls. For example, DGI scores below 19 (out of 24) are indicative of increased fall risk in older adults (Shumway-Cook et al., 1997).

The "Stops Walking When Talking" (SWWT) test examines the ability of the older adult to perform a secondary task, talking, while walking (Lundin-Olsson, Nyberg, & Gustafson, 1997). The examiner begins a conversation with the walking client and a positive test is defined if the client stops walking in order to talk. The SWWT has been found to be a predictor of falls among frail, institutionalized older adults (Lundin-Olsson et al., 1997).

Laboratory assessment of gait typically requires sophisticated and costly equipment, including high-speed digital video recording systems, floor-mounted force plates, and electromyography, and thus, it tends to be limited to the research setting. Although costly, this type of assessment allows the kinematic and **kinetic** (i.e., analysis of forces) qualities of the gait pattern, and the spatial and temporal qualities of muscle activation patterns (via electromyography) throughout the gait cycle to be captured. Studies that have used these sophisticated methods for evaluating gait have been extremely useful in providing an understanding of how age and pathology influence gait (e.g., see Winter et al., 1990). Portable walkways, consisting of a long strip of walking surface in which an array of embedded pressure-sensitive sensors run across and along the surface length, and foot-switch systems, pressure-sensitive switches placed either on the feet or inside or outside of the shoes, are less expensive but do allow more objective and reliable methods of evaluating temporal and spatial gait parameters and the timing, symmetry, and sequencing of gait events. These less-expensive methods of gait assessment are often used in rehabilitation settings where more comprehensive gait analysis is warranted.

Management of Neuromusculoskeletal Impairments in the Older Adult

Successful aging equates to sustaining a high quality of life, primarily through the maintenance of functional independence. Research evidence suggests that participation in physical activities may help control chronic conditions and decrease the impact of the normal changes associated with aging. In addition, resistance training exercises can reverse many of the age-related physiologic changes, in addition to improving strength and function.

Numerous benefits of participation in regular physical activity have been identified for older adults in the past two decades, and the extent to which changes related to aging, such as decreased muscle mass and strength, can be ameliorated with interventions, including specific exercise programs, have been the focus of numerous research studies. Examination of *successful aging* reveals factors extrinsic to aging and disease process (nutrition, lifestyle and daily routine, degree of social support, amount of exercise, and sense of autonomy and control) play a strong, positive role in enabling older individuals to maintain their health and independence, and research has shown that remaining active and productive is a critical component of successful aging (Berkman et al., 1993; Fisher, 1995; Seeman et al., 1995). Health care professionals play key roles in promoting healthy lifestyles in older adults. Health and quality of life can be promoted through specific exercise programs and management plans, and occupation-based interventions that include meaningful choices of activities and productive activities (Figure 6-9).

A variety of factors have been found to determine adherence to exercise in older adults. Some of these increase adherence (motivators), whereas others decrease adherence (barriers). One of the strongest motivators affecting exercise adherence in older adults is self-efficacy, the concept that a person is capable of controlling his or her own behavior (Burton, Shapiro, & German, 1999; Conn, 1998; Resnick, 2001; Resnick & Spellbring, 2000). Outcome expectation, the belief that specific consequences will result from specific personal actions, is another strong motivator (Burton et al., 1999; Resnick, 2001; Resnick & Spellbring, 2001). Barriers to exercise for older adults include fear of falling or injury; lack of time, social support, a physical space to exercise, transportation to the exercise site; and insufficient resources to either buy exercise equipment or join an exercise facility (King et al.,

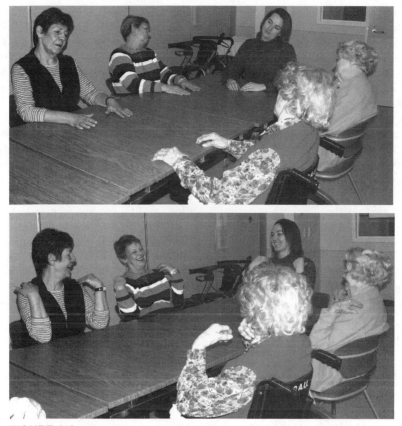

FIGURE 6-9 Regardless of physical abilities or function, exercising and remaining physically active are key to successful aging, especially when personally meaningful and enjoyable. (Courtesy of the Geriatric Day Hospital, Specialized Geriatric Services, Saskatoon Health Region, Saskatoon, Saskatchewan, with permission).

2002; Melillo et al., 1996; U.S. Department of Health and Human Services, 1996). In addition, increased stress and depression levels, increased age, decreased health status, and lack of enjoyment while exercising are associated with poor exercise adherence (Burton et al., 1999; Conn, 1998; Melillo et al., 1996; Resnick, 2001; Resnick & Spellbring, 2000).

Older adults will have very specific purposes and goals when seeking interventions or when beginning an exercise program, and these client-specific needs must be considered when developing a management plan. For example, some individuals may want to address the age-related changes that have manifested and that interfere with physical function, or may want to prevent further decline. Some older adults may seek to participate in an exercise program to improve overall fitness or for general health benefits, and others may be drawn by the social interactions

offered by group exercise programs. Because of the variability in personal preferences, lifestyle, fitness levels, and potential or actual comorbidities, it is important that exercise and activity programs be tailored and appropriate for the older individual. Areas of focus for intervention need to be based on the client's needs and interests in order for the intervention to be meaningful and purposeful to the client.

Because typical age related changes can cause impairments, older adults are at risk for functional decline and may have difficulty performing their daily occupations. Programs should be comprehensive and include exercises to increase or maintain strength, flexibility, postural stability, and endurance (see Chapter 4 for endurance exercise prescription). Activities should also be included that are tailored to the functional needs of the client. Any exercise or activity program should be designed to stress safety, in addition to meeting its goals and objectives. Age-related differences in response to exercise need to be taken into consideration, and modifications may be required when developing a program. Exercise prescription and training guidelines for older adults have been published (ACSM, 1998a, 1998b), are described briefly below, and are summarized in Table 6-4.

Strength and Resistance Exercises

Although there is no evidence to date suggesting that strength training halts the age-related loss of muscle fibers, it has been well documented that systematic strength training programs can be used to improve skeletal muscle strength in the older adult (Buchner et al., 1997a). Changes in the muscles of older adults following strengthening programs are similar to the gains observed in younger subjects who participate in exercise. In addition, a number of training methods, including endurance-training programs (see Chapter 4), have been used with varying degrees of success to accomplish an increase in strength in older persons (Sipilä et al., 1996).

Strength training has been found to be effective in both young-old and very-old adults (Buchner et al., 1997b; Fiatarone et al., 1990, 1994; Frischknecht, 1998; Frontera, Meredith, O'Reilly, Knuttgen, & Evans, 1988); in older adults who are healthy (Skelton et al., 1995) or living in institutional care (Fiatarone et al., 1994; McMurdo & Rennie, 1994); and in older adults following injury, such as post hip fracture (Mitchell, Stott, Martin, & Grant, 2001; Sherrington & Lord, 1997) or injurious fall (Hauer et al., 2001) (see Chapter 8).

Some of the research that has examined strength-training programs in older adults is summarized in Table 6-5, and readers are referred to the systematic review of progressive resistance strength training by Latham, Bennett, Stretton, and Anderson (2004) for additional information and references. In general, studies have found that both older men and women are able to safely engage in a strength-training exercise program with supervision, regardless of the type of exercise and the intensity of the program. Musculoskeletal injuries that have been reported were typically minor and did not interfere with participation in the exercise program (Judge, Whipple, & Wolfson, 1994; Pollock et al., 1991). Cardiovascular/pulmonary events include one incidence of shortness of breath (Jette et al., 1996) and one episode of fainting (Skelton & McLaughlin, 1996). Older adults who participate in strength-training research studies are typically carefully screened for risk factors and exercise contraindications, but some studies did not monitor and report adverse events, making it difficult to assess the risk of injury (Latham et al., 2004). Thus, it is not known whether or not participation in strength training increases an older adult's cardiovascular risk. Prior to the initiation of any vigorous exercise program, the older adult, especially if known cardiovascular risk factors are present, should undergo a medical evaluation and appropriate stress testing (ACSM, 2007).

Isometric, isotonic, and isokinetic programs, simple active exercises using body weight as resistance, and walking and aerobic programs have been found to be successful at increasing U/E and L/E strength in older men and women. Strengthening studies initially focused on low-intensity programs. However, in the past 10 years, the benefits of moderate- to heavy-resistance programs have been demonstrated, with remarkable gains. Strength gains achieved in the healthy, older adult are maintained for at least short periods after the formal exercise program is discontinued, and some studies have documented structural changes of the muscles, specifically increases in cross-sectional type IIB fiber areas, following formal exercise programs in older individuals. In addition, there is evidence that even frail older adults in long-term care or nursing home settings can tolerate heavy-resistance programs and can make similar gains as healthy, community-dwelling older adults.

Improvements extend beyond impairments. Significant functional benefits, such as improvement in gait speed (Judge, Underwood, & Gennosa, 1993), walking endurance (Ades et al., 1996), stair-climbing ability, and dynamic balance have been reported. However, effects of strengthening exercises on psychological well-being and participation restrictions remain unclear, as these areas have been not well studied, and with the few studies that do exist, results are inconsistent. A summary of points that should be considered when assisting an older person with a strengthening program are outlined in Box 6–7.

TABLE 6-4 Evidence-based Exercise Prescription for the Older Adult

Exercise Type	Exercise Parameters	Benefits	Precautions for the Older Adult
Stretching	• Static stretches—10 to 30 second hold for each major U/E and L/E muscle/tendon group • At least 4 repetitions for each muscle group • At least 2 to 3 days/week; every day is preferable	Documented benefits • Improved flexibility • Improved joint ROM Potential benefits • Improved function • Decreased risk of injury	• Stretching exercises should be performed through pain-free ROM only
Strengthening/Resistance	• Moderate (60% of 1 RM) to high intensity (70 to 80% of 1 RM) • 8 to 12 repetitions • 1 to 3 sets • 3 times/week	Documented Benefits • Increased strength • Increased walking endurance • Improved mobility • Increased stair-climbing endurance • Decreased functional/ADL decline • Increased functional ability Potential benefits • Improved quality of life • Improved sense of well-being	• Severely deconditioned older adults or those with known exercise risk factors require close supervision and an initial low intensity program • Exercises should be performed pain-free ROM • Movements should be controlled
Balance (also see Chapter 8)	• Dynamic exercises • Static exercises • Exercises for specific postural control problem • Tai Chi • Combined exercise programs	Documented Benefits • Improved balance performance • Improvement in fall risk scores • Decreased falls Potential Benefits • Improved agility • Improved quality of life • Improved sense of well-being	• A fall risk screen should be conducted prior to exercise prescription • Close supervision required for those at risk for falls • Need to sufficiently challenge balance, while ensuring safety • The older adult should use his/her typical assistive device while exercising, as needed
Endurance/Aerobic	• see Chapter 4		

ADL = activities of daily living; L/E = lower extremity; RM = repetition maximum; ROM = range of motion; U/E = upper extremity Data in part from ACSM. (1998). Position Stand: Exercise and Physical Activity for Older Adults. *Medicine and Science in Sports and Exercise, 30*(6), 992–1003; American College of Sports Medicine. (2006). ACSM's guidelines for exercise testing and prescription. 7th ed. (pp. 237–251). Philadelpnia, Lippincot, Williams & Wilkins.

TABLE 6-5 Summary of Selected Strengthening Studies in Older Adults

	Design			
Bamman et al. (2003)	RCT	Healthy M (mean age = 69) and F (mean age = 66)	3 x/week @ 80% 1 RM for 25 weeks	M = 82% ↑ 1-RM L/E strength F = 58% ↑ 1-RM L/E strength
Charette et al. (1991)	RCT	Healthy community-dwelling F (mean age = 69)	3 x/week @ 65–75% 1 RM for 12 weeks	28–115% ↑ 1-RM L/E strength; 7% ↑ in type 1 fiber area 20% ↑ in type 2 fiber area
Carmeli et al. (2000)	RCT	Ambulatory M and F in nursing home (mean age = 82)	2–5 kg free weights, 3 x/week for 12 weeks	10–15% ↑ isokinetic L/E strength ↑ in 3-minute walking distance
Ferri et al. (2003)	No control	Healthy, physically active M (mean age = 68)	3 x/week @ 80% 1 RM for 16 weeks	27% ↑ 1-RM L/E strength 11% ↑ isokinetic L/E strength
Fiatarone et al. (1990)	No control	Ambulatory M and F in nursing home (mean age = 90)	3 x/week @ 80% 1 RM for 8 weeks	174% ↑ 1-RM L/E strength
Fiatarone et al. (1994)	RCT	Ambulatory M and F in nursing home (mean age = 87)	3 x/week @ 80% 1 RM for 10 weeks	37–178% ↑ 1-RM L/E strength
Frontera (1988)	No control	Healthy, sedentary M (60–72)	3 x/week @ 80% 1 RM for 12 weeks	107% ↑ 1-RM L/E strength 11–15% ↑ in isokinetic L/E strength
Hruda, Hicks, & McCartney (2003)	RCT	M and F living in a LTC facility (75 to 94 years)	Progressive L/E exercises using body weight and bands (gradually performed more quickly—aimed at increasing power)	44% ↑ eccentric knee extensor power 60% ↑ eccentric knee extensor power 31% ↑ in 8-foot up-and-go test 66% ↑ in 30 s chair stand test 33% ↑ in walk time
Lexell et al. (1995)	RCT	Healthy community-dwelling M and F (70 to 77 years)	3 x/week @ 85% 1 RM for 11 weeks	163% ↑ in 1-RM L/E strength
Meuleman, Breuche, Kubilis, & Lowenthal (2000)	RCT	Debilitated M and F living in a nursing home setting (mean age = 75)	3 x/week using isokinetic dynamometer for 4 to 8 weeks	32.8% ↑ isometric strength across muscle groups (compared to 10.2% ↑ in control group) Significant increase in ADL score
Vincent et al. (2002)	RCT	Healthy, sedentary, community dwelling M (mean age = 68) and F (mean age = 67)	3 x/week @ 50% 1 RM for 24 weeks 3 x/week @ 50% 1 RM for 24 weeks	16% ↑ 1-RM L/E strength 20% ↑ 1-RM L/E strength ↓ time to ascend one flight of stairs

ADL = activities of daily living; F = female; LTC = long-term care; M = male; RCT = randomized control trial; RM = repetition maximum

> ### BOX 6-7 **Exercise Considerations for the Older Adult**
>
> - Use simple directions and gestures
> - Ensure adequate warm-up and cool-down
> - Take into consideration current and potential musculoskeletal problems, chronic conditions, and functional limitations
> - Institute short and graded exercise sessions, but apply the overload principle
> - Use a variety of muscle contractions: isometric, isotonic, isokinetic, concentric, and eccentric
> - Establish an exercise program with a focus on multiple components (low-impact aerobic, muscular strength, power, endurance and flexibility, and balance)
> - Monitor skin for signs of heat stress, respiration, and pulse rate in response to exercise
> - Exercise at an RPE of 12 to 14 ("somewhat hard") or use the *talk test:* the older adult should be able to engage in a conversation during the exercise
> - Older adults may gain less absolute strength
> - Older adults may gain strength slowly
> - Older adults may have less adaptability to exercise stress
>   - More susceptibility for injuries? Increased cramping during exercise?
> - Older adults may have decreased oxygen consumption
>   - May fatigue more easily?

Flexibility (Stretching) Exercises

Flexibility exercises increase the length and elasticity of periarticular tissues and muscle, increase joint mobility (Hubley, Kozey, & Stanish, 1984), prevent soft-tissue contractures, decrease risk of injury (Worrell, 1994a; 1994b), and are important to overall joint ROM. The following are main types of flexibility exercises:

- Static—a position is assumed, held for a period of time, and then relaxed
- Ballistic—repetitive bouncing motions where the muscle is rapidly stretched and immediately relaxed
- Proprioceptive neuromuscular facilitation (PNF)—alternating isometric muscle contraction and passive stretching through a series of movements
- Dynamic—the joint is moved through full ROM repetitively, such as with dancing or tai chi

Of all the types of programs, flexibility exercises have not been well studied in older adults, and the ideal type and duration of stretching exercises has yet to be determined. Studies have found that older adults who participate in a program of regular exercise or general exercise interventions can increase range of motion of various joints (Hubley-Kozey, Wall, & Hogan, 1995; Leslie & Frekany, 1975; Morey, Cowper, Feussner, Dipasquale, Crowley, & Sullivan, 1991). However, these studies also incorporated stretching exercises as part of the overall exercise program; thus, it is not known whether the stretching exercises or the general exercise are more beneficial for increasing flexibility (Hurley & Hagberg, 1998). Lan, Lais, Chen, and Wong (1998) studied the effects of a 12-month Tai Chi Chuan program and found the older males who participated increased their thoracic/lumbar flexibility by 11 degrees and the older females' increase in thoracic/lumbar flexibility was 8.8 degrees, compared to the control group. Rider and Daly (1991) studied the effects of specific stretching exercises in a group of older adults with a mean age of 71.8 years. The thrice-weekly, supervised exercise program focused on lumbar spine movements, and stretches were held for 10 seconds and repeated three times. After 10 weeks, the sit-and-reach test increased by 25% and spinal extension increased by 40% in the group that exercised, but the control group did not change. Static flexibility exercises are often prescribed for older individuals and may be performed independently or as part of a warm-up and cool-down for a strength or endurance exercise program.

Balance Exercises

Various types of balance exercises can be prescribed, and research has yet to find one form of balance exercise to be more beneficial than another. Several studies have examined the effects of a combination of types of exercises on balance, in addition to specific balance training (Hu & Woollacott, 1994; Tinetti et al., 1994; Wolf et al., 1996; Wolfson et al., 1996). Balance training programs that have emphasized postural stability have been shown to improve balance performance in older adults (Ledin et al., 1990; Rose & Clark, 2000; Wolfson et al., 1996). Combined exercise approaches that incorporate balance training in addition to flexibility, coordination, strength, and endurance exercises have also been shown to improve balance (Campbell, Robertson, Gardner, Norton, Tilyard, & Buchner, 1997; Campbell, Robertson, Gardner, Norton, & Buchner, 1999; Day et al., 2002; Hauer et al., 2001).

Balance programs should include a variety of elements and should sufficiently challenge individual abilities. Static balance exercises require no body movement, such as standing on one leg; dynamic balance exercises generally consist of moving the center of mass over the base of support, such as with walking or side-stepping. Decreasing the size of the base of support, incorporating U/E and head movements during balance activities, altering sensory demands, changing directions suddenly, and changing speed during a balance activity are methods of challenging the individual's balance. Because balance requires attentional resources and cognitive demands, balance activities with concurrent dual task activity may be beneficial, and balance activities that are closely related to everyday activities and function can also be incorporated into exercise programs. More recently, the effects of Tai Chi and balance training with a weighted vest have been studied in older adults. Both forms of exercises were found to be beneficial in decreasing fall risk (Shaw & Snow, 1998; Tsang & Hui-Chang, 2003, 2005).

Therapeutic intervention for balance dysfunction in the older adult should be specific to the cause or causes of the problem and the impact on function, as determined by a comprehensive assessment. With some older adults, simply changing shoes, altering the lighting or other environmental influences, applying a properly fitting orthosis, or using an assistive device may be all that is necessary. Other older adults may require a more focused management plan that addresses specific postural control problems identified in an evaluation. As described in Chapter 8 fall risk factors include impaired gait, decreased L/E muscle strength and flexibility, and decreased reaction times and coordination. Many of these impairments and functional limitations also impact on balance and can be remediated with exercise (Fiatarone et al., 1990; Probst, 1989; Whipple et al., 1987). In some cases, the factors that contribute to balance dysfunction may be less specific or undiagnosed; thus, the overall postural control mechanism must be "exercised."

Other Impairments
Coordination
Treatment of movement impairments relating to incoordination must take into consideration the cause. For example, alleviating musculoskeletal problems (e.g., decreased ROM, decreased flexibility) may improve coordination. Direct practice of functional activities, practice of non-functional movements, such as tracing a figure eight with a limb, weight-bearing activities for L/E incoordination, and environmental modifications to reduce performance deficits may assist in improving coordination. Because requirements for accuracy create increasing demands for coordination, selecting functional tasks with increasing accuracy demands may also train coordination (Shumway-Cook & Woollacott, 2007).

Skeletal Deformities and Postural Problems
Common postural problems in older persons may result from the age-related changes in the muscles and joints and may respond to an exercise program designed to increase both flexibility and strength. Educating the older adult in correct body posture during sedentary activities, such as reading or watching television, is important. The older adult should be educated regarding proper body mechanics during daily activities. Posture correction can be helpful in alleviating some of the problems that can occur with skeletal changes in the older adult. In addition, scoliosis (Brocklehurst et al., 1982) and leg-length discrepancy (Mahar et al., 1985) have been associated with increased postural sway in the older adult and may be corrected simply by providing a heel lift.

■ Summary

Clearly, changes that occur in the neuromusculoskeletal systems with aging can have negative consequences on functional abilities. There is no clear line between "normal" aging and what constitutes "disease" or "dysfunction." Most older adults manage their daily tasks quite well until some specific event, such as a fall or an acute illness, changes their physical status or until an accumulation of small decrements or chronic disease impairments reaches some breakpoint at which a particular activity or set of activities becomes impossible.

Although changes in the neuromusculoskeletal system may be a major factor associated with the loss of independence in ADLs, factors other than neuromuscular integrity, such as comorbidities (i.e., arthritis, impaired vision, changes in cognition and cardiorespiratory symptoms), may cause a decline in functional abilities. This chapter discussed the typical and expected age-related changes in the neuromusculoskeletal systems and the resulting impact on functional performance. It is important to recognize that these generalizations about change reflect an "average" and that individual variability is great. Physically active, older adults tend to have less disability than frail, older adults who are housebound or get out only infrequently.

Although not all-inclusive, a variety of assessments and intervention strategies were presented in this chapter. An exercise program consisting of strength, flexibility, balance, and endurance training can improve functioning of the neuromusculoskeletal system. The training response is dependent on a multitude of factors and requires a thorough understanding of all the subsystems involved, and several factors should be evaluated prior to establishing an appropriate program. If the goal of care is to return or to maintain the older adult at his or her highest functional level, it is paramount for health care providers to view each aging person as having unique life experiences that influence mobility.

Case Study

Mr. Stevens is a 78-year-old man who lives with his wife in a two-story home. The bedroom and bathroom are on the second floor and he has no home equipment. Mr. Stevens is a retired cattle farmer. When he retired from farming at the age of 70, Mr. Stevens decided he would "take life easy and let my son do all the hard work." He helps his wife with the gardening in the summer, but finds it difficult to find things to do "to keep busy" in the winter. He no longer goes golfing. He has quit his recreational curling team and no longer skates in the winter because he doesn't feel like he can keep up with his friends and is embarrassed that he might fall. His current hobbies include playing bridge once a week.

Other than the beginnings of cataracts in both eyes, he has no other health problems. Mr. Stevens states he is independent with mobility and all ADLs, with the exception of tub transfers—he needs minimal assistance from his wife with tub transfers. Mr. Stevens has difficulty getting up from low levels and soft surfaces. Mr. Stevens reports a history of imbalance during walking and states he loses his balance at least three or four times per week.

U/E mm strength was graded as 4 for all major muscle groups. L/E muscle strength was graded as 4– for all major muscle groups except bilateral hip flexion and abduction (graded 3 bilaterally) and bilateral ankle DF (graded as 3–).

TUG time was 12.8 seconds. Mr. Stevens used his arms to push up from the chair and rose from the chair very slowly. Slight postural instability was noted with immediate standing and turning. Stride length and foot clearance were decreased.

continued on page 168

Case Study (continued)

Questions

1. Using the ICF framework and the older adult continuum of function, describe Mr. Steven and his current scenario.
2. What assessment findings might be related to normal age-related changes?
3. What additional assessment information would you like to gather from Mr. Stevens?
4. What other tests and measures might you include in your evaluation? Why?
5. Based on the information provided in the scenario, what do you think the main focus of your intervention might include?

Review Questions

1. What are the most profound changes in the aging neuromusculoskeletal system? What are the functional implications of these changes in the everyday lives of older adults?
2. Mrs. Elena Sampson is a 73-year-old woman without chronic illness. How would you expect Mrs. Sampson's muscular system to differ from that of a 35-year-old individual? Be sure to include both structural and histochemical aspects.
3. Compare three different strength assessment procedures that are commonly used with the older individual. Under what circumstances should they be used?
4. Muscle strengthening programs in the older adult have been successful. Describe any special considerations that should be adhered to during strength training of an older adult.
5. What are the expected age-related changes in posture, balance, and coordination?
6. Define postural sway, postural control, postural orientation, postural stability, static posture, static balance, and dynamic balance. Why are each important? How are each assessed?
7. What components need to be considered when prescribing a comprehensive exercise program to an older adult?

Web-Based Resources

For helpful information about the experience of neuromusculoskeletal and movement function, visit:

www.acsm-msse.org/pt/re/msse/positionstandards.htm;jsessionid=
FqJbwQRJ8ZnSCcRDN1wpQvD7QGGQGNc5k2NDFsrDp4v5byz497W36!-1455700262!-
949856145!8091!-1,The American College of Sports Medicine, date last connected March 30, 2007. This website contains a listing of various full-text position stands that have been published in *Medicine and Science in Sports and Exercise,* the official journal of the American College of Sports Medicine. The Position Stand on **Exercise and Physical Activity for Older Adults** is found on this site.

www.arthritis.org, **The Arthritis Foundation,** date last connected March 30, 2007. This official website of the Arthritis Foundation contains numerous resources for people with arthritis.

www.nof.org, **National Osteoporosis Foundation,** date last connected March 30, 2007. This the official website of the National Osteoporosis Foundation contains numerous resources for people with osteoporosis and for health care professionals.

www.agingblueprint.org, **The National Blueprint: Increasing Physical Activity Among Adults Age 50 and Older,** date last connected March 30, 2007. This website houses numerous resources and links to other healthy aging websites. Content is geared toward health care professionals and older adults

www.phac-aspc.gc.ca/pau-uap/fitness/index.htm, **The Healthy Living Unit (Public Health Agency of Canada, Government of Canada),** date last connected March 30, 2007. This website contains numerous resources about the benefits of physical activity and the range of opportunities to be physically active in daily life, for different age groups, including older adults. A consumer guide that includes checklists, and a tracking chart about physical activity, *Canada's Physical Activity Guide to Healthy Active Living for Older Adults* (published by Health Canada, 2001) can be found on this site.

REFERENCES

Ades, P. A., Waldmann, M. L., Meyer, M. L., Brown, D. A., Poehlman, E. T., Pendleburgy, W. W., et al. (1996). Skeletal muscle and cardiovascular adaptations to exercise conditioning in older coronary patients. *Circulation, 94,* 323–330.

American College of Sports Medicine. (1998a). Stand. Exercise and physical activity for older adults. *Medicine and Science in Sports and Exercise, 30,* 992–1008.

American College of Sports Medicine. (1998b). Stand. The recommended quantity and quality of exercise for developing and maintaining cardiorespiratory and muscular fitness, and flexibility in healthy adults. *Medicine and Science in Sports and Exercise, 30*(6), 975–991.

American College of Sports Medicine. (2007). *ACSM's guidelines for exercise testing and prescription* (7th ed.). Philadelphia: Lippincott, Williams & Wilkins.

American Geriatrics Society Panel on Exercise and Osteoarthritis. (2001). Exercise prescription for older adults with osteoarthritis pain: Consensus practice recommendations. *Journal of the American Geriatrics Society, 49,* 808–823.

Anderson, J. L., Terzis, G., & Kryger, A. (1999). Increase in the degree of coexpression of myosin heavy chain isoforms in skeletal muscle fibers of the very old. *Muscle and Nerve, 22,* 440–454.

Aniansson, A., Grimby, G., & Hedberg, M. (1992). Compensatory muscle fibre hypertrophy in elderly men. *Journal of Applied Physiology, 73,* 812–816.

Aniansson, A., Grimby, G., Hedberg, M., & Krotkiewski, M. (1981). Muscle morphology, enzyme activity and muscle strength in elderly men and women. *Clinical Physiology, 1,* 73–86.

Aniansson, A., Hedberg, M., Henning, G. B., & Grimby, G. (1986). Muscle morphology, enzymatic activity, and muscle strength in elderly men: A follow-up study. *Muscle & Nerve, 9,* 585–591.

Baloh, R. W., Corona, S., Jacobson, K. M., Enrietto, J. A., & Bell, T. (1998). A prospective study of posturography in normal older people. *Journal of the American Geriatrics Society, 46,* 438–443.

Bamman, M. M., Hill, V. J., Adams, G. R., Haddad, F., Wetzstein, C. J., Gower, B. A., et al. (2003). Gender differences in resistance-training-induced myofiber hypertrophy among older adults. *Journal of Gerontology: Biological Sciences, 58A,* 108–116.

Bassey, E. J., Fiatarone, M. A., O'Neill, E. F., Kelly, M., Evans, W. J., & Lipsitz, L. A. (1992). Leg extensor power and functional performance in very old men and women. *Clinical Science, 82,* 321–327.

Bassey, E. J., Morgan, K., Dallosso, H. M., & Ebrahim, S. B. (1989). Flexibility of the shoulder joint measured as range of abduction in a large representative sample of men and women over 65 years of age. *European Journal of Applied Physiology, 58,* 353–360.

Bean, J. F., Kiely, D. K., Herman, S., Leveille, S. G., Mizer, K., Frontera, W. R., et al. (2002). The relationship between leg power and physical performance in mobility-limited older people. *Journal of the American Geriatrics Society, 50,* 461–467.

Bean, J. F., Leveille, S. G., Kiely, D. K., Bandinelli, S., Guralnik, J. M., & Ferrucci, L. (2003). A comparison of leg power and leg strength within the In CHIANTI study: Which influences mobility more? *The Journals of Gerontology: Biological Sciences, 58A*(8), 728–733.

Bendall, M. J., Bassey, E. J., & Pearson, M. B. (1989). Factors affecting walking speed of elderly people. *Age and Ageing, 18,* 327–332.

Berg, K. O., Wood-Dauphinee, S. L., Williams, J. I., & Maki, B. (1989). Measuring balance in the elderly: Validation of an instrument. *Canadian Journal of Public Health, 83,* S7–S11.

Berkman, L. F., Seeman, T. E., Albert, M., Blazer, D., Kahn, R., Mohs, R., et al. (1993). High, unusual and impaired functioning in community-dwelling older men and women: Findings from the MacArthur Foundation Research Network on Successful Aging. *Journal of Clinical Epidemiology, 46,* 1129–1140.

Blanke, D., & Hageman, P. (1989). Comparison of gait of young men and elderly men. *Physical Therapy, 69,* 144–148.

Bohannon, R. W. (1997). Comfortable and maximum walking speed of adults aged 20–79 years: Reference values and determinants. *Age & Ageing, 26*(1), 15–19.

Bohannon, R. W. (2006). Reference values for the Timed Up and Go Test: A descriptive meta-analysis. Bornstein, R. A. (1986). Normative data on intermanual differences on three tests of motor performance. *Journal of Clinical Experimental Neuropsychology, 8,* 12–20.

Brocklehurst, J. C., Robertson, D., & James-Groom, P. (1982). Skeletal deformities in the elderly and their effect on postural sway. *Journal of the American Geriatrics Society, 30,* 534–538.

Brown, M. (1993). The well elderly. In A. A. Guccionee (Ed.), *Geriatric Physical Therapy.* St. Louis, MO: Mosby.

Brown, M., Sinacore, D. R., & Host, H. H. (1995). The relationship of strength to function in the older adult. *Journal of Gerontology: Biological Sciences & Medical Sciences, 50,* 55–59.

Buchner, D. M., Beresford, S. A., Larson, E. B., LaCroix, A. Z., & Wagner, E. H. (1992). Effects of physical activity on health status in older adults. II. Intervention studies. *Annual Review of Public Health, 13,* 469– 488.

Buchner, D. M., Cress, M. E., de Lateur, B. J., Esselman, P. C., Margherita, A. J., Price, R., et al. (1997a). The effect of strength and endurance training of gait, balance, fall risk, and health services use in community-living older adults. *Journal of Gerontology: Medical Sciences, 52A,* M218–M224.

Buchner, D. M., Cress, M. E., de Lateur, B. J., Esselman, P. C., Margherita, A. J., Price, R., et al. (1997b). A comparison of the effects of three types of endurance training on balance and other fall risk factors in older adults. *Aging and Clinical Experimental Research, 9,* 112–119.

Burton, L. C., Shapiro, S. B., & German, P. S. (1999). Determinants of physical activity initiation and maintenance among community-dwelling older persons. *Prevention Medicine, 29,* 422–430.

Campbell, A. J., Robertson, M. C., Gardner, M. M., Norton, R. N., & Buchner, D. M. (1999). Falls prevention over 2 years: A randomized controlled trial in women 80 years and older. *Age and Ageing, 2*(6), 513–518.

Campbell, A. J., Robertson, M. C., Gardner, M. M., Norton, R. N., Tilyard, M. W., & Buchner, D. M. (1997). Randomised controlled trial of a general practice programme of home based exercise to prevent falls in elderly women. *British Medical Journal, 315,*1065–1069.

Campbell, W. C., Trappe, T. A., Wolfe, R. R., & Evans, W. J. (2001). The recommended dietary allowance for protein may not be adequate for older people to maintain skeletal muscle. *Journal of Gerontology: Medical Sciences, 56A,* M373–M380.

Capranica, L., Tessitore, A., Olivieri, B., Minganti, C., & Pesce, C. (2004). Field evaluation of cycled coupled movements of hand and foot in older individuals. *Gerontology, 50*(6), 399–406.

Carmeli, E., & Reznick, A. Z. (1994). The physiology and biochemistry of skeletal muscle atrophy as a function of age. *Proceedings of the Society for Experimental Biology and Medicine, 206,* 106–113.

Carmeli, E., Reznick, A. Z., Coleman, R., & Carmeli, V. (2000). Muscle strength and mass of lower extremities in relation to functional abilities in elderly adults. *Gerontology, 46*(5), 249–257.

Cesari, M., Kritchevsky, S. B., Penninx, B. W., Nicklas, B. J., Simonsick, E. M., Newman, A. B., et al. (2005). Prognostic value of usual gait speed in well-functioning older people—Results from the Health, Aging and Body Composition Study. *Journal of the American Geriatrics Society, 53*(10), 1675–1680.

Charette, S. L., McEvoy, L., Pyka, G., Snow-Harter, C., Guido, D., Wiswell, R. A., et al. (1991). Muscle hypertrophy response to resistance training in older women. *Journal of Applied Physiology, 70,* 1912–1916.

Chen, H. S., Ashton-Miller, J. A., Alexander, N. B., & Schultz, A. B. (1994). Effects of age and available response time on ability to step over an obstacle. *Journal of Gerontology: Medical Sciences, 49,* M227–M233.

Cieza, A., Brockow, T., Ewert, T., Amman, E., Kollerits, B., Chatterji, S., et al. (2002). Linking health-status measurements to the international classification of functioning. Disability and health. *Journal of Rehabilitation Medicine, 34*(5), 205–210.

Clark, G. S., & Siebens, H. C. (1998). Geriatric rehabilitation. In J. A. DeLisa & B. M. Gans (Eds.), *Rehabilitation medicine principles and practice* (3rd ed.). Philadelphia: Lippincott-Raven.

Conn, V. S. (1998). Older adults and exercise: Path analysis of self-efficacy related constructs. *Nursing Research, 47,* 180–189.

Cooper, C., Campion, G., & Melton, L. J., III. (1992). Hip fractures in the elderly: A world-wide projection. *Osteoporosis International, 2,* 285–289.

Cress, M. E., Buchner, D. M., Questad, K. A., Esselman, P. C., deLateur, B. J., & Schwartz, R. S. (1996). Continuous-scale physical functional performance in a broad range of older adults: A validation study. *Archives of Physical Medicine and Rehabilitation, 77*(12), 1243–1250.

Csuka, M., & McCarty, D. J. (1985). Simple method for measurement of lower extremity muscle strength. *American Journal of Medicine, 78,* 77–81.

Cummings, S. R., & Melton, J., III. (2002). Epidemiology and outcomes of osteoporotic fractures. *Lancet, 359,* 1761–1766.

D'Antona, G., Pellegrino, M. A., Adami, R., Rossi, R., Carlizzi, C. N., Canepari, M., et al. (2003). The effect of ageing and immobilization on structure and function of human skeletal muscle fibres. *Journal of Physiology, 552,* 499–511.

Day, L., Fildes, B., Gordon, I., Fitzharris, M., Flamer, H., & Lord, S. (2002). Randomised factorial trial of falls prevention among older people living in their own homes. *British Medical Journal, 325,* 128–134.

Desrosiers, J., Hebert, R., Bravo, G., & Dutil, E. (1995a). The Purdue pegboard test: Normative data for people aged 60 and over. *Disability and Rehabilitation, 17,* 217–224.

Desrosiers, J., Hebert, R., Bravo, G., & Dutil, E. (1995b). Upper extremity performance tests for the elderly (TEMPA): Normative data and correlates with sensorimotor parameters. *Archives of Physical Medicine and Rehabilitation, 76,* 1125–1129.

Doherty, T. J., Vandervoort, A. A., Taylor, A. W., & Brown, W. F. (1993). Effects of motor unit losses on strength in older men and women. *Journal of Applied Physiology, 74,* 868–874.

Duncan, P., Weiner, D. K., Chandler, J., & Studenski, S. (1990). Functional reach: A new clinical measure of balance. *Journal of Gerontology, 45,* M192–M197.

Eastlack, M. E., Arvidson, J., Snyder-Mackler, L., Danoff, J. V., & McGarvey, C. L. (1991). Inter-rater reliability of videotaped observational gait-analysis assessments. *Physical Therapy, 71,* 465–472.

Einkauf, D. K., Gohdes, M. L., Jensen, G. M., & Jewell, M. J. (1987). Changes in spinal mobility with increasing age in women. *Physical Therapy, 67,* 370–375.

Essen-Gustaysson, B., & Borges, O. (1986). Histochemical and metabolic characteristics of human skeletal muscle in relation to age. *Acta Physiologica Scandinavica, 126,* 107–114.

Ferri, A., Scaglioni, G., Pousson, M., Capodaglio, P., Van Hoecke, J., & Narici, M. V. (2003). Strength and power changes of the human plantar flexors and knee extensors in response to resistance training in old age. *Acta Physiologica Scandinavica, 177,* 69–78.

Ferrucci, L., Guralnik, J. M., Buchner, D., Kasper, J., Lamb, S. E., Simonsick, E. M., et al. (1997). Departures from linearity in the relationship between measures of muscular strength and physical performance of the lower extremities: The women's health and aging study. *Journal of Gerontology: Medical Sciences, 52A,* M275–M285.

Fiatarone, M. A., Marks, E. C., Ryan, N. D., Meredith, C. N., Lipsitz, L. A., & Evans, W. J. (1990). High-intensity strength training in nonagenarians: Effects on skeletal muscle. *Journal of the American Medical Association, 263,* 3029–3034.

Fiatarone, M. A., O'Neill, E. F., Ryan, N. D., Clements, K. M., Solares, G. R., & Nelson, M. E. (1994). Exercise training and nutritional supplementation for physical frailty in very elderly people. *New England Journal of Medicine, 330,* 1769–1775.

Fiatarone Singh, M. A., Ding, W., Manfredi, T. J., Solares, G. S., O'Neill, E. F., Clements, K. M., et al. (1999). Insulin-like growth factor I in skeletal muscle after weight-lifting exercise in frail elders. *American Journal of Physiology, 277,* E135–E143.

Fielding, J. W. (1985). The cervical spine. In T. P. Sculco (Ed.), *Orthopedic Care of the Geriatric Patient.* St. Louis, MO: Mosby.

Fisher, B. J. (1995). Successful aging, life satisfaction and generativity in later life. *International Journal of Aging and Human Development, 41,* 239–250.

Fitzgerald, G. K., Wynyeen, K. J., Rheault, W., & Rothschild, B. (1983). Objective assessment with establishment of normal values for lumbar spinal range of motion. *Physical Therapy, 63*(11), 1776–1781.

Foldvari, M., Clark, M., Laviolette, L. C., Bernstein, M. A., Kaliton, D., Castaneda, C., et al. (2000). Association of muscle power with functional status in community-dwelling elderly women. *Journals of Gerontology Series A-Biological Sciences & Medical Sciences, 55*(4), M192–M199.

Frischknecht, R. (1998). Effect of training on muscle strength and motor function in the elderly. *Reproduction, Nutrition, Development, 38,* 167–174.

Frolkis, V., Martynenko, O. A., & Zamostyan, V. P. (1976). Aging of the neuromuscular apparatus. *Gerontology, 22,* 244–279.

Frontera, W. R., Hughes, V. A., Fielding, R. A., Fiatarone, M. A., Evans, W. J., & Roubenoff, R. (2000). Aging of skeletal muscle: A 12-yr longitudinal study. *Journal of Applied Physiology, 88,* 1321–1326.

Frontera, W. R., & Larsson, L. (1999). Skeletal muscle function in older people. In T. L. Kauffman (Ed.), *Geriatric Rehabilitation Manual.* Philadelphia: Churchill Livingstone.

Frontera, W. R., Meredith, C., O'Reilly, K. P., Knuttgen, H. G., & Evans, W. (1988). Strength conditioning in older men: Skeletal muscle hypertrophy and improved function. *Journal of Applied Physiology, 64,* 1038–1044.

Gabell, A., & Nayak, U. (1984). The effect of age in variability in gait. *Journal of Gerontology, 39,* 662–666.

Gehlsen, G. M., & Whaley, M. H. (1990). Falls in the elderly: Part II. Balance, strength, and flexibility. *Archives of Physical Medicine and Rehabilitation, 71*(10), 739–741.

Genant, H. K., Cooper, C., Poor, G., Reid, I., Ehrlich, G., Kanis, J., et al. (1999). Interim report and recommendations of the World Health Organization Task-Force for Osteoporosis. *Osteoporosis International, 10,* 259–264.

Golding, L. A., & Lindsay, A. (1989). Flexibility and age. *Perspective, 15,* 28–30.

Goodkin, R., & Diller, L. (1973). Reliability among physical therapists in diagnosis and treatment of gait deviations in hemiplegics. *Perceptual and Motor Skills, 37,* 727–734.

Grimby, G. (1995). Muscle performance and structure in the elderly as studied: Cross-sectionally and longitudinally. *Journal of Gerontology (Special Issue) 50A,* 17–22.

Hageman, P., & Blanke, D. (1986). Comparison of gait in young women and elderly women. *Physical Therapy, 66,* 1382–1387.

Hakkinen, K., Newton, R. U., Gordon, S. E., McCormick, M., Volek, J. S., Nindl, B. C., et al. (1998). Changes in muscle morphology, electromyographic activity, and force production characteristics during progressive strength training in young and older men. *Journal of Gerontology: Biological Sciences, 53,* B415–B423.

Hale, S., Meyerson, J., & Wagstaff, D. (1987). General slowing of nonverbal information processing: Evidence for a power law. *Journal of Gerontology, 42,* 131–136.

Hauer, K., Rost, B., Rutschle, K., Opitz, H., Specht, N., Bartsch, P., et al. (2001). Exercise training for rehabilitation and secondary prevention of falls in geriatric patients with a history of injurious falls. *Journal of the American Geriatrics Society, 49,* 10–20.

Hay, L., Bard, C., Fleury, M., & Teasdale, N. (1996). Availability of visual and proprioceptive afferent messages and postural control in elderly adults. *Experimental Brain Research, 108*(1), 129–139.

Hikida, R. S., Staron, R. S., Hagerman, F. C., Walsh, S., Kaiser, E., Shell, S., et al. (2000). Effects of high-intensity resistance training on untrained older men. II. Muscle fiber characteristics and nucleo-cytoplasmic relationships. *Journal of Gerontology Series A-Biological Sciences & Medical Sciences, 55*(7), B347–B354.

Hill, K. D., Schwarz, J. A., Kalogeropoulos, A. J., & Gibson, S. J. (1996). Fear of falling revisited. *Archives of Physical Medicine and Rehabilitation, 77,* 1025–1029.

Hruda, K. V., Hicks, A. L., & McCartney, N. (2003). Training for muscle power in older adults: Effects on functional abilities. *Canadian Journal of Applied Physiology, 28*(2), 178–189.

Hu, M. H., & Woollacott, M. H. (1994). Multisensory training of standing balance in older adults: I. Postural stability and one-leg stance balance. *Journal of Gerontology: Medical Sciences, 49,* M52–M61.

Hubley, C. L., Kozey, J. W., & Stanish, W. D. (1984). The effects of static exercises and stationary cycling on range of motion at the hip joint. *Journal of Orthopaedic & Sports Physical Therapy, 6,* 104–109.

Hubley-Kozey, C. L., Wall, J. C., & Hogan, D. B. (1995). Effects of general exercise program on passive hip, knee, and ankle range of motion of older women. *Topics in Geriatric Rehabilitation, 10,* 33–44.

Hughes, V. A., Frontera, W. R., Wood, M., Evans, W. J., Roubenoff, R., & Dallal, G. E. (2001). Longitudinal muscle strength changes in older adults: Influence of muscle mass, physical activity and health. *Journal of Gerontology: Biological Sciences, 56A,* B209–B217.

Hultsch, D. F., MacDonald, S. W. S., & Dixon, R. A. (2002). Variability in reaction time performance of younger and older adults. *Journal of Gerontology: Psychological Sciences, 57B*(2), P101–P115.

Hunter, S., White, M., & Thompson, M. (1998). Techniques to evaluate elderly human muscle function: A physiological basis. *Journal of Gerontology: Biological Sciences, 53A,* B204–B216.

Hurley, B. F., & Hagberg, J. A. (1998). Optimizing health in older persons: Aerobic or strength training? *Exercise and Sports Reviews, 26,* 61–89.

Iannuzzi-Sucich, M., Prestwood, K. M., & Kenny, A. M. (2002). Prevalence of sarcopenia and predictors of skeletal muscle mass in healthy, older men and women. *Journal of Gerontology: Medical Sciences, 57A,* M772–M777.

James, B., & Parker, A. (1989). Active and passive mobility of lower limb joints in elderly men and women: Lower extremity range of motion. *American Journal of Physical Medicine and Rehabilitation, 68*(4), 162–167.

Jebsen, R. H., Taylor, N., Treischmann, R. B., Trotter, M. J., & Howard, L. A. (1969). An objective and standardized test of hand function. *Archives of Physical Medicine and Rehabilitation, 50,* 311–319.

Jette, A. M., Assmann, S. F., Rooks, D., Harris, B. A., & Crawford, S. (1998). Interrelationships among disablement concepts. *Journal of Gerontology: Biological Sciences & Medical Sciences, 53A,* M395–M404.

Jette, A. M., & Branch, L. G. (1981). The Framingham disability study: II. Physical disability among the aging. *American Journal of Public Health, 71,* 1211–1216.

Jette, A. M., Harris, B. A., Sleeper, L., Lachman, M. E., Heislein, D., Giorgetti, M., et al. (1996). A home-based exercise program for nondisabled older adults. *Journal of the American Geriatrics Society, 44,* 644–649.

Johnson, H. (1985). Is aging physiological or pathological? In H. A. Johnson (Ed.), *Relations Between Normal Aging and Disease.* New York: Raven Press.

Judge, J. O., Davis, R. B., III., & Ounpuu, S. (1996). Step length reductions in advanced age: The role of ankle and hip kinetics. *Journal of Gerontology Series A-Biological Sciences & Medical Sciences, 51*(6), M303–M312.

Judge, J. O., Underwood, M., & Gennosa, T. (1993). Exercise to improve gait velocity in older persons. *Archives of Physical Medicine and Rehabilitation, 74,* 400–406.

Judge, J. O., Whipple, R. H., & Wolfson, L. I. (1994). Effects of resistive and balance exercises on isokinetic strength in older persons. *Journal of the American Geriatrics Society, 42,* 937–946.

Kanis, J. A., & World Health Organization Study Group. (1994). Assessment of fracture risk and its application to screening for postmenopausal osteoporosis: Synopsis of a WHO report. *Osteoporosis International, 4,* 368–381.

Katzman, R., & Terry, R. (1992). Normal aging of the nervous system. In R. Katzman & R. Terry (Eds.), *The Neurology of Aging.* Philadelphia, PA: F.A. Davis.

Kauffman, T. (1982). Association between hip extension strength and standup ability in geriatric patients. *Physical and Occupational Therapy in Geriatrics, 1,* 39–45.

Kauffman, T. (1987). Posture and age. *Topics in Geriatric Rehabilitation, 2,* 13–28.

Kellor, M., Frost, J., Silberberg, N., Iverson, I., & Cummings, R. (1971). Hand strength and dexterity: Norms for clinical use. *American Journal of Occupational Therapy, 25,* 77–83.

Kendall, F. P., Kendall, E. M., Provance, P., Rodgers, M., & Romani, W. (1993). *Muscles, Testing and Function: With Posture and Pain.* Williams & Wilkins, Baltimore.

Kent-Braun, J. A., Ng, A. V., & Young, K. (2000). Skeletal muscle contractile and non-contractile components in young and elderly women and men. *Journal of Applied Physiology, 88,* 662–668.

Kiltgaard, H., Mantoni, M., Schiaffino, S., Ausoni, S., Gorza, L., Laurent-Winter, C., et al. (1990). Function, morphology and protein expression of ageing skeletal muscle: A cross-sectional study of elderly men with different training backgrounds. *Acta Physiologica Scandinavica, 140,* 41–54.

King, M. B., Whipple, R. H., Gruman, C. A., Judge, J. O., Schmidt, J. A., & Wolfson, L. I. (2002). The Performance Enhancement Project: Improving physical performance in older persons. *Archives of Physical Medicine and Rehabilitation, 83,* 1060–1069.

Kirkendall, D., & Garrett, W. (1998). The effects of aging and training on skeletal muscle. *American Journal of Sports Medicine, 26,* 598–602.

Kjeken, I., Dagfinrud, H., Slatkowsky-Christensen, B., Mowinckel, P., Uhlig, T., Kvien, T. K., et al. (2005). Activity limitations and participation restrictions in women with hand osteoarthritis: Patients' descriptions and associations between dimensions of functioning. *Annals of the Rheumatic Diseases, 64*(11), 1633–1638.

Klotzbuecher, C. M., Ross, P. D., Landsman, P. B., Abbott, T. A., 3rd, & Berger, M. (2000). Patients with prior fractures have an increased risk of future fractures: A summary of the literature and statistical synthesis. *Journal of Bone and Mineral Research, 15,* 721–739.

Krebs, D. E., Edelstein, J. E., & Fishman, S. (1985). Reliability of observational kinematic gait analysis. *Physical Therapy, 65,* 1027–1033.

Kressig, R. W., Gregor, R. J., Oliver, A., Waddell, D., Smith, W., O'Grady, M., et al. (2004). Temporal and spatial features of gait in older adults transitioning to frailty. *Gait and Posture, 20*(1), 30–35.

LaJoie, Y., Teasdale, N., Bard, C., & Fleury, M. (1993). Attentional demands for static and dynamic equilibrium. *Experimental Brain Research, 97,* 139–144.

Lan, C., Lais, J. S., Chen, S. Y., & Wong, M. K. (1998). 12-month Tai Chi training in the elderly: Its effect on health fitness. *Medicine & Science in Sports and Exercise, 30*(3), 345–351.

Larsson, L., Grimby, G., & Karlsson, J. (1979). Muscle strength and speed of movement in relation to age and muscle morphology. *Journal of Applied Physiology, 46,* 451–456.

Larsson, L., Sjodin, B., & Karlsson, J. (1978). Histochemical and biochemical changes in human skeletal muscle with age in sedentary males, age 22–65 years. *Acta Physiologica Scandinavica, 103,* 31–39.

Latham, N. K., Bennett, D. A., Stretton, C. M., & Anderson, C. S. (2004). Systematic review of progressive resistance training strength training in older adults. *The Journals of Gerontology, 59A*(1), 48–61.

Laufer, A. C., & Scheitz, B. (1968). Neuromuscular response tests as predictors of sensorimotor performance in aging individuals. *American Journal of Physical Medicine, 478,*250–263.

Laufer, Y. (2005). Effect of age on characteristics of forward and backward gait at preferred and accelerated walking speed. *Journal of Gerontology Series A-Biological Sciences & Medical Sciences, 60,* 627–632.

Ledin, T., Kronhed, A., Moller, C., Moller, M., Odkvist, L. M., & Olsson, B. (1990). Effects of balance training in elderly evaluated by clinical tests and dynamic posturography. *Journal of Vestibular Research, 1,* 129–138.

Leslie, D. K., & Frekany, G. A. (1975). Effects of an exercise program on selected flexibility measures of senior citizens. *Gerontologist, 4,* 182–183.

Lexell, J. (1995). Human aging, muscle mass, and fiber type composition. *Journal of Gerontology: Biological Sciences and Medical Sciences, 50A,* 11–15.

Lexell, J., Henriksson-Larsen, K., Winblad, B., & Sjöström, M. (1983). Distribution of different fiber types in human skeletal muscles: Effects of aging studies in whole muscle cross-sections. *Muscle & Nerve, 6,* 588–595.

Lexell, J., Taylor, C. C., & Sjöström, M. (1988). What is the cause of the ageing atrophy? Total number, size and proportion of different fiber types studied in whole vastus lateralis muscle from 15- to 83-year-old men. *Journal of Neurological Science, 84,* 275–294.

Lundin-Olsson, L., Nyberg, L., & Gustafson, Y. (1997). "Stops walking when talking" as predictor of falls in elderly people. *Lancet, 349,* 617.

Lynch, N. A., Metter, E. J., Lindle, R. S., Fozard, J. L., Tobin, J. D., Roy, T. A., et al. (1999). Muscle quality. I. Age associated differences between arm and leg muscle groups. *Journal of Applied Physiology, 86,* 188–194.

MacRae, P. G., Lacourse, M., & Moldavon, R. (1992). Physical performance measures that predict faller status in community-dwelling older adults. *Journal of Orthopedic and Sports Physical Therapy, 16,* 123–128.

Mahar, R. K, Kirby, R. L., & MacLeod, D. A. (1985). Simulated leg-length discrepancy: Its effect on mean center-of-pressure position and postural sway. *Archives of Physical Medicine and Rehabilitation, 66*(12), 822–824.

Maki, B. E., & McIlroy, W. E. (1996). Postural control in the older adult. *Clinics in Geriatric Medicine, 12,* 635–658.

Malatesta, D., Simar, D., Dauvilliers, Y., Candau, R., Borrani, F., Prefaut, C., et al. (2003). Energy cost of walking and gait instability in healthy 65- and 80-year-olds. *Journal of Applied Physiology, 95,* 2248–2256.

Martin, P. E., Rothstein, D. E., & Larish, D. D. (1992). Effects of age and physical activity status on the speed-aerobic demand relationship of walking. *Journal of Applied Physiology, 73*(1), 200–206.

Mathias, S., Nayak, U. S. L., & Isaacs, B. (1986). Balance in elderly patient: The "Get Up and Go" test. *Archives of Physical Medicine and Rehabilitation, 67,* 387–389.

Mathiowetz, V., Volland, G., Kashman, N., & Weber, K. (1985). Adult norms for the box and block test of manual dexterity. *American Journal of Occupational Therapy, 39,* 386–391.

Mbourou, G. A., Lajoie, Y., & Teasdale, N. (2003) Step length variability at gait initiation in elderly fallers and non-fallers, and young adults. *Gerontology, 49*(1), 21–26.

McComas, A. J. (1996). *Skeletal muscle.* Champaign, IL: Human Kinetics.

McMurdo, M. E., & Rennie, L. M. (1994). Improvements in quadriceps strength with regular seated exercise in the institutionalized elderly. *Archives of Physical Medicine and Rehabilitation, 75,* 600–603.

Melillo, K. D., Futrell, M., Williamson, E., Bourque, A. M., MacDonnell, M., & Phaneuf, J. P. (1996). Perceptions of physical fitness and exercise activity among older adults. *Journal of Advanced Nursing, 23,* 542–547.

Metter, E. J., Conwitt, R., Tobin, J., & Fozard, J. L. (1997). Age-associated loss of power and strength in the upper extremities in women and men. *Journal of Gerontology: Biological Sciences, 52A,* B267–B276.

Meuleman, J. R., Brechue, W. F., Kubilis, P. S., & Lowenthal, D. T. (2000). Exercise training in the debilitated aged: Strength and functional outcomes. *Archives of Physical Medicine and Rehabilitation, 81,* 312–318.

Milne, J. S., & Lauder, I. J. (1974). Age effects in kyphosis and lordosis in adults. *Annals of Human Biology, 1,* 327–337.

Mitchell, S. L., Stott, D. J., Martin, B. J., & Grant, S. J. (2001). Randomized controlled trial of quadriceps training after proximal femoral fracture. *Clinical Rehabilitation, 15,* 282–290.

Molbeck, S. (1976). Methods for measuring co-ordination and accuracy of muscular movements. *Scandinavian Journal of Rehabilitative Medicine, 6*(Suppl.), 127–132.

Montero-Odasso, M., Schapira, M., Soriano, E. R., Varela, M., Kaplan, R., Camera, L. A., et al. (2005). Gait velocity as a single predictor of adverse events in healthy seniors aged 75 years and older. *Journals of Gerontology Series A-Biological Sciences & Medical Sciences, 60*(10), 1304–1309.

Morey, M. C., Cowper, P. A., Feussner, J. R., Dipasquale, R. C., Crowley, G. M., & Sullivan, R. J. (1991). Two-year trends in physical performance following supervised exercise among community-dwelling old veterans. *Journal of the American Geriatrics Society, 38,* 549–554.

Morris, S., Morris, M., & Iansek, R. (2001). Reliability of measurements obtained with the timed "Up & Go" test in people with Parkinson's disease. *Physical Therapy, 81,* 81–88.

Murray, C. J., & Lopez, A. D. (1996). *Global health statistics, global burden of disease and injury series*(vol. II). Geneva: Harvard School of Public Health, World Bank and World Health Organization.

Murray, D. (1998). Surgery and joint replacement for joint disease. *Acta Orthopaedica Supplementum, 281,* 17–20.

Neiman, D. C. (2003). *Exercise testing and prescription.* Boston, MA: McGraw-Hill.

Newton, R. A. (2001). Validity of the Multi-Directional Reach Test: A practical measure for limits of stability in older adults. *Journal of Gerontology: Medical Sciences, 56A,* M248–M252.

NIH Consensus Development Panel on Osteoporosis Prevention. (2001). Diagnosis and therapy: Osteoporosis prevention, diagnosis and therapy. *Journal of the American Geriatrics Society, 285,* 785–795.

O'Brien, K. O., Culham, E., & Pickles, B. (1997). Balance and skeletal alignment in a group of elderly female fallers and nonfallers. *Journal of Gerontology: Biological Sciences, 52A,* B221–B226.

O'Gorman, H., & Jull, G. (1987). Thoracic kyphosis and mobility: The effect of age. *Physiotherapy Practice, 3,* 154–162.

Overend, T. J., Cunningham, D. A., Paterson, D. H., & Lefcoe, M. S. (1992). Knee extensor and knee flexor strength: Cross sectional area rations in young and elderly men. *Journal of Gerontology: Medical Sciences, 41,* M204–M210.

Podsiadlo, D., & Richardson, S. (1991). The timed "up and go": A test of basic functional mobility for frail elderly persons. *Journal of the American Geriatrics Society, 39,*142–148.

Pollock, M. L., Carroll, J. F., Graves, J. E., Leggett, S. H., Braith, R. W., Limacher, M., et al. (1991). Injuries and adherence to walk/jog and resistance training programs in the elderly. *Medical Science and Sports Exercise, 23,* 1194–1200.

Porter, M. M., Vandervoort, A. A., & Kramer, J. F. (1997). Eccentric peak torque of the plantar and dorsiflexors is maintained in older women. *Journal of Gerontology: Biological Sciences, 52,* B125–B131.

Porter, M. M., Vandervoort, A. A., & Lexell, J. (1995). Aging of human muscle: Structure, function and adaptability. *Scandinavian Journal of Medicine & Science in Sports, 5,* 129–142.

Potvin, A. (1980). Human neurologic function and the aging process. *Journal of the American Geriatrics Society, 28*(1), 1–9.

Potvin, A. R., Syndulko, K., Tourtelotte, W. W., Lemmon, J. A., & Potvin, J. H. (1980). Human neurologic function and the aging process. *Journal of the American Geriatrics Society, 28,* 1–9.

Powell, L. E., & Myers, A. M. (1995). The Activities-specific Balance Confidence (ABC) Scale. *Journal of Gerontology Series A-Biological Sciences and Medical Sciences, 50,* M28–M34.

Probst, C. (1989). *The influence of hip abduction strength on postural sway in elderly females.*Thesis, University of Pittsburgh, Pittsburgh, PA.

Rantanen, T., Guralnik, J. M., Ferrucci, L., Leveille, S., & Fried, L. P. (1999). Coimpairments: Strength and balance as predictors of severe walking disability. *Journal of Gerontology Series A-Biological Sciences & Medical Sciences, 54*(4), M172–M176.

Rantanen, T., Guralnik, J. M., Ferrucci, L., Penninx, B. W., Leveille, S., Sipilä, S., et al. (2001). Coimpairments as predictors of severe walking disability in older women. *Journal of the American Geriatrics Society, 49*(1), 21–27.

Rantanen, T., Guralnik, J. M., Foley, D., Masaki, K., Leveille, S., & Curb, J. D. (1999a). Midlife hand grip strength as a predictor of old age disability. *Journal of the American Geriatrics Society, 281*(6), 558–560.

Rantanen, T., Guralnik, J. M., Sakari-Rantala, R., Leveille, S., Simonsick, E. M., Ling, S., et al. (1999b). Disability, physical activity, and muscle strength in older women: The women's health and aging study. *Archives of Physical Medicine and Rehabilitation, 80,* 130–135.

Resnick, B. (2001). Testing a model of exercise behavior in older adults. *Research in Nursing Health, 24,* 83–92.

Resnick, B., & Spellbring, A. M. (2000). Understanding what motivates older adults to exercise. *Journal of Gerontological Nursing, 26,* 34–42.

Reuben, D. B., & Siu, A. L. (1990). An objective measure of physical function of elderly outpatients: The Physical Performance Test. *Journal of the American Geriatrics Society, 38,* 1105–1112.

Rice, C. L. (2000). Muscle function at the motor unit level: Consequences of aging. *Topics in Geriatrics and Rehabilitation, 15,* 70–82.

Richardson, J. (1999). Generalized peripheral neuropathy. In T. Kauffman (Ed.), *Geriatric rehabilitation manual.* Philadelphia: W.B. Saunders.

Rider, R. A., & Daly, J. (1991). Effects of flexibility training on enhancing spinal mobility in older women. *Journal of Sports Medicine and Physical Fitness, 31,* 213–217.

Rikli, R. E., & Jones, C. J. (2001). *Senior fitness test manual.* Champaign, IL: Human Kinetics.

Rooyackers, O. E., Adey, D. B., Ades, P. S., & Nair, K. S. (1996). Effects of age on in vivo rates of mitochondrial protein synthesis in human skeletal muscle. *Proceedings of the National Academy of Science U.S.A., 93,* 15364–15369.

Rose, D. J. (2003). *FallProof: A comprehensive balance and mobility program.* Champaign, IL: Human Kinetics.

Rose, D. J., & Clark, S. (2000). Can the control of bodily orientation be significantly improved in a group of older adults with a history of falls? *Journal of the American Geriatrics Society, 48*(3), 275–282.

Rosenhall, U., & Rubin, W. (1975). Degenerative changes in the human vestibular sensory epithelia. *Acta Oto-Laryngologica, 79,* 67–81.

Roubenoff, R., & Hughes, V. A. (2000). Sarcopenia: current concepts. *Journals of Gerontology Series A-Biological Sciences & Medical Sciences, 55*(12), M716–M724.

Schmitz, T. (2007). Coordination assessment. In S. O'Sullivan & T. Schmitz (Eds.), *Physical rehabilitation.* (5th ed.). Philadelphia: F.A. Davis.

Sculco, T. P. (1985). The lumbar spine. In T. P. Sculco (Ed.), *Orthopedic care of the geriatric patient.* St. Louis, MO: Mosby.

Seeman, T. E., Berkman, L. F., Charpentier, P. A., Blazer, D. G., Albert, M. S., & Tinetti, M. E. (1995). Behavioral and psychosocial predictors of physical performance. *Journal of Gerontology, 50A,* M177–M183.

Serrien, D. J., Swinnen, S. P., & Stemach, G. E. (2000). Age related deterioration of coordinated interlimb behavior. *Journal of Gerontology: Psychological Sciences, 55*(5), P295–P303.

Shaw, L. M., & Snow, C. M. (1998). Weighted vest exercise improves indices of fall risk in older women. *Journal of Gerontology: Biological Sciences, 53,* M53–M58.

Sheldon, J. (1963). The effect of age on the control of sway. *Gerontologia Clinica, 5,* 129–138.

Sherrington, C., & Lord, S. R. (1997). Fall risk factors following hip fracture: A randomized controlled trial of home exercise. *Archives of Physical Medicine and Rehabilitation, 78,* 208–212.

Sherwood, D. E., & Selder, D. J. (1979). Cardiorespiratory health, reaction time, and aging. *Medicine and Science in Sports and Exercise, 11,* 186–189.

Shkuratova, N., Morris, M. E., & Huxham, F. (2004). Effects of age on balance control during walking. *Archives of Physical Medicine and Rehabilitation, 85*(4), 582–588.

Short, K. R., & Nair, K. S. (2001). Muscle protein metabolism and the sarcopenia of aging. *International Journal of Sport Nutrition & Exercise Metabolism, 11,* S119–S127.

Shumway-Cook, A., Brauer, S., & Woollacott, M. (2000). Predicting the probability for falls in the community-dwelling older adults using the Timed Up & Go Test. *Physical Therapy, 80*(9), 896–903.

Shumway-Cook, A., Gruber, W., Baldwin, M., & Liao, S. (1997). The effect of multidimensional exercises on balance, mobility, and fall risk in community-dwelling older adults. *Physical Therapy, 77,* 46–57.

Shumway-Cook, A., & Horak, F. (1986). Assessing the influence of sensory interaction on balance. *Physical Therapy, 66,* 1548–1550.

Shumway-Cook, A., & Woollacott, M. (1995). *Motor control: Theory and practical applications.* Baltimore: Williams and Wilkins.

Shumway-Cook, A., & Woollacott, M. (2001). *Motor control: Theory and practical applications.* (2nd ed.). Philadelphia: Lippincott, Williams & Wilkins.

Shumway-Cook, A., & Woollacott, M. H. (Eds.). (2007). *Motor control: Translating research into clinical practice* (3rd ed.). Philadelphia: Lippincott, Williams & Wilkins.

Sipilä, S., Multanen, J., Kallinen, M., Era, P., & Suominen, H. (1996). Effects of strength and endurance training on isometric muscle strength and walking speed in elderly women. *Acta Physiologica Scandinavica, 156,* 457–464.

Skelton, D. A., Greig, C. A., Davies, J. M., & Young, A. (1994). Strength, power and related functional ability of healthy people aged 65–89 years. *Age and Ageing, 23*(5), 371–377.

Skelton, D. A., & McLaughlin, A. W. (1996). Training functional ability in old age. *Physiotherapy, 82,* 159–167.

Skelton, D. A., Young, A., Greig, C. A., & Malbut, K. E. (1995). Effects of resistance training on strength, power, and selected functional abilities of women aged 75 and older. *Journal of the American Geriatrics Society, 43,* 1081–1087.

Skelton, D. A., Young, A., Walker, A., & Hoinville, E. (1999). *Physical activity later in life: Further analysis of the Allied Dunbar National Fitness Survey and the Health Education Authority National Survey of Activity and Health.* Health Education Authority: London.

Skinner, H. B., Barrack, R. L., & Cook, S. D. (1984). Age-related decline in proprioception. *Clinical Orthopaedics and Related Research, 184,* 208–211.

Smith, K., Winegard, K., Hicks, A. L., & McCartney, N. (2003). Two years of resistance training in older men and women: The effects of three years of detraining on the retention of dynamic strength. *Canadian Journal of Applied Physiology, 28*(3), 462–474.

Sperling, L. (1980). Evaluation of upper extremity function in 70-year-old men and women. *Scandinavian Journal of Rehabilitative Medicine, 12,* 139–144.

Spirduso, W. W. (1975). Reaction and movement time as a function of age and physical activity level. *Journal of Gerontology, 30,* 435–440.

Spirduso, W. W., Francis, K., & MacRae, P. (2005). *Physical dimensions of aging.* Champaign, IL: Human Kinetics.

Stuart, M., Turman, A. B., Shaw, J., Walsh, N., & Nyugen, V. (2003). Effects of aging on vibration detection thresholds at various body regions. *BMC Geriatrics, 3*(1), 1–10.

Stucki, G., Ewert, T., & Cieza, A. (2003). Value and application of the ICF in rehabilitation medicine. *Disability and Rehabilitation, 24*(17), 932–938.

Sudarsky, L., & Ronthal, M. (1983). Gait disorders among elderly patients: A survey of 50 patients. *Archives of Neurology, 40,* 740–743.

Suzuki, T., Bean, J. F., & Fielding, R. A. (2001). Muscle power of the ankle flexors predicts functional performance in community-dwelling older women. *Journal of the American Geriatrics Society, 49*(9), 1161–1167.

Teasdale, N., Bard, C., LaRue, J., & Fleury, M. (1993). On the cognitive penetrability of postural control. *Experimental Aging Research, 19,* 1–13.

Tell, G. S., Lefkowitz, D. S., Diehr, P., & Elster, A. D. (1998). Relationship between balance and abnormalities in cerebral magnetic resonance imaging in older adults. *Archives of Neurology, 55,* 73–79.

Thelen, D. G., Brockmiller, C., Ashton-Miller, J. A., Schultz, A. B., & Alexander, N. B. (1998). Thresholds for sensing foot dorsi- and plantarflexion during upright stance: Effects of age and velocity. *Journal of Gerontology Series A-Biological Sciences & Medical Sciences, 53*(1), M33–M38.

Tiffin, J. (1968). *Purdue pegboard examiner manual.* Chicago: Science Research Associates.

Timiras, P. S. (1994). Aging of the nervous system: Functional changes. In P./S. Timiras (Ed.), *Physiological basis of aging and geriatrics.* Boca Raton, FL: CRC Press.

Tinetti, M. E. (1986). Performance-oriented assessment of mobility problems in elderly patients. *Journal of the American Geriatrics Society, 34,* 110–126.

Tinetti, M. E., Baker, D. I., McAvay, G., Claus, E. B., Garrett, P., Gottschalk, M., et al. (1994). A multifactorial intervention to reduce the risk of falling among elderly people living in the community. *New England Journal of Medicine, 331,* 821–827.

Topp, R., Mikesky, A. E., & Thompson, K. (1998). Determinants of four functional tasks among older adults: An exploratory regression analysis. *Journal of Orthopaedic & Sports Physical Therapy, 27*(2), 144–153.

Tremayne, A., Taylor, N., McBurney, H., & Baskus, K. (2002). Correlation of impairment and activity limitation after wrist fracture. *Physiotherapy Research International, 7*(2), 90–99.

Tsang, W. W. N., & Hui-Chan, C. W. Y. (2003). Effects of Tai Chi on joint proprioception and stability limits in elderly subjects. *Medicine and Science in Sports and Exercise, 35*(12), 1962–1971.

Tsang, W. W. N., & Hui-Chan, C. W. Y. (2005). Comparison of muscle torque, balance, and confidence in older Tai Chi and healthy adults. *Medicine and Science in Sports and Exercise, 37*(2), 280–289.

U.S. Department of Health and Human Services. (1996). *Physical activity and health: A report of the Surgeon General.* Atlanta, GA: U.S. Department of Health and

Human Services, Centers for Disease Control and Prevention, National Center for Chronic Disease Prevention and Health Promotion.

van Balen, R., Steyerberg, E. W., Polder, J. J., Ribbers, T. L., Habbema, J. D., & Cools, H. J. (2001). Hip fracture in elderly patients: Outcomes for function, quality of life, and type of residence. *Clinical Orthopedics and Related Research, 390,* 232–243.

Van Swearingen, M., Paschal, K. A., Bonino, P., & Yang, J. F. (1996). The modified Gait Abnormality Rating Scale for recognizing the risk of recurrent falls in community-dwelling elderly adults. *Physical Therapy, 76*(9), 994–1002.

Vandervoort, A. A. (2002). Aging of the human neuromuscular system. *Muscle and Nerve, 25,* 17–25.

Vandervoort, A. A., Chesworth, B. M., Cunningham, D. A., Paterson, D. H., Rechnitzer, P. A., & Koval, J. J. (1992). Age and sex effects of mobility of the human ankle. *Journal of Gerontology: Medical Sciences, 47,* M17–M21.

Vellas, B., Lauge, S., Andrieu, S., Nourhashemi, F., Rolland, Y., Baumgartner, R., et al. (2001). Nutrition assessment in the elderly. *Current Opinion in Clinical Nutrition and Metabolic Care, 4,* 5–8.

Verkek, R. H., Schouten, J. P., & Oosterhuis, H. J. G. H. (1990). Measurement of the hand coordination. *Clinical Neurology and Neurosurgery, 92,* 105–109.

Vincent, K. R., & Braith, R. W. (2002). Resistance exercise and bone turnover in elderly men and women. *Medical Science and Sports Exercise, 34,* 17–23.

Walker, J., Sue, D., Miles-Elkowusy, N., Ford, G., & Trevelyan, H. (1984). Active mobility of extremities in older subjects. *Physical Therapy, 64*(6), 919–923.

Wall, C., & Scarbrough, J. (1997). Use of a multimemory stopwatch to measure the temporal gait parameters. *Journal of Orthopaedic Sports and Physical Therapy, 199,* 277–281.

Wang, F. C., DePasqua, V., & Delwaide, P. J. (1999). Age-related changes in fastest and slowest conducting axons of thenar motor units. *Muscle and Nerve, 22,* 1022–1029.

Whanger, A., & Wang, H. S. (1974). Clinical correlates of the vibratory sense in elderly psychiatric patients. *Journal of Gerontology, 29,* 39–45.

Whipple, R. H., Wolfson, L. I., & Amerman, P. M. (1987). The relationship of knee and ankle weakness to falls in nursing home residents: An isokinetic study. *Journal of the American Geriatrics Society, 35,* 13–20.

Williams, M. E., Gaylord, S. A., & McGaghie, W. C. (1990). Timed manual performance in a community elderly population. *Journal of the American Geriatrics Society, 38,* 1120–1126.

Winter, D., Patla, A. E., Frank, J. S., & Walt, S. E. (1990). Biomechanical walking pattern changes in the fit and healthy elderly. *Physical Therapy, 70,* 340–347.

Wolf, S. L., Barnhart, H. X., Kutner, N. G., McNeely, E., Coogler, C., & Xu, T. (1996). Reducing frailty and falls in older persons: An investigation of Tai Chi and computerized balance training. *Journal of the American Geriatrics Society, 44,* 489–497.

Wolfson, L., Judge, J., Whipple, R., & King, M. (1995). Strength is a major factor in balance, gait, and the occurrence of falls. *Journal of Gerontology, 50A,* 64–67.

Wolfson, L., Whipple, R., Amerman, P., Kaplan, J., & Kleinberg, A. (1985). Gait and balance in the elderly: Two functional capacities that link sensory and motor abilities to falls. *Clinics in Geriatric Medicine, 1,* 649–659.

Wolfson, L., Whipple, R., Amerman, P., & Tobin, J. N. (1990). Gait assessment in the elderly: A gait abnormality rating scale and its relation to falls. *Journal of Gerontology, 45,* M12–M19.

Wolfson, L., Whipple, R., Derby, C. A., Amerman, P., & Kleinberg, A. (1986). Stressing the postural response: A quantitative method for testing balance. *Journal of the American Geriatrics Society, 34,* 845–850.

Wolfson, L., Whipple, R., Derby, C., Judge, J., King, M., Amerman, P., et al. (1996). Balance and strength training in older adults: Intervention gains and Tai Chi maintenance. *Journal of the American Geriatrics Society, 44,* 498–506.

Woo, J., Ho, C., Lau, J., Chan, G., & Yuek, K. (1995). Age-associated gait changes in the elderly: Pathological or psychological? *Neuroepidemiology, 14,* 65–71.

Woodhull-McNeal, A. P. (1992). Changes in posture and balance with age. *Aging—Clinical and Experimental Research, 4,* 219–225.

Woolf, A. D., & Pfleger, B. (2003). Burden of major musculoskeletal conditions. *Bulletin of the World Health Organization, 81*(9), 646–656.

World Health Organization. (2001). *ICF introduction.* Retrieved December 28, 2006, from www3.who. int/icf/intros/ICF-Eng-Intro.pdf.

Worrell, T. W., Smith, T. L., & Winegardner, J. (1994a). Factors associated with hamstring injuries: An approach to treatment and preventative measures. *Sports Medicine, 17,* 335–345.

Worrell, T. W., Smith, T. L., & Winegardner, J. (1994b). Effect of stretching on hamstring muscle performance. *Journal of Orthaepedic Sports and Physical Therapy, 20,* 154–159.

Wu, F., Mason, B., Horne, A., Ames, R., Clearwater, J., Liu, M., et al. (2002). Fractures between the ages of 20 and 50 years increase women's risk of subsequent fractures. *Archives of Internal Medicine, 162,* 33–36.

Wyke, B. (1979). Conference on the aging brain. *Age and Ageing, 8,* 251–258.

Yelin, E. (1998). *The economics of osteoarthritis* (pp. 23–30). New York: Oxford University Press.

Youndas, J. W., & Atwood, R. (2000). Measurement of temporal aspects of gait obtained with a multimemory stopwatch. *Journal of Orthopaedic Sports and Physical Therapy, 30,* 279–286.

Young, A., Stokes, M., & Crowe, M. (1985). The size and strength of the quadriceps muscles of old and young men. *Clinical Physiology, 5*(2), 145–154.

CHAPTER 7

Mental Function

Kathryn Perez Riley, PhD

Life has changed me greatly, it has improved me greatly,
but it has also left me practically the same.

Florida Scott Maxwell,
The Measure of My Days, Penguin Books,
New York, 1968, p. 17.

OBJECTIVES

By the end of this chapter, readers will be able to:

1. Discuss some primary findings from research in cognition and aging, identifying the strengths and limitations of the research methods most commonly used.
2. Describe the changes that occur in memory and attention with normal aging, including mild cognitive impairments.
3. Discuss the relationship between normal age-related cognitive change and occupational performance, leisure activities, and activities of daily living (ADLs).
4. Identify practical methods that can be used with older adults to permit job maintenance and enhance performance and satisfaction in leisure and daily life activities.

Does the aging process bring on inevitable waning of intellect, memory, and reason? Is the aging adult forced to give up work, leisure, and independence as a result of loss of cognitive ability? Those who have grown old or who have studied or worked with others who have grown old can answer "no" to both questions. Yet there are documented changes and losses that may require adaptation on the part of aging adults as they seek balance in lifestyle, occupation, and daily activities. (See Chapter 2 of this volume for a discussion of some of the biological changes that may accompany the aging process.)

This chapter addresses the issue of normal age-related changes in cognitive abilities as related to functional performance in older adults. The nature of these cognitive changes is reviewed, followed by a discussion of the relationship between cognition, activities, and occupational performance.

Cognitive Changes in Normal Aging

Researchers first began investigating and documenting the changes in cognition that accompany the aging process in the 1920s and 1930s, not long after the use of standardized intelligence tests became common. The early literature focused on performance on intelligence tests and gradually branched out into the study of other forms of cognitive activity, including problem solving, memory, attention, and language. The following sections discuss these areas of cognition, providing only a few highlights of a voluminous body of literature. Although this literature shows that changes and declines generally do occur in elderly persons and that older adults tend to perform more poorly on many laboratory tasks than do younger persons, it is important to note that the *individual* older adult may never experience these changes, or may never be affected by a decline in cognition that can be measured by laboratory tests.

It is essential that an actual assessment of an older adult's ability be obtained when working with the person in an applied setting, rather than relying on generalized findings about the cognitive function of older adults.

Methodological Considerations

To understand past and present research results in the area of cognition and aging, it is necessary to recall the basic methodologies employed in these investigations (Wilson, Bennett, & Swartzendruber, 1997). The cross-sectional design is by far the most common approach used to study age differences in most areas of inquiry. In this design, two or more age groups are compared with each other at one point in time. Thus, it is quite common to see studies that have examined cognitive test performance in 20-, 40-, 60-, and 80-year-olds. Although these studies yield information about differences between age groups, they cannot address the issue of actual maturational changes—that is, changes that accompany the aging process within an individual. A longitudinal design is required to address this question, involving the repeated testing of a group of individuals over an extended period of time.

An additional construct that is of relevance to both methods of investigation is the **cohort effect.** A cohort is generally defined as a group of individuals born within a certain time frame (e.g., a 5- or 10-year period). The differential effects of one's birth year on one's cognitive abilities or test performance can be great, in light of the importance of educational opportunities, life experience, access to medical care, and occupational opportunities.

Cross-sectional studies are limited in that they show differences between current cohorts

of adults, but they cannot predict the patterns of differences between future cohorts. These studies cannot report with any certainty that the older cohorts studied have actually declined (or improved) in any area of cognitive ability.

Longitudinal studies can better answer the question of maturational change but are able to address only the issue of change in the limited number of cohorts included in their sample. Past and future cohorts' experiences with intellectual change cannot reliably be predicted using longitudinal results (American Psychiatric Association [APA], 1994; Woods & Britton, 1985). This method is further complicated by dropout rates, resulting in bias. A partial solution to the limitations of these two methods of research is the cross-sequential design (Schaie & Eisdorfer, 1987) in which different age groups are tested at repeated intervals over a fairly extended period of time. In some cases, both new and old samples of subjects from the same pool are included in the retest samplings. Cross-sequential designs, then, can yield information about age differences and age changes, both within individuals and between cohorts. Unfortunately, the complexity of this design makes it difficult to carry out, and it is not without its methodological problems. Thus, the bulk of available literature on cognitive changes in aging is based primarily on cross-sectional designs and secondarily on longitudinal studies (Sliwinski, Hofer, & Hall, 2003).

Intelligence

The very early data on IQ test performance among older adults were based almost entirely on cross-sectional studies. These early findings, comparing young adults in their 20s to older persons aged 60 years and older, generally showed very large differences between young and old on tests such as the Army Alpha Test and later on the Wechsler Adult Intelligence Scale (WAIS and WAIS-Revised) (Albert & Heaton, 1988; APA, 1994; Schaie & Eisdorfer, 1987). In general, these early data were interpreted as showing a rather precipitous decline in intelligence beginning at about age 25 and continuing into the seventh and eighth decades.

More recent research has resulted in a major change in thinking about declines in intellectual abilities, with both cross-sectional and longitudinal studies showing consistent age-associated decline by about the sixth decade of life (Cunningham, 1987; Lindenberger, Mayr, & Kliegl, 1993). These studies also note, however, that the range of cognitive performance is greater among older than younger adults, with some older adults exhibiting superior performance in some areas of function (Ivnik, Smith, Malec, Petersen, & Tangalos, 1995).

Although general declines in the full-scale WAIS scores and other general measures of intelligence have been documented in the advanced years, it is important to note the differential rates of decline and stability seen in various categories of intellectual ability. The most prominent of these is the verbal-performance split seen on these two scales of the WAIS. Specifically, the Performance scale, which measures speed and accuracy in problem solving, and psychomotor and perceptual abilities, shows earlier and more significant decline than does the verbal scale, which measures abilities and knowledge acquired over a lifetime, including vocabulary skills, a general fund of information, and verbal comprehension and reasoning. This pattern of differential decline has been explained using Cattell's (1963; Horn & Cattell, 1967) model of crystallized and fluid intelligence. **Fluid intelligence,** which involves the ability to adapt to and use new information in reasoning, solving, and integrating problems or novel information, corresponds to the subtests of the WAIS Performance scale. **Crystallized abilities,** corresponding to the verbal scale, reflect the accumulated practical skills and knowledge of the individual. The decline in fluid intelligence has been postulated as due to biological changes in the central nervous system, a decline in speed of information processing, and slower psychomotor output (Hartley, 1992). Although none of these models or explanatory devices has been accepted as complete or definitive, it is clear that normative samples of older adults consistently show the verbal-performance split in both longitudinal and cross-sectional studies. The development of age based normative data for current versions of the WAIS-III and most standardized neuropsychological test batteries and measures makes it possible to detect the presence of cognitive decline that is more severe than would be expected based on chronological age alone (Riley, 1999). Thus, significant impairment, as documented by cognitive testing, or cognition-related declines in the older individual's ability to function in daily life should be taken as an indication of a pathological process

such as dementing illness or other central nervous system dysfunction that may require professional intervention.

A final general note concerning the measurement of cognitive function in older adults: Although most recent studies of cognition and aging take steps to ensure that the study participants are free from cognitive impairment, it is quite likely that a number of these participants were experiencing subtle cognitive decline that would later prove to be the early stage of a dementing disorder such as Alzheimer's disease. This is more likely to have been a problem in older research studies and in those that did not employ rigorous screening measures for signs of incipient dementia or possible causes of cognitive impairment. Thus, much of the early data on cognitive change with age may be exaggerated by the inclusion of data from older adults who were in the earliest stages of a dementing illness (Morgan, 2001; Riley & Snowdon, 1999; Sliwinski, Hofer, Hall, Buschke, & Lipton, 2003).

Cognitive Slowing

Of special relevance to this chapter is the finding that the rate at which an individual can process perceptual information (often referred to as perceptual speed) has been shown to decline with advancing age (Salthouse, 1993; Wilson, Bennett, & Swartzendruber, 1997). Although extraneous variables such as motivation, ecological validity of the tests used, depression, cautiousness, and motor skills all complicate the issue of measuring pure central-processing speed, the idea that generalized cognitive slowing occurs with advancing age remains as a dominant concept in the literature (Hartley, 1992). This slowing has been postulated as accounting for some of the age-related decline seen in many areas of cognitive function (Earles & Salthouse, 1995). However, this factor provides only a partial explanation for these deficits, and some studies have shown that even when older adults are given more time on these tests, their improved scores may still fail to reach the level of younger adults (Perlmutter et al., 1987). The relevance of these empirical findings to the older adults' daily functioning is discussed later in this chapter, because generalized cognitive slowing may in fact be perceived as troublesome by the older individual in his or her daily activities and vocational performance.

An important addition to the literature on cognitive function and aging is the finding that sensory functioning (e.g., visual and auditory acuity) has been shown to be a strong predictor of individual differences in intellectual functioning in older adults (Lindenberger & Baltes, 1994). Although more research is needed to understand fully the relationships between visual and auditory acuity among older adults, the data highlight the complex nature of age-related changes in cognitive function.

Other Cognitive Abilities

Reasoning and Problem Solving

Designing research to examine the reasoning or problem-solving abilities of older adults is a complex matter, given that factors such as speed of information processing, intelligence, memory, and relevance of test items all affect one's reasoning or problem-solving skills. Some studies that have taken these factors into account by using cross-sequential methodological approaches (Arenberg, 1982) indicate that there is a decline in the speed and efficiency of problem solving associated with the aging process (Rabbitt, 1982). The selection of inappropriate strategies, information overload, and poor organizational processes all may contribute to the observed declines in performance (Saczynski, Willis, & Schaie, 2002). One aspect of problem-solving skills is the ability to abstract. This ability is often assessed through the use of tests of concept formation, such as the similarities subtest of the WAIS and the Halstead-Reitan battery's Category test. Reasonably significant and consistent age differences have been found on these types of tests, suggesting that older adults are less proficient at abstract reasoning tasks than are young adults (Albert, 1988). Once again, the tasks used to evaluate this skill must be evaluated in terms of the amount of variance in performance that is accounted for by factors such as memory, attention, and lack of ecological validity—that is, the relationship between test content and functioning in daily life. Mental flexibility or set shifting in reasoning tasks also has been shown to decline somewhat with advanced age, even when memory demands are minimal (Albert, Duffy, & Naeser, 1987). Difficulties in the area of problem solving are not commonly cited by older adults as being of major concern, and it remains unclear whether laboratory-based tests designed to measure problem solving do in fact approximate real-life decision making to an adequate degree. The interested reader is directed to Salthouse (1992) for a thorough discussion of age and reasoning ability.

Memory and Attention

Of all the cognitive abilities, memory is the most discussed, studied, and evaluated by researchers and laypersons alike. Changes in memory functioning with advancing age are expected, feared, and exaggerated in common folklore, and similar biases are likely to have occurred in empirical investigations. The cross-sectional design has been predominant in memory research, although in recent years, a number of longitudinal studies of cognition and memory have been reporting interesting findings (Ivnik et al., 1995; Riley, 1999; Sliwinski, Hofer, Hall, Buschke, et al., 2003).

There are a variety of theoretical models of memory functioning, with different sets of terminology being used for the same memory functions (Craik & Jennings, 1992; Rockey, 1997). This has sometimes led to confusion as to which abilities decline with age and which remain stable (Kausler, 1989; Perlmutter et al., 1987). The following discussion will focus on memory storage systems, touching on selected findings from the literature on memory functioning in healthy older adults.

Before one can meaningfully discuss memory, the role of attention must be considered (Sweeney, Rosano, Berman, & Luna, 2001). The ability to focus on and attend to the information that is to be remembered is essential if a lasting memory is to be formed. Researchers have classified attention into a number of categories, including sustained attention, attentional capacity, and selective or divided attention (Hartley, 1992; Hasher & Zacks, 1979). Although some studies have found little significant decline in the older adult's sustained and selective attention abilities (Gilmore, Tobias, & Royer, 1985), the data are mixed, and it is impossible to make sweeping generalizations about the performance of older adults on laboratory-based tests of these subtypes of attention. Similarly, the results of investigations into the attentional capacity of older adults (the amount of information that can be successfully attended to at one time) are not uniform, with some studies indicating decline and others finding no age-related deficits. There may be a decrease in the maximum amount of attentional resources available and a decline in the ability to separate relevant material from the irrelevant, whereas sustained attention or vigilance may not be significantly affected by increasing age.

The concept of working memory (Baddeley, 1981; Van Gerven, Paas, Van Merrienboer, Hendriks, & Schmidt, 2003) is closely related to attention and provides a link between attention and the formation of lasting memory traces. **Working memory** can be thought of as simultaneously holding information in mind (storage) and using that information to perform a task (processing). A decrease in the storage component of working memory has been documented (Foos & Wright, 1992), which may help account for some portion of the overall decline in memory abilities seen in older adults.

Secondary Memory and Encoding Strategies

The largest and most consistent age differences are found in **secondary (long-term) memory** (Grady, 1998). This memory store is generally viewed as containing an unlimited amount of information for almost any length of time. In order for data to reach secondary memory, the information must be actively processed or transferred from primary or working memory. Older adults have been shown to have deficits in recall of information from the secondary memory store, with the deficits being more pronounced in tests of free recall than in tests of recognition. Although there is little evidence for reduced capacity of the secondary or long-term memory store in normal aging, there is strong evidence to support deficits in the encoding processes used to transfer data into this storage system. This rather large body of data (Craik & Jennings, 1992; Poon & Yesavage, 1986) documents the failure of older adults to use effective strategies spontaneously to encode to-be-learned material. That is, whereas younger adults are likely to use a variety of organizational, semantic, or "deep" processing strategies, older adults may fail to employ any such strategy, or they may use one that is less efficient. These deficits in the transfer of data from one storage system to the next can affect the amount of information stored as well as the efficiency with which it can be retrieved.

It is important to note that although older individuals may not employ **encoding** strategies spontaneously, when structure is imposed on the material or when older adults are trained to use mnemonic devices, the deficits previously seen in secondary memory are diminished (Smith, 1980; Zachs, 1982). Increasing the ecological validity or meaningfulness of the materials also may minimize age-related deficits (Poon & Yesavage, 1986). Thus, although there may be some degree of absolute decline in secondary or long-term memory accompanying the aging process, these deficits can be alternately exaggerated or reduced, depending on the nature of the to-be-remembered material, the instructions that accompany the learning task, and the manner in which memory is tested (i.e., free recall versus recognition). In addition, there is a good deal of data showing that, although initial learning may be impaired in healthy older adults, the ability to recall newly learned information is generally not impaired once the amount of information they actually have learned is taken into account (Petersen, Smith, Kokmen, Ivnik, & Tangalos, 1992).

Differences in test construction and administration procedures also may reflect differences in daily life memory demands, and it is not unusual for older adults to report that their memory for important or personally relevant information is better than their recall for uninteresting stories or events. In addition, although they may not be able to recall the name of a new acquaintance as readily as in the past, older adults are likely to report little trouble with facial recognition or remembering the names of old friends.

Everyday or Practical Memory

The preceding discussion of cognitive abilities and memory has focused on research conducted with traditional laboratory and clinical tests. In recent years, the ecological validity of some of these tests has been called into question as gerontologists began to examine the effects of older adults' motivation and interest on test performance. Some work has been conducted in the area of everyday or practical intelligence (West & Sinnott, 1992; Willis, 1987), and an increasing body of literature is available on the issue of **everyday memory** (Jobe et al., 2001; Riley, 1992; West, 1986). The goal of this work is to develop measures that will tap into those areas that are important in the older adult's daily life activities, including work, leisure, and interpersonal interactions.

Mild Cognitive Impairments

A final issue related to age-related changes in cognition is that of **mild cognitive impairments** (MCIs) (Luis, Loewenstein, Acevedo, Barker, & Duara, 2003; Petersen, Parisi, & Dickson, 2006), previously labeled as age-associated memory impairments and similar terms (Crook, Bartus, Ferris, & Whitehouse, 1986; Smith, Petersen, Parrisi, & Ivnik, 1996). These impairments describe the changes in memory and other areas of cognitive function that may be seen in healthy, older adults of at least average intellectual functioning. Progress in understanding mild cognitive impairments has been slowed by variations in the definitions of mild cognitive impairments across researchers, although there is some common ground (Bennett, Schneider, Bienias, Evans, & Wilson, 2005; Palmer, Fratiglioni, & Winblad, 2003; Peterson et al., 2001; Ritchie & Touchon, 2000). Essentially, mild cognitive impairment involves the relatively deficient performance in learning and recall of information, in conjunction with complaints of memory impairment in daily life (Peterson et al., 2001; Smith et al., 1996). Variant forms of mild cognitive impairment may involve cognitive abilities other than memory (Palmer et al., 2003; Perneczky et al., 2006; Riley, Snowdon, & Markesbery, 2002). Performance in activities of daily living is relatively well preserved, as compared to the declines in ADLs seen in dementia. The onset of these mild impairments is gradual and initially fairly subtle.

Although it is not clear how many older adults suffer from mild cognitive impairments, it seems to be a common condition, and the likelihood of developing this condition increases with age (Gauthier et al., 2006; Larrabee & Crook, 1994; Peterson et al., 2001). A crucial question is the extent to which the diagnosis of mild cognitive impairment predicts the eventual development of a dementing disorder such as Alzheimer's disease (Peterson et al., 2006; Riley et al., 2002; Turner, 2003). Some longitudinal studies have shown that nearly a third of the individuals classified as having this level of impairment no longer met the criteria after 18 months of follow-up (Helkala et al., 1997). However, other data have shown

high rates of conversion to clinical dementia after a longer follow-up period of more than 4 years, with over half of the individuals who were diagnosed with MCIs converting to dementia) (Bennett et al., 2005; Smith et al., 1996). However, the available data suggest that although mild memory impairment coupled with memory complaint is a predictor of more serious and widespread cognitive impairment in a substantial portion of adults older than 65 years of age, many older adults who are diagnosed with mild cognitive impairments remain stable without developing dementia. Finally, research findings in this area have been helpful in pointing out that subjective complaints of memory deficits in the absence of objective test data confirming impaired performance may point to other conditions such as depression (Helkala et al., 1997) or neurological disorders. The definition of this condition and subsequent research on mild cognitive impairments have led to remediation programs that show promise in improving the quality of life for many older adults (Crook et al., 1986; Jobe et al., 2001). As noted later in this chapter, this knowledge of the laboratory and everyday memory changes seen in healthy older adults can be usefully applied to considerations of the functional performance of older adults.

Cognition and Activities in Normal Aging

The previous discussion of normal age-related changes in cognition has largely been based on the performance of older adults in laboratory settings, although increasing numbers of studies are using clinical tests and measures or those that have been designed to have relevance to daily-life functions. Although the lab-based data show age-associated declines in many domains of cognitive function, there remains a substantial degree of stability in older adults' abilities throughout the life span, as well as great individual variability in the experience of cognitive change (Table 7-1).

The remainder of this chapter focuses on a discussion of the relevance of these cognitive changes to the older adults' occupational and daily life functioning. Of particular interest is the identification of those changes that may have a detrimental effect on functioning. In addition, the findings from cognitive aging

TABLE 7-1 Changes in Cognition with Normal Aging

Cognitive Abilities	Changes
Problem solving memory	Declines tend to be delayed until the 70s
Working memory retained	Some limitations minimize the amount of material that can be retained
Long term (secondary)	Some decline; deficits in encoding processes
Very long term (remote)	Little decline in remembering information such as details from personal childhood or early adulthood
Psychomotor skills	Decline may begin in early 50s
Speed of processing	Slowing may begin in early 50s and continue through late life
Verbal skills	Declines late in life, but changes are relatively minor
Reasoning	Older adults may be less proficient on laboratory tests but may not experience changes in daily life

literature are applied to a consideration of how best to optimize the fit between older individuals and their work or leisure environment.

The term "normal aging" has been employed in this chapter as a means of distinguishing physically and mentally healthy older adults from those who suffer from conditions and diseases that are likely to affect cognitive abilities. The remainder of this chapter will deal only with the occupational and daily life performance of essentially healthy older adults (Birren, Robinson, & Livingston, 1986).

Age, Vocational Performance, and Cognitive Change

Detailed consideration of general changes in vocational performance that accompany normal aging may be found elsewhere in this volume. As noted by Sterns and Alexander (1987), there has been a shortage of information concerning these age differences in job performance, although work is continuing in this area. The relationship between cognitive change and vocational skills has not been extensively studied either, although some investigators have addressed this issue (Baugher, 1978; Park, 1994; Rhodes, 1983; Salthouse, 1994; Waldman & Avolio, 1985; Welford, 1976).

In general, it may be stated that the available literature in industrial gerontology indicates little overall decline in the vocational performance of healthy older adults (Rhodes, 1983; Sterns, 1986; Waldman & Avolio, 1985). Increased job satisfaction, job involvement, and commitment, and decreased turnover rates all have been associated with the aging worker. The actual job performance of the older worker may be described as declining in a limited number of situations, specifically in jobs that are physically demanding or require extremely fast responses (Yokomizo, 1985). A number of researchers (Green, 1972; Rebok, Offermann, Wirtz, & Montaglione, 1985; Salthouse 1994) have noted the relative lack of evidence of negative changes in older workers' performance. A consistent conclusion drawn in the literature on industrial gerontology is that the greatest amount of age-related vocational deficits are seen in physically challenging jobs such as manual labor and some blue-collar jobs. The least decline may be expected in vocations in which the skills and information needed require extensive formal education, such as teaching. Moderate levels of change might be seen in jobs that require a combination of intellectual and physical skill or when new skills must be learned that cannot easily be integrated into previously developed habits of working. These data suggest that older workers are as able as younger workers to meet the demands of their work, providing they are physically able, and providing that sufficient time is allowed for the acquisition of new information and skills.

What, then, is the role of cognitive change in the vocational performance of older adults? Although only a few studies have directly addressed this issue, inferences may be drawn between the cognitive aging literature and the work of industrial gerontologists.

The Disuse Theory, Brain Reserve, and The Older Adult

It has been hypothesized that greater environmental complexity and stimulation may prevent or attenuate intellectual decline in older adults (Rebok et al., 1985). Some researchers (Singleton, 1983) have discussed the idea that older adults (as nonstudents or nonworkers) are less likely to encounter the types of situations that require active problem solving, memory, and other intellectual skills (see also Chapter 2 of this volume). This lack of environmental demand has been hypothesized, with limited empirical support, to account for the declines in fluid intelligence and secondary memory seen in older adults.

This form of "use it or lose it" theorizing has been used to explain the adequate performance of older workers who remain actively engaged in their vocation, to account for cognitive deficits seen in laboratory tasks (Singleton, 1983), and as the basis for remediation efforts in intellectual and memory skills. This concept, along with what is known about the nature and timing of age-related cognitive changes, combine to support the general findings that any deficits in cognitive abilities that would be significant enough to affect job performance are not likely to occur until after the age of 65 or 70 and, thus, after retirement age for most people.

In recent years, increasing attention has been paid to a concept researchers have called cognitive reserve (Scarmeas et al., 2003; Stern, 2002). This concept suggests that some people may have more reserve capacity in their cognitive function, allowing them to delay the signs of cognitive loss that may come with normal aging or with brain pathology due to a condition such as Alzheimer's disease. A number of studies have shown that participation in cognitively stimulating activities, such as reading or playing card games, may increase reserve capacity in older adults (Scarmeas et al., 2003; Wilson et al., 2003). These findings suggest that all adults, including those nearing retirement age and beyond, would benefit from continuing a pattern of engaging in cognitively stimulating activities. Those persons who have not engaged in such activities in early life should consider developing these kinds of activities in order to maintain optimal cognitive function.

When Does Cognitive Decline Affect Vocational Performance?

Although the preceding discussion has focused on continuity and adequacy of vocational performance in older workers, there may be some areas in which cognitive changes affect one's work. These changes include a decline in fluid intelligence, increased cautiousness, decreased speed of information processing, and the declines in secondary memory seen in mild cognitive impairments.

Some studies have shown some performance declines in older managers (Streufert, Pogash, Piasecki, & Post, 1990). For example, it has been noted that older managers may perceive declines in intellectual processing abilities (Rebok et al., 1985). This perceived decline is likely to be related to the laboratory-based findings of declines in fluid intelligence and slower information processing or response rates. It may be that the older worker whose job requires the active processing of a great deal of information or fast rates of output and decision making, or both, may in fact feel less effective in his or her job. However, as Rebok and associates (1985) and others (Singleton, 1983) have found, this type of older worker is also likely to use a variety of intellectual and instrumental coping strategies to compensate for any declines in cognitive ability, thus leading to an intact sense of competence and self-efficacy.

The normal age-related changes in memory and those deficits seen in mild cognitive impairments are potential sources of decline in the vocational performance of older adults. If one's job begins to involve a higher level of memorization than was previously required or if the need to transfer significant amounts of information into secondary memory begins to exceed the aging worker's capacity, then a decline in job capability may be seen. It is to be emphasized that most healthy older workers do not experience mild cognitive impairments or other forms of memory impairment that are severe enough to cause this kind of dysfunction. In addition, it is likely that older adults develop or maintain those coping and information management skills necessary to counteract any reduced efficiency in their memory abilities.

In summary, normal age-related cognitive changes are likely to have an adverse effect on vocational performance only when the amount of information exceeds the older worker's rate or capacity of processing (e.g., fluid intelligence; response speed), when quick responses are to be made in ambiguous situations (e.g., cautiousness), or when the memory demands of a particular job increase or exceed the memory capabilities of the older worker. A number of explanations have been offered for the general lack of evidence for a strong association between aging and reduced work performance (Park, 1994; Salthouse, 1994). These explanations include the suggestion that the increased experience that comes with age could affect both the preservation of cognitive abilities as well as the fund of accumulated knowledge necessary for high levels of performance. Another potential explanation is the idea that older adults have more environmental supports in place (such as assistants who gather and synthesize new information). Thus, it is likely that the stability of crystallized intelligence and the advantages of years of accumulated knowledge and vocational experience, along with job-related coping and time-management skills, result in an older worker whose competence is little diminished.

Job Training and Retraining: A Note on Cognitive Aging

One remaining area of interest to this discussion of vocational performance, cognition, and the older adult involves job training or retraining (Birren et al., 1986; Sterns & Alexander, 1987). Briefly, it has been suggested that we apply what is known about the intellectual and memory abilities of older adults (Auerback & Katz, 1988) to vocational training programs. One of the first issues to address should be the motivation of the older adult to engage in such training or retraining. Deficient self-esteem, negative expectations of (younger) others, and anxiety about new learning all must be allayed if the older worker is to be successfully trained. Literature on everyday memory and the meaningfulness of to-be-learned material indicates that the training sessions must involve information that is of relevance and interest to the older adult. Sterns and Alexander (1987) add that the use of familiar material and learning methods enhances the older worker's chance of being successfully trained. These authors also stress the importance of providing feedback on successes during the training program in order to bolster self-confidence and maintain motivation.

Additional considerations for the training or retraining of older workers are related to changes in speed of information processing and transfer of information into secondary or long-term memory. It has been recommended that older adults be given more time to learn new skills and that a self-paced format of learning be employed whenever possible. These strategies have been shown to improve performance on laboratory tasks as well as in real-life learning situations. Finally, the changes in memory that accompany normal aging and that are seen in mild cognitive impairments may be overcome if the older worker is instructed in or provided with organizational and other mnemonic strategies that enhance the effectiveness of encoding, transfer, storage, and retrieval of the material to be learned (Sterns & Alexander, 1987). For further discussion of work performance of older adults, see Chapter 13.

Cognitive Changes: Leisure and Daily Activities

There is little research to be found that addresses the issue of how cognitive abilities in healthy elderly people are related to leisure and daily activities. It is not likely that the cognitive changes associated with the normal aging process bring about significant deficits in instrumental and personal ADLs, such as shopping, cooking, managing daily financial matters, or performing personal care and hygiene activities. Instead, deficits in these areas are generally considered to be indicative of physical illness, dementia, or mental illness (Glass, Seeman, Herzog, Kahn, & Berkman, 1995). For example, cognitive impairments may have a direct impact on activities such as bathing, grooming, or cooking when planning, sequencing, and memory abilities are impaired (Raji et al., 2005).

Leisure Activities

Although a reasonably large body of literature on social and leisure activities among the elderly population is available (Carstensen, 1987; Kaufman, 1988; Nadler, Damis, & Richardson, 1997; Nilsson & Fisher, 2006), research linking cognitive abilities to these activities in healthy, community-dwelling older adults is a recently emerging field (Fabre, Traisnei, & Mucci, 2003; Wang, Karp, Winblad, & Fratiglioni, 2002). Much of the literature deals either with leisure, life satisfaction, or retirement without reference to the role of cognitive abilities (Kelly & Ross, 1989), or it is related to activities programs for the institutionalized, impaired older adult (Kaufman, 1988). The pursuit of leisure activities among healthy older individuals, whether retired or not, is likely to involve either continued involvement in well-established hobbies and interests or the development of new activities following retirement or other lifestyle changes, such as the retirement of a spouse (Purcell & Keller, 1989; Scarmeas, & Stern, 2003). If one recalls the concept of crystallized intelligence (Hayslip & Sterns, 1979), a stable form of cognitive ability composed of learned information and skills, then it is reasonable to assume that similar stability would be seen in the older adult's ability to pursue familiar hobbies and interests, such as playing cards, doing needlepoint, or repairing machinery. These activities, in which the older person may have engaged for as many as 40 or 50 years, should not be affected by the types of normal cognitive changes we have discussed. Possible exceptions to this general conclusion are presented in the next section.

It is not surprising to suggest stability in the pursuit of lifelong hobbies and leisure activities, but what of the older adult who chooses to learn a new skill in his or her efforts to find meaningful leisure activities? Although there may be little direct empirical data to answer this question, it is reasonable to apply what we know from the industrial gerontology and general cognitive aging literature to this question. Because older adults have repeatedly demonstrated the ability to be retrained in new job skills and to be able to maintain high levels of performance in changing work environments (Olson & Robbins, 1986), there is no reason to assume that older persons could not learn the new skills or information necessary to engage in novel forms of entertainment or leisure activity. Although some of the training principles discussed earlier may be as helpful in leisure as in work-related activities, most healthy older adults should be able to pursue any type of recreational pastime they desire, assuming they are physically and financially able to do so and have the requisite skills. As has been noted, participation in stimulating leisure activities, including physical, social, and cognitive pursuits, can help maintain cognitive functions in late life (Fabre et al., 2003; Wilson et al., 2003) and may reduce the risk of dementia (Wang et al., 2002)

Exceptions to the Rule

The normal changes in cognition that may be relevant to the older adults' functional performance in leisure activities are slowed speed of information processing and changes in memory abilities. This author (Riley, 1992) and others (West & Sinnott, 1992) have reported observational or self-report data suggesting that older adults may perceive the slowing of central processing and perceptual motor response time as a reduced ability to follow fast-paced news presentations and television programs or movies; similar age-related deficits could become evident to the older adult as he or she engages in challenging card games such as bridge or cribbage. Each of these leisure activities requires the kind of rapid information processing or decision making or both that has been documented to be problematic for older adults in a variety of settings. However, these cognitive changes should not lead to the older adult's inability to engage in the activities. Instead some adaptation of the activity such as making notes, requesting additional time in card games, or relinquishing some of the details in a film or news program may be necessary. Crombie, Irvine, Williams, McGinnis, Slane, Alder, and colleagues (2004) have conducted an interesting investigation into the factors that may prevent older adults from engaging in physical leisure activities. Their findings point to ways in which attitudes may be changed in order to increase such activities among older persons.

The other area in which leisure activities could be affected by cognitive change involves the deficits in secondary memory seen in many healthy elderly adults which have been subsumed under the category of mild cognitive impairments. Older adults who experience these cognitive changes may experience difficulty in remembering the names of new acquaintances, misplacing objects, forgetting newly learned telephone numbers, and difficulty remembering multiple items or tasks on a list (Crook et al., 1986). It is easy to see how these changes could lead to frustration and reduced enjoyment of leisure activities, particularly when these activities involve the learning and memorization of large amounts of new information, such as traveling with a group of new acquaintances, learning to play bridge, or keeping track of a busy schedule of social engagements. It is crucial to emphasize, however, that normal age-related memory deficits should not force older adults to give up these activities, unless their level of frustration tolerance is very low and they expect perfect memory performance in every situation. When an individual does voluntarily give up many previously enjoyed and well-practiced leisure (or occupational) interests, it is often a sign of true dementia or serious depression. The physically and emotionally healthy adult may alter activities in some way as a concession to memory deficits, but major lifestyle changes are rarely necessary (Table 7-2). For additional discussion of engagement in leisure activities, see Chapter 12.

The Use of Memory Aids and Intervention Programs

We have already discussed the application of findings from cognitive aging research to vocational issues related to job maintenance and retraining. Similar applications may be made if one desires to enhance performance and satisfaction in leisure and daily life activities of older adults. Literature on mild cognitive impairments, everyday memory, and cognitive intervention programs indicate that formal and informal methods of intervention and adaptation may help the older adult compensate for the effects of age-related memory changes. It has been this author's clinical observation that many older adults are experiencing frustration in their daily lives because they are reluctant to use the kinds of external memory aids that many younger people use and that they may well have used when they were younger. These aids are simple forms of reminders. These reminders include lists and note pads for shopping, errands, and telephone numbers or messages; a daily diary or calendar for social engagements or appointments; and various devices used for monitoring medication dosages and timing. Many older adults are afraid to use these aids because they fear that this means they are developing Alzheimer's disease. Others subscribe to the "use it or lose it" theory of cognitive aging and worry that if they rely on external aids, their memory will fail rapidly. It seems reasonable to encourage the active older adult, or one who takes many medications, to use concrete and simple assistive devices to help him or her remember and function well. It is helpful to remind worried older people who avoid these aids that they probably used them earlier in life and that there is no reason not to use them now.

In addition to these informal and concrete memory aids, some older persons may benefit from taking a class or reading a book on memory skills enhancement. Experimental evidence shows that a variety of training methods can improve the memory performance of older adults (Rasmusson, Rebok, Bylsma, & Brandt, 1999; Scogin, Storandt, & Lott, 1985; Sheikh, Hill, & Yesavage, 1986; Van Gerven et al., 2003; Yesavage & Jacob, 1984). Other cognitive abilities may be enhanced by training as well (Saczynski et al., 2002). The main problem with this kind of formal training is that motivation to continue to use the mnemonic strategies after training ends is low. However, recent research emphasizes practical training strategies that are designed to be "user-friendly" in an effort to help the older adult maintain the strategies they learn (Jobe et al., 2001; Mohs et al., 1998). Box 7-1 shows some strategies for using memory aides.

TABLE 7-2 Effects of Age-Related Changes in Cognition on Daily Activities of Older Adults

Components of Cognition	Effects on Daily Activities
Long-term memory	Difficulty in remembering newly learned facts such as telephone numbers, associating faces and names
	Problems may be experienced in the workplace if job requires high level of memorization
	Misplacing objects, forgetting appointments
Speed of processing	Some difficulty following and remembering the content of fast-paced television programs or movies
	Could lead to difficulties in reaction time or decision making while driving

---

BOX 7-1   **Strategies and Tools for Enhancing Memory Performance**

External Aids
- Carry a small notebook in purse or pocket to jot down reminders, notes, directions to unfamiliar destinations, etc.
- Leave messages on your own answering machine at home
- Keep a pocket calendar with you to help you remember dates and appointments
- Write reminders with a dry-erase marker on bathroom mirror

Internal training strategies
- Pay attention and really focus on material you want to remember

- Rehearse information and test yourself (for example, when trying to learn someone's name)
- Before trying to learn or remember something, use relaxation techniques
- Put easily misplaced objects in a visible "memory spot" *every time*
- Create a visual image or personally meaningful association when trying to remember names and faces
- Organize lists that you want to remember, such as alphabetizing the items creating a word from the first letters of the items
- Break lists into smaller chunks or groupings

■ Summary

As older individuals continue to live longer, healthier, and more productive lives, gerontologists will continue to study the changes and continuities in cognition, lifestyle, and occupational performance that accompany the aging process. Future research is likely to emphasize the practical importance of these issues as well as to grow more sophisticated in research design and methodology. The accumulation of data from longitudinal studies begun in recent years should provide valuable insights into the ways in which aging persons work, think, retire, and enjoy life. It is to be hoped that this kind of research, along with medical advances, will enable gerontologists to de-emphasize dysfunction and disability and focus instead on health and positive functioning in older adults.

C a s e   S t u d y

Mrs. Albert is an 86-year-old widow who lives alone in a one-bedroom high-rise condominium. Her home is located in a suburban area of a medium-sized city. She has two sons who live in the same city, both of them within about a 10 minute drive. She is a retired elementary school teacher who stays in contact with some of her former students and coworkers. She also has a large network of friends who live within a few minutes of her. She has always been very active in the community, particularly enjoying her volunteer work reading to inner-city children, and her efforts to promote adult literacy.

Recently, Mrs. Albert has begun to experience troubling difficulties with her memory. She finds that she cannot always recall the names of her former students when she is describing them to her sons. She also finds herself sometimes getting up to get something, and having difficulty remembering what she got up for. Her sons became concerned when she described leaving an evening meeting and getting lost when she found construction blocking her usual route home. However, both they and she feel that she manages most daily tasks without too much difficulty.

Questions

1. What do you think is Mrs. Albert's most likely problem?
2. How might you assess Mrs. Albert?
3. Based on what is presented here, what might you recommend for Mrs. Albert?

Review Questions

1. Research on age-related cognitive changes has used cross-sectional, cross-sequential, and longitudinal designs. What are the strengths and limitations of each of these designs?
2. Discuss the age-related changes that may be seen in secondary memory. How is the use of encoding strategies related to memory among older adults?
3. Define mild cognitive impairments. Give an example of how this condition might affect an older adult's daily functioning.
4. How might the job performance or leisure activities of the adult decline with normal aging?
5. What issues should be considered by a person devising job training or retraining for an older adult?
6. How might an older adult be instructed to compensate for the effects of age-related cognitive changes?

Web-Based Resources

For helpful information about the experience of Mental Function, visit:

www.asaging.org/asav2/mindalert/fitness.cfm, **American Society on Aging,** date connected October 26, 2007. Includes information about normal age-related changes in mental function, and various kinds of problems that arise in later life. Includes an overview of strategies for maintaining mental function, and links to resources about research.

http://nutritionandaging.fiu.edu/aging_network/aging_network, **National Resource Center on Nutrition, Physical Activity & Aging,** date connected October 26, 2007. Sponsored by Florida International University, this site provides a reasonably reliable summary of information about strategies for maintaining good cognitive function in later life. Readers should be careful to note that there are many unreliable sites, particularly commercial ones hawking various products as "the answer" to cognitive decline. The site also includes links to many government and university sites for additional information.

www.healthinaging.org/agingintheknow/chapters_ch_trial.asp?ch=3, **Foundation for Health in Aging,** date connected October 26, 2007. Another site with information about a large number of issues related to later life. Many resources and links, as well as summaries of research information.

REFERENCES

Albert, M. S. (1988). Cognitive function. In M. S. Albert & M. B. Moss (Eds.), *Geriatric neuropsychology* (pp. 33–58). New York: The Guilford Press.

Albert, M. S., Duffy, F. H., & Naeser, M. (1987). Nonlinear changes in cognition and their neurophysiologic correlates. *Canadian Journal of Psychology, 41,* 141–157.

Albert, M. S., & Heaton, R. K. (1988). Intelligence testing. In M. S. Albert & M. B. Moss (Eds.), *Geriatric neuropsychology* (pp. 13–32). New York: The Guilford Press.

American Psychiatric Association [APA]. (1994). *Diagnostic and statistical manual of mental disorders* (4th ed.). Washington, DC: American Psychiatric Association.

Arenberg, D. (1982). Changes with age in problem solving. In F. I. Craik & S. Rehub (Eds.), *Aging and cognitive processes* (pp. 221–235). New York: Plenum Press.

Auerback, S., & Katz, N. (1988). Assessment of perceptual cognitive performance. Comparison of psychiatric and brain injured adult patients. *Occupational Therapy in Mental Health, 54,* 57–68.

Baddeley, A. (1981). The concept of working memory: A view of its current state and probable future development. *Cognition, 10,* 17–23.

Baugher, D. (1978). Is the older worker inherently incompetent? *Aging and Work, 1,* 243–250.

Bennett, D. A., Schneider, J. A., Bienias, J. L., Evans, A., & Wilson, R. S. (2005). Mild cognitive impairment is related to Alzheimer disease pathology and cerebral infarctions. *Neurology, 64,* 834–841.

Birren, J. E., Robinson, P. K., & Livingston, J. (1986). *Age, health and employment*. Englewood Cliffs, NJ: Prentice Hall.

Carstensen, L. L. (1987). Age-related changes in social activity. In L. L. Carstensen & B. A. Edelstein (Eds.), *Handbook of clinical gerontology* (pp. 222–237). New York: Pergamon Press.

Cattell, R. B. (1963). The theory of fluid and crystalline intelligence. *Journal of Educational Psychology, 54,* 1–11.

Craik, F. I., & Jennings, J. M. (1992). Human memory. In F. I. Craik & T. A. Salthouse (Eds.), *Handbook of aging and cognition* (pp. 51–110). Hillsdale, NJ: Lawrence Erlbaum Associates.

Crombie, I., Irvine, L., Williams, B., McGinnis, A. R., Slane, P. W., Alder, E. M., & McMurdo, M. E. T. (2004). Why older people do not participate in leisure time physical activity: A survey of activity levels, beliefs and deterrents. *Age and Ageing, 33,* 287–292.

Crook, T., Bartus, R. T., Ferris, S. H., & Whitehouse, P. (1986). Age associated memory impairment: Proposed diagnostic criteria and measures of clinical change: Report of a National Institute of Mental Health work group. *Developmental Neuropsychology, 2,* 261–269.

Cunningham, W. R. (1987). Intellectual abilities and age. In K. W. Schaie & C. Eisdorfer (Eds.), *Annual review of gerontology and geriatrics* (Vol. 7, pp. 117–134). New York: Springer.

Earles, J., & Salthouse, T. (1995). Interrelations of age, health and speed. *Journals of Gerontology: Psychological Sciences, 50B,* P33–P41.

Fabre, C., Traisnei, C., & Mucci, P. (2003). Benefits of gymnastic activity on fitness, cognitive function and medication in elderly women. *Science and Sports, 18,* 196–201.

Foos, P. W., & Wright, L. (1992). Adult age differences in the storage of information in working memory. *Experimental Aging Research, 18,* 51–57.

Gauthier, S., Reisberg, B., Zaudig, M., Petersen, R., Ritchie, K., Broich, K., Belleville, S., Brodaty, H., Bennett, D., & Chertkow, H. (2006). Mild cognitive impairment. *Lancet, 367,* 1262–1270.

Gilmore, G. C., Tobias, T. R., & Royer, F. L. (1985). Aging and similarity grouping in visual search. *Gerontologist, 40,* 586–592.

Glass, T. A., Seeman, T. E., Herzog, A. R., Kahn, R., & Berkman, L. F. (1995). Change in productive activity in late adulthood: MacArthur studies of successful aging. *Journals of Gerontology: Social Sciences, 50,* S65–S76.

Grady, C. (1998). Brain imaging and age-related changes in cognition. *Experimental Gerontology, 33,* 671–673.

Green, R. F. (1972). Age, intelligence and learning. *Industrial Gerontology, 12,* 29–41.

Hartley, A. (1992). Attention. In F. I. Craik & T. A. Salthouse (Eds.), *Handbook of aging and cognition* (pp. 3–50). Hillsdale, NJ: Lawrence Erlbaum Associates.

Hasher, L., & Zacks, R. T. (1979). Automatic and effortful processes in memory. *Journal of Experimental Psychology, 108,* 356–388.

Hayslip, B., & Sterns, H. (1979). Age differences in relationships between crystallized and fluid intelligences and problem solving. *Journal of Gerontology, 34,* 404–414 .

Helkala, E. L., Koivisto, K., Hanninen, T., Vanhanen, M., Kuusisto, J., Mykkanen, L., Laasko, M., & Reikkinen, P., Sr., (1997). Stability of age-associated memory impairment during a longitudinal population-based study. *Journal of the American Geriatrics Society, 45,* 120–121.

Horn, J. L., & Cattell, R. B. (1967). Age differences in fluid and crystallized intelligence. *Acta Psychologica, 26,* 107–129.

Ivnik, R. J., Smith, G. E., Malec, J. F., Petersen, R. C., & Tangalos, E. G. (1995). Long-term stability and intercorrelations of cognitive abilities in older persons. *Psychological Assessment, 7,* 155–161.

Jobe, J., Smith, D. M., Ball, K., Tennstedt, S. L., Marsiske, M., Willis, S. L., Rebok, G. W., Morris, J. N., Helmers, K. F., Leveck, M. D., & Kleinman, K. (2001). ACTIVE: A cognitive intervention trial to promote independence in older adults. *Controlled Clinical Trials, 22,* 453–479.

Kaufman, J. E. (1988). Leisure and anxiety: A study of retirees. *Activities, Adaptation and Aging, 11,* 1–10.

Kausler, D. H. (1989) Impairment in normal memory aging: Implications of laboratory evidence. In G. C. Glimoar, P. Whitehouse, & M. Wykel (Eds.), *Aging, memory and dementia* (pp. 41–62). New York: Springer.

Kelly, J. R., & Ross, J. (1989). Later-life leisure: Beginning a new agenda. *Leisure Sciences, 11,* 47–56.

Larrabee, G. J., & Crook, T. H. (1994). Estimated prevalence of age-associated memory impairment derived from standardized tests of memory function. *International Psychogeriatrics, 6,* 95–104.

Lindenberger, U., & Baltes, P. B. (1994). Sensory functioning and intelligence in old age: A strong connection. *Psychology of Aging 9,* 339–355.

Lindenberger, U., Mayr, U., & Kliegl, R. (1993). Speed and intelligence in old age. *Psychology of Aging, 8,* 207–220.

Luis, C., Loewenstein, D. A., Acevedo, A., Barker, W. W., & Duara, R. (2003). Mild cognitive impairment: Directions for future research. *Neurology, 61,* 438–444.

Mohs, R., Ashman, T., Jantzen, K., Albert, M., Brandt, J., & Gordon, B. (1998). A study of the efficacy of a comprehensive memory enhancement program in healthy elderly persons. *Psychiatry Research, 77,* 183–195.

Morgan, D. (2001). The intersection of Alzheimer's disease and typical aging. *Neurobiology of Aging, 22,* 159–160.

Nadler, J. D., Damis, L., & Richardson, E. (1997). Psychosocial aspects of aging. In P. D. Nussbaum (Ed.), *Handbook of neuropsychology and aging* (pp. 44–62). New York: Plenum Press.

Nilsson, I., & Fisher, A. (2006). Evaluating leisure activities in the oldest old. *Scandinavian Journal of Occupational Therapy, 13,* 31–37.

Olson, S. K., & Robbins, S. B. (1986). Guidelines for the development and evaluation of career services for the older adult. Special issue: Career counseling of older adults. *Journal of Career Development, 13,* 53–64.

Palmer, K., Fratiglioni, L., & Winblad, B. (2003). What is mild cognitive impairment? Variations in definitions and evolution of nondemented persons with cognitive impairment. *Acta Neurologica Scandinavia, 107,* 14–20.

Park, D. C. (1994). Aging, cognition and work. *Human Performance, 7,* 181–205.

Perlmutter, M., Adams, C., Berry, J., Kaplan, M., Person, D., & Verdonik, F. (1987). Aging and memory. In K. W. Schaie & C. Eisdorfer (Eds.), *Annual review of gerontology and geriatrics* (Vol. 7, pp. 57–92). New York: Springer.

Perneczky, R., Pohl, C., Sorg, C., Hartmann, J., Komoss, K., Alexopoulos, P., Wagenpfeil, S., & Kurz, A. (2006). Complex activities of daily living in mild cognitive impairment: Conceptual and diagnostic issues. *Age and Ageing, 35,* 240–245.

Petersen, R. C., Doody, R., Kurz, A., Mohs, R. C., Morris, J. C., Rabins, P. V., Ritchie, K., Rossor, M., Thal, L., & Winblad, B. (2001). Current concepts in mild cognitive impairment. *Archives of Neurology, 58,* 1985–1992.

Petersen, R. C., Parisi, J. E., & Dickson, D. W. (2006). Neuropathologic features of amnestic mild cognitive impairment. *Archives of Neurology, 63,* 665–672.

Petersen, R. C., Smith, G., Kokmen, E., Ivnik, R. J., & Tangalos, E. G. (1992). Memory function in normal aging. *Neurology, 42,* 396–401.

Poon, L. W., & Yesavage, J. (Eds.). (1986). *Handbook for the clinical assessment of older adults.* Washington, DC: American Psychological Association.

Purcell, R. Z., & Keller, M. J. (1989). Characteristics of leisure activities which may lead to leisure satisfaction among older adults. *Activities, Adaptation and Aging, 13,* 17–29.

Rabbitt, P. (1982). How do old people know what to do next? In F. I. Craik & S. Trehub (Eds.), *Aging and cognitive processes* (pp. 79–98). New York: Plenum Press.

Raji, M. A., Kuo, Y., Snih, S. A., Markides, K. S., Peek, M. K., & Ottenbacher, K. J. (2005). Cognitive status, muscle strength, and subsequent disability in older Mexican Americans. *Journal of the American Geriatrics Society, 53,* 1462–1468.

Rasmusson, D. X., Rebok, G. W., Bylsma, F. W., & Brandt, J. (1999). Effects of three types of memory training in normal elderly. *Aging, Neuropsychology and Cognition, 6,* 56–66.

Rebok, G. W., Offermann, L. R., Wirtz, P. W., & Montaglione, C. J. (1985). Work and intellectual aging: The psychological concomitants of social organizational conditions. *Educational Gerontology, 12,* 359–374.

Rhodes, S. R. (1983). Age related differences in work attitude and behavior: A review and conceptual analysis. *Psychological Bulletin, 93,* 328–338.

Riley, K. P. (1992). Bridging the gap between researchers and clinicians: Methodological perspectives and choices. In R. L. West & J. Sinnott (Eds.), *Everyday memory and aging: Current research and methodology* (pp. 182–189). New York: Springer-Verlag.

Riley, K. P. (1999). Assessment of memory and dementia. In P. Lichtenberg (Ed.), *The handbook of geriatric assessment* (pp. 134–166). New York: John Wiley & Sons.

Riley, K. P., & Snowdon, D. A. (1999). The challenges and successes of aging: Findings from the Nun Study In P. Lichtenberg (Ed.), *Advances in medical psychotherapy and psychodiagnosis* (Vol. 10, pp. 1–12). New York: Kendall/Hunt.

Riley, K. P., Snowdon, D. A., & Markesbery, W. R. (2002). Alzheimer's neurofibrillary pathology and the spectrum of cognitive function: Findings from the Nun Study. *Annals of Neurology, 51,* 567–577.

Ritchie, K., & Touchon, J. (2000). Mild cognitive impairment: Conceptual basis and current nosological status. *Lancet, 355,* 225–228.

Rockey, L. S. (1997). Memory assessment of the older adult. In P. D. Nussbaum (Ed.), *Handbook of neuropsychology and aging* (pp. 385–393). New York: Plenum Press.

Saczynski, J. S., Willis, S. L., & Schaie, W. K. (2002). Strategy use in reasoning training with older adults. *Aging, Neuropsychology and Cognition, 9,* 48–60.

Salthouse, T. (1992). Reasoning and spatial abilities. In F. I. Craik & T. A. Salthouse (Eds.), *Handbook of aging and cognition* (pp. 167–212). Hillsdale, NJ: Lawrence Erlbaum Associates.

Salthouse, T. (1993). Speed mediation of adult age differences in cognition. *Developmental Psychology, 29,* 722–738.

Salthouse, T. (1994). Age-related differences in basic cognitive processes: Implications for work. *Experimental Aging Research, 20,* 249–255.

Scarmeas, N., & Stern, Y. (2003). Cognitive reserve and lifestyle. *Journal of Clinical and Experimental Neuropsychology, 25,* 625–633.

Scarmeas, N., Zarahn, E., Anderson, K. E., Hilton, J., Flynn, J., Van Heertum, R. L., Sackeim, H., & Stern, Y. (2003). Cognitive reserve modulates functional brain responses during memory tasks: A PET study in healthy young and elderly subjects. *Neuroimage, 19,* 1215–1227.

Schaie, K. W., & Eisdorfer, C. (1987). *Annual review of gerontology and geriatrics* (Vol. 7). New York: Springer.

Scogin, F., Storandt, M., & Lott, L. (1985). Memory skills training, memory complaints and depression in older adults. *Journal of Gerontology, 40,* 562–568.

Sheikh, J. I., Hill, R. D., & Yesavage, J. A. (1986). Long term efficacy of cognitive training for age associated memory impairment: A six month follow-up study. *Developmental Neuropsychology, 2,* 413–421.

Singleton, W. T. (1983). Age, skill and management. *International Journal of Aging and Human Development, 17,* 15–23.

Sliwinski, M. J., Hofer, S. M., & Hall, C. (2003). Correlated and coupled clinical change in older adults with and without preclinical dementia. *Psychology and Aging, 18,* 672–683.

Sliwinski, M. J., Hofer, S. M., Hall, C., Buschke, H., & Lipton, R. B. (2003). Modeling memory decline in older adults: The importance of preclinical dementia, attrition and chronological age. *Psychology and Aging, 18,* 658–671.

Smith, A. (1980). Age differences in encoding, storage and retrieval. In L. W. Poon, J. L. Fozard, L. S. Cermak, D. Arenberg, & L. W. Thompson (Eds.), *New directions in memory and aging* (pp. 23–47). Hillsdale, NJ: Lawrence Erlbaum Associates.

Smith, G. E., Petersen, R. C., Parrisi, J. E., & Ivnik, R. J. (1996). Definition, course, and outcome of mild cognitive impairment. *Aging, Neuropsychology and Cognition, 3*, 141–147.

Stern, Y. (2002). What is cognitive reserve? Theory and research application of the reserve concept. *Journal of the International Neuropsychological Society, 8*, 448–460.

Sterns, H. L. (1986). Training and retraining adult and older adult workers. In J. E. Birren, P. K. Robinson, & J. Livingston (Eds.), *Age, health and employment* (pp. 43–54). Englewood Cliffs, NJ: Prentice Hall.

Sterns, H. L., & Alexander, R. A. (1987). Industrial gerontology: The aging individual and work. In K. W. Schaie & C. Eisdorfer (Eds.), *Annual review of gerontology and geriatrics* (Vol. 7, pp. 243–264). New York: Springer.

Streufert, S., Pogash, R., Piasecki, M., & Post, G. M. (1990). Age and management team performance. *Psychology of Aging, 5*, 551–559.

Sweeney, J. A., Rosano, C., Berman, R. A., & Luna, B. (2001). Inhibitory control of attention declines more than working memory during normal aging. *Neurobiology of Aging, 22*, 39–47.

Turner, R. S. (2003). Biomarkers of Alzheimer's Disease and mild cognitive impairment: Are we there yet? *Experimental Neurology, 183*, 7–10.

Van Gerven, P. W. M., Paas, F., van Merrienboer, J. J. G., Hendriks, M., & Schmidt, H. G. (2003). The efficiency of multimedia learning into old age. *British Journal of Educational Psychology, 73*, 489–505.

Waldman, D., & Avolio, B. (1985). A meta-analysis of age differences in job performance. *Journal of Applied Psychology, 71*, 33–46.

Wang, H., Karp, A., Winblad, B., & Fratiglioni, L. (2002). Late-life engagement in Social and Leisure activities is associated with decreased risk of dementia: A longitudinal study from the Kungsholmen Project. *American Journal of Epidemiology, 155*, 1081–1087.

Welford, A. T. (1976). Thirty years of psychological research on age and work. *Journal of Occupational Psychology, 49*, 129–138.

West, R. L. (1986). Everyday memory and aging. *Developmental Neuropsychology, 2*, 313–322.

West, R. L., & Sinnott, J. J. (Eds.) (1992). *Everyday memory and aging: Current research and methodology.* New York: Springer-Verlag.

Willis, S. (1987). Cognitive training and everyday competence. In K. W. Schaie & C. Eisdorfer (Eds.), *Annual review of gerontology and geriatrics* (Vol. 7, pp. 159–188). New York: Springer.

Wilson, R. S., Bennett, D. A., & Swartzendruber, A. (1997). Age-related change in cognitive function. In P. D. Nussbaum (Ed.), *Handbook of neuropsychology and aging* (pp. 7–14). New York: Plenum Press.

Wilson, R. S., Bennett, D. A., & Swartzendruber, A. (2003). Assessment of lifetime participation in cognitively stimulating activities. *Journal of Clinical and Experimental Neuropsychology, 25*, 634–642.

Woods, R. T., & Britton, P. G. (1985). *Clinical psychology with the elderly.* Rockville, MD: Aspen Systems Corporation.

Yesavage, J. A., & Jacob, R. (1984). Effects of relaxation and mnemonics on memory, attention and anxiety in the elderly. *Experimental Aging Research, 10*, 211–214.

Yokomizo, Y. (1985). Measurement of ability in older workers. *Ergonomics, 28*, 843–854.

Zachs, R. T. (1982). Encoding strategies used by young and elderly adults in a keeping track task. *Journal of Gerontology, 37*, 203–211.

Interruptions in Function

CHAPTER 8

Falls

Rein Tideiksaar, PhD

This is the state of man: to-day he puts forth the tender leaves of hopes;
to-morrow blossoms, And bears his blushing honours thick upon him;
The third day comes a frost, a killing frost, And, when he thinks,
good easy man, full surely His greatness is a-ripening,
nips his root, And then he falls, as I do. And when
he falls, he falls like Lucifer, Never to hope again.

William Shakespeare, *Henry VIII*

OBJECTIVES

By the end of this chapter, the readers will be able to:

1. Define falls.
2. Discuss the frequency and consequences of falls for older adults.
   If agreed, other objectives would be renumbered.
3. Discuss the reasons for falls in older adults.
4. Describe the assessment of falls and fall risk.
5. Describe intervention strategies aimed at fall prevention.
6. Describe the best practice approach aimed at fall prevention.

Falls are among the most serious health problems faced by older people. They are a major cause of premature death, physical injury, immobility, psychosocial dysfunction, and nursing home placement. The rapidly growing population of people 75 years of age and older are those at greatest fall risk (Nevitt, 1997). To reduce the alarming rate of falls and related excessive mortality and morbidity, efforts must be made to detect persons at fall risk and to prevent or reduce the frequency of falls. To facilitate such approaches, it is essential to know why (and under what conditions) older people fall and the factors that are associated with fall risk. Of equal importance, it is necessary to have an organized approach to the clinical assessment of falls and fall risk. This chapter reviews the epidemiology of falls, their complications, and the various host and environmentally related causes of falls. An approach to clinical assessment of falls and fall risk is described. Multidisciplinary interventions aimed at reducing falls as well as a "best practice" approach to the clinical assessment of falls and fall risk are described.

Epidemiology

Approximately one-third of community-residing persons over age 65 fall each year; and of these, one half have multiple falls (Downton, 1998; O'Loughlin, Robitaille, Boivin, & Suissa, 1993). Falls are even more frequent in nursing homes, where up to 50% of older residents fall annually (Tideiksaar, 2002); over 40% of individuals experience recurrent falls (Rubenstein & Josephson, 1992). Older adults in the hospital also fall frequently, averaging about 1.5 falls per bed per year (Rubenstein & Powers, 1999). The likelihood of falling increases with age; the incidence of falls begins to rise steadily after the age of 75 years (Campbell, Spears, & Borrie, 1990; Rubenstein & Josephson, 2002).

The true extent of falling may be underestimated (Cwikel, Fried, & Galinsky, 1990; Rubenstein, Robbins, Josephson, Schulman, & Osterweil, 1990). Typically, only falls with injury requiring medical attention or causing problems with mobility are likely to be reported by older persons. Falls may not be reported if they are thought to be a consequence of "normal" aging, a reminder of increasing frailty,

or if there is a fear that reporting an event will lead to restriction of activities or placement in a nursing home. Even in institutional settings, many falls are not witnessed, and patients may fail to report them, perhaps because of underlying cognitive dysfunction or a fear of activity restrictions. Also, hospital and nursing home staff may underreport falls because they fear being blamed for falls; this occurs most often in organizations that do not practice a "culture of safety" (i.e., staff feel free to report falls without blame; when an organization does not have such a culture, staff members are often unwilling to report falls because they fear reprisal).

Complications

Falls are the leading cause of death due to "accidents" or unintentional injury in persons aged 65 years and older (Baker, Ginsburg, & O'Neill, 1992). About 10,000 deaths per year are attributable to falling (Tideiksaar, 2002). Of those persons hospitalized as a result of falling, only about one half will be alive 1 year later (Sattin, 1992). Mortality appears not to be the direct result of the fall because the majority of fatalities occur weeks to months after the fall (Dunn, Rudberg, Furner, & Cassel, 1992), but rather, it is a consequence of **comorbidity** (e.g., pneumonia, heart failure, and so on). The actual number of fall-related deaths is probably much higher because falls are not listed consistently on death certificates (Fife, 1987). For those who survive a fall, significant morbidity is likely to follow. An estimated 5% of falls by older persons both in the community and in institutions result in fractures, and an additional 10% of falls result in nonfracture injuries (Nevitt, 1997; O'Loughlin et al., 1993), including head injuries, **hematomas,** joint dislocations, and muscle sprains. Women experience a higher rate of fracture and nonfracture injuries than men (O'Loughlin et al., 1993). The most common fractures associated with falls are those of the forearm and hip (Griffin, Ray, Fought, & Melton, 1992). Distal forearm or **Colles' fractures** occur when an older person attempts to break a fall by extending the arms outward. The incidence of forearm fractures plateaus after the age of 65 years, at which time there is a steep increase in the incidence of hip fractures (Cummings et al., 1990).

Approximately 332,000 hip fractures occur annually in the United States; the overwhelming majority of hip fractures occur in persons 65 years of age and older (Stevens, 2002). The mortality and morbidity rates following hip fractures are substantial. Of all patients with hip fractures, 4% die in the hospital, and within 1 year after their injury, 23% are dead (Fisher et al., 1991); persons 75 years and older have the highest mortality rates (Davis, 1995). A high incidence of coexisting chronic diseases in persons with hip fracture contributes to this increased mortality rate (Sartoretti, Sartoretti-Schefer, Ruckert, & Buchmann, 1997). After a hip fracture, many older people never regain their **premorbid** level of ambulation. For persons who survive to 6 months, 60% recover their prefracture walking ability, half recover their prefracture ability to perform activities of daily living (ADLs), and about 25% recover their prefracture ability to perform instrumental activities of daily living (IADLs) (Magaziner, Simonsick, Kashner, Hebel, & Kenzora, 1990). However, after 1 year, only about 54% of surviving individuals can walk unaided, and only 40% can perform all physical ADLs independently (Magaziner et al., 1990). A small number of hip fractures (fewer than 1%) occur spontaneously as a result of **osteopenia,** causing a fall (Norton, Campbell, Lee-Joe, Robinson, & Butler, 1997). However, the majority of hip fractures are caused by a number of interacting factors (Birge, Morrow-Howell, & Proctor, 1994; Nevitt, Cummings, The Study of Osteoporotic Fractures Study Group, 1993). Although international comparisons of hip fracture incidence, mortality, and morbidity are likely to be affected by differences in coding and assignment of cause of death, as well as genetic differences, different levels of exposure to risk, susceptibility to injury, and interventions to reduce mortality and morbidity when falls occur, the extent and consequences associated with hip fracture are similar for many developed nations (Chang, Center, Nguyen, & Eisman, 2004; Kanis et al., 2002; Schwartz et al., 1999).

Height of the Fall and Impact Surface

In order to build sufficient momentum to produce injury (e.g., bone fracture), an individual must fall a considerable distance. For example, an unexpected fall from a standing height (e.g., a slip, loss of consciousness) or a fall from an elevated bed (e.g., over bed side rails) is more likely to result in injury because of the increased force of impact than a fall from a relatively low height, such as from a chair or toilet. Falls on hard, nonabsorptive ground surfaces, such as linoleum tile, concrete, and wood, are more likely to result in injury than falls onto absorptive surfaces, such as carpeting.

Protective Reflexes

The onset of a fall elicits several protective reflexes: extending the arms outward and initiating quick shifting movements of the feet in order to regain balance. Both may avert a fall or minimize the force of impact. Conversely, a loss of protective reflexes stemming from neuromuscular dysfunction that affects the extremities or from sedation induced by medication may increase the impact of falling and risk of fracture.

"Shock Absorbers"

Increased fat and muscle bulk surrounding vulnerable areas, such as the hip, are capable of absorbing the impact of a fall, and thereby decreasing the risk of fracture. Fractures are more likely to occur in people whose muscles have atrophied or those who have a decreased amount of fat padding (e.g., thin people).

Bone Strength

A loss of bone strength attributable to osteoporosis at the femoral neck may result in fractures that occur even with minimal ground impact against the bone. Bone loss is a particular problem in older women. By age 80 years, women may lose up to 50% of their bone strength, compared with 15% in men (Stevens, 2002).

Falls that do not result in physical injury can lead to a restriction of activities and self-imposed immobility related to fear of falling. Between 40% and 73% of older people who have had a recent fall admit to avoiding some activities because of fear of additional falls and injury (King & Tinetti, 1995). If the resulting avoidance of mobility leads to prolonged immobility, a host of complications may develop, including **deep venous thrombosis, decubitus ulcers,** urinary tract infections, **hypostatic pneumonia,** muscle atrophy, joint contractures, depression, and functional dependence (Tideiksaar, 2002). Long lies or the inability to get up from the floor by oneself is another common consequence of falling, occurring in up to 50% of individuals (King & Tinetti, 1995). Many individuals with long lies develop a fear of falling. Falling and instability are a leading contributor of nursing home placement, a factor in about 40% of admissions (Fuller, 2000).

Causes of Falling

Falls occur when an individual engages in an activity that results in a loss of balance and the body mechanisms responsible for compensation fail. In older people, falls often occur during routine activities, such as walking; descending or climbing steps; transferring on or off chairs, beds, toilets, or in or out of bathtubs; and reaching up or bending down. The fall may be a sign of an underlying problem indicative of intrinsic host factors, including age-related physiological changes, diseases, medications, or extrinsic factors or environmental hazards (King & Tinetti, 1995).

Age-Related Physiological Changes

Normal age-related physiological changes contribute to both falling and fall risk. The most important of these occur in the visual, neurological, cardiovascular, and musculoskeletal systems. See Chapters 4, 5, and 6 for additional information.

Vision

One of the most important functions of the eye in mobility is detecting cues in the surrounding environment. Elements of visual function related to occurrence of falls include declines in **visual acuity** (e.g., decreased ability to see clearly and particularly affects near objects), **contrast sensitivity** (e.g., difficulty seeing objects and ground surfaces that have low contrast, especially against a bright background), **accommodation** (e.g., inability to focus clearly on objects over a range of distances), lateral and upper visual fields (e.g., inability to detect hazardous situations or objects in field of vision), **dark adaptation** (e.g., inability of the eye to adjust to low levels of illumination), color perception (e.g., inability to perceive, differentiate, and distinguish colors of objects in environment), **glare recovery** (e.g., inability of the eye to recover from intense illumination, such as bright lighting), and **depth perception** (e.g., inability to judge distances and relationships among objects in the visual field) (Pinto et al., 1997; Tideiksaar, 1997b).

Balance

The body's ability to maintain balance or postural stability during standing and walking is dependent largely on feedback received from the vestibular, visual, and proprioceptive systems. With age, postural sway tends to increase to a level of unsteadiness (Alexander, 1994). Older persons who fall have more sway than nonfallers, and persons with multiple falls demonstrate greater sway than those with isolated falls (Tideiksaar, 1997b). Age-related disturbances of sway or balance have been attributed to visual, vestibular, and proprioceptive loss. People with a decline in visual acuity (Felson et al., 1989) or poor proprioception (Lord, Clark, & Webster, 1991) have increased sway. A loss of proprioception is also associated with impaired vibration sense (Lord et al., 1991). The vestibular righting response also declines with age (Alexander, 1994), which can lead to a failure to maintain balance during postural displacements.

Musculoskeletal

An older person's gait and balance are affected by a number of changes in the musculoskeletal system, as discussed in Chapter 6. With advancing age, there is a calcification of tendons and ligaments, a flattening of the disks between the vertebrae, and increased curvature of the spine. As a consequence, changes in posture occur. The trunk is frequently bent forward and the head is flexed at the neck. Such a stance places the body center of gravity forward at the outer limits of an older individual's stability. This increases the risk of balance loss and falls. Also, a decline in proximal muscle strength and hip extensor and flexor strength occur, which results in decreased walking speed, step length, and step height. The gait in older people who fall is even more compromised than that of normal elderly individuals (Alexander, 1996), resulting in a slower walk and shorter, shuffling steps.

Blood Pressure

Baroreflex activity, a mechanism of the cardiovascular system, plays a crucial role in the regulation of systemic blood pressure. With advancing age, there is a progressive decline in baroreflex sensitivity to both hypotensive and hypertensive stimuli (Lipsitz, 1991). As a result, heart rate in older people often fails to increase in response to postural changes in position (e.g., moving from supine to sitting position). Also, older people have less capacity for cardio-acceleration or increase in heart rate to compensate for the hypotensive effects of medications. This problem leads to **hypoxia** and accompanying falls.

Conditions

The risk of falling increases with the number of medical conditions or other intrinsic factors present. Virtually any chronic or transient medical problems that interfere with mobility may predispose an individual to falling. Visual, neurological, cardiovascular, musculoskeletal, and psychological disorders are some of the most important.

Visual Disorders

Diseases of the eye such as cataracts, **macular degeneration,** and glaucoma have been associated with fall risk (Tideiksaar, 1997b). Superimposed on age-related changes in vision, they can further impair visual function. Even without severe visual impairment, the decline in visual perception and acuity is sufficient to increase fall risk when combined with environmental factors. Objects (e.g., upended rug edges or step heights) are difficult to perceive.

Neurological Disorders

Neurological disorders such as dementia, neuropathy, stroke, cervical degeneration, and Parkinsonism are particularly important in predisposing older people to falls (Tideiksaar, 1997b). Dementia, including Alzheimer's disease, vascular dementia, and dementia with Lewy bodies (DLB), is associated with gait and balance changes, ataxia, and altered proprioception (Tideiksaar, 1998). As a consequence, people tend to walk more slowly, with shorter steps, increased double support time, and greater step-to-step variability (Tideiksaar, 1998). Also, people with dementia tend to have problems with the spatial recognition of objects in the environment (Tideiksaar, 1997b). This problem, along with poor judgment in perceiving hazards, commonly results in trips and slips. People with neuropathy as a result of diabetes, **pernicious anemia,** or nutritional disorders can have lower extremity weakness, hyperactive reflexes, and altered proprioceptive function, leading to poor balance and abnormal gait (Richardson & Hurvitz, 1995; Tideiksaar, 1997b). People with hemiparetic gait, especially with decreased ankle dorsiflexion, are susceptible to tripping falls. Cervical degeneration, the result of diseases such as **ankylosing spondylosis** and rheumatoid arthritis, is a common cause of proprioceptive dysfunction (Tideiksaar, 1998), which can lead to gait abnormalities and postural instability. People with Parkinsonism often display alterations of gait and postural control that contribute to balance loss and fall risk. Their gait becomes short-stepped and shuffling, with the feet barely clearing the ground. At times, gait initiation becomes difficult, and people stutter-step or take short, rapid, shuffling steps when they walk. Other gait changes include **"freezing"**— the feet suddenly come to a halt, but the body keeps moving forward, placing persons at risk for loss of balance. This type of gait can result in propulsion, an uncontrolled forward motion when walking, or retropulsion, falling backward. Loss of automatic postural reflexes can affect the ability to maintain upright posture and stability. To preserve balance, people compensate by assuming a stooped posture, with their neck, trunk, and limbs held in forward flexion with bent arms and knees (Alexander, 1996; Tideiksaar, 1998).

Cardiovascular Disorders

Any cardiovascular disorder that results in a reduction of cerebral perfusion can precipitate a fall. Common disorders include cardiac arrhythmias, **carotid sinus node disease,** and abnormalities in blood pressure regulation. Cardiac arrhythmias produce extremely slow or fast heart rates that can lead to cerebral hypoperfusion and dizziness. Carotid sinus node disease presents with **syncope** and is brought on by such common activities as turning the head to one side as if looking over one's shoulder or hyperextending the neck and head backward. This disorder is due either to carotid sinus sensitivity or to a mechanical obstruction (Lipsitz, 1991) that interferes with the supply of blood to the brain. Postural, or **orthostatic hypotension** can lead to instability following changes in body position (e.g., rising from the supine or sitting position). It has several causes, including autonomic dysfunction, **hypovolemia,** low cardiac output, Parkinsonism, and medications such as diuretics. Another abnormality of blood pressure homeostasis is **postprandial hypotension** (Lipsitz, 1991). This syndrome, which leads to profound declines in blood pressure after eating, has no known cause. People who have fainting spells following a meal should be suspected of having postprandial hypotension and should be cautioned against sudden rising or activities after dining.

Musculoskeletal Disorders

Diseases of the bone, muscle, and joints may contribute to the risk of falling (Tideiksaar, 1997b). Osteoarthritis of the hip and knee joints can limit the ability to walk, climb, or descend stairs and transfer effectively. Muscle weakness resulting from thyroid disease, **polymyalgia rheumatica, hypokalemia,** or deconditioning may lead to gait and transfer problems. Osteomalacia, characterized by deficient mineralization of bone, causes proximal muscle weakness and an unstable, waddling gait.

Psychological/Psychosocial Issues

Older people with depression may develop problems with concentrating, which can lead to judgment errors, a misperception of environmental hazards, and fall risk (Tideiksaar, 1997b). In those persons who fall frequently and have severe, prolonged depression, the falling episodes may be a sign of suicidal intent or need for attention.

Medications

Drugs are an important cause of falls in older people (Hanlon, Cutson, & Ruby, 1996; Thapa, Gideon, Fought, & Ray, 1995). Any drug that interferes with postural control, cerebral perfusion, or cognitive function (e.g., sedatives, antipsychotics, diuretics, antihypertensives, tricyclic antidepressants, or alcohol) (Hanlon et al., 1996) may induce a fall. Generally, fall risk is greater for those taking drugs with extended **half-lives** (i.e., greater than 24 hours) and increases with the number of medications a person receives (Hanlon et al., 1996). In both community and institutional settings, psychotropic medications (e.g., neuroleptics, benzodiazepines, and antidepressants) are consistently associated with increased fall risk.

Environmental Factors

The overwhelming majority of falls experienced by community-residing older people occur in the home (Tideiksaar, 1997b), especially the bedroom, bathroom, and stairway. In the hospital and nursing home, the bed and bathroom represent the most common locations where people fall (Tideiksaar, 2002). Several environmental obstacles, design factors, and host activities are associated with falling: transferring from low or high beds, chairs, or toilets; walking in poorly illuminated areas and tripping over low-lying objects or floor coverings, such as thick pile carpets or unsecured rug edges; slipping on waxed or wet ground surfaces; and climbing or descending steps that lack handrail support or are difficult to see (Carter, Campbell, Sanson-Fisher, Redmen, & Gillespie, 1997; Northridge, Nevitt, Kelsey, & Link, 1995; Tideiksaar, 1997a, 1997b). This list is by no means exhaustive. Its importance lies in the fact that it is evidence of a causal relationship between environmental hazards and falling. Ironically, assistive devices may contribute to falls. Bedrails may actually increase the risk as a result of attempts by the older adult to leave the bed without lowering the rails (Tideiksaar, 2002). Wheelchairs contribute to falls as a result of poor transfer techniques or forgetfulness about procedures (e.g., not locking wheel brakes) (Tideiksaar, 1997b). Canes and walkers can cause falls (Tideiksaar, 1997b), presumably because of improper size or application of these aids. The use of physical restraints to prevent falls in many instances contributes to further falls, especially injurious falls (Tideiksaar, 1997b).

Clinical Assessment and Intervention

The goals of fall prevention in both the community dwelling and institutionalized populations are similar. First, persons at risk must be identified, and for those with falls, the cause must be determined. Second, the risk of falling or sustaining further falls must be reduced by implementing interventions that maintain the older person's mobility.

Interaction among risk factors can increase risk of falls. Identifying those factors and defining fall etiology in persons who have fallen require a multidisciplinary approach directed toward assessing both intrinsic and extrinsic risk factors. Assessment components include a medical and medication history, physical examination, mobility evaluation, environmental assessment, and a fall history. A psychosocial assessment may uncover a history of substance abuse or related risk factors. Although the approaches to the assessment of fall risk and falls are similar, each is discussed separately and is followed by a consideration of potential intervention strategies.

Fall Assessment

The components of an assessment of falls in older people are shown in Figure 8-1. As a first step, persons who have fallen need to be identified. In the institutional setting, this can be done by simply recording falls on the incident report. For community-residing persons, this is best accomplished by asking during a clinical visit whether they have experienced any recent falls. Discovering falls that have occurred within the past 3 months is most useful because these are most predictive of future falls. Because older people tend to underreport falls, family members living with the person should be questioned.

It is important to ask people not only about completed falls—that is, episodes in which the individuals actually come to rest on the ground—but about near-falls as well. These include events in which people lose their balance but manage to avert a fall by grabbing an environmental object, such as a chair or bathroom towel bar, for support. Near-falls are as important as completed falls because, if the

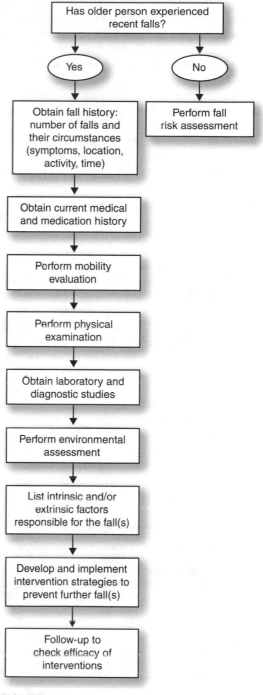

FIGURE 8-1   Fall assessment

environmental object were not available, the person would probably have fallen.

If the person has fallen, it is important to obtain a fall history. This includes asking about the precise number of completed and near-falls and, for each episode, the circumstances. A convenient acronym to help remember the components of the fall history is SPLAT (symptoms, previous falls, location, activity, and time). Family members and other witnesses can help provide a complete fall history. In the institutional setting, documentation of circumstances should be a part of the incident report. Staff who have opportunity to observe the resident should be questioned, including nurses and aides, therapists, and, depending on the setting, individuals in dietary and housekeeping departments.

When alert individuals are unable to remember the circumstances of their falls, determining the reasons for falling is difficult. For these individuals, the use of a fall diary (Figure 8-2) to record the circumstances of falls may provide a clearer account of falls and help identify causes.

This information can point to possible causes of falling. For example, falls associated with rising from a lying or seated position and experiencing symptoms of dizziness suggest orthostatic hypotension. If no such symptoms are present, the design of furniture may be a causative factor. If a person complains of tripping or slipping, a gait or balance disorder must be suspected, either by itself or in conjunction with an environmental hazard, such as an uneven or slippery floor surface or poor lighting. Other questions to ask during the history that might indicate the presence of psychosocial factors include the following: Does the person live alone? How long was the person on the ground after the fall or falls (i.e., long lie time)? Have physical injuries resulted? What effect did the fall have on the person's self-confidence? Does he or she fear further falls? Has he or she restricted activities as a result? Do families or caregivers have any concerns about safety?

Next, obtain a current and comprehensive history of medical problems, complaints, and medications. In particular, the relationship between prescription and over-the-counter medications (e.g., when medication started, when stopped, dosage changes, and compliance) and falls should be reviewed. An association may indicate that the fall is due to an adverse medication effect.

The physical assessment of the individual includes a mobility evaluation and an assessment of gait, balance, and ability to change position (e.g., standing up or sitting down). This is particularly helpful in providing clues to underlying causes of falling, localizing the organ systems involved, isolating potential environmental problems, and designing interventions. A number of simple mobility evaluations are available that require little time, special expertise, space, or equipment. These include the "get-up-and-go test" in which the person is asked to rise from a chair, stand still momentarily, walk a short distance, turn around, walk back, and sit down (Mathias, Nayak, & Isaacs, 1986). The test is scored on a five-point scale, with 1 being normal and 5 being severely abnormal. Another is the "Performance-Oriented Assessment of Mobility" (Tinetti, 1986). This assessment is a scored

FALLING DOWN IS NOT A NORMAL PART OF GROWING OLD. THERE ARE MANY CAUSES OF FALLING WHICH CAN BE TREATED. IN ORDER TO PREVENT FALLS, WE NEED TO KNOW AS MUCH ABOUT YOUR FALLS AS POSSIBLE. THIS DIARY WILL HELP YOU TO REMEMBER THE TIMES WHEN YOU FALL. EACH TIME YOU FALL, WRITE DOWN THE DATE, TIME OF DAY WHEN THE FALL OCCURRED, WHERE THE FALL OCCURRED (LOCATION), WHAT YOU WERE DOING AT THE TIME (ACTIVITY), AND HOW YOU FELT (SYMPTOMS). BELOW WE HAVE LISTED TWO EXAMPLES.

DATE	TIME	LOCATION	ACTIVITY	SYMPTOMS
4/8	8:00 AM	Bedroom	Getting out of bed	I felt dizzy
5/1	10:00 PM	Bedroom	I slipped while walking	None

1. _____ _____ _____ _____ _____
2. _____ _____ _____ _____ _____
3. _____ _____ _____ _____ _____
4. _____ _____ _____ _____ _____
5. _____ _____ _____ _____ _____

FIGURE 8-2 Fall diary

performance of balance and gait that examines the person's ability to rise from and sit down in a chair, standing balance, and gait with respect to step initiation, height, and symmetry, walking deviation, trunk stability, and turning ability.

Table 8-1 shows a mobility evaluation devised in part from existing tests. It can generally be administered in less than 5 minutes and is simple to understand, administer, and record. The evaluation is based on the

TABLE 8-1 Mobility Evaluation

Instructions: Ask the person to perform the following maneuvers. For each, indicate whether the person's performance is normal or abnormal.

Ask Person To:	Observe:	Response:
1. Sit down in chair. Select a chair with armrests that is approximately 16 to 17 inches in seat height	Able to sit down in one smooth, controlled movement without using armrests	Normal
	Sitting is not a smooth movement; falls into chair or needs armrests to guide self into chair	Abnormal
2. Rise up from chair	Able to get up in one smooth, controlled movement without using armrests	Normal
	Uses armrests and/or moves forward in chair to propel self up; requires several attempts to get up	Abnormal
3. Stand after rising from chair for approximately 30 seconds in place	Steady; able to stand without support	Normal
	Unsteady; loses balance	Abnormal
4. Stand with eyes closed for approximately 15 seconds in place	Steady; able to stand without support	Normal
	Unsteady; loses balance	Abnormal
5. Stand with feet together, push lightly on sternum two to three times	Steady; maintains balance	Normal
	Unsteady; loses balance	Abnormal
6. Reach up onto tiptoes as if attempting to reach an object	Steady, without loss of balance	Normal
	Unsteady; loses balance	Abnormal
7. Bend down as if attempting to obtain object from floor	Steady, without loss of balance	Normal
	Unsteady; loses balance	Abnormal

Instructions: If the person uses a walking aid such as a cane or walker, the following walking maneuvers are tested separately with and without the aid. Indicate type of aid used.

8. Walk in a straight line, in your "usual" pace (a distance approximately 15 feet); then walk back	Gait is continuous without hesitation; walks in a straight line and both feet clear the floor	Normal (with aid) Normal (without aid)
	Gait is noncontinuous with hesitation; deviates from straight path; feet scrape or shuffle on floor	Abnormal (with aid) Abnormal (without aid)
9. Walk a distance of 5 feet and turn around	Does not stagger; steps are smooth, continuous	Normal (with aid) Normal (without aid)
	Staggers; steps are unsteady, discontinuous	Abnormal (with aid) Abnormal (without aid)
10. Lie down on the floor and get up	Able to rise, without loss of balance	Normal
	Unable to rise, or loses balance in the process	Abnormal

performance of 10 activities, scored as either normal or abnormal. Difficulty in performing these maneuvers may indicate underlying myopathy, arthritis, Parkinsonism, postural hypotension or vestibular dysfunction, loss of proprioception, or balance problems.

The best method to assess a person's mobility is to observe the described maneuvers in his or her living environment (e.g., home or nursing home). This takes into account the relationship between performance and the environment (e.g., types of floor surface or chair design) (Tideiksaar, 1997a). In addition, activities such as bed, toilet, and bathtub transfer and stair climbing and descending maneuvers can be assessed. After the mobility evaluation, the next step is to conduct a physical examination and perform laboratory and diagnostic studies. Information gathered from the fall history and mobility evaluation serves as a guide to elements of the physical examination that deserve special attention. For example, if the fall history reveals that falls occur in association with dizziness during changes in position, orthostatic hypotension should be considered.

The extent of the laboratory and diagnostic studies is dictated by the information gathered from all previous evaluations. If the physical examination confirms the presence of orthostatic hypotension, blood and stool tests to evaluate volume-depletion states such as dehydration are ordered.

The next step is the environmental assessment. Under the best circumstances, all older people who have falls should have their living environment evaluated. Environmental assessment is essential for people whose fall history and mobility evaluation suggests the presence of an extrinsic cause of falling.

The goal of the environmental assessment is to determine a person's level of mobility function—that is, to identify environmental areas or design features that increase fall risk and the need for environmental modification and adaptive equipment.

In the home setting, the person should be observed walking through every room; transferring on and off beds, chairs, and toilet; getting in and out of the bathtub or shower; reaching to obtain objects from kitchen and closet shelves; bending to retrieve objects from the ground or low heights such as coffee tables; and negotiating stairs. The institutional assessment of the environment is similar; activities usually not performed independently by the person, such as stair climbing or bathtub transferring, can be omitted. Environmental obstacles that interfere with safe mobility should be noted and modifications recommended.

After all evaluations are complete, a list of factors responsible for the person's falls can be constructed and interventions to prevent further falls designed. Follow-up should ensure that intervention strategies are effective and needed changes are made.

Fall Risk Assessment

The components of an assessment program for fall risk are shown in Figure 8-3. Although

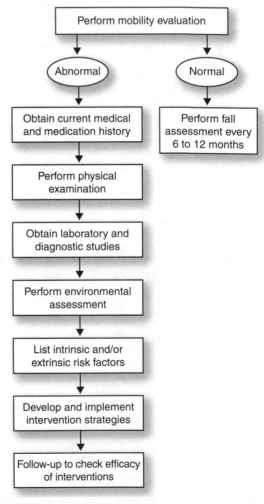

FIGURE 8-3 Fall risk assessment

these factors are easy to identify, their true risk is represented by their effects on an individual's mobility. Therefore, a mobility evaluation should be performed as a screening test. If it and the routine physical examination are normal, the person is probably not at elevated fall risk. In these individuals, the mobility evaluation should be repeated every 6 to 12 months. However, if an abnormality is detected, a complete fall evaluation should be performed and intervention planned to alleviate risk factors (Figure 8-4).

Interventions

Falls that occur in older people often have more than one etiology and require multiple intervention strategies. To be effective, interventions to reduce fall risk are based on assessment results (Tideiksaar, 1997b, 2002). Although it may not be practical to consider eliminating all falls, an interdisciplinary team-focused approach that concentrates on reducing fall risk is an achievable goal when caring for frail, elderly people. There are multiple comorbid conditions, as well as environmental factors, that contribute to fall risk, and when approached in a coordinated

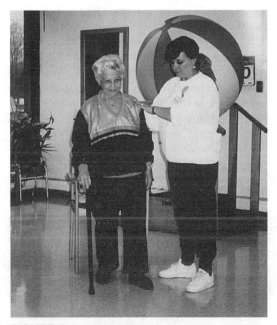

FIGURE 8-4 Careful assessment of balance and gait is important in designing falls prevention intervention (Courtesy of the Menorah Park Nursing Home, Cleveland, Ohio, with permission.)

manner, these conditions can be identified and interventions designed. Each member of the interdisciplinary team has a specific expertise that should be utilized when creating therapeutic approaches. In the end, it takes critical integration of all team members in a coordinated manner to reduce fall risk.

Medical Strategies

Because falls may be caused by underlying diseases, adverse medication effects, and resulting disabilities, all older people with falls should be referred to their primary care providers for evaluation. Diagnosing risk factors, such as visual disorders, cognitive impairment, postural hypotension, cardiovascular irregularities, discontinuing inappropriate or excessive medication and changing medication, managing existing chronic diseases, and referring the individual for treatment of gait, balance, and muscle impairments, are of great benefit in reducing fall risk. In addition, investigating and then treating osteoporosis by administering vitamin D, calcium supplementation, and bone-strengthening medications, and instituting weight-bearing exercises helps to reduce the risk of injurious falls.

Rehabilitative Strategies

Rehabilitative strategies include therapeutic exercise, wearing proper footwear, and utilizing appropriate ambulation devices to assist with mobility. Older people with impaired mobility resulting from medical disorders or deconditioning may benefit from a trial of exercises. Exercise programs can be grouped into two broad categories: general physical activity (e.g., walking, aerobic movements, and other endurance exercises) and specific physical activity (i.e., training geared specifically toward increasing balance and strength). To be effective, exercise needs to be tailored to the older individual's physical capabilities and needs (Figure 8-5). Although exercise has many proven benefits, the optimal type, duration, and intensity of exercise for falls prevention remains unclear. Tai Chi Chuan is a promising type of balance exercise which also helps to reduce fear of falling; its contribution to fall prevention requires further evaluation.

Paying attention to shoe type and fit is important, as it can either interfere with or

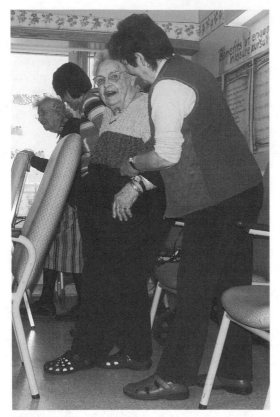

FIGURE 8-5 Participating in exercises designed to improve balance can be fun as well as therapeutic (Courtesy of the Geriatric Day Hospital, Specialized Geriatric Services, Saskatoon Health Region, Saskatoon, Saskatchewan, with permission.)

support safe gait and balance. Stability is improved with shoes that have a thin and firm sole, rather than footwear with thicker soles, such as sneakers or running shoes. For those individuals with gait and balance disorders, canes and walkers can be used to maintain or improve mobility. Ambulation devices, such as a cane or walker, increase the elder's standing and walking base of support and stability. The devices furnish proprioceptive feedback through the handle, and shift the load on weight-bearing joints (such as hips, knees, ankle, or foot) to the upper limb. Furthermore, devices provide the older person with a visual presence of support that can instill confidence during ambulation, and thereby may help to reduce fear of instability and falls.

Environmental Strategies

Extrinsic interventions consist of eliminating or modifying environmental conditions that interfere with safe mobility. For individuals residing in the community, health professionals can encourage elimination of such hazards as slippery floors, bathtub surfaces or rugs, and inadequate lighting. Checklists (Tideiksaar, 1986, 1987; United States Consumer Product Safety Commission, 1986) can serve as a guide in helping make homes safe. At the same time, people should be cautioned to avoid hazardous activities that may predispose them to falls, such as standing on chairs to reach objects from high shelves, walking across wet floors, or using stairways that are in ill repair or are poorly illuminated. This approach may not be effective, particularly for those people who have not fallen but are at risk.

Definitive studies that demonstrate the advantages of environmental modifications in reducing falls are lacking; nevertheless, conducting a safety assessment to identify unsafe activities and environments is a reasonable approach, particularly if targeted to specific functional impairments (e.g., bathroom grab bars for the elder with balance impairment).

Table 8-2 identifies environmental hazards and design features of furnishings and structures in both the home and the institutional setting that are most likely to be unsafe and addresses their modification (Tideiksaar, 1997b). A major point to consider when modifying the environment is whether the suggested adaptations are acceptable to the person. Compliance is enhanced if older people understand why the adaptation is being made; if the adaptation improves mobility and reduces falls and is at the same time in keeping with the aesthetic features of the environment; and if the adaptation is affordable and easy to obtain and apply.

Psychosocial Strategies

The problem of falls in older people is often associated with various psychosocial consequences. Foremost are the complications that accompany the fear of falling. Fear is an instinctive reaction to danger. Thus, older people with histories of falling tend to avoid situations they perceive as dangerous, recognize their physical limitations, and adjust their activities. In this sense, fear works to the person's advantage, functioning as a protective mechanism. However, fear of falling can work against the best interests of

TABLE 8-2 **Environmental Modifications to Reduce Risk of Falls**

Floors	1. Avoid polish or wet floors
	2. Use slip-resistant surfaces
	3. Add nonslip adhesive strips
	4. Use indoor–outdoor carpet
	5. Use slip-resistant floor wax
	6. Avoid thick or patterned carpet
	7. Use double-faced tape at carpet edges
Walls	Add grab bars, especially in bath, hall, stairs (round, 16 to 26 inches high, color contrasted to wall, 2 to 3 inches from wall)
Lighting	1. Increase intensity by two to three times, especially in baths and stairways
	2. Use three-way bulbs and rheostats
	3. Use full-spectrum, fluorescent light
	4. Add night lights and bedside lamps with secure bases
	5. Add easy-to-find switches (accessible, contrasting color, pressure sensitive)
	6. Use tinted windows, Mylar shades to reduce glare
	7. Add automatic turn-on timers
Tables	1. Avoid unsteady tables
	2. Avoid drop-leaf or pedestal styles
	3. Use nonslip tops
	4. Avoid low-lying, glass- and mirror-top tables
Shelves	1. Move frequently used items to middle shelves
	2. Use reachers
Bath	1. Use grab bars, securely fastened
	2. Use adjustable toilet seat, securely fastened, with vinyl with color contrast
	3. Use nonslip strips in tub or shower
	4. Install soap dispenser
	5. Add hand-held shower hose
Bed	1. Place at easiest transfer height
	2. If on wheels, lock and put on nonslip strips or immobilize legs
Stairs	1. Add rails, extended 12 inches beyond stairs and curved in at end
	2. Add nonslip adhesive
	3. Replace worn runners
	4. Mark edges
Chairs	1. Tailor height to person
	2. Feet should be firmly on floor; feet at 90 degrees; seat depth 15 to 18 inches
	3. Armrests should be 7 inches above seat
	4. Use sturdy chairs

an individual. Some older people become so frightened and preoccupied with fall avoidance that they limit activity unnecessarily. When they are asked what concerns them about falling, their common responses include a fear of not being able to get up by themselves and needing assistance, having prolonged long lie times, feeling embarrassed about falling in public places and displaying an image of frailty, and a fear that a fall will result in a hip fracture or placement in a nursing home (Tideiksaar, 1997b). If fear of falling is left untreated and unresolved, severe restriction of physical and social activities is likely to result, often with dire consequences.

People residing in the community may become increasingly immobile to the point of becoming house bound, eventually requiring long-term care. Hospitalized people may avoid discharge to their home and require nursing home placement, and in the nursing home, people may end up living their lives in a wheelchair or require excessive assistance.

Several terms have been coined to describe abnormal fear of falling: ptophobia (Bhala, O'Donnell, & Thoppil, 1982), fallaphobia (Tideiksaar, 1997b; Tideiksaar & Kay, 1986), and the 3-F syndrome—that is, fear of further falls (Overstall, 1983). Fear of falling is more common in persons who have a cluster of falls, increased post-fall or long lie time (Tideiksaar, 1997b), fall-related injury, or poor balance and gait, and persons who live alone. Fear of falling may be accompanied by panic attacks when attempting an activity that previously resulted in a fall. These attacks usually subside once the feared activity has either been accomplished successfully or abandoned. These persons display abnormal gait, typified by hesitancy and irregularity of steps when walking, usually the result of an underlying balance disturbance (Sudarsky & Tideiksaar, 1997). As a consequence, they ambulate by clutching or grabbing onto furniture or only attempt walking with the help of human assistance for support. They express great anxiety about their ability to walk safely.

The goal of treating fear of falling is to help these people regain confidence in their ability to achieve safe, independent mobility. This is accomplished by a multidisciplinary program that includes reducing identifiable fall risk factors, eliminating environmental hazards, education and counseling, and behavioral modification (Alexander, 1994; Sudarsky & Tideiksaar, 1997).

Behavioral modification to correct fear of falling is most successful if the approach is started early and fully explained. The approach involves progressively increasing involvement in the feared activity, with close supervision. The supervisor should ensure the person's physical safety and provide verbal reassurance to build confidence. The person should proceed at a pace that is comfortable and non–anxiety provoking. Clearly, the professional undertaking such an approach should have a good grasp of behavior-modification principles. As well, educating older individuals with fear of falling about falls and how they can reduce falls is important; Box 8-1 offers a cognitive and behavioral approach.

Caregiver Strategies

Family members and other caregivers who interact with an older person who is at risk for falling are likely to develop excessive physical and emotional burdens. Certain strategies are apt to be of equal benefit for older persons and their family caregivers. First, discuss in clear language the reasons for falling and why the elder is at risk for falling. Attempt to address the prognosis or anticipated course of the problem; whether it is expected to be of short or long duration; and the

various social and financial consequences that might arise. At the same time, allow all concerned parties to express their fears and concerns, and attempt to allay their apprehension. One method for accomplishing this is to discuss the plan for reducing the likelihood of further falls. This may consist of treating disease processes, modifying medications, and attempting rehabilitative and environmental interventions.

For those older people who live alone and who may not have family members or friends to help with daily mobility tasks, access to health services, shopping, and other errands, paid assistance either on a temporary or more permanent basis may help to alleviate fears. Similarly, for those older individuals with estranged family relationships, or those whose families cannot shoulder the responsibilities of caregiving, professional assistance should minimize mobility problems. Last, when appropriate, older people and their families need to be counseled about nursing home placement. Often, older adults are reluctant to accept residential care, and family members may experience guilt over "abandoning" a parent. Under these circumstances, discuss the benefits and risks involved in remaining at home, as opposed to entering a protective environment.

Educational Strategies

The lack of awareness about falls and fall risks by older people is a major risk factor. Consequently, the main purpose of fall preventive education for older people is to increase their awareness of falls, risk factors, and strategies to reduce risks. Education should focus on activities and behaviors aimed at risk reduction and health promotion, such as periodic medical visits; reporting all falls, near falls, and episodes of instability; a regular program of exercise; and home safety inspection and improvement. Orienting family caregivers as to what they can do to reduce the risk of falls is also beneficial. Educational materials should provide information on fall risk factors, fear of falling, risk mitigation strategies, and community resources. The information included in Box 8-1 can be used for this purpose.

Injury Reduction Strategies

Strategies aimed at injury reduction include hip protector garments, personal emergency

BOX 8-1 Cognitive and Behavioral Strategies Aimed at Reducing Fear of Falling

Cognitive Strategies

- Explain that falling is not a normal part of aging and that risk of falling can be reduced.
- Explain that falls can be due to certain medical problems, medications, and environmental hazards.
- Discuss possible home hazards and explain the need to correct any existing hazards (provide a home-hazard checklist that can be used by the individual or a family member to help identify fall hazards and to suggest corrective action).
- Explain that falls can be an early sign of illness that may require treatment and the importance of reporting all falling episodes.
- Explain that fear of falling is both a realistic and common fear.
- Discuss fear of falling and its impact on the quality of life.
- Explain the consequences of restricting mobility as a response to fear of falling.
- Explain the need to stay as active as possible, before and after a fall.
- Discuss the role of exercises aimed at improving neuromuscular performance (activities that improve strength, balance, and coordination can increase confidence and reduce the risk for fall-related injuries).
- Discuss the use of hip protectors to reduce fear of injury (and risk of hip fracture).
- Discuss the use of assistive ambulation devices and durable medical equipment to support safe balance and mobility.
- Discuss the need to wear sensible footwear.
- Discuss possible response to a fall emergency, including how to get up from a fall and acquiring a personal emergency response system (device designed to reduce the risk of down time on the floor following a fall; device also helps to reduce fear of downtime).

Behavioral Strategies

- Ask your doctor if you are at fall risk and why. Get regular physical exams even if you're feeling fine.
- Ask your doctor to suggest ways to decrease your risk for falling.
- Get regular physical exams even if you're feeling fine.
- Ask about the side effects of all medications you are taking. Do they affect your balance and coordination? Make sure your doctor knows about all the medications you're taking (prescription and over-the-counter) so you can prevent harmful combinations of drugs. Limit the amount of alcohol you drink.
- Report all falls and near falls or changes in balance to your doctor. He or she may want to evaluate you.
- Have your vision tested regularly. If you need glasses, use them. Wear sunglasses or a brimmed hat to cut down glare on sunny days.
- If you feel unsteady, use a cane or walker to help maintain balance. Be sure that assisted devices are fitted properly and you are trained to use them correctly.
- Avoid taking chances and putting yourself in high-risk situations. Minimize sudden movements, rushing, or quickly changing positions. You are more likely to fall when you are ill, tired, or emotionally upset.
- Watch where you walk. Look for uneven ground, rocks, or other obstructions that could cause you to trip.
- Be careful on wet and icy surfaces.
- Avoid carrying heavy loads. If you start to lose your balance, the weight will increase your chances of falling.
- Get up slowly from lying down and sitting.
- Wear sturdy walking shoes, avoiding backless shoes and strapless sandals. Wear low-heeled shoes with rubber soles.
- Make your home safe. For example, eliminate potential tripping hazards such as clutter and throw rugs, improve lighting, add nonslip floor surfaces, and install grab bars in bathrooms.
- Exercise regularly to keep muscles toned and joints flexible and bones strong. Try to include such activities as dancing, gardening, and stretching exercises to improve flexibility and balance. Weight-bearing activities, such as walking and going up steps, help to strengthen muscles and bones.
- It's important to talk to your doctor before starting any exercise program so you don't hurt yourself.

response systems (PERS), and fall alarms. Previously stated, more than 95% of hip fractures are caused by direct trauma against a hard surface following a fall. Hip protectors are designed to guard against hip fractures in the event of a fall. The principle of wearing a hip protector is to absorb the impact of a fall and reduce the risk of fracture by shunting the energy away from the hip region. Hip protectors are usually made of hard plastic pads or shields that are padded or constructed with foam-type materials. They fit into specially designed pockets in undergarments or pants. Hip protectors are highly effective in preventing hip fracture. The downside of hip protectors is noncompliance. Some older persons choose not to wear them for a variety of reasons, such as denial of injury risk, discomfort, and inconvenience, especially when toileting. Hip protectors are likely to be more acceptable to those individuals who are at risk for a second hip fracture.

For those people who live alone, the fear of not being able to get up from the floor following a fall can be especially traumatic. About 20% of falls experienced by community-dwelling elders result in lie times of 1 hour or more (Sattin, 1992). Personal emergency response systems are electronic devices designed to provide frail older persons with a means to summon assistance in the event of a fall, and thus prevent a lengthy lie time. They increase the older person's feelings of security and confidence as well as allay family fears regarding the safety of their loved one. Although PERS are generally well accepted, some elderly resist them because they find them inconvenient or difficult to operate, remind individuals of their frailty and dependency, or are too costly to purchase; consequently, nonadherence with PERS can be a problem. Adherence with PERS is more common in system users who obtain the system themselves (i.e., acceptance is less common in users who obtain the system at the request of a family member), had a history of recent falls, receives positive responses to alarm activations, uses an assistive mobility device, and receives instruction on the system (Levine & Tideiksaar, 1995).

Physical restraints (i.e., any appliance used to inhibit independent mobility by securing a person in a bed, chair, or wheelchair, including such devices as belts, sheets, harnesses, or bedrails) are sometimes used in hospitals and nursing homes to prevent falls. However, there is no scientific evidence that supports the use of physical restraints as a fall prevention strategy for older adults (Strumpf & Tomes, 1993; Tideiksaar, 2002). Although some care providers may believe that an older person is at less risk of falling and hurting himself or herself when wearing a restraint, the opposite is actually true. Individuals who are restrained are more likely to experience a fall than those who are not restrained (Tideiksaar, 2002). Restraints can also contribute to a host of untoward complications such as impaired circulation of legs and arms, breathing problems, skin abrasions, decubitus ulcers, and strangulation (Tideiksaar, 2002). In an attempt to guard against falls in older persons, restraint-free, fall alarms are sometimes used (Tideiksaar, 2002; Tideiksaar, Feiner, & Maby, 1993). The purpose of a fall alarm is to alert staff when an individual who is at risk for falls is rising from a bed or chair. The efficacy of a fall alarm is dependent on the response time of the nursing staff. Candidates for bed or chair alarms are older persons at risk for bed falls and restraint complications (Tideiksaar, 2002), including those with multiple bed or chair falls, those who need but do not ask for assistance in bed and chair transfers (e.g., individuals with dementia), and persons with congestive heart failure in whom restraints will interfere with physiological compensation to clear the lungs of fluid (i.e., sitting up from the supine position). Caution is advised in using fall alarms. Research about their effectiveness is conflicting (Tideiksaar, 1997b). The main objection is that they can cause false alarms (i.e., the alarm sounds when the person is not leaving the bed). Even when they sound appropriately, nurses on occasion feel that they don't have sufficient time to get to the patient; implementation requires adequate staffing to respond in a timely manner to the alarms.

Turning Evidence-Based Strategies into Best Practices

Randomized controlled trials provide the most reliable evidence of the efficacy of strategies aimed at preventing falls. Two studies provide the strongest evidence that interventions for older persons living in the community can prevent falls, especially if targeted at those who are the highest risk. Tinetti and colleagues (1994) conducted a randomized trial comparing the effectiveness of usual care and social visits with a multifactorial abatement strategy in reducing falls. Subjects included members of a health maintenance organization who were 70 years and over and had at least one risk factor. Subjects were visited at home and assessed by a nurse and physical therapist for the presence of risk factors (e.g., postural hypotension; psychotropic medications; more than three prescribed drugs; environmental hazards in the home; gait, balance, and transfer impairment; and leg or arm weakness. The intervention group received home-based gait, balance, and strength training exercises supervised by a physical therapist; a medication review by a nurse who discussed possible medication changes with subjects and their physicians; transfer skills training; and home modifications. The control group only received home visits by social work students; risk factors were not addressed. During follow-up, the intervention group experienced a 31% reduction in falls.

These findings are confirmed by Close and colleagues (1999) in another community-based study of elders who were at high risk for falls. Subjects were older patients at an accident and emergency department who had fallen. The intervention group had a comprehensive medical assessment by a geriatrician and a home visit by an occupational therapist, and a significant reduction in falls was experienced.

Because multiple risk factors are often involved in falls, a falls prevention program addressing more than one fall risk factor is more likely to be successful in reducing falls. Single strategies have not been found to be particularly effective in reducing falls. Even multiple interventions need to be targeted specifically to the needs of the older adult (American Geriatrics Society, British Geriatrics Society, and American Academy of Orthopedic Surgeons Panel on Falls Prevention, 2001; Feder, Cryer, Donovan, & Carter, 2000). The challenges to implementing evidence-based strategies under real-world conditions are many. Among the most problematic is a widespread lack of recognition that fall risk reduction is an ongoing process, one that is highly dependent upon structure (i.e., awareness by both health care providers and older people of why falls occur

and how to prevent falls) and process (i.e., identifying fall risk, implementing multidisciplinary risk reduction and health promotion activities, and evaluating outcomes of strategies). With an anticipatory system of risk management, the likelihood of reducing falls is greatly improved. As well, a better understanding of both fall risks and the sources of those risks, and enhanced risk identification and matching of interventions with need are realized. Educational programs for health care professionals to increase knowledge about falls in older persons and ways of promoting behavior changes can be extremely useful in increasing awareness. Clinical fall preventive guidelines (American Geriatrics Society et al., 2001; Feder et al., 2000) that translate research findings into clinically practical information, should be part of health care profession education.

The following steps in the process of care will enable health care professionals to develop the most effective approach to reducing falls.

Screening/Risk Assessment

Detecting a history of falls and performing a fall-related assessment are likely to reduce the future probability of falls when coupled with pertinent interventions. Lengthy fall risk assessments are time consuming. Consequently, a program of brief screening for lower-risk individuals and a more comprehensive and detailed assessment for those at fall risk is preferable. A stepwise approach to risk identification might include basic screening questions, such as asking older persons about recent falls and functional impairments (e.g., bathing, toileting, and transfer and walking ability), and observing their mobility (e.g., transfers, gait, and balance). Despite the presence of diseases or medications associated with fall risk, those individuals who have not fallen and have no functional impairments or mobility problems are at low fall risk. They should receive educational materials aimed at health promotion (i.e., disease and medication self-management; and how to maintain the current functional level, including home safety advice focused on common environmental hazards and modifications—"what's good for everyone!").

In contrast, those older persons who have fallen or who have functional impairments or mobility dysfunction are at significant fall risk and should receive a detailed risk assessment (e.g., identification of comorbid risk factors, modes of health care utilization and behaviors, fear of falling, social and caregiver situation). For those elders with functional impairments with or without altered mobility, a home safety evaluation focused on specific functional impairments and environmental problems can be of great benefit. The screening and assessment results should be provided to the older person's health care professionals. The patient and family should receive an explanation of specific risk factors and written recommendations of actions to take for every factor identified.

Care Planning

The plan of care should include the results of risk evaluation, findings from the home safety assessment, a prioritization of an older person's problems, and recommended actions specific to the elder's needs and goals. The patient and family should be involved in planning risk reduction and behavioral changes, ways of involving health care providers, plans for monitoring the older person's progress, and updates to the care plan as needed. The plan should also include ways of implementing home environmental modifications, medical interventions, possible use of assistive devices, and behavioral and educational programs. A given person may require multiple interventions or only single change. What really matters is that interventions should be targeted at modifiable risk factors and that the older person accepts the intervention.

Monitoring

Regardless of whether the older person has fallen, a telephone follow-up a month after intervention is useful to evaluate whether preventive strategies are working and acceptable to the elder. Thereafter, the older person should be contacted every quarter or more frequently depending on the extent of risk of falling. Follow-up "safety telephone calls" and "safety-grams" (i.e., providing the older person with fall prevention tips) encourage behaviors and activities aimed at reducing fall risk.

Post-Fall Assessment

Conducting an assessment for older persons who experience a fall is valuable to discover the cause of falls. The assessment should identify the circumstances of the fall (i.e., location of the fall, symptoms at the time of the fall, activity at the time of the fall, the time of the fall, any trauma resulting from the fall, and all previous falls). Inquiring about past falls and their circumstances is important because many older people experience "patterned falls" (i.e., multiple falls due to the same cause). Reassessment of fall risk factors, identification of gait and balance impairments, recording of changes in social supports and living situation, evaluation of caregiver status (i.e., willing and capable of providing care), and modification of the care plan as needed are other elements of the post-fall assessment.

Because primary care providers know their patients best, they should be involved in assessing and managing all falls experienced by older persons. However, for those "at-risk" elders (e.g., individuals with recurrent falls; multiple medical, psychological, functional, and social problems; gait and balance impairments; disabling fear of falling; and nonresponse to several attempts at intervention), specialty fall preventive clinics utilizing a multidisciplinary team can be very helpful.

■ Summary

Falls are an important health problem for older people, resulting in significant rates of mortality and morbidity. Most falls are not random "accidental" events but are the result of a cumulative effect of multiple intrinsic and extrinsic factors. Prevention requires a multifaceted and multidisciplinary approach aimed, first, at identifying and assessing older people who have sustained falls and are at fall risk and, second, at attempting realistic interventions focused on reducing fall risk factors.

Case Study

Glenda Landing is an 83-year-old woman who has experienced several noninjurious falls at home over the past 3 months. Her falls have taken place while walking to the bathroom, reaching up into her kitchen cabinets, getting in and out of her bathtub, and getting up from her toilet. After two of Ms. Landing's falls, she was unable to get up following falling and had to crawl on all fours to her living room, where she used the support of a chair to get up from the floor.

Medical History

Ms. Landing has a diagnosis of diabetes mellitus (treated with oral hypoglycemic medications), arthritis treated with high doses of nonsteroidal anti-inflammatory medications), frequent nighttime urination (approximately four to five trips every night), glaucoma and cataracts, and impaired hearing. Ms. Landing complains of a recent worsening of her hearing and occasional dizzy spells made worse with movement.

Psychological History

Ms. Landing is very fearful about falling. In particular, she is fearful of going outdoors by herself and fearful of environments and situations that may cause her to lose her balance and fall (e.g., walking at night, getting in and out of the bathtub, and moving to and from the toilet). She also expresses a fear that she will fall and be unable to get up, especially in her bathtub. As a result, she has restricted her activities. She does not leave her apartment by herself and no longer bathes in her tub. Ms. Landing complains of feeling depressed about her situation and not being able to go to church or visit with friends. Previously, Ms. Landing had been independent in her activities of

daily living, but now her falls have dramatically affected her feeling of safety.

Functional History

Ms. Landing exhibits both gait and balance impairments. She complains that her walking and balance are worse at night when she is going to the bathroom. Ms. Landing has a cane and two-wheeled walker, but she doesn't use either device. The cane does not help her balance, and the walker is difficult to use, particularly when she is walking outdoors, because its rear legs drag on the pavement, causing her to lose balance. Additionally, Ms. Landing has difficulty moving to and from her toilet and bathtub. She has no bathroom grab rails or other equipment to support her safe mobility.

Social History

Ms. Landing lives alone in a small, cluttered one-bedroom apartment. Before her falls, Ms. Landing enjoyed going to church on Sundays and visiting with friends who live in her apartment building. Ms. Landing has a 54-year-old married son who lives 10 miles away. Because of his busy job and family obligations, he is only able to visit with his mother once a week. During this time, he does his mother's grocery shopping and cleans her apartment. He is very worried about his mother's safety and is considering placing her in a nursing home.

Questions

1. What are Ms. Landing's risk factors for falling?
2. Based on her risk factors, what should Ms. Landing's plan of care include?

Review Questions

1. For what reasons might someone underreport falls? Why might they be overreported?
2. In what ways can environmental adaptations to the risk of falls be made more acceptable to the individual?
3. A client you are working with reports having fallen 2 weeks ago. How will you determine whether the individual is at risk of falling again?
4. Assuming that you determine the client's risk of falling is substantial, what strategies will you employ to help reduce the risk?
5. What are the potential negative outcomes if the individual falls again?

Web-Based Resources

For helpful information about functional performance in older adults, visit:

www.nice.org.uk/page.aspx?o=CG021, **The National Institute for Health and Clinical Excellence (NICE),** date connected March 28, 2007. NICE is an independent organization responsible for providing national guidance on promoting good health and preventing and treating ill health. The NICE clinical guideline on falls addresses older people who live in the community, either at home, in a retirement complex, or in a residential or nursing home.

www.stopfalls.org/international/index.shtml, **The Fall Prevention Center of Excellence,** date connected March 11, 2007. The center identifies best practices in fall prevention and helps communities offer fall prevention programs to older people who are at risk of falling. The international webpage provides links to global efforts to prevent falls.

www.premierinc.com/quality-safety/tools-services/safety/topics/falls/, **Premier, Inc.,** date connected April 10, 2007. Premier, Inc., develops resources for performance improvement. Fall prevention resources can be found on the following webpage, and within the webpage there are numerous links to other sources of information.

www.profane.eu.org/about/about.php, **The Prevention of Falls Network Europe (Profane),** date connected March 15, 2007. Profane brings together workers from around Europe to develop multifactorial prevention programs aimed at reducing the incidence of falls and fractures among older adults. Numerous resources are available in different languages.

www.americangeriatrics.org/products/positionpapers/Falls.pdf, **Guideline for the Prevention of Falls in Older Persons,** date connected March 20, 2007. This site is a link to the *Guideline for the Prevention of Falls in Older Persons* developed by the American Geriatrics Society, British Geriatrics Society, and American Academy of Orthopaedic Surgeons Panel on Falls Prevention and published in the *Journal of the American Geriatric Society* in 2001 (see References for complete reference).

REFERENCES

Alexander, N. B. (1994). Postural control in older adults. *Journal of the American Geriatrics Society, 42,* 93–108.

Alexander, N. B. (1996). Gait disorders in older adults. *Journal of the American Geriatrics Society, 44,* 434–451.

American Geriatrics Society, British Geriatrics Society, and American Academy of Orthopedic Surgeons Panel on Falls Prevention. (2001). Guideline for the prevention of falls in older persons. *Journal of the American Geriatrics Society, 49,* 664–672.

Baker, S. P., Ginsburg, M. J., & O'Neill, B. (1992). *The injury fact book* (2nd ed). New York: Oxford University Press.

Bhala, R. P., O'Donnell, J., & Thoppil, E. (1982). Phobic fear of falling and its clinical management. *Physical Therapy, 62,* 187–190.

Birge, S. J., Morrow-Howell, N., & Proctor, E. K. (1994). Hip fracture. *Clinics in Geriatric Medicine, 10*(4), 589–609.

Campbell, A. J., Spears, G. F., & Borrie, M. J. (1990). Examination by logistic regression modelling of the variables which increase the relative risk of elderly women falling compared to elderly men. *Journal of Clinical Epidemiology, 43*(2), 1415–1420.

Carter, S. E., Campbell, E. M., Sanson-Fisher, R. W., Redmen, S., & Gillespie, W. J. (1997). Environmental hazards in the homes of older people. *Age & Ageing, 26*, 195–202.

Chang, K. P., Center, J. R., Nguyen, T. V., & Eisman, J. A. (2004). Incidence of hip and other osteoporotic fractures in elderly men and women. *Journal of Bone and Mineral Research, 19*(4), 532–536.

Close, J., Ellis, M., Hooper, R., Glucksman, E., Jackson, S., & Swift, C. (1999). Prevention of falls in the elderly trial (PROFET): A randomized controlled trial. *Lancet, 353*, 93–97.

Cummings, S. R., Black, D. M., Nevitt, M. C., Browner, W. S., Cauley, J. A., Genant, H. K., et al. (1990). Appendicular bone density and age predict hip fracture in women: The study of osteoporotic fractures research group. *Journal of the American Medical Association, 263*(5), 665–668.

Cwikel, J., Fried, V., & Galinsky, D. (1990). Falls and psychosocial factors among community-dwelling elderly people: A review and integration of findings from Israel. *Public Health Reviews, 17*(1), 39–50.

Davis, A. E. (1995). Hip fractures in the elderly: Surveillance methods and injury control. *Journal of Nursing Trauma, 2*(1), 15–21.

Downton, J. (1998). Falls. In R. C. Tallis, H. M. Fillit, & J. C. Brocklehurst (Eds.), *Brocklehurst's textbook of geriatric medicine and gerontology* (5th ed., pp. 1359–1370). London: Churchill Livingstone.

Dunn, J. E., Rudberg, M. A., Furner, S. E., & Cassel, C. K. (1992). Mortality, disability, and falls in older persons: The role of underlying disease and disability. *American Journal of Public Health, 82*, 395–400.

Feder, G., Cryer, C., Donovan, S., & Carter, Y. (2000). Guidelines for the prevention of falls in people over 65. The Guidelines' Development Group. *British Medical Journal, 321*(7267), 1007–1011.

Felson, D. T., Anderson, J. J., Hannan, M. T., Milton, R. C., Wilson, P. W., & Kiel, D. P. (1989). Impaired vision and hip fracture: The Framingham study. *Journal of the American Geriatrics Society, 37*, 495–500.

Fife, D. (1987). Injuries and deaths among elderly persons. *American Journal of Epidemiology 126*, 936–941.

Fisher, E. S., Baron, J. A., Malenka, D. J., Barrett, J. A., Kniffin, W. D., Whaley, F. S., et al. (1991). Hip fracture mortality in New England. *Epidemiology, 2*(2), 116–122.

Fuller, G. F. (2000). Falls in the elderly. *American Family Physician, 61*(7), 2159–2168, 2173–2174.

Griffin, M. R., Ray, W. A., Fought, R. L., & Melton, L. J. (1992). Black–white differences in fracture rates. *American Journal of Epidemiology, 136*(11), 1378–1385.

Hanlon, J. T., Cutson, T., & Ruby, C. M. (1996). Drug-related falls in older adults. *Topics in Geriatric Rehabilitation, 11*(3), 38–54.

Kanis, J. A., Johnell, O., De Laet, C., Jonsson, B., Oden, A., & Ogelsby, A. K. (2002). International variations in hip fracture probabilities: Implications for risk assessment.

Journal of Bone and Mineral Research, 17(7), 1237–1244.

King, M. B., & Tinetti, M. E. (1995). Falls in community-dwelling older persons. *Journal of the American Geriatrics Society, 43*, 1146–1154.

Levine, D. A., & Tideiksaar, R. (1995). Personal emergency response systems: Factors associated with use among older persons. *Mount Sinai Journal of Medicine, 62*(4), 293–297.

Lipsitz, L. A. (1991). Cardiovascular risk factors for falls in older persons. In R. Weindruch, E. Hadley, & M. G. Ory (Eds.), *Reducing frailty and falls in older persons* (pp. 67–75). Springfield, IL: Charles C Thomas.

Lord, S. R., Clark, R. D., & Webster, I. W. (1991). Physiological factors associated with falls in an elderly population. *Journal of the American Geriatrics Society, 39*, 1194–2000.

Magaziner, J., Simonsick, E. M., Kashner, T. M., Hebel, J. R., & Kenzora, J. E. (1990). Predictors of future recovery one year following hospital discharge for hip fracture: A prospective study. *Journal of Gerontology, 45*, M101–M107.

Mathias, S., Nayak, U. S., & Isaacs, B. (1986). Balance in elderly patients: The "Get-Up and Go" test. *Archives of Physical Medicine & Rehabilitation, 67*, 387–389.

Nevitt, M. C. (1997). Falls in the elderly: Risk factors and prevention. In J. C. Madseu., L. Sudarsky, & L. Wolfson (Eds.), *Gait disorders of aging: Falls and therapeutic strategies* (pp. 13–36). New York: Lippincott-Raven.

Nevitt, M. C., Cummings, S. R., & The Study of Osteoporotic Fractures Study Group. (1993). Type of fall and risk of hip and wrist fractures: The study of osteoporotic fractures. *Journal of the American Geriatrics Society, 41*, 1226–1234.

Northridge, M. E., Nevitt, M. C., Kelsey, J. L., & Link, B. (1995). Home hazards and falls in the elderly: The role of health and functional status. *American Journal of Public Health, 85*, 509–515.

Norton, R., Campbell, A. J., Lee-Joe, T., Robinson, E., & Butler, M. (1997). Circumstances of falls resulting in hip fracture among older people. *Journal of the American Geriatrics Society, 45*, 1108–1112.

O'Loughlin, J. L., Robitaille, Y., Boivin, J. F., & Suissa, S. (1993). Incidence of and risk factors for falls and injurious falls among community-dwelling elderly. *American Journal of Epidemiology, 137*(3), 342–354.

Overstall, P. W. (1983). Determining the causes of falls in the elderly. *Geriatric Medicine Today, 2*, 63.

Pinto, M. R., De Medici, S., Zlotnicki, A., Bianchi, A., Van Sant, C., & Napoli, C. (1997). Reduced visual acuity in elderly people: The role of ergonomics and gerontechnology. *Age & Ageing, 26*, 339–344.

Richardson, J. K., & Hurvitz, E. A. (1995). Peripheral neuropathy: A true risk factor for falls. *Journal of Gerontology, 50A*, M211–M215.

Rubenstein, L. Z., & Josephson, K. R. (1992). Causes and prevention of falls in elderly people. In B. Vellas, M. Toupet, L. Rubenstein, J. L. Albarede, & Y. Christen (Eds.), *Falls, balance and gait disorders in the elderly* (pp. 21–38). Paris: Elsevier.

Rubenstein, L. Z., & Josephson, K. R. (2002). The epidemiology of falls and syncope. *Clinics in Geriatric Medicine, 18,* 141–158.

Rubenstein, L. Z., & Powers, C. (1999). *Falls and mobility problems: Potential quality indicators and literature review (the ACOVE project)* (pp. 1–40). Santa Monica, CA: Rand Corporation.

Rubenstein, L. Z., Robbins, A. S., Josephson, K. R., Schulman, B. L., & Osterweil, D. (1990). The value of assessing falls in an elderly population: A randomized clinical trial. *Annals of Internal Medicine, 113,* 308–316.

Sartoretti, C., Sartoretti-Schefer, S., Ruckert, R., & Buchmann, P. (1997). Comorbid conditions in old patients with femur fractures. *Journal of Trauma, 43*(4), 570–577.

Sattin, R. W. (1992). Falls among older persons: A public health perspective. *Annual Review of Public Health, 13,* 489–508.

Schwartz, A. V., Kelsey, J. L., Maggi, S., Tuttleman, M., Ho, S. C., Jonsson, P. V., et al. (1999). International variation in the incidence of hip fractures: Cross-national project on osteoporosis for the World Health Organization Program for Research on Aging. *Osteoporosis International, 9*(3), 242–253.

Stevens, J. (2002). Falls among older adults: Public health impact and preventive strategies. *Generations, 26*(4), 7.

Strumpf, N. E., & Tomes, N. (1993). Restraining the troublesome patient. A historical perspective on a contemporary debate. *Nursing History Review, 1,* 3–24.

Sudarsky, L., & Tideiksaar, R. (1997). The cautious gait, fear of falling, and psychogenic gait disorders. In J. C. Masdeu, L. Sudarsky, & L. Wolfson (Eds.), *Gait disorders of aging: Falls and therapeutic strategies* (pp. 283–295). New York: Lippincott-Raven.

Thapa, P. B., Gideon, P., Fought, R. L., & Ray, W. A. (1995). Psychotropic drugs and risk of recurrent falls in ambulatory nursing home residents. *American Journal of Epidemiology, 142,* 202–211.

Tideiksaar, R. (1986). Preventing falls: Home hazard checklists to help older patients protect themselves. *Geriatrics, 41,* 26–28.

Tideiksaar, R. (1987). Fall prevention in the home. *Topics in Geriatric Rehabilitation, 3,* 57–64.

Tideiksaar, R. (1997a). Environmental factors in the prevention of falls. In J. C. Masdeu, L. Sudarsky, & L. Wolfson (Eds.), *Gait disorders of aging: Falls and therapeutic strategies* (pp. 395–412). New York: Lippincott-Raven.

Tideiksaar, R. (1997b). *Falling in old age: Its prevention and treatment* (2nd ed.). New York: Springer.

Tideiksaar, R. (2002). *Falls in older persons: Prevention and management* (3rd ed.). Baltimore, MD: Health Professions Press.

Tideiksaar, R. (1998). Disturbances of gait, balance, and the vestibular system. In R. C. Tallis, H. M. Fillit, & J. C. Brocklehurst (Eds.), *Brocklehurst's textbook of geriatric medicine and gerontology* (5th ed., pp. 595–609). London: Churchill Livingstone.

Tideiksaar, R., Feiner, C. F., & Maby, J. (1993). Falls prevention: The efficacy of a bed alarm system in an acute-care setting. *Mount Sinai Journal of Medicine, 60,* 522–527.

Tideiksaar, R., & Kay, A. D. (1986). What causes falls? A logical diagnostic procedure. *Geriatrics, 41,* 32–50.

Tinetti, M. E. (1986). A performance-oriented assessment of mobility problems in elderly patients. *Journal of the American Geriatrics Society, 34,* 119–126.

Tinetti, M. E., Baker, D. I., McAvay, G., Claus, E. B., Garrett, P., Gottschalk, M., et al. (1994). A multifactorial intervention to reduce the risk of falling among elderly people living in the community. *New England Journal of Medicine, 331,* 821–827.

United States Consumer Product Safety Commission (USCPC). (1986). *Home safety checklist for older consumers.* Washington, DC: USCPC.

CHAPTER 9

Dementia

Susan Doble

I knew something was wrong when my ability to read slowed drastically. The final straw was when I couldn't memorize a brief anecdote from Reader's Digest. What should have been memorized in six minutes took me 45 minutes spread over three days. . . . I recognized the likelihood of Alzheimer Disease. . . . I find it necessary to dwell on what I am still able to do, rather than focus on what I have lost. I work hard to enjoy my somewhat limited abilities and take pleasure in my accomplishments.

Norma's Story,
Dementia Advocacy and Support Network (DANS)
(www.dasninternational.org/2005/norma.php)

OBJECTIVES

By the end of the chapter, readers will be able to:

1. Appreciate how our understanding of dementia and specific dementing conditions has changed over time.
2. Describe the impact of dementia on individuals, families, and society.
3. Describe unique features of common dementing conditions such as Alzheimer's disease, vascular dementia, dementia with Lewy bodies, frontotemporal dementia, and Parkinson's disease dementia.
4. Describe the dementia diagnosis process.
5. Identify how dementia is typically staged.
6. Appreciate how the traditional conceptualization of occupational and social functioning has influenced assessment and management approaches.
7. Define occupational and social functioning from a broader perspective than that of independent performance of activities of daily living.
8. Identify how the assessment of occupational and social functioning contributes to the diagnosis of dementia, the evaluation of the effectiveness of interventions, the design of therapeutic environments, and the development of strategies to support the occupational performance of persons with dementia.

continued on page 216

OBJECTIVES (continued)

9. Describe the role of the family in supporting the occupational and social functioning of persons with dementia.
10. Identify strategies that can be used to support the occupational and social functioning of persons with dementia.

Have you ever forgotten to pick up a specific item at the grocery store, experienced difficulty locating your house keys, or had trouble recalling an acquaintance's name? Such lapses in memory are common, particularly when we are busy and stressed. However, increasingly you will hear individuals, albeit sometimes jokingly, attribute such lapses to dementia or Alzheimer's disease (AD). These comments not only provide an indication of society's increased awareness of dementia as a medical condition, but they also highlight the many misconceptions about dementia that continue to exist. Dementia is *not* an inevitable part of normal aging. Memory loss is *not* always the first sign of dementia. Dementia is *not* always a progressive condition. Many forms of dementia *do* respond to treatment.

The purpose of this chapter is to provide health professionals with a better understanding of dementia, and how it is experienced in the context of the different conditions in which it arises. As a health care provider, it is critical that you be able to provide clients and their families with accurate information about dementia. Without this, they may delay or avoid seeking medical attention and adopt ineffective coping strategies that compromise the health and well-being both of those with dementia, and those providing care. This chapter is also designed to challenge health professionals to consider how persons with dementia can be supported to continue to participate in meaningful occupations and, thus, experience greater quality of life.

Defining Dementia

Dementia can be broadly defined as a deterioration in cognitive functioning that renders a person unable to meet the diverse intellectual demands of everyday life (American Psychiatric Association [APA], 2000). Dementia is "an

acquired, persistent impairment in multiple areas of intellectual function not due to delirium" (Mendez & Cummings, 2003, p. 4). Some forms of dementia are progressive, but others may plateau or be static. In some cases, onset may be insidious, as is typically the case in AD, but in other cases, onset of dementia may be acute, particularly if it occurs following head trauma or stroke. Although most dementias are the result of structural brain changes, infections and metabolic causes can be successfully addressed. As we delve into the area of dementia and the increasingly expanding area of dementia research, we are confronted with a myriad of terms and diagnostic criteria. In order to appreciate and recognize how our understanding and conceptualization of dementia and conditions that result in dementia have changed over time, it is important to gain some historical perspective.

Until the 1970s, it was generally assumed that cognitive changes were an inevitable part of the aging process, even though AD had been identified as a distinct clinical and pathological entity as early as 1907. Cognitive impairments of the elderly were termed "senility," but as interest and research into the concept of dementia increased, senility was transformed from an expected stage of life into a "disease" (Fox, Kelly, & Tobin, 1999). That is, dementia was no longer viewed as a part of "normal" aging but was identified as a behavioral syndrome. At the same time, efforts were made to differentiate AD from dementias that had a vascular basis (Blessed, Tomlinson, & Roth, 1968; Tomlinson, Blessed, & Roth, 1970). The idea that vascular dementia was related to chronic ischemia (i.e., atherosclerosis) was abandoned, and the importance of infarction was highlighted (Miller Fisher, 1968). Thus, the term "multiinfarct dementia" (Hachinski, Lassen, & Marshall, 1974) became more widespread. As the proportion of elderly adults in the population increased and average life spans were extended, the efforts of interest groups, as well as federal government initiatives, led to greater recognition of AD and "cerebrovascular disease as a cause of dementia was eclipsed" (Bowler & Hachinski, 2003, p. 1).

A consequence of the increased recognition of the prevalence and public health consequences of AD was an "Alzheimerization" of the concept of dementia. That is, the clinical case definition of dementia came to be based on the cognitive changes that typify AD, specifically, memory impairment. Today, this is reflected in the diagnostic criteria defined within the APA's *Diagnostic and Statistical Manual-IV (DSM-IV-TR)* (APA, 2000), in which the first and foremost symptom of dementia is defined as memory loss, even though individuals to be diagnosed with dementia must also demonstrate other cognitive impairments (i.e., aphasia, agnosia, apraxia, or a disturbance of executive function) and a decline in occupational or social functioning (APA, 2000). For vascular dementia (VaD), the criteria are virtually the same with the exception that their presence can be attributed to cerebral vascular disease.

Nevertheless, across the spectrum of disorders that can give rise to dementia, persons may present with a wide array of symptoms. Even though some areas of the brain are affected in their structure and function, other areas are spared. It is the resulting retention of specific cognitive abilities contrasted with the deterioration of others that gives rise to the identifiable patterns of cognitive impairments commonly associated with specific dementia syndromes, including not only AD and VaD, but also dementia with Lewy bodies (DLB), frontotemporal dementia (FTD), and Parkinson's disease dementia (PDD). However, in some instances, this pattern of cognitive impairment is best considered a clinical syndrome that reflects the regional onset of a disease process rather than a specific underlying neuropathological condition, per se (McMonagle, Deering, Berliner, & Kertesz, 2006). Furthermore, we need to keep in mind that although dementia is typically viewed as a disorder of cognition, not all symptoms of dementia are related to cognition (Lopez et al., 2003). In some dementia syndromes, behavioral symptoms (e.g., changes in mood, manifestations of agitation, and psychotic symptoms) may, in fact, precede any clinical evidence of changes in cognition.

This chapter will challenge the natural desire to simplify the concept of dementia to a single entity that is clearly defined by changes in neurological structures. It is important that we appreciate that dementia is a clinical diagnosis (Hogan, 2006) and, as such, is socially constructed (Whitehouse, 2006). Thus, we must recognize that our understanding of the causes and consequences of dementia will continue to change over time. As consensus diagnostic criteria have become more established and symptomatic treatments have become available, attention has now turned to early detection of dementia. Although concepts such as "age-associated memory impairment," "aging-related cognitive decline," and "mild cognitive impairment" (MCI) (Petersen et al., 1999) have been developed to identify those in the early stages of AD, these terms have been used and applied inconsistently. Mild cognitive problems may be conceptualized as part of the normal aging process or as part of an early or "prodromal" dementia (Davis & Rockwood, 2004). However, it is also true that individuals with MCI may not develop AD, that they may get better, or that all of the above are true (Fisk, Merry, & Rockwood, 2003; Ganguli, Dodge, Shen, & DeKosky, 2004; Geslani, Tierney, Herrmann, & Szalai, 2005; Morris, 2006).

Many questions remain unanswered despite the rapid growth in our scientific, medical, and sociological understanding of dementia. In 2003, Mendez and Cummings observed "at least 20 scientific papers a week are published on Alzheimer's disease (AD) alone, with a rapidly rising number on other dementing diseases" (p. xi). By now, this number is likely a significant underestimate. The scientific and medical issues being examined include the development of standard nomenclatures and clinical criteria for dementia, and the search for biological markers, modifiable risk factors, neuroimaging indicators of disease processes, and pharmacological interventions. Increased attention is also being paid to the experience of dementia from affected persons' own perspectives; the effects of dementia on family relations and social interactions; caregivers' experiences; and the effectiveness of education, support, and behavioral interventions at both individual and societal levels. Our efforts to differentiate dementia syndromes will ultimately be shaped by our understanding of epidemiology and biological processes, as well as our understanding of the impact on individuals' abilities to function within society. It is measurement of the latter on which our ability to measure treatment effectiveness and cost-effectiveness hinges.

Impact of Dementia

Dementia has been described as "a health care problem of epidemic proportions" (Mendez & Cummings, 2003, p. 2). Though uncommon among those younger than 60 years of age, the risks of developing dementia increase considerably with age. At least 7% of the world's population (4% to 12% of persons over the age of 65, and nearly half of those over 85) experience some form of dementia (Canadian Study of Health and Aging [CSHA], 1994a; Evans, Scherr, Smith, Albert, & Funkenstein, 1990; Henderson, 1990; Katzman, 1993). In industrialized countries such as those in North America and Western Europe where life spans are longer, the prevalence of dementia among the elderly is closer to 8% to 10% (Anderson et al., 1999; Breteler, Claus, van Duijn, Launer, & Hoffman, 1992; General Accounting Office Report, 1998). Moreover, it has been suggested that prevalence rates rise even more when very mild forms of dementia are considered (Fillenbaum et al., 1998). It has also been suggested that prevalence rates will continue to rise as life span is extended and as the proportion of the world's population that is elderly increases. Ferri and colleagues (2005) estimated that 24.3 million persons worldwide have dementia. This number, however, will double every 20 years such that by 2020 there will be 42 million, and by 2040, there will be 81.1 million persons in the world living with dementia. These estimates take into consideration findings of previous studies that have indicated that age-specific prevalence is not uniform, and that prevalence rates are not the same across the world. For example, the prevalence of dementia in sub-Saharan Africa (Hendrie et al., 1995) is much lower than in developed countries. Despite the lower prevalence rates in developing countries, about 60% of those with dementia live in developing countries (e.g., India, China, South Asian, and Western Pacific nations). By 2040, it is expected that 71% of those with dementia will live in developing countries.

Much effort is being directed toward delaying the onset of dementia and slowing its progression as well as preventing dementias, particularly those related to vascular changes in which the potential risk factors are more readily evident. The need for preventative strategies is clear. It has been suggested that if the mean age of onset of AD could be increased by even 5 years, the numbers of persons with AD in the population could be reduced by 50% by the year 2050 (Brookmeyer, Gray, & Kawas, 1998).

We may place our hopes on the fruits of future research developments, but the current reality is that individuals with dementia and their families continue to experience considerable stresses and losses. Depending on the type of dementia with which an individual has been diagnosed, different patterns of cognitive and behavioral deficits will be manifest. Regardless of how these changes are manifested, individuals will experience deterioration in their day-to-day functioning. Initially, some of the changes in behavior and function may not be apparent to their family, coworkers, friends, or even to the individuals themselves. However, as dementia progresses, the individuals' abilities to engage in meaningful occupations will diminish, and deficits will become increasingly apparent. Confronted with progressive changes in the ability to perform what previously may have been considered either particularly important tasks or relatively simple tasks, individuals will have varied emotional and behavioral reactions. Feelings of incompetence, frustration, and loss of control are not uncommon. These, in turn, will affect their interactions and relationships with others. Over time, safety will become an increasing concern, not only in relation to those with dementia (e.g., when cooking at a stove or when using power tools), but also in relation to others (e.g., when driving). Also, as dementia progresses, individuals will require increasing amounts of assistance, support, or supervision and become increasingly dependent on others for both physical care and emotional support. The need to adapt how things are done, simplify tasks, or give up meaningful tasks and valued roles poses significant adjustment challenges, particularly for persons who may also lack insight into their condition. Regardless of the specific diagnosis, individuals at the end stages of dementia tend to have a similar presentation;

that is, they are no longer able to communicate effectively, they are disoriented, and they may no longer recognize family and friends. However, the paths that they take to reach this end stage may vary dramatically.

Over time, family members (spouses, adult children, and other relatives) and friends may assume the role of unpaid informal caregiver. In addition to providing care and support, most caregivers have a number of other major responsibilities at home, work, and in the community. In a study of 1500 family caregivers, Ory, Hoffman, Yee, Tennstedt, and Schulz (1999) found that caregivers of persons with dementia spend significantly more time per week providing care than do caregivers of persons without dementia. It is important to recognize that the challenge of balancing these multiple roles can lead to stress that, in turn, may affect caregivers' own health, and physical, emotional, and social well-being (Bookwala, Yee, & Schulz, 2000; Light, Niederehe, & Lebowitz, 1994; Ory et al., 1999; Schulz, O'Brien, Bookwala, & Fleissner, 1995). In most cases, the caregiving role will be maintained in some way even when persons with dementia move to long-term care facilities (Hertzberg, Ekman, & Alexsson, 2001; Keefe & Fancey, 2000). When caregivers decide to move the person with dementia to a nursing home, the following are the most common reasons that caregivers cite:

- The need for the person with dementia to receive more skilled care
- A deterioriation in the caregivers' health
- Evidence of dementia-related behaviors in persons with dementia, specifically those related to behavior dysregulation and psychotic symptoms (Buhr, Kuchibhatla, & Clipp, 2006)

In many cases, caregiving also affects individuals' current and future financial well-being. Many family caregivers reduce their work hours, take extended leaves, or withdraw from the workforce completely to perform their caregiver responsibilities. Thus, the loss of income potential for those caring for family members with dementia is a significant financial burden. Although the majority of those with dementia may be retired by the time they are diagnosed, this is not always the case, and their loss of income is also a major problem, especially for younger persons with dementia. If and when caregivers determine that care in the home is no longer feasible, persons with dementia may be relocated to institutional care settings such as nursing homes. Even though such a move may reduce caregivers' physical and emotional stress, the economic costs of paying for or subsidizing costly institutionalized care are heightened. The societal costs of dementia are difficult to estimate because of the various perspectives that can be adopted in any such analyses (e.g., direct economic costs to government for subsidized nursing home care versus indirect societal costs that include reduced workplace productivity of caregivers). Regardless of the perspective taken, or the type of dementia considered, the costs are clearly substantial (Hux et al., 1998; Leon, Cheng, & Neumann, 1998; Ostbye & Cross, 1994; Rockwood, Brown, & Fisk, 2003).

Common Types of Dementia

Alzheimer's Disease

As described above, Alzheimer's disease (AD) is the most prevalent form of progressive dementia. Using the *DSM-IV-TR* diagnostic criteria (APA, 2000), AD is diagnosed when individuals demonstrate insidious onset of the hallmark feature of impaired memory (episodic and recent), as well as deficits in at least one other cognitive domain (i.e., aphasia, agnosia, apraxia, or executive dysfunction). In contrast, research criteria developed by the National Institutes of Neurologic and Communicative Disorders and Stroke and the AD and Related Disorders Associated Work Group (NINCDS-ADRDA) (McKhann et al., 1984) stipulate that for a diagnosis of dementia, individuals must demonstrate a decline in three or more of the following spheres of cognition:

- Memory
- Language
- Perception (especially visuospatial)
- Praxis
- Calculations
- Conceptual or semantic knowledge
- Executive functions
- Personality or social behavior
- Emotional awareness or expression

Memory impairment is not a "required" symptom for a diagnosis of dementia based on the NINCDS-ADRDA criteria. The NINCDS-ADRDA criteria also differentiate "clinically probable" AD from "possible AD." For a diagnosis of clinically probable AD to be applied, there must be evidence of impairment in any two areas of cognition (i.e., memory, language, visuospatial perception or constructions, calculations, praxis, and executive functions); the cognitive deficits must be sufficient to affect individuals' everyday activities; there must be no evidence of delirium; and there must be no evidence of other dementing diseases. When the temporal profile is atypical, when there is a systemic or brain disorder but it is not thought to be a cause of the dementia, or when there is a progressive deficit in only one cognitive domain, a diagnosis of "possible AD" is used. These criteria were developed not only to aid in clinical diagnoses, but also to help researchers studying AD to more accurately identify appropriate persons for their study groups. Importantly, when the NINCDS-ADRDA criteria (McKhann et al., 1984) are used, memory impairment may not be a primary presenting symptom. Instead, AD may be diagnosed when impairments in language, visual perceptual or constructional abilities, calculations, praxis, and executive functions are more prominent.

Although it is commonly believed that a diagnosis of AD can only be established at autopsy, there is no pathological "gold standard" for AD. Instead, a variety of pathological criteria exist. Nevertheless, in most settings, a diagnosis of AD can be confirmed at autopsy using published guidelines developed by the National Institute on Aging and the Reagan Institute Working Groups on Diagnostic Criteria for the Neuropathological Assessment of Alzheimer's Disease (1997). The two main criteria for a pathological diagnosis of AD include (1) a Consortium to Establish a Registry for Alzheimer's Disease (CERAD) "frequent" neuritic plaque score (Khacaturian, 1985; Mirra et al., 1991; Newell, Human, Growdon, & Hedley-Whyte, 1999) such that the number of neurofibrillary tangles and neuritic plaques, particularly in the cerebral cortex, is greater than what would be expected given the individual's age, and (2) evidence of Braak and Braak (1991) stage V or VI changes (i.e., evidence of extensive neurofibrillary tangles and neuropil threads in virtually all areas of the hippocampal formation). Despite some consensus on the use of these neuropathological markers, there remains debate as to whether amyloid plaques or neurofibrillary tangles are the cause of AD or merely the result of another, more basic process. Neurotransmitter deficits, primarily in the cholinergic system but also in noradrenergic and serotonergic systems, are also evident in AD.

The cause of AD remains unknown. The predominant risk factor is increasing age, with differential rates for diagnosis depending on gender (female) (Fratiglioni et al., 1997; Heyman, Peterson, Fillenbaum, & Pieper, 1996), ethnicity (African American) (Heyman et al., 1991), and positive family history (Amaducci, Falcini, & Lippi, 1992; Graves et al., 1990; Mendez et al., 1992). Serious head injury with a loss of consciousness has been found to increase the risk of a subsequent diagnosis of AD (Guo et al., 2000; Lye & Shores, 2000; Plassman et al., 2000). Genetic factors (including the presence of trisomy 21, presenilin 1 located on chromosome 14, presenilin 2 located on chromosome 1, amyloid precursor protein [APP] located on chromosome 21, and the E4 allele of the apolipoprotein [ApoE] gene on chromosome 19) have also been found to contribute to the development of AD (Brugge, Nichols, & Salmon, 1994; Dal Forno et al., 2002; Goldstein et al., 2001; Heyman et al., 1996; Kennedy et al., 1995; Levy-Lahad, Lahad, Wijsman, Bird, & Schellenberg, 1995; van Duijn et al., 1994). No strong evidence has been found to date to support potentially remediable factors such as the treatment of systolic hypertension, prescription of ASA (aspirin) and statin drugs, and consumption of fish, omega 3 fatty acids, and moderate wine consumption. Recently, a large randomized controlled trial provided some evidence that the use of estrogens alone or with progestins by perimenopausal or postmenopausal women increases the risk of a subsequent diagnosis of AD (Shumaker et al., 2004).

Vascular Dementia

Vascular dementia (VaD), as noted above, is a dementia syndrome that is a result of cerebral vascular damage, although the clinical case criteria have generally been similar to AD. Several different consensus criteria have been used to diagnose VaD but all suffer poor sensitivity at the cost of high specificity (i.e., they do not detect all cases of VaD). These consensus criteria include

- The National Institute of Neurologic Disorders and Stroke and the Association Internationale pour la Recherche et l'Enseignement en Neurosciences (NINDS-AIREN) criteria (Roman et al., 1993)
- The Hachinski Ischemic Score (HIS) (Hachinski et al., 1975)
- Those found in the *DSM-IV*
- The Alzheimer Disease Diagnostic and Treatment Centers (ADDTC; Chiu, Victoroff, Margolin, Jagust, Shankle, & Katzman, 1992) criteria
- The International Classification of Diseases, 10th Revision (ICD-10; World Health Organization, 1989)
- The *DSM-IV-TR* criteria (APA, 2000)

One problem common to most of the case definitions comes from the use of AD as a framework on which they are based (Bowler, 2000). For example, the *DSM-IV-TR* criteria (APA, 2000) for VaD are simply the same as the diagnostic criteria for AD with the addition of evidence of a temporally related cerebral vascular event (e.g., stroke). Although there is evidence that AD and VaD are separate diseases (Roman & Royall, 2004) with different clinical presentations (Erkinjuntii et al., 2000; McKhann et al., 1984), different neuropathological bases (Braak & Braak, 1991; Munoz, 2003), and different risk factor profiles (Klages, Fisk, & Rockwood, 2005), it is also the case that a person can have both AD and VaD, or what is commonly referred to as "mixed" dementia (Rockwood et al., 2000).

More recently, our understanding of cerebral vascular disease as a cause of dementia has been undergoing a conceptual change. In particular, this has meant the emergence of the concept of vascular cognitive impairment (VCI) as a diagnosis reflecting cognitive changes that can be attributed to vascular changes, most often due to cerebral vascular insufficiency, but that do not meet the criteria for dementia. Although VCI may progress and result in vascular dementia (VaD), if detected and its underlying causes treated, VaD may be prevented. This reinforces the importance of VCI as a construct, because, as with MCI and AD, recognition of VCI may allow for early diagnosis and intervention to avoid progression of cognitive impairment to dementia.

VCI and VaD can occur following a single strategically placed brain infarct, large or small, or may be the cumulative effect of numerous discrete, smaller, and often subcortical lesions, as is the case for the subtype of VaD referred to as subcortical ischemic vascular dementia (SIVD) (Erkinjuntti et al., 2000). Even though there is much debate as to what vascular changes and what severity of change are necessary to cause cognitive impairment, specific changes to white matter and lacunar infarcts (Chui, 2001) and hippocampal formation atrophy possibly due to hippocampal sclerosis (Vinters et al., 2000) are indications of cerebrovascular disease that can give rise to dementia.

The pattern of cognitive deficits and the nature of the course of cognitive decline will vary depending on subtype of VCI, reflecting the number, size, and location of infarction. However, the hallmark cognitive impairment for both VCI and VaD is a dysexecutive syndrome (Desmond et al., 1999). This means that individuals demonstrate particular impairments in attention, working memory, planning, sequencing, abstraction, and speed of mental processing rather than memory, per se (Desmond et al., 1999; Wolfe, Linn, Babikian, Knoefel, & Albert, 1990). As a result, individuals with VaD are more likely than those with AD to demonstrate perseverative behaviors (Lamar et al., 1997) and to have difficulties with verbal fluency on neuropsychological tests (Desmond et al.).

VaD accounts for between 10% and 30% of all dementias (Canadian Study of Health and Aging Working Group [CSHA], 1994a; Fratiglioni et al., 2000; Traykov et al., 1999). Epidemiological studies have suggested a variety of risk factors for VaD including advancing age, male gender, known history of strokes, and other vascular risk factors such as hypertension (Gorelick, 1997; Hébert & Brayne, 1995; Klages et al., 2005; Kokmen, Whisnant, O'Fallon, Chu, & Beard, 1996; Nyenhuis & Gorelick, 1998; Rockwood, Ebly, Hachinski, & Hogan, 1997; Skoog, 1998).

Dementia with Lewy Bodies

Demenita with Lewy bodies (DBL) is so named because of the presence of Lewy bodies in the brain. Lewy bodies, round neurofilament inclusion bodies that contain damaged nerve cells deposits, are the pathological hallmark of this disorder (Drach, Steinmetz, Wach, & Bohl, 1997). In addition to Lewy bodies, individuals diagnosed with DBL typically have amyloid pathology and senile plaques similar to those with AD. DBL represents another neurodegenerative dementia with core features that include (a) parkinsonism—that is, an extrapyramidal movement disorder characterized by rigidity and bradykinesia; (b) cognitive fluctuations with prominent deficits in attention; and (c) recurrent, well-formed, and detailed visual hallucinations (McKeith et al., 2005). Although prominent or persistent memory impairment is not necessarily evident in the early stages of DBL, it typically becomes apparent as the disorder progresses. Deficits on tests of attention, visuospatial ability, and executive function may be more prominent. Clinical diagnosis is strengthened if there are repeated falls, nonvisual hallucinations, delusions, syncope or transient losses of consciousness, and hypersensitivity to neuroleptics.

The population prevalence of DBL is not well established, but it is claimed by some to be the second or third most frequent cause of dementia after AD and vascular dementia, and accounts for about 14% to 20% of those with dementia (Drach et al., 1997; McKeith, O'Brien, & Ballard, 1999). Males are twice as likely to be diagnosed with DBL and are, most often, over the age of 65 years when diagnosed (Barber, Panikkar, & McKeith, 2001).

Frontotemporal Dementia

Frontotemporal dementia (FTD) is part of a heterogeneous group of frontal lobe dementias that in addition to FTD includes more focal conditions such as primary progressive aphasia, semantic aphasia, and frontal dementia with motor neuron disease. FTD is the most common neurodegenerative dementia syndrome after AD and DLB. Although the age of onset can vary widely, the average age of onset of FTD is 57 years with a typical range of 51 to 63 years (Pasquier & Delacourte, 1998). FTD typically has an insidious onset with slow progression. Gradual but prominent changes in personality, behavioral disturbances, and changes in social awareness are typically the early and most obvious impairments in FTD (Kertesz, Davidson, & Fox, 1997; Neary et al., 1998). Those with FTD may manifest lack of social tact, fail to demonstrate acceptable manners, violate others' interpersonal space, or touch others inappropriately. Emotional blunting may also be an early indication of FTD, with affected individuals demonstrating a lack of sympathy, empathy, emotional warmth, and awareness of the needs of others. Because they can fail to demonstrate basic emotions such as happiness, sadness, fear, and anger, they may be judged by others as emotionally shallow and indifferent. Individuals with FTD may be inactive and apathetic and demonstrate a loss of initiative, spontaneity, and interest. Neglect or loss of interest in maintaining personal hygiene (i.e., no longer washing, bathing, grooming, or dressing appropriately) can also be an indication of FTD. In contrast, some individuals may show signs of disinhibition and may display an inability to regulate their own behaviors. This may be manifest by hyper-oral or other eating behavior changes; unrestrained expression of sexual feelings; disinhibited verbal or physical acts; overt sexual comments; or compulsive-like, stereotypical, or repetitive behaviors. In contrast, other features may include prominent disturbances of speech and language.

In keeping with a frontal "dysexecutive" syndrome, persons with FTD often experience loss of insight and demonstrate difficulties in abstract thinking, planning, and problem solving (Kertesz et al., 1997; Neary et al., 1998). Although memory is impaired in persons with FTD, this is often a reflection of inefficient and inconsistent use of active strategies for learning and retrieval. Thus, despite impaired free recall, their cued recall and recognition tend to be better than that of persons with AD (Glosser, Gallo, Clark, & Grossman, 2002; Nestor, Graham, Bozeat, Simons, & Hodges, 2002; Pasquier, Grymonprez, Lebert, & Van der Linden, 2001).

Parkinson's Disease with Dementia

Although Parkinson's disease (PD) is typically thought of as a disorder of movement, a significant number of those diagnosed with PD will develop Parkinson's disease with dementia (PDD). The development of dementia in persons with PD is often very slow and insidious but, if present, usually becomes apparent about 10 years after the initial diagnosis of PD (Mendez & Cummings, 2003). This is in contrast to DLB in which the cognitive impairment typically precedes the onset of significant movement disorder.

Other than the time sequence in which symptoms appear, there are no distinguishing clinical features that can discriminate PDD and DLB at any one given point in time (Noe et al., 2004). Both present a pattern of cognitive deficits reflecting disruption of cortical–subcortical circuitry (Darvesh & Freedman, 1996). Cognitive changes in PDD include slowed performance on tests of psychomotor speed, problems with tasks that place demands on attention, and difficulties initiating activities (Peavy et al., 2001; Sawamoto, Honda, Hanakawa, Fukuyama, & Shibasaki, 2002). Other changes include deterioration on tasks of delayed recall, semantic knowledge, frontal-executive functions, speech and language, and visuospatial functions (Freeman et al., 2000; Portin, Laatu, Revonsuo, & Rinne, 2000; Zakzanis & Freedman, 1999). Persons with PDD develop problems with specific aspects of memory (i.e., short-term memory, effortful memory, incidental learning, retrieval of information, temporal ordering of learned information, and procedural memory) (Ivory, Knight, Longmore, & Caradoc-Davies, 1999; Kuzis et al., 1999). Changes in executive functioning are also evident. These include deficits in planning, set-shifting, response initiation, and the organization of retrieval for memory; deterioration in abstraction, concept formation, cognitive flexibility, categorization accuracy, and in developing successful approaches to problem solving; and markedly reduced rates of information processing and failure to initiate activities spontaneously. Visuospatial abilities and visual integration are also impaired. Speech production can also be affected.

Diagnosing Dementia

Dementia has been described as a "diagnostic challenge" (Mendez & Cummings, 2003, p. 6) and as a "difficult and time consuming" process (Rockwood & MacKnight, 2001, p. 9). That said, careful clinical examination and history-taking are usually sufficient to diagnose the most common types of dementia.

Because AD is the most common type of dementia, a concern about memory is what most often brings individuals to the attention of their physicians. Thus, the first step in the diagnostic process is to determine if an individual with a memory complaint actually has memory impairment (Rockwood & MacKnight, 2001). Any health professional attempting to establish a diagnosis of dementia, including family physicians, must take a careful patient history that includes a review of the individual's education and work history as well as their medical history and current symptoms. Follow-up studies have shown that when an individual's subjective complaints are not confirmed by either objective assessment findings or by family members' reports, depression or anxiety are more likely to be the cause (Jorm et al., 1997). Thus, efforts must be made to clarify important features of the presenting complaint so that other potential contributing factors such as depression and anxiety as well as delirium (Lipowski, 1989) or medication-induced problems can be ruled out as possible causes of the complaints. It is, however, important to recognize that symptoms of depression and dementia may have a shared pathophysiology, and that depression among those with mild dementia is common (Visser, Verhey, Ponds, Kester, & Jolles, 2000). Both AD and VCI in the early stages can be difficult to dissociate from each other and from changes that can occur with normal aging, but as described above, it is important to remember that memory complaints are not always the first indication of dementia.

Once the presence of memory impairment is established, the next step is to determine which type of memory impairment is present. Memory, however, is not a uniform construct. Two main distinctions are made between **short-term or immediate memory** and **long-term or delayed memory.** Short-term or immediate memory refers to the process whereby someone holds an idea in his or her mind for a brief period of time (30 seconds to a few minutes), often through active rehearsal. This active rehearsal is also involved in working memory, the process whereby someone holds information in mind for a brief period of time, manipulates it in some way, and then responds with an answer. In contrast, long-term or delayed memory can be thought of as including both **declarative (explicit) memory** (i.e., explicit memory that requires conscious effort and thought such as when remembering facts) and **procedural (nondeclarative) memory** (i.e., implicit memory in which skills or knowledge are obtained by observation or activity without conscious thought). **Declarative or explicit memory** can also be divided into the concepts of semantic and episodic memory. **Semantic memory** is involved in the recollection of facts or information, whereas **episodic memory** is involved in the autobiographical memory of our past (Lezak, Howieson, & Loring, 2004). In general, the successful use of declarative episodic memory involves taking in information, encoding it, retrieving it later, and expressing a response. Difficulty with any of those steps will result in memory impairment.

In addition to assessing memory, however, it is essential to determine what, if any, other cognitive impairments are present, how these impairments affect the person's everyday life, and if any behavioral problems are evident. The goal at this stage is to determine if a diagnosis of AD can be confirmed or if a different diagnosis can be made. Neuropsychological evaluations, designed to directly assess a person's cognitive abilities through the presentation of standardized questions and tasks, as well as neuroimaging studies, both can provide valuable information that will assist in the establishment of a differential diagnosis (Hentschel, Kreis, Damian, Krumm, & Frölich, 2005). Regardless of the underlying pathological process, an accurate and early diagnosis increases the likelihood that individuals will be able to access appropriate pharmacological treatment, which may prolong individuals' time at stages of higher levels of cognitive functioning and may maintain quality of life.

Staging

Our understanding of the progression of dementia is largely based on the natural history of AD (i.e., untreated AD). Left untreated, most persons with AD move through characteristic stages of disease progression that include a presymptomatic stage, an early symptomatic stage with evidence of some changes to cognition or affect, and then symptomatic mild, moderate, and severe stages (APA, 2000; Auer & Reisberg, 1997; Cohen-Mansfield et al., 1996; Reisberg, 1988). This staged progression has been substantiated in several longitudinal studies (e.g., Carswell & Eastwood, 1993; Galasko

et al., 1995; Green, Mohs, Schmeidler, Aryan, & Davis, 1993; Sclan & Reisberg, 1992; Stern, Hesdorffer, Sano, & Mayeux, 1990) as well as cross-sectional studies (e.g., Baum, Edwards, Morrow-Howell, 1993; Gélinas, Gauthier, McIntyre, & Gauthier, 1999). It is important to recognize that these stages generally reflect changes in individuals' occupational and social functioning. As such, staging can provide a context for defining realistic expectations when developing intervention strategies. However, it is also important to recognize that disease progression is not uniform, and that rates of decline may vary widely between individuals. Some individuals may experience slow deterioration over a period of 20 years or more, and others may experience rapid progression in as little as a 1-year time period despite the fact that the duration from onset of symptoms to death is usually 8 to 10 years (Hébert et al., 1995; Mann, Mohr, Gearing, & Chase, 1992).

Reisberg (1988) has described the pattern of decline experienced by those with AD in the Functional Assessment Staging (FAST) scale that is composed of seven stages. These stages correspond to the seven stages of cognitive and global deterioration described by Reisberg and colleagues (1988) in the Global Deterioration Scale (GDS).

Stage 1

Stage 1 represents no decrement in the functioning of normal adults.

Stage 2

As normal adults age, they begin to experience some subjective deficits in word-finding or recalling the location of objects.

Stage 3

Stage 3 is compatible with incipient AD. Individuals begin to note difficulties in demanding work settings, forget appointments, and may experience difficulty finding their way in unfamiliar environments. In the early stages of AD, individuals will typically experience difficulties maintaining their attention and remembering new information and may occasionally experience confusion and disorientation. They may go to great efforts to disguise or conceal any difficulties they experience by blaming others for misunderstandings; repeating things that have already been said; and dismissing forgotten tasks, appointments, or deadlines as being unimportant. If one listens carefully to their conversations, it will be evident that descriptions of situations or events provided by those with AD often lack detail and informational content. Word-finding difficulties may be evident. Unable to recall an individual's name, persons with dementia may instead refer to others as "she" or "he." Similarly, objects may be referred to as "that thing" or "thingamajig." Others may consider that their decisions reflect questionable judgment. Despite these difficulties, however, most individuals in the early stages of AD are still able to manage the activities that constitute their everyday lives. Thus, they can still care for themselves; independently perform instrumental activities of daily living (IADL) such as shopping, preparing meals, and cleaning the house; and if working, continue to carry out work-related tasks even though they may be done with greater effort and less efficiency and accuracy (Figure 9-1).

Stage 4

By the time individuals reach Stage 4, they will require assistance with performance areas reflecting more complex community or domestic tasks, such as handling finances or shopping. Impairments in orientation and memory become more pronounced. Affected individuals repeat stories more often and ask others the same questions repeatedly. When engaged in conversations with others, they experience difficulty staying on topic. Language difficulties in the form of impaired comprehension and word-finding difficulties will become more evident. Tasks will be performed with even less efficiency and even greater effort.

Stage 5

By Stage 5 (moderate AD), individuals are no longer able to live alone safely. Although still able to dress, their ability to select appropriate attire will become compromised. Moreover, their ability to perform simple over-learned tasks is adversely affected.

Although individuals' underlying motor abilities are not affected in the earlier stages of AD, by the later stages, changes in tone, reaction time, movement time, and gait may be evident (Franssen, Kluger, Torossian, & Reisberg, 1993;

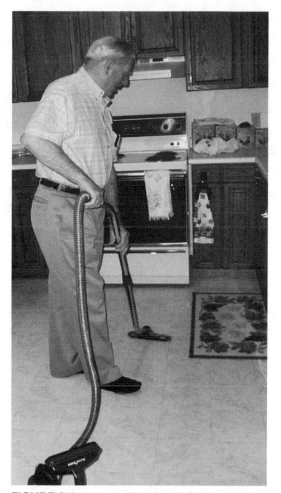

FIGURE 9-1 In the early stages of AD, most individuals are still able to perform familiar tasks such as vacuuming the floor.

Förstl et al., 1992; Funkenstein et al., 1993; Gordon & Carson, 1990; Kishka, Mandir, Ghika, & Growdon, 1993; Mahurin & Pirozzolo, 1993).

Stage 6

By Stage 6 (moderately severe AD), individuals will require assistance to perform even the most basic personal activities of daily living, such as dressing, eating, and the mechanics of toileting (e.g., wiping, flushing). Urinary and fecal incontinence begins at the end of Stage 6.

Stage 7

Individuals with severe dementia (Stage 7) generally demonstrate incoherent speech; disorientation for time, place, and person; failure to recognize close relatives; incontinence of urine and feces; and complete dependence on others for basic personal care. Regardless of whether dementia is due to AD, VaD, DBL, or PDD, individuals in the late stages require similar levels of assistance for self-care tasks such as dressing, grooming, and feeding.

It remains important to remember that the presentation and progression of non-AD dementias differ. For example, some studies have suggested that the rate of functional decline in those with VaD is slower than in those with AD (Black et al., 2003; Nyenhuis, Gorelick, Freels, & Garron, 2002; Wilkinson et al., 2003), although Rockwood, Wallack, and Tallis (2003) have suggested that the high costs of early-stage VCI reflected significant functional impairment in individuals with VCI and relatively mild cognitive impairment. At this point in time, our understanding of the rate and pattern of functional decline in non-AD dementias remains limited.

Thus, we still have much to learn about patterns of functional change (and changes in performance patterns) across different types of dementia. The context for understanding dementia is shifting dramatically now that pharmacological treatments are more widely available. However, current pharmacological treatments for dementia are symptomatic and do not reverse the disease process. Instead, if effective, they simply change the pattern of cognitive, behavioral, and functional deficits and lead to new "treated stages" of AD (Rockwood et al., 2003).

Defining and Measuring the Impact on Occupational and Social Functioning

As noted earlier, the APA (2000) diagnostic criteria for dementia requires that an individual demonstrate a "decline" in occupational or social functioning that can be attributed to changes in his or her cognitive abilities. However, our ability to clearly define occupational and social functioning and to articulate how these constructs can be operationalized and measured in clinical and research settings has been limited.

To a large extent, occupational and social functioning has been operationalized simply as the independent performance of activities of daily living (ADL) to the point that for some, these concepts have become synonymous. This conceptualization of occupational and social functioning has been reinforced by society's view that costly institutional and paid professional care should be avoided whenever possible. Thus, effort has been made to reduce the demands of caregiving or, as it is often referred to, caregiver burden. Caregiver burden has been found to increase when persons with dementia require greater levels of assistance to perform instrumental activities of daily living (IADL) (e.g., telephone use, meal preparation, housecleaning, money management, shopping) and personal activities of daily living (PADL) (e.g., feeding, dressing, toileting, grooming, bathing). Thus, attention has been directed more toward "independent" performance of IADL and PADL.

This simplistic conceptualization of occupational and social functioning, however, severely restricts our understanding of dementia, as well as our ability to support individuals with dementia. First, even though the ability to perform PADL and IADL is important, individuals need to engage in a variety of occupations that will provide them with opportunities to experience feelings of achievement, pleasure, rejuvenation, and social connection. Second, persons, for reasons of both personal preference and differences in performance skills, neither need nor want to do the same things as others. Instead, individuals perform different jobs, assume different roles, and engage in different recreational activities. Third, occupations vary in difficulty and complexity such that the demands that different occupations place on individuals' skills and underlying capacities vary considerably. As a result, even though two individuals may experience the same level of cognitive impairment, the impact of that impairment on their everyday lives can be markedly different. Although subtle changes in cognition may seriously disrupt one person's ability to function, those same changes may have little impact in the life of another.

The complexity of occupational roles has led some researchers to erroneously conclude that occupational and social functioning, as a construct, is "imprecise and not quantifiable" (Mendez & Cummings, 2003, p. 6) and, therefore, cannot be assessed in a standardized manner. Others have argued that this complexity makes it too difficult to apply the diagnostic criterion of impaired occupational and social functioning "in a uniform, meaningful way" (Evans et al., 1989, p. 2553). Consequently, clinical judgments about individuals' occupational and social functioning are often made on the basis of their neuropsychological and cognitive test scores. Although a relation between occupational and cognitive functioning has been demonstrated (Carswell & Eastwood, 1993; Doble, Fisk, MacPherson, Fisher, & Rockwood, 1997; Gélinas et al., 1999; Hershey, Jaffe, Greenough, & Yang, 1987; Reed, Jagust, & Seab, 1989; Robinson & Fisher, 1996; Teri, Borson, Kiyak, & Hamagishi, 1989), the strength of the relation varies considerably depending on the range of disease severity demonstrated by subjects, and the specific assessments used to evaluate both occupational functioning and cognitive functioning. Moreover, changes in cognition alone may not account for changes in individuals' occupational functioning. Other potential contributing factors to the specific pattern of functional loss experienced by individuals include changes in individuals' physical health status, perceptual abilities, behavior and motivation, as well as the availability of appropriate environmental supports (Borell, 1996; Doble et al., 1997; Josephsson, 1996; Josephsson, Bäckman, Borell, Bernspång, & Nygård, 1993).

Our inability to provide clear operational definitions of occupational and social functioning has affected our understanding of dementia. For example, prevalence estimates of dementia generated in different studies have varied considerably depending on how occupational and social functioning was operationalized. Evans and colleagues (1989) estimated the prevalence of dementia to be 10.3%, but the prevalence estimate for dementia obtained by the Canadian Study of Health and Aging (CSHA; 1994a), another population-based study, was considerably lower at 5.1%. Although a more general term of "functional impairment" was used in the CSHA in place of "occupational and social functioning," functional impairment was defined according to whether individuals were judged by a proxy to need assistance to do PADL and IADL. When Larrea, Fisk, Graham, and Stadnyk (2000) reexamined the CSHA data, they found that the prevalence of dementia was greater and similar to that found by Evans et al.

(1989) when estimates were based on impaired neuropsychological test performance only and not by a clinical consensus that considered "functional impairment." However, when proxy-report data from section H of the Cambridge Mental Disorder Examination (Roth et al., 1986) were combined with these neuropsychological test scores, the prevalence estimates were closer to those based on the CSHA clinical consensus opinions.

There are, no doubt, many challenges facing us as we try to determine how to best assess individuals' occupational and social functioning. However, some of the confusion may be reduced if we focus on the reasons *why* individuals' occupational and social functioning should be assessed. In the next section, the role of assessment of occupational and social functioning will be discussed in relation to four key issues:

- Supporting a diagnosis of dementia
- Evaluating the effectiveness of interventions
- Designing therapeutic environments
- Supporting the occupational performance of persons with dementia

Role of Assessment of Occupational and Social Functioning

Supporting a Diagnosis of Dementia

As noted earlier, the APA (2004) diagnostic criteria for dementia require that an individual demonstrate a "decline" in occupational or social functioning that can be attributed to changes in their cognitive abilities. The most effective way to determine if these criteria have been met is to adopt an individualized approach to assessment that incorporates the use of the dementia-specific assessments and the use of clinical judgment.

Given the heterogeneity of individuals' occupational and social lives, the first step is to identify an individual's occupational performance baseline. The insidious nature of many dementias means, however, that no single time frame can be used for all persons when determining a baseline. That said, it is essential to elicit specific information about the individual's premorbid levels of occupational and social functioning from the individual and other relevant informants. This means finding out what the individual needed and was expected to do given his or her roles within the home, at work, in the community, within social organizations, and as a family member and friend. Second, health professionals must determine what the individual is currently doing so that a comparison can be made between premorbid and current levels of occupational and social functioning. It is important to remember that a change in an individual's occupational and social functioning is not, however, an independent criterion for a diagnosis of dementia. Changes in occupational and social functioning may be related to changes in cognition, but they may also be related to medical conditions other than dementia (e.g., arthritis, depression) or even developmental role changes. For example, an individual may be adjusting to the loss of the work role after retirement or the loss of an occupational partner after the death of a spouse or friend. In addition, at the first sign of difficulty, family members whose tolerance for risk is limited may impose restrictions on what an individual is "allowed" to do. In such situations, judgments about an individual's occupational and social functioning that are based on what they are currently doing may overrepresent their level of disability. More often than not, changes in an individual's occupational and social functioning are related to a variety of factors. Thus, the use of clear and well-directed questions and observations, in conjunction with sound clinical reasoning and judgment, will help health professionals determine the impact that cognitive changes are having on an individual's occupational and social functioning. Dementia-specific assessments including the Alzheimer's Disease Cooperative Study ADL scale (Galasko et al., 1997), the Alzheimer's Disease Functional Assessment and Change scale (Mohs et al., 2001), the Bristol Activities of Daily Living Scale (Bucks, Ashworth, Wilcock, & Seigfried, 1996), the Disability Assessment for Dementia (DAD) scale (Gélinas et al., 1999), the Interview for Deterioration in Daily living activities in dementia (Teunisse, Derix, & van Crevel, 1991), and the Nurses Observation Scale for Geriatric patients (Spiegel et al., 1991) may prove valuable in the diagnostic phase. The DAD, for example, can be used to determine whether an individual demonstrates patterns of occupational performance characteristic of AD or of other dementias that reflect frontal–subcortical

system dysfunction (i.e., difficulty effectively initiating, planning, and organizing occupational performances).

The utility of these assessments for persons with other types of dementia, however, is questionable. Moreover, the DAD, like many other assessments, relies on informants' reports, which are inherently biased. In a study where a clinician's ratings of the overall level of ADL functioning of subjects with AD were compared with the proxy-reports of family caregivers, 46% of the caregivers overestimated their family members' ADL functioning (Doble, Fisk, & Rockwood, 1999). This overestimation was more likely to occur when family informants rated the ADL functioning of persons with mild cognitive impairment. Of the measures generated using standardized observational assessments, only 23% were discordant with the clinician ratings, and overestimation was as frequent as underestimation. Thus, the observational measures were more concordant, but of equal importance was their lack of systematic bias.

An alternative assessment approach to patient or informant report is to directly observe individuals' occupational performance. This can be done using informal observational approaches that have clinical application at the level of the individual patient, but this does not provide quantifiable data that allow for comparisons across individuals or across time. In contrast, standardized observational assessments, such as the Assessment of Motor and Process Skills (AMPS) (Fisher, 2006), provide health professionals with an opportunity to observe and measure an individual's skilled performance. In the case of the AMPS, this is done for a sampling of two or three PADL and IADL that are familiar and personally relevant to the individual. Although not designed specifically for persons with dementia, specific patterns of motor and process skill strengths and deficits have been identified using the AMPS (Figure 9-2). When 341 persons with AD and 287 nondisabled control subjects were assessed using the AMPS, Cooke, Fisher, Mayberry, and Oakley (2000) found that in comparison to the nondisabled control subjects, the AD sample demonstrated specific difficulties in many of the skills measured by the AMPS but also in some areas in which skill was relatively less affected. Box 9-1 shows those skills. One unfortunate limitation of Cooke and colleagues' study was that the authors did

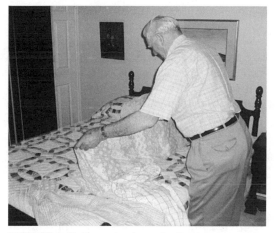

FIGURE 9-2 Example of standardized tasks used in the Assessment of Motor and Process Skills (AMPS).

not report the AD subjects' stages of dementia. It is likely that different patterns of occupational performance skill strengths and deficits will be evident across the different stages of AD. Nevertheless, this preliminary research suggested that patterns of skill strengths and deficits can be documented by observational measures of task performance, and with further research, these may help support the diagnosis process.

Evaluating the Effectiveness of Interventions

With the development of symptomatic pharmacological interventions for dementia, such as

---

> ### BOX 9-1   **ADL Process Skill Challenges**
>
> - *Heeding* the goal of the task
> - *Choosing* appropriate tools and materials
> - *Inquiring* when they need information
> - *Benefiting* from cues to prevent problems from recurring
>
> *Relative ADL Process Skill Strengths*
> - *Handling* and *using* tools and materials appropriately
> - *Navigating* obstacles within the task environment
> - *Gathering* tools and materials into their workspaces
> - *Organizing* their workspaces in a logical manner

---

cholinesterase inhibitors (ChEIs), the need for valid, reliable, and responsive assessments of occupational and social functioning has become more evident. Common disease milestones that provide potential endpoints for clinical trials include the emergence of cognitive symptoms, conversion from amnestic MCI to a diagnosis of dementia, emergence of behavioral and psychological symptoms of dementia, the decision that institutional care is required, and death (Gauthier & MacKnight, 2006). However, changes in individuals' occupational and social functioning can also serve as meaningful clinical endpoints.

As noted earlier, the challenges of dealing with the individualized nature of occupational and social functioning has led to these potential outcomes being largely ignored. Thus, our ability to evaluate the effect of interventions, both pharmacological and nonpharmacological, on the occupational and social functioning of persons with dementia has been constrained by our inability to clearly define and measure these constructs.

The focus of most assessments that rely on patient or informant reports is the independent performance of tasks within broadly defined categories of PADL and IADL, such as meal preparation and grooming. However, because no clear definition is provided as to what constitutes, for example, "meal preparation," the responses for different individuals or for the same individual over different periods of time may preclude meaningful comparisons. Efforts have been made to identify items that are applicable to a broad cross section of the population, but some items will not be relevant to some individuals, particularly when individuals may have never performed particular PADL or IADL. As Gauthier noted (2006), it is important that scales be designed so that there is some nonarbitrary means, other than denoting the item as "missing," for dealing with activities that may not be performed by individuals or may have never been a part of an individual's pattern of occupational performance.

In evidence-based reviews on the measurement of IADL and PADL in dementia, it has been argued that dementia-specific assessments should be used as outcomes in intervention studies (Gélinas & Auer, 2001; Gauthier et al., 1999; Lehnfeld & Erzigkeit, 2000; Lindeboom, Vermeulen, Holman, & DeHaan, 2003) such as those described in the previous section of this chapter. The assumption made when using such scales, however, is that if change is detected in any of the items making up these scales, that change can be attributed to a change in individuals' underlying cognitive abilities. Moreover, because many of these assessments utilize simple nominal rating criteria such as "independence/dependence" or "presence/ absence," they may prove to be insensitive to subtle changes in the quality of individuals' performances, such as in the effort required or the efficiency of actions used when performing occupations.

Furthermore, by limiting the focus of assessment to PADL and IADL, we ignore the ability of persons with dementia to engage in other types of occupations that may provide them with opportunities to experience achievement, pleasure, rejuvenation, and social connection. Even if standardized assessments of the ability of persons with dementia to participate in other occupations cannot be identified, other approaches to evaluation, such as **goal-attainment scaling (GAS)** can provide valid, reliable, and responsive measures. When using GAS, persons with dementia and their caregivers are provided with the opportunity to identify meaningful functional endpoints for improvement and worsening from their own personal perspectives. In an intervention study conducted by Rockwood, Graham, and Fay (2002), these GAS endpoints, identified by persons with dementia and their caregivers, reflected their own unique occupational lives and histories, and most importantly, those things that had personal meaning to them. For example, one individual identified his goal as being able to find his way safely to the corner store on most days. The advantage of the GAS approach is that these individualized endpoints can, nonetheless, be combined to provide quantifiable outcomes that can be compared across treatment groups (Kiresuk, Lund, & Larsen, 1982).

As noted earlier, most assessments used as outcome measures in intervention studies rely on proxy-reports of family members and caregivers rather than performance-based assessments completed by trained observers. One of the main reasons for researchers' reliance on proxy-reports is their desire to use assessments that are quickly and easily administered by personnel with no specialized training. What is ignored, however, is that the data generated using proxy-report assessments are inherently biased.

To accurately determine treatment effectiveness, a distinction must be made between individuals' **occupational performance potential** (i.e., what they are capable of doing) and their **actual occupational performance** (i.e., what they actually do). Even if interventions have a positive effect on individuals' occupational performance potential, changes in their actual occupational performance may not always be manifest. This has been termed "the tutoring effect" (Gauthier et al., 1999), meaning that once family members and caregivers have restricted an individual's opportunities to engage in meaningful occupations such as driving, balancing the checkbook, using the stove to prepare a meal, ironing a shirt, or using a power saw to cut wood, they may continue to restrict the individual's opportunities to engage in these activities, even if they become capable of performing them with less effort, greater efficiency, greater safety, and greater independence. Family members' unwillingness to tolerate the potential for risk is usually the primary reason for this. Standardized observational assessments such as the AMPS (Fisher, 2006) which assess the difficulty of the meaningful and personally relevant tasks they are observed performing may provide objective measures of ability and information about individuals' abilities to perform tasks safely and effectively.

Designing Therapeutic Environments

Recently, more attention has been directed toward contextual interventions such as the physical design of special care units for persons with dementia within long-term care facilities in order to promote not just the comfort and safety of residents but also the ability of residents to participate in meaningful occupations (c.f., Day, Carreon, & Stump, 2000, for review; Cooper & Day, 2003). These special care units are designed to reflect a more "home-like" physical setting in which small groups of residents with dementia reside in comfortable family-style units. This provides residents with more privacy, choices, and opportunities to participate in meaningful occupations and also supports family members' active participation in the lives of the residents. Residents' independent use of washrooms for toileting may be promoted by providing clear cues such as bright colors or graphics to encourage residents to enter the washrooms; residents' abilities to locate their own bedrooms may be enhanced by providing clear and meaningful room identification cues, such as large numbers, name plates, and areas of personal photographs (Cooper & Day, 2003).

In a prospective, matched-group design, Reimer and colleagues (Reimer, Slaughter, Donaldson, Currie, & Eliasziw, 2004) followed 185 residents with middle- to late-stage dementia from 24 long-term care centers and four designated assisted living environments over a 1-year period. Their intervention group included 62 residents of a 60-bed purpose-build specialized care facility where residents lived in bungalows designed to accommodate 10 residents. The 123 control subjects resided in traditional institutional facilities. Reimer and colleagues found that residents of the specialized care facility demonstrated less decline in ADL, more sustained interest in the environment, and less negative affect than residents in the traditional institutional facilities.

Supporting Occupational Performance

When a diagnosis of dementia is made and appropriate symptomatic pharmacological management is initiated, the focus of clinical attention should shift to ensure that individuals with dementia are supported in their attempts to remain active participants in meaningful occupations. Participation in meaningful occupation maintains occupational performance skills. This is essential if one is to derive feelings of satisfaction and enjoyment from doing, retain one's identity and dignity as an occupational being, and overcome the debilitating effects of inactivity.

In this next section, four strategies that health care professionals can use in their work with persons with dementia and their caregivers to support the occupational performance of persons with dementia will be discussed:

- Supporting family in their role as caregivers
- Identifying meaningful occupations
- Training caregivers to use compensatory strategies
- Training caregivers to manage "problem behaviors"

Supporting Family in Their Roles as Caregivers

For most people with dementia, occupational and social functioning will only be maintained with the support of family and friends who take on the role of caregiver. In Canada, about half of the population with dementia live in the community, and of these, over 90% receive some support and care from family and friends (CSHA, 1994b). Nevertheless, it is also important to keep in mind that of those in the community with dementia, about one third reside alone (Ebly, Hogan, & Rockwood, 1999). Caregivers of those living alone tend to provide less hands-on assistance, report less burden, and are less likely to be depressed than those living with persons with dementia, although they are also more likely to consider the option of institutionalization of the affected individual.

Health professionals must recognize that no two families are alike (Maheu & Cohen, 1999). Efforts should be made to work collaboratively with persons with dementia and their families, regardless of whether family members live with persons with dementia or not, but the way in which this is done may vary considerably from one family to another. However, it is only through collaborative efforts that health professionals can be confident that the care decisions made reflect the needs of both the caregivers and the person with dementia (Gwyther, 1990). It is important that the role of the person with dementia in the family is clearly identified (e.g., emotional supporter, mediator, social organizer) and that the family is able to recognize that these roles will change over time. Thus, the families need to be prepared to deal with shifting dynamics within the family. Relationship difficulties that existed prior to the diagnosis of dementia will, in all likelihood, continue to exist and, in many cases, will be further exacerbated. However, when persons with dementia and their families perceive that they have access to adequate and dependable support resources when needed, the stresses associated with caregiving can be buffered. See Chapter 15 for further discussion of family issues in later life.

To ensure that care decisions will meet the needs of persons with dementia and caregivers, everyone involved must be provided with opportunities to learn about dementia and about how the abilities of those with dementia change over time (Robinson, 1997). Valuable resources can be accessed through Alzheimer's Disease International (ADI), an umbrella organization for national Alzheimer's associations, as well as 75 national organizations and two regional ones (i.e., Europe and Latin America). Educational materials are available through ADI and their member organizations, as well as access to support programs. See Resources listed at the end of this chapter for contact information.

It is important to be cautious in expectations for families. Dementia is stressful for the whole family, and caregivers can be overwhelmed by the unremitting needs of the individual. Excessive stress can lead to illness for the caregiver, or can contribute to elder abuse. See Chapter 25 for more information regarding elder abuse.

Caregivers also need to be provided with emotional and esteem support from the time of diagnosis and throughout the course of the disease. Caregivers of persons with dementia are at increased risk for depression and anxiety, with reported rates being as high as 50% (Schulz et al., 1995). Advocacy organizations often provide opportunities for support, particularly emotional and esteem support, through support groups, through peer mentoring where caregivers meet face-to-face, and through telephone or computer networks in which caregivers can share their experiences and coping strategies. Health professionals should also be prepared to address the support needs of caregivers which are outlined in Box 9-2. These can be provided through psycho-educational

caregiver training offered on an individual basis or within a group format. However, even though programs that provide specialized dementia services, support groups, and community services have been shown to extend the time that caregivers are able to provide care within the home and community setting (Mittelman, Ferris, Shulman, Steinberg, & Levin, 1996), such community programs are not well utilized (CSHA, 1994b). The reasons for this are numerous:

- A reluctance on the part of caregivers to acknowledge that they are unable to manage until absolutely necessary
- A view that caregiving is an expected familial responsibility
- A lack of awareness of existing services
- Difficulty accessing services due to such factors as distance and costs

Although respite care programs have received considerable public attention as a means of supporting caregivers, a recent systematic review of studies of such programs provided no evidence of their efficacy (Lee & Cameron, 2004). It is assumed that when caregivers are provided with respite, they will use their time to engage in personally meaningful and satisfying occupations, but this may not always be the case. Instead, caregivers may use respite time to complete other required tasks such as shopping, dealing with financial issues, or even providing care to other family members. The effectiveness

---

BOX 9-2 **Examples of How Health Professionals Can Support Families**

- Support families to make care decisions in which they consider both their own needs and the needs and desires of the person with dementia
- Clarify how the diagnosis will affect the individual's occupational and social functioning
- Provide resources that will enable them to support the occupational functioning, well-being, and overall quality of life of their family member with dementia
- Support family to take steps when the person with dementia is still able to make decisions related to financial planning (e.g., making a will), care preferences, and end-of-life decisions (advanced directives) (Alzheimer Society of Canada, 1997; Cohen, 1994; Fisk et al., 1998)

- Share practical strategies for dealing with behavioral problems and other challenges
- Assist family in identifying what tangible supports they need and how they might elicit assistance from other family members, friends, neighbors, and available community resources
- Share information about community resources (e.g., Meals-on-Wheels, transportation assistance, housekeeping or chore services, adult day care, senior citizens' center activities, friendly visitors, respite programs)
- Validate family members' feelings and experiences as caregivers

of these studies is judged by determining whether there was a reduction in caregiver burden or an increase in the time to institutional care, but it is possible that these outcomes were simply not the most appropriate. Instead, it may be more appropriate to determine if, despite the challenges facing caregivers, they report experiencing a sense of well-being derived not just from time spent engaged in non-caregiving occupations, but also from caregiving efforts.

Identifying Meaningful Occupations

Caregivers, as much as health professionals, need to recognize how they can support the occupational and social functioning of individuals with dementia. Health professionals should encourage persons with dementia and their caregivers to define a "new normal" (Gwyther, 2000) by them to collaboratively identify what the person with dementia needs and wants to be able to do; and what others, including the caregiver, expect the person with dementia to do. In identifying meaningful occupations, the person with dementia and caregiver need to extend their thinking beyond self-care and household tasks, and consider occupations that had previously provided opportunities for the person with dementia to fulfill their needs for achievement (e.g., mowing the grass, volunteering at the local food bank), pleasure (e.g., playing badminton, reading with a grandchild), rejuvenation (e.g., walking in the woods, playing the piano), and social connection (looking at photos with a family member, playing a game of bridge with friends), and that have the potential to provide these same opportunities now.

There are some preliminary data that support that "activity-oriented" interventions including structured opportunities to engage in crafts, music, dance, drama, and pet therapy (e.g., Filan & Llewellyn-Jones, 2006; Holm, Lepp, & Ringsberg, 2005; Kinney & Rentz, 2005; Lepp, Ringsberg, Holm, & Sollersjo, 2003; Vink, Birks, Bruinsma, & Scholten, 2004) can positively affect individuals' feelings of satisfaction, achievement, and pleasure, and support their interactions with others. In a review of several small studies on the impact of pet therapy or animal-assisted therapy (AAT) on persons with dementia, Filan and Llewellyn-Jones (2006) concluded the presence of a dog not only reduces aggression and agitation but also promotes social behavior in people with dementia. Although the sample was small

(N = 12), Kinney and Rentz (2005) examined the effectiveness of participation in a "Memories in the Making" art program that encouraged persons in the early and middle stages of dementia to express their ideas and feelings using art. Each subject participated in the art program, as well as in more traditional adult day care programs (e.g., current events and crafts). When they participated in the "Memories in the Making" program, the participants were observed to demonstrate significantly more interest, sustained attention, pleasure, and self-esteem. Lepp and colleagues (2003) examined the responses of 12 adults with moderate to severe dementia and their seven caregivers to a drama program (i.e., weekly 1.5-hour sessions over a 2-month period of time). Caregivers reported feeling a greater sense of fellowship with other participants, and persons with dementia were observed to communicate with the leaders as well as other participants and to make associations with situations experienced earlier in their lives. The caregivers reported that in other daily life situations, the participants with dementia more openly expressed their feelings, conveyed a greater sense of confidence, and showed greater interest in their surroundings. In another small study (N = 6) of persons with intermediate and severe dementia and their three caregivers, Holm and colleagues (2005) examined reactions of the participants to a six-session, storytelling, drama program (i.e., weekly 1.5-hour sessions). Participation in this program reportedly stimulated those with dementia to communicate and interact with other people.

However, not everyone can be expected to respond in the same way to specific activities. The findings of a study conducted by Hutchinson and Marshall (2000) highlight how attempting to engage individuals in activities that they do not find meaningful can have negative repercussions. When they examined responses of persons with AD and their caregivers to an "activity kit" that contained 20 therapeutic activities, they found that although some caregivers reported that the activities helped fill time, inspired additional activities, and facilitated connections with the family member, for others it was perceived as just an additional burden. Moreover, although some persons with AD responded well to some of the activities, others found the activities to be "insulting."

Individuals' responses may, however, be more positive when they are provided with opportunities to engage in activities that they perceive as meaningful (i.e., reflecting their personal interests, goals, values, sense of competence and efficacy, and experiences). An example of this is provided by the study of Teri and Logsdon (1991) in which they developed an intervention program based on identifying a number of pleasant activities in which individuals could participate. Their findings suggested the intervention resulted in improvements in the mood of both the persons with dementia and of their caregivers.

Although also an "activity-oriented" therapy, reminiscence therapy is grounded in the idea of eliciting pleasant memories and creating opportunities for pleasurable interaction. Videotapes, photographs, possessions, archival material, and life-story books that will be perceived as meaningful to participants are reviewed with the goal of stimulating participants to share memories. Somewhat surprisingly, the findings of a recent systematic review of four randomized controlled trials with a total sample of 144 subjects suggested only limited success for this intervention (Woods, Spector, Jones, Orrell, & Davies, 2005). In contrast to the studies referred to above where the focus was placed on indicators that would suggest greater engagement and a higher level of satisfaction, these studies focused on outcomes of improved cognition, behavior, and mood. Thus, the use of outcomes that are more appropriately focused on satisfaction derived while engaged in specific occupations, as well as larger sample sizes, may yield stronger evidence of effectiveness of interventions, such as reminiscence therapy, that employ meaningful occupations.

Training Caregivers to Use Compensatory Strategies

By definition, dementia affects individuals' abilities to perform occupations in a skilled manner (i.e., efficiently, safely, and independently). As dementia progresses, individuals will need to perform occupations differently to compensate for the skill changes they experience and engage in tasks that are less demanding and challenging. They may choose to give up occupations that they now experience as difficult, frustrating, and unfulfilling. Alternatively, others, including family members, may require them to give up occupations that can no longer be performed in a competent or safe manner. To prepare for the

inevitability of giving up some occupations, health professionals need to support persons with dementia and their caregivers to engage in open discussions about these eventualities.

Concerns about the safety of the person with dementia and the extent to which the person's actions may place others at risk are real but need to be evaluated carefully. For example, according to consensus guidelines developed in Sweden (Lundberg et al., 1997), although a diagnosis of moderate to severe dementia should preclude driving, individuals with mild dementia need to be evaluated on an individual basis, ideally using a specialized assessment of their driving competence. Unfortunately, a diagnosis of dementia leads some persons with dementia and their caregivers to ignore what individuals can still do. Caregivers need to be aware that their efforts to restrict the participation of persons with dementia in some occupations may contribute to excess disability (Brody, Kleban, Lawton, & Silverman, 1971)—that is, the situation where individuals present as being less able than they really are. The challenge is to help persons with dementia and their caregivers recognize their occupational performance skill strengths and also identify strategies that can be used to compensate for their deficiencies. Plans should be developed, keeping in mind that changes need not and should not take place all at once. A diagnosis of dementia does not suddenly render someone incapable. Caregivers must also appreciate that when individuals are confronted with the need to give up former occupations, they need to be provided with the opportunities to grieve those losses.

Health professionals need to support caregivers to find a healthy balance between autonomy and safety while acknowledging that there are risks inherent in all occupations. There is no question that efforts need to be made to reduce risks. However, caregivers also need to recognize that the elimination of all risks is not only impractical but will severely threaten the quality of life of those living with dementia. Health professionals should be prepared to work with family members and persons with dementia to identify potential risk factors for accidents and injuries within the home and other relevant environments. Examples of structured checklists to guide a review of occupational performance environments include the Safety Assessment of Function and the Environment for

Rehabilitation (SAFER) (Oliver, Bathwayt, Brackley, & Tamaki, 1993), the Westmead Home Safety Assessment (WeHSA) (Clemson, Fitzgerald, & Heard, 1999), the Home Falls and Accidents Screening Tool (HOME FAST) (Mackenzie, Byles, & Higginbotham, 2000), and the Safety Assessment Scale (Poulin de Courval et al., 2006) which has been specifically designed for use with older adults with cognitive impairments.

The risks associated with some occupations can be reduced when the focus shifts from "independent" performance to "interdependence" or shared performance. For example, individuals with dementia may insist that they continue to dress themselves for as long as possible even if it takes a great deal of effort and the end result is less than ideal in the eyes of the caregiver. Others may be receptive to receiving direct assistance so that they can use their time, skills, and energies to engage in more personally meaningful occupations such as helping to prepare breakfast or working with the caregiver in the garden.

After identifying those occupations that persons with dementia and their caregivers decide are the ones that the person with dementia needs and wants to perform, an assessment of the individual's occupational performance strengths and deficits should be undertaken. Rather than making assumptions about the ability of persons with dementia on the basis of their diagnosis or even stage of dementia, individuals' occupational performance in real-life contexts should be evaluated and collaborative information sought. For example, performance-based assessments of driving should be conducted (Lundberg et al., 1997) with descriptions of individuals' actual driving behavior elicited from family and friends. Similarly, individuals' occupational performance potential within the context of personally relevant and meaningful PADL and IADL can be assessed using standardized assessments such as the AMPS (Fisher, 2006) with corroborating information from the caregiver using the DAD (Gélinas et al., 1999) in order to also determine their perception of the individual's occupational performance. Although not specifically designed for persons with dementia, occupational therapists can use the AMPS (Fisher, 2006) to identify those motor and process skills that are used effectively, as well as those that are not (Josephsson et al., 1993). One advantage of

the AMPS (Fisher, 2006) is that efforts are made to ensure that the individual is motivated to perform the tasks (i.e., that the tasks performed are both familiar and relevant to the individual's life), that the individual is provided with task options that will provide sufficient challenge, and that the individual has been familiarized with the environment in which the tasks are to be performed. Using this information, occupational performance skills strengths (e.g., the skills of attending to the task without distraction; choosing appropriate tools and materials for the task, sequencing the steps of the task in a logical order) and difficulties (e.g., difficulty searching and locating materials and tools needed for the task, and heeding the goal of the task) can be identified (Josephsson et al., 1993). Information obtained from the caregiver using the DAD (Gélinas et al., 1999) may provide essential additional information, such as identifying that, despite intact skills, the person with dementia does not initiate task performance independently. A similar assessment process or methodology can be used to evaluate the occupational performance strengths and limitations within the context of other meaningful occupations such as using the computer to e-mail friends, going to the local pool for a swim, or building and painting a birdhouse. Baum and Edwards (2003) have also developed the Functional Behavior Profile (FBP) to enable caregivers to structure the observations they make when persons with dementia complete everyday tasks. More specifically, the tool is used to guide caregivers to take note of what those with dementia are able to do rather than focusing on what they can no longer do. Drawing on the caregivers' observations, practitioners can then help caregivers identify strategies that will more effectively support the participation of persons with dementia in everyday tasks.

Once an assessment of the individual's occupational performance strengths and deficits has been completed, one can determine if observed skill difficulties in everyday occupations reflect problems related to the following:

• The individual's underlying impairments or capacity limitations (e.g., underlying cognitive impairments that hamper the individual's ability to recall where materials and tools are stored or how much coffee should be added for each cup being made)

- The demands of the specific task being performed (e.g., the expectation that after changing the sheets on the bed, the individual will place the soiled sheets in the laundry, or that the task of setting the table requires that all placemats and napkins selected match)
- Aspects of the physical task environment (e.g., cluttered workspace, materials being stored out of sight in cupboards, a coffee pot that is big and heavy and thus, awkward to fill and lift)
- The social environment (e.g., a family member who hovers nearby and makes comments while the person tries to complete the task)

Rather than setting up expectations that caregivers do tasks *for* persons with dementia, an approach that reinforces individuals' participation enables caregivers to support individuals to continue to engage in meaningful occupations (Figure 9-3). As Corcoran (1994) found in

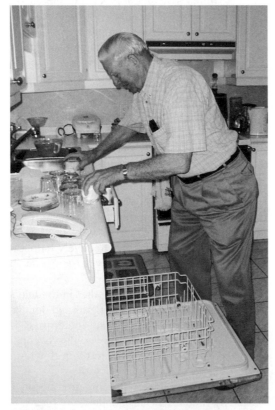

FIGURE 9-3 Participation in familiar tasks can be supported when task performance is shared. After the dishes have been removed and stacked, the caregiver can ensure they are returned to their appropriate places.

a study of spousal caregivers of persons with AD, the roles of caregivers in supporting the well-being of persons with AD are many and varied. This supports Bowers' (1987) earlier conceptualization of caregiving as consisting of anticipatory care, preventative care, supervisory care, instrumental care, and protective care.

Corcoran (1994) identified five categories of management strategies used by caregivers to maintain and support the well-being and dignity of those with AD. These strategies included

1. Engagement in productive activities
2. Distraction away from difficult topics or situations
3. Error-proofing the environment by adapting objectives or tasks, completing some steps of the task for the person with AD, and relaxing expectations about the "right" way to do tasks
4. Strategic time use through the use of routines and extending activities to fill as much time as possible
5. Maintained involvement with friends and family

These strategies, used intuitively by some spousal caregivers, are reflected in the compensatory strategies identified in Box 9-3. These strategies are conceptualized as

- Changing how the task is performed
- Changing the task expectations or demands
- Changing elements of the physical task environment
- Changing elements of the social task environment (i.e., the supports provided by caregivers within the context of the task performance)

Building on their earlier work, Gitlin and colleagues (2002) developed an assessment tool, the Task Management Strategy Index (TMSI). Preliminary evidence suggests that the TMSI can be easily administered and generate valid and reliable findings. The TMSI includes a list of actions caregivers might use to support the occupational performance of persons with dementia who are physically dependent and agitated. Such actions include introducing an activity that uses the same motion over and over such as sweeping, raking, and dusting; placing items out in the order in which they need to be used by the person with dementia; putting away items that aren't needed for what the person

BOX 9-3 Examples of Compensatory Strategies

Change how the task is performed
- Reduce number of task steps (e.g., eliminate need to wash, dry, and tear lettuce for a salad by using prepackaged salad greens; buy ready-to-serve soup in a tin with a pull-tab lid and avoid need to use a can opener and to do step of measuring and adding water to soup; use memory speed dial on phone for frequently called numbers)
- Gather all needed materials and tools at the beginning of the task
- Take a break
- Use adapted tools and materials (e.g., replace buttons with Velcro closings; use kettle that shuts off automatically)

Change task expectations or demands
- Redefine "successful" task completion or task engagement (change views on what is ideal or necessary)
- Reduce demands of task (e.g., vacuum but vacuum one room only)
- Share performance (e.g., one person washes dishes, other person dries and puts them away)
- Develop a routine—schedule tasks so performed at same time every day
- Give choices but limit number (e.g., no more than two should be offered)
- Reduce time pressures to complete the task

Change elements of the physical task environment
- Minimize visual and auditory distractions (visual and auditory)
- Reduce unnecessary clutter
- Create soothing atmosphere (e.g., low lights, warm water, and air temperature when bathing)
- Ensure all needed materials and tools are available and within sight and place in order will need to be used
- Label contents of cupboards, drawers, boxes
- Reduce number of tools and materials from which the individual needs to make selections
- Ensure tools and materials are returned to the same place each and every time

Change elements of the social task environment
- Emphasize the process of doing rather than quality of end-outcome
- Use short simple sentences
- Ask yes/no questions
- Provide single-step instructions
- Make direct eye contact when providing cues
- Use written, visual, or physical cues (touch) to avoid lengthy explanations
- Do with the person to serve as a role model
- Provide feedback in a calm, reassuring manner

with dementia is doing; and trying to ignore mistakes made by persons with dementia. In clinical practice settings, the TMSI might be used to provide caregivers with positive feedback about the strategies that they are effectively using. By identifying strategies that they are not currently using, practitioners could develop individually tailored educational sessions to meet the caregiver's unique needs.

An important aspect of "changing elements of the social task environment" relates to how the caregiver communicates with the person with dementia. Health professionals should be prepared to assist caregivers in identifying strategies that will enable them to communicate effectively with persons with dementia. Although empirical support for specific communication strategies is, in most cases, nonexistent (Small, Gutman, Makela, & Hillhouse, 2003), some small studies have been conducted in which the effectiveness of specific communication

strategies was examined. For example, Small and Perry (2005) examined the effects that different types of questions posed by caregivers had on their spouses with AD. They found that communication was more successful (i.e., persons with AD were able to respond appropriately) when caregivers used yes–no questions as opposed to open-ended questions and when the questions asked placed demands on their semantic memory (i.e., more general knowledge about the external world) rather than on their episodic memory (i.e., specific incidents in the individual's own life). In another study, 20 healthy older adults listened to prerecorded samples of interactions between caregivers and their spouses with dementia. Small, Perry, and Lewis (2005) found that the healthy older adults rated interactions more positively when they perceived that the content and manner of caregivers' speech was respectful, caring, and not controlling, and when the caregivers conveyed positive beliefs about their spouses' competence. Innovative research conducted by Dijkstra, Bourgeois, Youmans, and Hancock (2006) with adults with dementia highlights how relatively preserved skills can be tapped to support the participation of persons with dementia in different social roles. In their first study, 12 persons with dementia were asked to engage in social conversations (e.g., talk about their marriage, talk about their children, talk about their church) and during another session were asked to give advice in areas in which they had life experience (e.g., getting married, having children, joining a church). When in the "advice-giving" condition, participants generated more imperatives (e.g., you should, you have to, do this) and more discourse-building utterances than when they were in the "social conversation" condition. In a second study, Dijkstra and colleagues (2006) asked subjects (i.e., six persons with dementia and six persons without dementia) to "teach" another adult to complete a recipe by using a booklet that contained visual cues. No significant differences were found between the two groups. However, subjects with dementia demonstrated competence in the "teacher" role where they were required to give instructions and provide evaluative feedback, and use recipe-relevant discourse. Although preliminary, these findings provide some support for efforts made to provide opportunities for persons with dementia to engage in social situations where they can use their relatively preserved role-related and discourse abilities.

When recommending that caregivers try different strategies, health professionals need to recognize that caregivers will also need to go through a process of "trial-and-error" to find out what works best in their situation. In other words, health professionals should be prepared to encourage caregivers to try different strategies before deciding what works, what doesn't work, and how strategies might be modified. An important consideration in selecting possible compensatory strategies is whether they will be deemed acceptable or feasible to those with dementia, as well as their caregivers. As Gwyther (1998) highlighted, there is no "right" way to care for a person with AD. Each family must determine, with the help of health professionals, how they can best meet the needs of the person with dementia, as well as the needs of the caregiver and other family members.

There has been only limited research designed to examine the effect of caregiver training caregivers on the participation of persons with dementia in meaningful occupations, and the findings of this research have been inconsistent. For example, Martin-Cook and colleagues (2005) enrolled 24 caregivers of persons with dementia in a four-session training program. After observing their family member with dementia being administered the Texas Functional Living Scale (Cullum et al., 2001), a performance-based assessment of IADL, caregivers were then coached to provide cues that would support their family member's task performance. The findings of this randomized controlled trial suggested that this particular intervention was not effective in reducing the gap between caregivers' expectations and the performance abilities of persons with dementia. In contrast, Dooley and Hinojsa (2004) found a significant improvement in caregiver burden and quality of life of persons with AD (specifically, positive affect, activity frequency, and self-care status) in a study designed to examine the effectiveness of individualized occupational therapy home-based interventions. The 20 caregivers in the intervention group were provided with training on how to use compensatory strategies, including environmental modifications, and how to support their family members' occupational performance. Similar positive findings were reported by Gitlin and colleagues (2001) in their examination of the effects of a home environmental intervention on the self-efficacy and level of upset experienced by caregivers, as well as the daily function of dementia patients, using a much larger sample (N = 171). Those assigned to the intervention group received five 90-minute home visits by occupational therapists. Following the completion of an assessment, the occupational therapists provided education and worked collaboratively with the caregivers to identify appropriate compensatory strategies and physical and social environmental modifications that they might use to support the occupational performance of their family members with dementia. In contrast to caregivers in the control group, who received usual care, the caregivers in the intervention group reported being less upset and feeling more competent in their abilities to manage the behaviors of their family members with dementia. They also reported that their family members better maintained their ability to independently perform IADL and PADL, and demonstrated fewer behavior problems 3 months after the intervention. Thus, although there is some evidence that interventions designed to train caregivers to support the occupational and social functioning of persons with dementia can be beneficial, further research is needed. These efforts must ensure that the outcomes measured reflect the broad goal of supporting the occupational and social functioning of persons with dementia, however.

Training Caregivers to Manage "Problem Behaviors"

It is important for caregivers to recognize that although some "problem or negative behaviors" demonstrated by persons with dementia are a symptom of their specific type of dementia, other "problem behaviors" may arise from their confusion, frustration, fear, fatigue, and even pain. It has been suggested that at some point, 90% of all persons with dementia will demonstrate behaviors that their caregivers will identify as being problematic (Teri, Larson, & Reifler, 1988). Rather than reacting to the behavior as a negative attribute of the individual with dementia or a willful attempt to be difficult, health professionals can play an important role in enabling caregivers to view these "problem behaviors" as the consequence of individuals' inability to express their feelings verbally and directly. If caregivers can identify triggers or precipitants for behaviors, they will be more likely to identify effective strategies either for preventing or dealing with such problems when they appear. It is possible that actively engaging persons with dementia in meaningful occupations where they will have opportunities to experience a sense of achievement and mastery, pleasure and enjoyment, rejuvenation and relaxation, and connections with others will reduce such problem or negative behaviors.

■ Summary

As noted in this chapter, a diagnosis of dementia is contingent on evidence that supports that individuals demonstrate a decline in occupational or social functioning and that the decline can be attributed to changes in their cognitive abilities. In much of the research literature, occupational and social functioning has been operationalized simply as the independent performance of ADL such that these concepts have become synonymous. This operationalization has been reinforced by efforts to design interventions for persons with dementia and caregivers with the long-term goal being to delay or avoid the need for costly institutional or paid professional care. In this process, the need for persons with dementia to continue to participate occupations that provide them with opportunities to experience feelings of achievement, pleasure, rejuvenation, and social connections, including connections with their caregivers, has been largely overlooked. We now stand at a critical juncture in which there are clear opportunities for leadership that will move the agenda of dementia research forward and allow the occupational needs of persons with dementia and their caregivers to be addressed directly. Particular attention must be directed toward methodological issues such as clearly designed intervention protocols and the selection of appropriate outcome measures. This, however, requires that clinical and research efforts be directed toward the development and evaluation of interventions that embrace a broad and more individualized understanding of occupational and social functioning.

Case Study

Design of Long-Term Care Facility, Specific for Dementia

An architectural firm was commissioned to design a new long-term care facility for the elderly that would include a unit specifically for persons with dementia to replace the existing facility. An occupational therapist was hired to provide consultation services.

1. The occupational therapist's goal is to advise the architect on environmental factors that will meet the needs of individuals with AD. What assessment process should be used?
2. What might you anticipate that the family members would identify as problems?
3. What structural factors might the therapist suggest?

Review Questions

1. How has our understanding of dementia and specific dementing conditions changed over time?
2. What impact does dementia have on (a) individuals, (b) families, and (c) society?
3. What are the unique features of (a) Alzheimer's disease, (b) vascular dementia, (c) dementia with Lewy bodies, (d) frontotemporal dementia, and (e) Parkinson's disease dementia?
4. Describe the dementia diagnosis process.
5. Identify how dementia is typically staged.
6. How has the traditional conceptualization of occupational and social functioning influenced assessment and management approaches?
7. Define occupational and social functioning from a broader perspective than that of independent performance of activities of daily living.
8. Identify how the assessment of occupational and social functioning contributes to (a) the diagnosis of dementia, (b) the evaluation of the effectiveness of interventions, (c) the design of therapeutic environments, and (d) the development of strategies to support the occupational performance of persons with dementia.
9. How can family members support the occupational and social functioning of persons with dementia?
10. What strategies could be used to support the occupational and social functioning of persons with dementia?

Web-Based Resources

For helpful information about the experience of dementia, visit:

www.aarp.org, **AARP,** date connected March 18, 2007. This is an organization with a wide range of services for elders. This site describes those services, including information and resources for individuals with AD and their family members.

www.alz.org, **Alzheimer's Association,** date connected March 18, 2007. The leading U.S. consumer organization dedicated to providing resources and seeking a cure for AD. Local chapters have an array of support resources for individuals with dementia and their families.

www.alz.co.uk, **Alzheimer's Disease International,** date connected March 10, 2007. The international version of the U.S. Alzheimer's Association.

www.alzheimer.ca, **Alzheimer Society of Canada,** date connected March 10, 1997. The Canadian version of the U.S. Alzheimer's Association.

www.caps4caregivers.org, **Children of Aging Parents,** date connected March 10, 2007. A support group for adult children caring for their adult parents. Includes information about managing care for demented elderly relatives.

www.dasninternational.org/2005/norma.php, **Dementia Advocacy and Support Network (DASN),** date connected March 10, 2007. Efforts to fund services for and research on dementia requires advocacy. This is one of the many groups advocating for those resources.

www.ethnicelderscare.net, **Ethnic Elders Care Network,** date connected March 10, 2007. Contains helpful information about the cultural aspects of care for individuals with dementia.

www.caregiver.org, **Family Caregiver Alliance,** date connected March 10, 2007. Another advocacy group for adult caregivers of elderly individuals.

www.caregiving.org, **National Alliance for Caregiving,** date connected March 10, 2007. Another advocacy group for adult caregivers of elderly individuals.

www.nfcacares.org, **National Family Caregiver's Association,** date connected March 10, 2007. Another advocacy group for adult caregivers of elderly individuals.

REFERENCES

Alzheimer Society of Canada. (1997). *Tough issues: Ethical guidelines.* Toronto: Alzheimer Society of Canada.

Amaducci, L., Falcini, M., & Lippi, A. (1992). Descriptive epidemiology and risk factors for Alzheimer's disease. *Acta Neurologica Scandinavica, 139,* 21–25.

American Psychiatric Association (APA). (2000). *Diagnostic and statistical manual of mental disorders: DSM-IV-TR* (4th, text revision ed.). Washington, DC: American Psychiatric Association.

Anderson, K., Nielsen, H., Lolk, A., Andersen, J., Becker, I., & Kragh-Sorensen, P. (1999). Incidence of very mild to severe dementia and Alzheimer's disease in Denmark: The Odense Study. *Neurology, 52*(1), 85–90.

Auer, S., & Reisberg, B. (1997). The GDS/FAST staging system. *International Psychogeriatrics, 9* (Suppl. 1), 167–191.

Barber, R., Panikkar, A., & McKeith, I. G. (2001). Dementia with Lewy bodies: Diagnosis and management. *International Journal of Geriatric Psychiatry, 16*(Suppl. 1), S12–S18.

Baum, C., & Edwards, D. F. (2003). What persons with Alzheimer's disease can do: A tool for communication about everyday activities. *Alzheimer's Care Quarterly, 4*(2), 108–115.

Baum, C., Edwards, D. F., & Morrow-Howell, N. (1993). Identification and measurement of productive behaviors in senile dementia of the Alzheimer type. *The Gerontologist, 33*(3), 403–408.

Black, S., Roman, G. C., Geldmacher, D. S., Salloway, S., Hecker, J., Burns, A., et al. (2003). Efficacy and tolerability of donepezil in vascular dementia: Positive results of a 24-week, multicenter, international, randomized, placebo-controlled clinical trial. *Stroke, 34*(10), 2323–2330.

Blessed, G., Tomlinson, B. E., & Roth, M. (1968). The association between quantitative measures of dementia and of senile change in the cerebral grey matter of elderly subjects. *British Journal of Psychiatry, 114,* 797–811.

Bookwala, J., Yee, J. L., & Schulz, R. (2000). Caregiving and detrimental mental and physical health outcomes. In G. M. Williamson, D. R. Shaffer, & P. A. Parmelee (Eds.), *Physical illness and depression in older adults: A handbook of theory, research, and practice* (pp. 93–131). New York: Plenum.

Borell, L. (1996). Supporting functional behavior in Alzheimer's disease. *International Psychogeriatrics, 8*(Suppl. 1), 123–125.

Bowers, B. J. (1987). Intergenerational caregiving: Adult caregivers and their aging parents. *Advances in Nursing Science, 45*(1), M1–M2.

Bowler, J. V. (2000). Criteria for vascular dementia: Replacing dogma with data. *Archives of Neurology, 57*(2), 170–171.

Bowler, J. V., & Hachinski, V. (2003). Current criteria for vascular dementia—A critical appraisal. In J. V. Bowler & V. Hachinski (Eds.), *Vascular cognitive impairment: Preventable dementia* (pp. 1–11). Oxford: Oxford University Press.

Braak, H., & Braak, E. (1991). Neuropathological staging of Alzheimer-related changes. *Acta Neuropathologica, 82*(4), 239–259.

Breteler, M. M., Claus, J. J., van Duijn, C. M., Launer, L. J., & Hoffman, A. (1992). Epidemiology of Alzheimer's disease. *Epidemiologic Review, 14,* 59–82.

Brody, E. M., Kleban, M. H., Lawton, M. P., & Silverman, H. A. (1971). Excess disabilities of mentally impaired aged: Impact of individualized treatment. *The Gerontologist, 11*(2), 124–133.

Brookmeyer, R., Gray, S., & Kawas, C. (1998). Projections of Alzheimer's disease in the United States and the public health impact of delaying disease onset. *American Journal of Public Health, 88*(9), 1337–1342.

Brugge, K. L, Nichols, S. L., & Salmon, D. P. (1994). Cognitive impairment in adults with Down's syndrome: Similarities to early cognitive changes in Alzheimer's disease. *Neurology, 44*(2), 232–238.

Bucks, R. S., Ashworth, D. L., Wilcock, G. K., & Seigfried, K. (1996). Assessment of activities of daily living in dementia: Development of the Bristol Activities of Daily Living Scale. *Age and Ageing, 25*(2), 113 120.

Buhr, G. T., Kuchibhatla, M., & Clipp, E. C. (2006). Caregivers' reasons for nursing home placement: Clues for improving discussions with families prior to the transition. *The Gerontologist, 46,* 52–61.

CSHA (Canadian Study of Health and Aging). (1994a). Canadian Study of Health and Aging: Study methods and prevalence of dementia. *Canadian Medical Association Journal, 150*(6), 899–913.

CSHA (Canadian Study of Health and Aging). (1994b). Patterns of caring for people with dementia in Canada. *Canadian Journal of Aging, 13*(4), 470–487.

Carswell, A., & Eastwood, R. (1993). Activities of daily living, cognitive impairment and social function in community residents with Alzheimer disease. *Canadian Journal of Occupational Therapy, 60,* 130–136.

Chui, H. (2001). Dementia due to subcortical ischemic vascular disease. *Clinical Cornerstone, 3*(4), 40–51.

Chiu, H. C., Victoroff, D., Margolin, W., Jagust, R., Shankle, R., & Katzman, R. (1992). Criteria for the diagnosis of ischemic vascular dementia proposed by the State of California Alzheimer's Disease Diagnostic and Treatment Centers. *Neurology, 42,* 473–480.

Clemson, L., Fitzgerald, M. H., & Heard, R. (1999). Content validity of an assessment tool to identify home fall hazards: The Westmead Home Safety Assessment. *British Journal of Occupational Therapy, 62,* 171–179.

Cohen, D. (1994). A primary care checklist for effective family management. *Medical Clinics of North America, 78*(4), 795–809.

Cohen-Mansfield, J., Reisberg, B., Bonneman, J., Berg, L., Dastoor, D. P., Pfeffer, R. I., et al. (1996). Staging methods for the assessment of dementia. Perspectives. *Journal of Clinical Psychiatry, 57*(5), 190–198.

Cooke, K. Z., Fisher, A. G., Mayberry, W., & Oakley, F. (2000). Differences in activities of daily living process skills of persons with and without Alzheimer's disease. *Occupational Therapy Journal of Research, 20*(2), 87–105.

Cooper, B. A., & Day, K. (2003). Therapeutic design of environments for people with dementia. In L. Letts, P. Rigby, & D. Stewart (Eds.), *Using environments to enable occupational performance* (pp. 253–268). Thorofare, NJ: SLACK Inc.

Corcoran, M. A. (1994). Management decisions made by caregiver spouses of persons with Alzheimer's disease. *American Journal of Occupational Therapy, 48*(1), 38–45.

Cullum, C. M., Saine, K., Chan, L. D., Martin-Cook, K., Gray, K. F., & Weiner, M. F. (2001). Performance-based instrument to assess functional capacity in dementia: The Texas Functional Living Scale. *Neuropsychiatry, Neuropsychology and Behavioral Neurology, 14*(2), 103–108.

Dal Forno, G., Carson, K. A., Brookmeyer, R., Troncoso, J., Kawas, C. H., & Brandt, J. (2002). APOE genotype and survival in men and women with Alzheimer's disease. *Neurology, 58*(7), 1045–1050.

Darvesh, S., & Freedman, M. (1996). Subcortical dementia: A neurobehavioral approach. *Brain and Cognition, 31*(2), 230–249.

Davis, H. S., & Rockwood, K. (2004). Conceptualization of mild cognitive impairment. *International Journal of Geriatric Psychiatry. 19*(4), 313–319.

Day, K., Carreon, D., & Stump, C. (2000). The therapeutic design of environments for people with dementia: A review of the empirical research. *Gerontologist, 40*(4), 379–421.

Desmond, D. W., Erkinjuntti, T., Sano, M., Cummings, J. L., Bowler, J. V., Pasquier, F., et al. (1999). The cognitive syndrome of vascular dementia: Implications for clinical trials. *Alzheimer Disease and Associated Disorders, 13*(Suppl. 3), S21–S29.

Dijkstra, K., Bourgeois, M., Youmans, G., & Hancock, A. (2006). Implications of an advice-giving and teacher role on language production in adults with dementia. *The Gerontologist, 46*(3), 357–366.

Doble, S. E., Fisk, J. D., MacPherson, K. M., Fisher, A. G., & Rockwood, K. (1997). Measuring functional competence in older persons with Alzheimer's disease. *International Psychogeriatrics, 9*(1), 25–38.

Doble, S. E., Fisk, J. D., & Rockwood, K. (1999). Assessing the ADL functioning of persons with Alzheimer's disease: Comparison of family informants' ratings and performance-based assessment findings. *International Psychogeriatrics, 11*(4), 399–409.

Dooley, N. R., & Hinojosa, J. (2004). Improving quality of life for persons with Alzheimer's disease and their family caregivers: Brief occupational therapy intervention.

American Journal of Occupational Therapy, 58(5), 561–569.

Drach, L. M., Steinmetz, H. E., Wach, S., & Bohl, J. (1997). High proportion of dementia with Lewy bodies in the postmortems of a mental hospital in Germany. *International Journal of Geriatric Psychiatry, 12*(3), 301–306.

Ebly, E. M., Hogan, D. B., & Rockwood, K. (1999). Living alone with dementia. *Dementia and Geriatric Cognitive Disorders, 10*(6), 541–548.

Erkinjuntti, T., Inzitari, D., Pantoni, L., Wallin, A., Scheltens, P., & Rockwood, K., et al. (2000). Limitations of clinical criteria for the diagnosis of vascular dementia in clinical trials. Is a focus on subcortical vascular dementia a solution? *Annals of the New York Academy of Sciences, 903,* 262–272.

Evans, D. A., Funkenstein, H., Albert, M. S., Scherr, P. A., Cook, N. R., Chown, M. J., et al. (1989). Prevalence of Alzheimer's disease in a community population of older persons. *Journal of the American Medical Association, 262*(18), 2551–2556.

Evans, D. A., Scherr, P. A., Smith, L. A., Albert, M. S., & Funkenstein, H. H. (1990). The East Boston Alzheimer's Disease Registry. *Aging* (Milano), *2*(3), 298–302.

Ferri, C. P., Prince, M., Brayne, C., Brodaty, H., Fratiglioni, L., Ganguli, M., et al. (2005). Global prevalence of dementia: A Delphia consensus study. *Lancet, 336*(9503), 2112–2117.

Filan, S. L., & Llewellyn-Jones, R. H. (2006). Animal-assisted therapy for dementia: A review of the literature. *International Psychogeriatrics,* April 26, 1–15.

Fillenbaum, G. G., Heyman, A., Huber, M. S., Woodbury, M. A., Leiss, J., Scmader, K. E., et al. (1998). The prevalence and 3-year incidence of dementia in older Black and White community residents. *Journal of Clinical Epidemiology, 51*(7), 587–595.

Fisher, A. G. (2006). *Assessment of motor and process skills manual* (6th ed.). Fort Collins, CO: Three Star Press.

Fisk, J. D., Merry, H. R., & Rockwood, K. (2003). Variations in case definition affect prevalence but not outcomes of mild cognitive impairment. *Neurology, 61*(9), 1179–1184.

Fisk, J. D., Sadovnick, A. D., Cohen, C. A., Gauthier, S., Dossetor, J., Eberhart, A., et al. (1998). Ethical guidelines of the Alzheimer Society of Canada. *Canadian Journal of Neurological Sciences, 25,* 242–248.

Förstl, H., Burns, A., Levy, F., Cairns, N., Luthert, P., & Lantos, P. (1992). Neurologic signs in Alzheimer's disease: Results of a prospective clinical and neuropathologic study. *Archives of Neurology, 49,* 1038–1042.

Fox, P., Kelly, S., & Tobin, S. (1999). Defining dementia: Social and historical background of Alzheimer disease. *Genetic Testing, 3,* 13–19.

Franssen, E. H., Kluger, A., Torossian, C. L., & Reisberg, B. (1993). The neurologic syndrome of severe

Alzheimer's disease: Relationship to functional decline. *Archives of Neurology, 50,* 1029–1039.

Fratiglioni, L., Launer, L. J., Andersen, K., Breteler, M. M., Copeland, J. R., Dartigues, J. F., et al. (2000). Incidence of dementia and major subtypes in Europe: A collaborative study of population-based cohorts. Neurologic Diseases in the Elderly Research Group. *Neurology, 54,* S10–S15.

Fratiglioni, L., Viitanen, M., von Strauss, E., Tontodonati, V., Herlitz, A., & Winblad, B. (1997). Very old women at highest risk of dementia and Alzheimer's disease: Incidence data from the Kungshomen Project, Stockholm. *Neurology, 48,* 132–138.

Freeman, R. Q., Giovannetti, T., Lamar, M., Cloud, B. S., Stern, R. A., Kaplan, E., et al. (2000). Visuoconstructional problems in dementia: Contribution of executive systems functions. *Neuropsychologia, 14,* 415–426.

Funkenstein, H. H., Albert, M. S., Cook, N. R., West, C. G., Scherr, P. A., Chown, M. J. et al. (1993). Extrapyramidal signs and other neurologic findings in clinically diagnosed Alzheimer's disease. *Archives of Neurology, 50,* 51–56.

Galasko, D., Bennett, D., Sano, M., Ernesto, C., Thomas, R., Grundman, M., et al. (1997). An inventory to assess activities of daily living for clinical trials in Alzheimer's disease. *Alzheimer Disease and Associated Disorders, 11*(Suppl. 2), S33–S39.

Galasko, D., Edland, S. D., Morris, J. C., Clark, C., Mohs, R., & Koss, E. (1995). The Consortium to Establish a Registry for Alzheimer's disease (CERAD). Part XI. Clinical milestones in patients with Alzheimer's disease followed over 3 years. *Neurology, 45,* 1451–1455.

Ganguli, M., Dodge, H. H., Shen, C., & DeKosky, S. T. (2004). Mild cognitive impairment, amnestic type: An epidemiologic study. *Neurology, 63*(1), 115–121.

Gauthier, S. (2006). Functional outcomes. In K. Rockwood & S. Gauthier (Eds.), *Trial designs and outcomes: Dementia therapeutic research* (pp. 113–118). London: Taylor & Francis.

Gauthier, S., & MacKnight, C. (2006). Clinical trial designs and endpoint selection. In K. Rockwood & S. Gauthier (Eds.), *Trial designs and outcomes: Dementia therapeutic research* (pp. 37–44). London: Taylor & Francis.

Gauthier, S., Rockwood, K., Gélinas, I., Sykes, L., Teunisse, S., Orgogozo, J. M., et al. (1999). Outcome measures for the study of activities of daily living in vascular dementia. *Alzheimer Disease Association Disorders, 13*(Suppl. 3), S143–S147.

Gélinas, I., & Auer, S. (2001). Functional autonomy. In S. Gauthier (Ed.), *Clinical diagnosis and management of Alzheimer's disease* (2nd ed., pp. 213–226). London: Martin Dunitz.

Gélinas, I., Gauthier, L., McIntyre, M. C., & Gauthier, S. (1999). Development of a functional measure for persons with Alzheimer disease: The Disability Assessment for Dementia. *American Journal of Occupational Therapy, 53*(5), 471–481.

General Accounting Office Report. (1998). *Health, Education, and Human Services Division, Alzheimer's disease prevalence.* January 28.

Geslani, D. M., Tierney, M. C., Herrmann, N., & Szalai, J. P. (2005). Mild cognitive impairment: An operational definition and its conversion rate to Alzheimer's disease. *Dementia and Geriatric Cognitive Disorders, 19*(5–6), 383–389.

Gitlin, L. N., Corcoran, M., Winter, L., Boyce, A., & Hauck, W. W. (2001). A randomized, controlled trial of a home environmental intervention: Effect on efficacy and upset in caregivers and on daily function of persons with dementia. *The Gerontologist, 41*(1), 4–14.

Gitlin, L. N., Winter, L., Dennis, M. P., Corcoran, M., Schinfeld, S., & Hauck, W. W. (2002). Strategies used by families to simplify tasks for individuals with Alzheimer's disease and related disorders: Psychometric analysis of the Task Management Strategy Index (TMSI). *The Gerontologist, 42,* 61–69.

Glosser, G., Gallo, J. L., Clark, C. M., & Grossman, M. (2002). Memory encoding and retrieval in frontotemporal dementia and Alzheimer's disease. *Neuropsychologia, 16*(2), 190–196.

Goldstein, F. C., Ashley, A. V., Gearing, M., Hanfelt, J., Penix, L., Freedman, L. J., et al. (2001). Apolipoprotein E and age at onset of Alzheimer's disease in African American patients. *Neurology, 57*(10), 1923–1925.

Gordon, B., & Carson, K. (1990). The basis for choice reaction-time slowing in Alzheimer's disease. *Brain and Cognition, 13*(2), 148–166.

Gorelick, P. B. (1997). Status of risk factors for dementia associated with stroke. *Stroke, 28*(2), 459–463.

Graves, A. B., White, E., Koepsell, T. D., Reifler, B. V., van Belle, G., Larson, E. B., et al. (1990). A case-control study of Alzheimer's disease. *Annals of Neurology, 28*(6), 766–774.

Green, C. R., Mohs, R. C., Schmeidler, J., Aryan, M., & Davis, K. L. (1993). Functional decline in Alzheimer's disease: A longitudinal study. *Journal of the American Geriatrics Society, 41*(6), 654–661.

Guo, Z., Cupples, L. A., Kurz, A., Auerbach, S. H., Volicer, L., Chui, H., et al. (2000). Head injury and the risk of AD in the MIRAGE study. *Neurology, 54*(6), 1316–1323.

Gwyther, L. P. (1990). Clinician and family. A partnership for support. In N. L. Mace (Ed.), *Dementia care: Patient, family and community* (pp. 193–210). Baltimore: John Hopkins Press.

Gwyther, L. P. (1998). Social issues of the Alzheimer's patient and family. *American Journal of Medicine, 104*(4A), 17S–21S, 39S–42S.

Gwyther, L. P. (2000). Family issues in dementia: Finding a new normal. *Neurologic Clinics, 18*(4), 993–1010.

Hachinksi, V. C., Iliff, L. D., Zilhka, E., Du Boulay, G. H., McAllister, V. L., Marshall, J., et al. (1975). Cerebral blood flow in dementia. *Archives of Neurology, 32*(9), 632–637.

Hachinski, V. C., Lassen, N. A., & Marshall, J. (1974). Multi-infarct dementia: A cause of mental deterioration in the elderly. *Lancet, 2*(7874), 207–209.

Hébert, L. E., Scherr, P. A., Beckett, L. A., Albert, M. S., Pilgrim, D. M., Chown, M. J., et al. (1995). Age-specific incidence of Alzheimer's disease in a community population. *Journal of the American Medical Association, 273*(17), 1354–1359.

Hébert, R., & Brayne, C. (1995). Epidemiology of vascular dementia. *Neuroepidemiology, 14*(5), 240–257.

Henderson, A. S. (1990). Epidemiology of dementia disorders. *Advances in Neurology, 51,* 15–25.

Hendrie, H. C., Osuntokun, B. O., Hall, K. S., Ogunniyi, A. O., Hui, S. L., Unverzagt, F. W., et al. (1995). Prevalence of Alzheimer's disease and dementia in two communities: Nigerian Africans and African Americans. *American Journal of Psychiatry, 152,* 1485–1492.

Hentschel, F., Kreis, M., Damian, M., Krumm, B., & Frölich, L. (2005). The clinical utility of structural neuroimaging with MRI for diagnosis and differential diagnosis of dementia: A memory clinical study. *International Journal of Geriatric Psychiatry, 20*(7), 645–650.

Hershey, L. A., Jaffe, D. F., Greenough, P. G., & Yang, S. L. (1987). Validation of cognitive and functional assessment instruments in vascular dementia. *International Journal of Psychiatry and Medicine, 17*(2), 183–192.

Hertzberg, A., Ekman, S., & Alexsson, K. (2001). Staff activities and behaviours are the source of many feelings: Relatives' interactions and relationships with staff in nursing homes. *Journal of Clinical Nursing, 10,* 380–388.

Heyman, A., Fillenbaum, G., Prosnitz, B., Raiford, K., Burchett, B., & Clark, C. (1991). Estimated prevalence of dementia among elderly black and white community residents. *Archives of Neurology, 48*(6), 594–598.

Heyman, A., Peterson, B., Fillenbaum, G., & Pieper, C. (1996). The Consortium to Establish a Registry for Alzheimer's Disease (CERAD). Part XIV. Demographic and clinical predictors of survival in patients with Alzheimer's disease. *Neurology, 46*(3), 656–660.

Hogan, D. (2006). Inclusion and exclusion criteria. *Trial designs and outcomes in dementia therapeutic research* (pp. 65–74). London: Taylor & Francis.

Holm, A. K., Lepp, M., & Ringsberg, K. C. (2005). Dementia: Involving patients in storytelling—A caring intervention. A pilot study. *Journal of Clinical Nursing, 14*(2), 256–263.

Hutchinson, S. A., & Marshall, M. (2000). Responses of family caregivers and family members with Alzheimer's disease to an activity kit: An ethnographic study. *Journal of Advanced Nursing, 31,* 44–50.

Hux, M. J., O'Brien, B. J., Iskedjian, M., Goeree, R., Gagnon, M., & Gauthier, S. (1998). Relation between severity of Alzheimer's disease and costs of caring. *Canadian Medical Association Journal, 159*(5), 457–465.

Ivory, S. J., Knight, R. G., Longmore, B. E., & Caradoc-Davies, T. (1999). Verbal memory in non-demented patients with idiopathic Parkinson's disease. *Neuropsycholigia, 37*(7), 817–828.

Jorm, A. F., Christensen, H., Korten, A. E., Henderson, A. S., Jacomb, P. A., & MacKinnon, A. (1997). Do cognitive complaints either predict future cognitive decline or reflect past cognitive decline? A longitudinal study of an elderly community sample. *Psychological Medicine, 27*(1), 91–98.

Josephsson, S. (1996). Supporting everyday activities in dementia. *International Psychogeriatrics, 8*(Suppl. 1), 41–44.

Josephsson, S., Bäckman, L., Borell, L., Bernspång, B., & Nygård, L. (1993). Supporting everyday activities in dementia: An intervention study. *International Journal of Geriatric Psychiatry, 8,* 395–400.

Katzman, R. (1993). Education and the prevalence of dementia and Alzheimer's disease. *Neurology, 43*(1), 13–20.

Keefe, J., & Fancey, P. (2000). The care continues: Responsibility for elderly relatives before and after admission to a long term care facility. *Family Relations, 49,* 235–244.

Kennedy, A. M., Newman, S. K., Frackowiak, R. S., Cunningham, V. J., Roques, P., Stevens, J., et al. (1995). Chromosome 14 linked familial Alzheimer's disease. A clinio-pathological study of a single pedigree. *Brain, 118*(Part 1), 185–205.

Kertesz, A., Davidson, W., & Fox, H. (1997). Frontal lobe behavioural inventory: Diagnostic criteria for frontal lobe dementia. *Canadian Journal of Neurological Sciences, 24*(1), 29–36.

Khachaturian, Z. S. (1985). Diagnosis of Alzheimer's disease. *Archives of Neurology,42*(11), 1097–1105.

Kinney, J. M., & Rentz, C. A. (2005). Observed well-being among individuals with dementia: Memories in the Making, an art program, versus other structured activity. *American Journal of Alzheimer's Disease and Other Associated Dementias, 20*(4), 220–227.

Kiresuk, T. J., Lund, S. H., & Larsen, N. E. (1982). Measurement of goal attainment in clinical and health care programs. *Drug Intelligence & Clinical Pharmacy, 16,* 145–153.

Kishka, U., Mandir, A. S., Ghika, J., & Growdon, J. H. (1993). Electrophysiologic detection of extrapyramidal motor signs in Alzheimer's disease. *Neurology, 43* (3 Pt. 1), 500–505.

Klages, J., Fisk, J. D., & Rockwood, K. (2005). APOE genotype, vascular risk factors, memory test performance and the five-year risk of vascular cognitive impairment or Alzheimer's disease. *Dementia and Geriatric Cognitive Disorders, 20*(5), 292–297.

Kokmen, E., Whisnant, J. P., O'Fallon, W. M., Chu, C. P., & Beard, C. M. (1996). Dementia after ischemic stroke: A population-based study in Rochester, Minnesota (1960–1984). *Neurology, 46*(1), 154–159.

Kuzis, G., Sabe, L., Tiberti, C., Merello, A., Leiguarda, R., & Starkstein, S. E. (1999). Explicit and implicit learning in patients with Alzheimer disease and Parkinson disease with dementia. *Neuropsychiatry Neuropsychology and Behavioural Neurology, 1*(7), 265–269.

Lamar, M., Podell, K., Carew, T. G., Cloud, B. S., Resh, R., Kennedy, C., et al. (1997). Perseverative behaviour in Alzheimer's disease and subcortical ischaemic vascular dementia. *Neuropsychologia, 11,* 523–534.

Larrea, F. A., Fisk, J. D., Graham, J. E., & Stadnyk, K. (2000). The prevalence of cognitive impairment and dementia as defined by neuropsychological test performance. *Neuroepidemiology, 19,* 121–129.

Lee, H., & Cameron, M. M. (2004). Respite care for people with dementia and their carers. *The Cochrane Database of Systematic Reviews,* Issue 1. Art. No.: CD004396. DOI: 10.1002/14651858.CD004396.

Lehnfeld, H., & Erzigkeit, H. (2000). Functional aspects of dementia. In S. Gauthier & J. L. Cummings (Eds.), *Alzheimer's disease and related disorders annual* (pp. 155–178). London: Martin Dunitz.

Leon, J., Cheng, C. K., & Neumann, P. J. (1998). Alzheimer's disease care: Costs and potential savings. *Health Affairs (Millwood), 17,* 206–216.

Lepp, M., Ringsberg, K. C., Holm, A. K., & Sellersjo, G. (2003). Dementia—involving patients and their caregivers in a drama programme: The caregivers' experiences. *Journal of Clinical Nursing, 12,* 873–881.

Levy-Lahad, E., Lahad, A., Wijsman, E. M., Bird, T. D., & Schellenberg, G. D. (1995). Apolipoprotein E genotypes and age of onset in early-onset familial Alzheimer's disease. *Annals of Neurology, 38*(4), 678–680.

Lezak, M. D., Howieson, D. B., & Loring, D. W. (2004). *Neuropsychological assessment* (4th ed.). Oxford; New York: Oxford University Press.

Light, E., Niederehe, G., & Lebowitz, B. D. (1994). *Stress effects on family caregivers of Alzheimer's patients: Research and interventions.* New York: Springer.

Lindeboom, R., Vermeulen, M., Holman, R., & DeHaan, R. J. (2003). Activities of daily living instruments. Optimizing scales for neurologic assessments. *Neurology, 60*(5), 738–742.

Lipowski, Z. J. (1989). Delirium in the elderly patient. *New England Journal of Medicine, 320*(9), 578–582.

Lopez, O. L., Becker, J. T., Sweet, R. A., Klunk, W., Kaufer, D. I., Saxton, J., et al. (2003). Psychiatric symptoms vary with the severity of dementia in probable Alzheimer's disease. *Journal of Neuropsychiatry and Clinical Neurosciences, 15*(3), 346–353.

Lundberg, C., Johansson, K., Ball, K., Bjerre, B. Blomqvist, C., Braekhus, A. et al. (1997). Dementia and driving: An attempt at consensus. *Alzheimer Disease and Associated Disorders, 11*(1), 28–37.

Lye, T. C., & Shores, E. A. (2000). Traumatic brain injury as a risk for Alzheimer's disease. A review. *Neuropsychological Review, 10*(2), 115–129.

Mackenzie, L., Byles, J., & Higginbotham, N. (2000). Designing the Home Falls and Accidents Screening Tool (HOME FAST): Selecting the items. *British Journal of Occupational Therapy, 63,* 260–269.

Maheu, S., & Cohen, C. A. (1999). Support of families. In S. Gauthier (Ed.), *Clinical diagnosis and management of Alzheimer's disease* (2nd ed.) (pp. 307–318). London: Martin Dunitz.

Mahurin, R. K., & Pirozzolo, F. J. (1993). Application of Hick's law of response speed in Alzheimer and Parkinson diseases. *Perceptual and Motor Skills, 77*(1), 107–113.

Mann, U. M., Mohr, E., Gearing, M., & Chase, T. N. (1992). Heterogeneity in AD: Progression rate segregated by distinct neuropsychological and cerebral metabolic profiles. *Journal of Neurology, Neurosurgery, and Psychiatry, 55*(10), 956–1050.

Martin-Cook, K., Davis, B. A., Hynan, L. S., & Weiner, M. F. (2005). A randomized, controlled study of an Alzheimer's caregiver skills training program. *American Journal of Alzheimer's Disease and Other Dementias, 20*(4), 204–210.

McKeith, I. G., Dickson, D. W., Lowe, J., Emre, M., O'Brien, J. T., Feldman, H., et al. (2005). Diagnosis and management of dementia with Lewy bodies: Third report of the DLB Consortium. *Neurology, 65,* 1863–1872.

McKeith, I. G., O'Brien, J. T., & Ballard, C. (1999). Diagnosing dementia with Lewy Bodies. *Lancet, 354*(9186), 1227–1228.

McKhann, G., Drachman, D., Folstein, M., Katzman, R., Price, D., & Stadlan, E. M. (1984). Clinical diagnosis of Alzheimer's disease: Report of the NINCDS-ADRDA work group under the auspices of the Department of Health and Human Services Task Force on Alzheimer's disease. *Neurology, 34*(7), 939–944.

McMonagle, P., Deering, F., Berliner, Y., & Kertesz, A. (2006). The cognitive profile of posterior cortical atrophy. *Neurology, 66*(3), 331–338.

Mendez, M. F., & Cummings, J. L. (2003). *Dementia: A clinical approach* (3rd ed.). Philadelphia, PA: Butterworth-Heinemann (Elsevier).

Mendez, M. F., Underwood, K. L., Zander, B. A., Mastri, A. R., Sung, J. H., & Frey, W. H., 2nd. (1992). Risk factors in Alzheimer's disease: A clinicopathologic study. *Neurology, 42*(4), 770–775.

Miller Fisher, C. (1968). Dementia in cerebrovascular disease. In J. F. Toole, R. G. Kiekert, & J. P. Whisnant (Eds.), *Cerebral vascular diseases* (pp. 232–236). New York: Grune and Stratton.

Mirra, S. S., Heyman, A., McKeel, D., Sumi, S. M., Crain, B. J., Brownlee, L. M., et al. (1991). The Consortium to Establish a Registry for Alzheimer's Disease (CERAD). Part II. Standardization of the neuropathologic assessment of Alzheimer's disease. *Neurology, 41*(4), 497–486.

Mittelman, M. S., Ferris, S. H., Shulman, E., Steinberg, G., & Levin, B. (1996). A family intervention to delay nursing home placement of patients with Alzheimer's disease. A randomized controlled trial. *Journal of the American Medical Association, 276*(21), 1725–1731.

Mohs, R. C., Doody, R. S., Morris, J. C., Ieni, J.R., Rogers, S.L., Perdomo CA, et al. (2001). A 1-year, placebo-controlled preservation of function survival study of donepezil in AD patients. *Neurology, 57,* 481–488.

Morris, J. C. (2006). Mild cognitive impairment is early-stage Alzheimer disease: Time to revise diagnostic criteria. *Archives of Neurology, 63*(1), 15–16.

Munoz, D. G. (2003). Histopathology. In J. V. Bowler, & V. Hachinski (Eds.), *Vascular cognitive impairment: Preventable dementia* (pp. 57–75). Oxford, New York: Oxford University Press.

Neary, D., Snowden, J. S., Gustafson, L., Passant, U., Stuss, D., Black, S., et al. (1998). Frontotemporal lobar degeneration: A consensus on clinical diagnostic criteria. *Neurology, 51*(6), 1546–1554.

Nestor, P. J., Graham, K. S., Bozeat, S., Simons, J. S., & Hodges, J. R. (2002). Memory consolidation and the hippocampus: Further evidence from studies of autobiographical memory in semantic dementia and frontal variant frontotemporal dementia. *Neuropsychologia, 40*(6), 633–654.

Newell, K. L., Hyman, B. T., Growdon, J. H., & Hedley-Whyte, E. T. (1999). Application of the National Institute on Aging (NIA)—Reagan Institute criteria for the neuropathological diagnosis of Alzheimer disease. *Journal of Neuropathology and Experimental Neurology, 58*(11), 1147–1155.

Noe, E., Marder, K., Bell, K. L., Jacobs, D. M., Manly, J. J., & Stern, Y. (2004). Comparison of dementia with Lewy bodies to Alzheimer's disease and Parkinson's disease with dementia. *Movement Disorders, 19*(1), 60–67.

Nyenhuis, D. L., & Gorelick, P. B. (1998). Vascular dementia: A contemporary review of epidemiology, diagnosis, prevention, and treatment. *Journal of the American Geriatrics Society, 46,* 1437–1448.

Nyenhuis, D. L., Gorelick, P. B., Freels, S., & Garron, D. C. (2002). Cognitive and functional decline in African Americans with VaD, AD, and stroke without dementia. *Neurology, 8*(11), 56–61.

Oliver, R., Bathwayt, J., Brackley, C., & Tamaki, T. (1993). Development of the Safety Assessment of Function and the Environment for Rehabilitation (SAFER) tool. *Canadian Journal of Occupational Therapy, 60,* 78–82.

Ory, M. G., Hoffman, R. R., Yee, J. L., Tennstedt, S., & Schulz, R. (1999). Prevalence and impact of caregiving: A detailed comparison between dementia and nondementia caregivers. *The Gerontologist, 39,* 177–185.

Ostbye, T., & Cross, E. (1994). Economic costs of dementia in Canada. *Canadian Medical Association Journal, 51*(10), 1457–1464.

Pasquier, F., & Delacourte, A. (1998). Non-Alzheimer degenerative dementias. *Current Opinions in Neurology, 11*(5), 417–427.

Pasquier, F., Grymonprez, L., Lebert, F., & Van der Linden, M. (2001). Memory impairment differs in frontotemporal dementia and Alzheimer's disease. *Neurocase, 17*(2), 161–171.

Peavy, G. M., Salmon, D., Bear, P. I., Paulsen, J. S., Cahn, D. A., Hofstetter, C. R. et al. (2001). Detection of mild cognitive deficits in Parkinson's disease patients with the WAIS-R NI. *Journal of the International Neuropsychological Society, 7*(5), 535–543.

Petersen, R. C., Smith, G. E., Waring, S. C., Ivnik, R. J., Tangalos, E. G., & Kokmen, E. (1999). Mild cognitive impairment: Clinical characterization and outcome. *Archives of Neurology, 56*(3), 303–308.

Plassman, B. L., Havlik, R. J., Steffens, D. C., Helms, Newman, Drosdick, et al. (2000). Documented head injury in early adulthood and risk of Alzheimer's disease and other dementias. *Neurology, 55*(8), 1158–1166.

Portin, R., Laatu, S., Revonsuo, A., & Rinne, U. K. (2000). Impairment of semantic knowledge in Parkinson disease. *Archives of Neurology, 57*(9), 1338–1343.

Poulin de Courval, L., Gélinas, I., Gauthier, S., Gayton, D., Liu, L., Rossignol, M., et al. (2006). Reliability and validity of the Safety Assessment Scale for people with dementia living at home. *Canadian Journal of Occupational Therapy, 73*(2), 67–75.

Reed, B. R., Jagust, W. J., & Seab, J. P. (1989). Mental status as a predictor of daily function in progressive dementia. *The Gerontologist, 29*(6), 804–807.

Reimer, M. A., Slaughter, S., Donaldson, C., Currie, G., & Eliasziw, M. (2004). Special care facility compared with traditional environments for dementia care: A longitudinal study of quality of life. *Journal of the American Geriatrics Society, 52*(7), 1085–1092.

Reisberg, B. (1988). Functional assessment staging (FAST). *Psychopharmacology Bulletin, 24*(4), 653–659.

Robinson, K. M. (1997). The family's role in long-term care. *Journal of Gerontological Nursing, 23*(9), 7–11.

Robinson, S. E., & Fisher, A. G. (1996). A study to examine the relationship of the Assessment of Motor and Process Skills (AMPS) to other tests of cognition and function. *British Journal of Occupational Therapy, 47,* 298–301.

Rockwood, K., Brown, M., & Fisk, J. D. (2003). The cost of vascular cognitive impairment. In J. V. Bowler & V. Hachinski (Eds.), *Vascular cognitive impairment: Preventable dementia* (pp. 51–56). Oxford: Oxford University Press.

Rockwood, K., Ebly, E., Hachinsky, V., & Hogan, D. (1997). Presence and treatment of vascular risk factors in patients with vascular cognitive impairment. *Archives of Neurology, 54*(1), 33–39.

Rockwood, K., Graham, J. E., & Fay, S. Goal setting and attainment in Alzheimer's disease patients treatment with donepezil. (2002). *Journal of Neurology, Neurosurgery and Psychiatry, 73*(5), 500–507.

Rockwood, K., & MacKnight, C. (2001). *A primer of diagnosis and management: Understanding dementia.* Halifax: Pottersfield Press.

Rockwood, K., MacKnight, C., Wentzel, C., Black, S., Bouchard, R., Gauthier, S., et al. (2000). The diagnosis of "mixed" dementia in the Consortium of the Investigation of Vascular Impairment of Cognition (CIVIC).

Annals of New York Academy of Sciences, 903, 522–528.

Rockwood, K., Wallack, M., & Tallis, R. (2003). Treatment of Alzheimer's disease: Understanding success short of cure. *Lancet Neurology, 2*(10), 630–633.

Roman, G. C., & Royall, D. R. (2004). A diagnostic dilemma: Is "Alzheimer's dementia" Alzheimer's disease, vascular dementia, or both? *Lancet Neurology, 3*(3), 141.

Roman, G. C., Tatemichi, T. K., Erkinjuntti, T., Cummings, J. L., Masdeu, J. C., Garcia, J. H., et al. (1993). Vascular dementia: Diagnostic criteria for research studies. Report of the NINDS-AIREN international workshop. *Neurology, 43*(3), 250–260.

Roth, M., Tym, E., Mountjoy, C. Q., Huppert, F. A., Hendrie, H., Verma, S., et al. (1986). CAMDEX: A standardized instrument for the diagnosis of mental disorder in the elderly with special reference to the early detection of dementia. *British Journal of Psychiatry, 149,* 698–709.

Sawamoto, N., Honda, M., Hanakawa, T., Fukuyama, H., & Shibasaki, H. (2002). Cognitive slowing in Parkinson's disease: A behavioural evaluation independent of motor slowing. *Journal of Neurosciences, 22*(12), 5198–5520.

Sclan, S. G., & Reisberg, B. (1992). Functional assessment staging (FAST) in Alzheimer's disease: Reliability, validity, and ordinality. *International Psychogeriatrics, 4,* 55–69.

Schulz, R., O'Brien, A. T., Bookwala, J., & Fleissner, K. (1995). Psychiatric and physical morbidity effects of dementia caregiving: Prevalence, correlates and causes. *The Gerontologist, 35*(6), 771–791.

Shumaker, S. A., Legault, C., Rapp, S. R., Thal, L., Wallace, R. B., Ockene, J. K., et al. (2004). Estrogen plus progestin and the incidence of dementia and mild cognitive impairment in postmenopausal women: The women's Health Initiative Memory Study: A randomized controlled trial. *Journal of the American Medical Association, 289*(20), 2651–2662.

Skoog, I. (1998). Status of risk factors for vascular dementia. *Neuroepidemiology, 17*(1), 2–9.

Small, J. A., Gutman, G., Makela, S., & Hillhouse, B. (2003). Effectiveness of communication strategies used by caregivers of persons with Alzheimer's disease during activities of daily living. *Journal of Speech, Language and Hearing Research, 46*(2), 353–367.

Small, J. A., & Perry, J. (2005). Do you remember? How caregivers question their spouses who have Alzheimer's disease and the impact on communication. *Journal of Speech, Language and Hearing Research, 48*(1), 125–136.

Small, J. A., Perry, J., & Lewis, J. (2005). Perceptions of family caregivers' psychosocial behavior when communicating with spouses who have Alzheimer's disease. *American Journal of Alzheimers Disease and Other Dementias, 205,* 281–289.

Spiegel, R., Brunner, C., Ermini-Fünfschilling, D., Monsch, A., Notter, M., Puxty, J., et al. (1991). A new behavioural assessment scale for geriatric out- and

in-patients: The NOSGER (Nurses' Observation Scale for Geriatric Patients). *Journal of the American Geriatrics Society, 39,* 339–347.

Stern, Y., Hesdorffer, D., Sano, M., & Mayeux, R. (1990). Measurement and prediction of functional capacity in Alzheimer's disease. *Neurology, 40*(1), 8–14.

Teri, L., Borson, S., Kiyak, H. A., & Hamagishi, M. (1989). Behavioral disturbance, cognitive dysfunction and functional skill. Prevalence and relationship in Alzheimer's disease. *Journal of the American Geriatrics Society, 37*(2), 109–116.

Teri, L., Larson, E. B., & Reifler, B. V. (1988). Behavioral disturbance in dementia of the Alzheimer's type. *Journal of the American Geriatrics Society, 36*(1), 1–6.

Teri, L., & Logsdon, R. G. (1991). Identifying pleasant activities for Alzheimer's disease patients: The Pleasant Events Schedule-AD. *The Gerontologist, 31*(1), 124–127.

Teunisse, S., Derix, M. M., & van Crevel, H. (1991). Assessing the severity of dementia. Patient and caregiver. *Archives of Neurology, 48*(3), 274–277.

The National Institute on Aging and Reagan Institute Working Group on Diagnostic Criteria for the Neuropathological Assessment of Alzheimer's Disease. (1997). Consensus recommendations for the postmortem diagnosis of Alzheimer's disease. *Neurobiology of Aging, 18*(4 Suppl.), S1–S2.

Tomlinson, B. E., Blessed, G., & Roth, M. (1970). Observations on the brains of demented old people. *Journal of Neurological Sciences, 11*(3), 205–242.

Traykov, L., Rigaud, A. S., Caputo, L., Couderc, R., Coste, J., Michot, J. L., et al. (1999). Apolipoprotein E phenotypes in demented and cognitively impaired patients with and without cerebrovascular disease. *European Journal of Neurology, 6*(4), 415–421.

van Duijn, C. M., Clayton, D. G., Chandra, V., Fratiglioni, L., Graves, A. B., Heyman, A., et al. (1994). Interaction between genetic and environmental risk factors for Alzheimer's disease: A reanalysis of case-control studies. EURODEM Risk Factors Research Group. *Genetic Epidemiology, 11*(6), 539–551.

Vink, A. C., Birks, J. S., Bruinsma, M. S., & Scholten, R. J. (2004). Music therapy for people with dementia. *Cochrane Database Systematic Review, 3,* CD003477.

Vinters, H. V., Ellis, W. G., Zarow, C., Zaias, B. W., Jagust, W. J., Mack, W. J., et al. (2000). Neuropathologic substrates of ischemic vascular dementia. *Journal of Neuropathology and Experimental Neurology, 59*(11), 931–945.

Visser, P. J., Verhey, F. R., Ponds, R. W., Kesker, A., Jolles, J. (2000). Distinction between preclinical Alzheimer's disease and depression. *Journal of the American Geriatric Society, 48*(5), 479–484.

Whitehouse, P. (2006). The history of therapeutic trials in dementia. *Trial designs and outcomes in dementia therapeutic research* (pp. 11–24). London: Taylor & Francis.

Wilkinson, D., Doody, R., Helme, R., Taubman, K., Mintzer, J., Kertesz, A., et al. (2003). Donepezil in vascular dementia: A randomized placebo-controlled study. *Neurology, 61*(4), 479–486.

Wolfe, N., Linn, R., Babikian, V. L., Knoefel, J. E., & Albert, M. L. (1990). Frontal systems impairment following multiple lacunar infarcts. *Archives of Neurology, 47*(2), 129–132.

Woods, B., Spector, A., Jones, C., Orrell, M., & Davies, S. (2005). Reminiscence therapy for dementia. *The Cochrane Database of Systematic Reviews,* Issue 2. Art. No.: CD001120. DOI: 10.1002/14651858. CD001120.

World Health Organization. (1989). *International classification of diseases* (10th revised ed.). Geneva, Switzerland: World Health Organization.

Zakzanis, K. K., & Freedman, M. (1999). A neuropsychological comparison of demented and undemented patients with Parkinson's disease. *Applied Neuropsychology, 6*(3), 129–146.

CHAPTER 10

Depression

Kathryn Perez Riley, PhD

*In the middle of the journey of our life I found myself
in a dark wood, For I had lost the right path.*

Dante Alighieri,
The Divine Comedy, Inferno, canto I, I.1, circa 1310–1320

OBJECTIVES

By the end of this chapter, the reader will be able to:

1. Compare and contrast the symptoms and manifestations of depression in older adults, including major depressive disorder, subsyndromal depression, and dementia syndrome of depression.
2. Discuss assessment and evaluation of depressive and suicidal symptoms in older adults.
3. Discuss the relationship between depression and functional abilities in older adults.
4. Identify special factors in depression in special populations, including persons who are physically ill, diagnosed with a dementing disorder, or institutionalized, as well as caregivers.
5. Describe the major methods of treating depression through prevention, psychotherapy, medications, and electroconvulsive therapy (ECT).

Depression in older adults is often seen as a normal part of aging or as a reaction to the stressors and losses that most people associate with growing old. In fact, as this chapter shows, most elderly individuals do not ever experience a clinically significant depression, and when they do, it is rarely simply a result of the normative life events encountered during aging.

For those older adults who do become depressed, early diagnosis and treatment are essential. Depressive disorders are as treatable in the old as in the young, but when they are left undetected or untreated, they can lead to functional impairments and excess disabilities, lost jobs and relationships, institutionalization, and death.

This chapter includes an overview of the prevalence, symptoms, and detection of depressive syndromes in older adults; a discussion of the relationship between depression and social and daily function; and a review of major treatment options for depressed older adults.

Overview of Depressive Disorders in Older Adults

The term "depressive disorder" refers to the clinical symptoms listed in most diagnostic manuals as major depressive episode and dysthymic disorder. In addition, less severe or subclinical depressive syndromes are included here because they are frequently seen in older adults (Delano-Wood & Abeles, 2005; Djernes, 2006; Storandt & Van den Bos, 1994; Zarit & Zarit, 1998). Depression may present itself in a number of forms among older adults, including the traditional or formal depressive disorders, masked depression, subsyndromal or minor depression (Lyness et al., 2006), and depression with cognitive deficits, often referred to as the dementia syndrome of depression (Ganguli, Du, Dodge, Ratcliff, & Chang, 2006; Baldwin, 2002; Kaszniak & Christenson, 1994).

Traditional Depressive Disorders

The traditional symptoms of depression as described in the *Diagnostic and Statistical Manual of Mental Disorders* (*DSM-IV-TR*) (American Psychiatric Association, 2000) include the following:

- Depressed or sad mood
- Decreased interest of pleasure in activities
- Feelings of excessive guilt or worthlessness
- Apathy or lack of motivation
- Change (increase or decrease) in sleep, appetite, weight, energy, sexual desire
- Decline in attention, concentration, memory
- Thoughts of death or suicide

The criteria for a diagnosis of major depressive disorder include the presence of at least five of the symptoms listed earlier, presence of these symptoms for at least 2 weeks, and clinically significant distress or impairment in daily functioning. In many studies, this diagnosis may be referred to as a "clinically significant depressive disorder" (Djernes, 2006; Girling et al., 1995).

Dysthymic disorder is a less severe form of depression in which the symptoms have lasted for at least 2 years. Related to, but less chronic than, dysthymic disorders, it is a recurrent or transient pattern of depressive symptoms that older adults (like younger persons) may experience in response to stress, life events, loss (Fry, 1986), or physical illness (Harman, Edlund, Fortney, & Kallas, 2005; Norton et al., 2006). The terms "subsyndromal" or "minor depression" may be used interchangeably with dysthymic disorder. These conditions include complaints of symptoms such as insomnia, lack

of energy, anxiety, and feelings of sadness. These symptoms may cause significant levels of distress for the older adult and have warranted increased study in recent years (Elderkin-Thompson et al., 2003; Norton et al., 2006; Janzing, Naarding, & Eling, 2005; Lyness et al., 2006).

Depression is the most common psychiatric syndrome in older adults, both in the community and in institutions (Djernes, 2006; Norton et al., 2006; Smit, Ederveen, Cuijpers, Deeg, & Beekman, 2006). Most researchers conclude that although the prevalence rates of the most serious form of depression, major depressive disorder, are relatively low in older adults, there are high rates of **subsyndromal depression,** which is defined as a pattern of depressive symptoms that are not severe or pervasive enough to meet the diagnostic criteria for a depressive disorder. Estimates of prevalence vary, depending on the nature of the diagnostic tools used to define depression (Friedman, Heisel, & Delavan, 2005a; Hammond, O'Keefe, & Barer, 2000; Reynolds, Alexopolous, Katz, & Lebowitz, 2001). Rates vary from 1% to 5% for the diagnosis of major depressive disorder among community-dwelling adults older than the age of 65, but when all types of depressive disorders and syndromes are included, prevalence rates may be as high as 20% to 25% for community-dwelling older adults. The prevalence rates of major depressive disorder and other syndromes are higher for older adults who are medically ill or institutionalized (Djernes, 2006; Mulsant & Ganguli, 1999; Reynolds et al., 2001).

Variations in Patterns of Depressive Symptoms

Some of the symptoms of depression may be more prominent than others in older individuals. For example, themes of loss and hopelessness related to perceived and real losses are commonly seen in older individuals. Although hopelessness and perceived losses are also present among the depressive symptoms of young people, these symptoms may be more reality based in an older adult who in fact has little chance of replacing or restoring that which he or she has valued and lost, such as a spouse of 50 years or the occupational achievements of years past (Riley & Carr, 1989). Apathy, withdrawal, self-depreciating behavior, and slowing of cognitive and motor processes (**psychomotor retardation**) also may be prominent features of depression in older adults.

It is often difficult to determine when an older adult is suffering from a depressive disorder that should be treated, as opposed to an understandable reaction to bereavement, poor health, poverty and deprivation, or other cumulative losses that can come with advancing age. There are dangers in erring in either direction of misdiagnosis (Greenglass, Fiskenbaum, & Eaton, 2006; Reynolds et al., 2001; Ritchie, Touchon, & Ledesert, 1998; Zarit, Todd, & Zarit, 1986). If one determines that a merely distressed or unhappy individual is clinically depressed, unnecessary interventions may be instituted, with accompanying side effects and negative outcomes. On the other hand, the failure to detect and treat a depressive disorder can lead to extremely negative outcomes of excess functional disability, deterioration of physical health, and suicide (Conwell, Duberstein, & Caine, 2002). Well-designed assessment procedures used by trained individuals can prevent the overdiagnosis and inappropriate treatment of depression in older adults.

Grief reactions in older adults can sometimes appear indistinguishable from a depressive disorder, especially in older adults who have lost a spouse after decades of marriage. Increasing numbers of older adults are experiencing the death of an adult child, and these losses, as well as the deaths of close friends, all can lead to significant periods of mourning that may last for a year or longer. Hospice programs around the country offer support groups and counseling for grieving persons, which can aid in establishing a healthy grieving process. Professionals who run such support groups are often in the best position to determine if the grief reaction has led to a depressive disorder that requires medication or more intensive psychotherapy. More information about the grieving process and about the role of occupational therapy in working with people who are mourning can be found in Chapter 26.

There are a number of depression scales available (see "Web-Based Resource" section at the end of this chapter), and researchers have offered guidelines for the appropriate use of several of the better measures with older individuals (Carrete et al., 2001; Friedman, Heisel, & Delavan, 2005b; Fujisawa et al., 2005; Nguyen & Zonderman, 2006; Thompson et al., 1988). When these measures are used in conjunction with the criteria outlined in *DSM-IV-TR* (APA, 2000), mildly unhappy or temporarily distressed older adults will not meet all of the criteria for a depressive disorder, and those individuals who are clinically depressed will receive the appropriate diagnosis and can be referred for treatment.

Atypical Depression

Although it has been demonstrated that many depressed elderly do exhibit traditional symptoms and complaints, it also has been observed that older individuals may present only with symptoms of physical illness, without the expected emotional, cognitive, and behavioral manifestations of depression. This type of depressive illness has been called *somatic,* or *atypical,* depression (Baldwin, 2002; Smit, Ederveen, Cuijpers, Deeg, & Beekman, 2006). In this form of depression, the older adult is likely to complain about changes in sleep, appetite, weight, energy levels, and sexual functioning. However, when the elderly person presents with these symptoms, he or she may not be as likely to discuss feeling sad, blue, unhappy, or hopeless. Instead, additional complaints of physical dysfunction will be listed, including diffuse or localized pain, headaches, gastrointestinal upset, constipation, breathing problems, and other vague discomforts.

This form of depression is most likely to be seen in individuals who have their first depressive episode after the age of 65. If detected, these late-onset depressions respond well to treatment. However, older adults are likely to seek help from a family physician rather than a mental health professional even when they are experiencing emotional difficulties. This makes diagnosis of a masked or hidden depression more difficult, because the individual is presenting a medical professional with symptoms of physical illness, without any indication of psychological distress (Norton et al., 2006).

As primary care physicians receive more information about mental health needs of older adults and increased numbers of geriatric specialists are trained, misdiagnosis may become less likely. The emergence of multidisciplinary geriatric assessment centers has also resulted in better evaluation and treatment of psychiatric disorders in older adults. Nevertheless, the number of depressed older individuals who actually receive treatment may be as low as one in ten (Crabb & Hunsley, 2006; Harman et al., 2005;

Lawrence et al., 2006; Tai-Seale et al., 2005). This very low proportion of treated depression in late life points to the need for further education of professionals and laypersons.

Suicide

If the depressive illness of an older adult is dismissed as a "normal" reaction to growing old, there is a risk of increased disability, desperation, and death through passive or active suicide. Untreated depression can lead to a number of negative consequences, the most serious of which is, of course, an attempted or completed suicide (Dombrovski, Szanto, & Reynolds, 2005; Oyama et al., 2006; Reynolds et al., 2001; Yen et al., 2005). The risk of suicide in older adults is estimated as being nearly three times greater than the risk in younger persons (Friedman, Conwell, Delavan, Wamsley, & Eggert, 2005; Fry, 1986). Persons older than the age of 65 account for a disproportionately high number of suicides. This increased rate is partially due to older males (NIMH website, 2006), for whom the incidence of suicide peaks at the 80-years to 85-years age bracket. A slight decline in suicide rates is seen in women after the age of 65, although the risk remains significant. Older adults are more likely to be serious about their suicide attempts, with the ratio of attempts to completed suicides as high as 2 to 1. Older adults are also at risk for passive or indirect suicide. Passive suicide behaviors include refusing necessary medical treatments and surgeries, failing to take medications, failing to follow prescribed diet regimens, and refusing to eat. There are a number of clues and risk factors that may identify an individual who is at relatively high risk for suicide:

- The presence of depression
- Medical illness
- Intense feelings of hopelessness
- Single or widowed status
- Recent loss of a loved one
- Previous psychiatric illness or alcohol or drug abuse
- Previous suicide attempts or threats
- Diagnosis of terminal illness in self or spouse

A combination of these factors may lead the older adult to suicide, and all threats must be taken very seriously (Ganguli et al., 2006). Indirect references such as talk of wishing one were dead or feelings of being tired of living should

also be explored as potential indicators of suicidal intent. Not all individuals who commit suicide are recognizably depressed. Their suicide attempts or actions may be a deliberate and planned response to the diagnosis of a terminal illness or to the death of a spouse. Professionals need to be alert to all of the direct and oblique warning signs and signals of suicide intent in older adults in order to provide appropriate and effective interventions. Occupational therapists should immediately confer with their supervisor and client's physician if they have reason to believe their client is suicidal.

Depression and Cognitive Deficits

Reports of impaired cognitive function and memory occur in a significant proportion of depressed older adults. (Barnes, Alexopolous, Lopez, Williamson, & Yaffe, 2006; Burt, Zembar, & Niederehe, 1995; Ganguli et al., 2006). These complaints can outweigh the more traditional complaints of sadness or other symptoms included in the diagnosis of a depressive disorder. Many terms have been used to describe this pattern of reports, including **pseudodementia** (Wells, 1979), cognitive deficits of depression, and the dementia syndrome of depression (Folstein & McHugh, 1978). Individuals who exhibit this symptom pattern, like those with masked depression, may seek help for a condition that they believe is medical rather than psychological. This can lead to an inaccurate diagnosis of a dementing illness, such as Alzheimer's disease, resulting in inappropriate and ineffective interventions. Alternatively, the reports of poor concentration, memory, and other cognitive abilities may be dismissed as a normal part of the aging process, again leaving the depressive illness undetected and untreated (Elderkin-Thompson et al., 2003; O'Boyle, Amadeo, & Self, 1990). See Table 10-1 for the differences between depression and dementia.

Data on the differential diagnosis of depression from dementia (Kaszniak & Christenson, 1994; Holtzer et al., 2005) show that although attention, motivation, and initial learning curves may be impaired in depressed older adults, formal testing reveals the deficits to be limited in duration, severity, and variety when compared with the cognitive deficits seen in true dementia. The additional deficits in language, memory, perception, and problem solving seen

TABLE 10-1 **Differences Between Depression and Dementia**

Dementia	Depression
Generally, a gradual onset of cognitive impairments, over a period of years	Generally has a more sudden onset that coincides with onset of depressive symptoms
Limited awareness or reports of memory impairment	Many reports of memory impairment
Definite and global impairments seen in neuropsychological testing	Impairments more limited in scope and severity seen in testing results
Cognitive impairments become progressively worse with time	Reports of cognitive impairment generally do not become severe and will lift when depression is treated

in dementia (see Chapter 7) are not typically seen in depression. Furthermore, it is fairly clear that although dementia has a slow and insidious onset, the depressed person's cognitive impairments often have a sudden or easily identifiable onset. Although there may be a strong relationship between cognitive complaints and depression scale scores of depressed elderly patients, only minor correlations have been found between the depressed patients' cognitive complaints and scores on a mental status exam (O'Boyle et al., 1990).

A final distinction between a brain-based dementia and cognitive deficits associated with depression is the fact that although some cognitive changes do occur with depression, the older individual's complaints and distress concerning these changes can far outweigh the actual dysfunction seen in daily life functioning and on neuropsychological testing. In contrast, the truly demented individual is more likely to minimize or be unaware of his or her cognitive deficits in spite of actual dysfunction. The accurate differential diagnosis of the dementia syndrome of depression can be challenging and is crucial for the long-term well-being of the older adult. See Box 10-1 for the types and subtypes of depressive disorders.

BOX 10-1 **Types and Subtypes of Depressive Disorders**

- Major depressive disorder
  - Traditional
  - Masked
  - Dementia syndrome of depression
- Dysthymic disorder
- Subsyndromal or minor depression

The preceding discussion provided a very brief summary of a large body of literature. As has been shown, depression may be manifested in a variety of traditional and atypical forms in older adults, making accurate diagnosis and treatment problematic. Additional difficulties are created by the reluctance of older adults to seek help from mental health professionals and by the older adults' unfamiliarity with or inability to recognize signs and symptoms of emotional distress. Finally, the shortage of mental health professionals who specialize in geriatrics compounds the problem of inadequate treatment of depressive disorders in older adults, although this situation is improving.

Depression and Functional Status: An Interactive Relationship

Depressive syndromes present a significant threat to the well-being and life satisfaction of a substantial number of older adults. Impaired social, occupational, and interpersonal functioning are integral components of most clinically significant depressive disorders (APA, 2000). This dysfunction in daily activities can be severe enough to result in total withdrawal, isolation, and inability to care for even the most basic of personal needs. The following sections of this chapter examine this critical link between depression and daily functioning in several subgroups of older adults.

Research on functional status in older persons with depression has focused on activities of daily living (ADL), social and interpersonal activities, and recreational or leisure activities

(Djernes, 2006; Greenglass, Fiskenbaum, & Eaton, 2006; Smit et al., 2006). The literature leads to two conclusions: First, there is a negative relationship between depressive symptoms and activities of almost any kind. Second, although depression can lead to impaired function, deficits in functional abilities may also lead to depression.

Thus, decreases in daily activities are related to symptoms of depressed mood in older adults. This may be the result of lack of access to pleasurable or instrumental activities, lack of ability to engage in these activities due to physical or mental deficits, or lack of motivation. There is evidence that occupational therapy to increase occupational engagement can reduce the incidence of depression (Clark et al., 1997), and that occupational therapy interventions focused on providing meaningful occupations can ameliorate depressive symptoms.

A clearer understanding of the reasons for severe depression in older adults may result from an examination of depression in physically ill, demented, institutionalized, and other groups of older adults.

Physical Illness and Depression

It is clear that depression and medical illness commonly coexist in older adults (Harman et al., 2005; Whooley, Stone, & Soghikian, 2000). The kinds of activities that may be affected by depression and illness are quite varied but can be grouped into ADL, instrumental activities of daily living (IADL), vocational activities, and social and recreational activities (Crabb & Hunsley, 2006; Doan and Wadden, 1989; Dombrovski et al., 2005; Hunkeler et al., 2006; Lawrence et al., 2006).

Berkman and her colleagues (1986) examined the relationship between physical health, depressive symptoms, and functioning in the elderly population. They found a strong, although not causal, relationship between functional disability and symptoms of depression. In some cases, functional impairment may be more strongly associated with higher rates of depression than the actual medical illness.

Some researchers have suggested that a causal pattern may involve a medical condition leading to a depressive reaction which, in turn, leads to functional disability. Depression may prevent individuals from seeking or following through on rehabilitation and other services,

resulting in additional functional disability (Cacioppo, Hughes, Waite, Hawkley, & Thisted, 2006; Holtzer et al., 2005; Motl et al., 2005). For example, Doan and Wadden (1989) found significant levels of depression in a sample of patients with chronic pain from headaches, arthritis, and back pain, with depression proving to be a better predictor of functional limitation in daily activities than the amount of perceived pain. Symptoms of depression are often related either to loss of ability or desire to participate in social and recreational abilities. Thus, medical illness, pain, and functional disabilities are linked to depression in what may be thought of as a circular and amplifying relationship. Physical illness may first lead to dysfunction in the ability to carry out ADL or to participate in leisure and social activities, and these limitations can then cause a depressive reaction that can exacerbate the illness (or perceived impact of the illness). The depression then may result in excess disability through decreased motivation to perform or engage in activity (Figure 10-1). Findings in this area point to the need to take a comprehensive or holistic approach to the care of the older adult, incorporating medical illness, depression, and functional status in assessment and treatment approaches (Hunkeler et al., 2006; Schoevers et al., 2003; Smit et al., 2006).

Depression and Dementia

An additional group for whom depression and illness may coincide includes older adults who have been diagnosed with one of the dementing disorders, such as Alzheimer's disease, multi-infarct (vascular) dementia, Parkinson's disease, and other less common forms of dementing illness. A substantial percentage of patients with dementia experience symptoms of depression (Barnes et al., 2006; Bortz & O'Brien, 1997; Elderkin-Thompson et al., 2003; Ritchie et al., 1998; Teri and Wagner, 1992). By its very nature, dementia leads to dysfunction in daily activities, first affecting more complex and demanding activities such as occupational functioning and some forms of leisure activities (e.g., playing bridge, golfing) and then having an impact on the more basic functions involved in IADL and ADL. Given the effects of depression on these same activities, it is likely that persons who become depressed as a result of their awareness of declines in cognitive abilities will

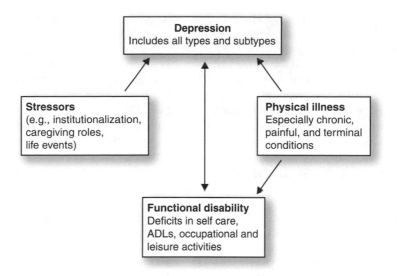

FIGURE 10-1 Relationships between stressors, physical illness, depression, and functional disability.

also suffer from increased functional disability (Holtzer et al., 2005; Janzing et al., 2005).

Pearson and colleague (1989) evaluated this potential for **double disability** in a small sample of patients with Alzheimer's disease. These investigators noted that IADL are most susceptible to the effects of depression, because shopping, housework, and cooking require levels of motivation and initiative that may be beyond the capability of the depressed older adult. When depressed Alzheimer's patients are compared to persons with dementia who are not depressed, the depressed patients are generally found to be more functionally impaired than those who suffer only from dementia (Barnes et al., 2006). Although it is not clear if the depressive condition is a cause or result of decreased functional capacity, it is likely that active treatment of depression in patients with dementia will prevent excess disability from occurring. In addition to new medications designed to treat the cognitive symptoms of Alzheimer's disease and other forms of dementia, the opportunity to treat the accompanying depression may offer valuable hope and improved functioning for the patient with dementia. Riley (Riley, 1989; Riley and Carr, 1989) and others (Bonder, 1994) have discussed interventions designed for patients with dementia and their caregivers which can help ameliorate the depressive reactions likely to occur in the early stages of dementing illnesses.

Caregiver Burden, Stress, and Depression

Thus far, this chapter has focused on identifying and treating depression in medically ill and demented patients in order to prevent unnecessary disability and other negative outcomes. The caregiving literature also makes it very clear that this attention to mental health issues should be extended to the spouse or other individual who plays the primary caregiving role for the identified patient. The caregiver has been identified as the "second victim," with depression ranking as one of the most common negative outcomes of the caregiving process (Pruchno & Resch, 1989). In addition, much has been written about the elderly caregiver's burden, with accompanying increases in stress, physical illness, and psychological distress (Malone-Beach & Zarit, 1991; Zarit et al., 1986). Risk factors in older adults which may have special relevance for caregivers include loneliness, dispositional tendencies such as optimism, and past history of depression (see Cacioppo et al., 2006; Giltay, Zitman, & Kromhout, 2006; Schoevers et al., 2003).

Caregivers of demented and frail older adults are likely to be older individuals whose physical strength and stamina may be overburdened by the caregiving role (Koizumi et al., 2005). If the disabling effects of depression complicate this physical burden, then the ability to carry out daily activities and engage in social interactions will be negatively affected, and the ability to perform the caregiving role will be diminished. Interventions designed for caregivers alone or in conjunction with the chronically ill older adult (Pruchno & Kleban, 1993; Riley & Carr, 1989) can reduce the sense of perceived burden and depressive symptoms of caregivers, which, in turn, can increase their ability to function in all of their roles.

Depression in the Institutionalized Older Adult

A final group of older adults to be considered in this discussion of depression in special populations is those who are institutionalized (Lichtenberg, 1998; Teresi, Abrams, Holmes, Ramirez, & Eimicke, 2001). It has been estimated that at least one-fourth of nursing home residents older than the age of 65 suffer from a depressive disorder (Djernes, 2006). Although many individuals may be depressed before they enter the nursing home, the social and emotional losses brought about as a result of institutionalization also are likely to lead to depressive reactions. Furthermore, nursing home environments appear to reinforce passive, apathetic, and dependent behaviors (Kahana et al., 1988) which can aggravate the motivational and affective problems that characterize the depressive disorders. Learned helplessness stemming from a sense of lack of control or inadequate reinforcement for independent behaviors can add to the severity of depressive reactions in the institutionalized older adult.

This high proportion of older nursing home residents who either enter the institution with a depressive disorder or become depressed after moving to the home should be of great concern to health care professionals. Although psychotropic medications are provided to nursing home residents, the fact that only a small proportion of facilities have consulting psychiatrists or psychologists means that intervention often does not occur. Unfortunately, the availability of mental health services in institutional settings may be quite limited (Kahana et al., 1989; Teresi et al., 2001).

Although the issues of depression and dysfunction in the institutional environment are complex and defy simple solutions, the basic principles of comprehensive assessment of emotional disorders followed by individualized treatment plans can prevent and diminish depressive disorders in institutionalized older adults. Assessment of depression and counseling can be provided in these settings, using resources like the Minimum Data Set for Nursing Homes and other brief rating scales (see "Web-Based Resources" section). Consulting psychiatrists and psychologists, social workers, and nursing staff can play an important role in detecting and treating depressive disorders in institutionalized older adults. Occupational therapists may recognize a loss of pleasure in daily activities, social withdrawal, and other signs of depression in the course of efforts to sustain occupational engagement.

Taken in combination with the nursing home environment's emphasis on compliance and routine, the depressed elderly resident is at great risk for slipping into a withdrawn, apathetic, and even vegetative state. The lack of meaningful interpersonal relationships and daily activities can exacerbate depression in elderly nursing home residents. In addition to medical and psychotherapeutic interventions, treatment of depression in these residents may involve increasing their social interactions and fostering more independent behaviors to the greatest extent possible. Examining occupational patterns and ensuring meaningful activity and participation is an essential role for occupational therapists.

One example of an innovative and successful approach to creating an environment in nursing homes that reduces social isolation and increases social stimulation is the Eden Alternative (Thomas, 1999). Long-term care facilities that employ this model work to reduce loneliness, helplessness, and boredom of their residents by providing a "habitat" that includes intergenerational interactions, opportunities to give as well as receive care, and the presence of pets in the facility. The use of this approach may have a positive impact on nursing students and care professionals (Rosher & Robinson, 2005). Approaches that pay attention to the continuing needs for human interaction, friendship, and a variety of stimulating occupations among older adults (Bell & Troxel, 2002, 2003) in long-term care facilities should prove valuable in reducing the likelihood that they will develop depressive disorders, and can also improve overall quality of life.

Treatment of Depression

It has been repeatedly noted that depression in older adults is a treatable condition, one that should not be ignored or dismissed as a normal part of aging or as a lost cause. First, preventive and early intervention efforts are crucial (Conn & Steingart, 1997; Gareri et al., 1998; Hay et al., 1998; Hunkeler et al., 2006; Motl et al., 2005). Second, two major forms of treatment for depression—psychotherapy and antidepressant medications—are highly successful methods of intervention. In addition, although less frequently used, electroconvulsive therapy (ECT) has been shown to be a safe and effective treatment in severely depressed older adults (Delano-Wood & Abeles, 2005; Mulsant & Sweeney, 1997; Reynolds et al., 2001; Smit et al., 2006).

Prevention and Early Intervention

In general, active, involved older adults have greater life satisfaction, higher morale, and lower incidence of depression than those who are isolated, withdrawn, and inactive. Although some older adults are content with solitary or inactive lifestyles, increasing the amount of meaningful activity and involvement seems to reduce depressive symptoms in many others. Ensuring that the older adult has access to and is able to participate in vocational, volunteer, or leisure activities may either prevent a depressive reaction or reduce its severity and duration. The key is for the professional, whether a psychologist, social worker, occupational therapist, activity therapist, or other specialist, to be certain that the activities suggested to the elderly person are interesting and meaningful to that individual. Simply pushing older persons into activities without exploring their interests is not likely to yield positive results. Occupational therapists often work with clients to complete an occupational profile and to identify the constellation of activities that will support meaningful activity and participation.

Next to prevention, early detection of depression in older adults is the most important function of professionals in geriatric practice (Gum et al., 2006; Harris et al., 2006; Oyama et al., 2006). Awareness of the "triggers" of depression, risk factors, and common symptoms and manifestation of depression should help mental health and allied professionals recognize the problem in the earliest stages, leading to formal assessment, diagnosis, and development of an intervention plan.

The preceding section on physically ill older adults has important implications for health care professionals. First, both affective and medical illnesses must be evaluated in older adults who complain of one or the other of the conditions. When depressive symptoms are discovered, active intervention should be instituted in order to prevent the downward spiral of increasing functional disability, poor health, and worsening depression. In addition, efforts need to be made to improve functional abilities directly, because improved functional status can lead to improvements in mood. A comprehensive approach to assessment and intervention in geriatric patients that emphasizes both emotional and physical symptoms should maximize the positive outcomes desired by elderly clients and their health care professionals.

Psychotherapy

A variety of therapeutic approaches have been described as being successful in the treatment of depression in older adults (Crabb & Hunsley, 2006; Gatz, 1994; Hunkeler et al., 2006). Psychodynamic (Riley & Carr, 1989; Steuer et al., 1984) and behavioral (Teri, 1994) approaches have been successful in ameliorating depression in later life; however, cognitive-behavioral therapies also have received considerable attention in the gerontological literature. Supportive approaches emphasizing reassurance, encouragement, and direct social service–type interventions are also commonly used with older adults. Both group therapy and individual approaches have been used, and although specific therapeutic approaches differ in style and content, some commonalities emerge. Themes of loss, illness, death, and uncontrollable change must be dealt with, regardless of theoretical orientation. An emphasis on positive coping skills and adjusting to or finding substitutes for losses is helpful to the older individual. Short-term treatment (6 months or less) of late-life depression has been most commonly described, although some long-term work also has been done. Couples and family therapy are important in the treatment of depressive disorders in older adults, and these modalities may be especially helpful when dealing with reactions to chronic medical illnesses such as cancer, Parkinson's disease, or dementia.

Consideration of psychotherapeutic interventions for older adults must also include a note on support groups. Although these groups are not designed to provide formal therapy and are not generally led by professional therapists, they do provide a valuable service to many older adults who may be experiencing mild or chronic depressive reactions to loss, illness, or ongoing stress. There is a large network of specialty support groups in the United States including groups for caregivers for patients with Alzheimer's disease and other caregivers, cancer and other chronic illness support groups, as well as groups for the recently bereaved. These groups are often a valuable adjunct or follow-up to individual psychotherapy with the depressed elderly.

Medications and Electroconvulsive Therapy

Antidepressant medications can be safely and effectively used with older individuals, if the prescribing physician is aware of the special cautions and considerations related to the older adult's reactions. There are a number of physiological changes accompanying the aging process that affect the choice and dosage of antidepressant medications. In particular, the older adult often needs lower doses than those prescribed for young persons in order to reach the desired therapeutic level. A second issue is the fact that older adults as a group have twice the incidence of side effects and negative drug interactions as do younger persons, making the prescription of psychotropic medications a job best handled by a psychiatrist who is familiar with geriatrics (Gum et al., 2006; Lyness et al., 2006; Reynolds et al., 1999; Streim et al., 1997).

There are three major classes of antidepressants: the tricyclics, monoamine oxidase inhibitors (MAOIs), and the selective serotonin uptake inhibitors (SSRIs), as well as a number of newer medications that do not fit into one of these categories. Each class of medication has its own set of side effects, and a careful assessment of the individual's pattern of symptoms and other medical conditions must be conducted in order to choose the medication with the greatest potential for efficacy with the lowest side effect profile. Common side effects of antidepressant medications include confusion and cognitive impairment, as well as sleeplessness, agitation, vivid dreams, dry mouth, and constipation. See Box 10-2 for a list of frequent side effects of antidepressant medications in the elderly population. An additional consideration of great concern when antidepressant medications are prescribed for older individuals is the fact that these drugs can cause a drop in blood pressure on standing (a condition known as orthostatic hypotension), which can lead to dizziness and falls.

Used with care, antidepressants can result in dramatic recovery from the severe depression experienced by many older adults. Psychotropic medications may be especially helpful in recurrent depression or in suicidal and profoundly withdrawn patients. The use of both medications and psychotherapy can be a very potent treatment program for many depressed older adults who may not respond to only one of the treatment modalities. For those individuals who do not improve after medications and therapy have been tried, ECT may be the treatment of choice (Delano-Wood & Abeles, 2005). There is no reason to avoid the use of this procedure in older adults, unless there are serious medical illnesses or other major contraindications, and in fact severely depressed older adults may be among the best candidates for this type of treatment. These include depressed individuals who are imminently suicidal, for whom the 3- to 6-week waiting period involved in noting the effects of antidepressant medications involves too great a risk. ECT may be particularly helpful in depressive disorders with psychotic or delusional features. Finally, when ECT has been successful in treating an elderly individual's earlier episode of major depression, it may be expedient to use this treatment again. Although ECT has been shown to cause transient cognitive impairment, there is little research data to indicate that it causes significant, enduring cognitive loss. However, it has been noted that persons who have undergone ECT may experience a subjective sense of permanent memory loss. Additional research will be needed to determine the nature and causes of such potential cognitive loss attributed to ECT.

Occupational Therapy

Occupational therapy has an important contribution to make in the treatment of depression in older adults in every intervention setting. Clark and her colleagues (1997) found that

BOX 10-2 Frequent Side Effects of Antidepressant Medications in the Elderly

- Confusion and disorientation
- Dry mouth
- Urinary retention or constipation
- Blurred vision
- Sleep disturbances and nightmares
- Agitation
- Cardiovascular changes, including increased blood pressure or orthostatic hypotension and change in heart rate

providing well elders with occupational therapy intervention focused on creating meaningful occupational lives was effective in promoting health and life satisfaction. At the same time, such intervention reduced the likelihood of depression. Such preventive intervention can enhance later life. At the same time, occupational therapy has been demonstrated to be successful in home health intervention (Gitlin et al., 2006), short-term rehabilitation (Sood, Cisek, Zimmerman, Zaleski, & Fillmore, 2003), and for individuals whose depression is secondary to a major health event such as hip fracture (Elinge et al., 2005). Both individual and group interventions are effective (McWha, Pachana, & Alpass, 2003).

The primary emphasis of occupational therapy in all these settings is to assist individuals in identifying constellations of occupations that engage their interest and have meaning. As discussed in Chapter 3, such occupations contribute to life satisfaction and quality of life. In this way, they maximize individuals' positive feelings about their lives and prevent or reduce depression in later life. Once those activities have been identified, occupational therapy can assist the individual to continue the occupation as their functional capacity diminishes either as a result of age or a debilitating illness. Alternatively, therapy may be helpful in enabling the individual to substitute other activities that are meaningful. This process of selection–optimization–compensation was described in Chapter 3. It is, of course, important to keep in mind cultural factors that might mediate occupational therapy interventions with individuals with depression. The process of selecting occupations, optimizing them, and compensating is affected by individuals' perception of culturally appropriate occupations (Bonder, 2001).

Cultural Factors in Depression

A brief mention of cultural factors in depression among elderly people is made here. There is a small but significant body of literature on racial, ethnic, and cultural differences in the symptoms, correlates, diagnosis, and treatment of depression in older adults (Fujisawa et al., 2005; Leo et al., 1998; Lichtenberg, 1997; Steffens et al., 1997; Tai-Seale et al., 2005). The largest body of literature deals with African Americans and includes studies that compare groups of African Americans with whites or other racial and ethnic groups (Baldwin, 2002; Djernes, 2006; Husaini, 1997; Okwumabua et al., 1997). Some studies examine the nature of depressive symptoms and related factors only in African Americans. Although a number of studies show racial differences in the clinical presentation of depressive symptoms (Black et al., 1998; Carrete et al., 2001; Leo et al., 1998), other studies report minimal differences in symptoms between African Americans and whites (Blazer, Landerman, Hays, Simonsick, & Saunders, 1998). There also may be differences in how frequently African Americans are referred for evaluation of symptoms or in the likelihood that these individuals will receive a diagnosis of a depressive disorder (Okwumabua et al., 1997). Additional studies report that African Americans are less likely than other racial or ethnic groups to seek or receive treatment for depression (Tai-Seale et al., 2005).

Studies are beginning to emerge that examine depressive disorders in older adults of other cultural or ethnic groups, such as Mexican Americans, Asian Americans, and others (Black et al., 1998; Black & Markides, 1999; Carrete et al., 2001; Iwamasa & Hilliard, 1999; Oyama et al., 2006; Zhang et al., 1997). Questions have arisen as to the validity of measures of depression with cultural and racial groups other than whites (Tran, 1997; Yen et al., 2005), and the predictors and correlates of depression may differ among these groups. This body of research points to important considerations in the assessment and treatment of depressive disorders in the major ethnic and racial groups in the United States and abroad.

■ Summary

This chapter has presented a brief overview of the symptoms, assessment, daily functioning, and treatment of depressive disorders in older adults. The interactions between physical illness, dementia, life events, and emotional well-being have been discussed, and it should be clear that it is not always possible to determine the first link in the causal chain of depression and dysfunction in social, occupational, and daily activities. Work in the area of late-life depression has moved from an initial focus on the detection and assessment of the various forms and manifestations of this cluster of disorders to investigation of the most effective methods of treating depressed older adults. The next phase should involve efforts aimed at preventing depression in older adults to the greatest extent that this is possible. The further development of second, late-life careers, voluntary work, meaningful social interactions, and community programs can help prevent some reactive depressions. Support groups and wider availability of mental health services designed for the isolated, bereaved, ill, or disabled older adult should also result in a lowered incidence or severity of late-life depression. Given the negative consequences of the depressive disorders on the independent function of the growing population of aged persons, this emphasis on prevention could reduce the ultimate cost to society while enhancing the quality of life for older adults and those who care for them.

Case Study

Mr. Arthur is a 74-year-old African American who was widowed 18 months ago. Since that time, his three daughters have noted a significant decline in his hygiene and grooming. This worries them because he was always an immaculate dresser who took pride in his appearance. In addition, he appears to have lost weight and seems lethargic. The pastor of his church called one of the daughters recently to express his concern that Mr. Arthur has not been attending Sunday services, although he used to come regularly.

Questions

1. What issues would a clinician have to consider to accurately diagnose Mr. Arthur?
2. What strategies might assist in diagnosing the underlying problem?
3. What might an occupational therapist address in this situation?
4. What modalities might the occupational therapist use?

Review Questions

1. Discuss the major symptoms of depressive disorders and describe how some of these symptoms are emphasized in atypical or minor forms of depression in older adults.
2. Describe some of the factors that may trigger a depressive or suicidal condition in the older adult, commenting on how a professional might assess these conditions in an elderly patient.
3. Explain what is meant by the "circular" relationship between depression and functional disability in older adults.
4. Describe and compare the nature of depression and functional impairment in two of the following special populations: physically ill, demented, or institutionalized elderly.

5. How might a professional work to prevent depression in older patients?
6. Discuss two different methods of treating an older adult who is depressed. Include the possible advantages and disadvantages of each method.

Web-Based Resources

For helpful information about the experience of depression, visit:

http://harcourtassessment.com/HAIWEB/Cultures/en-us/Productdetail.htm?Pid=015-8018-370&Mode=summary **Harcourt Assessments,** date connected May 2, 2008. BDI can be purchased from this site.

http://counsellingresource.com/quizzes/cesd/index.html, **Center for Epidemiologic Studies- Depression Scale (CES-D) Counseling Resource,** date connected August 28, 2007. This site describes the test and includes the questions.

http://mqa.dhs.state.tx.us/qmweb/Depression/CSDD.htm, **Cornell Scale for Depression in Dementia (CSDD),** date connected August 28, 2007. This site includes the questions and scoring for the Cornell Scale.

www.stanford.edu/~yesavage/GDS.html, **Geriatric Depression Scale (GDS),** date connected August 28, 2007. This site includes access to the questions as well as a reference list and other resources.

www.stanford.edu/~yesavage/GDS.english.short.score.html, **GDS—Short form,** date connected August 28, 2007. This short form includes the questions and the scoring system.

www.columbia.edu/cu/ssw/projects/pmap/docs/mui_gds.pdf, **Columbia University,** date connected August 28, 2007. Information about both the long and short forms of the GDS.

http://www.measurecme.org/resources/MEASURE_HAMD.pdf?PHPSESSID=e8eb56719704de17df88aaee85f7e93d **Hamilton Rating Scale for Depression Rating Scale,** date connected May 2, 2008. The questions and scoring are available here.

www.who.int/substance_abuse/research_tools/zungdepressionscale/en/index.html, **Zung Self-Rating Depression Scale,** date connected August 28, 2007. A World Health Organization site that provides the instrument and its scoring.

Links and resources for diagnosis and treatment

www.agingresearch.org/section/topic/depressionresources, **Alliance for Aging Research,** date connected August 28, 2007. This site provides a wide array of links to reputable sources for information about diagnosis and treatment of depression in later life.

http://hsl.mcmaster.ca/tomflem/aging.html, **McMaster University** date connected August 28, 2007. This site, hosted by the Head of Public Services in the McMaster University Health Sciences Library, has a wide array of resources for working in later life. They include many focused on depression.

REFERENCES

American Psychiatric Association (APA). (2000). *Diagnostic and statistical manual of mental disorders (DSM-IV-TR)* (4th ed. Text Revision). Washington, DC: Author.

Baldwin, R. (2002). Research into depressive disorders in later life: Who is doing what? A literature search from 1998–2001. *International Psychogeriatrics, 14,* 335–346.

Barnes, D., Alexopolous, G., Lopez, O., Williamson, J., & Yaffe, K. (2006). Depressive symptoms, vascular disease, and mild cognitive impairment: Findings from the cardiovascular health study. *Archives of General Psychiatry, 63*(3), 273–280.

Bell, V., & Troxel, D. (2002). *A dignified life: The best friends approach to Alzheimer's care. A guide for family caregivers.* Baltimore: Health Professions Press.

Bell, V., & Troxel, D. (2003). *The best friends approach to Alzheimer's care.* Baltimore: Health Professions Press.

Berkman, L. F., Berkman, C. S., Kasl, S., & Freeman, D. H. (1986). Depressive symptoms in relation to physical health and functioning in the elderly. *American Journal of Epidemiology, 124,* 372–388.

Black, S. A., & Markides, K. S. (1999). Depressive symptoms and mortality in older Mexican Americans. *Annals of Epidemiology, 9,* 45–52.

Black, S. A. Goodwin, J. S., & Markides, K. S. (1998). The association between chronic diseases and depressive symptomatology in older Mexican Americans. *Journal of Gerontology: Biological Sciences and Medical Sciences, 53,* M188–M194.

Blazer, D. G., Landerman, L. R., Hays, J. C., Simonsick, E. M., & Saunders, W. B. (1998). Symptoms of depression among community-dwelling elderly African-American and white older adults. *Psychological Medicine, 28,* 1311–1320.

Bonder, B. R. (1994). Psychotherapy for individuals with Alzheimer's disease. *Alzheimer Disease and Related Disorders, 8*(Suppl. 3), 75–81.

Bonder, B. R. (2001). Culture and occupation: A comparison of weaving in two traditions. *Canadian Journal of Occupational Therapy, 65,* 310–319.

Bortz, J. J., & O'Brien, K. P. (1997). Psychotherapy with older adults: Theoretical issues, empirical findings and clinical applications. In P. D. Nussbaum (Ed.), *Handbook of neuropsychology and aging* (pp. 431–451). New York: Plenum Press.

Burt, D. B., Zembar, M. J., & Niederehe, G. (1995). Depression and memory impairment: A meta-analysis of the association, its pattern, and specificity. *Psychological Bulletin 117*(2), 285–305.

Cacioppo, J., Hughes, M., Waite, L., Hawkley, L., & Thisted, R. (2006). Loneliness as a specific risk factor for depressive symptoms: Cross-sectional and longitudinal analysis. *Psychology and Aging, 21*(1), 140–151.

Carrete, P. , Augustovski, F., Gimpel, N., Fernandez, S., Di Paolo, R., Schaffer, I., et al., 2001). Validation of a telephone-administered geriatric depression scale in a Hispanic elderly population. *Journal of General Internal Medicine, 16,* 446–450.

Clark, F., Azen, S. P., Zemke, R., Jackson, J., Carlson, M., Mandel, D., et al. (1997). Occupational therapy for independent-living older adults. A randomized controlled trial. *Journal of the American Medical Association, 278,* 1321–1326.

Conn, D. K., & Steingart, A. B. (1997). Diagnosis and management of late life depression: A guide for the primary care physician. *International Journal of Psychiatry Medicine, 27,* 269–281.

Conwell, Y., Duberstein, P. R., & Caine, E. D. (2002). Risk factors for suicide in later life. *Biological Psychiatry, 52,* 193–204.

Crabb, R., & Hunsley, J. (2006). Utilization of mental health care services among older adults with depression. *Journal of Clinical Psychology, 62,* 299–312.

Delano-Wood, L., & Abeles, M. (2005). Late-life depression: Detection, risk reduction and somatic intervention. *Clinical Psychology: Science and Practice, 12,* 207–217.

Djernes, J. K. (2006). Prevalence and predictors of depression in populations of elderly: A review. *Acta Psychiatrica Scandinavica, 113,* 372–387.

Doan, B. D., & Wadden, N. P. (1989). Relationship between depressive symptoms and description of chronic pain. *Pain, 36,* 75–84.

Dombrovski, A., Szanto, K., & Reynolds, C. F. (2005). Epidemiology and risk factors for suicide in the elderly: 10-year update. *Aging Health, 1,* 135–145.

Elderkin-Thompson, V., Kumar, A., Bilker, W., Dunkin, J., Minz, J., Mesholam, R., et al. (2003). Neuropsychological deficits among patients with late-onset minor and major depression. *Archives of Clinical Neuropsychology, 18*(5), 529–549.

Elinge, E., Stenvall, M., von Heideken Wågert, P., Löfgren, B., Gustafson, Y., & Nyberg, L. (2005). Daily life among the oldest old with and without previous hip fractures. *Scandinavian Journal of Occupational Therapy, 12*(2), 51–58.

Folstein, M. F., & McHugh, P. (1978). Dementia syndrome of depression. *Aging 7,* 87–93.

Friedman, B., Conwell, Y., Delavan, R., Wamsley, B., & Eggert, G. (2005). Depression and suicidal behaviors in Medicare primary care patients under age 65. *Journal of General Internal Medicine, 20*(5), 397–403.

Friedman, B., Heisel, M. J., & Delavan, R. L. (2005a). Psychometric properties of the 15-item Geriatric Depression Scale in functionally impaired, cognitively intact, community-dwelling elderly primary care patients. *Journal of the American Geriatrics Society, 53,* 1570–1576.

Friedman, B., Heisel, M. J., & Delavan, R. L. (2005b). Validity of the SF-36 five-item Mental Health Index for major depression in functionally impaired, community-dwelling elderly patients. *Journal of the American Geriatrics Society, 53*(11), 1978–1985.

Fry, P. S. (1986). *Depression, stress and adaptations in the elderly.* Rockville, MD: Aspen.

Fujisawa, D., Tanaka, E., Sakamoto, S., Neichi, K., Nakagawa, A., & Ono, Y. (2005). The development of a brief screening instrument for depression and suicidal ideation for the elderly: The Depression and Suicide Screen. *Psychiatry and Clinical Neurosciences, 59,* 634–638.

Ganguli, M., Du, Y., Dodge, H., Ratcliff, G., & Chang, C. (2006). Depressive symptoms and cognitive decline in late life. *Archives of General Psychiatry, 63,* 153–160.

Gareri, P. Stilo, G., Bevacqua, I., Mattace, R., Ferreri, G., & De Sarro, G. (1998). Antidepressant drugs in the elderly. *General Pharmacology, 30,* 465–475.

Gatz, M. (1994). Application of assessment to therapy and intervention with older adults. In M. Storandt, & G. R. VandenBos (Eds.), *Neuropsychological assessment of dementia and depression in older adults: A clinician's guide* (pp. 155–176). Washington, DC: American Psychological Association.

Giltay, E., Zitman, F., & Kromhout, D. (2006). Dispositional optimism and the risk of onset of depressive symptoms during 15 years of follow-up: The Zutphen Elderly Study. *Journal of Affective Disorders, 91*(1), 45–52.

Girling, D., Barkley, C., Paykel, E., Gehehaar, E., Brayne, C., Gill, C., et al. (1995). The prevalence of depression in a cohort of the very elderly. *Journal of Affective Disorders, 34,* 319–329.

Gitlin, L. N., Winter, L., Dennis, M. P., Corcoran, M., Schinfeld, S., & Hauck, W. W. (2006). A randomized trial of a multicomponent home intervention to reduce functional difficulties in older adults. *Journal of the American Geriatrics Society, 54,* 809–816.

Greenglass, E., Fiskenbaum, L., & Eaton, J. (2006). The relationship between coping, social support, functional disability and depression in the elderly. *Anxiety, Stress and Coping, 19,* 15–31.

Gum, A., Arean, P., Hunkeler, E., Tang, L., Katon, W., Hitchcock, P., et al. (2006). Depression treatment preferences in older primary care patients. *Gerontologist, 46*(1), 14–22.

Hammond, M. F., O'Keefe, S. T., & Barer, D. H. (2000). Development and validation of a brief observer-rated screening scale for depression in elderly medial patients. *Age and Ageing, 29,* 511–515.

Harman, J. S., Edlund, M., Fortney, J., & Kallas, H. (2005). The influence of comorbid chronic medical conditions on the adequacy of depression care for older Americans. *Journal of the American Geriatrics Society, 53,* 2178–2183.

Harris, T., Cook, D. G., Victor, C., De Wilde, S., & Beighton, C. (2006). Onset and persistence of depression in older people—Results from a 2-year community follow-up study. *Age and Ageing, 35,* 25–32.

Hay, D. P., Rodriguez, M. M., & Franson, K. L. (1998). Treatment of depression in late life. *Clinical Geriatric Medicine, 14,* 33–46.

Holtzer, R., Scarmeas, N., Wegesin, D., Albert, M., Brandt, J., Dubois, B., et al. (2005). Depressive symptoms in Alzheimer's disease: Natural course and temporal relation to function and cognitive status. *Journal of the American Geriatrics Society, 53*(12), 2083–2089.

Hunkeler, E., Katon, W., Tang, L., Williams, J., Kroenke, K., Lin, E., et al. (2006). Long term outcomes from the IMPACT randomized trial for depressed elderly patients in primary care. *British Medical Journal, 332,* 1–5.

Husaini, B. A. (1997). Predictors of depression among the elderly: Racial differences over time. *American Journal of Orthopsychiatry, 67,* 48–58.

Iwamasa, G. Y., & Hilliard, K. M. (1999). Depression and anxiety among Asian American elders: A review of the literature. *Clinical Psychology Review, 19,* 343–357.

Janzing, J., Naarding, P., & Eling, P. (2005). Depressive symptoms predict slow cognitive decline in mild dementia. *Dementia and Geriatric Cognitive Disorders, 20*(2–3), 77–81.

Kahana, E., Kahana, B., & Riley, K. P. (1988). Contributions of qualitative research issues to studies of institutional settings for the aged. In G. D. Rowles & G. Reinharts (Eds.), *Qualitative gerontology* (pp. 197–216). New York: Springer.

Kahana, E., Kahana, B., & Riley, K. (1989). Learned helplessness and dependency in the institutionalized aged. In P. S. Fry (Ed.), *Psychology of helplessness and control* (pp. 121–153). New York: North Holland.

Kaszniak, A. W., & Christenson, G. T. (1994). Differential diagnosis of depression and dementia. In M. Storandt & G. R. VandenBos (Eds.), *Neuropsychological assessment of dementia and depression in older adults: A clinician's guide* (pp. 81–118). Washington, DC: American Psychological Association.

Koizumi, Y., Awata, S., Kuriyama, S., Ohmori, K., Hozawa, A., Seki, T., et al. (2005). Association

between social support and depression status in the elderly: Results of a 1-year community-based prospective cohort study in Japan. *Psychiatry and Clinical Neurosciences, 59,* 563–569.

Lawrence, V., Murray, J., Banerjee, S., Turner, S., Sangha, K., Byng, R., et al. (2006). Concepts and causation of depression: A cross-sectional study of the beliefs of older adults. *The Gerontologist, 46*(1), 23–32.

Leo, R. J., Sherry, C., & Jones, A. W. (1998). Referral patterns and recognition of depression among African American and Caucasian patients. *General Hospital Psychiatry, 20,* 175–182.

Lichtenberg, P. A. (1997). The DOUR project: A program of depression research in geriatric rehabilitation minority patients. *Rehabilitation Psychology, 42,* 103–114.

Lichtenberg, P. A. (1998). *Mental health practice in geriatric health care settings.* New York: Haworth Press.

Lyness, J., Heo, M., Datto, C., Ten Have, T., Katz, I., Drayer, R., et al. (2006). Outcomes of minor and subsyndromal depression among elderly patients in primary care settings. *Annals of Internal Medicine, 144,* 496–504.

MaloneBeach, E. E., & Zarit, S. H. (1991). Current research issues in caregiving to the elderly. *International Journal of Aging and Human Development, 32,* 103–114.

McWha, J. L., Pachana, N. A., & Alpass, F. (2003). Exploring the therapeutic environment for older women with late-life depression: An examination of the benefits of an activity group for older people suffering from depression. *Australian Occupational Therapy Journal, 50,* 158–169.

Motl, R., Konopack, J., McAuley, E., Elavsky, S., Jerome, G., & Marquez, D. (2005). Depressive symptoms among older adults: Long-term reduction after a physical activity intervention. *Journal of Behavioral Medicine, 28,* 385–395.

Mulsant, B. H., & Ganguli, M. (1999). Epidemiology and diagnosis of depression in late-life. *Journal of Clinical Psychology, 60*(Suppl.), 9–15.

Mulsant, B. H., & Sweeney, J. A. (1997). Electroconvulsive therapy. In P. D. Nussbaum (Ed.), *Handbook of neuropsychology and aging* (pp. 508–514). New York: Plenum Press.

National Institute of Mental Health (NIMH). (2006). Suicide in the U.S.: Statistics and Prevention. http://www.nimh.nih.gov/health/publications/suicide-in-the-us-statistics-and-prevention.shtml; Accessed May 2, 2008.

Nguyen, H., & Zonderman, A. (2006). Relationship between age and aspects of depression: Consistency and reliability across two longitudinal studies. *Psychology and Aging, 21*(1), 119–126.

Norton, M., Skoog, I., Toone, L., Corcoran, C., Tschanz, J., Lisota, R., et al. (2006). Three-year incidence of first-onset depressive syndrome in a population sample of older adults: The Cache County study. *American Journal of Geriatric Psychiatry, 14,* 237–245.

O'Boyle, M., Amadeo, M., & Self, D. (1990). Cognitive complaints in elderly depressed and pseudodemented patients. *Psychology and Aging, 5*(3), 467–468.

Okwumabua, J. O, Baker, F., Wong, S., & Pilgram, B. (1997). Characteristics of depressive symptoms in elderly urban and rural African Americans. *Journal of Gerontology: Biological and Medical Sciences, 52,* M241–M246.

Oyama, H., Ono, Y., Watanabe, N., Tanaka, E., Kudoh, S., Sakashita, T., et al. (2006). Local community intervention through depression screening and group activity for elderly suicide prevention. *Psychiatry and Clinical Neurosciences, 60*(1), 110–114.

Pearson, J. R., Teri, L., Reifler, B. V., & Taskind, M. A. (1989). Functional status and cognitive impairment in Alzheimer's patients with and without depression. *Journal of the American Geriatrics Society, 37,* 1117–1121.

Pruchno, R., & Kleban, M. H. (1993). Caring for an institutionalized parent: The role of coping strategies. *Psychology and Aging, 8,* 18–25.

Pruchno, R., & Resch, N. L. (1989). Husbands and wives as caregivers: Antecedents of depression and burden. *Gerontologist, 29,* 159–165.

Reynolds, C. F., Alexopolous, G., Katz, I., & Lebowitz, B. (2001).Chronic depression in the elderly: Approaches for prevention. *Drugs and Aging, 18,* 507–514.

Reynolds, C. F., Frank, E., Perel, J. M., Imber, S. D., Cornes, C., Miller, M. D., et al. 1999). Nortriptyline and interpersonal psychotherapy as maintenance therapies for recurrent major depression: A randomized controlled trial in patients older than 59 years. *Journal of the American Medical Association, 281,* 39–45.

Riley, K. P. (1989). Psychological interventions with Alzheimer's disease. In G. C. Gilmore, P. J. Whitehouse, & M. L. Wykle (Eds.), *Memory impairment and aging: Theory, testing and treatment.* New York: Springer.

Riley, K. P., & Carr, M. (1989). Group psychotherapy with older adults: The value of an expressive approach. *Psychotherapy: Theory, Research and Practice, 26,* 366–371.

Ritchie, K., Touchon, J., & Ledésert, B. (1998). Mixed cognitive and affective disorders in the elderly: A longitudinal study of related disability. *Archives of Gerontology and Geriatrics, 26,* 443–450.

Rosher, R., & Robinson, S. (2005). The Eden Alternative: Impact on student attitudes. *Educational Gerontology, 31,* 273–282.

Schoevers, R. A., Beekman, A. T., Deeg, D. J., Hooijer, C., Jonker, C., & van Tilburg, W. (2003). The natural history of late-life depression: Results from the Amsterdam study of the elderly (AMSTEL). *Journal of Affective Disorders, 76,* 5–14.

Smit, P., Ederveen, A., Cuijpers, P., Deeg, D., & Beekman, A. (2006). Opportunities for cost-effective prevention of late-life depression. *Archives of General Psychiatry, 63,* 290–296.

Sood, J. R., Cisek, E., Zimmerman, J., Zaleski, E. H., & Fillmore, H. H. (2003). Treatment of depressive symptoms during short-term rehabilitation: An attempted replication of the DOUR project. *Rehabilitation Psychology, 48,* 44–49.

Steffens, D. C., Artigues, D. L., Ornstein, K. A., & Krishnan, K. R. R. 1997). A review of racial differences in geriatric depression: Implications for care and clinical research. *Journal of the American Medical Association, 89,* 731–736.

Steuer, J., Mintz, J., Hammen, C. L., Hill, M. A., Jarvik, L. F., McCarley, T., et al. (1984). Cognitive-behavioral and psychodynamic group psychotherapy in treatment of geriatric depression. *Journal of Consulting and Clinical Psychology, 52,* 180–189.

Storandt, M., & VandenBos, G. R. (Eds.). (1994). *Neuropsychological assessment of dementia and depression in older adults: A clinician's guide.* Washington, DC: American Psychological Association.

Streim, J. E., Oslin, D., Katz, I. R., & Parmelee, P. A. (1997). Lessons from geriatric psychiatry in the long-term care setting. *Psychiatric Quarterly, 68,* 281–307.

Tai-Seale, M., Bramson, R., Drukker, D., Hurwicz, M., Ory, M., Tai-Seale, T., et al. (2005). Understanding primary care physicians' propensity to assess elderly patients for depression using interaction and survey data. *Medical Care, 43*(12), 1217–1224.

Teri, L. (1994). Behavioral treatment of depression in patients with dementia. *Alzheimer Disease and Related Disorders, 8,* 66–74.

Teri, L., & Wagner, A. (1992). Alzheimer's disease and depression. *Journal of Consulting and Clinical Psychology, 60,* 379–391.

Teresi, J., Abrams, R., Holmes, D., Ramirez, M., & Eimicke, J. (2001). Prevalence of depression and depression recognition in nursing homes. *Social Psychiatry and Psychiatric Epidemiology, 36*(12), 613–620.

Thomas, W. H. (1999). *The Eden Alternative handbook: The art of building human habitats.* Sherburne, NY: Summer Hill Company.

Thompson, L. W., Futterman, A., & Gallagher, D. (1988). Assessment of later life depression. *Psychopharmacology Bulletin, 24,* 577–586.

Tran, T. (1997). Exploring the equivalence of factor structure in a measure of depression between black and white women: Measurement issues in comparative research. *Research on Social Work Practice, 7,* 500–517.

Wells, C. E. (1979). Pseudodementia. *American Journal of Psychiatry, 136,* 895–900.

Whooley, M. S., Stone, B., & Soghikian, K. (2000). Randomized trial of case-finding for depression in elderly primary care patients. *Journal of General Internal Medicine, 15,* 293–300.

Yen, Y.-C., Yang, M. J., Yang, M. S., Lung, F., Shih, C., Hahn, C., et al. (2005). Suicidal ideation and associated factors among community-dwelling elders in Taiwan. *Psychiatry and Clinical Neurosciences, 59,* 365–371.

Zarit, S., Todd, P. A., & Zarit, J. M. (1986). Subjective burden of husbands and wives as caregivers: A longitudinal study. *The Gerontologist, 26*(3), 260–266.

Zarit, S. H., & Zarit, J. M. (1998). *Mental disorders in older adults.* New York: Guilford Press.

Zhang, A. Y., Yu, L. C., Yuan, J., Tong, Z., Yang, C., & Foreman, S. E. (1997). Family and cultural correlates of depression among Chinese elderly. *International Journal of Social Psychiatry, 43,* 199–212.

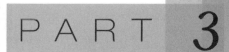

PART 3

Activities
and Participation

*T*his book is not focused on disease, except insofar as disease affects function. More central to our considerations are data about functional limitations. The rate of functional limitation is decreasing, but at least 20% of those over 65 are chronically disabled (Federal Interagency Forum on Aging-Related Statistics [FIFARS], 2004). These figures represent a snapshot at a specific point in time; over time, the majority of older adults experience at least some short-term disability.

An understanding of underlying capacities and the kinds of interruptions in body structures and functions that can occur in later life is essential to grasping the kinds of changes that occur in activities and participation. Chapters 11 through 16 focus on major areas of participation for everyone, emphasizing changes in later life. These changes can occur for many reasons: normal development (e.g., children grow and grandchildren are born); personal preference (changing interests, new experiences); and uncontrollable external events (loss of a spouse, mandatory retirement from principal employment). Elders must be prepared to deal with all of these—and most are. Chronic diseases hover in the background, perhaps with exacerbations that intrude on day-to-day activity, or perhaps with minimal impact on performance. For health-care providers trying to enhance well-being, these chronic diseases can pose challenges when their effects are conflicting. For example, an individual may have both osteoporosis and arthritis. For osteoporosis, weight-bearing exercise would typically be recommended, but such a regimen must be undertaken carefully for an individual with arthritis as it can aggravate joint pain. These types of interactions among conditions, when added to social and environmental factors, create situations of considerable complexity.

The seriousness of diseases is different in elders than in younger individuals. Some kinds of cancer that are relatively lethal in younger individuals may be much less aggressive in older adults. One elderly man was diagnosed with prostate cancer on his 65th birthday. Twenty-five years later, it appears he will die *with* prostate cancer, rather than *of* prostate cancer. On the other hand, influenza, which is merely unpleasant for younger people, may be lethal to elders. Older adults require a longer time to return to baseline physical capacity following illness, as well. And, of course, they are not immune to problems like substance abuse that are more typically described for younger populations.

For older adults, interruptions in function may relate to individual changes (i.e., loss of physiological function or onset of a disease process), or they may relate to the social milieu. Loss of family and friends may have as profound an impact on function as loss of physical capacity. To get a feel for the effect of such a loss, imagine that you do not know how to drive, and that your roommate, who has always served as chauffeur, decides to move out. If an older individual has never learned to drive, cook, or manage money, independence may be compromised by loss of important services, in addition to loss of emotional support, when a spouse or sibling dies. Environmental factors have an effect on function as well. Supportive environments can enhance performance regardless of loss of physical ability; unsupportive environments can impair function in the most able of individuals. Taking a walk on an icy day will give you some sense of the potential impact of an unsupportive environment. Imagine that you are an elder with some degree of osteoporosis and diminished visual acuity, and consider the additional difficulties such an individual might have taking the same walk.

Federal Interagency Forum on Aging-Related Statistics (FIFARS). (2004). *Older Americans 2004: Key indicators of well-being.* Washington, DC: U.S. Government Printing Office.

CHAPTER 11

Self-Care

Charles H. Christiansen • Kristine Haertl • Lauren Robinson

The capacity to do something useful for yourself or others is key to personhood, whether it involves the ability to earn a living, cook a meal, put on shoes in the morning, or whatever other skill needs to be mastered at the moment.

Mary Catherine Bateson, Enfolded activity and the concept of occupation.
In R. Zemke & F. Clark (Eds.), *Occupational science:
The evolving discipline*, F.A. Davis, Philadelphia, 1996, p. 11.

OBJECTIVES

By the end of this chapter, readers will be able to:

1. Define self-care activities within the domains of everyday occupations.
2. Identify the symbolic and practical meanings of self-care activities.
3. Understand the performance of self-care activities as a function of the individual and the environment.
4. Define conceptual elements necessary for viewing self-care performance.
5. Understand the relationship between self-care performance and perceptions of competence and control.
6. Summarize research findings on limitations in self-care.
7. Identify common assessments of activities of daily living (ADL) used for older adults.
8. Identify intervention strategies for enabling self-care performance.

A complete understanding of the functional performance of older adults includes the importance of daily activities and how they contribute to overall health and well-being. Self-care skills are affected by declining function, including sensory limitations, cognitive declines, reduced strength and agility, and restricted mobility. These often accompany chronic disease and expected physiological changes that occur through the aging process. This chapter considers self-care a special category of the domain of everyday human activity that has important implications for the health and well-being of elderly persons.

The chapter begins with a definition of self-care and description of a framework for understanding how daily living tasks often present challenges to elderly people in their attempt to fully engage in life and participate in society in order to achieve a sense of well-being. Within this framework, self-care may be viewed as a foundation to social participation. This discussion is followed by a brief review of common limitations to functional performance and how they can be assessed. The chapter concludes with a description of the possibilities for intervention, including requirements for assistance in performing self-care tasks.

Defining Self-Care

Self-care is daily activity composed of duties and chores ranging from personal care (e.g., bathing, dressing, grooming) to personal business (e.g., using the telephone, managing medications, banking, shopping for food). These tasks are fundamental to living in a social world; they enable basic survival and sustained health and create a sense of self-efficacy and greater life satisfaction. They are sometimes referred to as **activities of daily living** (ADL) (Figure 11-1).

Health care providers differ in their opinions as to what specific tasks to include under this heading, but basic ADL nearly always include the personal requirements of toileting (bowel and bladder functions), bathing, dressing, eating, and grooming (including oral hygiene). The *Occupational Therapy Practice Framework* (OTPF) of the American Occupational Therapy Association (2002) also includes functional mobility, sexual activity, and personal device care as part of taking care of one's self in ADL; managing basic self-care needs, however, is not sufficient for living alone in the community. Living alone also requires the ability to maintain the living environment and to conduct service transactions, such as shopping for groceries or using a checking account to pay bills.

The late M. Powell Lawton (1971), a noted U.S. gerontologist, used the term **instrumental activities of daily living** (IADL) to describe these additional requirements for community living. He identified use of the telephone, food preparation, housekeeping, doing laundry, shopping, managing money, using transportation, and managing medication as tasks constituting this category of IADL. In recent years, the Practice Framework (AOTA, 2002) has included personal health maintenance, household management, caregiving (e.g., pets, children, dependents), and safety and emergency response in the realm of IADL.

Together, basic or personal self-care activities and IADL may be viewed as forming a

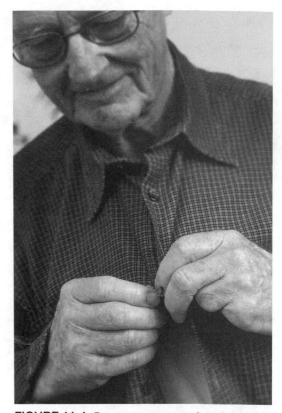

FIGURE 11-1 Because appearance is an important aspect of social life, basic self-care requires dressing or grooming, whether performed independently or with the assistance of other people or assistive technologies. Because of impairments affecting vision or eye–hand coordination, buttoning shirts can become a challenge. To compensate for impairments, there are devices such as button aids that can make the process easier. Another alternate is to use fasteners that avoid the demands of buttoning, such as Velcro® closures. (Source: Photos To Go Unlimited, with permission.)

foundation for survival and for participation in the community. Participation, here, is conceptualized in its richest sense, as embracing routine performance of everyday interactive tasks and the social and symbolic implications of those interactions for community participation. Not only is independence in performing self-care ADL a significant aspect of life satisfaction in older persons (Sato, Demura, Kobayashi, & Nagasawa, 2002), but continued participation in one's personal care routine is viewed as essential to avoiding disability and maintaining independence (Raia, 1999; Vogelpohl, Beck, Heacock, & Mercer, 1996). These three elements—the person, his or her transactions within the physical and social environment, and the successful performance of the specific tasks necessary to those interactions—are referred to repeatedly in the description of a general conceptual framework for self-care.

Models to Explain Everyday Functional Abilities

There are many models in the social and behavioral sciences to explain the factors that influence everyday actions. Most usually consider the individual person as well as the environments in which a person transacts the business of living. Such "contextual or ecological" models are often described in terms of "person–environment fit." The implication is that people best meet the demands of living when their capabilities fit well with those demands (Deci & Ryan, 1991; Lawton, Windley, & Byerts, 1982).

Health care providers have been most concerned with the circumstances in which declining function leads to a disruption in the balance between the demands of living and a person's capabilities. Several taxonomies of function have evolved over the years, beginning with work by Nagi (1976) and extending to efforts by the World Health Organization (2000), The National Center for Medical Rehabilitation Research (1993), and more recently, work by Brandt and Pope (Brandt, Pope, & U.S Institute of Medicine Committee on Assessing Rehabilitation Science and Engineering, 1997). As these models have evolved, they have included environmental and psychological factors to the point of becoming specialized variations of person–environment-fit frameworks. Figure 11-2 consolidates the ideas within the models by Brandt and Pope (Brandt et al., 1997) and that of Willis (Tousignant, Arsenault, Corriveau, & Philippe, 2000), thus focusing on the continuing interaction of meeting the immediate requirements of daily living while coping with limitations in meeting those demands.

White (1959) defined "competence" as the ability to meet demands successfully. More contemporary ecological or person–environment-fit models view competence as dependent both on the individual's capabilities and skills, and on the nature of the task and the environment in which it is performed. The term *environment,* here includes not only physical aspects, such as natural terrain or the man-made, "built" environment (such as buildings, tools, and other objects), but also the less apparent sociocultural environment that influences the attitudes and expectations of performance, through policies, customs, or societal prejudices.

Aspects of the physical environment may facilitate or hinder task performance. For

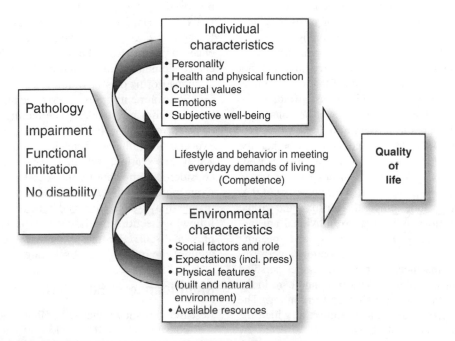

FIGURE 11-2 Person–environment-enablement framework.

example, people need quiet places to concentrate and locations with adequate lighting to perform tasks requiring visual acuity. When physical limitations are present, the environment can create significant barriers to competence. The Americans with Disabilities Act of 1990 reflected awareness of this problem through its legislative requirements to construct public places according to design standards that do not limit access or use for persons with physical limitations (Adamkin, 1997). As a result, using principles of universal design, architects may design working and living environments to make them usable by all individuals, regardless of any physical limitations they may have (Story, 1998). These features also apply to the design of products, outdoor recreational facilities, and transportation systems. Chapter 24 provides additional information about environmental modifications.

Prior to 1990, the term **everyday competence** appeared in the gerontological literature to refer to a person's ability to perform a broad array of activities considered essential for independent living, even though an individual may not perform these tasks on a regular basis or may do so only infrequently. A comparison of "everyday competence" with White's narrow definition, notes that this modern usage describes potential or capability rather than actual behavior, and involves multiple domains and components. The standard for this evaluation involves physical, psychological, and social functioning, which are dependent on a host of underlying factors.

Investigators have discovered that it is not sufficient to view competent function as simply the performance of a given task. Rather, the physical and social context must be considered part of the appraisal of an individual's task performance in order to understand whether the actions of his or her life lead to a sense of well-being. Conceptualizations of context have been extended within the Practice Framework (AOTA, 2002) to include temporal, spiritual, and virtual considerations as integral to individual engagement in society. Personal value and meaning within a context affect occupational performance. For instance, a person who values personal appearance may take extra time and care in the self-care tasks of dressing and grooming. The nature, type of dress, and context in which the grooming takes place is further affected by cultural norms and social expectations. The

successful completion of the dressing and grooming, therefore, would contribute to an individual's self-perception and personal satisfaction.

An individual's ability to competently carry out daily activities is also affected by client factors, context, and task requirements. Personal competence is unique for each individual and is constantly changing. Diehl (1998) asserted that everyday competence is not only dynamic but also recursive. This means that physical health and psychological functioning are not only requirements of everyday competence but also consequences of such competence. People's self-appraisal, morale, and subjective sense of well-being are influenced by their ability to participate in the world by performing tasks that are personally meaningful. Although everyday competence may involve instrumental tasks that are viewed as mundane or as less meaningful than discretionary activities, these tasks are nonetheless foundations for participation in a social world and are important symbols of personal competence and efficacy.

Society looks at each individual and evaluates status by his or her ability to do things—physically, intellectually, or artistically. A person's experience of this expectation of ability has been termed **environmental press.** This term is often included in theories of adaptation and aging (Lawton, 1982). The idea of press, first proposed by the personality theorists (Murray, Barrett, & Hamburger, 1938) and extended by Lawton (1982), is important because it influences or motivates behaviors by creating perceived demands. Social approval is one of the strongest forms of motivation.

Environmental press exerts social expectations (or informal standards) pertaining to levels of performance for the tasks of self-care. These expectations influence behavior, because unless social expectations are met, we may not be considered competent by the social community. Even before society deems us incompetent, people may sense failing competence. In the following section, the issue of expectations or press is discussed as part of an overall consideration of the importance of self-care.

Significance of Self-Care

Research has shown that self-maintenance activities consume about 10% to 15% of the average able-bodied person's waking day (Badke, 2000).

Research also indicates that elderly people with disabilities require a higher proportion of the day to accomplish their self-maintenance activities (Lawton, 1990). Decline in the ability to perform ADL and IADL may lead to increased dependence on the health care system and increased need for in-home supports. Self-care factors including personal mobility, fall risk, malnutrition, and cognitive impairment have been shown to predict prolonged hospital stays in the elderly (Lang et al., 2006).

The extent of an individual's ability to perform self-care tasks independently affects decisions about the need for personal care assistance or special environments, including the need for home health services or placement in long-term-care facilities. For example, a chronically ill individual is defined by the Health Insurance Portability and Accountability Act (HIPAA) as any individual who has been certified by a licensed health care practitioner as being unable to perform (without substantial assistance from another individual) at least two activities of daily living for a period of at least 90 days due to loss of functional capacity (United States Department of Health and Human Services Centers for Medicare and Medicaid Services [USDHHS], 2005). As older adults experience a decline in function, increased assistance or a change in residence may be required in order to provide supports needed to manage daily self-care requirements.

Almost 75% of nursing-home residents over age 65 need personal assistance with three or more ADL, and 96% need assistance with bathing or showering (Sundin, Norberg, & Jansson, 2001). Forty-four percent of residents have difficulty with bowel and bladder continence (Sundin et al., 2001). As might be expected, these percentages are considerably higher than the proportion of the general population over age 65 who require self-care assistance as indicated in Figure 11-3. The need for assistance increases dramatically for persons who are 85 years and older.

Practical Importance of Self-Care: Nutrition, Safety, and General Health

Self-care activities are important because they are necessary for survival, safety, and general health. One of the primary health and survival requirements is adequate nutrition. Without nourishment, health declines rapidly. The

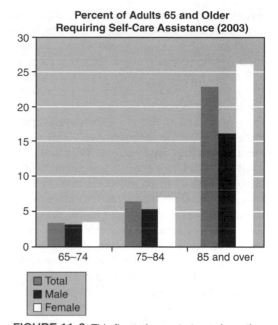

FIGURE 11-3 This figure demonstrates a dramatic increase in need for assistance for individuals age 85 years and over. (Source: National Health Interview Survey, 2003.)

popularity of social programs designed to provide regular nourishment to seniors living in the community can be attributed to the public's recognition of the importance of regular and well-balanced meals. Good nutrition requires the ability to plan menus and prepare food, as well as the ability to eat independently, or "self-feed." In addition to motor, sensory, and cognitive disabilities that limit meal preparation, some elderly people have dental problems or lack the teeth to eat regular meals. Additional factors affecting nutritional intake in the elderly include a lack of appetite and willingness to eat.

As a result of these factors, elderly persons may be at risk for poor nutrition. A study of homebound elderly persons found poor dietary quality was universal; half or more consumed diets that deviated from recommended standards for at least 13 of the 24 nutritional guidelines studied (Millen et al., 2001). Challenges also exist to maintain adequate nutrition in supported living environments given the limitations on choice and dietary restrictions placed on an individual receiving care. A qualitative study of 15 elderly individuals living in Swedish retirement homes identified mood, personal values, food, wholesomeness, eating environment, and meal fellowship as factors influencing personal appetite and willingness to eat (Wikby & Fägerskiöld, 2004). Clearly, nutrition is an important public health issue among seniors which relates directly to self-care activities in both meal preparation and meal consumption.

Safety is another concern for the elderly. The inability to maintain a safe living environment may lead to injury. The normal aging process often results in diminished visual acuity due to macular degeneration. Diabetes may result in visual loss from degeneration of the retina as well as from peripheral sensory loss. Joint inflammation, insomnia, and side effects of medications, such as benzodiazepines, can diminish coordination and balance, reduce reaction times, and impair judgment. These factors make it essential that potential environmental hazards be minimized. Steps and passageways within living environments for community-dwelling elders must be well lit, glare free, and without unnecessary obstacles or hazardous surface conditions. The most common type of home injury among elderly persons involves fractures or head injuries resulting from falls (Commodore, 1995). Studies have shown that the risk of poorer quality of life, morbidity, and mortality is greatly increased following hip fracture in both men and women (Pande & McCloskey, 2006). See Chapter 8 for additional discussion on falls and falls prevention.

Finally, the ability to perform self-care activities promotes better general health. Adequate personal hygiene and sanitation protect the individual from germs that spread disease. Laws protecting public health are based on awareness that neglect of hygiene results in unsanitary conditions that can contribute to unhealthy conditions. The media occasionally report accounts of community-dwelling individuals who, because of emotional or cognitive impairment, are unable to address important self-care needs or maintain living quarters in a manner that is healthful.

Self-care performance has practical importance because it enables people to maintain their personal health and the environments in which they live. It also has symbolic importance as it enables social relationships, fosters and reflects self-identity, and promotes psychological well-being.

Importance of Self-Care for Self-Identity

Functional capacity and personal self-care have been shown to relate to self-esteem and life satisfaction (Backman & Hentinen, 2001). Western cultural norms place value in meeting self-care needs and fitting in with society. Meeting social expectations requires competent role performance that extends to dress, appearance, speech, mannerisms, and other elements of symbolic communication in the culture. In his theory of personality, Hogan and Sloan (1991) noted that people loathe rejection and strive for acceptance by the social group. As a result, their self-esteem and sense of social identity are determined by the reactions of others. Finding one's level of acceptance in the eyes of others is a fundamental notion of symbolic interactionism (Mead, 1934), a theory deeply rooted in the perceived influence of peoples' keen awareness of the imagined and actual reactions of others to their behavior. An individual's roles, relationships, and perceived competence are all integral to the formation of identity, or how they wish to portray themselves to themselves and others.

Importance of Self-Care for Social Relationships

Maintaining competence is necessary for performance of daily living tasks, but it is also an important aspect of an individual's self-esteem, social acceptance, and, ultimately, social well-being. Social and individual perception of competence is important; to be perceived as incompetent may erode self-confidence and self-esteem. Goffman (1959) described how social acceptance is tied to the ability to perform roles within the range that meets expectations of one's cultural group. Talcott Parsons (1975) extended this idea of a range of expectation to the context of the sick role. He noted that persons viewed as "sick" were temporarily exempted from normal role expectations as long as they demonstrated good-faith efforts to regain their health. Parson's work suggested that illness is beyond personal control, yet the individual has a duty to try to get well (Young, 2004). Malingering or other behaviors that deviate from social norms violate role expectations and result in forms of reduced social acceptance, which in the extreme are labeled **"stigma"** (Goffman, 1963). In order to provide quality health services, the social, psychological, and personal cultural effects of illness behaviors should be understood in the realm of the individual and society (Young, 2004). An awareness of societal role expectations and the effects of disabling conditions on personal identity and social relationships is important in delivering comprehensive services to the elderly.

Importance of Self-Care for Psychological Well-Being

Studies have shown that the inability to perform everyday tasks, such as self-care and IADL, has a negative impact on psychological well-being (Badke, 2000). Drageset (2004) found that as competence in ADL declined among seniors in nursing homes, their loneliness and social isolation tended to increase. Lawton (1990) found that elderly persons with higher levels of everyday competence (i.e., the ability to perform self-care and ADL) spent more time in diverse leisure and social activities, which, in turn, resulted in a greater sense of psychological well-being.

Part of this psychological effect is related to perceptions of competence and **agency,** or the ability to act on the environment. Being able to remain in the home setting conveys to elderly people that they have a sense of control over the environment, and this contributes to feelings of efficacy and well-being (Zingmark, Norberg, & Sandman, 1995). Research has demonstrated a relationship between perceived control and other health factors related to survival and well-being (Chipperfield, Campbell, & Perry, 2004). This work suggests that when older people's personal control of activities is restricted, there are detrimental effects to their sense of efficacy and self-esteem.

It is generally accepted that despite a greater awareness and understanding of institutional conditions that promote well-being for residents, seniors are best served when they are assisted to remain outside nursing home environments as long as they are physically and mentally capable (Rosow, 1985). In 2003, 18.8% of men and 31.7% of women over age 65 lived alone in the United States (Wan, Sengupta, Velkoff, & DeBarros, 2005). Although research shows that living alone is desirable because such conditions offer more autonomy, it may also increase social isolation and reliance upon formal social supports (Wilmoth, 2001).

Physiological changes associated with the aging process often create conditions that decrease performance or enjoyment of daily activities. For example, macular degeneration reduces close vision, often forcing an individual to limit reading because of the need to use magnifying lenses, or may cause a person to fail to take note of drug warning labels or precautions, thus creating safety hazards. In these instances, the secondary consequences of the impairment may be as problematic as the direct effects. The following section will address the impact of various impairments on daily function.

Specific Categories of Declining or Impaired Function Leading to Self-Care Limitations

Conditions associated with aging have more profound effects when they impose limitations on movement, sensation, or language. Boult and colleagues reported that the best predictors of functional limitations in ADL and IADL were cerebrovascular disease, arthritis, and coronary artery disease (Boult, Kane, Louis, Bould, & McCaffrey, 1994). These three disease categories, which are prevalent in the elderly population, result in significant limitations because they restrict functional movement and sensation.

Stroke

Cerebrovascular disease can result in weakness or paralysis of extremities on one side of the body, visual limitations, vestibular and sensory problems, and loss of the ability to communicate. The variety and extent of impairments possible following stroke may have a devastating impact on the ability of an individual to perform self-care tasks. Although recovery following stroke can be nearly complete, it often leaves those affected with serious residual disability. This is particularly true if the individual has impaired perceptual functioning, because body image dysfunction (e.g., unilateral neglect, somatoagnosia) interferes with self-care tasks such as dressing and grooming.

Kwakkel and colleagues reviewed the literature to determine variables capable of predicting functional ADL outcomes following stroke (Kwakkel, Wagenaar, Kollen, & Lankhorst, 1996). Their analysis of 78 studies suggested that paralysis, sitting balance, level of social support, urinary continence, and cognitive factors that influence orientation to time and place are the factors most predictive of ADL function following stroke.

Joint Inflammation and Disease

Joint diseases, particularly osteoarthritis (OA) and rheumatoid arthritis (RA), are prevalent in older segments of the population, with nearly all individuals older than 75 years showing some evidence of osteoarthritis (Hochberg, 1991). These conditions typically result in pain and restriction of joint movement, with RA characterized by systemic changes and severe inflammation, and OA marked by degeneration of cartilage, often due to wear and tear.

Because of pain and restriction in joint range of motion, both ADL and IADL are significantly affected by RA and require additional time and energy. Katz (1995) studied the impact of RA on the life activities of a sample of persons over a 5-year period, finding that, on average, the individual subjects studied could no longer perform 10% of valued activities. Losses occurred in every performance area, including work, nurturing, cultural, leisure, and social participation activities. A study by Badley (1995) showed that 25% of persons with arthritis have significant difficulties with mobility.

Sensory Problems

Sensory problems impact the daily functioning of older adults. These problems are covered in detail in Chapter 5 but are briefly described here in relation to their impact on self-care performance.

Vision Problems

Nearly one in five adults in the United States age 70 years or older has a vision impairment; data indicate that this frequently limits activity and participation in valued social activities, particularly with advancing age and comorbidity (Cambell, Crews, Moriarity, Zack, & Blackman, 1999). Branch, Horowitz, and Carr (1989) found that elderly persons with vision problems experience lower levels of everyday competence and are twice as likely as those without vision difficulties to report needing assistance with shopping and paying bills, and are less likely to leave their residence and travel by car. Studies of community-dwelling elders indicate that visual impairment is highly correlated with the need for assistance in ADL and IADL, and this results in higher levels of loneliness and poorer self-rated health (Jacobs, Hammerman-Rozenberg, Maaravi, Cohen, & Stessman, 2005; Williams, Brody, Thomas, Kaplan & Brown, 1998).

Hearing

The impact of hearing deficits on the quality of life is well understood, but there is some evidence that hearing impairments can also influence performance of ADL. Diehl (1998) found significant relationships among general health, cardiovascular health, and hearing impairment when measuring an older adult's performance on a set of observed tasks of daily living.

Disease, injury, and the aging process may cause hearing loss resulting in auditory disability. Throughout life, people experience a gradual loss of auditory sensitivity, particularly in the higher frequencies. This makes sound localization more difficult. Higher frequency loss also affects the ability to understand speech, because many consonants have high-frequency components. Although the use of assistive listening devices helps with many types of hearing loss, this solution is not without problems, including the need for maintenance and regular evaluation.

The acoustic treatment of surfaces to reduce extraneous sounds and rearrangement of furniture can be useful in reducing the consequences of hearing loss (McNair, Brown, Stone, & Sims, 2001). Therefore, these characteristics should be given careful attention and consideration by those who have the ability to modify living environments.

Taste and Smell

Receptors sensing taste and smell decline throughout life but may not begin to be significant until age 70. Conditions such as Alzheimer's disease and the effects of drugs can intensify this lower sensory awareness and lead to a reduced or distorted sense of taste and smell. The impact of these sensory declines on nutrition is readily apparent. If food is enjoyed less, appropriate intake may become problematic. Additionally, olfactory deficits can increase the risk of ingesting spoiled food for those elderly people living in the community (Ripich, 1995).

Cognition

Studies have verified that cognition and memory play a critical role in the performance of everyday tasks. A decline in cognitive functioning and processing is inherent in the aging process and lessens the rate at which older adults process information, thereby reducing their ability to perform ADL in a timely manner and thus diminishing the time available for other perhaps more meaningful activities (Lawton, 1994; Owsley, Sloane, McGwin, & Ball, 2002). A reduction in memory function may be the first indicator of reduced capacity that an elderly person encounters. Types of dementia, particularly the Alzheimer's type, are associated with aging and can have a significant impact on cognitive functioning in terms of memory, orientation, initiation, sequencing, and judgment. Safe, functional performance of self-care and IADL can be greatly reduced when cognitive functioning decreases, because the initiation or sequencing of tasks may be forgotten (Abreu, 2000). Chapter 9 provides a detailed discussion of the impact of cognitive disorders on function.

Measuring Self-Care Performance

Self-care and IADL assessments for the elderly population are performed for several reasons. Assessment of self-care gives a better understanding of geriatric medical problems. Often a decline in function is an early indicator of disease or illness. Self-care assessments also identify the level of impairment or disability. The assessment process and assessment selection are covered in detail in Chapter 17. The following provides a brief discussion on the assessment of self-care.

According to the World Health Organization International Classification of Function (ICF) (WHO, 2000), activity refers to the individual's function, while participation refers to the individual in the environment, and his or her ability to fully engage with society. The results of self-care assessments can help professionals identify the individual's potential level of functioning in terms of both activity and participation, and develop effective treatment interventions. Determining an elderly person's ability to live independently and the supports (internal and external) needed to do so can be ascertained, in part, through an assessment of self-care and IADL skills.

In accordance with the Practice Framework (AOTA, 2002), client evaluation includes development of an occupational profile that considers individual performance patterns along with client values and needs. Areas of occupational performance (including ADL and IADL) are assessed along with client factors, contextual areas, skills, performance, and activity demands. Within the Practice Framework, a holistic client-centered approach to assessment is integral to designing intervention plans. Consideration of current habits and routines, daily ADL requirements, and present and possible future living situations serve to identify personal strengths, areas of difficulty, available resources, and future resource needs.

Because self-care and IADL are multifaceted, it is necessary to use assessment measures that are multidimensional. Often, therapists use more than one type of method to gain a greater understanding of an individual's capabilities. A review of a person's history supplies demographic information (e.g., age, sex, religion) as well as information about past and present medical issues, current and desired occupations, and changes in occupational performance. Interviews with the individual and the caregivers are useful to obtain additional information about past and present roles, abilities, and disabilities. This serves to clarify the picture of the whole individual. Direct observation of task performance supplies objective data in addition to drawing on the clinical expertise of the therapist. This approach adds detail about the individual's performance, and when used with a variety of evaluation techniques, the sum of these methods leads to the clearest determination of where and why limitations in function occur.

In the event of a failure of performance, the complexity of everyday tasks demands that the evaluator pay careful attention to the factors underlying the individual's inability to perform. For example, a person involved in a cooking task may have difficulty following written directions because of visual impairment, or problems with verbal directions because of hearing impairment. The person may also have memory deficits that make it difficult to recall the correct sequence of steps he or she just finished reading in order to execute a task successfully. Persons with aphasia may have difficulty with reception or expression of language, causing poor comprehension or communication resulting in impaired daily function. For example, someone with receptive aphasia might be able to fry an egg with written directions but not with verbal directions, or vice versa. The impairment is, therefore, not necessarily in frying the egg— at least not until the egg is tasted. Determining the underlying cause of the functional deficit is necessary for successful intervention planning.

Assessment of the aged population warrants special attention and revision of focus. Much of the gerontology literature on assessment has focused on prediction of ADL function to assist in determining the need for residential placement. There is somewhat less emphasis on measures that guide possible remediation or compensatory strategies. The importance of this distinction was made evident in the enabling–disabling model offered by Brandt et al. (1997). The model described the relationship between pathology and impairment as evidenced in specific components of function (such as cognition or sensation) and other factors related to the quality of life.

Determining the relationship between specific performance skills such as movement, cognition, or sensation, and performance of the task has been the subject of continuing controversy among rehabilitation scientists who want to provide for an objective assessment of function while also identifying directions for intervention. It is useful to discuss functional assessment approaches in terms of top-down versus bottom-up strategies. The top-down approach to assessment focuses on occupational tasks and roles specific to the individual, whether the tasks can be performed now, and what might be the possible reasons for not being able to carry them out. In contrast, a bottom-up approach is concerned with the performance components that are considered prerequisites to carrying out tasks (e.g., range of motion, strength). Although each approach has advantages and disadvantages when compared with the other, neither approach is wholly effective in assessing self-care and IADL performances in the elderly population. Thus, many practitioners favor a combined approach.

When evaluating the elderly population, it is important to be aware of the normal aging process and related losses in capabilities. The relationship between performance capacity and the demand of the task requires added sensitivity when assessing elderly people. For example, some evidence suggests that when the focus is on the performance of familiar tasks in familiar environments, the effects of the aging process

on measurement of capability are reduced and task performance is improved (Rogers, Holm, & Stone, 1997). However, this is not always the case. Loss of visual and auditory acuity, sensory functioning, cognitive processes, and motor performance caused by aging can have a significant negative impact on the elderly person's performance during assessment. The resulting decreased performance may not indicate deficits in the actual task performance, as we have stated earlier, but may be due to underlying issues.

Assessing Visual and Perceptual Deficits

The majority of self-care and IADL assessments require adequate vision. The Rivermead Perceptual Assessment Battery (RPAB) was initially designed to assess visual perceptual skills following head injury or stroke and later was used to assess older adults as well (Whiting, Lincoln, Bhavani, & Cockburn, 1985). The test does not accommodate for possible visual deficits in the elderly person, and modifications may need to be made to adjust for visual deficits and adjust measurements of performance during the assessment. Strategies may include adjusting the quantity and quality of light, changing background surfaces and color to provide contrast, and enlarging the size and boldness of the test items or written materials. A newer test of ADL for persons with visual impairment, the Melbourne Low Vision ADL Index, has been developed and demonstrates satisfactory reliability and validity (Haymes, Johnston, & Heyes, 2001a, 2001b, 2001c). The test is not only a measure of ADL, but is also useful for measuring the impact of disability on ADL function (Haymes et al., 2001a).

Assessing Activities of Daily Living in Individuals with Auditory Deficits

Hearing loss distorts any assessment process because of potential difficulty hearing the instructions and misinterpretation of the information. To compensate for hearing impairments, excess noise should be minimized during the assessment. If necessary, the evaluator might move closer to the individual or face the person to allow the person to read lips. Improving visual cues, adjusting lighting, and minimizing glare can also maximize the person's visual abilities in order to accommodate for hearing loss. Various self-care instruments may be used to assess individuals with hearing impairment. In addition to tools designed by occupational therapy, research has demonstrated the validity of the WHO DASII (World Health Organization, 1999) as an effective tool for assessing activity limitations for persons with adult acquired hearing loss (Chisolm, Abrams, McArdle, Wilson, & Doyle, 2005).

Assessing Sensorimotor Disorders

Many assessments for self-care and IADL skills include tasks with motor components. These tasks frequently require the manipulation of objects or the use of pen and paper. Because of musculoskeletal changes associated with the aging process, elderly people often experience decreased strength, flexibility, coordination, and sensation. Often, the motor components of assessments are not directly related to functional everyday tasks; therefore, decreased performance in speed and accuracy does not automatically imply a deficit in self-care or IADL functioning. The Assessment of Motor and Process Skills (AMPS) can be used to assess observable motor skills required to carry out IADL (Fisher, 1993). However, the training and costs of administering this assessment limit its practicality in many settings.

Assessing Self-Care in Individuals with Cognitive Impairment

In administering assessments to elderly persons with cognitive impairments, the length and complexity of instructions may need to be adjusted, the instructions repeated, or additional information or assistance provided. If administering norm-referenced or standardized tests, such as the RPAB (Whiting et al., 1985), the validity of the results may be compromised when elderly people with cognitive deficits do not correctly follow the standardized instructions. The evaluator needs to be aware of and compensate for this problem. In addition, the individual may have trouble describing the sequence of a task with a pen and paper; yet perform better when engaged in the actual activity. Finally, because of decreased processing speed, the elderly person may require increased time to complete the assessment task. If adjustments and compensations are made to standardized tests, it is crucial

that the rationale, type of change, and results are clearly documented.

Bucks, Ashworth, Wilcock, and Siegfried (1996) described a special ADL assessment, the Bristol Activities of Daily Living Scale, which is designed especially for persons with dementia. The instrument consists of caregiver ratings for 20 daily living activities. The scale's psychometric properties indicate satisfactory reliability, and it correlates well with the Mini Mental Status Examination.

Assessing Instrumental Activities of Daily Living

Several assessments have been designed specifically to measure IADL functioning in older adults. Examples include Tappen's (1994) Refined ADL (RADL) Assessment Scale and the Older Americans Resource and Services (OARS) (Pattic, 1988). The Assessment of Living Skills and Resources (ALSAR) combines 11 IADL tasks with varying available resources to determine the level of risk when comparing current resources available to resource needs for the individual (Baer & Smith, 2001). Observation of performance is necessary with this and other IADL measures in order to validly assess everyday competence, as client self-reports often overestimate ability (Hilton, Fricke, & Unsworth, 2001).

Home-based assessments may be advantageous because they allow the individuals evaluated to perform tasks in their natural environments and the contexts in which they typically occur and have been shown to yield more accurate results (Bottari, Dutil, Dassa, & Rainville, 2006). These assessments take the environment into account when assessing the elderly person's ability to carry out day-to-day activities safely. They provide a firsthand account of actual performance. In addition, they allow recommendations for equipment, modifications, and adaptations specific to each individual's home. This allows any intervention to compensate for disabilities and to enhance current abilities for safe, independent living.

Due to physiological, psychological, and social changes associated with aging, many individuals experience an alteration in the roles they assume, in their abilities to engage in them, and in their level of participation. Assessing these changes is critical to determining the barriers to healthy social functioning and the elderly person's abilities to overcome them (Lawton, 1988). The Role Checklist (Oakley, 1986) assesses perceived life roles, role balance, and value. For elderly individuals dealing with grief and loss, The Role Adaptation Bereavement Inventory (Meyer et al., 1998) focuses on the elderly person's adaptation to new roles as a result of the loss of a loved one or spouse.

Several assessments evaluate self-care (ADL) and IADL performance in adults, and an increasing number evaluate the older adult population. A newer tool, the Performance Assessment of Self-Care Skills (PASS) is a criterion-referenced, performance-based observational tool that helps therapists to determine safety aspects, independence, and outcomes of functional mobility; basic ADL; and IADL performance tasks (Holm & Rogers, 1999). The Functional Independence Measure (FIM) was initially designed to assess basic ADL (e.g., bathing, dressing, toileting) in adults; however, a recent study has proved it to be a valid measure of functional performance in older adults as well (Claesson & Svensson, 2001). The Arnadottir OT-ADL Neurobehavioral Evaluation (A-One) (Arnadottir, 1990) is a carefully defined scale to measure performance and underlying cognitive processes. Within this assessment, client neurobehavior is assessed through observation of the following ADL: dressing, grooming, hygiene, transfer, mobility, feeding, and communication.

Assessing Environmental Factors

When assessing function in the elderly population, evaluators often overlook environmental factors—the physical environment (e.g., living space and the objects therein) and the social and cultural environment (e.g., group memberships and interactions) in which the individual performs life tasks. The level of assistance, support, and adaptations individuals require to carry out self-care and IADL within their identified roles is also a component of the environment. The availability of such support may enhance the manner in which tasks are carried out, just as lack of support can hinder the individual's level of functioning. Assessing the individual environments in which specific tasks take place can be difficult, because the environment is often a home, a workplace, or another location in the community.

According to Rogers and colleagues (1997), assessment of the physical environment should focus on the architectural barriers and beneficial features of a living environment, as well as its safety and the degree to which assistive technology may benefit the individual.

Assessment of the social environment concerns the care receiver and the *caregiver,* which in this context can be defined as a knowledgeable person who is able to provide assistance to elderly people and receive training in their care. It is important that the caregiver is able to manage the burden and have a healthy attitude regarding functional independence. In addition, it is important to assess the care receiver's ability to engage in life tasks and meaningful roles, and to be accepted in the social world by peers and friends. Involvement by the elderly population in social activities may be compromised by a decline of independence, by the inability to perform self-maintenance tasks, or by poor mobility. Cultural factors, such as the individual's health, beliefs, values, roles, education, experiences, and family makeup, need to be taken into account to ensure that the assessment is relevant to the individual being assessed.

There are several assessments available to evaluate the impact of elderly persons' environments on their level of functioning and ability to maintain roles. Because the environment is not an isolated component of everyday functioning, many environmental assessments also address cognitive, self-care, and IADL function.

Safety

Ensuring safety within the physical environment is crucial to maintaining the elderly person's current level of functioning and to preventing further disability. Two useful assessments that address safety include Darzins' (1994) Functional Assessment and Safety Tool (FAST) and the Safety Assessment of Function and the Environment for Rehabilitation (SAFER) (Oliver, Blathwayt, Brackley, & Tamaki, 1993). Both the FAST and the SAFER were designed to evaluate elderly persons' ability to perform functional activities safely within their home environments; however, the FAST also addresses available support systems (Box 11-1).

A summary of some of the more common self-care assessments can be found in Table 11-1.

TABLE 11-1   Examples of Self Care Assessments

Assessment Tool	Type	Description
A-One (Arnadottir, 1990)	Observation	Test of neurobehavior through observation of grooming, transfer, mobility, feeding, and communication
Assessment of Living Skills and Resources (Williams et al., 1991)	Interview/ Rating scale	Measure of IADL that compares skill level to resources available to determine a combined risk score related to level of assistance that may be needed for care
Assessment of Motor & Process Skills (Fisher, 1993)	Observation	Structured assessment of motor and processing skills based on observation of client chosen ADL tasks. The assessment provides options of over 60 ADL items. (formal training required)
Bristol Activities of Daily Living Scale (Bucks et al., 1996)	Caregiver checklist	Caregiver checklist designed to detect functional change in persons with dementia
Functional Independence Measure (*Guide for the Uniform Data System for Medical Rehabilitation: The FIM Instrument,* Buffalo-SUNY, 1997)	Observation	Measure of functional status, and disability on the individual and caregiver
Katz Index (Katz et al., 1963)	Observation	Quick assessment of basic ADL including bathing, dressing, toileting, continence, Transferring and feeding
Klein-Bell Activities of Daily Living Scale (Klein & Bell, 1982)	Observation	Fairly comprehensive assessment of ADL in areas of dressing, elimination, mobility, bathing, hygiene, eating, and emergency phone
Melbourne Low Vision ADL (Haymes, Johnston, & Heyes, 2001)	Observation	Test of ADL specifically designed for persons with low vision. The assessment may be used to monitor current function and rehabilitative outcomes.
Performance Assessment of Self Care Skills (Holm & Rogers, 1999)	Observation	Comprehensive structured measure of ADL and IADL in four domains including functional mobility, personal care, physical IADL, and cognitive IADL
Role Checklist (Oakley, 1986)	Personal Checklist	Assesses productive and meaningful roles, and role balance from the client's perspective.
Structured Assessment of Independent (Mahurin et al., 1991)	Observation	Assessment of daily activities in ten different areas including ADL and IADL.
Structured Observational test of Function (Laver & Powell, 1995)	Observation	Screening tool of function related to ADL and underlying neurophysiological deficits.
*World Health Organization Disability Assessment Schedule II (WHO, 1999)	2 Versions: Self Administered/Structured Interview	Health status instrument that assesses function on 6 domains: communication, mobility, self-care Interpersonal, life activities and participation

*Used primarily for research

BOX 11-1 **Best Practices in Assessment of Self-Care**

- Only validated, standardized scales should be used
- Choose measures that are sensitive to change in client status
- Performance-based measures are best
- Measure performance in the actual living setting
- Include IADL in any comprehensive assessment
- Incorporate living area assessments into overall evaluation
- Consider the client's needs, lifestyle, and living setting before setting intervention goals based on assessment

Prevalence and Type of Limitations of Activities of Daily Living Among Elderly Persons

Data from the National Health Interview Survey in 2003 showed that 3.3% of adults from the ages of 65 to 74, 6.4% of those 75 to 84, and 22.9% of those 85 and older required help with personal care needs (Schiller, Martinez, Hao, & Barnes, 2005). Nearly one half of the older people living in the community have a limitation in performing basic or instrumental ADL. Nearly half have at least one limitation, and nearly 40% have limitations affecting their performance of both ADL and IADL. As demonstrated in Figure 11-3, individuals age 85 or over have a much higher level of need for assistance with ADL and IADL than those who are younger.

Levels of disability and impact on ADL performance increase both nationally and internationally for the lowest socioeconomic groups (Ahmed, Tomson, Petzold, & Kabir, 2005; Lei, Chen, & Kuo, 2005; Shoeini, Martin, Andreski, & Freedman, 2005). However, data have shown a declining rate of disability among elderly persons across all age categories that may be accounted for by improvements in technology, improvements in general health and life expectancy, or both (Spillman, 2003). The estimated percentages of elderly persons in the total population of the United States requiring assistance with specific ADL based on a National Long Term Care survey done in 1999 indicated that 5.8% of community-dwelling seniors required human assistance for bathing, 3.3% required assistance with toileting, and 2.3% required assistance for eating. Percentages are lower for elderly persons residing in institutional settings.

Activity of Daily Living Intervention

As previously described, progression of normal aging, pathological conditions, and trauma can create impairments and limitations in function that interfere with the performance of ADL and IADL. In many cases, intervention techniques can address these difficulties. In accordance with the Occupational Therapy Practice Framework (AOTA, 2002), strategies are formulated based on collaboration with the client in order to develop an intervention plan and work toward the overarching outcome of occupational engagement in support of participation and achievement of client goals.

The Occupational Therapy Guide to Practice (Moyers, 1999) suggested that intervention techniques involve remediation/restoration, compensation/adaptation, disability, prevention, and health promotion. Restoration or remediation strategies may be applied in cases where there is a possibility of significant reduction in impairments that leads to

> prevention of further activity limitations and participation restrictions or resolution of activity limitations that enable increased participation in occupations. For example, following mild strokes, it is sometimes possible for restorative intervention to normalize patterns of voluntary movement and enable the individual to resume basic and instrumental activity of daily living. Since there is not a linear relationship between sensory or motor restoration and performance of tasks, best practice requires the therapeutic intervention to be contextually relevant.
>
> Often, teaching or training, as a means of remediation, is necessary to re-learn or learn alternative approaches to accomplishing tasks, such a with assistive devices or in supervising others for assistance. (Moyers, 1999, p. 281)

With an aging population, often the limitations of function are due to the result of chronic and progressive disorders or injuries due to falls and accidents. Intervention strategies often include compensation or adaptation. Compensatory strategies focus on adaptation of the environment, task, or the use of residual function. In changing the context of performance, the individual may be provided with assistive devices, or modifications can be made in the physical environment. If the current living situation does not promote optimal occupational performance, the individual may choose to move to a congregate home or an apartment complex designed for older adults. In cases of significant inability to perform ADL, the individual may be placed in an assisted living environment or may require placement in a skilled nursing facility. This is the most extreme type of environmental or contextual change.

Remediation strategies are directed at correcting the underlying pathology or physiological change. If this is accomplished successfully, performance of ADL requirements usually improves. The decision of whether to incorporate remedial or adaptive strategies includes clinical judgment, prognosis, and expectations for physiological improvement. For instance, if an individual has a cognitive impairment due to a stroke or head trauma as a result of a fall, the timing of the incident, the amount and type of damage, and physician prognosis for improvement have a bearing on intervention planning. In general, however, within cognitive rehabilitation of persons that have endured head trauma, adaptation has been shown to be more efficacious in promoting improvement than remedial therapies (Carney et al., 1999).

In addition to limitations brought on by illness and disability, the normal aging process often cause declines that impact occupational performance in ADL and IADL. Rogers, Meyer, Walker, and Fisk (1998) studied the constraints to daily living described by a sample of healthy, active adults aged 65 to 88 years. They found that more than half of the problems reported had the potential to be improved through environmental changes, use of assistive technologies, or task modifications. The following sections provide brief summaries of environmental changes, assistive technologies, and task modification approaches useful for enabling people to perform self-care tasks.

Environmental Modifications

Environmental modifications range from curb cuts to major alterations in the design of rooms or dwellings. The Americans with Disabilities Act (ADA) in the United States (Adamkin, 1997) heightened public awareness of the need to design environments and to make other accommodations so that persons with functional limitations might enjoy full societal participation. Unfortunately, bureaucratic obstacles, such as reimbursement restrictions, often preclude the timely completion of environmental modifications or the acquisition of devices to facilitate adaptation. An additional problem is lack of public awareness about the kinds of easily accomplished home modifications that can greatly assist the performance of everyday tasks. In this section, we briefly discuss environmental modifications for self-care activities related to mobility, food preparation and eating, and bathroom and dressing areas. Environmental modifications may be particularly problematic in low-income areas or in developing nations where other health care concerns take priority.

Mobility

Community mobility and the performance of some IADL, such as shopping, often depend on the presence of curb cuts, ramps, and signage that permit travel by persons with motor and sensory deficits. Store- and street-located automated teller machines (ATMs) must be available at an accessible height, but drive-through ATMs can often be a problem because they are exempted from the legislation.

Within the home, individuals with deficits affecting mobility often require ramps, widened doorways, or other accommodations for facilitating wheelchair access. In multistory homes, environmental modifications may require the conversion of downstairs rooms to bedrooms or bathrooms. In general, mobility can be made safer without area rugs or carpets with long pile. Rugs and carpets should be replaced with tile, wood, or linoleum for easier access. Leg extenders can be added to low chairs or beds to improve the ease with which people can transfer to or from them. They may also be used to adjust furniture for persons with movement difficulties. High legs on beds or chairs can be cut to lower the height. Often, simply removing interior doors provides sufficient access for wheelchair users. If privacy is not an issue, this approach avoids costlier modifications.

Bathroom and Dressing Areas

Bathroom modifications for safety and access include higher toilet seats and shallow sinks positioned in lowered counters. Grab bars should be installed for showers and tubs, and insecure towel racks removed or replaced. Glass shower doors should be replaced with shower curtains. All areas need adequate lighting and nonskid surfaces (Christensen, 2004). Cabinets may be lowered and cabinet doors removed to make them accessible for persons with physical limitations. Within the bedroom, electric beds, which can be purchased or rented, can improve accessibility to persons with physical limitations. Control systems to operate lights, drapes, fans, televisions, stereos, and heat are available and can greatly reduce the physical demands of adjusting the environment.

Kitchen Modifications

Common kitchen modifications include lowered counters and sinks, and the installation of microwave ovens as adaptations for persons with varying mobility restrictions. The choice of appliances (side-by-side refrigerators, bottom or top freezers) depends on the limitations of the person using the environment. In all rooms, lighting and color contrast should be planned to improve visibility without glare.

Although modifications such as those described earlier may be made to create better, safer, and easier home environments for self-care and everyday living, only a small percentage of elderly persons who need such modifications have had them installed. Although in some cases this is due to financial restrictions, it is more frequently the result of lack of awareness or inadequate intervention strategies. Wylde (1998) argues that an improved knowledge of consumer preferences and more concerted public education can make such improvements part of the mainstream consumer marketplace.

In all cases in which environmental modifications are proposed, the service provider should take care to consider the impact of the change on other inhabitants of the environment and to recognize that such modifications may restrict task performance to specific environments. No modifications should be completed without considering the aesthetic preferences of the user. Table 11-2 lists a sample of environmental modifications recommended by Christensen (2004).

Assistive Devices for Self-Care

The use of assistive devices as an intervention strategy can help elderly people overcome impairment, promote safety through the prevention of accidents, and enhance independence and quality of life. Assistive devices are defined by the Technology-Related Assistance for Individuals with Disabilities Act of 1988 (Public Law 100-107, "the tech act") as "any item, piece of equipment, or product system, whether acquired commercially off the shelf, modified, or customized, that is used to increase, maintain, or improve functional capabilities of individuals with disabilities." This act was amended in 1998 (PL 105-394) to extend national support for AT programs and reaffirm the importance of devices for enabling participation in important life activities. Technological advances have signif-icantly broadened the scope, sophistication, and availability of assistive devices as described in Chapter 24. Figure 11-4 shows an assistive device that can be helpful to individuals in accomplishing ADL and IADL in the home or in an institutional setting.

Task Modifications

Task modification strategies, a final category of intervention, may successfully address some self-care limitations in older adults with intact cognition and endurance, who have caregiver support, and the motivation to practice. Modification means substituting one act for another or a device to replace a lost ability. For example, adults who cannot reach or bend because of balance deficits or restricted range of motion may use

TABLE 11-2   Environmental Modifications

Conditions	Suggested Environmental Modifications
Visual aids	Use large, contrasting letters on signs and written materials; large-face clocks and watches; large-print calendars, books, playing cards, and bingo cards; magnifying glasses; and large telephone dials.
Lighting	Increase illumination; use nonglare glass, indirect lighting, awnings, roof overhangs, sunscreens, recesses, and night lights; avoid glossy paint and shiny surfaces.
Color perception	Contrast color of floor and wall; contrast between toothbrush and sink, slippers and floor, food and plate, handrail and wall; clothing colors should clearly contrast each other; avoid patterned tablecloths.
Hearing	Hearing aids; allow increased processing time; speak slowly and distinctly; repeat information or reword sentences; use sound amplifiers on telephones; decrease background noise; move into person's field of vision to get their attention before beginning to speak; look directly at the person; do not shout; include visual cues (e.g., flashing light) on fire and smoke alarms; use furnishings and materials to absorb sound (i.e., acoustical ceiling tile, carpets, drapes, insulated Sheetrock, tight window weather seals) to decrease exterior noise; earth berms, trees, and large plant material to divert and absorb traffic sounds.
Taste	Use safe substitutes for sugar and salt such as herbs and spices; host tasting parties (i.e. wine, cheese, ice cream); serve ethnic food along with music, costumes, dances, and visuals.
Smell	Incorporate familiar odors such as popcorn, coffee, smell of baking, flowers, and plants into the environment.
Tactile/touch	Course wall hangings made from burlap, carpet, and heavy yarns; large raised or recessed letters and numbers give tactile input; wear street clothes as opposed to institutional garments; use one dominant texture as opposed to combining textures; vary textures for orientation (i.e. handrails, different rooms).
Proprioception	Do not rush the person while walking; use vinyl floors as opposed to carpets; floor surfaces should be free of obstacles; there should be no throw rugs, no trailing telephone and extension cords.
Ambulation	Use handrails, sturdy tables, and shallower steps (4" as opposed to 8").
Balance	Stairs may be better than ramps for ambulatory individuals; move slowly; avoid quick movements; position TV, signs, and directional information in field of vision (i.e., from wheelchair level); decrease height of clothing rods and shelves; use rocking chairs and porch swings to provide vestibular input.

Source: Christenson, MA: Adaptations of the physical environment to compensate for sensory changes. Physical and Occupational Therapy in Geriatrics 8:3–30, 1990.

a reacher to pick up objects on the floor. Use of the reacher, however, requires upper extremity coordination, wrist and grip strength, and adequate cognitive skills.

This type of intervention is often referred to as compensation. Typically, compensation strategies are coupled with remediation strategies. Alteration of the task involves teaching the adult new, more efficient, or more effective ways of completing the task, ways that more closely correspond with the client's remaining capacities and that do not require the use of those performance components with deficits (Holm, Rogers, & James, 1997).

Task modifications are appropriate if there is a desire or need for immediate success, if there is little expectation for improvement in the adult's sensory or motor deficits, if the person prefers this method, or if there are problems with safety. A simple example of self-task modification might be recommending that the adult with limited standing tolerance sit down to perform activities typically performed while standing, such as washing dishes. Older adults with fatigue or limited endurance can perform more difficult IADL earlier in the day, thus avoiding the exertion, stress, or cognitive errors when they have the least energy (Box 11-2).

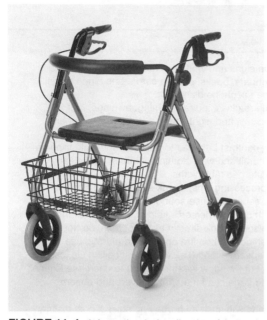

FIGURE 11-4 A four-wheeled walker is a frequently used **assistive technology device** to compensate for diminished balance, strength, or endurance. (Photo courtesy of Abledata.)

■ Summary

The self-care activities of older adults discussed in this chapter are of vital importance to meaningful participation in the home environment and in the larger social world. The normal aging processes as well as various health conditions can cause sensory, motor, and cognitive losses that limit self-care performance.

Assessment of an individual's performance in his or her environment can identify potential interventions to help older adults manage needed ADL and IADL performance. Environmental modifications, assistive technologies, and modifications in task performance may reduce the need for institutionalization (and loss of control and self-esteem) by preserving self-care functions. If, with this help, elders can successfully remain at home, or if they can live productively in a community, this may foster the self-esteem and sense of well-being that we all cherish as adults.

BOX 11-2 Important Questions for Setting Self-Care Intervention Goals

- How important is the activity to the client and his or her well-being?
- Is the time and effort required for self-performance worth the benefit?
- What assistive technologies are available to facilitate the task?
- Does the living environment support safe performance?

- To what extent will the activity contribute to the individual's sense of identity and social participation?
- Have the perspectives of family members or caregivers been considered?

Case Study

Occupational Profile

Mr. G is a 74-year-old man who was admitted to the acute care unit of the local hospital after he was found by his wife with slurred speech and significant weakness on the left side of his body. He stayed in the acute care unit for 10 days before being transferred to the inpatient rehabilitation unit for more intensive therapy to address his decreased ADL functioning. His past medical history includes a right CVA 7 years prior to this admission, hypertension, coronary artery disease, and mild dementia. Mr. G presented to the inpatient rehabilitation unit with residual left limb weakness, left-sided paresis, incoordination, and slight left neglect. He stated that he was independent in ADL prior to hospitalization. Mr. G lives with his wife and son in a one-story home with a ramped entry. He already had a raised toilet with arms, a handheld shower, a wheelchair, and also a tub bench and rolling walker that he does not use. Mr. G was employed as a manager of a bank for 36 years before retiring. He enjoys going to the park, exercising, spending time with friends, watching TV, and going to church.

Problem Areas

- Requires supervision with ADL (needs help with lower extremity dressing) and transfers
- Has decreased strength, balance, and endurance to perform basic ADL
- Has decreased coordination (difficulty with snaps on a shirt)
- Needs verbal cues to use affected side and to modify actions when problems arise in task performance

Goals

Mr. G will:

- Demonstrate stand pivot transfers for toilet, tub, wheelchair, and bed with supervision
- Perform feeding, grooming, dressing, and bathing with supervision and minimal cuing
- Demonstrate proper positioning of trunk and affected limb while seated in the wheelchair, during transfers, and when repositioning in bed
- Demonstrate safe use of recommended assistive devices
- Perform left upper extremity home exercise program for coordination with supervision

Mr. G's Family will demonstrate the following:

- Assist with self-care activities
- Verbally communicate understanding of home exercise program
- Provide encouragement to attend to the affected side

Treatment Plan and Discharge Status

The treatment plan for Mr. G's 2-week stay in the inpatient rehabilitation unit included an activity program that focused on ADL training to address bilateral coordination, proper management of the left upper extremity for positioning, and attending to and scanning of the left visual field. In addition, client and family education that emphasized safety awareness, guided supervision to Mr. G during his daily activities, and recommended compensatory strategies and modifications that support Mr. G's functional independence were provided.

At discharge, Mr. G was able to perform dressing, feeding, and grooming activities with supervision and setup and with minimal cuing to modify his actions when a problem arose. Mr. G's trunk alignment was fair, and attention to the position of his affected arm required minimal to moderate cuing at times. Stand pivot transfers improved and required minimal assistance. Mr. G was discharged to his home with his wife and son. Both his wife and son attended family education sessions prior to discharge to familiarize them with the home exercise program, provide information on the use of the recommended assistive devices, and make suggestions to assist with the supervision of self-care activities as well as modifications that may promote participation and independence in his desired leisure activities. Written and printed handouts that covered the material addressed in the family education sessions were provided.

Reflect and Discuss

1. What frame(s) of reference would you use if Mr. G was your client?
2. How does the family's understanding of the situation and the recovery process influence Mr. G's potential for functional improvement?
3. If Mr. G admitted that he would not use the assistive devices that were recommended for him, what other adaptive strategies can you suggest that would assist him in performing his daily activities? Do any of these strategies require training and instruction to the family members? If so, what are some instructions that you might give?
4. Consider Mr. G's problems of left neglect. Do you have any thoughts or concerns about his return to his home environment? If so, what are they and what can be done about them?
5. What assessment tools could be used to assess this client's skills in self-care?
6. How would you incorporate Mr. G's leisure interests into your intervention?

Review Questions

1. Distinguish between basic self-care and IADL activities.
2. Describe factors that interact to influence the ability of seniors to perform ADL and IADL.
3. Define the concept of "environmental press."
4. List common environmental modifications that can increase or support performance of basic self-care and IADL in the major rooms of a home.
5. Describe the relationship between the performance of self-care and psychological well-being.
6. List significant predictors of limitations in ADL and IADL function.
7. Discuss factors especially important to the self-care assessment of older adults.
8. Differentiate between remediation and compensation in planning interventions for self-care limitations.

Web-Based Resources

For helpful information about the experience of self-care visit:

www.resna.org, **Rehabilitation Engineering and Assistive Technology Society of North America,** date connected March 26, 2007. This society presents information about training opportunities, as well as links to resources.

www.usdoj.gov/crt/ada/adahom1.htm, **Americans with Disabilities Act,** date connected March 26, 2007. This is a government website that describes the provisions of the ADA and interprets important aspects of the Act. Also provided are links to resources and publications.

www.infinitec.org, **Assistive Technology Resource Site (Infinitec),** date connected March 26, 2007. This site is a resource of the United Cerebral Palsy Association of Greater Chicago. It provides a wealth of links to assistive technologies and other resources to enhance function for people with disabilities.

www.abledata.com, **Abledata,** date connected March 26, 2007. This site is sponsored by the National Institute of Disability and Rehabilitation Research. It provides a great deal of information about products, including evaluation of the value of many of them.

www.homemods.org, **Environmental Modifications, National Resource Center on Supportive Housing and Home Modifications,** date connected March 26, 2007. This resource center is a university-based, nonprofit organization dedicated to promote aging in place and independent living for persons of all ages and abilities. This site provides links, resources, and information about training events and research.

REFERENCES

Abreu, B. C. (2000). Meeting self care needs with cognitive deficits. In C. Christiansen (Ed.), *Ways of living: Self care needs for special persons* (2nd ed., pp. 257–282). Bethesda, MD: American Occupational Therapy Association.

Adamkin, D. H. (1997). Nutrition report. Enteral and total parenteral nutrition in the very low birth weight infant: Part I—Enteral nutrition [originally published by Scientific Publishers OWN, Polish Academy of Sciences, Wienawskiego, Poznan]. *Neonatal Intensive Care, 10*(5), 19–23.

Ahmed, S. M., Tomson, G., Petzold, M., & Kabir, Z. N. (2005). Socioeconomic status overrides age and gender in determining health seeking behaviour in rural Bangladesh. *Bulletin of the World Health Organization, 83,* 109–117.

American Occupational Therapy Association (AOTA). (2002). Occupational therapy practice framework: Domain and process. *American Journal of Occupational Therapy, 56*(5), 609–639.

Arnadottir, G. (1990). *The brain and behavior. Assessing cortical dysfunction through activities of daily living.* St. Louis, MO: Mosby.

Backman, K., & Hentinen, M. (2001). Factors associated with the self care of home-dwelling elderly. *Scandinavian Journal of Caring Sciences, 15,* 195–202.

Badke, M. B. (2000). The Health and Activity Limitation Index: Determinants of health-related quality of life in persons with stroke. *Journal of Rehabilitation Outcomes Measurement, 4*(3), 1–16.

Badley, E. M. (1995). The impact of disabling arthritis. *Arthritis Care and Research, 8,* 221–228.

Baer, G., & Smith, M. (2001). The recovery of walking ability and subclassification of stroke. *Physiotherapy Research International, 6*(3), 135–144.

Bottari, C., Dutil, E., Dassa, C., & Rainville, C. (2006). Choosing the most appropriate environment to evaluate independence in everyday activities: Home or clinic. *Australian Occupational Therapy Journal, 53*(2), 1–9.

Boult, C., Kane, R., Louis, T. A., & McCaffrey, D. (1994). Chronic conditions that lead to functional limitations in the elderly. *Journal of Gerontology: Medical Sciences, 490,* M28–M36.

Branch, L. G., Horowitz, A., & Carr, C. (1989). The implications for everyday life of incident self-reported visual decline among people over age 65 living in the community. *The Gerontologist, 29*(3), 359–365.

Brandt, E. N., Pope, A. M., & U.S. Institute of Medicine, Committee on Assessing Rehabilitation Science and Engineering. (1997). *Enabling America: Assessing the role of rehabilitation science and engineering.* Washington, DC: National Academy Press.

Bucks, R. S., Ashworth, D. L., Wilcock, G. K., & Siegfried, K. (1996). Assessment of activities of daily living in dementia: Development of the Bristol Activities of Daily Living Scale. *Age and Ageing, 25,* 113–120.

Cambell, V., Crews, J., Moriarity, D., Zack, M., & Blackman, D. (1999). *Surveillance for sensory impairment, activity limitation and health related quality of life among older adults, United States, 1993–1997.* Atlanta, GA: Centers for Disease Control and Prevention.

Carney, N., Chesnut, R. M., Maynard, H., Mann, N. C., Patterson, P., & Helfand, M. (1999). Effect of cognitive rehabilitation on outcomes for persons with traumatic brain injury: A systematic review, *Journal of Head Trauma Rehabilitation, 14*(3), 277–307.

Chipperfield, J., Campbell, D., & Perry, R. (2004). Stability in perceived control. *Journal of Aging and Health, 16*(1), 116–147.

Chisolm, T. H., Abrams, H. B., McArdle, R., Wilson, R. H., & Doyle, P. J. (2005). The WHO DASII: Psychometric properties in the measurement of functional health status in adults with acquired hearing loss. *Trends in Amplification, 9*(3), 111–126.

Christensen, M. (2004). Environmental adaptations: Foundation for daily living. In C. Christiansen & K. Matuska (Eds.), *Ways of living: Adaptive strategies for special needs* (pp. 423–444). Bethesda, MD: AOTA Press.

Claesson, L., & Svensson, E. (2001). Measures of order consistency between paired ordinal data. Application to the Functional Independence Measure and Sunnaas index of ADL. *Journal of Rehabilitation Medicine, 33*(3), 137–144.

Commodore, D. (1995). Falls in the elderly population: A look at incidence, risks, healthcare costs, and preventative strategies. *Rehabilitation Nursing, 20,* 84–89.

Darzins, P. (1994). Functional assessment and safety tool user's manual. Hamilton, Ontario, Canada: McMaster University/Hamilton Civic Hospitals. www.aihw.gov.au/publications/dis/icfaugv1/modules/ugmod_108.pdf. Accessed May 30, 2006.

Deci, E. L., & Ryan, R. (1991). A motivational approach to self: Integration in personality. In R. Dienstbier (Ed.), *Nebraska symposium on motivation: Vol. 38. Perspectives on motivation* (pp. 237–288). Lincoln: University of Nebraska Press.

Diehl, M. (1998). Everyday competence in later life: Current status and future directions. *The Gerontologist, 38,* 422–433.

Drageset, J. (2004). The importance of activities of daily living and social contact for loneliness: A survey among residents in nursing homes. *Scandinavian Journal of Caring Sciences, 18,* 65–71.

Fisher, A. G. (1993). The assessment of IADL motor skills: An application of the many faceted Rasch analysis. *American Journal of Occupational Therapy, 47,* 319–329.

Goffman, E. (1959). *The presentation of self in everyday life.* New York: Doubleday.

Goffman, E. (1963). *Stigma: Notes on the management of soiled identity.* Englewood Cliffs, NJ: Prentice Hall.

Guide for the Uniform Data System for Medical Rehabilitation: The FIM Instrument. (1997). Version 5.1. Buffalo, NY: State University of New York at Buffalo.

Haymes, S. A., Johnston, A. W., & Heyes, A. D. (2001a). A weighted version of the Melbourne low-vision ADL index: A measure of disability impact. *Optometry and Vision Science, 78*(8), 565–579.

Haymes, S. A., Johnston, A. W., & Heyes, A. D. (2001b). Preliminary investigation of the responsiveness of the Melbourne Low Vision ADL Index to low-vision rehabilitation. *Optometry and Vision Science, 78*(6), 373–380.

Haymes, S. A., Johnston, A. W., & Heyes, A. D. (2001c). The development of the Melbourne Low-Vision ADL Index: A measure of vision disability. *Investigative Ophthalmology & Visual Science, 42*(6), 1215–1225.

Hilton, K., Fricke, J., & Unsworth, C. (2001). A comparison of self-report versus observation of performance using the assessment of living skills and resources (ALSAR) with an older population. *British Journal of Occupational Therapy, 64*(3), 135–143.

Hochberg, M. (1991). Epidemiology of osteoarthritis: Current concepts and new insights. *Journal of Rheumatology, 18*(Suppl. 27), 4–6.

Hogan, R., & Sloan, T. (1991). Socioanalytic foundations for personality psychology. *Perspectives in Personality, 3*(Part B), 1–15.

Holm, M. B., Rogers, J., & James, A. (1997). Treatment of occupational performance areas. In M. Neistadt & E. Crepeau (Eds.), *Willard and Spackman's occupational therapy* (pp. 322–369). Philadelphia: Lippincott-Raven.

Holm, M. B., & Rogers, J. C. (1999). Performance assessment of self care skills. In B. J. Hemphill-Pearson (Ed.), *Assessments in occupational therapy mental health: An integrative approach* (pp. 117–128). Thorofare, NJ: Slack.

Jacobs, J., Hammerman-Rozenberg, R., Maaravi, Y., Cohen, A., & Stessman, J. (2005). The impact of visual impairment on health, function and mortality. *Aging Clinical and Experimental Research, 17*(4), 281–286.

Katz, P. P. (1995). The impact of rheumatoid arthritis on life activities. *Arthritis Care and Research, 8*(4), 272–278.

Kwakkel, G., Wagenaar, R. C., Kollen, B. J., & Lankhorst, G. J. (1996). Predicting disability in stroke—A critical review of the literature. *Age & Ageing, 25*(6), 479–489.

Lang, P. O., Heitz, D., Hedelin, G., Drame, M., Jovenin, N., Ankri, J., et al. (2006). Early markers of prolonged hospital stays in older people: A prospective multicenter study of 908 inpatients in French acute hospitals. *Journal of the American Geriatrics Society, 54,* 1031–1039.

Lawton, M. P. (1971). The functional assessment of elderly people. *Journal of the American Geriatric Society, 19*(6), 465–481.

Lawton, M. P. (1982). Competence, environmental press and the adaptation of older people. In M. P. Lawton, P. G. Windley, & T. O. Byerts (Eds.), *Aging and the environment: Theoretical approaches* (pp. 33–59). New York: Springer.

Lawton, M. P. (1988). Scales to measure competence in everyday activities. *Psychopharmacology Bulletin, 24*(4), 609–614.

Lawton, M. P. (1990). Age and the performance of home tasks. *Human Factors, 32,* 527–536.

Lawton, M. P. (1994). Quality of life in Alzheimer Disease. *Alzheimer Disease and Associated Disorders, 8*(Suppl. 3), 138–150.

Lei, I. C., Chen, Y., & Kuo, H. (2005). The health status and health promotion behavior of low income elderly in the Taipei area. *Journal of Nursing Research, 13*(4), 305–312.

McNair, R., Brown, R., Stone, N., & Sims, J. (2001). Rural interprofessional education: Promoting teamwork in primary health care education and practice. Papers from the Australian College of Rural and Remote Medicine Inaugural Scientific Forum "Steps Along the Pathway," Brisbane, Queensland, 10 June 2001. *Australian Journal of Rural Health,* S19–S26.

Mead, G. H. (1934). *Mind, self and society: From the standpoint of a social ever.* Chicago: The University of Chicago Press.

Meyer, K., Schwaibold, M., Hajric, R., Westbrook, S., Ebfeld, D., Leyk, D., et al. (1998). Delayed VO2 kinetics during ramp exercise: A criterion for cardiopulmonary exercise capacity in chronic heart failure. *Medicine & Science in Sports & Exercise, 30*(5), 643–648.

Millen, B., Silliman, R., Cantey-Kiser, J., Copenhafer, D., Ewart, C., Ritchie, C., et al. (2001). Nutritional risk in an urban homebound older population. The nutrition and healthy aging project. *Journal of Nutritional Health and Aging, 5*(4), 269–277.

Moyers, P. A. (1999). The guide to occupational therapy practice. *American Journal of Occupational Therapy, 53*(3), 247–322.

Murray, H. A., Barrett, W. G., & Hamburger, E. (1938). *Explorations in personality.* New York: Oxford University Press.

Nagi, S. Z. (1976). An epidemiology of disability among adults in the United States. *Milbank Quarterly, 54,* 439–467.

National Center for Medical Rehabilitation Research. (1993). *Research plan for the National Center for Medical Rehabilitation Research.* Bethesda, MD: U.S. Department of Health and Human Services.

Oakley, F. (1986). The role checklist: Development and empirical assessment of reliability. *Occupational Therapy Journal of Research, 6*(2), 157–170.

Oliver, R., Blathwayt, J., Brackley, C., & Tamaki, T. (1993). Development of the safety assessment of function and the environment (SAFER) tool. *Canadian Journal of Occupational Therapy, 60,* 78–82.

Owsley, C., Sloane, M., McGwin, G., & Ball, K. (2002). Timed instrumental activities of daily living tasks: Relationship to cognitive function and everyday performance assessments in older adults. *Gerontology, 48*(4), 254–265.

Pande, K., & McCloskey, E. (2006). Quality of life, morbidity and mortality after low trauma hip fracture in men. *Annals of Rheumatic Disease, 65*(1), 87–92.

Parsons, T. (1975). The sick role and the role of the physician reconsidered. *Health and Society: Milbank Memorial Fund Quarterly, 51,* 257–278.

Pattie, A. (1988). Measuring levels of disability. The Clifton Assessment Procedures for the elderly. In J. P. Watts & I. Hindmarch (Eds.), *Psychological assessment of the elderly* (pp. 61–75). London: Churchill-Livingstone.

Raia, P. (1999). Habilitation therapy: A new starscape. In L. Volicer & L. Bloom-Charette (Eds.), *Enhancing the quality of life in advanced dementia* (pp. 21–37). Philadelphia: Brunner/Mazel.

Ripich, D. N. (1995). Serving sensory impaired elderly in long term care. In Z. Harel & R. E. Dunkel (Eds.), *Matching people with services in long term care* (pp. 243–260). New York: Springer.

Rogers, W. A., Meyer, B., Walker, N., & Fisk, A. (1998). Functional limitations to daily living tasks in the aged: A focus group analysis. *Human Factors, 40*(1), 111–125.

Rosow, I. (1985). Status and role change throughout the lifecycle. In R. H. Shanas & E. Shanas (Eds.), *Handbook of aging and the social sciences* (pp. 62–91). New York: Van Nostrand Reinhold.

Sato, S., Demura, S., Kobayashi, H., & Nagasawa, Y. (2002). The relationship and its change with aging between ADL and life satisfaction characteristics in independent Japanese elderly living at home. *Journal of Physiological Anthropology and Applied Human Science 21,* 195–204.

Schiller, J. S., Martinez, M., Hao, C., & Barnes, P. (2005). Early release of selected estimates based on data from the January–September 2004 National Health Interview Survey. National Center for Health Statistics.

http://www.cdc.gov/nchs/data/nhis/earlyrelease/insur200503.pdf. Accessed April 24, 2008.

Shoeini, R. F., Martin, L. G., Andreski, P. M., & Freedman, V. A. (2005). Persistent and growing socioeconomic disparities in disability among the elderly: 1982–2002. *American Journal of Public Health, 95*(11), 2065–2070.

Spillman, B. (2003). *Changes in elderly disability rates and the implications for health care utilization and cost.* Washington, DC: Urban Institute.

Story, M. (1998). Maximizing usability: The principles of universal design. *Assistive Technology, 10*(1), 4–12.

Sundin, K., Norberg, A., & Jansson, L. (2001). The meaning of skilled care providers' relationships with stroke and aphasia patients. *Qualitative Health Research, 1*(3), 308–321.

Tappen, R. M. (1994). Development of the refined ADL assessment scale for patients with Alzheimer's and related disorders. *Journal of Gerontological Nursing, 6,* 35–42.

Tousignant, M., Arsenault, A. B., Corriveau, H., & Philippe, P. (2000). Clinical evaluation of patient following stroke: Proposed stroke patient taxonomy based on cluster analysis method. *Physiotherapy Theory & Practice, 16*(2), 81–93.

United States Department of Health and Human Services Centers for Medicare and Medicaid Services (USDHHS). (2005). Health Insurance Portability and Accountability Act of 1996. www.cms.hhs.gov/HIPAAGenInfo. Accessed May 30, 2006.

Vogelpohl, T. S., Beck, C. K., Heacock, P., & Mercer, S. O. (1996). "I can do it!" Dressing: Promoting independence through individualized strategies. *Journal of Gerontological Nursing, 22,* 39–42.

Wan, H., Sengupta, M., Velkoff, V., & DeBarros, K. (2005). *65+ in the United States.* Retrieved From http://www.census2010.gov/prod/2006pubs/p23-209.pdf Accessed April 24, 2008.

White, R. W. (1959). Motivation reconsidered: The concept of competence. *Psychological Review, 66,* 297–333.

Whiting, S., Lincoln, N., Bhavani, G., & Cockburn, J. (1985). *RPAB—Rivermead Perceptual Assessment Battery—Manual.* Windsor: NFER-Nelson.

Wikby, K., & Fägerskiöld, A. (2004). The willingness to eat: An investigation of appetite in the elderly. *Scandinavian Journal of Caring Sciences, 18,* 120–127.

Williams, R., Brody, B. L., Thomas, R. G., Kaplan, R. M., & Brown, S. I. (1998). The psychosocial impact of macular degeneration. *Archives of Ophthalmology, 16*(4), 514–520.

Wilmoth, J. (2001). Living arrangements among older immigrants in the United States. *The Gerontologist, 41*(2), 1014–1130.

World Health Organization. (1999). *The World Health Organization disability assessment schedule phase II field trial instrument.* Geneva: Author.

World Health Organization. (2000). *International classification of impairment, disability, and handicap* (2nd ed.). Geneva: Author.

Wylde, M. A. (1998). Consumer knowledge of home modifications. *Technology and Disability, 8,* 51–68.

Young, J. T. (2004). Illness behavior: A selected review and synthesis. *Sociology of Health and Illness, 26,* 1–31.

Zingmark, K., Norberg, A., & Sandman, S. (1995). The experience of being at home throughout the lifespan. Investigations of persons aged from 2 to 102. *International Journal of Aging and Human Development, 41,* 47–62.

CHAPTER 12

Leisure

Anita C. Bundy, ScD, OTR, FAOTA • Lindy M. Clemson, PhD, MAppSc (OT), BAppSc (OT), Dip OT

Life should not be a journey to the grave with the intention of arriving safely in an attractive and well-preserved body. Better to skid in sideways, champagne in one hand, strawberries in the other, body thoroughly used up, totally worn out and screaming WOO HOO—what a ride!

Anonymous (adapted from Hunter S. Thompson)

OBJECTIVES

By the end of this chapter, readers will be able to:

1. Define leisure.
2. Discuss current issues relating leisure to aging and age-related disability.
3. Discuss leisure as a statement of identity.
4. Define four important elements of leisure: control, motivation, disengagement, and engagement.
5. Discuss the assessment of leisure.
6. Understand the importance of the elements of leisure for intervention.

Leisure, like many terms used in occupational therapy, is a "fuzzy" word. Although each of us may recognize leisure when it occurs in our own lives, its definition is elusive (Driver, Brown, & Peterson, 1991). Generally, **leisure** is defined in one of three ways (Csikszentmihalyi & Kleiber, 1991):

• *Discretionary time*—time not obligated to work, self-care, or instrumental activity (e.g., shopping, child care)

• *Culturally sanctioned activity*—an activity readily recognized as leisure (e.g., fishing, golfing)
• An *experience*—the perception that leisure "activities" are intrinsically motivated and freely chosen and allow one to disengage from some of the concerns of real life

None of these ways of defining leisure is, by itself, sufficient. Much unobligated time is not leisure. On the other hand, leisure is much more than unobligated time. Defining leisure by listing culturally sanctioned activities fails to capture the myriad activities an individual might consider as leisure (e.g., bathing, baking, caring for a grand-child) (Allen & Chin-sang, 1990; Hillman & Chapparo, 1995). Leisure defined as freely cho-sen, intrinsically motivating activities freed from some of the unnecessary constraints of reality comes closer to a definition that is useful to occu-pational therapists. However, this definition includes activities that are potentially harmful to the individual (e.g., drinking, drug use), society, or the environment (Csikszentmihalyi & Kleiber, 1991; Mannell, 1993). Potentially harmful activ-ities may not be ones that occupational therapists seek to promote with their clients. In contrast, desirable leisure activities embody these traits and lead to self-actualization (Csikszentmihalyi & Kleiber, 1991; Hogg, 1993; Mannell, 1993). In this chapter, we adopt a model of leisure that emphasizes traits of leisure leading to self-actualization.

Because it is freely chosen, individuals can use leisure to make statements to themselves and others about who they are. That is, leisure is a statement of identity. Thus, when at risk of losing a valued leisure pursuit, that individual also risks losing an important part of himself or herself.

Researchers (Atchley, 1989, 1993; Kelly, 1993) have suggested that individuals maintain a core set of leisure activities across the life span. Some of these activities are learned early in life and derive their meaning from a host of sources, including culture and association with significant others (Csikszentmihalyi & Kleiber, 1991; Iso-Ahola, Jackson, & Dunn, 1994; McGuire, 2004). At the same time, individuals also seek new leisure pursuits, either as replacement for relinquished activity or as a means to increase their leisure repertoire (Csikszentmihalyi & Kleiber, 1991; Iso-Ahola et al., 1994; Mobily, 1991; Zimmer, 1997).

The meanings contained within various leisure activities may differ from person to per-son and may change across the life span (Lawton, 1993). In contrast, the meaning may be retained even if the activity changes (Lawton, 1993). In the next sections, we examine various meanings potentially associated with leisure.

Leisure is an important issue for older adults for a variety of reasons. Many of them no longer have a primary identity that comes from their work (Bevil, 1993). Leaving one's professional or work role also results in significant unobligated time (McPherson, 1991; Mobily, 1991). For some people, these changes can be disconcerting. Many older adults have been socialized to believe that "being idle is the devil's work" (Goodale & Cooper, 1991). Further, older adults are prone to age-related disability (e.g., arthritis, stroke, dementia) that may result in the need to abandon or replace cherished leisure activities (Corr & Bayer, 1992; Fex, 1998; Husaini & Moore, 1990; Mansson, 1995; McGuire, 2004). Finally, leisure is commonly linked with life satisfaction and quality of life for men and women with and without disabilities (Beck & Page, 1988; Bevil, 1993; Gabriel & Bowling, 2004; Griffin & McKenna, 1998; Kinney & Coyle, 1992; Lau, Chi, & McKenna, 1998; Lindberg, 1995; Pereira & Stagnitti, 2006; Riddick & Stewart, 1994; Zoerink, 2001) Leisure is thought by some (Coleman & Iso-Ahola, 1993; Fabrigoule, 1995; Kleiber, Hutshinson, & Williams, 2002) to pro-vide a "buffer" against some forms of age-related disability (e.g., dementia). Thus, leisure is an important concern for occupational therapists who enable older adults to do what they want and need to do in their daily lives (Bevil, 1993; Freysinger, 1993; Griffin & McKenna, 1998; Lau, Chi, & McKenna, 1998; Mishra, 1992; Pereira & Stagnitti, 2006; Tatham & McCree, 1992; Voelki, 1993).

This chapter is composed of five major sections:

1. We review some current issues raised by major theorists and researchers related to leisure and aging.
2. We describe leisure as a statement of identity.
3. We probe four important elements of leisure: control, motivation (meaning), disengage-ment from some constraints of "real life," and the ability of the individual to become completely "absorbed."
4. We offer a tentative model of leisure designed particularly for use by occupational therapists who seek to assess and promote leisure with older clients.
5. We provide suggestions and case studies in which we use this model.

Leisure and Aging

There is a plethora of literature on leisure and aging. Leisure in aging individuals has been studied, for example, from the perspective of

- Its psychological benefits (e.g., well-being, life satisfaction) (Bevil, 1993; Gabriel & Bowling, 2004; Griffin & McKenna, 1998; Lau, Chi, & McKenna, 1998; Lawton, 1993; Pereira & Stagnitti, 2006; Zoerink, 2001)
- Its form and meaning (Kelly, 1982; Lawton, 1993)
- The ways in which it is affected by demographic and cohort characteristics (McGuire, 2004; Timmer, Bode, & Dittmann-Kohli, 2003)

A number of authors (McPherson, 1991; Riddick & Stewart, 1994) have pointed out that aging is a woman's issue because the number of older women is far greater than the number of older men. The ratio of women to men over the age of 85 years in the year 2002 was more than 2 to 1. Thus, leisure for aging individuals also is a woman's issue; however, until the 1980s, relatively little was done to describe women's leisure (Riddick, 1993). Even less is known about the leisure of nonwhite men or women (Allen & Chin-sang, 1990; Chin-Sang & Allen, 1991; Riddick & Stewart, 1994) or individuals from any "marginalized" group (e.g., people with disabilities, lesbians, and gay men) (Jacobson & Samdahl, 1998). Furthermore, although many previous cohorts of older women have had little experience with or value for leisure (Riddick & Stewart, 1994), current and future generations of women will have had significant leisure experiences throughout their lives. Thus, we can expect that they will continue their interests into retirement. Some may even develop new interests.

Elaine is a 73-year-old "semiretired" geologist. About 4 years ago, Elaine began running as support for her partner, who was training for a marathon. When her partner was injured, Elaine entered, and finished, her first marathon. She has been running ever since and now is ranked as one of the best in her age group.

Leisure wears many faces. Although many authors have offered classifications of leisure activities, there is little agreement among them (Lawton, 1993). For the most part, activities considered to be leisure are self-determined. What one individual calls leisure might be called work by another, and vice versa. There is no clear demarcation between work, self-care, and leisure, especially for older individuals (Hillman & Chapparo, 1995). Although many elderly people prefer home-based, sedentary leisure, there is no age at which individuals can be presumed to cease involvement in active or outdoor activities. Friendship and social interaction are a crucial part of some leisure activity (Adams, 1993). Other important activities are solitary (Bevil, 1993).

There is little agreement as to how health and perceived health affect leisure participation in older individuals (Bevil, 1993). Furthermore, little is known about how disabilities affect leisure, except that many older people who experience stroke, arthritis, or other age-related disability are likely to decrease their participation in leisure activities and to be unhappy about their loss (Corr & Bayer, 1992; Lindberg, 1995; Mansson, 1995). Clearly, some older individuals with or without disabilities are forced to change the pattern of their involvement in leisure activity (ceasing some, replacing others) because of factors beyond their control. A relatively recent tradition of research has examined these intrapersonal patterns with both healthy individuals and individuals with arthritis (Iso-Ahola et al., 1994; Jackson, 1990; Jackson & Dunn, 1988; McGuire, 1989; Zimmer, 1997).

Iso-Ahola, Jackson, and Dunn (1994) found that the percentage of healthy older adults (64 and over) and healthy middle-aged adults (44 to 63) who added new activities to their repertoires was essentially the same (approximately 20%). Similarly, approximately 20% replaced former activities with new ones and 20% quit activities without replacing them. The largest percentage of their sample (approximately 40%) continued with the same activities. Men were more likely than women to add, replace, and continue activities; the number of men and women who ceased an activity did not differ.

In contrast, Zimmer, Hickey, and Searle (1997) found that older adults who have arthritis were much more likely to replace (approximately 40%) or quit (approximately 48%) activities and much less likely to add new (approximately 7%) or continue with (approximately 5%) former activities. (The majority [74%] of the sample examined by Zimmer and associates was female.) Although ceasing activity was associated with the severity of arthritis, nonforfeiture of activity was related to a complex pattern that included social structure. Those with a strong social structure were more likely to continue or replace activities. The relationship between social structure and leisure with old people is a common finding (e.g., Coleman & Iso-Ahola, 1993). Potentially, professionals might become a part of a social structure that enables older adults to retain participation in satisfying leisure activities.

Although little is known empirically about the factors that contribute to loss of leisure in the elderly population, with few notable exceptions, even less is known about the effectiveness of intervention to minimize that loss. In one study, Searle, Mahon, Iso-Ahola, Srolias, and van Dyck (1995) implemented an extensive leisure education program with 13 older adults (2 males, 11 females) who had recently ceased, or were experiencing problems that were limiting their participation in, their favorite leisure activity. Following participation in a modified version of the Community Reintegration Program (Bullock & Howe, 1991), these individuals experienced higher levels of perceived leisure control, leisure competence, and life satisfaction and reduced levels of boredom with their leisure than a control group who did not receive any intervention. Although the participants in the study conducted by Searle and colleagues were not able to generalize their

increased feelings of control to their lives in general, the authors indicated that the intervention did not adequately target generalization. They suggested that future interventions could address this problem easily.

The program implemented by Searle and associates (1995) consisted of 12 units. Clients met individually with a therapist once a week. The average number of weeks spent in the program was 17 (range 14 to 25). An important part of the program was that after clients identified desired leisure activities, they met with the therapist in the place in which the activity took place (if it was outside the home). A summary of the units of the Leisure Education Program is shown in Table 12-1.

In another intervention study, Drummond and Walker (1996) examined the effect of a leisure rehabilitation program (as compared with no intervention and a "conventional" occupational therapy group). Participants who received leisure rehabilitation had significantly better skills in leisure and mobility (6 months after intervention) and psychological well-being

---

TABLE 12-1 **Leisure Education Program Units**

Unit	Title	Content
1	What do you do for leisure?	The client explores the potential benefits of leisure on physical and mental well-being and his or her personal recreation interests.
2	Why you do what you do.	Based on the list of interests identified in Unit 1, the therapist helps the client decide what motivates him or her to participate in specific leisure activities.
3	How do you do it?	The client learns to conduct an activity analysis of each of his or her leisure interests.
4	Can you do it?	Clients are taught to realistically assess current and potential physical and mental capabilities and how they may affect future recreation involvement.
5	Can or will you adapt?	The client is exposed to the concepts of activity adaptation and equipment modification, and is taught how to use the procedures to facilitate satisfactory leisure participation.
6	What are the barriers?	The client explores the variety of barriers he or she may face as well as ways and means of overcoming barriers to enable participation in chosen leisure pursuits.
7	What plans do you have for your future leisure?	The client is taught to make realistic short- and long-range leisure plans.
8	What else is there?	The client explores other potential leisure pursuits, determines what skills he or she must acquire to participate in those activities, and develops plans for participation.
9	Resources.	The client is taught to identify who may act as a support for him or her to carry out leisure goals and how to make clear and assertive requests for assistance.
10	Personal resources.	The client is taught to assess personal resources including such things as finances, transportation, and equipment as they relate to the leisure plans.

continued on page 294

TABLE 12-1 Leisure Education Program Units (continued)

Unit	Title	Content
11	Community resources.	The client is exposed to community resources and is taught how to assess such resources as a means of facilitating community based participation.
12	Before you are through with us.	The client reassesses and, if necessary, revises participation goals (In part, this is to ensure that the client is able to continue to reassess leisure goals in the future.)

Source: Adapted from Searle, MS, et al: Enhancing a sense of independence and psychological well-being among the elderly: A field experiment. Journal of Leisure Research 27:107, 1995, with permission.

(3 months after intervention) than those in the other groups. The leisure rehabilitation program involved individually prescribed interventions grouped by the authors into the following categories:

- Treatment (e.g., practice of transfers needed for leisure pursuits)
- Positioning
- Provision of equipment
- Advice on attaining financial assistance and transportation
- Liaison with specialist organizations
- Provision of physical assistance (e.g., referral to voluntary agencies)

Participation in leisure rehabilitation was contrasted with conventional occupational therapy in that conventional occupational therapy did not involve help or advice related to leisure activity. The duration of both interventions was at least 30 minutes every 2 weeks for 3 months.

Few other programs have been as successful. For example, in the largest randomized controlled trial conducted by an occupational therapist, neither improvements in mood nor increases in the number of leisure activities were noted after 6 or 12 months. In this trial, Parker and colleagues (Parker et al., 2001) compared a control group with two groups who received occupational therapy interventions, one leisure based and the other activities of daily living (ADL) based. A number of limitations were associated with the report of this trial. For example, although the protocols stipulated a minimum of 10 visits, a mean of only 8.5 was conducted. Further, neither the type nor the nature of the interventions was defined, apart from specifying goal setting and practice. This study confirmed that usual practice is not

sufficient for promoting leisure and greater attention needs to be paid to the nature and intensity of intervention. Perhaps it also highlights a need to evaluate leisure in more ways than simply how often it is performed, including examining clients' experience of and satisfaction with leisure (Bullock & Howe, 1991; Mactavish & Mahon, 2005; Meakins, Bundy, & Gliner, 2005).

Garcia-Martin, Gomez-Jacinto, and Martimportugues-Goyenechea (2004) showed that intrinsically motivated activities carried out in small groups of voluntary participants enhanced social support, perceived control, and self-efficacy. However, centers and adult day programs where leisure-related programming is most likely to occur get participants out of the house and keep them occupied but rarely involve real leisure (Tse & Howie, 2005). This is particularly true for the younger old (Pardasani, 2004) and minority groups (Bigby & Balandin, 2005; Pardasani, 2004).

Leisure as a Statement of Identity

Our actions help to shape our selves (Clark, 1991). Each activity we perform is associated with a self-specific experience of that activity. Each individual experiences the same activity very differently (Lawton, 1993; McGuire, 2004). The experience associated with any activity is likely to be more important than the activity itself in contributing to development (Kelly, 1996).

Conversely, we do what we are (Clark, 1991; Wilson, 1981). That is, our actions reflect ourselves; they are outward manifestations or statements of who we are. Through our actions, we tell others, and ourselves, about ourselves (Samdahl, 1988).

Each activity in which we engage reflects one or more life roles or identities (Kelly, 1982; Kielhofner, 1995). Furthermore, leisure roles and identities seem more important:

• To some people than others
• In certain periods of life than in others (Kelly, 1982)

However, because leisure experiences are freely chosen, they seem to make very important statements of who we are (Kelly, 1982; Neulinger, 1974; Scraton & Holland, 2006). It is common to decorate our homes with mementos of leisure experiences and pictures or other reminders of leisure companions (Csikszentmihayli & Rochberg-Halton, 1981; Rockwell-Dylla, 1991). Older people, in particular, enjoy displaying those objects and reminiscing. In so doing, they make statements about their accomplishments and identities.

Leisure identities and activities, perhaps in part because of their significant relationship with the perceived self, also seem to be particularly vulnerable to age-related barriers and disability. "If I can't do it the way (often translated 'as well as') I used to, I don't want to do it at all," is a comment frequently made by older people who no longer engage in particular leisure pursuits.

Rockwell-Dylla (1991) related the story of Stan, a 62-year-old man who had been an avid golfer before suffering a stroke. Following the stroke, he was unwilling even to hit whiffle balls in the yard, despite the urgings of his wife. Rockwell-Dylla wrote:

> Stan didn't take [his wife] up on her suggestions because he knew he wouldn't be able to hold the golf club like he used to do with ease. He wasn't afraid of having to learn to do something in a new way, but what did concern him was how he appeared in front of other people. Stan shared with me how he thought the neighbors would make comments like "what's he trying to do, he's a disabled person, we don't want anything to do with him." (p. 85)

Golfing once made a statement about Stan's physical prowess; however, following his stroke, he perceived that golfing would make a statement about his physical disability. Stan seemed to worry about looking foolish. Perhaps he feared that his neighbors would generalize his physical disability to a mental impairment. He seemed to fear that his neighbors' memories of Stan, the athlete, would be replaced by visions of Stan the "cripple" or Stan "the fool." Stan feared he could no longer make desirable statements about himself through golf, so he gave it up. Perhaps he would have benefited from having someone help him "change the frame" around golf. Rather than a statement of his incapacity, he might have been helped to transform golf into a "psychological triumph" (Lawton, 1993, p. 37).

In contrast, engagement in leisure activities that had previously been an important part of her life was integral to 74-year-old Sarah's recovery following a stroke. Sarah had been depressed, not only because of the loss of physical capability but because her children wanted her to go into a retirement village to receive "the kind of care they felt she needed." Sarah chose instead to attend a Day Therapy Center where she was introduced to Sailability. Becoming a "sailing grandmother," winning a championship race, and being featured in a local newspaper were turning points in her recovery. She did not have the strength or movement to handle the sails, but she said, "I'm the captain. I choose who rolls the sails and tell them how to do it. You have to think. Or you might hit another boat." When Sarah was a child, her family had sailed and many years later sailing renewed her identity and self-confidence. Sailability kept her independent and mentally alert. She went every week.

Elements of Leisure

Leisure both contributes to and reflects identity. Furthermore, leisure is more aptly characterized as experience than activity. However, the experience of leisure generally occurs in the context of activity. Thus, in order to promote leisure, it is necessary to separate leisure from nonleisure. We propose that four factors particularly contribute to leisure. These are control, motivation, freedom from some unnecessary constraints of reality, and engagement. Each factor represents a complex interaction between an individual, his or her life experiences, and the environment. Furthermore, these factors mutually influence one another (Neumann, 1971). For example, when one feels in control, he or she can determine how to act on his or her motivations

(Neumann). Each of these proposed elements of leisure requires further discussion.

Control

Control is a complex phenomenon. *Being in control* means that an individual can predict and feel power over certain aspects of the environment (Purcell & Keller, 1989). The individual is free to choose what to do and with whom (Neumann, 1971). Being in control also refers to some ability to determine the outcome of an activity. Leisure activities may be an important way to fulfill an individual's needs for control (Purcell & Keller, 1989). In the absence of control, one may feel helpless or as though powerful others or forces outside the self determine events and outcomes (Purcell & Keller, 1989). Feelings of helplessness may result in depression and decreased motivation, reasoning ability, or self-esteem (Abramson, 1978). In this section, we discuss multiple aspects of control as they apply to the determination of a leisure experience. These include the following:

- Freedom of choice
- Determination of outcomes
- Matching challenges to skill
- Psychological comfort
- Optimal levels of choice
- Reciprocity

We also discuss briefly using leisure to take control of one's life.

Freedom of Choice

Freedom of choice typically is the most important determinant of whether an activity is experienced as leisure (Gunter, 1980; Iso-Ahola, 1980; Neulinger, 1974). Generally, if individuals must, or feel they must, perform an activity, it is not leisure (Lawton, 1993; Neulinger, 1974). By this criterion, all activities can be leisure under certain circumstances (Hillman & Chapparo, 1995). What may be among the most mundane of tasks for some people, for example, bathing, can become leisure for the individual who chooses to "steal" some time away from the concerns of daily life for a long, restful bubble bath.

Freedom of choice seems a fairly simple criterion for distinguishing leisure from nonleisure; however, its very simplicity may make freedom of choice confusing when trying to analyze the leisure value of complex activities for particular individuals. For example, is the grandmother who offers freely to care for her grandchildren, even though her son and daughter-in-law had no previous plans, experiencing leisure? Using the criterion of free choice alone, she is. It is likely that she actually does experience leisure during some, or even most, moments of the weekend. However, it is equally likely that there will be moments in that weekend when what the woman experiences is far from leisure, even though she has freely chosen to care for her grandchildren. Control entails more than making an initial decision to engage in an activity.

In the course of an activity, one must also feel in control of all the various aspects. Control is not an all-or-none phenomenon. Rarely is a person in total control of any activity or event; in fact, total control may not be desirable. What is desirable is that the individual feel that his or her skills and abilities are matched to the challenges of the activity (Csikszentmihayli, 1975, 1985). Many things contribute to feelings of control or lack of control; these include such dimensions as

- Complexity of the activity
- Number of other people involved
- Duration of the activity

In general, the more complex the activity, the more other people are involved, and the longer the duration, the less likely a person is to feel in control, and hence, to experience leisure. Because control is such a complex issue, a freely chosen activity often is not determined to be leisure until it has been completed. That is, until the individual can reflect on the experience and weigh the relative amount of control experienced, the determination of whether leisure was experienced cannot be made definitively. Sometimes, based on past experience or anticipation of relative lack of control, an individual may decide not to engage in a particular activity, or to alter it significantly, in order to increase the chances that leisure will be experienced.

For example, consider Barbara, a 60-year-old woman who lives alone in a high-rise apartment in Chicago (Figure 12-1). She has three daughters and several grandchildren who live locally and visit frequently. Although she enjoys their company, she often wishes she could get away from their demands. Recently, Barbara received two plane tickets as a gift, enabling her to make two trips anywhere in the country or to take a companion with her on a single trip. As Barbara made plans to travel to Houston to visit a cousin for the Christmas holidays, she entertained the notion of taking Cherie, one of her older grandchildren, with her. In the end, however, she decided to take two trips by herself. In her words, "For a minute, I lost my mind. I thought it would be fun to take Cherie, but then I started thinking, 'I'm doing this for me. How much fun will I have if I take an 8-year-old along?' I'll go by myself to Houston. And I made a reservation to go to Atlanta for Thanksgiving. I have another cousin in Atlanta. She has a house there. I always have fun in Atlanta."

Barbara opted to use her tickets in a way that increased the chances she would experience leisure. She saw that if she traveled with an 8-year-old, she might have fewer opportunities to do what she wanted to do. Barbara might have experienced just as much leisure had she taken Cherie with her, but her past experiences suggested that having the responsibility for an 8-year-old significantly reduced her choices; thus, the chance for a leisure experience was also reduced.

Determination of Outcomes

For some leisure experiences, being in control extends to determining the outcome of an activity (Neumann, 1971). This is particularly true for creative endeavors; however, the need to determine the outcome of an activity is not always a part of the leisure experience. In fact, certain leisure activities are selected particularly for their lack of predictability. Many games fall under this rubric (Caillois, 1979). Older adults often list bingo and card games as favorite leisure activities (Havighurst, 1979). Yet when players are certain of the outcome (i.e., the winner), they throw in the chips or the hand, and they begin a new game, thereby reintroducing unpredictability (Caillois, 1979).

Even within activities in which lack of predictability is a part of the appeal, a certain amount of control must be present if the experience is to be leisure. The individual must feel in control of the necessary materials (e.g., cards) and other aspects of the situation (e.g., able to hear a partner's bid). In creative endeavors such as knitting, woodworking, and cooking, control includes the ability to manage materials in such a way as to construct a pleasing product. Activities vary widely in their demand for skill. The degree to which activities are experienced as leisure depends, in part, on the individual's physical skills and abilities (e.g., dexterity, strength). However, even the most physically skilled individual may lack the aesthetic sense to combine colors, shapes, or spices into a pleasing product; thus, physical skill alone does not ensure that an individual will have sufficient control in an activity to experience leisure.

Matching Challenges to Skill

With regard to control, what all the aforementioned activities have in common when they are

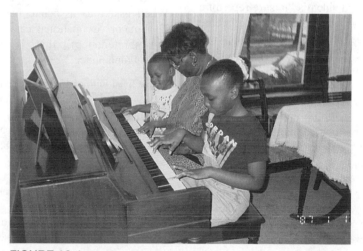

FIGURE 12-1 Barbara enjoys spending time with her grandchildren. (Courtesy of Anita Bundy, with permission.)

experienced as leisure is that the challenges presented match the skills of the individual (Csikszentmihayli, 1975, 1985; Mobily, Lemke, & Gisin, 1991). If that is not the case, no matter what the activity, the person engaging in it cannot be experiencing leisure. The grandmother caring for her grandchildren must feel that she can skillfully manage the range of events that she might encounter while babysitting. The older man who experiences leisure in woodworking must feel that he can manage the materials he will need to create a visually pleasing and, perhaps, utilitarian object. This may entail more than using tools and managing wood; it also may mean visualizing an object in a block of wood or creating jigs for completing some aspect of the project. Similarly, the older woman knitting an afghan or a sweater must be able to control the needles and the yarn and, perhaps, follow a pattern easily.

Psychological Comfort

Frequent participation in an activity often leads to psychological comfort with that activity. This concept is related to competence (matching skills to challenges); however, psychological comfort reflects internal rather than external standards for comparison. Mobily and colleagues (1991) offered the example of a competent reader confronted with very complex reading material. Although the individual might be competent by external standards (e.g., as good as others his age), he likely would feel psychological discomfort with the material. Thus, he is not likely to feel he is engaging in leisure. Mobily and associates were concerned with identifying activities that compose an individual's "leisure repertoire" and thus could be substituted one for another. They recommended that professionals helping an individual replace valued leisure activities evaluate perceived competence first, followed by perceived psychological comfort.

Beverly is 69 years old. She has always had a wide leisure repertoire encompassing both sedentary (e.g., reading) and physically active (e.g., cross country skiing, biking) or outdoor (e.g., camping) pursuits. Although reading is her passion, until recently, the number of strenuous activities in her repertoire far exceeded the sedentary ones. Within the last 2 years, Beverly had a number of health-related problems, including the development of bone spurs on her heels that have precluded her participation in strenuous activity. These bone spurs were treated with only partial success, and Beverly continues to experience pain from prolonged standing and walking. A friend suggested that Beverly take up in-line skating as an alternative to hiking. As much as she misses strenuous physical activity, Beverly balked. She did not believe she would have any more difficulty with in-line skating than any other woman her age; rather, she had never tried it. Her reaction was one of psychological discomfort.

Optimal Levels of Choice

To be experienced as leisure, any activity must contain an optimal level of choice. Optimal choice is determined by the individual and is a function of that person's level of skill and experience in that activity. For example, the inexperienced painter, or the painter who perceives himself or herself as lacking certain skills or abilities, may be more likely to experience leisure with a paint-by-number picture than with a blank easel. On the other hand, the established artist probably would be bored with a paint-by-number picture.

Reciprocity

Reciprocity in a relationship means the relationship is balanced or symmetrical. Individuals feel that, overall, the amount they receive is similar to the amount they give. Otherwise, a state of indebtedness develops (Goodman, 1984). Indebtedness alters the relationship. Hillman and Chapparo (1995) relayed the story of a participant in their study of occupational role performance in elderly men who had experienced a stroke. When asked to associate his role as a father in a major occupational category (e.g., leisure, self-maintenance), this participant selected "self-maintenance."

> He lived with his daughter, and seemed to be saying that, although his children cared for him, he did not reciprocate by doing anything for them. Their relationship with him seemed to focus on checking on his ability to care for himself successfully.
>
> "I seem to have more of a relationship with them than I have with them. Do you understand?"
>
> Interviewer: "No, say that again."
>
> "Well, they're always . . . seeking to see how I am . . . and I haven't bothered about them!"

Interviewer: "Oh, I see what you mean. So you think the relationship's a bit one way?"

"Well, it is . . . Because after all, they've got their own relationships." (p 94)

Although the relationship between reciprocity and control, motivation, or leisure is not clear, individuals may need to feel sufficient control to be *able* to give to another. Feeling as though one is giving to another is often believed to be an important motivator for leisure for older individuals (Allen & Chin-sang, 1990; Havighurst, 1979; Jacobson & Samdahl, 1998; Lawton, 1993). Given that, it is fairly surprising that Timmer, Bode, and Dittman-Kohli (2003) found that after age 54, older Germans were significantly less likely to express interest in helping their children or being there for their grandchildren.

Reciprocity can involve caring for anything or anyone that, in turn, makes one feel needed. Muriel, an 83-year-old woman, living alone since the death of her husband and then a long-time companion, was asked about her leisure pursuits. She thought a long time until "her birds and her lizard" came to mind. Her face lit up and her words conveyed her joy as she described the wild animals in her yard. She loves the "chatter and squabbling of the birds as they push each other to get to the food." When her beloved butcher birds are gone for the winter, she "misses the beautiful trill that announces their presence." "The brazen black and white magpies seem to stamp their feet" when she does not come quickly enough. Her blue-tongue lizard is "such a treasure." She has to watch he does not come in the house in his enthusiasm to reach her.

Leisure as Means of Taking Control of One's Life

Jim is 87 and, because of cardiac and orthopedic problems, has severely reduced mobility. His new scooter has given back some of his most important leisure. Each year Jim and his wife Jean take a holiday to the seaside. A merchant Navy man in his youth, Jim has retained his love of the sea. He and Jean get an apartment overlooking the sea and, with the scooter, meander along the long promenade, experiencing the fresh breezes and the smell and the sounds of the sea. He says, "I'm self-powered again. Otherwise I would be stuck." The scooter has allowed Jim to regain control over where, when,

and with whom he goes. In turn, he has reclaimed a leisure event that maintains his identity and gives him great pleasure.

Older people are at risk for feeling little control over their lives (Mobily, 1991; Savell, 1991). This is particularly true for institutionalized persons, individuals with disabilities, and members of other marginalized groups (Jacobson & Samdahl, 1998). Leisure is an important context for the exercise of control (Iso-Ahola, 1980; MacNeil & Teague, 1987). In classic studies of nursing home residents, numerous authors (Langer & Rodin, 1976; Perlmuter & Langer, 1982; Schulz, 1976) have associated control with increased self-esteem, happiness, activity level, and hopefulness for the future, as well as decreased pain, need for medication, loneliness, boredom, and mortality (Rodin & Langer, 1977; Schulz & Hanusa, 1978). Similarly, both Menec and Chipperfield (1997) and Timmer et al. (2003) have reported considerable evidence for a relationship between locus of control and activity in older people. Structural equation modeling allowed Menec and Chipperfield to hypothesize a causal relationship. Jacobson and Samdahl (1998) described leisure as a context in which their old lesbian participants, who felt ignored, invisible, or personally at risk in their "public lives," could create "safe spaces" for social interaction and to meet their needs for leaving the world a better place than they found it. Clearly, leisure can be a powerful tool for helping older people take control of their lives and express their identities.

Motivation

Motivation is the reason one chooses to engage in an activity. It is synonymous with meaning. Typically, motivation is an element discussed as a determinant of leisure. According to some leisure theories, motivation must be intrinsic; that is, the activity must be done only for its own sake, for the pleasurable experience associated with it, and not for any long-term gains by the individual, payment, or the benefit of someone else (Csikszentmihalyi, 1975, 1985; Mannell, Zuzanek, & Larson, 1988; Neulinger, 1974).

Although motivation clearly is an important factor in the determination of leisure, the degree to which motivation must be intrinsic is not clear. What is certain is that the activity must have an **autotelic aspect.** That is, the individual must experience most or all of the various aspects of the activity as pleasurable, whether or not the activity was originally undertaken for its intrinsic value (Csikszentmihayli, 1975). A number of authors (Allen & Chin-sang, 1990; Kaufman, 1993; Mannell, 1993) have suggested that helping another or doing an activity because it is "good for me" (e.g., exercise) are both powerful motivators. In fact, Mannell (1993) found that freely chosen, extrinsically motivated activities produced greater involvement from participants than did intrinsically motivated activity. Losier, Bourque, and Vallerand (1993) found that intrinsic motivation and self-determined extrinsic motivation were equally correlated with leisure satisfaction.

The lack of clarity about whether or not the motivation for leisure activities is always intrinsic can be seen throughout the leisure-related literature. Many authors (Allen & Chin-sang, 1990; Crandall, 1980; Donald & Havighurst, 1959; Havighurst, 1979; Havighurst & Feigenbaum, 1968; Kleiber, 1985; Mannell, Zuzanek, & Larson, 1988; Menec & Chipperfield, 1997) have examined and discussed older individuals' motivations for leisure in general or for specific leisure activities. Typically, many motivations or meanings are listed. Havighurst's list is representative; he and his colleagues included the following as motivations or meanings typically associated with leisure activities:

- Just for the pleasure of it
- Welcome change from work
- New experience
- Contact with friends
- Chance to achieve something
- Make time pass
- Allows creativity
- Benefit to society
- Helps financially
- Promotes self-respect
- Gives me more standing with others
- Makes me popular

Further, Havighurst (1979) and his colleagues (Donald & Havighurst, 1959; Havighurst & Feigenbaum, 1968) have indicated, not surprisingly, that certain motives or meanings are more commonly associated with certain leisure activities than with others, and that certain individuals experience different motivations or meanings for the same activity. Havighurst and colleagues are among the few researchers and theorists (Allen &

Chin-sang, 1990; Henderson & Rannells, 1988; Lawton, 1993; McGuire, 2004) who have attempted to examine individual differences in activity-specific motivations. These researchers have provided significant insight to occupational therapists seeking to promote leisure with elderly clients (Kelly, 1982).

Clearly, not all the motivations or meanings for leisure activities listed by Havighurst (1979) and his colleagues (Donald & Havighurst, 1959; Havighurst & Feigenbaum, 1968), Lawton (1993), or McGuire and his colleagues (2004) can be considered intrinsic; however, there is no indication that the subjects of these investigations did not also experience intrinsic reward in their activities or found their activities to be less rewarding because of the relatively extrinsic character of the motivations associated with them.

In fact, Mannell, Zuzanek, and Larson (1988) found that elderly people experienced the greatest "flow" in activities they performed for their own long-term gain or for another's benefit. However, when the subjects indicated that they primarily performed particular leisure activities for extrinsic motivations, they may have been responding as much to perceived social acceptability as to their true motivations. The notion of justifying one's pleasure by the long-term gains associated with an activity or by the possibility of another's gain has been suggested by Ekerdt (1986) in his discussion of the "busy ethic" and by Cohen (1987) in his descriptions of adults playing with children.

Interestingly, senior citizens frequently report gambling as a valued leisure activity (McNeilly & Burke, 2001). Outings to a casino offer low-stress leisure for depression-era adults who might once have thought of such activity as frivolous or even sinful. McNeilly and Burke observed how "once inside a casino, older adults are entertained in a very friendly, receptive and anonymous environment, where age seems to make little difference to one's inclusion and participation (p. 26)." There clearly are many motivations for such activity, and the possible thrill of winning must be among them.

Complexity of Motivation

The motivation to engage in, or the meaning associated with, a particular activity clearly is a complex phenomenon. As Havighurst (1979) noted, the experience of leisure is strongly associated with one's personality. What "drives" one individual is very different from what drives another. Some individuals are clearly more people oriented than others. Thus, some people perceive service to others as an important motivation for leisure (Donald & Havighurst, 1959; Havighurst, 1979; Havighurst & Feigenbaum, 1968) and derive meaning from it (Allen & Chinsang, 1990; Henderson & Rannells, 1988). Some do not (Timmer, Bode, & Dittmann-Kohli, 2003).

Activities that stress interaction with the environment are more readily observable than inwardly focused activity (e.g., meditation, reminiscing, creative thought, aesthetic appreciation). They also are more commonly included on leisure activity questionnaires. However, Lawton (1994) cautioned researchers and practitioners that "there is a great void in probing what types of affect occur as a person engages in inner-oriented activities such as daydreaming, listening to music, or gazing at a loved one" (p. 154). Are inwardly directed activities not leisure? "New research is needed to probe further the place of what have been called 'introverted activities' and to understand better how personality and mental health outcomes are related to leisure activity choice" (p. 155). Furthermore, practitioners must consider how personality variables affect the leisure choices of individuals.

Havighurst's (Donald & Havighurst, 1959; Havighurst, 1979; Havighurst & Feigenbaum, 1968) and Lawton's (1994) statements that leisure activities are associated with different motives or meanings for different people suggest a certain degree of complexity in the relationship between leisure and motivation. There may be many more motivations associated with a particular activity than are immediately apparent, and many powerful motivations may not appear on lists such as those developed by Havighurst. Uncovering an individual's motivation for a leisure activity is particularly important when the need arises to substitute one activity for another.

Ron is a 72-year-old retired engineer. As long as anyone can remember, Ron has built things. He spends a significant amount of time creating small pieces of furniture and repairing objects in his home. He enjoys these activities thoroughly; he expressed pleasure both in the completed project and with all steps of the process. He particularly enjoys figuring out how to do a project and creating the necessary jigs and devices.

Several years ago, Ron experienced an illness that was exacerbated by the dust and chemical fumes associated with woodworking. He was urged by his physician to replace woodworking with another activity. Ron chose painting as an alternative because it seemed to offer many of the same benefits (being creative, working with his hands) without the negative consequences.

For approximately 1 year, Ron painted instead of doing woodworking; he became a good painter. However, he also became increasingly disenchanted with his new leisure activity. Painting, while capturing some of the same benefits of woodworking, apparently was not a suitable substitute. After that year, Ron put away his paints permanently and, once again, took out his woodworking tools. "If I'm going to die," he expressed, "I'm going to die happy."

Clearly, the motivations for woodworking most salient to Ron were not captured in painting. Perhaps if Ron had worked with a professional trained to help him examine his motivations and recapture them in a suitable substitute, he might have been able to adopt a leisure activity that did not have the negative consequences associated with woodworking. Unfortunately, that did not happen.

Certainly, it sometimes is possible to capture the most salient motivations for one activity in another and thus to help a person substitute a new leisure activity for one in which he or she can no longer engage. Rockwell-Dylla (1991) related the story of Les, a 90-year-old white man who had survived two strokes and about with cancer. Les was the retired owner of a paint company. Before his illnesses, he spent much of his leisure time decorating the interior of his home. As a result of both his age and his disability, Les was no longer able to move furniture and perform other activities required for interior decorating. Although he might have elected to direct others in the interior decoration, this apparently did not hold the same motivation for Les (or perhaps for the others in his life). At the suggestion of an occupational therapist, Les got involved in decoupage. He created dishes and other decorative objects, mixing and matching colors and patterns as he desired. This substitution of decoupage for home decorating was highly successful. Although many of the most obvious traits of home decoration were not present, one important motivation for Les was "playing" with colors; that activity could be recaptured in decoupage. Or, perhaps decoupage captured another motivation or meaning for Les.

Losier, Bourque, and Vallerand (1993) offered a model of leisure participation that may be useful to professionals interested in understanding or promoting leisure involvement with elderly individuals. Motivation was an important aspect of their model, which was based in self-determination theory (Donald & Havighurst, 1959; Havighurst, 1979; Havighurst & Feigenbaum, 1968). They described three broad types of motivation: intrinsic, extrinsic, and amotivation (not knowing why you are engaging in a particular activity). Furthermore, they subdivided extrinsic motivation into two types: self-determined and non-self- (other) determined. They described these four types of motivation as representing a continuum from most to least self-determined.

Using path analysis, Losier, Bourque, and Vallerand (1993) found that leisure opportunities and constraints determined leisure motivation. Furthermore, intrinsically motivated leisure was highly satisfying, and both intrinsic motivation and leisure satisfaction led to greater participation.

Freedom from Unnecessary Constraints of Reality

Kleiber (1985) defined *disengagement* as a space/time context created by removing constraints. Freedom from unnecessary constraints of real life (disengagement) is a necessary component of leisure. Constraints may be real or perceived, and they take many forms (e.g., family demands, financial constraints, pain, poor health, or disability) (Burrus-Bamel & Bammel, 1985; Havighurst, 1979; McAvoy, 1979). If an individual is to experience leisure, he or she must be able to disengage temporarily from those constraints.

As Kleiber (1985) noted, disengagement alone may be sufficient to produce leisure. However, many individuals find it extraordinarily difficult to maintain their disengagement from real-life concerns unless they engage in activity in which they become totally absorbed.

Engaging in activity that allows one to disengage from some of life's demands does not necessarily ensure leisure. When individuals find that they are motivated to engage primarily in activities that depend on certain abilities or resources that are constrained, they have extraordinary difficulty experiencing leisure.

Mary is 79 years old. Her vision has become progressively more limited over the past 15 years, in part as a result of excessive drinking. Throughout her life, reading has been a primary leisure source for Mary; she often read for several hours a day. However, Mary's vision has now worsened to the point that she can no longer read even large print. Mary expresses no interest in talking books, tapes, or the radio as a substitute for reading. In fact, she has been able to find no activity, except drinking, that enables her to disengage from the constraints of her life. The only activities in which she expresses interest are visually dependent. Thus, her "leisure" pursuits only serve to remind her continually of the constraints of her life that most concern her. As she attempts to disengage, she actually becomes more aware of her difficulties. Mary succeeds in disengaging by drinking, but drinking exacerbates her visual impairments and contributes to her decreased ability to seek alternative and true leisure experiences. Mary is caught in a vicious circle. She is motivated to engage in a leisure pursuit for which she lacks a critical ability; because she has little "control" of the written word, she is unable to disengage from the constraints of her visual impairment. To succeed in developing alternative leisure options, Mary will need help to examine the benefits she once derived from reading and to devise activities that provide some of the most important benefits without depending heavily on vision. Alternatively, Mary might be helped to examine other important motivations that, if satisfied through activity, might enable disengagement and opportunities for leisure.

Engagement

Numerous authors (Csikszentmihayli, 1975, 1985; Gunter, 1980; Kleiber, 1985; Mannell, 1993; Wilson, 1981) have used various terms (e.g., **flow, involvement, serious leisure, committed leisure**) to describe the total engagement in an activity that characterizes leisure. Loss of self-consciousness, the open cognitive set, and the pleasurable sensations associated with total engagement in a leisure activity are crucial to the experience of an activity as leisure (Csikszentmihayli, 1975, 1985; Kleiber, 1985). Leisure activity in which one becomes totally involved leads to self-actualization (Csikszentmihalyi & Kleiber, 1991).

The concept of total engagement is particularly powerful in examining and seeking to promote leisure with older individuals. Asking older adults, "Tell me about the activities you do (or have done in the past) in which you become totally absorbed (forget about everything else)" has been much more successful in identifying the experience of leisure for an individual than asking people what they do in their leisure.

In response to the latter, people often indicate that they have no leisure. If they attempt to answer the question, they seem constrained by listing activities that have been socially sanctioned as leisure, for example, golf, gardening, games, or television. In contrast, when people talk about activities in which they become totally absorbed, they often relate thick narrative accounts (Geertz, 1973) of their experiences. It is then quite easy to elicit further information about the benefits that they derive from those pursuits. In the case of individuals who have lost the ability to engage in those absorbing activities, one also can examine whether or not it is possible, or desirable, to adapt the previously enjoyed activity or a suitable substitute.

Desiree is a 78-year-old traditional Navajo woman. In addition to all of the traditional activities in which she has engaged since a very young age, Desiree works several hours each week as a volunteer in a day care center supported by the Navajo tribal government. When Desiree was asked (through an interpreter) what she did in her leisure, she laughed aloud. She indicated that even as a child she had not had time to play. She lived with her disabled grandmother and was responsible for all the home maintenance tasks that required mobility (including cooking and cleaning) and for tending the sheep. All of her life, chores took up most of her time; there was always something that needed to be done. Play and leisure were "a waste of time"; she rarely even sat down to rest. Desiree clearly was not interested in talking about leisure. Throughout the dialogue, her tone of voice remained stern, and at one point, she asked why the interviewer was asking such silly questions.

In contrast, when Desiree was asked what she did, now or in the past, in which she became totally absorbed, her voice took on warmth and she became involved and interested in the conversation. Desiree began to talk about weaving. She indicated that she learned to spin yarn when she was about 3 years old and to weave as soon as she was old enough. When she was engaged in spinning or weaving, she forgot everything else.

Navajo women do not weave their rugs from patterns; rather, they create the patterns they envision in their heads on the loom. Desiree recounted that as the pattern of the rug began to emerge and the rug "took on a life of its own," she became more and more involved in its creation. Csikszentmihayli (1985) and his colleagues (Csikszentmihayli & Graef, 1980; Larson & Csikszentmihayli, 1983) described similar benefits when they asked adults about times they experienced total engagement in an activity.

For professionals seeking to promote leisure with older individuals, examining leisure as an experience in which one becomes totally absorbed is particularly valuable (Krefting & Krefting, 1991). Rowles (1991) noted that older people respond particularly well to interview. Interview for the purposes of developing intervention is most useful when it elicits rich narrative description and the opportunity to seek additional detail as needed.

Total engagement can occur in the context of virtually any activity, as long as the person engaged in the activity feels a sense of control and is able to disengage from his or her real-life concerns (Csikszentmihayli, 1975, 1985; Kleiber, 1985) and when that activity is sufficiently motivating. We do not seek to help older individuals to conform to socially accepted classifications of leisure activity. Rather, we seek to enable individuals to become totally engaged in, and reap the accompanying benefits of, self-defined leisure. In so doing, we seek to help them make the statements they want to make about who they are as individuals.

A Tentative Model

We described four concepts related to leisure:

1. Control
2. Motivation
3. Disengagement from unnecessary constraints of reality
4. Total engagement in leisure

None of these elements can be described as all-or-none phenomena; each is much better described with a continuum. We propose that control, motivation, and disengagement from unnecessary constraints of reality, collectively, determine whether or not a person becomes totally absorbed in, and self-actualized from, an activity—that is, whether or not the person experiences leisure. The summative contributions of control, motivation, and disengagement to total engagement in leisure are illustrated schematically in Figure 12-2.

The elements of leisure are mutually influencing. That is, an individual engaging in an activity in which he or she feels little control is unlikely to be able to disengage from the constraints of real life. The converse also is likely to be true. Thus, our model will require further refinement. However, we find it useful to conceptualize leisure in this way when planning intervention with older people.

The desired outcome of intervention is that people develop a repertoire of activities:

- In which they can become totally engaged
- That allow them to attain self-actualization and make desired statements of self-identity

Consideration of the elements of leisure as a continuum enables us to

- Reflect with individuals on their relative positions on each line in the content of a particular activity.
- Determine which of the elements will yield most productively to intervention—Where can or should we begin in intervention to enable this person to experience leisure in daily life?

Promotion of Leisure: Application of the Model

Applied models of leisure are useful only to the extent that they allow therapists to explain relationships among constructs, make meaningful predictions, and implement successful interventions with individuals. Successful intervention depends on thorough assessment. Assessment of leisure is more likely to be thorough (i.e., to capture the most salient aspects) when it reflects an organized conceptualization of the elements of leisure. Discussed in Box 12-1 is the assessment of leisure. In Box 12-2, the focus is on intervention to promote the leisure aspects of occupational engagement.

We suggested that leisure can be defined as the experience of total engagement in an activity. We proposed that three elements contribute to that leisure experience: control, motivation, and the ability to disengage from the constraints of real life. Assessment based on this conceptual model of leisure entails the examination, with the individual, of each of these elements and of particular activities. There are many ways to go about gathering this information, including using checklists such as the Leisure Diagnostic Battery (Witt & Ellis, 1989), the Leisure Satisfaction Scale (Ragheb & Beard, 1980), and the

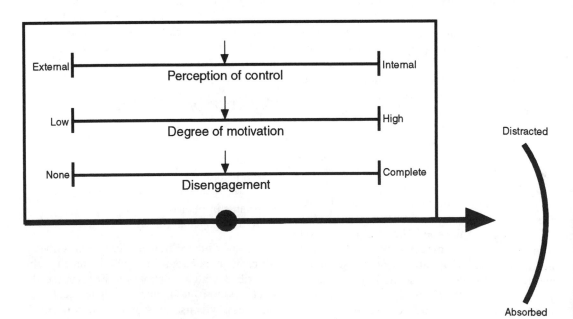

FIGURE 12-2 Summative contribution of the elements of leisure to total engagement in a leisure activity.

BOX 12-1 **Assessment**

- Assessment of leisure seeks to determine if an individual experiences leisure
- Assessment is more likely to lead to intervention that promotes leisure if it examines for the presence of intrinsic motivation, internal control and freedom from unnecessary constraints of within activities.
- Interview is essential for examining leisure in older people. These questions should be included:
  - What activities keep you totally engaged, allowing you to forget about everything else (now or in the past)?
  - What do you get from this particular activity? Why do it instead of others?
  - How able do you feel to make these activities come out the way you want them to?
- Asking clients to rate themselves along a continuum that reflects intrinsic motivation, internal control, freedom from unnecessary constraints of reality can be helpful for gaining their perceptions.

Experiences of Leisure scale (Meakins et al., 2005). We believe that interview is an essential tool, particularly given that little is known about the psychometric properties of most checklists with older people (Chang & Card, 1994).

We recommend that clinicians assess leisure by

- Inquiring about activities in which the individual is or was able to become totally absorbed (forgets everything else)
- Examining the individual's motivations for, degree of control in, and disengagement opportunities in each activity
- Asking the individual to rate himself or herself along the continuum reflecting the leisure elements can also be helpful

In the assessment, the clinician seeks to determine

- Whether or not an individual experiences leisure

- The relative presence, in the context of particular activities, of the elements contributing to the leisure experience
- The interrelationships among these elements

When this information has been gathered, it is possible to plan and evaluate the effectiveness of intervention. Intervention must be individually tailored and targeted toward promoting the leisure experience and eliminating barriers associated with it. We will illustrate this process with two case studies.

■ Summary

In this chapter, we considered leisure to be experiences through which older people make important statements about their identities. We proposed that leisure is experienced in the context of activities in which a person becomes totally engaged. We delineated three elements that contribute to the leisure experience: control, motivation, and freedom from unnecessary constraints of real life. We offered a methodology for examining and promoting leisure with older individuals. It is our hope that

- Professionals who seek to promote leisure experiences with their clients will find our model useful for framing their assessments and interventions.
- This model will spark research that will lead, in turn, to its refinement.

BOX 12-2 **Intervention**

- Leisure is an important lifelong occupation and its promotion is a worthy goal for intervention.
- Because leisure is self-determined, intervention to promote leisure must be tailored to the needs and desires of individual clients.
- Leisure may be experienced alone or in groups of any size, depending on the individual.

Case Study

Anna is an 83-year-old woman who lives alone. She suffered a mild *cerebrovascular accident* (CVA) 6 months before intervention. Anna said that cooking for her family was the activity in which she became most absorbed. When she cooked big meals, she forgot everything else and became totally "caught up" in timing events and creating the perfect combination of ingredients. However, Anna complained that since her stroke, she was no longer able to "cook like she used to." Although she still cooked, she did it only for herself, rather than for her family, and she was forced to use mixes, rather than begin from "scratch." These adaptations made cooking less enjoyable and failed to provide Anna with the same leisure experience she once enjoyed. Anna's profile for cooking is shown in Figure 12-3.

Anna was highly motivated to do a particular kind of cooking; she enjoyed the experience and saw it as a means of giving of herself to her family. The problem for Anna in cooking from scratch was with control. Because of

mild weakness on her left side and abnormal movements in her arm, she no longer felt comfortable lifting and carrying pans. Furthermore, her timing seemed off, and she worried about having one thing burn on the stove while she was attending to another thing at the sink. These concerns prevented her from disengaging from real life because she was continually reminded of the constraints imposed on her by her physical limitations. The combination of lack of control and inability to disengage prevented Anna from experiencing total engagement (leisure).

The occupational therapist working with Anna intervened by facilitating more normal patterns of movement in Anna's arm and helping her move more quickly. The therapist intervened in the context of complex cooking activities that Anna selected. The occupational therapist understood that the purpose of her intervention was to enable Anna to experience leisure by gaining greater control for cooking in a particular way. Thus, when she made decisions with

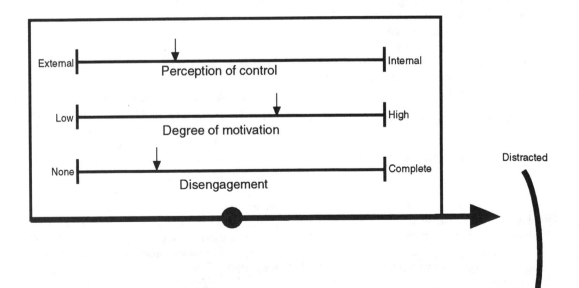

FIGURE 12-3 Anna's profile of the elements of leisure as they relate to cooking complex meals for her family.

regard to intervention, she framed her decisions in the context of leisure, rather than in the context of motor control.

Intervention with Anna was highly successful and took place over a reasonably short period of time (6 weeks). When the occupational therapist contacted Anna by phone several weeks after the last intervention session, Anna was too busy to talk; she was involved in preparing Thanksgiving dinner for her family.

Anna's problems with cooking related to physical limitations that reduced her feelings of control and prevented her from disengaging from the constraints of real life. Individuals like Anna typically receive intervention from occupational therapists.

However, intervention often centers on gaining control of movement rather than facilitating leisure experiences. Although intervention centered on motor control might have been effective with Anna, we believe that her intervention was much more meaningful (and perhaps of shorter duration) because it focused on enabling her to experience leisure.

Questions

1. Why did the therapist start by assessing what Anna found most engaging?
2. How did the limitations caused by Anna's CVA interact with her values around occupational enactment?
3. Why did the therapist not choose to focus on remediating Anna's physical limitations?

Review Questions

1. Define leisure.
2. What characteristics are most important to identifying an activity as a leisure activity?
3. In what ways are leisure activities important to elderly people?
4. In what ways does leisure represent an expression of identity?
5. What considerations are important in intervening to support an older person's optimal engagement in leisure?
6. Observe a group leisure activity in a retirement setting or nursing home. Describe participants' reactions to the event using the four factors of control, motivation, disengagement, and environment. Map these using the model described in this chapter.

Web-Based Resources

For helpful information about the experience of leisure, visit:

www.agingblueprint.org, **National Blueprint for Aging,** date connected March 27, 2007. This site pertains to active lifestyles.

www.csuchico.edu/kine/tasp, **The Association for the Study of Play,** date connected March 27, 2007. This site features a multidisciplinary group interested in the study of play and leisure across the life span in humans and animals. Included are environments for play and leisure and related topics.

REFERENCES

Abramson, L. Y. (1978). Learned helplessness in humans: Critique and reformulation. *Abnormal Psychology, 87*(1), 49–74.

Adams, R. G. (1993). Activity as structure and process. Friendships of older adults. In J. R. Kelly (Ed.), *Activity and aging* (pp. 73–85). Newbury Park, CA: Sage.

Allen, K. R., & Chin-sang, V. (1990). A lifetime of work: The context and meanings of leisure for aging black women. *The Gerontologist, 30*(6), 734–740.

Atchley, R. C. (1989). A continuity theory of normal aging. *The Gerontologist, 29,*183–190.

Atchley, R. C. (1993). Continuity theory and the evolution of activity in later adulthood. In J. R. Kelly (Ed.), *Activity and aging* (pp. 5–16). Newbury Park, CA: Sage.

Beck, S. H., & Page, J. W. (1988). Involvement in activities and the psychological well-being of retired men. *Activities, Adaptation & Aging, 11*(1), 31–47.

Bevil, C. A. (1993). Leisure activity, life satisfaction, and perceived health status in older adults. *Gerontology and Geriatrics Education, 14*(3), 3–19.

Bigby, C., & Balandin, S. (2005). Another minority group: Use of aged care day programs and community leisure services by older people with lifelong disability. *Australasian Journal on Ageing, 24*(1), 14–18.

Bullock, C. C., & Howe, C. Z. (1991). A model therapeutic recreation program for the reintegration of persons with disabilities into the community. *Therapeutic Recreation Journal, 25*(1), 7–17.

Burrus-Bammel, L. L., & Bammel, F. (1985). Leisure and recreation. In J. E. Birren & K. W. Schaie (Eds.), *Handbook of the psychology of aging* (2nd ed., pp. 848–863). New York: Van Nostrand Reinhold.

Caillois, R. (1979). *Man, play, and games.* New York: The Free Press.

Chang, Y. -S., & Card, J. A. (1994). The reliability of the Leisure Diagnostic Battery Short Form Version B in assessing healthy older individuals: Preliminary study. *Therapeutic Recreation Journal, Third Quarter,* 163–167.

Chin-Sang, V., & Allen, K. R. (1991). Leisure and the older black woman. *Journal of Gerontological Nursing, 17*(1), 30–34.

Clark, F. (1991, June). *The occupations of Seward Johnson.* Paper presented at the The Second Annual Research Colloquium of The American Occupational Therapy Foundation, Cincinnati.

Cohen, D. (1987). *The development of play.* New York: New York University Press.

Coleman, D., & Iso-Ahola, S. (1993). Leisure and health: The role of social support and self-determination. *Journal of Leisure Research, 25*(2), 111–129.

Corr, S., & Bayer, A. (1992). Poor functional status of stroke patients after hospital discharge: Scope for intervention? *The British Journal of Occupational Therapy, 55*(10), 383–385.

Crandall, R. (1980). Motivations for leisure. *Journal of Leisure Research, 12*(1), 45–54.

Csikszentmihayli, M. (1975). *Beyond boredom and anxiety.* San Franciso: Jossey-Bass.

Csikszentmihayli, M. (1985). Emergent motivation and evolution of the self. In D. A. Kleiber & M. L. Maehr (Eds.), *Advances in motivation and achievement* (pp. 93–119) (Vol. 4). Greenwich, CT: JAI Press.

Csikszentmihayli, M., & Graef, R. (1980). The experience of freedom in daily life. *American Journal of Community Psychology, 8*(4), 401–414.

Csikszentmihalyi, M., & Kleiber, D. A. (1991). Leisure and self-actualization. In B. L. Driver (Ed.), *Benefits of leisure* (pp. 91–102). State College, PA: Venture.

Csikszentmihayli, M., & Rochberg-Halton, E. (1981). *The meaning of things.* New York: Cambridge University Press.

Donald, M. N., & Havighurst, R. J. (1959). Meanings of leisure. *Social Forces, 37,* 355–360.

Driver, B. L., Brown, P. J., & Peterson, G. L. (1991). Research on leisure benefits: An introduction to this volume. In B. L. Driver (Ed.), *Benefits of leisure* (pp. 3–12). State College, PA: Venture.

Drummond, A., & Walker, M. (1996). Generalisation of the effects of leisure rehabilitation for stroke patients. *British Journal of Occupational Therapy, 59*(7), 330–334.

Ekerdt, D. J. (1986). The busy ethic: Moral continuity between work and retirement. *The Gerontologist, 26*(3), 239–244.

Fabrigoule, C. (1995). Social and leisure activities and risk of dementia: A prospective longitudinal study. *Journal of the American Geriatrics Society, 43*(5), 485–490.

Fex, E. (1998). Effect of rheumatoid arthritis on work status and social and leisure time activities in patients followed 8 years from onset. *Journal of Rheumatology, 25*(1), 44–50.

Freysinger, V. J. (1993). The community, programs, and opportunities: Population diversity. In J. R. Kelly (Ed.), *Activity and aging* (pp. 211–230). Newbury Park, CA: Sage.

Gabriel, Z., & Bowling, A. (2004). Quality of life from the perspectives of older people. *Ageing and Society, 24,* 675–691.

Garcia-Martin, M. A., Gomez-Jacinto, L., & Martimportugues-Goyenechea, C. (2004). A structural model of the effects of organized leisure activities on the well-being of elder adults in Spain. *Activities, Adaptation & Aging, 28*(3), 19–34.

Geertz, C. (1973). *The interpretation of cultures.* New York: Basic.

Goodale, T. L., & Cooper, W. (1991). Philosophical perspectives on leisure in English-speaking countries. In B. L. Driver (Ed.), *Benefits of leisure* (pp. 25–36). State College, PA: Venture.

Goodman, C. C. (1984). Natural helping among older adults. *The Gerontologist, 24*(2), 138–143.

Griffin, J., & McKenna, K. (1998). Influences on leisure and life satisfaction of elderly people. *Physical and Occupational Therapy in Geriatrics, 15*(4), 1–16.

Gunter, B. G. (1980). Leisure styles: A conceptual framework for modern leisure. *Sociological Quarterly, 21*(3), 361–374.

Havighurst, R. J. (1979). The nature and values of meaningful free-time activity. In R. W. Kleemeier (Ed.), *Aging and leisure* (pp. 309–344). New York: Arno Press.

Havighurst, R. J., & Feigenbaum, K. (1968). Leisure and lifestyle. In B. L. Neugarten (Ed.), *Middle age and aging: A reader in social psychology* (pp. 347–353). Chicago: University of Chicago Press.

Henderson, K. A., & Rannells, J. S. (1988). Farm women and the meaning of work and leisure: An oral history perspective. *Leisure Sciences, 10*(1), 41–50.

Hillman, A. H., & Chapparo, C. J. (1995). An investigation of occupational role performance in men over sixty years of age following a stroke. *Journal of Occupational Science, 2*(3), 88–99.

Hogg, J. (1993). Creative, personal and social engagement in the later years: Realisation through leisure. *The Irish Journal of Psychology, 14*(1), 204–218.

Husaini, B. A., & Moore, S. T. (1990). Arthritis disability, depression, and life satisfaction among black elderly people. *Health Social Work, 15*(4), 253–260.

Iso-Ahola, S. E. (1980). *The social psychology of leisure and recreation.* Dubuque, IA: W.C. Brown.

Iso-Ahola, S. E., Jackson, E. L., & Dunn, E. (1994). Starting, ceasing, and replacing leisure activites over the life-span. *Journal of Leisure Research, 26*(3), 227–249.

Jackson, E. (1990). Variations in the desire to begin a leisure activity. Evidence of antecedent constraints? *Journal of Leisure Research, 22*(1), 55–70.

Jackson, E., & Dunn, E. (1988). Integrating ceasing participation with other aspects of leisure behavior. *Journal of Leisure Research, 20*(1), 31–45.

Jacobson, S., & Samdahl, D. M. (1998). Leisure in the lives of old lesbians: Experiences with and responses to discrimination. *Journal of Leisure Research, 30*(2), 233–255.

Kaufman, S. R. (1993). Values as a source of the ageless self. In J. R. Kelly (Ed.), *Activity and aging* (pp. 17–24). Newbury Park, CA: Sage.

Kelly, J. R. (1982). Leisure in later life: Roles and identities. In N. J. Osgood (Ed.), *Life after work* (pp. 268–292). New York: Praeger.

Kelly, J. R. (1993). Theory and issues. In J. R. Kelly (Ed.), *Activity and aging* (pp. 5–16). Newbury Park, CA: Sage.

Kelly, J. R. (1996). *Leisure.* Englewood Cliffs, NJ: Prentice Hall.

Kielhofner, G. (1995). *A model of human occupation: Theory and application* (2nd ed.). Baltimore: Williams & Wilkins.

Kinney, W. B., & Coyle, C. P. (1992). Predicting life satisfaction among adults with physical disabilities. *Archives of Physical Medicine and Rehabilitation, 73*(9), 863–869.

Kleiber, D. A. (1985). Motivational reorientation in adulthood and the resource of leisure. In D. A. Kleiber & M. L. Maehr (Eds.), *Advances in motivation and achievement* (pp. 217–250). Greenwich, CT: JAI Press.

Kleiber, D. A., Hutshinson, S. L., & Williams, R. (2002). Leisure as a resource in transcending negative life events: Self-protection, self-restoration, and personal transformation. *Leisure Sciences, 24,* 219–235.

Krefting, L., & Krefting, D. (1991). Leisure activities after a stroke: An ethnographic approach. *American Journal of Occupational Therapy, 45*(5), 429–436.

Langer, E. J., & Rodin, J. (1976). The effects of choice and enhanced personal responsibility for the aged: A field experiment in an institutional setting. *Journal of Personality and Social Psychology, 34*(2), 191–198.

Larson, R., & Csikszentmihayli, M. (1983). The experience sampling method. In Reis, H. T. (Ed.), *Naturalistic Approaches to Studying Social Interaction. (New Directions for Methodology of Social and Behavioral Science, no. 15)* (pp. 41–56). San Francisco, CA: Jossey-Bass.

Lau, A., Chi, I., & McKenna, K. (1998). Self-perceived quality of life of Chinese elderly people in Hong Kong. *Occupational Therapy International, 5*(2), 118–139.

Lawton, M. P. (1993). Meanings of activity. In J. R. Kelly (Ed.), *Activity and aging* (pp. 25–41). Newbury Park, CA: Sage.

Lawton, M. P. (1994). Personality and affective correlates of leisure activity participation by older people. *Journal of Leisure Research, 26*(2), 138–157.

Lindberg, M. (1995). Quality of life after subarachnoid haemorrhage and its relationship to impairments, disabilities. *Scandinavian Journal of Occupational Therapy, 2*(3–4), 105–112.

Losier, S. F., Bourque, P. E., & Vallerand, R. J. (1993). The motivational model of leisure participation in the elderly. *Journal of Psychology, 127*(2), 153–170.

MacNeil, R., & Teague, M. (1987). *Ageing and leisure: Vitality in later life.* Englewood Cliffs, NJ: Prentice Hall.

Mactavish, J., & Mahon, M. J. (2005). Leisure education and later-life planning: A conceptual framework. *Journal of Policy and Practice in Intellectual Disabilities, 2*(1), 29–37.

Mannell, R. C. (1993). High-investment activity and life satisfaction among older adults: Committed, serious leisure, and flow activities. In J. R. Kelly (Ed.), *Activity and aging* (pp. 125–145). Newbury Park, CA: Sage.

Mannell, R. C., Zuzanek, J., & Larson, R. (1988). Leisure states and flow experiences: Testing perceived freedom and intrinsic motivation hypothesis. *Journal of Leisure Research, 20*(4), 289–304.

Mansson, M. (1995). On life satisfaction and activity preferences in long-term survivors after stroke. *Scandinavian Journal of Occupational Therapy, 2*(2), 51–55.

McAvoy, L. H. (1979). The leisure preferences, problems, and needs of the elderly. *Journal of Leisure Research, 11*(1), 40–60.

McGuire, F. A. (1989). Integrating ceasing participation with other aspects of leisure behavior. A replication and extension. *Journal of Leisure Research, 21*(4), 316–326.

McGuire, F. A. (2004). *Leisure and aging: Ulyssean living in later life* (2nd ed.). Champaign, IL: Sagamore.

McNeilly, D. P., & Burke, W. J. (2001). Gambling as a social activity of older adults. *International Journal of Aging and Human Development, 52*(1), 19–28.

McPherson, B. D. (1991). Aging and leisure benefits: A life cycle perspective. In B. L. Driver (Ed.), *Benefits of leisure* (pp. 423–430). State College, PA: Venture.

Meakins, C., Bundy, A. C., & Gliner, J. (2005). Reliability and validity of The Experience of Leisure scale (TELS). In F. McMahon, D. E. Lytle, & B. Sutton-Smith (Eds.), *Play: An interdisciplinary synthesis* (Vol. 6, pp. 255–267). Lanham, MD: University Press of America.

Menec, V. H., & Chipperfield, J. G. (1997). Remaining active in later life: The role of locus of control in seniors' level participation, activity, health, and life satisfaction. *Journal of Aging and Health, 9*(1), 105–125.

Mishra, S. (1992). Leisure activities and life satisfaction in old age. A case study of retired government employees living in urban areas. *Activities, Adaptation & Aging, 17*(4), 7–26.

Mobily, K. E., Lemke, J. H., & Gisin, G. J. (1991). The idea of leisure repertoire. *The Journal of Applied Gerontology, 10*(2), 208–223.

Neulinger, J. (1974). *The psychology of leisure: Research approaches to the study of leisure.* Springfield, IL: Charles C Thomas.

Neumann, E. A. (1971). *Elements of play.* New York: MSS Information.

Pardasani, M. P. (2004). Senior centers: Focal points of community-based services for the elderly. *Activities, Adaptation & Aging, 28*(4), 27–44.

Parker, C. J., Gladman, J. R. F., Drummond, A. E. R., Dewey, M. E., Lincoln, N. B., Barer, D., et al. (2001). A multicentre randomized controlled trial of leisure therapy and conventional occupational therapy after stroke. *Clinical Rehabilitation, 15*(1), 42–52.

Pereira, R. B., & Stagnitti, K. (2006). *The relationship between leisure experiences and health in an ageing Italian community in Australia.* Paper presented at the 14th World Federation of Occupational Therapists Congress, Sydney, Australia.

Perlmuter, L. C., & Langer, E. J. (1982). The effects of behavioral monitoring on the perception of control. *Clinical Gerontologist, 1*(2), 37–43.

Purcell, R. Z., & Keller, M. J. (1989). Characteristics of leisure activities which may lead to leisure satisfaction among older adults. *Activities, Adaptation & Aging, 13*(4), 17–29.

Ragheb, M. G., & Beard, J. G. (1980). Leisure satisfaction: Concept, theory, and measurement. In S. Iso-Ahola (Ed.), *Social psychological perspectives on leisure and recreation* (p. 261–289). Springfield, IL: Charles C Thomas.

Riddick, C. C. (1993). Older women's leisure activity and quality of life. In J. R. Kelly (Ed.), *Leisure in later life. Roles and identities* (pp. 75–87). Newbury Park, CA: Sage.

Riddick, C. C., & Stewart, D. G. (1994). An examination of the life satisfaction and importance of leisure in the lives of older female retirees: A comparison of blacks to whites. *Journal of Leisure Research, 26*(1), 75–87.

Rockwell-Dylla, L. A. (1991). *Older adults' meaning of environment: Hospital and home.* Chicago: University of Illinois.

Rodin, J., & Langer, E. J. (1977). Long term effects of a control-relevant intervention with the institutionalized aged. *Journal of Personality and Social Psychology, 35*(12), 897–902.

Rowles, G. D. (1991). Beyond performance: Being in place as a component of occupational therapy. *American Journal of Occupational Therapy, 45*(4), 265–271.

Samdahl, D. M. (1988). A symbolic interactionist model of leisure: Theory and empirical support. *Leisure Sciences, 10*(1), 27–39.

Savell, K. S. (1991). Leisure perceptions of control and well-being: Implications for the institutionalized elderly. *Therapeutic Recreation Journal, 25*(3), 44–59.

Schulz, R. (1976). Effects of control and predictability on the physical and psychological well-being of the institutionalized aged. *Journal of Personality and Social Psychology, 33*(5), 563–573.

Schulz, R., & Hanusa, B. H. (1978). Long-term effects of control and predictability-enhancing interventions: Bindings and ethical issues. *Journal of Personality and Social Psychology, 36*(11), 1194–1201.

Scraton, S., & Holland, S. (2006). Grandfatherhood & leisure: Meanings and values across different ethnicities. *Leisure Studies, 25,* 223–251.

Searle, M. S., Mahon, M. J., Iso-Ahola, S. E., Sdrolias, H., & van Dyck, J. (1995). Enhancing a sense of independence and psychological well-being among the elderly: A field experiment. *Journal of Leisure Research, 27,* 107–124

Tatham, M. G., & McCree, S. (1992). The role of the occupational therapist in senior housing. *Journal of Housing for the Elderly, 10*(1–2), 125–138.

Timmer, E., Bode, C., & Dittmann-Kohli, F. (2003). Expectations of gains in the second half of life: A study of personal conceptions of enrichment in a lifespan perspective. *Ageing and Society, 23,* 3–24.

Tse, T., & Howie, L. (2005). Adult day groups: Addressing older people's needs for activity and companionship. *Australasian Journal on Ageing, 24*(3), 134–140.

Voelki, J. E. (1993). Activity and aging. In J. R. Kelly (Ed.), *Activity and aging.* Newbury Park, CA: Sage.

Wilson, R. N. (1981). The courage to be leisured. *Social Forces, 60*(2), 281–303.

Witt, P. A., & Ellis, G. D. (1989). *The Leisure Diagnostic Battery users' manual.* State College, PA: Venture.

Zimmer, Z., Hickey, T., & Searle, M. S. (1997). The pattern of change in leisure activity behavior among older adults with arthritis. *The Gerontologist, 37*(3), 384–392.

Zoerink, D. A. (2001). Exploring the relationship between leisure and health of senior adults with orthopedic disabilities living in rural areas. *Activities, Adaptation & Aging, 26*(2), 61–73.

ACKNOWLEDGMENTS

The authors wish to acknowledge Jean Cannella, MEd, OTR, for her contributions to an earlier version of this chapter.

CHAPTER 13

Work and Retirement

Harvey L. Sterns, PhD • Greta A. Lax, MS • Boin Chang, MA

Each of us brings to our job, whatever it is, our lifetime of experience and our values.

Sandra Day O'Connor

OBJECTIVES

By the end of the chapter, readers will be able to:

1. Describe the characteristics of the older work force.
2. Discuss forms of employer-sponsored wellness programs for older workers and their value in enhancing work performance.
3. Discuss issues of work performance of older workers.
4. Describe characteristics that contribute to continuing competence of older workers.
5. Describe mechanisms for retraining older workers.
6. Describe issues related to decisions to retire and adjustments to retirement.
7. Discuss the development of retirement preparation programs and alternatives to retirement.
8. Discuss issues related to unemployment among older workers.

The study of aging and work, focusing on the employment and retirement issues of middle-aged and older workers, is called industrial gerontology (Sterns & Alexander, 1987). The aging of the work force creates unique issues—choosing to work longer, early retirement options, staffing shortages, career patterns, training and retraining, performance, productivity, and health and disability (Sterns & Huyck, 2001).

Whether older workers continue to occupy their present jobs or change jobs will be determined by their career choices, retraining, experience, health, and retirement preferences. Older workers are in direct competition with younger workers for some positions and will be needed to fill positions when there is a shortage of younger workers. Competent, able, older workers who desire to continue to work need to be competitive in the workplace of the future.

In this chapter, issues and research relevant to enhancing the work and retirement experience of older adults are explored. Current data regarding the employment patterns of older workers are provided. The role of health as a determinant of employment and retirement and related research issues are discussed next. Interventions such as wellness programs are also described.

Discussion then turns to issues such as older worker performance, obsolescence, and competence. Training and retraining and other interventions are discussed. Retirement is considered, and the role of retirement preparation and alternative approaches to work and retirement are analyzed. In addition, the complex factors that determine vocational and retirement outcomes are examined. Also, some of the cross-cultural issues will be briefly discussed.

The Older Labor Force

When the oldest baby boomers become age 65 in 2011, the labor force will age more rapidly (Johnson, 2004). According to the Bureau of Labor Statistics, the group of those age 55 and older will grow five times more than the growth of the overall labor force as well as that of younger groups. The projection for 2014 indicates that the 55-and-older age group will make up 21.2% of the labor force, which was 15.6% in 2004. Although the age group between 25 and 54 made up 69.3% of the labor force in 2004, this group will have decreased by 2014 to 65.2% (Bureau of Labor Statistics, 2005).

The increase in the labor force participation rates for women has been the most significant trend of the past 50 years. The labor force participation rate of women was 34% in 1950 and increased to 60% by 2000 (Toossi, 2002). Older women's labor force participation has constantly increased since 1955, from 32% to about 50% in 2005 (Table 13-1; Barth, McNaught, & Rizzi, 1995; Rix, 2006).

In addition, the workforce is anticipated to become more diverse. Minorities have become a rapidly emerging work population and their participation rate is increasing (Toossi, 2002). Toossi suggests that the share of Hispanics will double from 11% of the total workforce in 2000 to 24% in 2050. The share of blacks will be

increased from 12% to 14% between 2000 and 2050, and that of Asians will be expanding from 5% in 2000 to 11% in 2050.

The 1991 Commonwealth Fund Productive Aging Survey, which drew on interviews with 2999 older Americans, indicated that 8% (75 years of age and older), 13% (65 to 74 years of age), and 9% (55 to 64 years of age) of nonworking older adults were willing and able to work (Barth et al., 1995). Approximately 5.4 million older Americans report being willing and able to work (Barth et al., 1995; Sterns & Sterns, 1995).

A 2004 AARP report revealed that almost 80% of baby boomers reported that they want to continue working either part-time or full-time in their retirement years, while only 16% reported that they will not work at all. The reason for willingness to work varies; 35% are willing to work out of interest and enjoyment, and 23% want to work for financial reasons.

Many older workers will have some sort of postcareer employment before they retire, which include those working reduced or flexible schedules (Doeringer, 1990; Schultz, 2003). Most workers are employed at one job for the majority of their working lives (Ruhm, 1990). Retirement at a bridge job or jobs appears to fill the period from the end of the longest job to the point of retirement.

A recurrent theme in work for the older adult is health (Quinn & Burkhauser, 1990; Sterns & Sterns, 1995). Health changes that affect functional capacity are important variables affecting the behavior of older workers. It is somewhat difficult to determine the impact of age-related health changes on work because most health measures reflect poor health (presence of disease or disability) rather than good health. Among other concerns, older adults have

TABLE 13-1 **Labor Force Participation by Age and Gender: 2004 and 2005**

Age Group	Both Sexes		Males		Females	
	2004	2005	2004	2005	2004	2005
55–64	62.3	62.9	68.7	69.3	56.3	57.0
65–69	27.7	28.3	32.6	33.6	23.3	23.7
70–74	15.3	16.3	19.4	20.7	12.0	12.8
75+	6.1	6.4	9.0	9.4	4.3	4.5

Source: Rix, S. (2006). *Update on the aged 55+ worker: 2005*. Washington, DC: AARP.

greater variability in work-related functional ability than younger people. Reporting older adults as a single group distorts the reality of their functional ability, with the result that young-old people are portrayed as less functional than they actually are (Newquist, 1986). Functional capacity is difficult to assess, and needed databases for research are not available. Research is needed to develop indexes that incorporate variables such as sickness, impairment, and limitation, as well as functional capacity, as they relate to work (Newquist, 1986). Robinson (1986) suggests two pertinent questions related to the effects of age on health and job performance. First, "Is the job performance of middle-age and older workers adversely affected by age-related factors," and second, "if so, how can these age-related effects be minimized through workplace interventions?" As the working population ages, employers must pay attention to the relationship of aging to health and performance. Age-related health changes affecting job performance may be attributed to genetic predisposition, environmental influences, lifestyle, behavior, and stress.

Although there are some general trends, older people differ greatly on measures of health and functional capacity. Aging research suggested that physical and cognitive abilities tend to decline with age, but those declines may not result in lower levels of job performance (Salthouse & Maurer, 1996). In addition, numerous other factors that affect job performance within age groups far outweigh differences between age groups, and age differences are more obvious in some occupations such as airline pilots than others such as clerical work (Robinson, 1986). According to Sterns, Sterns, and Hollis (1996), people who are over 65 are more likely to have more health problems than the middle-aged, but the differences are small.

Health and functioning do not inevitably decline in the middle and later working years, and interventions such as reducing work hazards and promoting health-related behaviors can prevent or reduce health decrements. The workplace is a reasonable site for interventions because of the large amount of time spent at work. Workplace interventions include assessments (which may reveal reduced capabilities), workplace accommodations (such as environmental modifications), and retraining. However, these interventions may be threatening to workers

concerned about revealing deficits. Employers may fail to implement these programs because of lack of awareness of their potential benefits and lack of published data on health and job performance.

Workplace interventions offer numerous benefits for business in terms of reducing health hazards, promoting good health, assessing change, providing alternate working arrangements, redesigning jobs, and maintaining and retraining a skilled and committed workforce (Robinson, 1986; Sterns, Sterns, & Hollis, 1996). Furthermore, the current trend of the aging workforce emphasizes that we need to continue to examine the issues regarding aging as well as work-related processes and outcomes. Current groups of older workers may be different from earlier cohorts of older workers (Hedge, Borman, & Lammlein, 2006).

Occupational therapists have a significant role to play in terms of assisting employers and employees to maximize worker abilities through training and other employee-specific interventions. They also have an important role in helping employers structure tasks and environments that support all workers, but can have particular value in enhancing performance for older workers.

Older Worker Performance

In view of the elimination of mandatory retirement for most occupations, the increasing numbers of older workers, and the increasing number of age-discrimination cases (Snyder & Barrett, 1988; Sterns, Doverspike, & Lax, 2005), there has been a burgeoning need for an understanding of the relationship between age and work performance (Avolio, Waldman, & McDaniel, 1990; Sterns & Gray, 1999; Waldman & Avolio, 1986). However, studies of age and work performance are plagued by poor designs and inadequate analyses. They tend to ignore variations in job demands, individual experience, and measures of performance (Rhodes, 1983; Warr, 1994). Following a qualitative review of the literature, Rhodes (1983) concluded that an equal number of studies support a decline, an increase, and stability in performance with age. Warr (1994) suggested that there are several issues to consider when interpreting the findings of relationship between age and job performance. These include potentially unreliable or invalid job performance criteria, ignorance of cohort differences, and relevant experience. He also suggested that age differences in performance should be examined within a specific job category to assess whether a job requires capacities that decline with age and whether job performance can be enhanced by experience.

Waldman and Avolio (1986) conducted a meta-analysis of 40 studies and found the relationship between age and performance to vary with the type of job performance measure. Supervisory ratings of employees' performance showed a slight decline with age. With more objective measures, employees' performance increased slightly with age. These researchers also found that ones' profession may act as a moderator of the age and work performance relationship. The relationship between age and supervisor's rating of performance was more positive in professionals than nonprofessionals. McEvoy and Cascio (1989) performed a meta-analysis on 96 studies. Like Waldman and Avolio, they found a slight correlation between age and work performance but did not find the performance criterion and type of work to affect the relationship.

Researchers' inability to find a consistent linear relationship between age and work performance may suggest that such a relationship does not exist. Waldman and Avolio (1986) developed a nonlinear model that illustrates the compounding effects of individual characteristics, such as personality, ability, and motivation, and contextual characteristics, such as organizational policies, reward systems, and job demands. These characteristics may influence a worker's motivation, professional competence, and overall performance (Miller, 1990; Sterns & Gray, 1999).

Another reason for inconsistent findings could be the interactions between experience and age; experience has been found to be a better predictor of performance than age (Sterns & Gray, 1999). Czaja and Sharit (1998) conducted a study with computer-based data entry tasks and found that previous computer experience was the biggest predictor of the performance. But after controlling for previous computer experience, older participants performed significantly slower than the younger due to their slower psychomotor speed, which, it is important to note, can be enhanced by training

(Czaja & Sharit, 1998). In addition, Beehr and Bowling (2002) emphasized the importance of moderators among job characteristics, which might be either decreased or increased with age. Depending on the job characteristics, the effect of aging may vary. Thus, it is hard to tell the relationship between age and job performance in general.

Qualitative experience, though, is rarely examined and may be as important as quantitative experience. Workers with an equal number of years of experience may perform differently owing to the individual and contextual experiences, such as more effective supervision or more challenging work assignments. Based on the literature review, Hedge et al. (2006) recently suggested that older workers are as effective as younger workers especially when they have a relatively higher level of expertise or experiences, motivation on the given jobs, as well as some flexibility and managerial support at work. The life-span approach may enable us to understand individual and contextual factors that impact on continued productivity in later years. In sum, functional performance should be individually examined not based on age, but based on the individual characteristics and contextual factors (Sterns & Gray, 1999; Sterns & Huyck, 2001).

Obsolescence Versus Maintaining Competence

A major issue for the 2000s is the question of how long a worker's skills will remain current. With rapid technological changes, workers may find it necessary to continually update their knowledge, skills, and abilities (KSAs) or they may become obsolete. **Obsolescence** occurs when the demands of a job become incongruent with a worker's KSAs (Fossum, Arvey, Paradise, & Robbins, 1986). There have been a variety of approaches to the study of obsolescence (Willis & Dubin, 1990). Insightful writings on the topic have focused on the process of maintaining professional competence (Fossum et al., 1986). As Figure 13-1 demonstrates, older workers are capable of learning to use new technologies to maintain competence.

Professional competence has been defined as "the ability to function effectively in the tasks considered essential within a given profession"

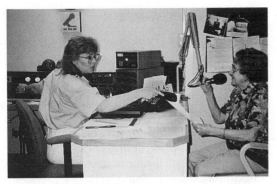

FIGURE 13-1 Continuation of work roles is important to many older adults. Here we see an elder with her own radio show. (Courtesy of the Menorah Park Center for Aging, Cleveland, Ohio, with permission.)

(Fossum et al., 1986). A developmental approach suggests that maintaining professional competence through updating is a continual process, starting as soon as an individual enters the work force and continuing throughout the individual's career (Sterns & Doverspike, 1989). This approach is contrasted with a remedial approach, which views updating as a process done to compensate for obsolescence after it occurs (Fossum et al., 1986). The developmental perspective seems more effective as a means for avoiding obsolescence and suggests that as workers age, they must continually develop new KSAs. Aspects of both the individual (e.g., age) and the job setting (e.g., organizational climate) are related to obsolescence.

Occupational therapists emphasize performance skills, performance patterns, and client factors (American Occupational Therapy Association, 2002), which reflect the knowledge, skills, and attitudes required to accomplish all tasks, including those associated with work. Recognition of typical age-associated changes in these areas can inform the kinds of strategies and interventions needed to maximize worker performance.

Individual Characteristics

Age

Older workers may face a greater risk of obsolescence because they have been out of school for a longer period of time. Empirical studies of this assumption, however, have produced inconsistent results. In the 1970s, studies in engineering found obsolescence to increase as early as the mid-30s (Dalton & Thompson, 1971; Shearer &

Steger, 1975). Willis and Tosti-Vassey (1990) found no age differences between up-to-date college professors and those less up to date. This may mean that age is related to obsolescence only in specific occupations. Additionally, Shearer and Steger (1975) found an increase in obsolescence with age for a civilian sample of engineers but the opposite effect in air force engineers. There was a negative relationship between age and obsolescence for the air force personnel. These results suggest that maintaining competence through updating is critical for workers of all ages.

Training and development programs may be the most common means by which individuals maintain professional competence (AARP, 1990). Older workers underuse training opportunities, possibly because they have not been afforded as many opportunities as younger workers (Lillard & Tan, 1992). Although special issues need to be considered when developing training programs for older workers (Sterns, 1986; Sterns & Doverspike, 1989), the fact remains that older workers benefit from training. Why, then, don't they participate in as much training as younger workers?

The answer to this question may lie in the older workers themselves or in the organizations where they work. Individual factors, such as motivation and values, impact on engagement in training or other updating, such as reading and networking. Additionally, external forces (in the organization or elsewhere) can influence workers at all stages of their careers and help determine the amount of updating and other career-development activities that they participate in (Farr & Middlebrooks, 1990; Fossum et al., 1986).

Motivation and Ability

Motivation may be one of the most important determinants of whether or not someone remains up to date at work. Current baby boomers who are age 50 or older reported a strong sense of personal motivation to succeed on the job; in addition, 88% of employees ages 45 to 74 reported that the opportunity to learn something new was an essential part of their ideal job (AARP, 2005). This strong motivation of older workers might encourage them to overcome certain training barriers. Motivation alone, however, does not guarantee this outcome. The worker must also possess the ability to execute successfully the behaviors necessary to remain professionally competent. Therefore, adequate ability and motivation are both critical for maintaining competence (Farr, Tesluk, & Klein, 1998).

External Factors

Although the ultimate responsibility for maintaining professional competence rests on the individual employee, the organization can foster or discourage the necessary updating behaviors to the extent that they provide opportunities for updating and enhance motivation through challenging work assignments and opportunities for interaction between peers and management. An organization should remain flexible and committed to professional development (Farr & Middlebrooks, 1990; Farr et al., 1998; Fossum et al., 1986). As is true for all workers, these factors can influence the likelihood that an older worker will engage in various activities to update his or her skills. The issues to consider include

- Challenging work coupled with security
- Interaction with coworkers and management
- Flexibility on the part of the organization, accompanied by an understanding that change may occur slowly
- Organizational support for continued training
- An effective system of rewards, both formal and informal

(Forisha-Kovach, 1984; Fossum & Arvey, 1990; Kaufman, 1990; Lawrence, 1985; Sterns & Huyck, 2001; Votruba, 1990). The environment and the policies of the organization can influence the likelihood that all workers, old and young alike, will take the necessary steps to maintain competence. Although professionals of all ages may be threatened by obsolescence, special issues need to be considered when training older workers.

In addition, it may be possible to focus on the context and the activity demands of particular work-related situations. Reconfiguring the physical environment, increasing the number of breaks, improving the lighting, and other modifications external to the worker can make task completion more feasible. Chapter 24 describes some of the kinds of environmental modifications that occupational therapists might recommend.

Training Older Workers

Although older workers may be more in need of training due to obsolescence, statistics show that they receive less training than younger workers (Farr et al., 1998). According to Barth, McNaught, and Rizzi (1996), large companies tended to invest more on training younger employees, under age 35, than older employees, age 51 or older. Cross (1982) cites three barriers to older adult participation in training: situational, dispositional, and institutional.

Barriers to Training
Situational Barriers. These barriers include lack of information, lack of money, and lack of time. Older workers may be unaware of community-based, job-related training. When training is on site, managers may fail to tell older workers about the opportunity because of stereotypes managers may have about older managers' learning abilities (Cross, 1982; Peterson, 1980). Education of management and workers can minimize these stereotypes and increase participation in training (Noe, 2001). Paid release time from work and tuition reimbursement are powerful incentives for participation in training (Cross, 1982).

Dispositional Barriers. Dispositional barriers include those related to self-perception (e.g., lack of confidence). Older workers may have internalized the negative stereotype that they are too old to learn. This may be one reason why older workers are those least likely to volunteer for training (Peterson, 1987). Success in training can also be affected by negative self-perceptions (Reed, Doty, & May, 2005). Thus, encouragement from managers can minimize this barrier. However, a recent study illustrated that older workers reported being actively involved in various training activity, especially training off the job or work (Simpson, Geller, & Stroh, 2002). Their research indicates that older workers do have interests in training.

Institutional Barriers. Institutional barriers include logistical policies and procedures such as difficult registration procedures, limited course offerings, inaccessible sites, or inconvenient times. Training scheduled right after work or at deadline times may cause fatigue or poor attendance. Policies that do not reward older workers through benefits and incentives for acquiring skills may actually encourage retirement (Cooperman & Keast, 1983; Sterns & Kaplan, 2003). The upcoming workforce has more formal education than the present older workforce. Fear of education may also be lower among future older workers, and managers may be better educated about the value of older workers to the company.

Designing the Training Program

As with the development of any training program, the initial step must be a needs analysis, which includes an analysis of the organization, the job, and the person (Noe, 2001). In developing a training program for workers of all ages, factors to consider include motivation, structure, active participation, familiarity, organization, time, and learning strategies (Sterns, 1986). With older workers, special sensitivity to these dimensions may be important.

Motivation

Older workers are least likely to volunteer for instruction, so trainers may need to encourage them more than others (Peterson, 1987). Both motivation and belief in one's own abilities can influence training involvement and success, especially in older workers (Belbin & Belbin, 1972; Colquitt, LePine, & Noe, 2000). Their desire to learn may be impeded by fear of failure or feelings of inadequacy as compared with younger workers. Older workers who have had little formal schooling may have particularly low self-esteem. Trainers can help alleviate feelings of fear if support is being given by managers and coworkers. The physical environment also affects motivation. Lighting, noise, and temperature should be adjusted to maximize comfort. Frequent rest periods help alleviate fatigue.

Structure

The training program should be relevant to the job based on a careful job analysis. This analysis can assist in the arrangement of training sequences. Anxiety of participants can be reduced by ensuring that the trainee masters each simple component of a task before moving on (Sterns, 1986). This mastery also gives trainers opportunities to provide positive feedback.

Active Participation

Active participation is desirable for older trainees, because lecture or rote memorization formats may cause difficulty (Sterns, 1986). Active participation through case studies, simulations, and role-plays may reduce cautiousness and hesitancy (Fisk & Rogers, 2000). Additionally, older workers' wealth of experience should enhance group discussion and learning.

Familiarity

If possible, trainers should use former skills of the trainees and build on their past knowledge, skills, and abilities. Providing relevant or generalizable examples during training may also increase participants' attention, which would improve training effectiveness.

Organization

Cognitive research has shown that older adults have difficulty organizing information effectively (Sterns, 1986). As a result, trainers should organize the material being presented to help retention and comprehension by placing material into meaningful groupings (Noe, 2001). Teaching older trainees organizational strategies, including rehearsal and learning strategies, is another effective option in training (Sterns & Doverspike, 1989; Warr, 1994).

Time

Behavioral research consistently indicates slowing of reaction time and increases in learning time with age. Thus, slower presentation of training material and provision of longer study and test periods should aid older workers (Czaja, 2001; Noe, 2001). Given sufficient time, older learners perform as well or better than younger learners (Sterns & Doverspike, 1989).

Strategies

Provision of learning strategies such as mnemonic techniques is the final critical component to be included in training older workers. Trainers expect trainees to learn but often fail to teach them how to learn. Older learners may never have learned strategies for retention, recall, and application, or they may have forgotten them.

Design may actually be of more importance in the success or failure of training than content (Valasek & Sterns, 1981). Morrell and Echt (1997) emphasized the importance of training instructions that reduce cognitive demands as well as reflect age-related physical changes, which will improve performance for individuals of all ages eventually. A design that addresses the factors identified here will facilitate success of the older learner by enhancing motivation and self-esteem and decreasing feelings of failure and anxiety.

Some of the factors listed here stem from **andragogy** (Knowles, 1989; Sterns, 1986), the term used to describe the instructional process for adults. Five andragogical assumptions are

1. Adults are increasingly self-directed.
2. Adults are rich in experience.
3. Adults' choice of learning depends on the stage of development.
4. Adults are problem centered.
5. Adults are motivated internally.

To apply these andragogical assumptions, Knowles (1989) suggests that trainers share their authority with the adults and allow the adults to be active participants in the determination of training content, method, goals, and evaluation. The result should be greater job relevance of training content and increased motivation of trainees. Participation in evaluation techniques may also reduce fear of failure. With this approach, trainers can also gain insight into the trainees' expectations, problems, functioning, and knowledge.

Knowles (1989) also highlights the importance of positive environment. Support from trainers, managers, and peers increases self-confidence, risk taking, and participation. Knowles adds, though, that the situation is the best determinant of instructional technique.

Pedagogical approaches (i.e., approaches used with children) may be the best if the topic is extremely technical. If the adults do not know anything about the material to be discussed, it will be difficult for them to develop training content.

Training or Retraining Applications

Numerous examples of effective training programs can be found in the literature (Belbin & Downs, 1964; Sterns & Doverspike, 1989). In one example, researchers trained younger (18 to 28 years), middle-aged (37 to 46 years), and older volunteers (55 to 67 years) in word-processing skills over a 2-week period (Elias, Elias, Robbins, & Gage, 1987). The design of the program was

chosen to be optimal for older adults; the seven 3½ hour training sessions were self-paced, and a trainer was available at all times for assistance. Participants of all ages learned the fundamentals of word processing, but older adults took longer to complete the subunits, evaluation protocol, and examination than the young and middle-aged groups. They also needed more trainer interventions, even though they did not request them. Requesting assistance might have reduced training time for the older trainees. Among the recommendations that emerged was the strategy of comparing new methods to those familiar to the older employee (Elias et al., 1987).

In another example, Gist, Rosen, and Schwoerer (1988) conducted a 3-hour workshop to enhance the acquisition of computer skills, comparing younger (under 45 years) and older trainees (over 45 years) as well as the effects of two training conditions: tutorial and modeling. The tutorial was a self-paced set of a spreadsheet exercise and problems, with immediate feedback on performance. The modeling condition had subjects observe a man demonstrate and discuss the steps involved in making a spreadsheet. After observing the model, subjects practiced the steps and were given feedback. The authors found that on the posttest, the younger adults significantly outperformed the older adults. The 3-hour time constraint may have limited the performance of the older subjects. The modeling condition was found to be superior for both age groups. Gist et al. (1988) provide two possible explanations for this finding. Realistic expectations of actions required for performing each step may have been developed, or vicarious reinforcement may have existed.

Finally, two studies by Czaja and Sharit (1998; Sharit & Czaja, 1999) examined age differences in the performance of computer tasks reflective of real-life job situations. They divided participants into three age groups, younger (20 to 39 years), middle-aged (40 to 59 years), and older (60 to 75 years). Examining 3 days of task performance, they found that older participants completed less work than the other age groups. In the 1998 study, when they controlled for differences in the amount of work, however, no age differences in errors were found; visuomotor skills and memory were more likely to predict the quantity or quality of work than age. Experience was the most important factor for older worker performance in the second study. An important consideration for training applications is that each age group had a different pattern of improvement over the 3 days of learning and performing the tasks. These differences must be considered when developing and implementing training programs. Czaja (2001) concluded that we need to identify the job component that may hinder older workers' performance and use interventions, such as redesigning the workplace or job.

Even though no single method has been determined to be best for training older adults, the most successful programs are sensitive to older workers' needs (Czaja, 2001). Training is a growing need for all workers, and added research should help improve methods.

Wellness Programs for Older Adults

Health promotion on the part of employers can maintain health and possibly even slow the changes associated with the aging process (Rowe & Kahn, 1998). There are many economic and social benefits for organizations that promote wellness.

Wellness programs typically emphasize a holistic approach to health. Preventive efforts may be directed at reducing the risk of illness through physical fitness, nutrition, weight control, stress management, hypertension control, and smoking cessation programs (Pfeiffer, 1989). Studies that have empirically evaluated the effectiveness of health promotion programs have found them to be effective in increasing fitness levels, decreasing health risk factors, lowering absenteeism rates, and reducing medical costs (Hollander & Hale, 1987). In a study of a work site health promotion program, a Midwestern paper company reported saving over $200,000 in 2003, and reported benefits included decreased reports of soft-tissue injuries, decreased days away from work, and continually decreasing workers' compensation claims over a 3-year period (Halls & Rhodes, 2004). Employer-sponsored programs specifically designed for older workers have been developed but are somewhat uncommon (Levin, 1987; Yen, Schultz, McDonald, Champagne, & Edington, 2006).

Retirees are often overlooked in an organization's health promotion efforts. Deobil (1989) suggests that one possible reason for the dearth of health promotion programs for retirees is the attitude, held by both employers and older employees and retirees, that it may be too late to develop preventive behaviors. Deobil suggests that the scope of wellness programs be expanded to include not only prevention but also maintenance and rehabilitation of functional capacity (the ability to carry out daily activities).

Health promotion efforts directed toward older workers and retirees are worthwhile. With the recent increases in health care costs and the increased usage of health care with age (Deobil, 1989; Pfeiffer, 1989), wellness programs are an attractive method for controlling escalating costs (Deobil, 1989). Several research findings support that the health risks of employees are reduced, and health status improves, which results in reducing health care costs when employees participate in a health promotion programs (Edington, Karjalainen, & Edington, 2002; Musich, Adams, & Edington, 2000; Yen, Edington, McDonald, Hirschland, & Edington, 2001). The implementation of wellness programs may enable older adults to remain functional in the workforce longer (Pohjonen, 2001). If health is maintained, with the aid of health promotion programs, employees may be able to increase their tenure at work. Benefits include decreased risk for disease, improved general fitness and health, and better maintenance of physical functioning (Delecluse et al., 2004; Hillsdon, Brunner, Guralnik, & Marmot, 2005; Pohjonen, 2001). One work site health program in a large telecommunications company was tied to a reduction in days spent on short-term disability (Serxner, Gold, Anderson, & Williams, 2001). Health promotion may be particularly important for employers as a way to decrease the number of days away from work due to injury or illness, because even though specific instances of absenteeism for older workers are lower overall, the number of days absent per instance (for example, 2 to 3 days in a row) tends to increase with age (Figure 13-2).

Older adults, both workers and retirees, have shown a great interest in wellness programs. Areas of expressed interest include weight management, physical fitness and exercise, avoiding workplace injuries, vision and hearing testing, health after retirement, and nutrition (Carter, Gaskins, & Shaw, 2005; Connell, Davies, Rosenberg, & Fisher, 1988).

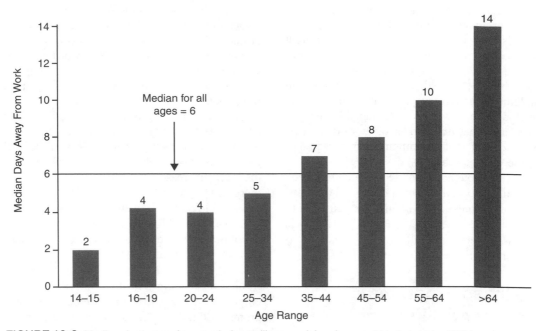
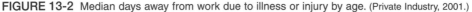

FIGURE 13-2 Median days away from work due to illness or injury by age. (Private Industry, 2001.)

Current Approaches to Wellness Programs

Methods for providing health information include appraisals of health risk (e.g., medical screenings), written health-related information (e.g., newsletters), classes and seminars on health and aging-related subject matter, and modified fitness programs for older workers and retirees (e.g., senior aerobics classes; Deobil, 1989; Pfeiffer, 1989; Rowe & Kahn, 1998).

Approaches that are most likely to be successful are easily accessible, offered at no cost, promise new information, and require minimal time (Connell et al., 1988; Yen et al., 2006). These factors and those that follow should be considered in developing wellness programs for older adults.

Considerations for Developing Wellness Programs

When designing the wellness program's goals, the needs, desires, and health levels of the participants need to be considered. Social, psychological, and physical needs must be addressed (Deobil, 1989; Sofie, 2000; Wood, Olmstead, & Craig, 1989). Three important psychological factors are motivation, safety, and confidence.

Any concern about engaging in exercise may be reduced through careful instruction about monitoring the intensity of exercise and making needed modifications. Positive feedback and an enjoyable atmosphere can enhance older participants' confidence and motivation to continue in the exercise program (Deobil, 1989). In order to encourage physical activity in older employees at work, several strategies should be considered:

1. Provide an environment where they can incorporate daily activities
2. Provide health insurance cost reductions to employers providing programs
3. Provide tools for employers to educate employees about a healthy lifestyle (Robert Wood Johnson Foundation, 2001).

Ethical issues must also be considered. These issues include the question of responsibility (who is responsible for an individual's health—the organization or the individual?), voluntary participation, and confidentiality (Hollander & Hale, 1987). Assurance that these factors have been addressed will reduce participant concerns about such factors as invasion of privacy.

Work site wellness programs can clearly benefit older workers and retirees. The programs have been shown to be empirically effective (Fitch & Slivinske, 1988; Yen et al., 2006) and offer many potential benefits to older workers, retirees, and the organization.

Retirement

Retirement creates many life changes for older adults. For the vast majority of people, with retirement comes an increase in free time as well as a decrease in income. Although these are not the only changes that result from retirement, they may be the most dramatic (Robinson, 1986; Sterns & Gray, 1999; Sterns & Kaplan, 2003). Occupational therapists may need to help elders focus on identifying meaningful constellations of occupations to address personal needs previously met by engagement in work.

Retirement today is characterized by changing transition patterns and ages of labor force exits. The transition from work to retirement is no longer clear cut. Retirement is not necessarily a complete withdrawal from the workforce and work activities (Sterns & Subich, 2005). An estimated one-third of retirees reenter the workforce, although the likelihood of reentry decreases with age (Hayward, Hardy, & Liu, 1994). Postcareer "bridge employment" may involve changes in industry, occupation, hours, or salary (Ruhm, 1990). Multiple pathways from work to retirement highlight the importance of thinking of retirement as a process and studying the process over time. The retirement process may include an anticipatory period of the retirement decision (may take place many years before), the decision itself, the act or acts of retirement, and continual adjustment to retirement (Atchley, 1976; Ekerdt, 1998; Sterns & Subich, 2005). Decisions regarding one's life and activities continue for the rest of the life span.

The multiple pathways of the retirement process were examined in a study of the different exit patterns in a sample of 2226 white and black men aged 55 to 74 years (Mutchler, Burr, Pienta, & Massagli, 1997). Patterns of continuous work, continuous nonwork, crisp exits, and blurred exits were examined over a period of 28 months. A crisp transition is a single, nonreversed, clear-cut exit from the labor force. A blurred pattern is a gradual role transition marked by repeated reentries and exits over

months or years. In this initial research, 10% of the sample was categorized as crisp transition, 15% as blurred transition, 34% continuous labor force participation, and 41% nonparticipation.

Crisp and blurred transitions were also found to differ in terms of age, financial resources, and health status. Crisp transitioners tended to be younger than 65. Although they were not associated with any particular ages, blurred transitions tended to be uncommon past the age of 68 years. Limited financial resources (i.e., pension availability, nonwage income) were associated with a blurred as opposed to a crisp exit pattern. Inadequate income seemed to cause people to maintain continued, although sporadic, labor force participation. Individuals with poor health were more likely to demonstrate blurred transition as opposed to continuous labor force participation. Individuals with the poorest health were more likely to demonstrate crisp exits or no labor force participation over the time course of the study. This research highlights the importance of looking at exit patterns as opposed to single transitions in understanding the retirement process. Retirement can no longer be seen as a single transition. We now know that there is much more complexity to the dynamics of the process (Sterns & Gray, 1999).

Factors Influencing the Retirement Experience

The effects of retirement are largely determined by an individual's specific experience. One factor is whether the decision to retire is voluntary. In addition, four personal characteristics have been linked to retirement satisfaction: health, income, attitudes, and preparedness for retirement (Beehr, 1986; Feldman, 1994; Sterns & Gray, 1999).

Voluntary Versus Nonvoluntary Retirement

The negative effects of retirement may be more pronounced for those who do not choose to retire. Voluntary retirees have reported higher life satisfaction, income, health, and occupational status than involuntary retirees (Palmore, Burchett, Fillenbaum, George, & Wallman, 1985; Quinn & Burkhauser, 1990). Involuntary retirees, in contrast, have shown signs of poor adaptation (Kimmel, Price, & Walker, 1978; Richardson, 1993; Sterns & Kaplan, 2003).

In 1986, amendments to the Age Discrimination in Employment Act eliminated mandatory retirement policies in most occupations. However, mandatory retirement legislation is only one cause of involuntary retirement; another cause is poor health (Sterns & Gray, 1999). Those forced to retire because of poor health are more likely to suffer negative consequences than those who retire as a consequence of mandatory retirement laws. Palmore and associates (1985) analyzed data from three longitudinal studies and discovered that retiring for compulsory reasons other than health had no significant effects on life satisfaction, whereas health-related retirement was related to lower living standards, poorer health, and lower satisfaction (with life, leisure, activity, and retirement).

Kimmel, Price, and Walker (1978) found that health and preretirement attitudes were the most significant predictors of retirement satisfaction, whether retirement was voluntary or not. Therefore, the elimination of mandatory retirement may not greatly improve retirement satisfaction. Rather, it may be the factors that influence the retirement decision, such as health, income, and preretirement attitudes, that determine adjustment (Richardson, 1993).

Health

Health is a pervasive force that affects the experiences of older adults. Although health may not be the primary factor in the decision to retire, poor health is probably the most salient reason for poor adjustment to retirement. Healthier retirees have higher life satisfaction and an easier retirement transition than do unhealthy persons (Sterns & Gray, 1999).

Income

Another personal variable that influences adjustment to retirement is income level (Sterns & Gray, 1999). The loss of money in retirement has been regarded as a primary stressor in retirement (Richardson, 1993). On the other hand, Maxwell (1985) found that life satisfaction was related to the absolute level of retirement income, as opposed to the level of income relative to preretirement income. Although the loss of money may be a stressor in retirement, what may be more important is the adequacy of the older person's present income. In order to adapt successfully to retirement, individuals need adequate financial resources in addition to the other factors discussed.

Attitudes

Positive attitudes toward retirement are related to better adjustment to retirement in some samples (Beck, 1983; Morrison & Jedrziewski, 1988) but have been shown to be unrelated to adjustment for women (Belgrave, 1988) and blacks (Behling & Merves, 1985). Additionally, people with positive attitudes toward retirement are not always prepared for the changes that occur with retirement. Behling and Merves found that white professionals were better prepared financially for retirement than were blacks or Puerto Ricans, in spite of similar attitudes toward retirement. What may be more important than a positive attitude is a realistic appraisal of the retirement situation (Ekerdt, 1998), coupled with adequate preparation.

Preparation for Retirement

People who plan for major life changes tend to be more successful in dealing with them (Dennis, 1989; Feit & Tate, 1986; Singleton, 1985). Because retirement is a major life change, those who are prepared for retirement will be better able to adapt to the retirement process (Kamouri & Cavanaugh, 1986). Research suggests that this is so (Richardson, 1993; Sterns & Gray, 1999).

Demographic characteristics influence the degree to which an individual is prepared for retirement. For example, research has indicated that people with higher incomes are better prepared and have a greater number of resources to use in retirement. However, regardless of income, active planning for retirement can ease the transition. Planning for retirement not only can enhance financial circumstances and contribute to a healthier lifestyle but also can provide an opportunity to explore new leisure, education, social participation activities, possible transitional work opportunities including volunteering, and alternative housing (Singleton, 1985; Sterns & Subich, 2005). So, the sooner planning is begun, the better!

Retirement Preparation Programs

Formal retirement preparation programs, provided by an employer, a nonprofit organization, a consulting firm, or an independent retirement specialist may be helpful (Dennis, 1989; Sterns & Gray, 1999). Unfortunately, only a small percentage of workers participate in formal preretirement preparation programs, and research at the organizational level suggests that few employers provide such programs (Richardson,

1993; Sterns & Subich, 2005). Fortunately, the situation may be improving. It is hoped that the increasing number of opportunities will result in better planning on the part of all workers, especially those who are approaching retirement age.

Comprehensiveness of Programs

Preretirement programs range from single sessions, with individual employees discussing benefits, to several group sessions covering a broad array of topics (Feit & Tate, 1986). The most common topic covered in preretirement programs is financial planning (Rowen & Wilks, 1987). Other topics commonly covered in comprehensive programs include health issues, leisure, housing, interpersonal relationships, legal issues, the use of time, and adjustment to changing roles (Dennis, 1989; Feit & Tate, 1986; Rowen & Wilks, 1987).

As noted above, the whole issue of meaningful occupational constellations is a vital one for occupational therapists to address. Many elders are not interested in spending the remainder of their years in leisure pursuits. They may need help identifying transitional work opportunities, social participation, educational activities, and the many other kinds of activities that contribute to a rich occupational life. Further, elders may need assistance determining how they can locate opportunities, and what resources (transportation, training, etc.) may facilitate their involvement. Research suggests that occupational therapy interventions with well-elders focused on their occupational choices can promote good physical and mental health (Clark et al., 1997).

Do Retirement Planning Programs Work?

Although there has not been a great deal of research, there is some evidence that these programs improve the retirement experience. They have been effective in improving participants' attitudes toward retirement (Richardson, 1993), increasing the amount of planning, increasing retirement knowledge, and enhancing satisfaction with retirement over time. The benefits of these programs, however, may not be sustained over time. In some cases, it may be necessary for the individual to address personal retirement issues with a retirement counselor (Sterns & Subich, 2005).

Informal Preparation

It is clear that some form of planning is essential. However, people do not have to attend formal programs to prepare for retirement. Informal methods, such as consulting with advisors and getting support from retired friends and family members, are much more common than participating in formal programs and can improve satisfaction, expectations, and knowledge (Kamouri & Cavanaugh, 1986). In fact, informal means may be more effective than formal ones (Parnes, 1989).

Alternatives to Retirement

A recent survey suggests that 42% of baby boomers would like to be able to cycle through periods of work and nonwork (Harris Interactive & Dychtwald, 2005). Other surveys estimating the preference for continued work after retirement suggest that more than half of retirees would like to continue some part-time work rather than retire totally (Sheaks, Pitt-Catsouphes, & Smyer, 2006; Sterns & Sterns, 1995). Far fewer actually do so. There are several possible explanations for this (Parnes, 1989). Alternative work schedules are not readily available (ASPA/CCH, 1988; Sheaks et al., 2006), and individuals may be unable to find part-time work in their area of expertise. However, a variety of options exist (ASPA/CCH, 1988; Newstrom & Pierce, 1979), and employers may retain highly skilled workers by providing one or more of these. Examples of such alternatives include allowing employees to remain with the company on a regular part-time schedule, or using retiring workers on a contractual basis (Sheaks et al., 2006). Job-sharing, extended leaves of absence, and gradually reducing hours worked over a period of time may also be alternatives.

Many advantages for older employees result from these options. They can continue to earn an income and remain productive. Phased or alternative work options also enable the older person to adjust psychologically to life without constant work demands, and the shorter or flexible work hours make it possible for workers to take care of personal matters more easily. The major barriers for older employees had been the social security earnings test, as well as tax penalties, and pension plans that preclude working or limit hours. Additionally, job coordination may be difficult (Morrison & Jedrziewski, 1988), and many of these options fail to provide benefits for the older workers.

Advantages for employers include decreased absenteeism, turnover, and tardiness; increased productivity; and decreased overtime costs

(Newstrom & Pierce, 1979; Paul, 1988; Rosow, 1990; Hedge et al., 2006). Older workers have fewer voluntary absences, less turnover, and fewer accidents (Rhodes, 1983; Hedge et al., 2006), and they can be ideal role models to younger employees. They can also help train younger employees and may attract older consumers. Disadvantages for employers include supervision and scheduling difficulties (Paul, 1988), and the potential for higher benefit costs.

Unemployed Older Workers

The unemployment rate of older adults 60 and over is the lowest among all age ranges (Sincavage, 2004). These rates are often just estimates, though, because older discouraged workers may choose to retire rather than continue a frustrating job search. It takes an average of 7 weeks longer for an older worker to find employment compared with a younger worker, and if one is a black male, a male with health problems, or one with less formal education, this period is even longer (Feit & Tate, 1986). When the numbers of discouraged workers are added into the unemployment rates, the rate becomes much higher (Sandell, 1987; Sandell & Baldwin, 1990). These rates are closer to those of younger workers.

Displaced Workers

With the many company buyouts, layoffs, and closings and increases in technology, the number of displaced workers increased dramatically in the late 1980s and throughout the 1990s and into the 2000s (Hall & Mirvis, 1995; Hedge et al., 2006). Job displacement has been found to be related to decreases in income and future job status, loss of pension benefits, increases in drug abuse, suicide, divorce, depression, illness, and homicide (Frese & Mohr, 1987; Kinicki, Bracker, Kreitner, Lockwood, & Lemak, 1987).

In many cases, older workers are less likely to be displaced and more likely to be recalled for employment. Yet, when additional training is required due to technological changes, older workers are more likely to be displaced (Sandell & Baldwin, 1990). Federal employment and training programs are available for displaced or disadvantaged workers 14 years of age and over. The Senior Community Service Employment Program, under Title V of the Older Americans Act, is a program specially designed for older workers. There is a great disparity, though, between the number of eligible older people and the number participating in such programs. The current need for workers at all levels has provided a climate more favorable for older workers.

Cross-Cultural Issues

Although most of the research findings and theories have been focused on Western cultures, the current trend of globalization requires us to consider whether the same approach regarding the place of older workers can be applied to the non-Westernized cultures. Researchers found that there were differences in value systems among members of other countries (Hofstede, 2001; Triandis, 1994). In addition, there are gender inequality issues within, as well as across, cultures. In some Asian countries, like Japan and South Korea, women are still expected to take primary care of domestic issues, such as child care and household chores, while men are more likely to be expected to work (Silverthorne, 2005). Current research in Western cultures has found that women are less likely to be promoted to the leader position compared to their male counterparts (Eagly & Karau, 2002).

Usually the dimensions of culture include power distance (the extent to which the less powerful members accept that power is distributed unequally), uncertainty avoidance (the extent to which members feel comfortable in ambiguous situations), individualism/collectivism (the degree to which members look after themselves or other members), and masculinity/femininity (the distribution of emotional roles between genders). Values and thinking processes may vary depending on the degree of each dimension within the culture (or country). For example, the way that employees seek feedback regarding their performance differs, for example, dependent on a culture's perceptions of appropriate relationships with authority figures, or power distance (Sully DeLuque & Sommer, 2000). Also, managers' perceptions of their subordinates in terms of moviation at work were different among North American, Latin American, and Asian managers, which resulted in differential performance ratings (DeVoe & Iyengar, 2004).

In addition, perception or definition of issues related to older workers, such as retirement timing and training issues, can be different.

Few countries provide incentives for retirement before age 60, and among countries with formal pension systems, incentives vary considerably for those between ages 60 and 65 (Antolin et al., 2003). Population aging influences on health care and pension costs have led some countries to explore more flexible retirement options in order to keep people in the workforce longer (Antolin et al., 2003; Taylor, 2002). Pension and retirement systems that do exist, mostly in industrialized countries, may be privately or publicly run. For some of the non-Westernized cultures, there are no institutionalized retirement concepts or timing. Rather, older people keep working as long as they are able. Alternatively, members in other cultures may transfer their roles from economic contribution to spiritual contribution (Luborsky & LeBlanc, 2003). Thus, unique cultural conditions should be considered when issues of older workers are discussed.

■ Summary

In the future, older workers are expected to represent a growing proportion of the workforce, and their absolute workforce number will increase.

The decision to retire or continue working reflects a complex array of factors, including economic well-being, personal preference, subjective health, attitudes regarding leisure, and the desire to continue work.

Contradictions in the research literature must continue to be clarified. Emphasis needs to be placed on individual differences in the nature of life and work experience. Satisfaction and ability to work reflect normative aging, generational differences, and unique life events of the older adult worker. Intervention in the workplace in such areas as wellness promotion, training and retraining, and human resources management may make work life extension a more frequent choice.

The ultimate responsibility for maintaining professional competence rests on the individual employee. At the same time, an organization can foster competence by updating opportunities, providing challenging work assignments, and providing interaction with coworkers and management.

Research on retirement indicates that in the future we will need to weigh carefully the importance of voluntary and involuntary decisions to retire and relevant factors related to satisfaction. For over 35 years, a major emphasis has been on the positive aspects and normalcy of retirement and approaches to facilitate the transition. At the same time, the United States was the first in its advocacy for the rights of older adult workers to continue to work if they are capable and able. A serious question for the future is what efforts will be made to make the workplace more attractive to adult and older adult workers who are in the process of exploring a change in how they view the working years and the choice to work longer either full or part time.

Cultural differences or similarities regarding older workers need to be given careful consideration. The aging workforce will be more diverse in every way in the future. This reminds us that each older worker needs to be considered on an individual basis.

Case Study

Sam Brown is a computer programmer for a medium-sized company. Three weeks ago, at age 58, Sam suffered a stroke. At this point in his recovery, Sam is having some difficulty with his speech, but all of the test results indicate that there is no cognitive impairment. Sam has started a program of speech therapy.

Sam's employer is concerned about his ability to return to work. Although they wish to support him, they are concerned that keeping him may lead to increased errors and the need to check his work, and may end up costing them more in the long run than hiring a new employee to take over his duties. However, recruiting, hiring, and training a new employee is expensive. In addition, Sam has knowledge and experience with both the job and the company which his employer recognizes as a valuable asset. Finally, the company lawyers recognize their

continued on page 326

Case Study (continued)

legal responsibility to allow Sam the opportunity to get back into the position he already occupies, and to provide reasonable accommodations for employees with disabilities.

The employer has chosen to consult with an industrial gerontologist, a specialist in issues concerning older workers, about their options. Sam's immediate supervisor is concerned about meeting company needs in a timely fashion and how to ensure that Sam is able to perform the duties necessary for his job. The specialist asks questions to determine what the essential duties of the job are, and what skills and abilities are required in order to perform these duties. These questions may help to determine ways in which the job might be modified, while still accomplishing the essential job tasks. In addition, answers to these questions can provide information on how Sam and the therapist he is working with can approach the rehabilitation of any other losses he experienced relevant to his job that might become apparent. The specialist

recommends testing Sam on a work sample, made up of the actual work tasks that are required as essential duties of his job, and refers Sam to an occupational therapist to do both the task analysis and a careful assessment of Sam's performance skills, performance patterns, and client factors. The results from this work sample can then be assessed by the employer, the specialist, and Sam's therapist to determine Sam's current ability to perform the job, potential rehabilitation needs, and ways in which the job might be modified, if necessary. A retraining program can be developed to deal with any special concerns.

Questions

1. What specific aspects of Sam's performance might the occupational therapist be concerned about?
2. What specific aspects of the task might be of particular concern?
3. What are some accommodations that might be of help to Sam?

Review Questions

1. In what ways are the capabilities and needs of older workers different from those of younger workers?
2. What person-centered interventions might assist elders to remain productive in the workplace?
3. How might contextual interventions assist elders to remain productive in the workplace?
4. How might employers modify activity demands to enhance worker performance for older adults?
5. An employer in a midsize company is interested in retaining her older workers for as long as possible. She is considering implementing both wellness and retraining programs for those workers but is unsure about potential benefits and the best structure for these programs. As a consultant to the company, what information would you gather, and what considerations would you advise her to review before making a decision?
6. You are working with an older person who is trying to decide whether or not to retire. What factors would you encourage him or her to consider?
7. You have a client who does not want to retire but is no longer interested in working full time. What alternatives might be available?

Web-Based Resources

For helpful information about work and retirement visit:

www.aarp.org/research/work, **AARP,** date connected May 23, 2007. AARP has many resources focused on work and retirement, including information about age discrimination, employment opportunities, satisfying retirement, and other topics.

www.bc.edu/centers/crr/pub_wor.shtml, **The Center for Research Retirement at Boston College,** date connected May 23, 2007. This site has links to a wide array of research reports about retirement.

www.urban.org/publications/900985.html, **The Urban Institute,** date connected May 23, 2007. The Urban Institute has published an extensive report focused on work and retirement.

REFERENCES

AARP. (1990). *The aging workforce: Managing an aging work force. Older employees instructional resources for instructors of higher education.* Washington, DC: Author.

AARP. (2004, May). *Baby boomers envision retirement II: Survey of baby boomers' expectations for retirement.* Washington, DC: Author.

AARP. (2005, December). *The business case for workers age 50+: Planning for tomorrow's talent needs in today's competitive environment.* Washington, DC: Author.

American Occupational Therapy Association. (2002). Occupational therapy practice framework: Domain and process. *American Journal of Occupational Therapy, 56,* 609–639.

American Society for Personnel Administration and Commerce Clearing House. (1988). *ASPA/CCH survey human resources management.* Chicago: Commerce Clearing House.

Antolin, P., Casey, B., Oxley, H., Whitehouse, E., Duval, R., & Leibfritz, W. (2003). Policies for an ageing society: Recent measures and areas for further reform. *OECD Economics Department Working Papers,* No. 369, OECD Publishing.

Atchley, R. C. (1976). *The sociology of retirement.* Cambridge, MA: Schenkman.

Avolio, B. J., Waldman, D. A., & McDaniel, M. A. (1990). Age and work performance in nonmanagerial jobs: The effects of experience and occupational type. *Academy of Management Journal, 33,* 407–422.

Barth, M., McNaught, W., & Rizzi, P. (1995). Older Americans as workers. In S. A. Bass (Ed.), *Older and active: How Americans over 55 are contributing to society* (pp. 35–70). New Haven, CT: Yale University Press.

Barth, M., McNaught, W., & Rizzi, P. (1996). The costs and benefits of older workers. In W. H. Crown (Ed.), *Handbook of employment and the elderly* (pp. 324–348). Westport, CT: Greenwood Press.

Beck, S. H. (1983). Position in the economic structure and unexpected retirement. *Research in Aging, 5,* 197–216.

Beehr, T. A. (1986). The process of retirement: A review and recommendations for future investigation. *Personnel Psychology, 39,* 31.

Beehr, T. A., & Bowling, N. A. (2002). Career issues facing older workers. In D. Feldman (Ed.), *Work careers: A developmental perspective* (pp. 214–241). San Francisco: Jossey-Bass.

Behling, J. H., & Merves, E. S. (1985). Pre-retirement attitudes and financial preparedness: A cross-cultural and gender analysis. *Journal of Sociology and Social Welfare, 12*(1), 113–128.

Belbin, E., & Belbin, R. I. (1972). *Problems in adult retraining.* London, UK: Heineman.

Belbin, E., & Downs, S. M. (1964). Activity learning and the older worker. *Ergonomics, 7,* 429–437.

Belgrave, L. L. (1988). The effects of race differences in work history, work attitudes, economic resources, and health or women's retirement. *Research in Aging, 10,* 383–398.

Bureau of Labor Statistics. (2005). *BLS release 2004-14 employment projections* (USDL 05-2276). Retrieved March 27, 2006, from http://www.bls.gov/news.release/ecopro.nr0.htm.

Carter, M., Gaskins, S., & Shaw, L. (2005). Employee wellness program in a small rural industry: Employee evaluation. *American Association of Occupational Health Nursing Journal, 53,* 244–248.

Clark, F., Azen, S. P., Zemke, R., Jackson, J., Carlson, M., Mandel, D., et al. (1997). Occupational therapy for independent-living older adults. A randomized controlled trial. *Journal of American Medical Association, 278,* 1321–1326.

Colquitt, J. A., LePine, J. A., & Noe, R. A. (2000). Toward an integrative theory of training motivation: A meta-analytic path analysis of 20 years of research. *Journal of Applied Psychology, 85,* 678–707.

Connell, C. M., Davies, R. M., Rosenberg, A. M., & Fisher, E. B. (1988). Retirees: Perceived incentives and barriers to participation in health promotion activities. *Health Education Research, 3,* 325–330.

Cooperman, L. F., & Keast, F. D. (1983). *Adjusting to an older workforce.* New York: Van Nostrand Reinhold.

Cross, K. P. (1982). *Adults as learners.* San Francisco: Jossey-Bass.

Czaja, S. J. (2001). Technological change and the older worker. In J. E. Birren & K. W. Schaie (Eds.), *Handbook of the psychology of aging* (5th ed., pp. 547–568). New York: Academic Press.

Czaja, S. J., & Sharit, J. (1998). Ability-performance relationships as a function of age and task experience for a data entry task. *Journal of Experimental Psychology: Applied, 4,* 332–351.

Dalton, G. W., & Thompson, P. H. (1971). Accelerating obsolescence of older engineers. *Harvard Business Review, 49,* 57–67.

Delecluse, C., Colman, V., Roelants, M., Verschueren, S., Derave, W., Ceux, T., et al. (2004). Exercise programs for older men: Mode and intensity to induce the highest possible health-related benefits. *Preventive Medicine, 39,* 823–833.

Dennis, H. (1989). The current state of retirement planning. *Generations, 13,* 38–41.

Deobil, S. J. (1989). Physical fitness for retirees. *American Journal of Health Promotion, 4,* 85–90.

DeVoe, S. E., & Iyengar, S. S. (2004). Managers' theories of subordinates: A cross-cultural examination of manager perceptions of motivation and appraisal of performance. *Organizational Behavior and Human Decision Processes, 93,* 47–61.

Doeringer, P. B. (1990). Economic security, labor market flexibility, and bridges to retirement. In P. B. Doeringer (Ed.), *Brides to retirement: Older workers in a changing labor market* (pp. 3–19). Ithaca, NY: ILR Press.

Eagly, A. H., & Karau, S. J. (2002). Role congruity theory of prejudice toward female leaders. *Psychological Review, 109,* 573–598.

Edington, M. P., Karjalainen, T., & Edington, D. W. (2002). The UAW-GM health promotion program: Successful outcomes. *American Association of Occupational Health Nursing Journal, 50*(1), 26–31.

Ekerdt, D. J. (1998). Workplace norms for the timing of retirement. In K. W. Schaie & C. Schooler (Eds.), *Impact of work on older adults* (pp. 101–123). New York: Springer.

Elias, P. K., Elias, M. F., Robbins, M. A., & Gage, P. (1987). Acquisition of word-processing skills by younger, middle-age, and older adults. *Psychology and Aging, 2,* 340–348.

Farr, J. L., & Middlebrooks, C. L. (1990). Enhancing motivation to participate in professional development. In S. L. Willis & S. S. Dubin (Eds.), *Maintaining professional competence* (pp. 195–213). San Francisco: Jossey-Bass.

Farr, J. L., Tesluk, P. E., & Klein, S. R. (1998). Organizational structure of the workplace and the older worker. In K. W. Schaie & C. Schooler (Eds.), *Impact of work on older adults* (pp. 143–185). New York: Springer.

Feit, M. D., & Tate, N. P. (1986). Health and mental health issues in preretirement programs. *Employee Assistance Quarterly, 1,* 49–56.

Feldman, D. C. (1994). The decision to retire early: A review and conceptualization. *Academy of Management Review, 19,* 285–311.

Fisk, A. D., & Rogers, W. A. (2000). Influence of training and experience on skill acquisition and maintenance in older adults. *Journal of Aging and Physical Activity, 8,* 373–378.

Fitch, V. L., & Slivinske, L. R. (1988). Maximizing effects of wellness programs for the elderly. *Health and Social Work, 13,* 61–67.

Forisha-Kovach, B. (1984). *The flexible organization.* Englewood Cliffs, NJ: Prentice Hall.

Fossum, J. A., & Arvey, R. D. (1990). Market place and organizational factors that contribute to obsolescence. In S. L. Willis & S. S. Dubin (Eds.), *Maintaining professional competence* (pp. 44–63). San Francisco: Jossey-Bass.

Fossum, J. A., Arvey, R. D., Paradise, C. A., & Robbins, N. E. (1986). Modeling the skills obsolescence process: A psychological/economic integration. *Academy of Management Review, 11,* 362–374.

Frese, M., & Mohr, G. (1987). Prolonged employment and depression in older workers. A longitudinal study of intervening variables. *Social Science & Medicine, 25,* 173–178.

Gist, M., Rosen, B., & Schwoerer, C. (1988). The influence of training method and trainee age on the acquisition of computer skills. *Personnel Psychology, 41,* 255–265.

Hall, D. T., & Mirvis, P. H. (1995). The new career contract: Developing the whole person at midlife and beyond. *Journal of Vocational Psychology, 47,* 269–289.

Halls, C., & Rhodes, J. (2004). Employee wellness—and beyond. *Occupational Health & Safety, 73,* 46–50.

Harris Interactive, & Dychtwald, K. (2005). The Merrill Lynch new retirement survey. A perspective from the baby boom generation. Retrieved April 1, 2006, from www.totalmerrill.com/retirement.

Hayward, M. D., Hardy, M. A., & Liu, M. (1994). Work after retirement: The experiences of older men in the U.S. *Social Science Research, 23,* 82–107.

Hedge, J. W., Borman, W. C., & Lammlein, S. E. (2006). *The aging workforce.* Washington, DC: American Psychological Association.

Hillsdon, M., Brunner, E., Guralnik, J., & Marmot, M. G. (2005). Prospective study of physical activity and physical function in early old age. *American Journal of Preventive Medicine, 28,* 245–250.

Hofstede, G. (2001). *Culture's consequences: Comparing values, behaviors, institutions and organizations across nations.* Thousand Oaks, CA: Sage.

Hollander, R. B., & Hale, J. F. (1987). Work site health promotion programs: Ethical issues. *American Journal of Health Promotion, 2,* 37–43.

Johnson, R. W. (2004, July). Trends in job demands among older workers, 1992–2002. *Monthly Labor Review, 127,* 48–56.

Kamouri, A. L., & Cavanaugh, J. C. (1986). Research note: The impact of preretirement education programmes on workers' preretirement socialization. *Journal of Occupational Behavior, 7,* 245–256.

Kaufman, H. G. (1990). Management techniques for maintaining a competent professional workforce. In S. L. Willis & S. S. Dubin (Eds.), *Maintaining professional competence* (pp. 249–261). San Francisco: Jossey-Bass.

Kimmel, D. C., Price, K. F., & Walker, J. W. (1978). Retirement choice and retirement satisfaction. *Journal of Gerontology, 33,* 575–585.

Kinicki, A., Bracker, J. S., Kreitner, B., Lockwood, C. A., & Lemak, D. J. (1987). Socially responsible for plant closing. *Personnel Administrator, 32,* 116–128.

Knowles, M. S. (1989). *The modern practice of adult education.* Chicago: Association Press.

Lawrence, J. H. (1985). Developmental needs as intrinsic incentives. In R. G. Baldwin (Ed.), *Incentives for faculty vitality* (pp. 59–68). San Francisco: Jossey-Bass.

Levin, R. (1987). *Wellness programs for older workers and retirees.* Washington, DC: Business Group on Health.

Lillard, L., & Tan, H. (1992). Private sector training: Who gets it and what are its effects? *Research in Labor Economics, 13,* 1–62.

Luborsky, M., & LeBlanc, I. (2003). Cross-cultural redefinition of the retirement concept. *Journal of Cross-Cultural Gerontology, 18,* 251–271.

Maxwell, N. (1985). The retirement experience: Psychological and financial linkages to the labor market. *Social Science Quarterly, 66,* 22–33.

McEvoy, G. W., & Cascio, W. F. (1989). Cumulative evidence of the relationship between employee age and job performance. *Journal of Applied Psychology, 74,* 11–17.

Miller, D. B. (1990). Organizational, environmental, and work design strategies that foster competence. In S. L. Willis & S. S. Dubin (Eds.), *Maintaining professional competence* (pp. 214–232). San Francisco: Jossey-Bass.

Morrell, R. W., & Echt, K. V. (1997). Designing written instructions for older adults: Learning to use computers. In A. D. Fisk & W. A. Rogers (Eds.), *Handbook of human factors and the older adult* (pp. 335–362). San Diego, CA: Academic Press.

Morrison, M., & Jedrziewski, M. K. (1988). Retirement planning: Everybody benefits. *Personnel Administration, 33*(1), 74–80.

Musich, S., Adams, L., & Edington, D. W. (2000). Effectiveness of health promotion programs in moderating medical costs in the USA. *Health Promotion International, 15*(1), 5–15.

Mutchler, J. E., Burr, J. A., Pienta, A. M., & Massagli, M. P. (1997). Pathways to labor force exit: Work transitions and instability. *Journal of Gerontology: Social Sciences, 52B,* S4–S12.

Newquist, D. D. (1986). Toward assessing health and functional capacity for policy development on work-life extension. In J. E. Birren, P. K. Robinson, & J. E. Livingston (Eds.), *Age, health and employment* (pp. 27–44). Englewood Cliffs, NJ: Prentice Hall.

Newstrom, J. W., & Pierce, J. L. (1979). Alternative work schedules: The state of the art. *Personnel Administrator, 24,* 19–23.

Noe, R. A. (2001). *Employee training and development.* Boston, MA: Irwin.

Palmore, E. B., Burchett, B. M., Fillenbaum, G. G., George, L. K., & Wallman, L. M. (1985). *Retirement: Causes and consequences.* New York: Springer.

Parnes, H. S. (1989). Postretirement employment: How much is there: How much is wanted? *Generations, 13,* 23–26.

Paul, C. E. (1988). Implementing alternative work arrangements for older workers. In H. Dennis (Ed.), *Fourteen steps in managing an an aging work force* (pp. 113–132). Lexington, MA: Lexington Books.

Peterson, D. A. (1980). *The older worker: Myths and realities.* Los Angeles, CA: Andrus Gerontology Center, USC.

Peterson, D. A. (1987). *Facilitating education for older learners.* San Francisco, CA: Jossey-Bass.

Pfeiffer, G. J. (1989). Health promotion programs for older workers. *Generations: Journal of the American Society on Aging, 8,* 28–29.

Pohjonen, T. (2001). Perceived work ability of home care workers in relation to individual and work-related factors in different age groups. *Occupational Medicine, 51,* 209–217.

Quinn, J. F., & Burkhauser, R. V. (1990). Work and retirement. In R. H. Binstock & L. K. George (Eds.), *Handbook of aging and the social sciences* (3rd ed., pp. 307–327). San Diego: Academic Press.

Reed, K., Doty, D. H., & May, D. R. (2005). The impact of aging on self-efficacy and computer skill acquisition. *Journal of Managerial Issues, 17,* 212–228.

Rhodes, S. R. (1983). Age-related differences in work attitudes and behavior: A review and conceptual analysis. *Psychological Bulletin, 93,* 328–367.

Richardson, V. E. (1993). *Retirement counseling.* New York: Springer.

Rix, S. (2006). *Update on the aged 55+ worker: 2005.* Washington, DC: AARP.

Robert Wood Johnson Foundation. (2001). *National blueprint: Increasing physical activity among adults age 50 and older.* Princeton, NJ: Author.

Robinson, P. K. (1986). Age, health, and job performance. In J. E. Birren, P. K. Robinson, & J. E. Livingston (Eds.), *Age, health, and employment* (pp. 63–77). Englewood Cliffs, NJ: Prentice Hall.

Rosow, J. M. (1990). Extending working life. In I. Bluestone, R. J. V. Montgomery, & J. D. Owen (Eds.), *The aging of the American work force* (pp. 399–418). Detroit, MI: Wayne State University Press.

Rowe, J., & Kahn, R. (1998). *Successful aging.* New York: Pantheon Books.

Rowen, R. B., & Wilks, C. S. (1987). Pre-retirement planning, a quality of life issue for retirement. *Employee Assistance Quarterly, 2,* 45–56.

Ruhm, C. J. (1990). Career jobs, bridge employment and retirement. In P. B. Doeringer (Ed.), *Brides to retirement: Older workers in a changing labor market* (pp. 92–107). Ithaca, NY: ILR Press.

Salthouse, T. A., & Maurer, J. J. (1996). Aging, job performance, and career development. In J. E. Birren & K. W. Schaie (Eds.), *Handbook of the psychology of aging* (4th ed., pp. 353–364). New York: Academic Press.

Sandell, S. H. (1987). *The problem isn't age: Work and older Americans.* New York: Praeger.

Sandell, S. H., & Baldwin, S. E. (1990). Older workers and employment shifts. Policy responses to displacement. In I. Bluestone, R. J. V. Montgomery, & J. D. Owen (Eds.), *The aging of the American work force* (pp. 126–148). Detroit: Wayne State University Press.

Schultz, K. S. (2003). Bridge employment: Work after retirement. In G. A. Adams, & T. A. Beehr (Eds.), *Retirement* (pp. 214–241). New York: Springer.

Serxner, S., Gold, D., Anderson, D., & Williams, D. (2001). The impact of a worksite health promotion program on short-term disability usage. *Journal of Occupational and Environmental Medicine/ American College of Occupational and Environmental Medicine, 43*(1), 25–29.

Sharit, J., & Czaja, S. J. (1999). Performance of a computer-based troubleshooting task in the banking industry: Examining the effects of age, task experience, and cognitive abilities. *International Journal of Cognitive Ergonomics, 3,* 1–22.

Sheaks, C., Pitt-Catsouphes, M., & Smyer, M. A. (2006). Legal and research summary sheet: Phased retirement. Boston: Alfred P. Sloan Foundation. Retrieved August 16, 2006, from http://agingandwork.bc.edu/documents/Center_on_AgingandWork_Phased_Retirement.pdf.

Shearer, R. L., & Steger, J. A. (1975). Manpower obsolescence: A new definition and empirical investigation of personal variables. *Academy of Management Journal, 18,* 263–275.

Silverthorne, C. P. (2005). *Organizational psychology in cross-cultural perspective.* New York: New York University Press.

Simpson, P. A., Geller, M. M., & Stroh, L. K. (2002). Variations in human capital investment activity by age. *Journal of Vocational Behavior, 61,* 109–138.

Sincavage, J. R. (2004). The labor force and unemployment: Three generations of change. *Monthly Labor Review, 127,* 34–41.

Singleton, J. F. (1985). Retirement: Its effects on the individual. *Adaptation and Aging, 6,* 1–7.

Snyder, C. J., & Barrett, G. V. (1988). The Age Discrimination and Employment Act: A review of court decisions. *Experimental Aging Research, 14,* 3–47.

Sofie, J. K. (2000). Creating a successful occupational health and safety program. *American Association of Occupational Health Nursing Journal, 48,* 125–147.

Sterns, A. A., Sterns, H. L., & Hollis, L. A. (1996). The productivity and functional limiations of older adult workers. In W. H. Crown (Ed.), *Handbook on employment and the elderly* (pp. 276–303). Westport, CT: Greenwood Press.

Sterns, H. L. (1986). Training and retraining adult and older workers. In J. E. Birren, P. K. Robinson, & J. E. Livingston (Eds.), *Age, health, and employment* (pp. 93–113). Englewood Cliffs, NJ: Prentice Hall.

Sterns, H. L., & Alexander, R. A. (1987). Industrial gerontology: The aging individual and work. *Annual Review of Gerontology and Geriatrics* (pp. 93–113). New York: Springer.

Sterns, H. L., & Doverspike, D. (1989). Aging and the training and learning process in organizations. In I. L. Goldstein (Ed.), *Training and development in work organization* (pp. 299–332). San Francisco: Jossey-Bass.

Sterns, H. L., Doverspike, D., & Lax, G. A. (2005). The Age Discrimination in Employment Act. In F. S. Landy (Ed.), *Employment discrimination litigation:*

Behavioral quantitative and legal perspectives (pp. 256–293). San Francisco: Jossey-Bass.

Sterns, H. L., & Gray, J. H. (1999). Work, leisure, and retirement. In J. C. Cavanaugh & S. K. Whitbourne (Eds.), *Gerontology* (pp. 355–390). New York: Oxford Univerity Press.

Sterns, H. L., & Huyck, M. H. (2001). The role of work in midlife. In M. E. Lachman (Ed.), *Handbook of midlife development* (pp. 447–486). New York: Wiley.

Sterns, H. L., & Kaplan, J. (2003). Self-management of career and retirement. In G. A. Adams, & T. A. Beehr (Eds.), *Retirement* (pp. 188–213). New York: Springer.

Sterns, H. L., & Sterns, A. (1995). Health and employment capability of older Americans. In S. A. Bass (Ed.), *Older and active: How Americans over 55 are contributing to society* (pp. 10–34). New Haven, CT: Yale University Press.

Sterns, H. L., & Subich, L. M. (2005). Counseling for retirement. In S. D. Brown & R. W. Lent (Eds.), *Career development and counseling: Putting theory and research to work* (pp. 506–521). Hoboken, NJ: Wiley.

Sully DeLuque, M. F., & Sommer, S. M. (2000). The impact of culture on feedback-seeking behavior: An integrated model and propositions. *Academy of Management Review, 25,* 829–849.

Taylor, P. (2002). Improving employment opportunities for older workers: Developing a policy framework. Presented at the Ninth EU–Japan Symposium, *Improving employment opportunities for older workers,* Brussels, Belgium.

Toossi, M. (2002, May). A century of change: The U.S. labor force, 1950–2050. *Monthly Labor Review, 125,* 15–28.

Triandis, H. C. (1994). Cross-cultural industrial and organizational psychology. In H. C. Triandis, M. D. Dunnette, & L. M. Hough (Eds.), *Handbook of industrial and organizational psychology* (Vol. 4, 2nd ed., pp. 103–172). Palo Alto, CA: Consulting Psychologists Press.

Valasek, D. L., & Sterns, H. L. (1981, November). Task analysis and training: Applications from lab to field. Paper presented as part of the "Symposium on Industrial Gerontological Psychology: Why Survive?" 34th Annual Meeting for the Gerontological Society of America. Toronto, Ontario.

Votruba, J. C. (1990). Strengthening competence and vitality in midcareer faculty. In S. L. Willis & S. S. Dubin (Eds.), *Maintaining professional competence: Approaches to career enhancement, vitality, and success throughout a work life* (pp. 214–232). San Francisco: Jossey-Bass.

Waldman, D. A., & Avolio, B. J. (1986). A meta-analysis of age differences in job performance. *Journal of Applied Psychology, 71,* 33–38.

Warr, P. (1994). Age and employment. In H. C. Triandis, M. D. Dunnette, & L. M. Hough (Eds.), *Handbook of industrial and organizational psychology* (Vol. 4, 2nd ed., pp. 487–550). Palo Alto, CA: Consulting Psychologists Press.

Willis, S. L., & Dubin, S. S. (1990). *Maintaining professional competence.* San Francisco: Jossey-Bass.

Willis, S. L., & Tosti-Vasey, J. L. (1990). How adult development, intelligence, and motivation affect competence. In S. L. Willis & S. S. Dubin (Eds.), *Maintaining professional competence* (pp. 64–84). San Francisco: Jossey-Bass.

Wood, E. A., Olmstead, G. W., & Craig, J. I. (1989). An evaluation of lifestyle risk factors and absenteeism after two years in a work site health promotion program. *American Journal of Health Promotion, 4,* 128–133.

Yen, L., Edington, M. P., McDonald, T., Hirschland, D., & Edington, D. W, (2001). Changes in health risks among the participants in the United Auto Workers-General Motors LifeSteps health promotion program. *American Journal of Health Promotion, 16*(1), 7–15.

Yen, L., Schultz, A. B., McDonald, T., Champagne, L., & Edington, D. W. (2006). Participation in employer-sponsored wellness programs before and after retirement. *American Journal of Health Behavior, 30,* 27–38.

CHAPTER 14

Community Mobility

Beth A. Ekelman, JD, OTR/L • Wendy Stav, PhD, OTR/L, SCDCM • Pat Baker, MHS, OTR/L, CLVT, CDRS • Pam O'Dell-Rossi, MPA, OTR/L • Steven Mitchell, OTR/L, ATP

*W*ith full-span lives the norm, people may need to learn
how to be aged as they once learned to be adult.

Ronald Blythe, The View in Winter: Reflections on Old Age,
Harcourt Brace Jovanovich, New York, 1979, p. 22.

OBJECTIVES

By the end of the chapter, readers will be able to:

1. Describe the national statistics on elderly drivers and the types of motor vehicle violations most commonly performed by elders.
2. Define Driving as an Occupation using the Occupational Therapy Practice Framework.
3. Explain the age-related physiological changes and disease-related changes associated with driving difficulties among elderly drivers.
4. Identify the clinical assessment and interventions used in driving rehabilitation programs for older drivers using evidence-based practice.
5. Discuss the psychosocial implications of driving and the inability to drive.
6. Explore alternative methods of community mobility recommended for the older adult.

Overview of National Statistics on Violations, Crashes, and Fatalities

According to the most recent report by the National Highway Traffic Safety Administration (NHTSA), there are 19.8 million older licensed drivers in the United States, ages 70 and older, representing a 27% increase from 1993. This group of drivers made up 10% of all licensed drivers in 2003 (NHTSA, 2004a). It is projected that this number will grow in the future due to several factors. First, as baby boomers age, the population of persons older than 55 years is expected to grow, resulting in an increase in the number of older persons eligible to drive. Second, the number of elderly women who drive is likely to increase because contemporary middle-aged women, accustomed to driving during their younger years, will grow older and continue to drive. Third, there is the potential influence that improved functional status, combined with a culture that endorses an independent lifestyle, will expand the elderly driver population even further (Retchin & Anapolle, 1993). Similar trends exist in Canada where it is expected that the number of older drivers will double over the next few years (Tuokko & McGee, 2002).

In 2004, there were 6.2 million police reported motor vehicle crashes (MVCs) in the

United States (NHTSA, 2004b). This represents a decline of 0.06% from 2003, and the fatality rate was at an historic low of 1.44 fatalities per 100 million vehicles. Fatality and injury rates were highest among drivers 16 to 24 years, and third highest among drivers 74 and older. In 2004, drivers 70 and older caused 12% of all traffic fatalities and 16% of all pedestrian fatalities (NHTSA, 2004a). Interestingly, older drivers involved in fatal crashes had the lowest proportion of intoxication of all adult drivers. Additionally, when involved in a two-vehicle fatal crash with a younger driver, the older driver was twice as likely to be the one struck (NHTSA, 2004a).

MVCs are reportedly the leading cause of accidental deaths for persons aged 65 to 74 years and the second leading cause (after falls) of any type of death for older people (Keplinger, 1998; Underwood, 1992). Most 2004 traffic fatalities involving the older driver occurred during the daytime (81%), on weekdays (72%), and involved another vehicle (74%) (NHTSA, 2004a). The most common causes of crashes involving the older driver include pulling out from the side of the road; changing lanes improperly; careless backing up; and difficulty with giving the right-of-way and with the reading of traffic signs. Elderly drivers also tend to have difficulty performing maneuvers requiring a series of rapid judgments (Underwood, 1992).

Driving as an Occupation

In accordance with occupational therapy literature, driving is an important occupation. Occupation is an "activity of everyday life, named, organized, and given value and meaning by individuals and a culture. Occupation is everything people do to occupy themselves, including looking after themselves, . . . enjoying life, . . . and contributing to the social and economic fabric of their communities" (Law, Polatajko, Baptiste, & Townsend, 1997, p. 32). Driving is an activity in which people participate on a daily basis and give meaning to based on personal and cultural values. Driving has value as a means of transportation to a destination, and it has value and meaning as an occupational enabler by contributing to engagement in other occupations within the community, including shopping, social participation, and self-care.

The occupation of driving is a complex task that requires one to receive multiple sensory stimuli simultaneously from the environment through visual, auditory, proprioceptive, kinesthetic, and vestibular functions. Extraneous stimuli must be filtered so that only relevant stimuli are attended to. Processing of relevant stimuli leads to the identification of objects and events, and a perception of their relationships in space to one another and the overall environment. Integration of this information with past experience provides meaning and context in relation to driving. In the environment, cues may be detected that have been associated with overlearned behaviors, which may result in the automatic and habitual performance of that behavior. For example, when one drives to work daily on a familiar route, the process of driving becomes routine and automatic. Higher-level processing skills regulate the performance of automatic behaviors and are necessary to learn new skills or deal with situations that are not routine.

The American Occupational Therapy Association's (AOTA) Practice Framework (AOTA, 2002) is used as a guideline to describe how the various client factors, performance skills, performance patterns, contexts, and activity demands influence one's ability to participate in the occupation of driving. The Driving as an Occupation model (Figure 14-1), adapted from Mitchell's Neurosensory Model of Driving (Ekelman, Mitchell, & O'Dell-Rossi, 2000), is a systems-based approach that provides a comprehensive overview of the relative contributions of the motor, process, and communication/interaction skills, as well as client factors that are required for safe driving. It incorporates many of the key concepts from models developed specifically for driving by Michon (1987) and Galski, Bruno, and Ehle (1992) with clinical models used to evaluate and treat cognitive (Sohlberg & Mateer, 1989) and visual processing (Warren, 1993a, 1993b) dysfunction in specific skill areas central to driving.

Figure 14-1, which should be referred to throughout the following discussion, represents the multidimensional construct of engagement in the occupation of driving. According to the Occupational Therapy Practice Framework (AOTA, 2002), the occupation of driving is one aspect of community mobility classified within the Instrumental Activities of Daily Living

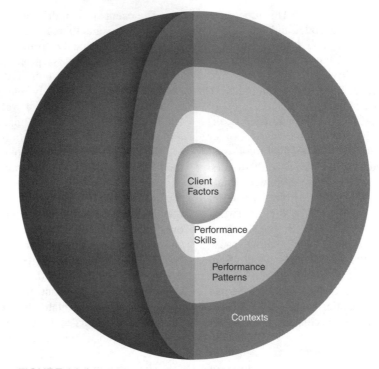

FIGURE 14-1 Driving as an Occupation Model

category of Areas of Occupation. Participation in driving has activity demands that are inherent in occupation that are a constant. These activity demands include the objects used and their properties, such as the vehicle, the space demands of the roadway, the social demands of sharing the road, sequencing and timing of vehicle operations and turntaking, and the required actions to operate the vehicle controls. Although these activity demands are relatively constant, the application of interventions such as changing the context or implementing adaptive equipment alters the activity demands of engaging in the occupation of driving for that person.

At the center of the engagement in driving are client factors, which represent the foundational underlying capacities including mental functions (attention, memory, and visuospatial perception), sensory functions (vision), and neuromusculoskeletal and movement-related functions. People enact their client factors into small units of performance called performance skills that include motor and process skills and impact the ability to operate a vehicle safely, interpret objects within the environment, and respond to environmental stimuli. Performance occurs in specific ways called performance

patterns that include automatic habitual behaviors associated with driving. Performance patterns can be safe habits (putting on seat belt or turn signal), routine (taking the same route to volunteer at the hospital), and facilitate role performance (a husband fulfills the role of primary driver in a married couple). Not all performance patterns are positive, and some can be portrayed as negative habits (speeding) or unsafe routines (completing weekly business calls on the cell phone while driving). All of this performance takes place within contexts that culturally determine the value of driving; physically dictate where one will drive; temporally identify when one drives with regard to time of day, in the life span or along the continuum of a progressing illness; socially provide networks to support alternative methods of driving; and control how safely or accurately driving occurs.

The aging process and age-associated conditions may lead to declines in any of the client factors and performance skill areas represented in the model. Because these client factors and performance skill areas are interdependent, dysfunction that exists in one client factor or skill area may influence the demands placed on other skill areas. When an older adult may no longer drive, alternative community mobility methods may need to be explored. At the same time, it is important to be cognizant of the individual's context or contexts and performance patterns, particularly life roles. Therefore, clinical evaluation of driving ability requires one to be aware of potential dysfunction that may exist in all of these areas. To be able to evaluate and diagnose dysfunction formally in the various areas, the health care professional needs to understand each of these areas and how they are interrelated.

Client Factors

According to the Occupational Therapy Practice Framework (AOTA, 2002), client factors consist of body functions and structures. Body functions

most relevant to driving are the sensory, mental, and neuromusculoskeletal functions. The body structures that support these body functions would be the eye, ear, and related structures, as well as structures related to movement. The next section will provide further detail about important body functions that impact one's ability to participate in the occupation of driving (Table 14-1).

Sensory Functions

Driving is a complex task that requires one to receive multiple sensory stimuli simultaneously through several modes of sensory input. Vision is the primary mode of sensory input, accounting for up to 90% of the sensory information necessary for driving (Hills, 1980). Visual acuity,

TABLE 14-1 Summary of Client Factors Affecting Driving Performance

Body Functions and Structures that Impact Driving Performance	
Mental functions	*Global mental functions,* such as global attention, consciousness, orientation, emotional stability, and impulse control are needed to drive. *Specific mental functions,* such as attention, memory, visuospatial perception, higher-level cognitive functions for judgment, and the ability to plan, impact motor and process skills.
Sensory functions and pain	Visual acuity and visual field functions are important for driving performance. The ability to hear sounds and horns, as well as ability to maintain balance are important. Appreciating pain and whether or not it interferes with driving performance is important to consider.
Neuromusculoskeletal and movement-related functions	It is important to consider an individual's ability to move his or her joints and bones to maneuver a vehicle safely and whether he or she has the strength to operate the controls. Individuals also need to have good voluntary motor control and reactions to drive.
Other functions, such as cardiovascular, hematological, immunological, respiratory, digestive, metabolic, endocrine, genitourinary, reproductive, skin and related structures	These functions should be considered if they interfere with performance skills and participation in driving, especially as these relate to safety and energy levels.
Body structures	It is important to consider which anatomical parts of the body are needed to drive: eyes, ears, structures related to movement, and structures of the nervous system are the primary structures. Other structures need to be considered in relation to how may impact performance skills they necessary for safe driving.

contrast sensitivity, visual fields, oculomotor control, and depth perception are important visual functions that form the foundation on which higher levels of process skills are based (Warren, 1993a, 1993b; Zoltan, 1996).

Visual Acuity

Visual acuity is a measure of the clarity of one's vision and can be defined as the ability to distinguish the details of an object and resolve its spatial properties (Strano, 1989; Warren, 1993a, 1993b; Zoltan, 1996). Cones are the sensory receptors that bear the primary responsibility for visual acuity. They function in bright light, are responsible for color vision, and are concentrated in the fovea of the retina. The American Association of Motor Vehicle Administrators recommends a minimum standard of 20/40 vision for unrestricted driving. To distinguish an object with the same degree of detail as a driver with 20/20 vision, the driver with 20/40 vision must be within half the distance of the object. Consequently, the driver with 20/40 vision will have only half the time to distinguish the same degree of detail as will the driver with 20/20 vision. Interestingly, road signs are designed on the basis of this minimum 20/40 vision standard (Strano, 1989). **Dynamic acuity** is the measure of one's ability to distinguish details of objects in motion and should play a supplemental role in providing a better overall picture of functional visual acuity.

Contrast Sensitivity

Contrast sensitivity is the ability to see a target when there is limited contrast between the target and the background (Hyvarinen, 1996). The need for intact contrast sensitivity is particularly important when driving at night or in the rain. In addition to interpreting visual information in low contrast, contrast sensitivity contributes to visual acuity and enhances the perception of the target image. Instead of traditional eye charts that measure acuity by the ability to distinguish high-contrast letters or symbols by reducing size, contrast sensitivity charts look at the ability to distinguish differences in letters or symbols of a constant size, but with a lesser degree of contrast or with images of sine waves that look like a series of stripes or bars that slant in different directions and become increasingly faint.

Peripheral Vision

Peripheral vision refers to the ability to perceive the presence or movement of stimuli in the periphery beyond the area of immediate focus that constitutes one's central vision (Warren, 2006). Rods are the sensory receptors primarily responsible for peripheral vision. They sense black and white, are sensitive to motion, and are denser in the areas farther away from the fovea. However, they are less adept at distinguishing detail or color. Peripheral vision has two essential functions. First, it is necessary to alert one to the location of potentially relevant stimuli outside the immediate area of focus. Second, it is integrated with information from other senses to provide a spatial orientation to the environment (Warren, 2006). Peripheral vision allows one to monitor areas of the driving environment that are outside the driver's central field of vision for motion or the presence of stimuli that warrant further inspection. It also assists in providing the driver with an orientation to lane markings and other characteristics of the road that are needed to perceive lane position of the vehicle.

Surprisingly, only 65% of states have visual field standards for driving (Fishbaugh, 1995). Measurements used as standards reflect either the maximum number of degrees in which stimuli can be perceived in the nasal and temporal fields of each eye individually, or a single value representing the total horizontal field in which stimuli can be perceived laterally to the left and right with both eyes looking straight ahead. Many states use a total horizontal field of 140 degrees as a minimum standard.

Oculomotor Skills

Oculomotor skills are frequently overlooked or underestimated by health care professionals concerned with visual skills and driving. In addition, no visual oculomotor standards exist in motor vehicle laws. Oculomotor skills are responsible for the coordinated use of extraocular eye muscles necessary for binocular vision and the efficient performance of conjugate eye movements (Warren, 2006). When one drives, the eyes must continually shift the focus of vision from one object to another. The object must be viewed from a vehicle in motion, and the object may be moving, requiring the driver to shift the focus of vision efficiently from one source to another. Oculomotor movement consists of two types: saccadic eye movements and smooth-pursuit eye movements. *Saccadic movements* change the line of sight to enable inspection of detail by the fovea. *Smooth-pursuit movements* are used when the eyes are following a moving object, and they maintain a steady image on the retina (Warren, 1993a, 1993b). Saccades and pursuits can be screened quickly in the clinical setting. One should observe the smoothness, range, accuracy, and speed of these movements, and document potential problems in terms of how saccades and smooth pursuits appear upon evaluation.

Depth Perception

Depth perception is a monocular skill that allows one to judge distances away from the self and is important in driving in order to judge how close the driver's vehicle is to other vehicles, objects, and roadway boundaries (Zoltan, 1996). The monocular nature of depth perception allows drivers with vision in only one eye to drive safely by using other environmental cues to judge distance from other objects. *Stereopsis* also is the ability to judge depth but relies on perception of the stimulus from two separate angles and therefore is a binocular skill (Zoltan, 1996). Clients having vision in only one eye or having only one eye can still perceive depth using other cues but do not have true stereopsis.

Other Sensory Functions

Although vision is the primary mode of sensory input, sources of auditory, tactual, and vestibular stimuli also may have a significant influence on motor skills needed for driving. Kinesthesia, proprioception, and the ability to sense pressure in one or both upper or lower extremities are essential for the safe operation of vehicle pedals, steering wheel, and other controls, such as the turn signal or windshield wipers. Horns, sirens, warning buzzers and chimes, and sounds from the vehicle may be important sources of auditory input. Therefore, dysfunction affecting the ability to perceive sensory stimuli from these sources may deny the driver essential information about the driving environment.

Mental Functions

Mental functions include both global and specific mental functions (AOTA, 2002). Mental functions play an integral role in the occupation of driving and are particularly relevant when discussing safety issues. In a moving vehicle, the environment is in a constant state of change, leaving little time to receive the input and identify stimuli that could be potentially relevant. **Global attention**—subdivided into **focused attention, sustained attention,** and **selective attention**—is largely responsible for the initial phase of sensory information processing. These subdivisions represent the lower levels in a hierarchy of attentional skills and are responsible for the ability to focus on relevant stimuli, filter extraneous or distracting stimuli, and sustain focus over time (Sohlberg & Mateer, 1989). Specific mental functions, such as higher-level attention and short- and long-term memory, are functions necessary for safe driving. Attention is needed so the driver is aware of the environment inside and outside the vehicle. Memory is essential for learning and provides an underlying foundation, which allows for the integration of perceptual and cognitive skill areas leading to the performance of specific driving behavior. Several functions of memory have various degrees of importance in the driving task.

Attention

Driving requires higher-level skills to shift the focus of attention among several sources in the driving environment. External environments to the front, rear, and sides of the vehicle are potential sources of critical information but cannot be viewed at the same time. Within the vehicle, the driver must receive information from dials, warning lights, auditory warnings, as well as tactual feedback coming from primary vehicle controls, such as the steering wheel and pedals. The driver also must be able to receive and interpret information from the interaction of the vehicle suspension with the road, for instance, if the vehicle hits a pothole or skids. **Alternating attention** is the capacity for mental flexibility, which enables one to shift the focus of attention and move between tasks having different cognitive requirements (Parente & Anderson, 1991). Driving also requires the allocation of attention to monitor stimuli simultaneously or to be able to perform multiple component tasks at the same time. This is the function of **divided attention** and represents the highest level of skill (Sohlberg & Mateer, 1989).

Although it may be influenced by the functioning of skills required for global attention, the term **visual attention** refers to a specific ability required to shift the focus of vision efficiently from one stimulus to another (Warren, 1993a, 1993b, 2006). Like global attention, visual attention is defined (in most models) as having inherent concepts of selectivity, ability to be shifted or allocated to monitor stimuli simultaneously, and finite capacity. Scanning represents the next level of the visual search, allowing for the thorough and systematic recording of visual information from the environment onto the retina (Warren, 1993a, 1993b, 2006). Scanning ability should not be equated with the oculomotor movements used for saccades and smooth pursuits. Rather, *scanning* is a cognitive process that requires oculomotor movements as well as the integration of visual acuity, peripheral vision, and visual attention skills.

Much of the research discusses visual attention in terms of the **"useful field of view"** (UFOV). This is the spatial area within which an individual can be quickly alerted to visual stimuli in a variety of situations (Keplinger, 1998). UFOV relies on both visual and mental functions and thus provides a more global measure of visual functional status than either sensory or cognitive tests alone. A dynamic measure, UFOV is a function of three test variables:

1. The duration of target presentation
2. The level of complexity of a secondary central task
3. The salience of a peripheral target

Short-Term Memory

Short-term memory, often referred to as immediate memory or working memory, is of limited capacity and frequently is considered to be a function of attention. It is brief in duration (15 to 30 seconds), is highly susceptible to decay, and requires rehearsal to retain information (Parente & Anderson, 1991). It functions to provide a "mental workspace" from which to analyze information and direct the performance of a task foundation for perceptual and cognitive processing of information.

Long-Term Memory

Long-term memory is a term that has different meanings to different professionals. When attempting to understand the role of memory in driving, it is useful to discuss longer-term forms of storage in the context of what is being stored.

Semantic memory, procedural memory, and prospective memory are the three forms of long-term memory most relevant to driving.

Semantic memory is the term used to describe the ability to store and recall meaning (Harrell et al., 1992). It is responsible for the storage of knowledge, learned concepts, and operating principles, which provide the foundation from which to carry out functional tasks. This form of memory has particular relevance to driving because it constitutes one's fund of driving-related information that has been learned through experience and any formal instruction. Semantic memory places little importance on the context of when the information was stored and is resistant to decay. An experienced driver will know the meaning of a "Yield" sign but will probably have no recall of when that meaning was learned.

Procedural memory refers to the ability to learn rule-based or automatic behavioral sequences. These include motor skills, conditioned responses, and perceptual-motor tasks (Harrell et al., 1992; Sohlberg & Mateer, 1989). This type of memory is largely subcortical and forms the basis for the performance of most routine functional tasks. Learning occurs through repetition. Once learned, performance of the behavior occurs automatically in response to a given stimulus. Although repetition serves to reinforce and maintain the behavior, procedural memory represents a relatively permanent form of storage that is resistant to decay. Driving habits and routines are developed from both semantic and procedural memory.

Prospective memory refers to the ability to remember future intentions (Sohlberg & Mateer, 1989). This ability to "remember to remember" is reinforced through repetition and from contextual cues in the environment. Diminished ability to recall recent events and information, and "forgetfulness" associated with breakdowns in prospective memory, are commonly the forms of "memory loss" noticed by older persons in daily activities. Age-associated dysfunction in these areas may have little effect on driving safety in the experienced driver who takes routine trips to familiar destinations. Manifestations may result in navigational inefficiency when driving in unfamiliar areas and having to rely on information from maps, written directions, or verbal instructions.

Performance Skills

Performance skills include motor, process, and communication/interaction skills. These are features of what one does, are observable, and have functional purposes (AOTA, 2002). Of course, certain activity demands and contexts may vary the extent to which certain performance skills are required to drive, such as size of the vehicle, whether one is driving on a busy road or highway, the lighting within the vehicle, and the design of the console, to name a few (Table 14-2).

Motor Skills

In order to drive safely, one needs certain motor skills to be able to maintain proper sitting posture and balance and be able to position the body, arms, and legs in relation to the driving controls to promote efficiency in movement during the driving process. Reaching for the controls within the vehicle and being able to flex and rotate one's trunk and neck are also important skills needed to operate the vehicle safely. Coordinating both sides of the body, arms, and legs, and being able to grasp and release vehicle

TABLE 14-2 Summary of Performance Skills Affecting Driving Performance

Motor Skills	
Posture	Able to maintain trunk control and balance while driving; maintains an upright sitting position; and is able to position body, arms, and legs in relation to the driving controls to promote efficiency in movement during performance.
Mobility	Able to reach for controls within the vehicle and flex, rotate, and twist trunk to operate the vehicle safely.
Coordination	Able to coordinate both sides of body (arms and legs) to safely operate the vehicle. Able to grasp and release vehicle controls, and movements are smooth and fluid during performance.
Strength and effort	Able to move vehicle controls and regulate the force, speed, and grade of movement to operate vehicle controls safely. Able to properly grip controls.
Energy	Able to participate in driving without obvious fatigue and is able to maintain a consistent tempo of performance throughout the entire driving process.

Process Skills	
Energy	Able to maintain a consistent tempo of performance throughout the entire driving process and maintain focused attention throughout the task when presented with extraneous auditory or visual stimuli.
Knowledge	Operates the vehicle safely and appropriately, adheres to goal-directed plans of action (able to follow directions, stay on designated route), asks questions or reads directions using map, road signs, and does not ask unnecessary information questions, such as how to turn on the car or put the car in gear.

continued on page 340

TABLE 14-2 **Summary of Performance Skills Affecting Driving Performance**
(continued)

Process Skills	
Temporal organization	Able to initiate the process of driving, follow appropriate steps in proper order to safely operate the vehicle, and appropriately terminates or stop the vehicle in the designated location when destination is reached.
Organizing space and objects	Able to locate and store keys, vehicle, and safety items (spare tire, jack, flashlight); aware of where all controls and safety items are located; able to maneuver vehicle around obstacles and on the road safely while adhering to driving laws.
Adaptation	Able to notice/respond to environmental cues while driving and makes an effective and efficient response, makes appropriate accommodations and adjustments in anticipation of environmental stimulus, anticipates and prevents undesirable circumstances from recurring or persisting. Able to problem solve.

Communication/Interaction Skills	
Physicality	Appropriately makes eye contact, gestures, and assumes appropriate physical postures necessary for participation in driving.
Information exchange	Able to effectively communicate (give and receive) information when communicating with others during driving (e.g., asking for directions, paying toll, communicating with police officer).
Relations	Able to follow the rules of driving and respectfully interact with others on the road.

controls with smooth and fluid movements are essential skills. One also needs to be able to regulate the force, speed, and grade of movement to operate vehicle controls safely (e.g., to know how much force to apply to the brakes to stop the vehicle). An individual also must be able to participate in driving without obvious fatigue and be able to maintain a consistent tempo of performance throughout the entire driving process.

Process Skills

After relevant stimuli from the various modes of sensory input are detected and filtered through attentional mechanisms, efficient processing is necessary to identify objects and changes in spatial relationships, perceive events in a temporal context, and form an overall sensory representation of the driving environment. Process skills are "used in managing and modifying actions en route to the completion of daily life tasks" (Fisher & Kielhofner, 1995, p. 120; AOTA, 2002, p. 621). Although most processing skills involve visual information, auditory, proprioceptive, kinesthetic, and vestibular information also are integrated to develop a multidimensional sensory representation of the driving environment.

Process skills begin with the ability to maintain focused attention while driving.

Temporal organization also is necessary to initiate the process of driving, to follow the appropriate steps to operate the vehicle safely, and to know when and where to stop the vehicle once the destination is reached. *Organizing space and objects* is another important process skill needed for driving. The dynamic nature of the driving environment requires the central nervous system to be able to identify objects based on incomplete information regarding configural aspects and specific details of the object. The position in space of stop signs, traffic signals, surrounding vehicles, and other objects in the driving environment must be appreciated relative to both the driver and to one another. Changes in the spatial relationships between the vehicle, pavement markings, and surrounding traffic are in a constant state of change and need to be monitored continually. The driver also needs to be able to locate and store keys, the vehicle, and safety items, such as the spare tire, jack, and flashlight, and be able to maneuver the vehicle safely around obstacles on the road while adhering to driving laws. Meaning may be attributed to a set of objects that appear in a given context leading to their perception as a specific event in the driving environment.

Knowledge and adaptation or **metacognition** refer to higher-level processing skills that are used in the implementation, verification, and regulation of goal-directed activity (Nelson & Narens, 1994). Knowledge skills include goal selection, planning, initiation, self-regulation, self-monitoring, and use of feedback (AOTA, 2002; Sohlberg & Mateer, 1989). Self-monitoring may refer to task-oriented behavior but also includes the ability to be aware of one's current cognitive status. Knowledge skills also are the ability to formulate strategies to accomplish aspects of driving that are goal oriented (for example, choice of destination and route selection, ability to read a map). Cognitive processing at this level occurs primarily in the gray matter of the frontal lobes, but information from areas throughout the brain also is integrated. Although its capabilities are much greater than automatic-level processing, executive-level processing requires a substantially greater degree of neural processing. As a result, it requires higher levels of attention to perform, more time to complete, and is subject to sensory overload.

Higher-level adaptation skills are critical so that the driver is able to notice and respond to environmental cues while driving and is able to make appropriate adjustments in anticipation of environmental stimulus (AOTA, 2002). Adaptation is the use of executive functions in the driving task to monitor and regulate the performance of automatic-level behaviors and predict events in the driving environment. It is essential to problem solving, judgment, and decision making when encountering nonroutine situations. Executive functions monitor and regulate the habitual performance of driving skills, anticipate conditions in the driving environment, and carry out volitional driving behaviors. They also are necessary to allocate available attentional skills to best meet the internal demands of the cognitive-perceptual operations in use and the external demands of the environment.

Communication/Interaction Skills

Communication and interaction skills are important to consider when describing driving as an occupation. In order to drive safely, one needs to assume appropriate physical postures to drive and be aware of appropriate and inappropriate gestures used while driving. One also needs to be able to ask for directions or help if needed, or understand when another driver may be asking for assistance and when it is appropriate to offer help. Most importantly, the driver needs to be able to follow the rules of driving and demonstrate respectful interactions with others on the road.

Performance Patterns

Performance patterns are "patterns of behavior related to daily life activities that are habitual or routine" (AOTA, 2002, p. 623). These are described in terms of habits, routines, and roles. Habits are automatic behaviors that are "integrated into more complex patterns that enable people to function on a day-to-day basis" (Neistadt & Crepeau, 1998, p. 869; AOTA, 2002, p. 623). Habits can be useful, such as always placing car keys in the same place, or impoverished, such as inconsistently looking both ways when crossing an intersection. Routines are occupations that have established sequences (Christiansen & Baum, 1997, p. 16; AOTA, 2002, p. 623), and roles are a "set of behaviors that have some socially agreed upon function and for which there is an accepted code of norms" (Christiansen & Baum, 1997, p. 603; AOTA, 2002, p. 623) (Table 14-3).

The experienced driver performs most component tasks with little conscious awareness. Automatic-level driving refers to the stimulus-bound initiation of overlearned processing skills and rule-based behavioral sequences used to accomplish component tasks of driving and perform routine driving functions. This level of processing is largely subcortical and relies heavily on procedural memory and semantic memory. Although the overlearned behavior may be associated with a specific environmental stimulus, component tasks of driving most often occur in response to a specific set of contextual cues, which have been identified during perceptual processing. The overall repertoires of component tasks performed at this level are a function of the driving experience and are maintained in procedural memory through repetition. Automatic-level processing requires mostly lower levels of attention and allows for the rapid processing of routine information. Examples of habitual or automatic-level driving include most "mechanical driving skills" required for basic vehicle control, navigating familiar routes when driving to routine destinations, and the many initial reactions performed in response to immediate driving hazards.

Stimulus-bound impulses are constantly generated during automatic-level driving. Most of the time, these impulses result in the efficient, automatic, and habitual performance of a component driving task. In fact, an experienced driver could be described as one who drives mostly on impulse! Occasionally, the impulse generated is inappropriate for the circumstances, and the role of executive-level driving is to detect and inhibit these habitual impulses and modify an automatic-level response before it occurs. For example, a driver's visual attention may alert him or her to motion sensed in the left temporal field via peripheral vision. Perceptual processing identifies the object as another vehicle moving forward in the adjacent area. The detection of forward motion in the context of stopping for a red light results in an impulse to move the right lower extremity from the brake pedal to the accelerator. The executive-level functions are triggered, and thus, the driver begins to scan the environment. The driver determines that a green left-turn arrow is present, although the light for the through lanes is still red. Executive-level driving inhibits the driver's impulse to drive into the intersection with a red light.

Driving routines, such as common routes or time of day one drives, are important to consider, because these will impact the performance skills required to drive safely. Although the complexity of road tests varies greatly among states, many state road tests consist of less than 5 miles of driving in a residential neighborhood with one-step verbal instructions provided for navigation. Such road tests may require little

---

TABLE 14-3 Summary of Performance Patterns Affecting Driving Performance

Performance Patterns	
Habits	Automatic behaviors associated with driving (e.g., "autopilot" driving on a familiar route, putting car keys in the same place so they can be found easily). Some habits are not safe or impoverished, (e.g., talking on the cell phone while driving, putting on makeup while driving, inconsistently looking both ways when crossing an intersection, driving while intoxicated, etc.).
Routines	Examples of driving routines are: common routes taken, time of day usually drive.
Roles	The individual may be the only driver in the household, responsible for carpooling, providing transportation for members of the household, or drives as a part of his or her work.

more than automatic-level processing for an experienced driver to pass.

Roles will influence how important driving is in the context of one's life. Whether or not there are other members in the household who can drive or why one needs to drive are all relevant considerations in determining the value placed on the ability to participate in driving as an occupation or the magnitude that loss of the ability to drive will have on an individual.

Contexts

The Occupational Therapy Practice Framework describes seven different types of contexts that should be considered when assessing a client's driving (AOTA, 2002). *Cultural contexts* are imposed by family, society, and one's culture (AOTA, 2002). For example, in the United States, driving is valued and viewed as a symbol of independence. In many cultures, men are the primary drivers and women are the passengers. Parents often must act as chauffeurs for their children, driving them to and from extracurricular activities. Some communities are more open to alternative modes of transportation, such as well-developed subway or train systems. *Physical contexts* are also important to consider, such as the physical layout of the vehicle or whether the vehicle has been adapted with devices such as hand controls, the environment where the person will be driving, the roadway markings, the presence of construction, and so forth. *Social contexts,* such as whether there are other family members available to drive, the social participation generated from transporting one's peers, or whether driving cessation will impact social participation, will impact the value and meaning placed on the ability to engage in the occupation of driving. Certain *personal contexts* are important to consider, such as age and socioeconomic factors that may impact one's ability to drive. For example, is the person old enough to get a driver's license; can the person afford to purchase a car, adaptive devices, and insurance; or should the person take public transportation? Driving may also be highly valued and meaningful to the person and contribute to perception of self and feeling like a whole person, which is relevant to the *spiritual context. Temporal contexts* need to be considered as well. For example, how long has the person been driving,

where did the person learn to drive, what time of day or night does the person usually drive, where is the person in the course of a progressive illness, what is the timing relevant to the peak medication times and when the person must drive, and what distances are usually driven? *Virtual contexts,* such as voice-activated controls or other computer devices used to facilitate driving performance, may be used as well (Table 14-4).

Age-Related Physiological and Disease-Related Changes Affecting Driving Performance

Age-related changes, common medical conditions, and medications can affect a driver's client factors and performance skills, thus compromising driving safety (Table 14-5) (Copeland, 1989; Keplinger, 1998; Morgan & King, 1995).

Sensory Functions

Visual Input

Several changes in visual function associated with aging affect driving performance. Mild changes in static visual acuity, although usually the only function tested for licensing in many states, have been found to have little effect on the risk of MVCs in the older driver (Keltner & Johnson, 1987; Keplinger, 1998). However, **dynamic visual acuity,** the ability to distinguish fine detail for objects moving relative to the observer, shows the strongest correlation to the driving record of the elderly driver.

Peripheral vision also deteriorates with aging. The total horizontal peripheral visual field typically drops from 170 degrees in the young adult to 140 degrees by age 50 (Retchin & Anapolle, 1993). Peripheral vision decreases with age as a result of normal age-related changes occurring within the eye. Peripheral vision also may be reduced functionally by structural changes affecting the location of the eye within the orbit and in surrounding skin folds. This is important to consider when assessing the older adult's driving performance.

The health care professional who has a role in assessing the skills of an older driver should not assume that the ability to renew one's driver's license represents proof of adequate

TABLE 14-4 **Summary of Contextual Issues that May Impact Driving Performance**

Contexts	
Cultural	Expectations to drive imposed by family, society, and culture, (e.g., in the United States, individuals may obtain a license at the age of 16, and driving is valued and viewed as a way of achieving independence). Why must the individual drive, (e.g., go to the grocery store for food, the bank for money)? Are there opportunities to explore alternative methods of community transportation or access to food, banking, and so forth?
Physical	What is the environment like where the individual will be driving (e.g., highway, country, suburbs)? What is the physical layout of the vehicle and adaptations? What distances does the person drive or need to drive?
Social	Are others in the family or social network available to drive? Are others depending on the individual to drive? Does the inability to drive impact social participation opportunities?
Personal	Age, gender, socioeconomic status, and educational status of client.
Spiritual	Is driving meaningful to the individual?
Temporal	When did the individual learn to drive, how long has he or she driven, what time of day does he or she drive?
Virtual	Does the individual use any voice-activated systems or other environmental controls to operate the vehicle? How does the client perform on the driving simulator?

peripheral vision for safe driving. A recurrent theme in the literature is that the most significant visual skills necessary for safe driving (i.e., contrast sensitivity, visual acuity in low-contrast conditions, dynamic visual acuity, and effective visual fields) are not the ones routinely examined for driver licensing (Zur & Shinar, 1998). Because licensing guidelines and screenings measure peripheral vision along only the horizontal plane at eye level, they may not detect visual upper- and lower-quadrant field deficits that may be of sufficient severity to prevent safe driving. For example, a residual upper-quadrant deficit that may have occurred as a result of a "mini-stroke" might make that driver susceptible to missing traffic signals in the affected quadrant.

Older adults have a smaller UFOV than young adults. Results indicate that the UFOV is highly sensitive and specific in predicting which older drivers are at risk for crash involvement (Ball, Owsley, Sloane, Roenker, & Bruni, 1993). Older drivers with a severe restriction in the spatial area over which they could rapidly use visual information were six times more likely to have incurred one or more crashes in the previous 5-year period than were those with minimal or no such restriction (Ball et al., 1993). In a more recent study of 295 drivers aged 55 to 87 years, subjects experiencing a 40% or greater reduction in UFOV were 2.2 times more likely than those with a less than 40% reduction to have incurred a crash over a 3-year period. Seventy percent of these crashes involved failure to yield the right-of-way, failure to heed a stop signal, or inadequate stopping distance (Owsley, Ball, Thomas, & Graves, 1995).

Other visual problems facing older drivers include an increased difficulty with glare from

TABLE 14-5 **Summary of Skill Areas and Changes Affecting Driving Performance of Older Adults**

Skill Area and Diseases Affecting Skill Area	Subskill	Driving Performance
Visual input (cataracts,	Dynamic visual acuity	Difficulty distinguishing fine detail (reading road signs), problems with glare in bright sunlight
glaucoma with peripheral field	Peripheral vision	Difficulty at intersections and changing lanes
loss, macular degeneration,	UFOV	Failure to identify potential hazards, failure to yield the right-of-way, failure to heed a stop sign, inadequate stopping distance
diabetic retinopathy)	Hearing	Difficulty hearing sirens, horns, and whistles
Other sensory input (peripheral vascular disease)	Tactual	Difficulty feeling pedals and modulating pressure on pedals
Cognitive function (Alzheimer's disease, multi-infarct dementia, Parkinson's disease, diabetes with transient cognitive impairment, cerebra-vascular accident)	Memory, attention, judgment, central information processing	Slowed reaction time Difficulty with traffic sign recognition, searching for hazards, executing evasive actions, identifying hazards Difficulty aligning car with side of road, entering and leaving the highway, dealing with traffic in roundabouts, performing two tasks at the same time in an emergency

overhead road lights or oncoming vehicles and markedly impaired vision in low-illumination situations (Keltner & Johnson, 1987; Marottoli, 1993). Much of this difficulty is from the decreased pupillary reaction time as a person ages. As a person ages, the speed at which the pupil can constrict and dilate slows, leaving longer periods of time for intense light to enter the eye which had been dilated during low-light driving conditions. However, there is only a weak relationship found between measures of disability glare and highway safety (Keplinger, 1998).

Several ocular diseases increase in prevalence with age and can result in irreversible or progressive visual impairment that can affect driving performance. Cataracts, glaucoma, age-related macular degeneration, diabetic retinopathy, and corneal disease can all interfere with driving safety (Underwood, 1992). Early cataracts may cause little decrease in visual acuity but can affect light scattering, glare sensitivity, color perception, and night vision. An individual who has a diffuse sclerotic cataract, with a daytime visual acuity of 20/25, will complain of glare in bright sunlight and may have difficulty seeing when looking into the headlights of an oncoming car at night. Individuals

with open-angle glaucoma with peripheral field loss may have difficulty seeing cars or pedestrians approaching from the side. Those individuals with age-related macular degeneration may have difficulty reading road signs or seeing cars. Persons with diabetic retinopathy may experience alternating periods of poor and good visual acuity and permanent loss of vision that could affect driving safety (Klein, 1991). Some medications used to treat visual conditions, particularly those used to treat glaucoma, can cause localized blurring of vision and pupillary changes affecting vision during suboptimal illumination conditions (Keplinger, 1998; Underwood, 1992).

Because many of these conditions have an insidious onset with gradual progression, patients may drive for years without being aware of significant visual disability and the associated increased crash risk (Underwood, 1992). Most visual field deficits do not affect central vision, and perceptual completion is a response of the brain to the absence of sensory stimuli to fill in the involved area with predictable environmental patterns (Warren, 1993a, 1993b). Therefore, the older driver's self-appraisal may not be a reliable means of identifying potential dysfunction in peripheral vision.

Changes in Other Sensory Functions

Although vision is the primary mode of sensory input, sources of auditory, proprioceptive, kinesthetic, and vestibular functions also have a significant influence on driving ability. Hearing loss affects one-third of all elderly persons. *Presbycusis,* the inability to hear high-frequency cues, is the main cause of hearing loss in older adults and can make it difficult for them to hear sirens, horns, and whistles (Underwood, 1992). Age-associated medical conditions also can result in impairment in tactual abilities. Diabetic neuropathy and peripheral vascular disease may result in impairment in distal lower-extremity sensation, which may make operating the pedals of the vehicle dangerous.

Changes in Mental Functions and Performance Skills

Age-related changes in mental function that can affect driving ability in older adults are memory loss, diminished attention, impaired judgment, and slowed central information processing (Underwood, 1992). As adults age, they initiate and execute movements more slowly and less precisely. Of particular interest is psychomotor slowing or reaction time. The literature on movement slowing with age indicates that alterations in motor and process skills are due to

1. Failure to use advance preparatory information
2. Difficulty in processing stimuli and making responses that are spatially incompatible
3. Initiation deficit in dealing with increased task complexity
4. Inability to regulate performance speed (Stelmach & Nahom, 1992)

Although some experts believe that reaction time is too complex to measure accurately (Marottoli, 1993), multiple studies indicate that there is a difference in reaction time between young and older drivers (Stelmach & Nahom, 1992). *Reaction time,* a measure of the speed of response to the onset of a single stimulus, often is defined in the context of driving as the time taken for the subject to release a simulated accelerator and depress a brake pedal after the light changes from green to red (Stelmach & Nahom, 1992). In the assessment of the older driver, reaction-time testing may be more valuable in assessing sustained attention and speed

of information processing than as a determinant of motor function. Welford (1984) measured total simple reaction time and varied the choice of stimuli, noting that the reaction time tended to increase disproportionately with age when the number of choices was increased or made more difficult. However, Olson & Sivak (1986) compared younger and older drivers in a real-world setting and found relatively little difference in reaction time.

Alzheimer's Disease

Studies relating cognition to driving abilities of older adults focus primarily on the effects of dementia or Alzheimer's disease (AD) on driving safety. Some studies show an excessive crash rate by persons with dementia; however, these studies are weakened by methodological shortcomings, such as small sample size, lack of appropriate control groups, and self-reporting of crash data (Trobe, Waller, Cook-Flannagan, Teshima, & Bieliauskas, 1996). These prior studies (Coyne, Feins, Powell, & Joslin, 1990; Friedland et al., 1988; Kaszniak, Nussbaum, & Allender, 1990; Lucas-Blaustein, Filipp, Dungan, & Tune, 1988) indicate that approximately 29% to 47% of older drivers with dementing illness, mostly AD, are involved in crashes following the onset of dementia.

Available empirical data appear to support the conclusion that dementia is accompanied by increased crash risk. Studies indicate a rate of between 17 and 19.3 crashes per million miles driven by the older driver with dementia, compared with estimates of 3.6 (Friedland et al., 1988), 9.0 (Williams & Carsten, 1989), and 12.1 crashes per million miles driven for adults without dementia in the same age range (Kaszniak et al., 1990). The American Academy of Neurology (Dubinsky, Stein, & Lyons, 2000) conducted a meta-analysis of studies of automobile accident frequency among drivers with AD and concluded that drivers with AD at a severity of Clinical Dementia Rating (CDR) 1 were found to pose a significant traffic safety problem both from crashes and from driving performance measurements, a crash risk that is higher than for drivers 16 to 19 years old. Drivers with early AD, at CDR stage 0.5, have an increased risk of accidents similar to that for drivers 16 to 19 years old and for those drivers intoxicated with alcohol at a blood alcohol level of less than 0.08%.

Although symptoms are progressive, the rate of progression and the clinical features prominent at particular stages of AD in a given individual vary (Donnelly & Karlinsky, 1990). The majority of experts feel that the diagnosis of AD alone is not sufficient to cause the immediate withdrawal of driving privileges. Not only is there a possibility of misdiagnosis, particularly in the early stages of dementia, but also driving performance in some persons in the milder stages of AD still may be satisfactory (Drachman & Swearer, 1993; Hunt, Morris, Edwards, & Wilson, 1993). For example, Drachman and Swearer studied the risk of auto crashes among individuals with AD who continued to drive after the onset of AD compared with normal age-matched control subjects. They concluded that patients with AD who drive present a slightly increased risk for crashes compared with drivers of all ages, but a lower risk than young, unimpaired drivers.

During the first 2 to 3 years after the onset of AD, the magnitude of crash risk is well within the accepted risk for other registered drivers. However, the annual crash rate for these individuals more than doubled in the fourth year. Noting that there is a marked variability in the degree of disability due to AD and its rate of progression, Drachman and Swearer (1993) recommend that direct tests of driving competence be administered to ensure the continued licensure is safe and that there be sufficiently frequent retesting to identify the expected decline over the years. Although there is no consensus on how frequently driving skills need to be tested, Duchek et al. (2003) recommend a driver examination every 6 months. Adler, Rottunda, and Dysken (2005) recognize that some clients with more rapidly progressive dementia may require more frequent assessments than every 6 months and suggest that a family member also take responsibility for monitoring driving performance and communicating any declines to the client's provider.

Current studies focus on how AD affects the performance of specific performance skills necessary for safe driving. Brashear and colleagues (1998) used the Traffic Sign Recognition Test (TSRT), comparing patients with dementia who continue to drive with normal elderly volunteers. Although the screening tool did not assess driving safety, drivers with dementia performed worse on the traffic sign recognition than normal elderly drivers, suggesting that these individuals may not recognize common traffic signs and may thus pose a risk to society. Carr, Shead, and Storandt (2005) designed a brief test of traffic sign naming that would discriminate between cognitively intact older drivers and drivers with mild to moderate AD. They concluded that the 10-item sign-naming test, which can be completed in 2 minutes or less, may be useful in identifying older drivers in need of further assessment of their driving competence.

Rebok, Keyl, Bylsma, Blaustein, and Tune (1994) evaluated 10 patients with AD and 12 healthy elderly adult controls on two tests of driving-related abilities and correlated severity of dementia as determined by a battery of neuropsychological tests with driving performance. They used two driving assessments: (1) the Driver Performance Test (DPT), which consists of a videotaped presentation of 40 driving situations with varying degrees of danger or hazard; and (2) the Driving Advisement System (DAS), a computer-based assessment of some aspects of cognition considered necessary for driving, such as reaction time, decision making, perceptual motor tracking, and self-appraisal. Although the elderly adult control subjects scored at an average level in all five skill areas tested on the DPT, the patients with AD scored in the average range in two of five skill areas (predicting the effects of a hazard and deciding how to avoid it); below average in two areas (searching for a hazard and executing evasive actions); and poorly in one area (identifying hazards). On the DAS, patients with AD also were significantly slower than the elderly adult control subjects on simple, two-choice, and conditional reaction-time tests and were much slower than drivers in general.

Research shows that some cognitive domains assessed by neuropsychological testing have a stronger correlation with driving performance than others (Adler et al., 2005; Reger et al., 2004). In a meta-analysis of the literature on the older driver with dementia, Adler et al. recommended that any assessment of driving include measures that assess visual spatial skills, attention, and reaction time, noting that neuropsychological testing taken as a whole is not strongly correlated to driving performance. However, the correlation between driving performance and cognitive testing improved when tests measuring specific areas such as visual spatial and attention skills were separated from the battery (Adler et al., 2005; Reger et al., 2004). Richardson &

Marottoli (2003) identified 25 of 36 driving behaviors that were associated with visual attention, noting that key driving maneuvers involving interaction with other vehicles and pedestrians, such as yielding right-of-way and negotiating safe turns or merges, have the greatest association with visual attention. Recognizing that researchers have argued that selective attention is more specific to driving deficits in dementia than other components of attention, such as divided and sustained attention, Reger et al. (2004) suggest that specific aspects of attention as related to driving ability should be studied further.

Other Medical Conditions Affecting Mental Function and Performance Skills

Other medical conditions common in the older adult may also affect mental function. Parkinson's disease (PD) is another cause of dementia and, combined with bradykinesia, can lead to an increased risk for MVAs (Keplinger, 1998). Grace et al. (2005) found that axial rigidity and postural instability correlated with driving safety and should be monitored, but fine motor bradykinesia or tremor did not necessarily relate to unsafe driving. Cerebrovascular disease is another cause of cognitive dysfunction. Legh-Smith, Wade, and Hewer (1986) conducted a study that concluded that individuals who have had a stroke may display difficulty aligning their cars with the side of the road, entering and leaving the highway, dealing with traffic in roundabouts, and performing two tasks at the same time in an emergency (Keplinger, 1998).

Individuals who are diabetic, especially those needing insulin or oral hypoglycemic drugs, have a higher risk for MVAs (Holmes, 1990; Keplinger, 1998; Koepsell et al., 1994). Because these individuals have more severe diabetes, they are at risk for hypoglycemia, which can cause transient cognitive impairment.

Alcohol and Medications

Alcohol, which is the number one contributor to fatal automobile accidents, can impair cognitive functions and motor and process skills of all drivers (Marottoli, 1993). In addition, certain medications that affect the central nervous system reportedly can impair psychomotor function and place older adults at increased risk for injurious motor vehicle collisions. For example, drivers using benzodiazepines for anxiety and insomnia had a 50% higher accident rate than nonusers

(Morgan & King, 1995; Ray, Fought, & Decker, 1992). The American Medical Association identifies several medication categories including anticholinergics, anticonvulsants, antidepressants, antiemetics, antihistamines, antihypertensives, antiparkinsonians, antipsychotics, benzodiazepines, sedatives, muscle relaxants, narcotic analgesics, and stimulants that can affect driving ability (Wang, Kosinski, Schwartzberg, & Shanklin, 2003). It is important for drivers to discuss with their doctors how new medications and interactions with existing medications may impact their ability to drive.

Changes in Neuromusculoskeletal Functions and Motor Skills

Aging can lead to decreased strength, coordination, reaction time, extremity range of motion, and trunk and neck mobility, all of which are necessary components of driving ability (Marottoli, 1993). Neuromusculoskeletal problems such as osteoarthritis (OA) are common in elderly adults. Driving problems due to OA are derived from pain that produces involuntary hesitancy and absolute restriction of range of motion (Roberts & Roberts, 1993). Most common neuromusculoskeletal changes due to OA are impaired cervical rotation, which can impair motor skills affecting the individual's ability to back up, park, or turn the vehicle, as well as limit peripheral vision. Painful finger joints may impede the elderly driver's ability to grip the steering wheel. Finally, pain or decreased range of motion in knees or hips may make it difficult to step on the brake or accelerator (Morgan & King, 1995; Roberts & Roberts, 1993).

Other medical conditions that can affect motor skills are neurological diseases, such as stroke, PD, or peripheral neuropathy, as well as diabetes mellitus. Whether cardiovascular disease can impair motor abilities necessary for driving is debatable, although congestive heart failure can impair alertness and stamina (Keplinger, 1998; Reuben, Silliman, & Traines, 1988).

Clinical Assessment and Intervention

Clinical practice with a focus in the area of driving rehabilitation is considered a specialized area of practice. Due to the complexities of diagnosis, equipment, policies, stakeholder involvement, and high risk to the client and the public, driving rehabilitation is not entry-level practice. Efforts to distinguish practitioners who specialize in driving rehabilitation from generalists have resulted in certification programs. The Association of Driver Rehabilitation Specialists (ADED), an interdisciplinary organization, enacted the first certification program in 1995 (ADED, 2006). The program designates individuals as certified driver rehabilitation specialists and awards a credential of CDRS. The CDRS credential identifies health care providers, driver educators/instructors, and equipment dealers who have met the certification requirements to plan, develop, coordinate, and implement driver rehabilitation services for individuals with disabilities (ADED, 2006). Individuals who meet the educational and experiential criteria and pass the certification exam are awarded the CDRS credential.

The second certification program for therapists in the practice area was developed by the American Occupational Therapy Association (AOTA) and initiated in 2006. The certification, available only to occupational therapists and occupational therapy assistants, designates individuals as specialty certified in driving and community mobility and awards a credential of SCDCM or SCADCM for occupational therapy assistants (AOTA, 2006). The SCDCM or SCADCM identifies occupational therapy practitioners who focus their practice on driving and community mobility as opposed to generalist practice. Earning the credential requires individuals to meet the experiential criteria and complete the reflective portfolio application according to the established competencies in the practice area (AOTA, 2006). The SCDCM or SCADCM certification program is based on a professional development program grounded in the AOTA Standards of Continuing Competence (AOTA, 2005). Neither the CDRS nor the SCDCM/SCADCM is required to practice clinically in the area of driving rehabilitation. Although not required, a specialization credential is important as it demonstrates focused knowledge, skills, and experience and adds credibility when working with other team members and state agencies.

Typically, clinical screenings consist of an assessment of motor function and reaction time, a screening of visual skills, and various tests to determine possible cognitive-perceptual dysfunction. Although not considered diagnostic in nature, the screening tools are designed to determine the possible presence of dysfunction in a given skill area and whether the identified dysfunction has the potential to affect driving ability. Although there is no evaluation tool that can clinically determine safe driving to a reasonable certainty, the Maryland Older Driver Project (NHTSA, 2003) reviewed a large number of tests and screening tools and found several that show some correlation to scores on the tests and increased driving risk (Staplin, Gish, & Wagner, 2003). These are listed in detail in Table 14-6.

Formalized evaluation of each skill area can be accomplished by a multidisciplinary team and can determine whether an individual has sufficient function in a given skill area to drive. Most driver rehabilitation specialists have acquired additional training to be able to screen areas that are beyond the scope of their particular discipline. Referral to other professionals occurs when formal assessment becomes necessary.

Clinical determinations based solely on these screening tools are usually made with a degree of certainty when a relatively severe degree of impairment exists. When there is lesser dysfunction in the evaluated skill, the impact on driving performance may not be clear. Although some programs may make a determination based solely on clinical data, most programs use this information to identify areas of concern that may need to be ruled out during a behind-the-wheel assessment.

Medical and Driving History and Performance Patterns

Clinical evaluations generally start with a medical and driving history, which may consist of a questionnaire or be part of the initial interview. By the conclusion of the interview and history, the evaluating professional should have obtained an impression about the older driver's general medical status, his or her driving experience, the role of driving in fulfilling life roles, any significant on-road incidents, and self-awareness of limitations and the impact of these factors on driving patterns. Figure 14-2 shows a summary of the recommendations based on a comprehensive driving assessment.

Medical information obtained as part of the medical history should include any diagnosed

TABLE 14-6 Maryland Older Driver Project's Recommended Assessments

Assessment	Purpose	Relevance to Driving
Cognitive Perceptual Measures		
Motor-Free Visual Perceptual Test (visual closure subtest)	Visual pattern perception Ability to visualize missing information	Sign recognition Traffic-control devices and safety threats that are partially hidden
Delayed recall	Working memory	Recognize and remember meaning of traffic-control devices and roadway features Remember and apply rules of the road and safe driving practices Navigational tasks that require sequential recall of route
Scan Chart Test	Scan pattern Rule out neglect	Visual search of road
Trailmaking Test, Part B	Ability to perform a directed visual search and divided attention	Navigational skills in an information-rich complex environment
Dynamic trails	Divided attention	Navigational skills
Useful field of vision	Visual attention: detection, localization, and identification of targets	Relevant to crash risk
Physical Measures		
Rapid Pace Walk Foot Tap	Leg strength, endurance and coordination	Sustained pedal control Ability to shift back and forth from accelerator to brake pedal Fall risk which correlates with crash risk
Arm reach	Upper body flexibility	Turn steering wheel
Head–neck rotation		Look to the sides and over shoulder
Mobility questionaire	Driving habits and levels of driving exposure	Relationship between self-regulating behaviors and indicators of functional status

medical conditions that could have implications for driving safety. Relevant conditions include common vision disorders such as cataracts, glaucoma, diabetic retinopathy, and macular degeneration. Systemic disorders may include diabetes mellitus, arthritis, cardiovascular disorders, atherosclerosis, and chronic obstructive pulmonary disease. Particular emphasis should be placed on identifying any history of neurological dysfunction such as transient ischemic attack, cerebrovascular accident, PD, AD, or seizures. Efforts also should be taken to determine the existence of any conditions affecting the individual's psychosocial function, especially with respect to depression and substance abuse.

The examiner also should inquire about prescription medications currently being taken by the individual. Not only does this information help determine the medications that could make driving hazardous because of their potential for sedation, but also it can yield clues to the presence of medical conditions that may not have been disclosed by the client in the interview (inadvertently or otherwise). For example, if a client with no known diagnosis arrives for an evaluation with little more than a physician's referral and reports taking donepezil hydrochloride, there is a significant possibility that an "unofficial" diagnosis of dementia may exist. It is often difficult for the occupational therapist or driver rehabilitation specialist to stay current

Occupational Therapy Driving Evaluation

Summary and Recommendations

Name:

Date:

Diagnosis: _____   Onset: _____

Medical History: _____

Referring Physician: _____

DRIVING HISTORY   STATE   LICENSE NUMBER   EXPIRES   RESTRICTIONS / ENDORSEMENTS

License/Permit Info: ___ _____ _____ _____ _____

5 Yr. Violation HX: _____   _____   **5 Yr. MVA HX:**   _____   _____

_____

CLINICAL SUMMARY

Sensorimotor Function   ☐ Compatible With Driving   ☐ Marginal For Driving   ☐ Not Sufficient For Driving

Visual Function   ☐ Compatible With Driving   ☐ Marginal For Driving   ☐ Not Sufficient For Driving

Cognitive/Perceptual   ☐ Compatible With Driving   ☐ Marginal For Driving   ☐ Not Sufficient For Driving

BEHIND-THE-WHEEL SUMMARY

Modifications: _____

Traffic Exposure: _____   **Cuing Provided:** _____

_____

_____

_____

ASSESSMENT OF DRIVING RISK: ☐ *High-Risk*   ☐ *Moderate-Risk*   ☐ *Low-Risk*

RECOMMENDATIONS   (To Be Submitted To Physician For Approval)

☐ **Resume Independent Driving Of Passenger Vehicles**

☐ **Refrain From Driving At This Time Under Any Circumstances**

☐ **Begin _____ Sessions Of Extended Behind-The-Wheel Assessment**

☐ **Begin _____ Sessions Of OT Driver Rehabilitation**

☐ **Reevaluate**

☐ _____

PROGNOSIS (For Independent Driving Following Treatment)   ☐ *N/A*   ☐ *Good*   ☐ *Fair*   ☐ *Poor*

I acknowledge that my evaluation performance and recommendations have been reviewed with me by the evaluating therapist

Client Signature

PLAN _____

_____

_____

_____

SIGNATURE _____

FIGURE 14-2 Summary and recommendations

with medications and the potential effects these may have on cognitive functions. The driving evaluator should never hesitate to discuss medications with the physician to ensure that driving performance will not be compromised by a particular medication. Figure 14-3 summarizes the medical information that should be obtained.

The person's driver's license number also should be noted so that the evaluator can document the existence of a valid driver's license or permit that allows the individual to operate a motor vehicle on public roads. Therapists working in states with online or telephone license verification should utilize that resource, as physical

**Occupational Therapy /Driver Rehabilitation Services
Intake Form**

Date _____

Name _____ Date Of Birth _____ Age _____ Sex _____

Address _____ Soc.Sec. No. _____

_____ Contact Person _____

_____ Relationship _____

Phone ( ) _____ Contact Phone ( ) _____

Other Phone ( ) _____ ☐ Call This Person To Schedule Appointments

---

Medical History

1. List Any Medical Condition, Disability, Illness, Or Injury For Which You May Have Been Referred.

_____ Date Of Onset: _____

_____ Date Of Onset: _____

2. Are You Diabetic? ☐ YES ☐ NO

3. Do You Have Glaucoma, Cataracts, or Other Eye Problems? ☐ YES ☐ NO

4. Have You Ever Had Any Seizures Or Loss Of Consciousness? ☐ YES ☐ NO

5. Do You Take Any Medications? List Names and Reason Prescribed (If Known) ☐ YES ☐ NO

_____   _____

_____   _____

_____   _____

6. Do You Experience Problems In Any Of These Areas?

a) *Weakness, Incoordination, or Limited Motion In An Arm Or Leg* ☐ YES ☐ NO

b) *Spasms, Tremors, Or Involuntary Movement In An Extremity* ☐ YES ☐ NO

c) *Decreased Balance* ☐ YES ☐ NO

d) *Loss Or Impaired Sensation (Numbness or Tingling)* ☐ YES ☐ NO

e) *Pain* ☐ YES ☐ NO

f) *Difficulty Turning Head Side To Side* ☐ YES ☐ NO

g) *Fatigue / Poor Endurance* ☐ YES ☐ NO

h) *Blurred Vision* ☐ YES ☐ NO

i) *Loss Of Peripheral Vision* ☐ YES ☐ NO

j) *Double Vision Or Scanning Problems* ☐ YES ☐ NO

k) *Problems Concentrating Or Filtering Out Distractions* ☐ YES ☐ NO

l) *Difficulty Doing More Than One Thing At A Time* ☐ YES ☐ NO

m) *Difficulty Remembering New Information* ☐ YES ☐ NO

n) *Difficulty Remembering Distant Events* ☐ YES ☐ NO

o) *Impulsivity (Acting Too Quickly Before Thinking Things Through)* ☐ YES ☐ NO

p) *Getting Lost Frequently Or Forgetting Routes* ☐ YES ☐ NO

FIGURE 14-3 Medical intake form

possession of a driver's license does not guarantee the individual is legally licensed. General information about the client's personal vehicle should be obtained, along with any assistive devices used while driving, such as cushions, auxiliary mirrors, or special sunglasses.

The driving history as shown in Figure 14-4, should include basic information about the individual's driving record. With the exception of a person's years of driving experience and any formal driver's education, the driving history should generally be limited to the previous

Occupational Therapy /Driver Rehabilitation Services
Intake Form

Name _____   Date _____

1. How Many Years Have You Been Driving?   _____

2. When Was The Last Time You Were Behind The Wheel?   _____

3. *Over The Past 5 Years,* What Was Your Annual Mileage?

☐ *< 5,000*   ☐ *5-10,000*   ☐ *10-20,000 (Average Range)*   ☐ *> 20,000 miles/year*

4. *Over The Past 5 Years,* How Many Accidents Have You Had, Regardless Of Fault?
Include Minor "Fender Benders" Or Parking Lot Incidents.

☐ *None*   ☐ *One*   ☐ *Two*   ☐ *Three*   ☐ *More Than Three*

5. *Over The Past 5 Years,* How Many Moving Violations Have You Had? (Parking Tickets Are Not Moving Violations)

☐ *None*   ☐ *One*   ☐ *Two*   ☐ *Three*   ☐ *More Than Three*

6. Has Your License <u>Ever</u> Been Suspended Or Revoked?   ☐ YES ☐ NO

7. Why Do You Want To Drive?   _____

_____

8. List Your Personal Vehicle (Year, Make & Model). List Any Adapted Driving Aids Used.

_____

9. How Concerned Are You About These Driving Conditions?

	No Concerns. Comfortable	Drive More Cautiously	Try To Avoid. Will Drive If Necessary	Totally Avoid. Will Not Drive.
Night Driving	☐	☐	☐	☐
Congested Traffic	☐	☐	☐	☐
Expressway Driving	☐	☐	☐	☐
Unfamiliar Areas	☐	☐	☐	☐
Slippery Roads	☐	☐	☐	☐
Trips Over 2 Hours	☐	☐	☐	☐

10. Are There Any Other Driving Situations Which Cause You Concern?   ☐ YES ☐ NO

_____

11. Do You Feel Your Illness/Disability Will Affect Your Driving *In Any Way?*   ☐ YES ☐ NO

If "Yes", How?   _____

_____

12. Are You As Good A Driver Now As Before Your Illness/Disability?   ☐ YES ☐ NO ☐ Uncertain

13. If You Are 65 or Older, Do You Feel Your Age Affects Your Driving?   ☐ YES ☐ NO ☐ N/A

If "Yes", How?   _____

FIGURE 14-4 Driving intake form

3- to 5-year period and should focus on the person's behavioral patterns with respect to driving, any means of self-regulation, and on-road incidents. Any crashes or moving violations occurring in recent years should also be explored. Encouraging the inclusion of all crashes regardless of fault, as well as any parking lot incidents, can provide a more complete picture. Those incidents occurring within the previous 6 to 12 months should be explored in detail. Inquiring about any recent near misses and the frequency of encountering motorists who sound their horns can also be revealing.

The Driving Habit Questionnaire by Owsley, Stalvey, Wells, and Sloane (1999) is a valuable tool that can determine whether or not the client is currently driving, how often he or she drives, and the approximate annual mileage accrued. An occupational profile also should be gathered to determine the client's interest and needs related to driving as well as other occupational engagement that is dependent upon driving. Driving is often required for successful performance of other activities of daily living (ADLs) that take place in the community and may be necessary to access socialization opportunities. This is especially true if the older person lives alone or has a spouse who does not drive. Destinations to which the individual drives on a regular basis should be identified along with any driving conditions that may be of particular concern to the individual. The examiner should identify conditions that might create excessive anxiety for the individual so that these can be avoided during a behind-the-wheel assessment. The development of new ADL dependencies may provide strong evidence that an individual with a dementing illness may encounter difficulty driving. A breakdown in the ability to perform ADLs suggests deterioration in lower-level cognitive skills, such as procedural memory, that are responsible for the performance of overlearned tasks. Because skills performed at this level are largely subcortical and resistant to deterioration, it is logical to assume when there is a breakdown in one overlearned activity, similar breakdowns may occur in other overlearned activities, such as driving (Carr et al., 1991; Foley & Mitchell, 1997).

Another key objective is to determine the level of insight the person has into his or her limitations and the effects of those limitations on driving performance. Particular attention should be paid to whether the individual self-regulates his or her driving in any way (for example, he or she avoids expressways, rush-hour traffic, left-hand turns, or unfamiliar areas). Complete reliance on the older driver's self-perception of driving ability may not be a reliable way to verify whether or not problems will manifest themselves in driving ability. The older person may deny any difficulties for fear of losing driving privileges or may lack awareness of any driving problems. This can often have a neurological basis due to deterioration of function in the frontal lobes. If significant visual dysfunction is present, the older driver may be unaware of near misses where other motorists may have taken evasive action to accommodate a significant observational error. Without this awareness of potential risks, the prognosis will be poor for the person to correct or compensate for any problems identified later in the evaluation. If the client consents, it may be helpful to obtain input from family members to assist in clarifying these issues. Even the seemingly innocuous observation that a family member or friend has to assist in filling out the questionnaire and medical forms for the client can be an indicator of visual or cognitive deficits.

In addition to medical and driving history, the clinician should spend time in this portion of the evaluation simply getting to know the client. As will be discussed more in depth in another section, the psychosocial aspect of driving is very important to most individuals. The loss of driving privileges can have a devastating impact on one's life roles, independence, and self-esteem, and the prospect of losing driving privileges may create great anxiety within the client. The clinician should explore why driving is important to the client, where he or she needs to drive, and what alternative means of transportation are available to this person. Most importantly, the clinician should explain the evaluation process, and while acknowledging that the recommendation of driving cessation is possible, indicate that the goal of the evaluation is to promote continued independence on the road, as long as the client is safe. It is important that the evaluator observe typical driving ability, insofar as it is possible, given the circumstances. Most elderly drivers come to the evaluation anxious and "psyched up" for the "test." It should be expected that the driver would and should provide his or her best effort in order to "pass the test." Observing what should be his or her "best" effort is important, but understanding what is "typical" driving performance is more likely to produce a more effective recommendation. Taking the time to listen to and reassure the client should decrease any fears or concerns, permitting a more realistic assessment of actual driving performance.

Clinical Assessment of Client Factors and Performance Skills

Key questions to answer during assessment are whether or not the individual possesses adequate sensory and neuromusculoskeletal functions and performance skills to safely drive a vehicle. The clinician needs to evaluate the client's mobility, posture, coordination, strength, effort, energy, and knowledge in relation to the activity demands of driving.

The first criteria to explore is the client's *functional mobility*. Factors to consider are the client's ability to travel to and from the vehicle; whether the client uses an assistive device for mobility, such as a wheelchair, walker, or cane, and whether he or she needs assistance from another person to travel to the vehicle. The Rapid Pace Walk developed as a subset of the Gross Impairment Screen (GRIMPS) is useful as a quickly administered assessment and has been shown to be predictive of driving performance (NHTSA, 2003). Even though the evaluator may be able to assist the client in traveling to and from the evaluation vehicle, the evaluator needs to consider whether or not the driver actually will be able to do this in his or her own environment. Another issue to consider is whether the client can transfer the mobility device in and out of the vehicle independently. If there are unresolved issues regarding mobility outside the vehicle, these will need to be a part of the intervention plan. If the prospective driver cannot get to the vehicle, transfer himself or herself and his or her mobility device in or out, or ambulate in some form to a desired location, then the issue of whether driving is an appropriate goal needs to be assessed. Likewise, the prospective driver who is found capable of returning to independent driving should either have access to a vehicle or have a plan to obtain a vehicle. If a client does not have access to a vehicle or cannot afford to purchase a vehicle, there may be ethical considerations to consider whether it is appropriate to conduct the evaluation in the first place if the client cannot participate in driving for these reasons.

The clinician also needs to evaluate the client's *posture and trunk stability*. In order to efficiently reach the gas, brake, and steering wheel, and to provide a stabile platform from which to operate the equipment, one has to have sufficient posture and trunk stability. If this is an issue, seating options will need to become part of the intervention plan. Many postural deficits can be overcome with the correct seating.

Coordination and strength/effort play a key roll in successful driving. Driving requires the smooth coordination of movements of both the upper and lower extremities, frequently simultaneously. Movements have to be graded for effort. For example, the driver might have to barely "tweak" the wheel to move around a small object in the road, or make a dramatic series of hard turns to avoid another vehicle while maintaining some control of the vehicle's direction so that a safe path can be resumed. The driver may have to steer, brake, turn on the windshield wipers, and glance in the rearview mirror, all at the same time. Ataxic movements, or tremors, such as might be evident in a person with PD or other neurological disease or brain injury, may or may not affect driving skills. When well positioned in the driver's seat, with the hands on the wheel, many drivers are sufficiently supported so that the tremor is not an issue. If the driver has difficulty repositioning his or her hands on the wheel while turning, a spinner knob may solve the problem. If the ataxia or tremor is of sufficient strength to physically cause uncontrolled wheel motion, or increases with purposeful activity, returning to independent driving may be more difficult but can truly be assessed only on the road.

Formal clinical assessments of client factors, such as manual muscle testing and passive range-of-motion measurements of individual joints, may be unnecessary when evaluating most older drivers. However, any functional limitations in active range of motion should be determined. Commonly, the older driver will have limitations in active range of motion in shoulder movements. Because of their potential to interfere with steering ability, any limitations in the range or strength of shoulder joint motions should be examined more closely, especially those movements involving the rotator cuff. In addition, if the individual's shoulder exhibits sufficient impairment to interfere with steering, the function of the opposite upper extremity will need to be examined in more detail to determine if sufficient function exists for the client to steer with adaptations. For example, a client's use of a steering spinner knob will place additional demands on upper extremity strength and range of motion to be able to grasp the knob, move it through the full circumference of the steering wheel, and overcome the additional torque required to turn the wheel because of loss of the other extremity.

Active range of motion for movements of the head and neck also require screening to determine whether arthritis or other degenerative changes have affected the driver's ability to turn his or her head sufficiently to check blind spots during lane changes. This can be especially important when evaluating the driver who has peripheral visual field deficits, as the combination of decreased cervical rotation and decreased peripheral vision can significantly impact the ability to check blind spots. As these conditions frequently occur slowly over time, the driver may not be aware of how limited he or she has become. Drivers with cervical spine issues might benefit from a physical therapy referral to maximize range of motion in the head and neck.

Although clinical measures of reaction time have not been found to be a strong indicator in determining driving ability, reaction-time testing is frequently measured as part of clinical driving evaluations. Devices such as the AAA Brake Reaction Timer are frequently used in clinical settings, although many driving simulators provide some measure of reaction time as well. As a measure of motor skills, reaction-time tests may indicate whether problems exist in the accuracy or speed of movement, but they are not sensitive to the ability to modulate the degree of force being applied to the pedals. Therefore, they may not predict whether the older driver with mild sensory impairment will be prone to abrupt braking or acceleration, or if they may unintentionally "ride" the gas or brake pedal if driving with both feet. In addition, caution should be used in generalizing results in determining the individual's physical ability to operate the pedals of an actual vehicle. Although simulated pedals are used during reaction-time tests, the client's seated position in a clinic chair is frequently much different than the position he or she assumes when sitting in a vehicle. In addition, the degree of offset of the simulated pedals may be significantly different than that encountered in a real-life automobile. For example, reaction-time tests usually require more antigravity movement and more effort from proximal lower-extremity musculature than do actual pedals. The implications may be especially significant in those older drivers with a history of hip fractures or joint replacement because the pattern of movement required to move from one pedal to the other, as well as the effects of gravity, will also be different.

Observation of subjects with slow reaction times reveals that delayed acknowledgement of the stimulus accounts for the majority of the overall response time, and that the actual motor response, once initiated, occurs relatively quickly. This is especially true in cases of dementia—where significant lapses in attention may be observed. These lapses, and any instances of becoming disoriented to the test-taking procedure once testing is underway, should be noted. These often correspond with significant problems in driving during the behind-the-wheel assessment.

Because reaction-time tests fail to simulate fully the demands required to operate vehicle pedals requiring both motor and cognitive skills, these tests do not adequately assess function. However, they are valuable measures as a general indication of speed of response because there are normative data available which allow for comparison of performance. The primary advantage to this test is that the clinician has the opportunity to observe efficiency of foot movement, note whether there is a delay in acknowledgement of the stimulus, and gauge how well the client can follow directions to complete a familiar task. Figure 14-5 summarizes neuromusculoskeletal and sensory factors needing assessment.

The clinician also needs to evaluate whether or not the client has the *energy* required to participate in all aspects of driving. The successful driver has to be capable of tolerating extended periods of physical and mental "work." The driver must be able to ambulate to the vehicle, transfer himself or herself and any devices such as canes or walkers into the vehicle, physically operate the automobile at an acceptable level to reach the desired destination, exit the vehicle, accomplish the desired goal for the trip, return to the vehicle, drive home, and reenter the home. The driver must also be capable of expending the required cognitive energy to accomplish these tasks, without losing focus or, worse, falling asleep.

A successful and safe driver needs a fund of knowledge regarding a number of topics including general knowledge about the vehicle, such as how to open the door, adjust the seat, and turn on the vehicle, and what secondary controls are available. General knowledge of vehicle operation is easily observed during the course of the evaluation, although whether the driver can locate specific secondary controls in a strange vehicle is not nearly as important whether he or she asks during the assessment, "how do I turn

| Occupational Therapy Driving Evaluation | Name: |
| Sensorimotor Assessment | Date: |

SENSORIMOTOR FUNCTION   Dominant Hand ☐ Right   ☐ Left

LEVEL OF FUNCTION RELEVANT TO DRIVING
(Includes Strength, A/PROM, Coordination, Tone & Sensation)

Right UE Function	☐ Sufficient	☐ Marginal	☐ Insufficient
Left UE Function	☐ Sufficient	☐ Marginal	☐ Insufficient
Right LE Function	☐ Sufficient	☐ Marginal	☐ Insufficient
Left LE Function	☐ Sufficient	☐ Marginal	☐ Insufficient
Sitting Balance	☐ Sufficient	☐ Marginal	☐ Insufficient
Head/Neck	☐ Sufficient	☐ Marginal	☐ Insufficient
Ambulation	☐ Independent	☐ Requires Device	☐ Requires W/C
Transfers	☐ Independent	☐ Requires Assistance	
Loading Device	☐ Independent	☐ Requires Assistance	☐ N/A

R	SHOULDER	L
	Flexion	
	Extension	
	Abduction	
	Adduction	
	Horiz. Abduction	
	Horiz. Adduction	
	Int. Rotation	
	Ext. Rotation	
	ELBOW	
	Flexion	
	Extension	
	FOREARM	
	Pronation	
	Supination	
	WRIST	
	Flexion	
	Extension	

AAA BRAKE REACTION TIMER

	RIGHT		LEFT	
	LE	UE	LE	UE
MEAN (sec)				
NORM				
PERCENTILE				
COGNITIVE ERRORS				
PHYSICAL ERRORS				
PRACTICE TRIALS	☐☐☐☐☐		☐☐☐☐☐	

R		L
	1	
	2	
	3	
	4	
	5	
	6	
	7	
	8	
	9	
	10	

ASSESSMENT OF SENSORIMOTOR FUNCTION:

☐ **Compatible With Driving**   ☐ **Marginal For Driving**   ☐ **Compatible With Adapted Driving**

☐ **Marginal For Adapted Driving**   ☐ **Not Suggestive Of Safe Driving Potential**

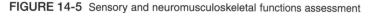

SIGNATURE

FIGURE 14-5 Sensory and neuromusculoskeletal functions assessment

on the wipers" if it begins to rain. In this situation, the evaluator should observe whether the driver fails to address the need to use the wipers entirely, or becomes completely distracted attempting to find the proper switch. Second, the driver must have knowledge of routes to familiar places as well as know how to find information regarding the route to unfamiliar locations. When possible, the evaluation route should

cover some territory familiar to the driver, such as driving from his or her home to the grocery store or church. When this is not possible, trying to replicate the environment may provide some insight into driving ability. For example, if the evaluator is familiar with the town in which the client lives, he or she might select the types of roads that are similar to those the driver would travel at home, for example, mostly residential or four-lane main thoroughfares with lots of stop-and-go traffic and many business entrances and complex intersections. Drivers also must have knowledge of the state motor vehicle laws. Clinically, many evaluators use a Road Signs identification tool to assess knowledge. Even though it would be possible to develop a test of motor vehicle laws, if the evaluator feels that this is a significant issue, he or she should recommend retesting with the Bureau of Motor Vehicles. If the client cannot pass this test, then the decision not to drive is in the hands of the appropriate authority.

Clinical Assessment of Visual Functions

The primary purpose of the vision screening should be to determine the possible presence of visual dysfunction that may have the potential to affect driving ability. It is not diagnostic in nature. At a minimum, distant visual acuity, visual fields, contrast, and oculomotor control should be screened. In her review of visual dysfunction on the ability to drive, Strano (1989) described the objective of an evaluation of visual skills with respect to driving in terms of two distinct tasks: (1) to determine whether vision meets legal visual requirements and (2) to determine what additional problems exist and what effect they may have on driving ability. Baker (2006) provides an extensive review of the visual system and the evaluation and treatment of potential dysfunction relevant to driving.

The ability to renew one's driver's license does not represent proof of adequate vision for safe driving. Most vision screenings are performed by state licensing agencies and are administered by employees who may have little, if any, medical training. Therefore, the screenings may be improperly performed, results may be misinterpreted, and license restrictions may be arbitrarily determined. There is no standardized requirement for visual ability for driving in the United States. Each state sets its own requirements through the Bureau of Motor Vehicles or other licensing agency. Most states require a minimum of 20/40 distance acuity for unrestricted driving, but the cutoff for driving varies greatly, from 20/70 to 20/200 (Pellertio, 2006). The other most frequently used criterion, peripheral visual fields, is equally variable, from no criteria in several states, to 140 degrees

binocularly, which is the more popular minimal standard. Various standards exist as well for monocular vision. The International Council of Ophthalmology (2006) recommends that a measurement of 20/40 distant acuity or better should be the standard for unrestricted driving, and that acuity measurements worse than 20/40 to 20/200 should be individually considered. Peripheral field recommendations state that 120 degrees horizontally and 40 degrees vertically should be the minimum standard, with peripheral fields less than this left to individual consideration.

Visual functions may be assessed using various methods. These visual assessments are summarized in Table 14-7. Eye charts, such as the Snellen "E" chart, traditionally are used to measure distant visual acuity. Although they are commonly thought of as wall charts, their format is also replicated on slides, allowing their use in industrial vision-screening devices. The black-and-white traditional eye chart used in the clinical setting represents a "static" measure of acuity under high-contrast conditions. Because such conditions rarely exist in the driving environment, eye charts are helpful to determine whether visual acuity meets state licensing standards, but they have inherent limitations as functional measures of visual acuity in real-world conditions. The "Tumbling E" chart is a useful supplement to the standard Snellen "E" chart in determining distant visual acuity in subjects who may be illiterate or aphasic. Common industrial vision-screening devices such as the OPTEC (www.stereooptical.com) or Titmus Vision Screener (www.titmus.com) are used in many driver assessment programs. These machines facilitate easy screening of distant visual acuity, color perception, and the oculomotor skills responsible for alignment of the eyes and depth perception. They can also screen peripheral vision in temporal and nasal fields if equipped with optional perimetry modules. Depth perception can be assessed functionally. Color perception screenings are frequently included with many industrial vision-testing devices. On the surface, color perception may appear to be a critical area to driving. Red-green color deficiency is the most common type of "color blindness." The term "red-green" means one color *or* the other has been affected (not both). Therefore, this type of color blindness would not result in the inability to distinguish a

TABLE 14-7 **Visual Skills Assessments**

Assessment	Purpose
Snellen "E" chart	Distant acuity
Tumbling "E" chart	Distant visual acuity for individuals who are aphasic or illiterate
Industrial vision-testing device	Distant acuity, color perception, oculomotor skills, temporal and nasal fields, contrast sensitivity, or sensitivity to glare, color perception, peripheral vision
Laser pointer	Peripheral vision
Pelli-Robson Chart, Functional Acuity Contrast Test (FACT), or LEA Low Contrast Flip Chart	Contrast sensitivity

red light from a green light in a traffic signal. Whatever the method used to assess vision clinically, the evaluator should remember that these tests are given under more or less "optimal" conditions. During the behind-the-wheel assessment, the evaluator should be observant of how the client's vision impacts his or her driving ability. Figure 14-6 summarizes issues relevant to vision screening.

Visual field deficits in upper or lower quadrants can be screened via confrontation testing or by acknowledgment of stimuli presented by a laser pointer. In this latter test, the client fixates on a central target and acknowledges the appearance of stimuli from a laser presentation pointer as shown in Figure 14-7. The clinician may also request a formal exam of visual fields from a physician, using devices such as the Humphreys Visual Field Exam, which is a computerized perimetry exam. Functionally, the evaluator should observe how well the client identifies relevant information in the periphery, including incorporation of cervical rotation to check blind spots while lane changing. Peripheral visual fields may be affected by changes in the physical structure of the face. As one ages, eyelids may become "droopy," known as ptosis. This may occur as part of a neurological disease or simply from loss of weight. Weight loss also may cause the eye to recede into the orbit of the eye slightly, giving a "sunken" appearance to the eyes. When testing is done with a device similar to those used by licensing agencies, even thick or wide eyeglass frames can conceal the tiny light cue in the device.

The clinician can quickly screen smooth pursuits in the clinical setting by observing the subject's ability to pursue a moving object along nine cardinal gaze positions. To screen saccadic movements, the clinician asks the subject to alternately shift his or her gaze between two targets approximately 6 inches apart at a distance of 16 inches from the bridge of the nose. The clinician should observe the smoothness, range, accuracy, and speed of these movements and document potential problems in nondiagnostic terms reflecting the appearance of these movements (Warren, 1993a, 1993b). On the road, the evaluation vehicle should have a small mirror mounted on the dash that can permit the evaluator to observe eye movements of the client, without having to take his or her eyes off the road.

Contrast sensitivity is the measure of the ability of the visual system to distinguish various shades of gray or shades of colors. Most printed material is (more or less) black print on a white background. Visual acuity tests are given using black symbols on a white background with optimal lighting. Functional activity is rarely completed in "optimal" conditions, especially when pertaining to driving. Lighting conditions and the backdrop of what is before the driver change continually. The quality of painted lane markings on the roadway may vary significantly, especially in winter months. Even the color of other vehicles can have some impact on the ability of drivers to see them efficiently. Persons with cataracts, glaucoma, optic neuritis, or other diseases affecting the cornea, lens, or retina of the eye may have increased difficulty with poor lighting conditions, even when they test well for acuity clinically. Contrast sensitivity declines as part of the natural aging process. Contrast sensitivity testing is conducted using a vision chart similar to a Snellen chart with color

Occupational Therapy Driving Evaluation	Name:
Vision Screening	Date:

☐ No Corrective Lenses   ☐ Wears Glasses/Contact Lenses For Driving   ☐ Not In Possession

DISTANT ACUITY

	LEFT	BOTH	RIGHT
20/200	Z N	R O	H K
20/100	R K S	H N C	Z O D
20/70	H C D V	S K Z O	R N D S
20/50	Z R O D	N S C H	V Z K N
20/40	K H S C	O Z N R	D N V C
20/30	O N R Z V	D K H C S	K D S O N
20/20	S D C H N	V R Z K O	H S N R D

20 / _____   BINOCULAR

20 / _____   RIGHT   20 / _____   LEFT

COLOR PERCEPTION

☐ PASS   ☐ FAIL   ____ / 8   (PASS: ≥ 5/8)

A (1 2) B (5) C (2 6) D (6) E (1 6) F (XX)

FUSION

☐ PASS   ☐ FAIL

☐ 3 Cubes   ☐ 4 Cubes   ☐ 2 Cubes   Suppressed ___ Image

LATERAL PHORIA

☐ PASS   ☐ FAIL

Esophoria 1 2 3 | 4 5 6 7 **8** 9 10 11 12 | 13 14 15 Exophoria

VERTICAL PHORIA

☐ PASS   ☐ FAIL

Left Hyperphoria   1 2 | 3 **4** 5 | 6 7   Right Hyperphoria

STEREOPSIS

☐ PASS   ☐ FAIL   _____ Angle Stereopsis (deg)

				400	200	100	70	50	40	30	25	20	A. S.
				1	2	3	4	5	6	7	8	9	
				B	L	B	T	T	L	R	L	R	

FUNCTIONAL DEPTH

☐ PASS   ☐ FAIL   _____ mm discrepancy aligning objects at 7 Feet

PERIPHERAL VISION

		NASAL		TEMPORAL	
		35°	55°	70°	85°
RIGHT EYE	Acknowledged	☐	☐	☐	☐
	Failed To Acknowledge	☐	☐	☐	☐
LEFT EYE	Acknowledged	☐	☐	☐	☐
	Failed To Acknowledge	☐	☐	☐	☐

TEMPORAL NASAL   NASAL TEMPORAL

LEFT EYE   RIGHT EYE

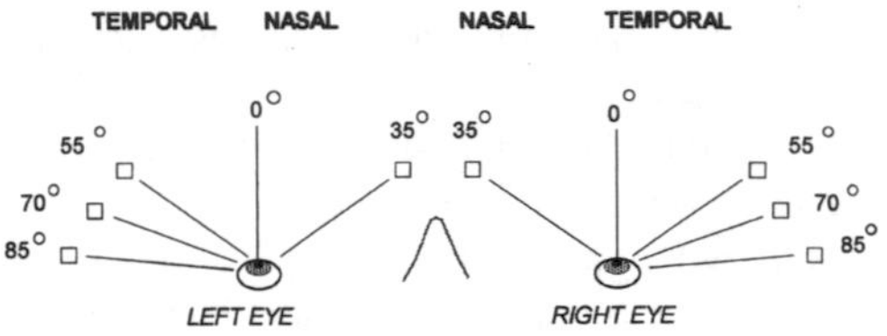

OCULOMOTOR SKILLS   *Observation Of Eye Movements Requiring These Skills Suggests...*

PURSUITS

☐ No Problems Apparent   ☐ Appeared Irregular/Slow   ☐ Loses Fixation   ☐ Asymmetry   ☐ Difficulty Crossing Midline

SACCADES

☐ No Problems Apparent   ☐ Inaccurate/Overshoots   ☐ Decreased Speed   ☐ Asymmetry   ☐ Difficulty Crossing Midline

NYSTAGMUS

☐ Not Apparent   ☐ May Be Present With Lateral Gaze   ☐ May Be Present During Pursuits   ☐ May Be Present At Midline

DIPLOPIA

☐ No Complaint Noted   ☐ Reported During Testing   ☐ Reported Under Specific Conditions   ☐ Reported H/O Diplopia

ASSESSMENT OF VISUAL FUNCTION:

☐ **Compatible With Driving**   ☐ **Marginal For Driving**   ☐ **Not Suggestive Of Safe Driving Potential**

SIGNATURE

FIGURE 14-6 Vision screening

of the text in decreasing shades of gray or with images of sine waves that look like a series of stripes or bars that slant in different directions and become increasingly faint. The Pelli-Robson Chart employs the letter chart with same-size letters but decreasing contrast levels from top to bottom and right to left (Pelli, Robson, & Wilkins, 1988). The chart was designed to test middle to low spatial frequencies and determines the contrast required to read large letters. Another method of testing contrast sensitivity is the Functional Acuity Contrast Test (FACT). The FACT chart, developed by Arthur Ginsburg, tests five spatial frequencies

Occupational Therapy Driving Evaluation	Name:
Visual Field Screening	Date:

NOTE: Screenings are performed to determine the possible presence of visual field dysfunction with potential to affect driving ability.   Findings are not intended to be diagnostic in nature.

OPTEC 2000 VISION TESTER

Ability To Identify Pinhole-Sized Flashing Lights. Similar To The Screening Used By The Bureau of Motor Vehicles

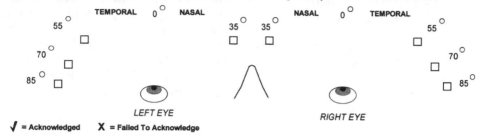

√ = Acknowledged   X = Failed To Acknowledge

LASER POINTER STIMULI

(Size Of Room Limits Presentation Of Stimuli To A Maximum Of Approximately 70 Degrees Laterally To Either Side.)

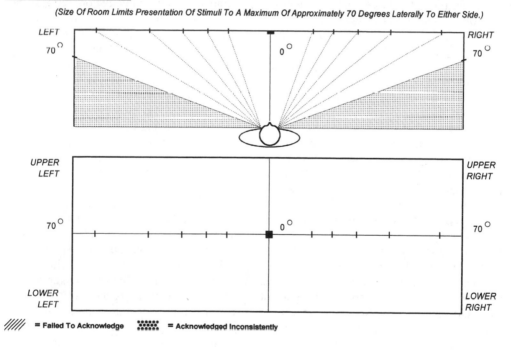

///// = Failed To Acknowledge   ⠿ = Acknowledged Inconsistently

SIGNATURE

FIGURE 14-7 Visual field screening

(sizes) and nine levels of contrast. Additional options may be available to screen contrast sensitivity or glare sensitivity. Because these devices often are used by state licensing agencies, they also may indicate whether the person will be able to renew his or her license. Due to the design of these devices, it is difficult or impossible to assess depth perception and contrast when the client has monocular or bi-ocular vision. There are various handheld charts that can address contrast, such as the LEA Low Contrast Flip Chart. There are presently no standardized limitations for driving with reduced contrast, but the evaluator should discuss limitations in contrast with the client, and the relevance to driving. Reductions in contrast sensitivity can be a symptom of eye diseases, such as cataracts and glaucoma. Sometimes the client may be unaware of these conditions, so the clinician should refer the client to his or her eye specialist for follow up.

Clinical Assessment of Client Factors and Performance Skills

The objective of the cognitive-perceptual screenings is to determine the potential presence of dysfunction in mental functions, such as attention and memory or processing skills that may potentially affect driving ability. Although there are multiple ways of assessing for potential dysfunction in processing skills that are necessary for driving, no single test or combination of tests can predict with certainty whether the degree of dysfunction measured will adversely affect driving ability. Unless test results indicate a severe degree of dysfunction, any concerns identified during the process skills screening should either be confirmed or ruled out during a behind-the-wheel assessment. In addition, results from processing skill screenings are used to determine whether significant errors committed behind the wheel are consistent with clinically noted concerns and whether these errors are amenable to treatment. Figure 14-8 shows cognitive/perceptual factors to be assessed in the driving evaluation process.

The specific tests constituting the mental functions and process skills component of clinical driving assessment vary from program to program but typically include assessments from three general categories: psychometric tests, driving simulators, and a separate category of "functional" assessments. No single category of assessment has been proven to be the most predictive of driving ability, and each has limitations with respect to both driving ability and use with the older population, in particular.

Frequently, assessments may be selected from more than one category. Several factors can influence which tests may be selected, including clinical space, financial resources, one's professional training, and the length of time needed to complete the evaluation. A battery of tests should be diverse enough to assess as many cognitive-perceptual skill areas as possible. However, no screening will be perfect.

One must understand both the strengths and limitations of the particular mental functions and process skills assessments and account for any identified dysfunction during the behind-the-wheel assessment.

Psychometric Tests

Psychometric tests have been found in various combinations to correlate with driving ability. In some settings, only psychologists or neuropsychologists can administer psychometric tests. Driver rehabilitation specialists should consult the psychologists or neuropsychologists in their facility before administering any psychometric test. If there is no objection to the use of a given test, the psychologist or neuropsychologist may wish to ensure that the test is administered in the standardized manner, or may permit its use only with supervision. Although it may be possible to arrange for a psychologist or neuropsychologist to administer these tests as part of every clinical driving evaluation, it is not practical to do this in many settings. It may be more efficient to investigate other means of measuring cognitive-perceptual skills. It should be noted that even with the extensive use of psychometric tests, the occupational therapist or driving rehabilitation specialist is using them only as screening tools. Any indications of cognitive deficits should be reported to the referring physician, or a referral made for follow-up with an appropriate medical doctor.

As with other types of assessments, psychometric batteries should not be used as the sole determinant of an older person's driving ability. In fact, psychometric tests may be of less value when determining the driving potential of older drivers than that of younger populations. One factor that limits the utility of many psychometric tests concerns the quality of normative data with respect to older age groups. Some of these tests may provide norms in 10-year increments for persons younger than 65 years, but for those aged 65 and older, the tests categorize subjects as a single group. Age-specific norms for those older than age 79 are uncommon. Therefore, the performance of the older driver who is 80 years old may be compared against a normative sample including subjects as much as 15 years younger. Although comparison of a test score with these norms may provide an indication of whether a score is within normal limits, it may be difficult to determine

Occupational Therapy Driving Evaluation

Cognitive/Perceptual Assessment

Name:

Date:

Road Sign Recognition:

	Correct	Partially Correct	Incorrect		Correct	Partially Correct	Incorrect
SCORE: [ ] Stop	☐	☐	☐	Merge (From Right)	☐	☐	☐
Yield	☐	☐	☐	School Crossing	☐	☐	☐
No Right Turn	☐	☐	☐	Slippery When Wet	☐	☐	☐
Do Not Enter	☐	☐	☐	Down Grade	☐	☐	☐
Divided Highway Begins	☐	☐	☐	Traffic Signal Ahead	☐	☐	☐

Motor-Free Visual Perception Test:

RAW SCORE: [ ] /36

PROCESSING TIME: [ ] Sec.

Age	Norm	SD	+/- 1 SD	- 2 SD
__ 18-49	35/36	(1)	(34-36)	(33)
__ 50-69	34/36	(2)	(32-36)	(28)
__ 70-79	30/36	(5)	(25-35)	(20)
__ 18-49	3.2 sec	(0.8 s)	(2.5-4.0 s)	(4.8 s)
__ 50-69	4.2 sec	(1.2 s)	(3.0-5.4 s)	(6.6 s)
__ 70-79	5.8 sec	(1.3 s)	(4.5-7.1 s)	(8.4 s)

_____

_____

_____

Driving Advisement System:

	Error %	Time	S. D.	Right	Left	-3.0	-2.5	-2.0	-1.5	-1.0	-0.5	Median	+0.5	+1.0
BRAKE:	[ ]	[ ]	[ ]	[ ]	[ ]	.97	.89	.81	.75	.67	.59	**.51**	.43	.35
DECIDE:	[ ]	[ ]	[ ]	[ ]	[ ]	1.22	1.14	1.06	.98	.90	.82	**.74**	.62	.58
INHIBIT:	[ ]	[ ]	[ ]	[ ]	[ ]	2.08	1.90	1.73	1.55	1.38	1.20	**1.03**	.86	.68

_____

_____

_____

Other:

☐ **Symbol Digit Modalities**

Score	Norm	S. D.
[ ]	[ ]	[ ]

☐ **Trail Making A & B**

	Score	Norm	Percentile		Score	Norm	Percentile
A	[ ]	[ ]	[ ]	**B**	[ ]	[ ]	[ ]

Visual Inattention / Spatial Neglect:

☐ Not Apparent   ☐ Possible--Inconsistent Findings   ☐ Probable--Findings On Multiple Screenings

_____

_____

_____

ASSESSMENT OF COGNITIVE/PERCEPTUAL FUNCTION:

☐ **Compatible With Driving**   ☐ **Marginal For Driving**   ☐ **Not Suggestive Of Safe Driving Potential**

_____

SIGNATURE

FIGURE 14-8 Cognitive/perceptual assessment

whether the value obtained from performance of the test is above average or below average, especially when the subject is of advanced age. For example, Strano (1991) studied the relationship between the Motor-Free Visual Perceptual Test (MVPT) scores and behind-the-wheel evaluation performance for 153 subjects who were diagnosed with brain injury, stroke, or cerebral palsy. In the 18 to 49 year age group and the 50 to 69 year age group, all subjects with MVPT raw scores within normal limits passed a behind-the-wheel evaluation. In the 70 to 79 year age group, however, only half those subjects having raw scores within normal limits passed the behind-the-wheel evaluation.

Other psychometric tests commonly used in driver rehabilitation settings and found to correlate with some measure of behind-the-wheel performance include the Useful Field of View Visual Analyzer, Uttl Letter Cancellation Test, Trailmaking Test, Parts A and B from the Halstead-Reitan Battery (Gouvier et al., 1989), the Symbol Digit Modalities Test (Sivak, Olson, Kewman, Won, & Henson, 1981), and the Picture Completion subtest from the Wechsler Adult Intelligence Scale (Gouvier et al., 1989; Sivak et al., 1984). The Physician's Guide to Assessing and Counseling Older Drivers (Wang et al., 2003), developed by the American Medical Association and the National Highway Transportation Safety Administration, recommend the use of the Fruend Clock Drawing Test and Trails Making Part B. Both assessments have shown some clinical correlation to driving performance. The MVPT is a frequent component of the clinical driving assessment and has shown some correlation to on-the-road performance. This screening tool assesses one's ability to interpret spatial relationships, visual discrimination, figure-ground, visual closure, and visual memory.

Functional Measures. Road sign recognition tests, the DAS, and the elemental driving simulator (EDS) are commonly used in combination with psychometric tests. As discussed previously, the UFOV is a functional description of visual field. A computer-based test by the same name provides a quick assessment of central vision and processing speed, selective and divided attention, and has been shown to be a significant indicator of increased crash risk.

Road Sign Recognition Tests. Screenings of road sign recognition represent one functional method of assessing potential deterioration of process skills related to driving that may have some value in predicting driving safety. Multiple studies have noted a correlation between various screenings of road sign recognition and road test performance (Hunt et al., 1993; Odenheimer et al., 1994). If the client cannot recall the correct name of the sign, the evaluator should permit the client to describe what a particular sign requires the driver to do. Many older drivers who have difficulty correctly identifying road signs in the clinic react to the same ones appropriately on the road. As these are separate cognitive functions, recalling the name of an object versus responding correctly to a particular navigational marker in a functional situation, the evaluator must consider this information when making his or her final assessment.

Driving Advisement System and Elemental Driving Simulator. The DAS (Gianutsos, Campbell, Beattie, & Mandriota, 1992) and EDS (Gianutsos, 1994) are two computer-based tasks that may play a meaningful role in a screening of mental functions and process skills needed for driving. These tests use simulated pedals, a steering wheel, and turn signal stalk to respond to events on a computer screen. Although they may be described as driving simulators, the tasks performed embody assessment concepts resembling those of neuropsychological tests used to measure various cognitive-perceptual skills. They may be more a simulation of psychometric tests of skills necessary for driving than a simulation of actual driving. These assessments place significant demands on selective, alternating, and divided attention skills, as well as visual attention skills. They are particularly beneficial in assessing executive-level functions, especially with regard to self-appraisal, mental flexibility, self-regulation, and impulse inhibition. These standardized assessments compare the subject's performance against norms, although they are not age specific. Their relationship to driving performance and other cognitive-perceptual driving tests have been validated to some degree through research (although most of the research published has been authored by one of the developers of these tests).

Driver Performance Test. The Driver Performance Test (Weaver, 1990) consists of a series of 40 videotaped driving scenes. Scores are obtained on five scales of driving performance, which reflect processing skills: scan, identify, predict, decide, and execute. After viewing each scene, the subject is required to answer a question about the scene. Using a multiple-choice format, the subject must select the most appropriate of four possible responses. The DPT has been identified as having significant value in one major study of psychometric tests as a predictor of driving performance (Sivak et al., 1984) and was found to correlate with the severity of dementia in another study (Rebok et al., 1994). The nonstop videotape format of the test and the rapid presentation of multiple-choice answers on the monitor place significant demands on language-processing abilities, which can adversely affect the performance of older drivers for reasons that are unrelated to driving. For example, if a driver has poor reading skills, he or she may have difficulty answering the questions because the DPT requires the driver to respond quickly. In addition, a driver with a small degree of receptive aphasia may struggle with the DPT but may be able to safely operate a motor vehicle.

Driving Simulators. There are a variety of devices marketed for use in clinical settings that are referred to as "driving simulators." If these devices truly simulated the task of driving, it would be possible to determine driving ability based entirely on clinical evaluation. The additional expense and risks associated with a behind-the-wheel assessment would become unnecessary. In fact, many facilities have purchased simulators and marketed themselves as providing "driver assessment" services based on these assumptions. In reality, however, none of the present-day driving simulators provide realistic, interactive simulation of on-road driving that can measure all of the skill involved in driving. Therefore, although simulators may provide useful information as part of a comprehensive evaluation, they should not be used as the sole determinant of an older person's driving ability. The health care professional who assumes responsibility for assessing the skills of the older driver should understand the potential benefits and inherent limitations of today's "driving simulators" in determining what role they may play in their particular setting.

For purposes of analysis, commonly used driving simulators can be divided into two types: the traditional driving simulators and the computer-based driving simulations. Most simulators consist of a module containing a driver's seat, a dashboard with instruments, a steering wheel, a turn signal, pedals, and other secondary controls. Simulators also can be equipped with common adapted-driving aids, such as a left-foot gas pedal, steering devices, or hand controls. The subject watches a film projected on a screen and responds to the information presented by moving the primary and secondary controls.

Clients tested in traditional driving simulators view a film from the perspective of the driver's seat in a moving vehicle. Although data from the steering wheel, pedals, turn signal stalk, or speedometer may be obtained and matched to the events on the film, the film is not influenced by the input provided by operating the controls. For example, turning the steering wheel has no effect on path of travel, and operation of the pedals will not have an effect on acceleration, speed, or braking as depicted in the film. The only mechanism of instantaneous feedback may be the speedometer reading or turn-signal indicator lights.

Traditional driving simulators may have value in assessing the ability to respond in emergency situations, which is often difficult to determine during a behind-the-wheel assessment. They may be of particular benefit in testing older drivers who must learn how to use adapted equipment to compensate for lower-extremity dysfunction by providing opportunities for repetition in a safe environment. In addition, traditional simulators may be of some benefit in teaching defensive driving strategies, although this is not a main function of many medically oriented driver rehabilitation programs.

Many older drivers have difficulty generalizing their skills from the context of driving on public roads to the context of the simulation environment. It is common for experienced drivers to complain that the simulator did not provide them with a true driving experience and to state their performance was not an accurate reflection of their driving skills. Several studies have examined the value of driving simulators in assessing the abilities of experienced drivers with neurological dysfunction. Some studies focus primarily on prediction of behind-the-wheel performance, but most also consider their relationship to other psychometric assessments that are commonly used (Cimolino & Balkovec, 1988; Galski, Bruno, & Ehle, 1993; Gouvier et al., 1989; Monga, Osterman, & Kerrigan, 1997; Nouri & Tinson, 1988; Quigly & DeLisa, 1983). Although the degree to which they predicted behind-the-wheel performance ranged from being an important part of a more comprehensive assessment to having almost no value at all, none of the studies advocated that simulation be used as a sole determinant of driving ability. Those studies that included an analysis of their predictive value versus that of psychometric tests varied and are at best inconclusive (Galski et al., 1992; Galski et al., 1993; Gouvier et al., 1989).

Although traditional driving simulators provide a driving environment that appears realistic but lacks much of the dynamic interaction between the driver, controls, and environment, computer-based driving simulators may be able to simulate the interactive aspects of driving required to control movement of a vehicle in a dynamic environment. Computer-based simulations, such as the STISIM Drive Simulation (www.systemstech.com), use a format similar to driving video games designed for entertainment. They simulate the visuospatial and perceptual motor demands required for a driver to control a moving vehicle and provide the simultaneous feedback necessary to affect the driver's actions. Present-day examples that are commercially available have greatly improved their ability to depict a realistic driving environment of sufficient complexity to simulate the demands normal driving places on scanning, interacting with traffic, and identifying hazards. First-time users of driving simulators are often instructed that it may take some practice to "get the feel" of the steering and so forth, and that some people experience nausea during the "driving" session. These factors must be considered when contemplating the use of a driving simulator.

Technological advances in computer graphics, artificial intelligence, and virtual reality, coupled with faster computers, have led to the development of more sophisticated driving simulators. However, use of these sophisticated simulators has been limited to research settings, and their cost would be prohibitive for most clinical health care settings.

In summation, driving simulators may provide useful information as part of a comprehensive evaluation. Traditional driving simulators provide a driving environment that appears realistic, but they lack the dynamic interaction between the driver and environment. Conversely, computer-based driving simulators allow for this dynamic interaction, but they lack sufficient realism and complexity necessary to assess many skills. Both types require the older person to generalize his or her driving skills to a simulation environment, which is imperfect in its ability to replicate the normal driving experience. Until state-of-the-art technology becomes sufficiently affordable to allow for the development of a cost-effective simulator that can evaluate all of the necessary skills in a realistic context, driving simulators should not be used as the sole determinant of an older person's driving ability.

Another factor to consider is that many elderly drivers are not familiar or comfortable with "computers." If, at the end of the evaluation, the recommendation is that the client discontinue driving, the best result would be that the client is able to accept and abide by the recommendation without the need to inform the state bureau of motor vehicles. Reaching a conclusion of driving cessation based on "some computer gizmo," or by looking at pictures and completing pencil-and-paper tests, may be difficult for the driver to accept, especially for a driver who has successfully operated a motor vehicle for 50, 60, or 70 years.

On-the-Road Assessment of Cognition

As discussed elsewhere in this chapter, the cognitive requirements for successful driving are among the most high-level cognitive skills we employ. Routine driving for the experienced driver is an "automatic" function, with little conscious thought given to the details for safe operation of the vehicle. It is so automatic that drivers routinely (though not necessarily wisely) talk on the cell phone, eat, read, carry on conversations with other passengers, daydream, and sing while negotiating complex, continually changing environmental conditions. The experienced driver in his or her fifties and sixties may notice some physical and or visual changes in function which have an impact on driving but are able to compensate for these due to his or her extensive driving experience. For example the 55-year-old executive who has some arthritic changes in his right leg may keep a greater distance between himself and the next vehicle, because he realizes it takes slightly longer to react and brake for sudden stops. The older driver may report limiting driving at night, to familiar places, or accepting rides from others when possible. Unfortunately, when cognition becomes an issue of driving performance, frequently decreased insight into actual functional performance is common. Adult children of elderly drivers report forgetfulness, unexplained dents and scrapes on their parent's vehicle, and forgetting to turn off the stove or lock the house. The parent vehemently denies these reports or tries to dismiss them as unimportant. Persons with memory deficits, almost by definition, do not remember what it is they are forgetting. Drivers with cognitive deficits may not notice or recall near misses, difficulty maintaining lane position, or difficulty interpreting navigational signs.

Behind-the-Wheel Assessment

Even if it were possible to formally test every skill area using specialized assessments having the highest degree of predictability of driving, the validity of any clinical assessment of driving potential would still be limited because of the complexity of the driving tasks, interdependence of skill areas, and personal variations in baseline driving skills. With the exception of those instances in which a severe degree of dysfunction has been identified on clinical testing, a behind-the-wheel assessment will almost always be necessary to determine the actual ability to operate a motor vehicle and whether the effects of any clinically noted dysfunction may be amenable to treatment.

Frequently, only one evaluator conducts the entire driving evaluation. However, some programs use a licensed driving instructor for the behind-the-wheel component. Ideally, the evaluator should be present during the behind-the-wheel assessment, even if riding in the back seat. Although published research provides valuable information regarding the relationship of clinical assessments to driving performance, an evaluator will not have a full appreciation of this relationship until he or she has sufficient behind-the-wheel experience to be able to associate specific problems identified during the clinical assessment with specific errors in behind-the-wheel performance.

Behind-the-wheel assessments (Figure 14-9) should be performed in a sedan that has been modified with equipment allowing the evaluator to monitor surrounding traffic and intervene if necessary. At a minimum, this equipment should include a trainer brake and an evaluator rearview mirror mounted on the windshield on the passenger side of the vehicle. Most evaluation sedans allow evaluators to physically intervene only at the trainer brake or by reaching over to turn the standard steering wheel. An electronic turn-signal switch, if installed, can be oriented toward the evaluator when not in use by the client. Assessment sedans may be customized to enable operation of the accelerator or to include a passenger-side steering wheel, although sedans having these modifications are comparatively rare.

The assessment sedan should contain basic items frequently needed to accommodate drivers of different size and stature, in order to provide the most comfortable "fit" between driver and vehicle. In vehicles having seats that do not allow a significant amount of adjustment, seat cushions may need to be provided to allow shorter drivers to attain an appropriate line of sight or access to vehicle pedals. Pedal extenders may be temporarily installed to further accommodate the shorter driver. In addition, a device may be needed to reposition the shoulder belt for a proper fit. Such devices can be found in most stores that sell automotive accessories.

In most cases, the same driving route should be used for each behind-the-wheel assessment. This enables the evaluator to provide instructions in a consistent manner, minimizes the possibility of a particular skill being overlooked, and allows the evaluator to compare the performance of one client to that of previous clients who have encountered the same situations. The route should be representative of normal driving conditions, include all routinely performed driving tasks, and it should take at least 45 to 60 minutes to complete. Over the course of the route, traffic congestion, maximum speed, and overall complexity of the driving environment should gradually increase. Atypical situations that may be confusing to any driver during the initial encounter should be excluded from the route. The route also must be sufficiently flexible to provide "escape routes" for those drivers who experience problems in less-complex environments or to eliminate

text continues on page 370

Occupational Therapy Driving Evaluation

Name:

Behind-The-Wheel Evaluation

Date:

AREA COVERED	☐ Residential	☐ Urban	☐ Expressway	MILES DRIVEN: _____	MODIFICATIONS:	☐ None	☐ Electronic Turn Signal Switch
TRAFFIC	☐ Light	☐ Moderate	☐ Heavy			☐ Steering Device	Knob Single-Pin V-Grip
WEATHER	☐ Clear	☐ Rain / Snow	☐ Overcast / Fog			☐ Hand Controls	Twist/Push Right Angle Pull
ROAD CONDITIONS	☐ Dry	☐ Wet	☐ Snow / Ice			☐ Left Side Accelerator ☐ Seat Cushion	

		Low-Risk / Technical	Moderate-Risk	High-Risk
USE OF CONTROLS/				
ADAPTATIONS	Improper Operation Of Controls	_____	_____	_____
	Used Turn Signal Early / Late	_____	_____	_____
	Failed To Use Turn Signal	_____	_____	_____
	Abrupt Acceleration / Braking	_____	_____	_____
LIMIT LINE /	Insufficient Braking	_____	_____	_____
STOPPING	Rolled Beyond Stop Sign/Line	_____	_____	_____
	Excessively Slow Proceeding From Stop	_____	_____	_____
	Failed To Attain Clear View For Possible Traffic	_____	_____	_____
OBSERVATION/	Flashing School Zone	_____	_____	_____
JUDGMENT	Essential Road Sign	_____	_____	_____
Failed To Identify /	Long-Standing Caution Light	_____	_____	_____
Acknowledge...	Change In Status Of Traffic Light	_____	_____	_____
	Stop Sign/Traffic Light	_____	_____	_____
	Navigation Landmark Or Sign	_____	_____	_____
	Sign Or Markings Needed To Identify Lane	_____	_____	_____
	Failed To Attain Clear View For Possible Traffic	_____	_____	_____
GAP ACCEPTANCE	Rejected Safe Gap In Traffic	_____	_____	_____
	Maintained Unsafe Fwd Distance	_____	_____	_____
	Accepted Marginal Gap	_____	_____	_____
	Attempted To Accept Unsafe Gap	_____	_____	_____
Lane Changing/	Omitted Signal	_____	_____	_____
Merging	Delayed Activating Turn Signal	_____	_____	_____
	Rejected Safe Opportunity To Change-Lanes	_____	_____	_____
	Failed To Check Appropriate Mirror	_____	_____	_____
	Failed To Turn Head To Check Blind Spot	_____	_____	_____
	Slowed Excessively/Veered	_____	_____	_____
	Accepted Marginal Gap	_____	_____	_____
	Attempted To Accept Unsafe Gap	_____	_____	_____
SPEED	Over Posted Limit > 5 MPH	_____	_____	_____
	Under Posted Limit > 5 MPH	_____	_____	_____
	Over/Under Posted Limit (>10-15 MPH)	_____	_____	_____
	Slowed Excessively In A Manner Difficult To Predict	_____	_____	_____
	Fast Turn (>10-15 MPH)	_____	_____	_____
	Inadequate Acceleration Exiting Turn	_____	_____	_____
PATH OF TRAVEL	Excessively Wide/Sharp Turn	_____	_____	_____
	Failed To Turn Into Proper Lane	_____	_____	_____
	Failed To Turn From Proper Lane	_____	_____	_____
	Straddled Unmarked Lane	_____	_____	_____
	On / Over Lane Dividing Line To Right	_____	_____	_____
	On / Over Lane Dividing Line To Left	_____	_____	_____
	Tire Briefly On Center Line	_____	_____	_____
	Over Center Line	_____	_____	_____
	Erratic Path Of Travel Within Lane	_____	_____	_____
	Off-Road/Made Contact With Curb	_____	_____	_____
MANEUVERABILITY/PARKING		_____	_____	_____
	TOTALS	[ ]	[ ]	[ ]

_____

SIGNATURE

FIGURE 14-9 Behind-the-wheel assessment

Occupational Therapy Driving Evaluation	Name:
Behind-The-Wheel Evaluation	Date:

Comments:

_____
_____
_____

Assessment:

_____
_____
_____
_____
_____
_____
_____

Goals:

_____
_____
_____
_____
_____
_____
_____
_____
_____

Plan:

_____
_____
_____
_____

_____

SIGNATURE

FIGURE 14-9 (continued)

conditions that the driver reports he or she normally avoids, such as expressway driving.

Errors in performance are recorded on a worksheet in either checklist or narrative format. The criteria for scoring behind-the-wheel assessments vary greatly among programs, and there is no standardized format used by a significant number of programs. However, information should be collected in a manner that allows for analysis of performance in terms of the driver's frequency of errors, the severity of errors, the ability to self-correct errors, as well as any strengths observed in the individual's performance.

Although cueing should be provided after initial instances of a particular error, the degree of subsequent cueing should be limited during an initial behind-the-wheel assessment. Even if a driver demonstrates a minor deficiency in technical driving skills, such as a minor infraction of a motor vehicle law, the repeated occurrence of a technical error despite feedback may raise concerns about executive-level skills used to anticipate circumstances and self-regulate the performance of automatic-level driving behaviors that are inappropriate under the circumstances. An inability to benefit from initial feedback may also suggest a poor prognosis; that is, the older driver may not benefit from additional therapeutic intervention.

Based on this information and data obtained during the clinical assessment, the evaluating therapist provides recommendations, which are reviewed with the older driver and forwarded to the referring physician for approval. Typical recommendations given may include the following:

- *Resume Independent Driving of Passenger Vehicles.* This recommendation is made when clinical testing and demonstrated behind-the-wheel performance yield no concerns regarding a driver's risk.
- *Participate in Additional Driver Rehabilitation Treatment Sessions.* If errors are potentially correctable, or when adapted equipment is used, treatment may be recommended and typically takes place behind the wheel. Specific goals should be set indicating successful performance outcomes, and the prognosis of attainment of low-risk driving should be determined before treatment begins.

- *Refrain From Driving Under Any Circumstances.* This recommendation is made when the driver demonstrates severe physical, cognitive-perceptual, or visual dysfunction; a high degree of risk when behind the wheel; and little or no potential to correct or compensate for the identified problems.
- *Other Recommendations.* These may include periodic reevaluations for drivers with marginally adequate performance or with a progressive condition.

Adapted Driving

The evaluation sedan also should accommodate equipment for those with common physical disabilities, if necessary—and this adapted equipment should be removed or installed easily. Although the fabrication of special brackets and other custom modifications by the vendor will result in additional costs, the ability to eliminate the vehicle's adapted equipment, so that outcomes of behind-the-wheel assessments are not compromised, is worth the expense.

Steering spinner devices and electronic turn-signal switches can be used to compensate for loss of function in one or both upper extremities. Left-foot accelerator pedals can compensate for loss of right lower-extremity function, and hand controls can enable driving using only the upper extremities. Adapted mirrors can be used to monitor blind spots or areas adjacent to the vehicle to compensate for limitations in cervical range of motion (Figure 14-10). Most of this equipment's design appears to be fairly simplistic. However, learning to use this equipment safely and proficiently is much more complex than the equipment's appearance might suggest. An experienced driver using adapted equipment for the first time is no longer performing a largely automatic task. Rather, the driver is performing a task that requires a greater degree of executive-level processing, places significantly greater demands on divided attention, and requires frequent inhibition of automatic-level responses that are no longer appropriate.

Although using adaptive equipment for driving should eventually become as automatic as normal driving, it is not unusual for these demands initially to lead to errors in equipment use or breakdowns in the performance of previously learned driving skills. Because the consequences of such breakdowns may have extremely serious implications, adapted equipment should

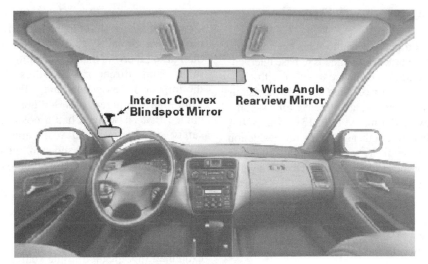

FIGURE 14-10 Mirrors within the driving sedan

never be recommended based solely on clinical evaluation results. Furthermore, when adaptations are necessary for a client to operate primary vehicle controls, evaluators should supervise the learning program and environment. Many states require some form of approval for the use of adaptive equipment, such as a restriction placed on the drivers' license, just as one might have a restriction for wearing corrective lenses. The clinician should be familiar with the state requirements and process for obtaining this approval and provide the client with this information. Many programs guide the client through the process, facilitating where necessary, even providing the use of the adapted vehicle for testing with the state licensing agency. Some states require that the driver with a medical condition that may potentially affect driving performance inform the state licensing agency of this condition.

If adaptive equipment is recommended for a client and he or she has demonstrated the ability to successfully transition to adaptive driving, the client usually will require some information regarding the purchase and installation of equipment for his or her vehicle. Most cities will have a garage or dealership that specializes in selling and installing adaptive equipment, and resources can be found online. Automobile dealers, although they may not do the work, often know of businesses that can perform this service. There are some businesses that may sell and install the adaptive equipment, without ensuring that the buyer has or

will receive sufficient training. This practice at the least is a disservice to the buyer and, given the potential for injury, would seem to be an unethical practice, which should be a red flag to the buyer to avoid such a business operator. Most adaptive equipment dealers require the potential purchaser to provide evidence of training with the equipment prior to installation. The clinician should provide the client with the exact type and brand of device required and discuss this with the installer. Although some devices are similar, brand-to-brand, offering a device significantly different from the style used in training can have a negative impact on performance.

Unfortunately, there are not many options for financial assistance for the purchase of adaptations. Adaptations may cost a few hundred dollars or well over a thousand dollars or more, depending on the type and sophistication of the device. The Bureau of Worker's Compensation and the Bureau of Vocational Rehabilitation Services, or similar organizations, may provide funding on a case-by-case basis for those who may be able to return to work or school. The major vehicle manufacturers provide a rebate for the purchase of adaptive equipment based on medical necessity for the purchase of a new vehicle. Some organizations such as the Multiple Sclerosis Society may provide some assistance, but this is likely to be a local practice, which varies by city or region. No insurance companies assist with the purchase of adaptive equipment, even though it is a medical necessity.

Evidence-Based Practice

In today's competitive health care environment, the health care practitioner needs to base intervention using "research evidence together with clinical knowledge and reasoning to make decisions about interventions that are effective for a specific client" (Law & Baum, 1998, p. 131). The AOTA has published in-depth guidelines for evaluation and intervention of driving. Within this guideline is a review of the evidence relevant to driving and the older adult. Level I, II, and III studies focused on six different intervention approaches:

1. Skills-based intervention
2. Education
3. Modification to the vehicle
4. Infrastructure design
5. Policy
6. Community mobility programs (Stav, Hunt, & Arbesman, 2006)

Studies focusing on skills-based intervention looked at visual training, psychomotor ability such as response time and anticipation time, and range-of-motion home exercise training (Stav et al., 2006). In general, UFOV intervention using a computerized visual attention analyzer seems to be more effective in improving performance on either a behind-the-wheel assessment or speed of processing outcome measure than traditional visuoperceptual treatment or driving simulator training as applied to clients who were poststroke, particularly those with right-sided lesions (Mazer et al., 2003; Roenker, Cissell, Ball, Wadley, & Edwards, 2003). In addition, after 18 months, the effect of the UFOV persisted but the effect of the simulator training did not (Roenker et al., 2003). Another study (Klavora et al., 1995) examined older adults poststroke who had impaired visual attention, using a Dynavision apparatus and behind-the-wheel driving test as the outcome measure. Six of the 10 participants earned a rating of safe to resume driving or to receive driving lessons. Finally, another study determined that older adults who participated in the exercise program to improve head and neck flexibility were more likely to have improved on handling position and observing while driving (Ostrow, Shafron, & McPherson, 1992).

Education-based studies concentrated on the use of auditory navigational systems or the influence of the presence of passengers on driving safety (Stav et al., 2006). Llaneras, Swezey,

Brock, Rogers, and Van Cott (1998) found that clients using the Simulated Prescriptive Auditory Navigational System (SPANS) made fewer navigational errors than those using paper-based maps and directions. Studies looking at the impact of passengers and safety are mixed. Vollrath, Meilinger, and Krüger (2002) concluded that passengers had a positive effect on safety when drivers 50 years and older were driving at night, in slow and standing traffic, and at crossroads. However, Hing, Stamatiadis, and Aultman-Hall (2003) determined that drivers over the age of 75 years are even more likely to cause a crash with two or more passengers when traveling on curves, grades, and two-lane roads.

Stav et al. (2006) reviewed studies that examined modification to the vehicle, looking at window tinting, windshield glare, and use of adapted cruise control system. These studies concluded that tinted windows negatively impact the older adult's ability to see low-contrast objects and maneuver the vehicle backwards (Burns, Nettelbeck, White, & Wilson, 1999; Freedman, Zador, & Staplin, 1993; LaMotte, Ridder III, Yeung, & De Land, 2000). In addition, decreased contrast sensitivity due to the angle of the windshield and dashboard reflectance is an important factor to consider when recommending the type of car that best meets the needs of the older driver (Schumann, Flannagan, Sivak, & Traube, 1997). Other studies have shown that older drivers take longer to locate controls and display systems (Laux, 1991), and they favored the use of an adapted cruise control device, especially to allow for more space between cars (Fancher et al., 1998).

Infrastructure studies focused primarily on signage, specifically color, reflectiveness, location, fonts, and familiarity (Stav et al., 2006). The evidence supports specific colors and fonts (Carlson, 2001; Chrysler, Carlson, & Hawkins, 2002; Ho, Scialfa, Caird, & Graw, 2001), but the studies were not conducted in real-life driving environments. Kline, Buck, Sell, Bolan, and Dewar (1999) determined that legibility thresholds were lower for familiar signs compared to unfamiliar signs and that older drivers used compensatory strategies to read signs.

Policies concerning license renewal usually include one or more of the following: vision testing, in-person renewal, and medical review (Stav et al., 2006). Studies suggest that as drivers age, renewal criteria should increase as a way to reduce motor vehicle accidents (Grabowski, Campbell, & Morrisey, 2004; Hakamies-Blomqvist, Johansson, & Lundburg, 1996; Marshall, Spasoff, Nair, & Walraven, 2002; Shipp 1998).

Finally, few studies have been conducted concerning the effectiveness of community mobility programs for older adults. One study supports the use of an integrative transportation program for seniors designed to meet the needs of the older adult, family members who were concerned about community mobility, and merchants. Paid transportation services were provided to transport older adults to area businesses. Participants were satisfied with the program (Freund, 2002). More needs to be done in this area to explore different models of community mobility programs and the efficacy on how these impact the quality of life, community integration, and social participation of the older adult (Stav et al., 2006).

Losing the Ability to Drive—A Psychosocial Perspective

In Western industrialized society, the ability to drive and hold a driver's license is very important psychologically because it is equated with freedom, choice, identity, independence and autonomy, and status. Because decisions to go out can be spontaneous and made independently, driving allows people to attend to their own needs on their own personal schedule. At various life stages, there is a certain excitement about being mobile and being able to attend to one's own needs. Teenagers look forward to the day when they obtain a driver's license and with it a new sense of freedom. A driver's license is a "rite of passage into adulthood" (Gillins, 1990).

Functionally, having a driver's license means you can go shopping, visit a friend, keep appointments, go to your place of worship, or just take a drive whenever and wherever you choose. Residential and commercial development, as well as the creation of suburbia, has led to the idea that owning an automobile and being able to drive are essential to the enjoyment of daily life (Hare, 1992). Grocery stores, convenience stores, and houses of worship are often not within walking distance, and public transportation is not easily accessible. Therefore, driving becomes a critical instrumental ADL, which must be considered when looking at a person's functional mobility status.

The decision to stop driving has both emotional as well as practical consequences. Driving cessation can decrease a person's social network, thereby increasing both isolation and loneliness. Marottoli et al. (1997) demonstrated that driving cessation has been associated with depressive symptoms, which, in turn, are associated with disability and mortality. Legh-Smith et al. (1986) studied patients who stopped driving after having a stroke. These ex-drivers did less local shopping and traveling and decreased their social interactions, resulting in an increased likelihood of experiencing depressive symptoms. Through a qualitative study, Johnson (1998) demonstrated that the decision to stop driving was not only depressing but also stressful, and that this decision process and outcome could cause anxiety and decreased morale.

Because driving is associated with autonomy and competence, giving up a driver's license can make a person feel embarrassed, inadequate, and incompetent. Driving cessation threatens one's self-esteem and personal dignity because it implies social disability and dependency on others. There is also a sense of loss of power, especially when having to use alternate forms of transportation. Gillins (1990) notes that losing the ability to drive is usually associated with other losses as well, such as vision or limb function. Usually some type of physical disability makes driving no longer an option for an elderly person. This adds to the person's feelings of anger and helplessness as he or she has lost an important piece of his or her identity (Gillins, 1990).

Family members and caregivers find the issue of driving to be a very difficult topic to discuss with a loved one, especially if the reason the family member needs to stop driving is related to impaired cognition. Often, physical disabilities are easier to discuss and resolve than cognitive deficits, especially if the elderly driver lacks an awareness of his or her limitations (Gillins, 1990). Other times, a family member may raise the issue indirectly by mentioning newspaper articles in which an elderly driver was involved in an accident, by discussing the cost of driving (gas, maintenance, repairs, and insurance), or by calling the elderly person (or asking him or her to call) when he or she is expected to return home after a driving excursion (Persson, 1993). Family members may develop excuses to keep an elderly loved one off the road (Gillins, 1990). Some family members have resorted to hiding the keys and disabling the car or actually selling it to keep a family member from driving. Other caregivers have solicited expert opinions by having their loved one assessed by a driver rehabilitation specialist, believing that their family member may heed that advice more readily.

Before giving up driving altogether, most elderly people restrict themselves to driving under certain conditions. However, driver rehabilitation specialists do not consider some of these modifications effective. Examples of self-regulation techniques employed by the elderly driver are driving only during daylight hours and on familiar streets, or avoiding inclement weather and heavy traffic times. Some elderly individuals report they do not want passengers with them because either the conversation is distracting or they are fearful they may injure a family member, especially a grandchild. Others prefer to have a second person in the car with them believing that two sets of eyes are better than one. However, most driver rehabilitation specialists do not recommend this modification. According to a study by Persson (1993), most elderly individuals decide to stop driving because their physician advises them to do so, they are increasingly nervous behind the wheel, or they have trouble seeing pedestrians and cars.

Another method used by the state to limit driving of elderly adults is *graded licensing*, which allows elderly people to drive as long as possible, provided they are safe (Malfetti & Winter, 1991). The license may impose some types of restrictions based on the driver's functional and cognitive abilities. Currently, many states have restricted licenses that allow the person to drive only with corrective lenses. However, other restrictions could be based on the elderly person's capabilities and may indicate that special equipment is required or that the individual may drive only during daylight hours. Restrictions based on functional and cognitive limitations can be more controversial because it is difficult to determine whether a dysfunction

that increases a driver's risk in one setting will negatively affect the driver's ability in another setting. For example, a driver who runs a stop sign on a behind-the-wheel evaluation route may attribute this error to being unfamiliar with the route. Although the driver may know the location of stop signs or other traffic signals on a familiar route, the driver's deficient performance during the behind-the-wheel evaluation may indicate the driver is at risk for failing to make an observation while driving. Although the driver may drive in familiar areas, the risk of this observation error may increase if there is an unpredictable traffic event or if the familiar route is somehow altered for construction or roadwork.

Community Mobility: Some Alternative Solutions

More than 30 years ago, the White House Conference on Aging recognized that transportation was the third greatest problem for the elderly after lack of good health and poverty. Access to public transportation for older adults continues to be a major challenge. By 2010, adults age 60 and older will represent 20% of the nation's population. With the aging of the baby boomers there will be an even greater need for reliable and easily accessible alternative forms of community transportation so that our elderly do not become isolated. Affordable, accessible, and flexible transportation options are essential for the elderly so they can access health care appointments and services, continue to independently obtain groceries and other household items, and prevent isolation and depression by maintaining contacts with family, friends, and social organizations (AARP, 2004).

For people who have used a car as their sole source of transportation, being forced to use alternate forms of transportation can be challenging, frustrating, and anxiety provoking. Seeking and using alternative transportation options may require mastery of new skills, which may elicit even more fear and frustration. For example, if an elderly person has never taken a bus, learning to read the schedule, finding the bus stops, and managing entering and exiting the bus can be challenging. Although buses may not be a good alternative to driving, special transportation designed for elderly persons, such as taxi or van services, is often too expensive, and most people can use this mode of transportation only for trips they consider critical, such as medical appointments. Issues with community mobility and the elderly can vary greatly depending upon where the elderly person lives. Rural areas certainly present different issues than the inner city and the suburbs. Rural and minority elderly are the most likely to feel isolated when they can no longer drive in comparison to their urban and suburban counterparts.

Studies have shown that few older adults use public transportation. One study concluded that 89% of older drivers made their trips in a private vehicle, whether they were the driver or the passenger, and only 8% chose to walk (Houser, 2005). Most notable was the fact that only 2% stated that they used public transportation or another means of transportation. Based on these statistics, that leaves perhaps as many as 7 million adults age 65 an older who do not drive (Houser, 2005). Exposure to inclement weather also is a concern for elderly adults when using public transportation. Both walking to and waiting for the bus in bad weather can increase exposure and lead to health problems. Also, if an individual is unable to operate a motor vehicle because of a physical impairment, chances are good that he or she will be unable to ambulate the distance necessary to get to the bus stop or carry purchases home from the bus stop. Gillins (1990) notes that many elderly people are concerned about their personal safety and fear harassment when taking public transportation.

The U.S. Department of Transportation recognized the challenges of safe mobility for the aging population in the United States. In its 2003 vision statement, the U.S. Department of Transportation (2003) placed a focus on safe and reliable mobility for the aging population.

> A transportation system that offers safe mobility to all people and allows older persons to remain independent and to age in place. Investments in highway and pedestrian infrastructure and public transportation services support independent. Medical and social service communities, transportation manager, motor vehicle administrators, and caregivers work together to extend safe driving and to offer other convenient and affordable transportation options when

driving and walking must be curtailed. Public and private organizations form new partnerships to enable all citizens to enjoy safe mobility for life. (p. 6)

Stated goals to achieve this vision include the following:

1. Safer, easier-to-use roadways and walkways
2. Safer, easier-to-use automobiles
3. Improved systems for assessing competency of older drivers and pedestrians
4. Better, easier-to-use public transportation services
5. Targeted state and local action plans
6. Better public information
7. Basic and social policy research (U.S. DOT, 2003)

Pilot programs have begun to emerge which attempt to address community mobility issues of the older adult. For example, the American Public Transportation Association (APTA) launched the Easy Rider Program in 2005. The focus of this program was to improve community mobility of America's aging population. The program included the following components:

1. New service designs and infrastructures
2. Application of new technologies
3. Transit user training and outreach programs
4. Strategies for engaging allies and supporters
5. Execution of broad-based communications activities
6. Strategies for engaging the media on behalf of mobility for seniors (APTA, 2005)

In Canada, Tuokko and McGee (2002) conducted focus groups with older adult drivers and individual interviews with health care professionals to identify ways to improve the driving condition for older adults. Although participants identified that there needs to be a societal shift in attitude toward the acceptance of alternative modes of transportation, as well as improved road engineering and transportation methods, education of the general public and professionals was identified as a priority. The group recommended that a mandatory defensive driving course should be offered through senior centers and that health care professionals could recommend nonmandatory self-assessments that would alert people of factors that may impact driving safety and provide suggested actions people could take. Public education that encourages people to plan ahead and provide strategies on how to manage without a vehicle could lessen the impact that driving cessation may have on an individual. Driving safety should be a discussion point in any health problem where the health problem might impact driving.

Important to the success of any community mobility program would be to promote the development of new skills to allow older adults to participate in actual activities involving the use of available transportation and community resources. The Well Elderly Program, developed by Jackson, Carlson, Mandel, Zemke, and Clark (1998), would be appropriate as a method of encouraging community mobility of the elderly through the acquisition of new skills within contexts. Using occupation in lifestyle redesign, these researchers enabled the participants, community-dwelling older adults, to explore their community transportation options by first discussing individualized obstacles and inhibitory fears regarding the use of transportation. After gathering practical knowledge about their traveling options, the participants embarked on several trips using buses, cabs, and the Metro subway system. They shared their experiences, traded tips, and motivated each other to continue using the available transportation options. These activities were completed with trained occupational therapists throughout. Noting that many of the participants also were afraid to even walk across the street to the market to buy food or to the library a few blocks away, the Well Elderly Program included safety education by having the participants practice safe community mobility techniques within the security of occupational therapy outings. This type of programming is essential to the successful community integration of older adults who cannot drive.

Kinsler (1999) offers additional suggestions for older adults who can no longer drive a car. She recommends that the transition be gradual when changing from a personal automobile to alternate forms of transportation. This is possible when dealing with the normal aging process but becomes more difficult when the transportation change is indicated because the individual has suffered a sudden physical change, such as a stroke. Additional suggestions offered to the caregiver by Kinsler are

- Offer to drive the older adult as much as possible. Ask other friends and family members to do the same so that the older adult will not feel he or she is relying on or burdening one particular person, and so that he or she will have a variety of options if one person is not available.
- When purchasing a new car, consider whether or not the older adult can get into and out of it comfortably. Cars that are too low to the ground or vans that are too high may be difficult for elderly passengers to enter and exit.
- Find other people with whom the elderly person can carpool. For example, people who attend the same worship service or social function may be willing to drive the elderly person to those events.
- Locate organizations and medical facilities that have vans available to pick up and drop off people for their social functions or appointments.
- Tell friends and family members to buy gift certificates for cab companies as holiday and birthday presents. They are practical and very helpful to an elderly person on a fixed income. Some cab companies offer discounted rates for seniors, so be sure to ask.
- Help the elderly person obtain schedules for other forms of public transportation in their community. Show them where stops are located.
- Look into hiring a driver. There is a listing of services in the phone book, and many community senior centers have lists of persons who will drive an elderly person either as a courtesy or for a nominal fee.
- If the elderly person is considering a move— sometimes to get out of a multilevel home— look for a place that is close to the things they like to do or to public transportation, or consider retirement communities.
- Look for vacations for them where the transportation is included or take them with you on vacation. Ask friends and family members to consider doing this as well.
- Call the local senior center in the community. Many senior centers or municipal Departments of Human Resources have shuttle services available to seniors.

Hare (1992) suggests that in addition to alternate transportation arrangements made through friends, family, or public transportation, changes in driver assessment, driver modification, vehicle modification, and highway modification can greatly increase the number of elderly people who can continue to safely drive.

For example, car dashboards, which are difficult to read with bifocals, could be redesigned with consideration of vision changes that occur with normal aging (for example, enlarged symbols and greater illumination of controls). In addition, road signs, designed for persons with 20/40 vision, could be made larger with better choices of contrasting colors to make them more visible. Although highways are designed with the young male driver in mind, Hare suggests that experts on aging study the needs of older adults to determine the most effective highway designs to help these individuals drive safely for a longer period of time. Other modifications to motor vehicles that would be beneficial to the elderly driver are being considered by automobile manufacturers:

1. Adjustable pedal extenders to allow the elderly driver suffering from osteoporosis to reach the pedals without being too close to the driver's side airbag
2. Night-vision systems that would help the elderly driver see at night
3. Heads-up displays that would allow the instrument panel to be reflected on the hood of the automobile so the driver would not have to look down to see the instruments
4. Warning sensors that will sound to alert the driver who is backing up that there is an obstacle behind the vehicle

There is overwhelming evidence provided by many sources ranging from medical professionals and health care providers, to social scientists, policy makers, and government officials, that addressing the transportation and mobility needs of an ever-increasing aging population has emerged as an issue that demands well-designed and purposeful solutions. Despite the overwhelming need, there is evidence of only slight change and progress on this issue; however, efficacy studies of existing programs need to be conducted. Considerations of how any solution would be administered and paid for are of paramount concern, but perhaps the greater challenge will be confronting the fact that we live in a society and culture that is built around private-care ownership. Our roadways and community development have been designed with the assumption that Americans own and operate their own vehicles. Addressing the community mobility issues of the older adult will call for a major paradigm shift. The costs involved in these changes are relatively small compared to the cost of providing transportation for this growing segment of the population. These types of improvements would help preserve the aging person's independence and dignity, and at the same time, allow them a more active role in society.

Suggestions for Clinicians in Geriatic Practice

By interviewing the elderly client or the client's family members or caregiver, the geriatric clinician can determine whether a referral to a driver rehabilitation specialist is indicated. Several factors should be considered as signs that the elderly client may be experiencing difficulties in driving. If any of the following factors are present, the geriatric clinician should recommend that the elderly client undergo a formal driving evaluation:

• If the client is experiencing difficulties performing ADLs, there is a good chance that driving is problematic as well.
• Although the self-report of an elderly driver is not usually reliable, the individual may have his or her own concerns about driving safety.
• Certainly, the family or caregiver should be asked if they have any concerns about the elderly client's ability to drive.
• If the elderly client reports episodes of getting lost on the way to appointments or meetings or an increased incidence of other drivers honking at him or her, a driving evaluation should be conducted.
• Physical limitations such as neck pain or limited upper or lower extremity range of motion are indications that the driver may have difficulty operating a motor vehicle safely.

If any of these indicators are reported or apparent clinically, the geriatric clinician should recommend that the elderly client receive a driving evaluation from a driver rehabilitation specialist. Under no circumstances should a geriatric clinician recommend adaptive equipment for a motor vehicle without having the elderly client undergo a thorough driving evaluation and training in the use of the equipment. Even the simplest adaptive device requires training to use safely because the slightest modification may require a more complex adjustment by the driver to ensure the safe operation of the vehicle.

The geriatric clinician also needs to consider alternative solutions available to the client should driving privileges be taken away and how the inability to drive may impact the client's ability to participate in valued activities. Community resources should be easily accessible to the client. Optimally, a program should exist to help the older adult explore alternatives and to develop new skills necessary to successfully utilize alternative community mobility options. This type of client-centered and community-based practice will help assure the safety of the older adult and facilitate successful participation in meaningful occupations within the community.

■ Summary

Driving is an important occupation, as well as a symbol of freedom and independence. As the elderly population ages, difficulties in driving arise as a result of normal physiologic and disease-related changes affecting the skills necessary to drive safely. Assessment of the elderly driver's functions, client factors, performance skills, performance patterns, and contexts is necessary to help determine whether the driver will be safe on the road. Ultimately, a behind-the-wheel assessment may be necessary to help identify skill-area deficiencies and to provide future recommendations. Psychosocial implications must be considered as well when evaluating and determining whether the elderly driver should continue to drive with restrictions or cease driving altogether. Proactive legislation and public policy initiatives to improve community mobility of the elderly will facilitate the independence and dignity of America's older adults by promoting continued participation in the community.

Case Study

Susie's 80-year-old father occasionally forgets where the keys are or what day it is. One day she rides to the grocery store with her parents, and discovers that her mother directs her father while he is driving, because he has difficulty remembering the route to take. Susie becomes sufficiently concerned so she makes an appointment with her father's physician to assess his cognitive skills. His daughter tells the physician that her father has forgotten to turn off the stove, forgets to take his medications, never knows what the date is, and occasionally asks for directions to what should be familiar places. Mr. Smith, who just turned 80, has never had an accident or ticket and feels he is a safe driver. He drives alone to the hardware store and to a local restaurant to "meet the boys" for breakfast. He and his wife go to the grocery and drug stores; he takes her to the beauty parlor, and to church. "Not at night, mind you," and avoids "downtown." He takes her because "she can't see well anymore." He reluctantly agrees to come in for an occupational therapy driving evaluation.

The occupational therapist completes several types of assessments. At the end of the testing the OT notes that Mr. Smith has some arthritis, which slows his walking, and he has trouble doing his woodworking, but otherwise does well physically. He is independent in all his self-care and his wife has always done all the housework. He has less than ideal vision, but within the parameters set by the state BMV, and he appears to have some mild cognitive issues. From Mr. Smith's perspective, he is faced with the prospect of not driving and loss of independence. As driving is such an integral part of our society, loss of driving privileges is a very real sign of "getting old," a prospect few people care to face.

The next portion of the driving assessment is taking an actual vehicle on the public streets. Unfortunately, the driver rehab car is not the same type that Mr. Smith owns, and he is unfamiliar with the public streets in the area of the OT clinic. The route used by the driving rehabilitation program was chosen to incorporate as many potential variables as possible that might be encountered while driving. After safety, the most important goal the OT has is to put the driver at ease. In addition, the OT driving evaluator needs to separate "poor driving habits," or simply differences in personal driving styles between the driver and evaluator, from errors associated with a medical condition

Overall, Mr. Smith did well, some small errors, or maybe some errors that were not risky, but could have been high or moderate risk, if the situation had been different. He demonstrates some obvious memory impairments throughout the entire evaluation but does not have any memory-related errors on the road during testing. He was able to drive in an environment similar to his own and there were no atypical situations that arose, and he was able to negotiate his usual routes. From experience, reports of the family, and just a "gut" feeling, the evaluator senses that this driver has the potential to have an accident, or become lost, but Mr. Smith did not demonstrate any significant errors during the driving evaluation.

Based on the information available, what are your recommendations for Mr. Smith? In determining your recommendations consider the following:

Questions

1. If Mr. Smith does continue driving, what could he do to improve his safety? Are there some self-limiting strategies with regard to certain driving situations that would help or some modifications that could be imposed?
2. Should there be a follow-up OT Driving Assessment in 6 or 12 months? Why? What needs to be monitored?
3. How do you communicate your recommendations to Mr. Smith or his family (remember patient confidentiality)?
4. Will Mr. Smith remember the evaluation or recommendations?
5. Why is driving so important to Mr. Smith? Consider loss of independence for Mr. Smith and his wife, the safety of other drivers on the road, self-esteem issues for Mr. Smith, and isolation issues that can lead to depression and further cognitive problems.
6. Knowing that the day Mr. Smith will need to completely give up his keys is quickly approaching, what recommendations could you offer the family about other alternatives? How would you go about informing him of these alternatives? What training might you provide and how would you go about doing this?
7. What if Mr. Smith does not have any family members with him for the OT Driving Assessment? Should concerns be addressed with the family members? If so, how should the evaluator go about doing this?

Review Questions

1. Describe the relationship between motor vehicle violations and crash rates and the elderly population.
2. Describe the different aspects of the Driving as an Occupation model.
3. How do the normal aging process and disease processes affect the elderly driver's ability to drive?
4. What information is important to obtain during the initial interview portion of a driver evaluation?
5. What are the pros and cons of functional measures used to assess driving performance?
6. Which is the most effective way to assess a driver's abilities: a driving simulator or a behind-the-wheel assessment? When is either of these assessments indicated?

Web-Based Resources

For helpful information about the experience of community mobility visit:

www.aaafoundation.org, **American Automobile Association (AAA) Foundation for Traffic Safety,** date connected May 23, 2007. This site includes information about safe driving and strategies for improvement.

www.seniordrivers.org/home/toppage.cfm, **AAA Foundation Older Drivers,** date connected May 23, 2007. Focuses on strategies older drivers can use to assess their ability to drive and to improve their skills.

www.thehartford.com/alzheimers/index.html, **Alzheimer's, Dementia and Driving,** date connected May 23, 2007. May help individuals and families decide when it's time to give up the car keys when the individual has Alzheimer's disease.

www.aarp.org/55alive, **American Association for Retired Persons (AARP), 55 ALIVE Driver Safety Program,** date connected May 23, 2007. AARP's driving program has helped many elders improve their driving. Information here includes sites for obtaining training.

www.ama-assn.org/ama/pub/category/8925.html, **American Medical Association—Older Driver Safety,** date connected May 23, 2007. Discusses impact of aging on driving and strategies for keeping older drivers safe.

www.driver-ed.org, **Association for Driver Rehabilitation Specialists (ADED),** date connected May 23, 2007. Discusses how to find a driver rehabilitation specialist to do a comprehensive assessment, what qualifications such individuals should have, and what kinds of recommendations to expect.

www.aota.org/olderdriver, **American Occupational Therapy Association Older Drive Microsite,** date connected May 23, 2007. Driver evaluation and safety strategies are included here.

www.ctaa.org, **Community Transportation Association of America,** date connected May 23, 2007. Discusses alternative transportation for individuals who cannot safely drive.

http://safety.fhwa.dot.gov/older_driver/older_resources.htm, **Federal Highway Administration—Older Drivers,** date connected May 23, 2007. Factors associated with safe driving, resources for improving driving.

www.nhtsa.dot.gov, **National Highway Traffic Safety Administration,** date connected May 23, 2007. Includes data with regard to driving for all drivers.

www.nhtsa.dot.gov/people/injury/olddrive/index.html, **National Highway Traffic Safety Administration—Older Road Users,** date connected May 23, 2007. Focuses on safety data for older adults.

www.nhtsa.dot.gov/people/injury/olddrive/Driving_macular/, **National Driving and Macular Degeneration,** date connected May 23, 2007. Discusses the impact of macular degeneration on driving and suggests strategies for evaluating safety to drive.

www.nhtsa.dot.gov/people/injury/olddrive/Driving_glaucoma/, **National Highway Traffic Safety Administration—Driving and Glaucoma,** date connected May 23, 2007. Discusses the impact of glaucoma on ability to drive and strategies for evaluating safety.

www.nhtsa.dot.gov/people/injury/olddrive/Driving_cataract/, **National Highway Traffic Safety Administration—Driving and Cataracts,** date connected May 23, 2007. Discusses the impact of cataracts on driving and strategies for evaluating safety.

REFERENCES

Adler, G., Rottunda, S., Dysken, M. (2005). The older driver with dementia: An updated literature review. *Journal of Safety Research, 36,*399–407.

American Association for Retired Persons (AARP): Aging Americans: Stranded without options (2004). Retrieved May 24, 2006 from www.transact.org/report.asp?id=232.

American Occupational Therapy Association (AOTA). (2002). Occupational therapy practice framework: Domain and practice. *American Journal of Occupational Therapy, 56,* 609–639.

American Occupational Therapy Association (2005). AOTA Standards for Continuing Competence. *American Journal of Occupational Therapy, 59,* 661–661.

American Occupational Therapy Association (2006, June 9). AOTA Board and Specialty Certification. Retrieved December 29, 2006, from www.aota.org/nonmembers/area15/links/link12.asp.

American Public Transportation Association (APTA): Easy rider program guide for public transportation organizations. (2005). Retrieved on May 24, 2006, from www.apta.com/easyrider/programguide.html.

Association of Driver Rehabilitation Specialists (ADED). (2006). *Certification.* Retrieved December 29, 2006, from www.aded.net/i4a/pages/index.cfm?pageid=120.

Baker, P. (2006). The clinical evaluation: Section II: The clinical evaluation of vision. In J. Pellertio (Ed.), *Driver rehabilitation and community mobility: Principles and practice.* (pp. 116–140). St. Louis, MO: Mosby.

Ball, K., Owsley, C., Sloane, M. E., Roenker, D. L., & Bruni, J. R. (1993). Visual attention problems as a predictor of vehicle crashes in older drivers. *Investigative Ophthalmology & Visual Science, 34*(11), 3110–3123.

Brashear, A., Farlow, M. R., Glazier, B. S., Hui, S. L., Kuhn, E. R., Perkins, A. J., et al. (1998). Impaired traffic sign recognition in drivers with dementia. *American Journal of Alzheimer's Disease, 13*(3), 131–137.

Burns, N. R., Nettelbeck, T., White, M., & Willson, J. (1999). The effects of car window tinting on visual performance: A comparison of elderly and young drivers. *Ergonomics, 42,* 428–443.

Carlson, P. J. (2001). Evaluation of Clearview alphabet with microprismatic retroreflective sheetings. FHWA Report #FHWA/TX-02/4049-1. Springfield, VA: National Technical Information Service.

Carr, D. B., Shead, V., & Storandt, M. (2005). Driving cessation in older adults with dementia of the Alzheimer's type. *The Gerontologist, 45*(6), 824–827.

Carr, D., Schmader, K., Bergman, C., Simon, T. C., Jackson, T. W., Haviland, S., et al. (1991). A multidisciplinary approach in the evaluation of demented drivers referred to geriatric assessment centers. *Journal of the American Geriatrics Society, 39*(11), 1132–1136.

Christiansen, C., & Baum, C. (Eds.). (1997). *Occupational therapy: Enabling function and well-being.* Thorofare, NJ: Slack.

Chrysler, S. T., Carlson, P. J., & Hawkins, H. G. (2002). Nighttime legibility of ground-mounted signs as a function of font, color, and retroreflective sheeting type. FHWA Report #FHWA/TX-03/1796-2. Springfield, VA: National Technical Information Service.

Cimolino, N., & Balkovec, D. (1988). The contribution of a driving simulator in the driving evaluation of stroke and disabled adolescent clients. *Canadian Journal of Occupational Therapy, 55*(3), 119–125.

Copeland, A. (1989). Traffic fatalities among the elderly population: The Metro Dade county experience from 1981–1983. *Medicine, Science, and the Law, 29*(2), 159–161.

Coyne, A. C., Feins, L. C., Powell, A. L., & Joslin, B. L. (1990 March). The relationship between driving and dementia. Paper presented at the Third Biennial Cognitive Aging Conference, Atlanta, GA.

Donnelly, R. E., & Karlinsky, H. (1990). The impact of Alzheimer's disease on driving ability: A review. *Journal of Geriatric Psychiatry and Neurology, 3*(2), 67–72.

Drachman, D., & Swearer, J. (1993). Driving and Alzheimer's disease: The risk of crashes. *Neurology, 43*(12), 2448–2456.

Dubinsky, R., Stein, A., & Lyons, K. (2000). Practice parameters: Risk of driving and Alzheimer's disease (an evidence-based review). *Neurology, 54,* 2205–2211.

Duchek, J. M., Carr, D. B., Hunt, L., Roe, C. M., Xiong, C., Shah, K., et al. (2003). Longitudinal driving performance in early-stage dementia of the Alzheimer type. *JAGS, 51,* 1342–1347.

Ekelman, B., Mitchell, S., & O'Dell-Rossi, P. (2000). Driving and older adults. In B. Bonder & M. Wagner (Eds.), *Functional performance of older adults* (2nd ed., pp.448–486). Philadelphia: F.A. Davis.

Fancher, P., Ervin, R., Sayer, J., Hagan, M., Bogard, S., Bareket, Z., et al. (1998). Intelligent Cruise Control Field Operational Test (Final Report). Report No. UMTRI-98-17. Ann Arbor, MI: Transportation Research Institute, University of Michigan.

Fishbaugh, J. (1995). Look who's driving now—Visual standards for driver licensing in the United States. *Insight, 20*(4), 11–20.

Fisher, A., & Kielhofner, G. (1995). Skills in occupational performance. In G. Kielhofner (Ed.), *A model of human occupation: Theory and application* (2nd ed., pp. 113–128). Baltimore: Williams & Wilkins.

Foley, K. T., & Mitchell, S. J. (1997). The elderly driver: What physicians need to know. *Cleveland Clinic Journal of Medicine, 64*(8), 423–428.

Freedman, M., Zador, P., & Staplin, L. (1993). Effects of reduced transmittance film on automobile rear window visibility. *Human Factors, 35*(33), 535–550.

Freund, K. (2002). *Pilot testing innovative payment operations for independent transportation for the elderly (final report for Transit-IDEA Project 18).* Washington, DC: Transportation Research Board.

Friedland, R. P., Koss, E., Kumar, A., Gaine, S., Metzler, D., Haxby, J. V., et al. (1988). Motor vehicle crashes in dementia of the Alzheimer type. *Annals of Neurology, 24*(6), 782–786.

Galski, T., Bruno, R. L., & Ehle, H. T. (1992). Driving after cerebral damage: A model with implications for evaluation. *American Journal of Occupational Therapy, 46*(4), 324–332.

Galski, T., Bruno, R. L., & Ehle, H. T. (1993). Prediction of behind-the-wheel driving performance in patients with cerebral brain damage: A discriminant function analysis. *American Journal of Occupational Therapy, 47*(5), 391–396.

Gianutsos, R. (1994). The driving advisement with the elemental driving simulator (EDS): When less suffices. *Behavior Research Methods, Instruments, & Computers, 26,* 183–186.

Gianutsos, R., Campbell, A., Beattie, A., & Mandriota, F. (1992). The driving advisement system: A computer-augmented quasi-simulation of the cognitive prerequisites for resumption of driving after brain injury. *Assistive Technology, 4*(2), 70–86.

Gillins, L. (1990). Yielding to age: When the elderly can no longer drive. *Journal of Gerontological Nursing, 16*(11), 12–15.

Gouvier, W. D., Maxfield, M. W., Schweitzer, J. R., Horton, C. R., Shipp, M., Neilson, K., et al. (1989). Psychometric prediction of driving performance among the disabled. *Archives of Physical Medicine and Rehabilitation, 70*(10), 745–750.

Grabowski, D. C., Campbell, C. M., & Morrisey, M. A. (2004). Elderly licensure laws and motor vehicle fatalities. *Journal of the American Medical Association, 291,* 2840–2846.

Grace, J., Amick, M., D'Abreu, A., Festa, E., Heindel, W., & Ott, B. (2005). Neuropsychological deficits associated with driving performance in Parkinson's and Alzheimer's disease. *Journal of the International Neuropsychological Society, 11,* 766–775.

Hakamies-Blomqvist, L., Johansson, K., & Lundburg, C. (1996). Medical screening of older drivers as a traffic safety measure: A comparative Finnish-Swedish evaluation study. *Journal of the American Geriatrics Society, 44,* 650–653.

Hare, P. (1992). Frail elders and the suburbs. *Generations: Journal of the American Society on Aging, 16,* 35–39.

Harrell, M., Parenté, F., Bellingrath, E.G., & Lisica, K.A. (1992). *Cognitive rehabilitation of memory: A practical guide.* Gaithersburg, MD: Aspen.

Hills, B. L. (1980). Vision, visibility and perception in driving. *Perception, 9*(2), 183–216.

Hing, J. Y. C., Stamatiadis, N., & Aultman-Hall, L. (2003). Evaluating the impact of passengers on the safety of older drivers. *Journal of Safety Research, 34,* 343–351.

Ho, G., Scialfa, C. T., Caird, J. K., & Graw, T. (2001). Visual search for traffic signs: The effects of clutter, luminance, & aging. *Human Factors, 43,* 194–207.

Holmes, C. (1990). Neuropsychological sequelae of acute and chronic blood glucose disruption in adults with insulin-dependent diabetes. In C. Holmes (Ed.), *Neuropsychological and behavioral aspects of diabetes* (pp. 122–154). New York: Springer-Verlag.

Houser, A. (2005). *Community mobility options: The older person's interest. Research report.* Retrieved May 24, 2006, from www.aarp.org/research/housing-mobility/transportation/fs44r_com_mobility.html.

Hunt, L., Morris, J. C., Edwards, D., & Wilson, B. S. (1993). Driving performance in persons with mild senile dementia of the Alzheimer type. *Journal of the American Geriatrics Society, 41*(7), 747–752.

Hyvarinen, L. (1996). *Vision testing manual.* Villa Park, IL: Precision Vision.

International Council of Ophthalmology: International Standards: Vision Requirements for Driving Safety. (2006). Retrieved May 24, 2006, from www.icoph.org/standards/driving.html.

Jackson, J., Carlson, M., Mandel, D., Zemke, R., & Clark, F. (1998). Occupation in lifestyle redesign: The well elderly study occupational therapy program. *American Journal of Occupational Therapy, 52,* 326–336.

Johnson, J. (1998). Older rural adults and the decision to stop driving: The influence of family and friends. *Journal of Community Health Nursing, 15*(4), 205–216.

Kaszniak, A. W., Nussbaum, P., & Allender, J. A. (1990). Driving in elderly patients with dementia or depression. Paper presented at the annual meeting of the American Psychological Association, Boston, MA.

Keltner, J., & Johnson, C. (1987). Visual function, driving safety, and the elderly. *Ophthalmology, 94,* 1180–1188.

Keplinger, F. (1998). The elderly driver: Who should continue to drive? *Physical Medicine and Rehabilitation: State of the Art Reviews, 12*(1), 147–155.

Kinsler, S. (1999). Transportation options for older parents and friends. Retrieved May 22, 2006, from www.womanmotorist.com/index.php/news/main/2214/event=view.

Klavora, P., Gaskovski, P., Martin, K., Forsyth, R. D., Heslegrave, R. J., Young, M., et al. (1995). The effects of dynavision rehabilitation on behind-the-wheel driving ability and selected psychomotor abilities of persons after stroke. *American Journal of Occupational Therapy, 49*(6), 534–542.

Klein, R. (1991). Age-related eye disease, visual impairment, and driving in the elderly. *Human Factors, 33*(5), 521–525.

Kline, D. W., Buck, K., Sell, Y., Bolan, T. L., & Dewar, R. E. (1999, September). Older observers' tolerance of optical blur: Age differences in the identification of defocused text signs. *Human Factors, 41*(3), 356–364.

Koepsell, T. D., Wolf, M. E., McCloskey, L., Buchner, D. M., Louie, D., Wagner, E. H., et al. (1994). Medical conditions and motor vehicle collision injuries in older adults. *Journal of the American Geriatrics Society, 42*(7), 695–700.

LaMotte, J., Ridder III, W., Yeung, K., & De Land, P. (2000). Effect of aftermarket automobile window tinting films on driver vision. *Human Factors, 42*(2), 327–336.

Laux, L. F. (1991). *Locating vehicle controls and displays: Effects of expectancy and age.* Washington, DC: AAA Foundation for Traffic Safety.

Law, M., & Baum, C. (1998). Evidence based occupational therapy. *Canadian Journal of Occupational Therapy, 65,* 131–135.

Law, M., Polatajko, H., Baptiste, W., & Townsend, E. (1997). Core concepts of occupational therapy. In E. Townsend (Ed.), *Enabling occupation: An occupational therapy perspective* (pp. 29–56). Ottawa, ON: Canadian Association of Occupational Therapists.

Legh-Smith, J., Wade, D. T., & Hewer, R. L. (1986). Driving after a stroke. *Journal of the Royal Society of Medicine, 79*(4), 200–203.

Llaneras, R. E., Swezey, R. W., Brock, J. F., Rogers, W. C., & Van Cott, H. P. (1998). Enhancing the safe driving performance of older commercial vehicle drivers. *International Journal of Industrial Ergonomics, 22*(3), 217–245.

Lucas-Blaustein, M. J., Filipp, L., Dungan, C., & Tune, L. (1988). Driving in patients with dementia. *Journal of the American Geriatrics Society, 36*(12),1087–1091.

Malfetti, J. L., & Winter, D. (1991). Concerned about an older driver? A guide for families and friends. Washington, DC: AAA Foundation for Traffic Safety.

Marottoli, R. (1993). Driving safety in elderly individuals. *Connecticut Medicine, 57*(5), 277–280.

Marottoli, R. A., Mendes de Leon, C. F., Glass, T. A., Williams, C. S., Cooney, L. M., Jr., Berkman, L. F., et al. (1997). Driving cessation and increased depressive symptoms: Prospective evidence from the New Haven EPESE. *Journal of the American Geriatrics Society, 45*(2), 202–206.

Marshall, S. C., Spasoff, R., Nair, R., & Walraven, C. (2002). Restricted driver licensing for medical impairments: Does it work? *Canadian Medical Association Journal, 167,* 747–751.

Mazer, B., Sofer, S., Korner-Bitensky, I., Gelinas, I., Hanley, J., & Wood-Dauphinee, S. (2003). Effectiveness of a visual attention retraining program on the driving performance of clients with stroke. *Archives of Physical Medicine and Rehabilitation, 84*(4), 541–550.

Michon, J. A. (1987). Dealing with danger: Summary report of a workshop in the traffic research center, State University, Groningen, 1979. Cited in van Zomeren, A. H., Brouwer, W. H., & Minderhoud, J. M. Acquired brain damage and driving: A review. *Archives of Physical Medicine and Rehabilitation, 68,* 697–705.

Monga, T. N., Osterman, H. J., & Kerrigan, A. J. (1997). Driving: A clinical perspective on rehabilitation technology. *Physical Medicine and Rehabilitation: State of the Art Reviews, 11*(1), 69.

Morgan, R., & King, D. (1995). The older driver—A review. *Postgraduate Medical Journal, 71,* 525–528.

National Highway and Traffic Safety Administration *Traffic Safety Facts 2004 Older Population (NHTSA).* (2004a). Retrieved May 24, 2006, from www-nrd. nhtsa.dot.gov/pdf/nrd-30/NCSA/TSF2004/ 809910.pdf.

National Highway and Traffic Safety Administration *Traffic Safety Facts 2004 Overview (NHTSA).* (2004b). Retrieved May 24, 2006, from www-nrd. nhtsa.dot.gov/pdf/nrd-30/NCSA/TSF2004/ 809911.pdf.

National Highway and Traffic Safety Administration: *Model driver screening and evaluation program: Final technical report: Volume II Maryland pilot older driver study.* (2003). Retrieved May 24, 2006 from www.nhtsa.dot.gov/people/injury/olddrive/ modeldriver/.

Neistadt, M. E., & Crepeau, E. B. (Eds.). (1998). *Willard & Spackman's occupational therapy* (9th ed.). Philadelphia: Lippincott.

Nelson, T. O., & Narens, L. N. (1994). Why investigate metacognition? In J. Metcalfe & P. Shimarmura (Eds.), *Metacognition: Knowing about knowing* (pp. 1–26) Cambridge: MIT Press.

Nouri, F. M., & Tinson, D. J. (1988). A comparison of a driving simulator and road test in the assessment of driving ability after stroke. *Clinics in Rehabilitation, 2,* 99–104.

Odenheimer, G. L., Beaudet, M., Jette, A. M., Albert, M. S., Grande, L., & Minaker, K. L. (1994). Performance-based driving evaluation of the elderly driver: Safety, reliability, and validity. *Journal of Gerontology, 49,* M153–M162.

Olson, P., & Sivak, M. (1986). Perception-response time to unexpected roadway hazards. *Human Factors, 28*(1), 91–96.

Ostrow, A. C., Shaffron, P., & McPherson, K. (1992). The effects of a joint range-of-motion physical fitness training program on the automobile driving skills of older adults. *Journal of Safety Research, 23*(4), 207–219.

Owsley, C., Ball, K., Thomas, B., & Graves, M. (1995). Driving avoidance, functional impairment and crash risk in older drivers [Special issue]. *The Gerontologist, 35,* 211.

Owsley, C., Stalvey, B., Wells, J., & Sloane, M. E. (1999). Older drivers and cataract: Driving habits and crash risk. *Journal of Gerontology A: Biological Sciences Medical Sciences, 54A,* M203–M211.

Parente, R., & Anderson, J. (1991). *Retraining memory: Techniques and applications.* Houston: CSY Publishing.

Pellertio, J. (Ed.). (2006). *Driver rehabilitation and community mobility: Principles and practice.* St. Louis, MO: Mosby.

Pelli, D. G., Robson, J. G., & Wilkins, A. J. (1988). The design of a new letter chart for measuring contrast sensitivity. *Clinical Vision Science, 2,* 187–199.

Persson, D. (1993). Elderly driver: Deciding when to stop. *The Gerontologist, 33,* 88–91.

Quigly, F. L., & DeLisa, J. A. (1983). Assessing driving potential of cerebral vascular accident patients. *American Journal of Occupational Therapy, 37*(7), 474–478.

Ray, W. A., Fought, R. L., & Decker, M. D. (1992). Psychoactive drugs and the risk of injurious motor vehicle crashes in elderly drivers. *American Journal of Epidemiology, 136*(7), 873–883.

Rebok, G., Keyl, P. M., Bylsma, F. W., Blaustein, M. J., & Tune, L. (1994). The effects of Alzheimer disease on driving-related abilities. *Alzheimer Disease and Associated Disorders, 8*(4), 228–240.

Reger, M., Welsh, R., Watson, G., Cholerton, B., Baker, L., & Craft, S. (2004). The relationship between neuropsychological functioning and driving ability in dementia: A meta-analysis. *Neuropsychology, 18,* 85–93.

Retchin, S., & Anapolle, J. (1993). An overview of the older driver. *Clinics in Geriatric Medicine, 9*(2), 279–296.

Reuben, D. B., Silliman, R. A., & Traines, M. (1988). The aging driver—Medicine, policy and ethics. *Journal of the American Geriatrics Society, 36*(12), 1135–1142.

Richardson, E., & Marottoli, R. (2003). Visual attention and driving behaviors among community-living older persons. *Journal of Gerontology, 58,* 832–836.

Roberts, W. N., & Roberts, P. (1993). Evaluation of the elderly driver with arthritis. *Clinics in Geriatric Medicine, 9*(2), 311–322.

Roenker, D. L., Cissell, G. M., Ball, K. K., Wadley, V. G., & Edwards, J. D. (2003). Speed-of-processing and driving simulator training result in improved driving performance. *Human Factors, 45,* 218–233.

Schumann, J., Flannagan, M. J., Sivak, M., & Traube, E. C. (1997). Daytime veiling glare and driver visual performance: Influence of windshield rake angle and dashboard reflectance. *Journal of Safety Research, 28*(3), 133–146.

Shipp, M. D. (1998). Potential human and economic cost-savings attributable to vision testing policies for driver license renewal, 1989–1991. *Optometry and Vision Science, 75,* 103–118.

Sivak, M., Hill, C. S., Henson, D. L., Butler, B. P., Silber S. M., & Olson, P. L. (1984). Improved driving performance following perceptual training in persons with brain damage. *Archives of Physical Medicine and Rehabilitation, 65*(4), 163–167.

Sivak, M., Olson, P. L., Kewman, D. G., Won, H., & Henson, D. L. (1981). Driving and perceptual/cognitive skills: Behavioral consequences of brain damage. *Archives of Physical Medicine and Rehabilitation, 62*(10), 476–483.

Sohlberg, M. M., & Mateer, C. A. (1989). *Introduction to cognitive rehabilitation.* New York: Guilford.

Staplin, L., Gish, K. W., & Wagner, E. K. (2003). Mary-PODS revisited: Updated crash analysis and implications for screening program implementation. *Journal of Safety Research, 34,* 389–397.

Stav, W. B., Hunt, L. A., & Arbesman, M. (2006). *Occupational therapy practice guideline: Driving and community mobility for older adults.* Bethesda, MD: AOTA Press.

Stelmach, G., & Nahom, A. (1992). Cognitive-motor abilities of the elderly driver. *Human Factors, 34*(1), 53–65.

Strano, C. (1989). Effects of visual deficits on ability to drive in the traumatically brain-injured population. *Journal of Head Trauma and Rehabilitation, 4*(2), 35–43.

Strano, C. (1991). Visual perception assessment for driver potential. *Occupational Therapy Practice, 3*(1), 3–4T.

Trobe, J., Waller, P. F., Cook-Flannagan, C. A., Teshima, S. M., & Bieliauskas, L. A. (1996). Crashes and violations among drivers with Alzheimer's disease. *Archives of Neurology, 53*(5), 411–416.

Tuokko, H., & McGee, P. (2002). *Improving conditions for older adults.* University of Victoria, Canada: Center on Aging.

Underwood, M. (1992). The older driver. Clinical assessment and injury prevention. *Archives of Internal Medicine, 152*(4), 735–740.

U.S. Department of Transportation. (2003). *Safe mobility for a maturing society: Challenges and opportunities.* Washington, DC: Author.

Vollrath, M., Meilinger, T., & Krüger, H. (2002). How the presence of passengers influences the risk of a collision with another vehicle. *Accident Analysis and Prevention, 34*(5), 649–654.

Wang, C. C., Kosinski, C. J., Schwartzberg, J. G., & Shanklin, A. V. (2003). Physician's guide to assessing and counseling older drivers. Washington, DC: National Highway Traffic Safety Administration.

Warren, M. (1990). Identification of visual scanning deficits in adults after cerebrovascular accident. *American Journal of Occupational Therapy, 44*(5), 391–399.

Warren, M. (1993a). A hierarchical model for evaluation and treatment of visual perceptual dysfunction in adult acquired brain injury, part 1. *American Journal of Occupational Therapy, 47*(1), 42–54.

Warren, M. (1993b). A hierarchical model for evaluation and treatment of visual perceptual dysfunction in adult acquired brain injury, part 2. *American Journal of Occupational Therapy, 47*(1), 55–66.

Warren, M. (2006). Evaluation and treatment of visual deficits following brain injury. In L. Pedretti (Ed.), *Occupational therapy practice skills for physical dysfunction* (6th ed., pp. 532–572). St. Louis, MO: Mosby.

Weaver, J. K. (1990). *Driver Performance Test II.* Palm Harbor, FL: Advanced Driving Skills Institute.

Welford, A. T. (1984). Psychomotor performance. In C. Eisdorfer (Ed.), *Annual review of gerontology and geriatrics* (pp. 237–273). New York: Springer.

Williams, A., & Carsten, O. (1989). Driver age and crash involvement. *American Journal of Public Health, 79,* 326–327.

Zoltan, B. (1996). *Vision, perception, and cognition* (3rd ed.). Thorofare, NJ: SLACK.

Zur, A., & Schinar, D. (1998). Older people's driving habits, visual abilities, and subjective assessment of daily visual functioning. *Work, 11,* 339–348.

ACKNOWLEDGMENT

The authors wish to thank Aaron Zinck for assisting with the Driving as an Occupation model graphic, and Steven Mitchell for contributing the illustrations regarding occupational therapy driving evaluations.

CHAPTER 15

Interactions and Relationships

Bette R. Bonder, PhD, OTR/L, FAOTA

He was wonderful to take care of . . . and [his wife] was a wonderful caregiver which also helped. She was the kind of person that would call a lot because she needed counseling or someone to re-affirm that what she was doing was okay. But also we learned from her because she did so much above and beyond the call of duty it seemed.

Alzheimer's Day-Care Center
Staff Member

OBJECTIVES

By the end of this chapter, readers will be able to:

1. Discuss the importance of social occupations in the lives of older adults.
2. Describe typical networks of older adults in terms of both family and other social interactions.
3. Discuss the concept of reciprocity.
4. Describe typical family occupations in later life.
5. Understand the dimensions of therapeutic interactions in working with elders and their families.
6. Explain external (institutional) pressures that complicate therapeutic relationships with families.
7. Describe techniques to promote family participation (e.g., ethnographic interviewing, levels of questioning).

Social interactions and occupations play a prominent role in the lives of elders. A huge body of literature discusses the importance of family and friends in promoting successful aging, quality of life, and well-being (Connidis, 2001). To be effective in providing services for older adults, it is essential to understand the diversity of social networks and families that include older adults, both in terms of structure and occupations. Factors associated with positive social interaction in later life include long-standing good relationships with family and friends (Krause, 2006), ability to engage in reciprocal interaction (Davey & Eggebeen, 1998), sense of spirituality (Krause, 2003), and established intergenerational networks (Hamilton et al., 1999).

It is clear that elders with strong social networks age best, but it is also clear that they face a number of challenges in maintaining satisfying relationships and coping with the inevitable changes wrought by the aging process. Friends and family move away or die. Elders become more limited in the abilities required to sustain relationships, including community mobility that facilitates interaction, hearing required to communicate effectively, and cultural stereotypes about aging that may affect both their own self-concepts and the perceptions of others. Further, social and family dynamics change not only because of events within individual families, but also because of societal changes (Connidis, 2001). Increased mobility means that adult children may live far away. Financial limitations that result from policy and pension changes may lead to reduced opportunities for interaction.

There are many misconceptions about the relationships between older adults and younger people (Cantor, 2000). **Dependency ratios** (i.e., the number of older people dependent on younger adults) are often used as a way to indicate who provides help and who receives it. Some projections indicate that as the population ages, the dependency ratio will grow. This assumes, however, that everyone older than 65 years of age is dependent, an assumption that is patently false. In fact, as noted in Chapter 1, individuals now reaching their later years are healthier and more functional than those who preceded them (Velkoff, He, Sengupta, & DeBarros, 2006). If this trend continues, the dynamics of family interactions will also continue to change.

An example of this misunderstanding is a misperception many hold about demographics of nursing home use. Many people believe that most older people as they grow frail are cared for in nursing homes. In reality, the majority of care for older people (70% to 80%) is provided in the community by family members (Tennstedt, 1999). Only 4% to 5% of older adults are in nursing homes at any given time. In addition, older adults provide considerable reciprocal care for younger generations, in terms of

financial, emotional, and instrumental support (Bonder, 2006).

The importance of family to all generations is reflected in the many descriptions and studies of family dynamics (Cantor, 2000; Connidis, 2001). However, there is a temptation for health care providers and researchers to focus on caregiving, usually framed in terms of care received by the older adult and provided by adult children or spouses (Miller & Lawton, 1997). Although at some point in the life cycle elderly persons may require care as a result of growing dependency, they also provide care for each other and for younger generations (Cantor, 2000). And although demographically many middle-aged individuals are "caught in the middle," in point of fact, relatively few are providing active care for their older family members at any given time (Brody, 2004).

The issue of intergenerational relations is crucial, given the tendency of the popular press to focus on intergenerational tensions (Connidis, 2001). Bengtson and colleagues (1996) noted that there is considerable evidence that the idea of intergenerational conflict is overblown; the vast literature on caregiver stress and burden may contribute to this misconception. Miller and Lawton (1997) called for a more balanced picture of caregiving that emphasizes both positive and negative aspects. Family members who provide care may find their contributions to the well-being of elders to be emotionally satisfying as this provides an opportunity for more balance in relationships (Connidis, 2001).

An emerging body of literature has begun to describe in detail the reverse caregiving that is increasingly common. Throughout history, grandparents have had responsibility for looking after young children in their families (Cole, 1992). A recent survey profiling grandparent involvement with grandchildren found that 6.8% of grandparents were serving as extensive caregivers (including custodial care), 23.3% were occasional caregivers, and 24.2% were "intermediate" caregivers (Fuller-Thompson & Minkler, 2001). There is growing recognition of the importance of this role, and the contribution it makes to the functioning of the family (Falk & Falk, 2002; Musil, Warner, Zauszniewski, Jeanblanc, & Kercher, 2006).

Because social interaction generally, and family in particular, is so central to older adults, effective care can be provided only when social interactions and their dynamics are well understood. This chapter considers first the research on social and family constellations and occupations in later life. It then considers strategies for helping elders sustain or build effective social networks with friends, neighbors, and, especially, families, when supportive care becomes necessary.

Building and Sustaining Social Relationships

Social networks are vital in later life. Adequate social support is important to avoiding depression (Okun & Keith, 1998) and loneliness (Koropeckyj-Cox, 1998), assistance with instrumental needs (Stoller, 1998), sustaining a sense of connection through the ability to provide reciprocal support (Litwin, 1998), and personal control (Bisconti & Bergeman, 1999). Elders who have strong social networks also enjoy better health (Bisconti & Bergeman, 1999) and are less likely to experience cognitive decline (Holtzman et al., 2004). Social networks are associated with lower rates of functional decline (Taylor & Lynch, 2004; Unger, McAvay, Bruc, Berkman, & Seeman, 1999). Social relationships can ameliorate some of the negative effects of low socioeconomic status, even though there is evidence that individuals from lower socioeconomic circumstances have somewhat smaller networks than better-educated and more affluent individuals (Ajrouch, Blandon, & Antonucci, 2005).

Social networks vary by age, as well as by socioeconomic status (SES) (Ajrouch et al., 2005). As people grow older, their social networks shrink, and their interactions with friends and families shift. It is important to keep in mind, though, that elders not only lose relationships, but also forge new ones over time

(van Tilburg, 1998). In particular, elders report the importance of intergenerational social relationships (Hamilton et al., 1999). Having younger friends and neighbors helps ensure that one's network is sustained in spite of death of peers. The Convoy Model of social engagement (Antonucci & Akiyama, 1987) suggests that over time, roles of various individuals in the network will shift so that at the beginning of late life, elders may provide more care than younger adults, while as the elders age, the balance shifts.

Litwin (2001) described a model including five network types: diverse, friends, neighbors, family, and restricted (Table 15-1). Diverse networks reflect the widest array of relationships among friends, family, and neighbors and are associated with high morale, as are friends networks. Individuals who have exclusively family networks or restricted networks have the lowest morale. These findings support the importance for elders of establishing a variety of relationships.

Social networks are important both because of the support they can provide for the elder and because of the opportunities they afford for elders to help others (Krause & Shaw, 2000). Such opportunities contribute to elders' self-esteem. This mutuality or reciprocity is an important component of social occupations both with family members and with other social contacts (Greenberg, 1994; Silverstein, Conroy, Wang, Giarrusso, & Bengtson, 2002), a finding that is consistent across cultures (Becker, Beyene, Newson, & Mayen, 2003).

In contrast, some social interaction can have negative consequences (Ingersoll-Dayton, Morgan, & Antonucci, 1997; Rook, 1997). Elders whose social exchanges are dysfunctional or problematic can experience resultant negative affect. However, the absence of social networks is likely to be more problematic, as loneliness can be a significant problem for elders who

---

TABLE 15-1 **Family Network Typology**

Diverse: Social network includes a wide array of individuals with varying relationships to the individual.
Friends: Social network includes primarily of unrelated friends.
Neighbors: Social network includes primarily of unrelated individuals living in close proximity.
Family: Social network includes primarily of related individuals (blood relations, in-laws)
Restricted: Social network is limited, without relationships to friends, neighbors, or family.

Source: Litwin (2001).

never had strong social ties or whose networks diminish substantially in later life (Fees, Martin, & Poon, 1999). Lone men tend to have the greatest difficulty in building social networks (Davidson, 2004). For these elders, physical health is likely to deteriorate as is mental health and sense of well-being.

Building and sustaining social relationships require a number of skills that hopefully have been acquired over the life course. However, late life presents unique challenges, particularly in terms of ongoing loss. Elders may find themselves constantly mourning deaths of friends and neighbors and may lose not only emotional support but also specific instrumental assistance that enabled them to live in familiar and desired settings. As will be discussed later in this chapter, interventions to assist elders in adding to their social networks as they cope with loss can be a meaningful and sometimes vital contribution of occupational therapy.

Family Occupations

For most older adults, family is at the center of the social network. There is no question that elders look to family for a variety of important purposes (Bonder, 2006). They value opportunities to pass along a legacy, to enjoy time together, and to continue to feel valued and useful. At the same time, they tend to look first to family at times when they need support, either emotional or instrumental. Family relationships in later life are affected by individual histories with family, gender, cultural values, and many other factors. Positive family relationships convey many benefits to elders and to their younger family members, including better health, including mental health (Davey & Eggebeen, 1998), subjective well-being, and enhanced function.

On the other hand, not all family interactions are positive, and in some circumstances, family can be a source of considerable stress and burden. Krause and Rook (2003) found that unpleasant family and interpersonal interaction is quite stable over long periods of time. Not all researchers agree. Some believe that it is possible to change family dynamics later in life (Akiyama, Antonucci, Takahashi, & Langfahl, 2003). If true, this may be relevant in health care settings where the goal is to improve function. The differing findings may be the result of different strategies for examining family dynamics, as Fingerman and Birditt (2003) found that elders are more likely than younger individuals to perceive interactions as positive. Thus, it is possible that adult children are dissatisfied with family interactions that elders find acceptable or even good.

Gender differences in roles and experiences are important issues for aging families (Carstensen, 2001). These differences can be seen both in family interaction where the elder is giving to others, and in interactions where they are in need of support. Over their life span, women tend to experience more personal disability and need more personal assistance than their male counterparts (Brody, 2004). They are also more likely to be sole caregivers for spouses, grandchildren, and other family members and less likely to hire assistants to help with these tasks. Although role flexibility has increased in the United States, women still experience considerable role strain and conflict as they juggle responsibilities as workers, parents, and caregivers for their own parents. To some extent, the women's movement and the increased likelihood that women will be in the workforce have complicated these tasks. As women's roles continue to evolve, it will be important to continue the process of identifying emerging concerns.

Other social issues change the nature of family interactions and social support. The growth of new family constellations including "stepfamilies" has increased the complexity of family dynamics (Ganong & Coleman, 2006). Even though some of these relationships may be of relatively long duration, it is increasingly common for elders to marry or remarry, introducing new relationships to the family late in life. Initial research suggests that adult children may not be as available to support these newcomers. Another trend that alters family dynamics is the increase in cohabitation among older adults (Brown, Lee, & Bulanda, 2006). Some elders choose this option because of policy limitations on pension funds from a previous marriage if a remarriage takes place. Others do so because they worry about the estate implications of a remarriage. Adult children and other family members may be uncomfortable or even hostile about the arrangement.

Cultural and ethnic backgrounds also affect family dynamics and expectations (Mahoney,

Cloutterbuck, Neary, & Zahn, 2005). There are differences among cultural groups in terms of the experience of aging (McIntosh & Danigellis, 1995), assistance received (Norgard & Rodgers, 1997), and the experience of caregiving (Aranda & Knight, 1997; Fingerman, 1996). So, for example, among Asian Indian families, daughters are expected to provide care for aging parents. This expectation may be disappointed if the daughter has moved to the United States and become acculturated to the lower expectation for supporting elders that typifies mainstream U.S. culture.

Culture and Family

Family expectations differ considerably in different cultures and countries. For example, the norm in the United States is to have nuclear families co-reside, with elders living elsewhere, sometimes even at considerable distance. In contrast, in Maya villages in Highland Guatemala, I observed extended families living together in homes that are expanded to accommodate multiple generations. Elders in these settings have responsibility for assisting with child care and household tasks for as long as they are physically able to do so. When they become unable to contribute, their adult children and grandchildren provide the care they need.

Draper (Draper & Keith, 1992) has studied the circumstances of older adults in two tribes in Botswana, the !Kung and the Herero. She found that among the !Kung, everyone able to do so was expected to make instrumental contributions to society (Draper, 1976). The relative poverty of the tribe, and the low birthrate, meant that elders could not count on support from younger individuals, and they could not stop helping with the many tasks required to sustain the community, including farming activities, household upkeep, child care, and so on. The Herero were more affluent, and elders in this community typically assumed more ceremonial roles. The availability of more resources meant that elders could expect more assistance from others.

The belief that many Asian cultures revere elders is accurate historically (Sung, 2000). However, current social trends have diminished the respect and the support afforded by family members to these individuals. In Scandinavia, by contrast, the existence of a social welfare system has reduced the extent to which family members may feel responsible for caring for family members (Lin, 2005).

Although most of the information in this chapter focuses on families in the United States, it is important to remember that in other places, family values may differ. And in a country that is as diverse as the United States, significant differences can be seen from community to community and among various culturally defined groups.

Family Constellations

Among the relationships that must be considered for older adults are spousal units, siblings, **nuclear families** including adult children and grandchildren, **extended family** (nieces, cousins, aunts), and **fictive kin** (neighbors and friends who have both instrumental and emotional relationships with the individual) (Cantor, 2000; C.L. Fry, 2004). In some cultures, family may include honorary members with particular roles—godparent, for example. Each of these relationships has unique characteristics and the potential to provide support to all the individuals involved. Each of these relation-ships is also fluid, with individuals intermittently providing and requiring assistance and emotional support.

In addition, family structures are not static. New people enter families through marriage, birth, and expanding networks of friends. Contrary to some stereotypes, many older adults take on new activities and expand their social groups. As noted above, this can include remarriage or cohabitation. On the other hand, people die, divorce, and drop out of sight. Such losses are characteristic of the family lives of elders and can be quite stressful for the individual. On the other hand, as grief over a loss is managed, memories of family members (**family of origin**) can become an important source of comfort.

Growing older does not alter long-standing family interactions (Connidis, 2001). Families that were characterized by close relationships will continue to have such interaction, even when they are geographically distant (Climo, 1992). Family members may call or write

TABLE 15-2 Family Relationships

Nuclear: Parents and their children
Extended: All relatives, including grandparents, siblings, nieces and nephews, in-laws, and so on
Fictive: Individuals who assume family-like interactions by choice, through long-standing friendships and other
   close interaction
Family of origin: One's parents, siblings, and other older relatives, living and dead

frequently, visit often, and incorporate into their lives memories of or allusions to family far away. In families in which conflict has been long-standing or interpersonal relationships strained, these difficulties will persist and will characterize family relationships in later life as well, unless active steps are taken by at least one family member to resolve them (Clarke, Preston, Raksin, & Bengtson, 1999) (Table 15-2 summarizes family structures).

A number of societal trends are changing family constellations in ways that affect the extent to which elders can rely on family support and can engage in meaningful reciprocal occupations (Velkoff et al., 2006). One significant factor is the increase in the divorce rate over the past several decades. Because spouses are typically the first family members to whom individuals look for support, the fact that elders (most often women) may find themselves divorced in later life can have profound impact.

Another societal trend that affects late-life family interactions is the reduction in family size. The current generation of elders often had three or more children, but the more typical pattern for the baby boom generation is one or two children. This will result in fewer adult children being available to provide care. Of course, this also means fewer adult children and grandchildren to whom elders may be responsible. As was noted in Chapter 1, the impact of these kinds of societal trends is difficult to ascertain, because many factors interact. The reduced availability of adult children to provide care may well be counterbalanced by the increased physical health and reduced disability of the generation about to enter later life.

The increasing geographic mobility of individuals and families has significant consequences for family interactions. Older adults may migrate to more moderate climates or may choose to live in two places (e.g., "snowbirds"). Some elders also migrate back to their original places of residence when it becomes necessary to secure instrumental support, because families are so often seen as the first resort when such care is needed. Adult children also move, as educational and work opportunities require. Thus, families may be quite far-flung, and whatever geographic realities are true at a given point in time may change.

Family Occupations

In the United States, elders engage in a wide array of occupations with their families (Bonder, 2006). These incorporate most performance areas of occupation as well as the patterns in which these occupations are clustered. In all of these occupations, there is the potential for exchange and reciprocity. So, for example, in the area of activities of daily living, elders might help their grandchildren learn to manage self-care. This older adult might need assistance washing his or her hair, or cutting toenails, with an adult child (most often a daughter or daughter-in-law) providing this help. In the area of instrumental activities of daily living, elders might need to rely on adult children for transportation or to manage home maintenance. The same elder might teach an adult child to cook a favorite family recipe. Shopping together might be considered an instrumental activity of daily living, or might be a leisure outing for both the elder and his or her family members.

In the area of education, a grandparent might be pressed into service helping a grandchild do homework, or an adult child might be pressed into service to help an elder decipher health materials provided by a physician. Here, too, leisure opportunities may also be present. Many travel companies now offer family trips that incorporate an element of education. Grandparent/grandchild trips are increasingly popular.

Play and leisure occupations are common among families. Spending time together engaged in pleasurable activities is a frequently identified aspect of family that is mentioned by family members of every generation. Going to movies, traveling, playing games with grandchildren, and sharing holiday meals are all areas of occupational performance that are often shared. And these performance areas offer many opportunities for reciprocity, as the elder may host a gathering or may be invited to join children and grandchildren on an outing.

Social participation is an aspect of all these occupations, and it is one of the most salient elements of family engagement for every generation. As adults grow older, their social circle almost inevitably constricts (Connidis, 2001) with the loss of spouse, siblings, and friends. Thus, interaction with younger family members becomes particularly important. But here, too, there is the opportunity for reciprocity, as children and grandchildren may benefit from the wisdom and experience of their older family members. Adult children often enjoy spending time with their parents, and grandparent/grandchild ties can be highly valued (Reitzes & Mutran, 2004a). Grandparenting takes on different character in different cultures (Weibel-Orlando, 2000; Williams, 1998). In Native American families, an important role for grandparents is as a "ceremonial grandparent" (Weibel-Orlando, 2001), while in Mexican American families, the grandparent may label himself or herself a "provider" rather than a grandparent (Williams, 1998).

Many of these occupations carry elements of habits and routines (Silverstein, 2006). For every generation, there may well be important family traditions that provide emotional comfort and an element of predictability and safety in an unpredictable world. Family gatherings for holidays, for example, are frequently treasured by family members of every generation. Even family disagreements may carry an element of tradition. So, a holiday spent together, complete with family friction, can be deeply meaningful to each generation.

Family occupations require shifting roles over time. Becoming a grandparent, a caregiver, or a widow all convey particular meanings.

Some of these roles must be learned through experimentation or observation. The observational aspect of this learning may reflect family members long dead, as new grandparents remember their own grandparents and the ways in which they interacted.

The reciprocal nature of family interactions in the United States and in other countries needs emphasis (Legge & O'Loughlin, 2000; Ong & Phillips, 2003). Elders provide finances as well as an array of support services to their adult children, grandchildren, and extended family. It is not unusual to find that family members of several generations enjoy social interaction (Bonder, 2006; Fingerman, 2000) and other pleasurable activities together. Immigrant families may have particularly strong family ties, and traditional models of intergenerational support (Usita, 2001; Usita & Bleszner, 2002).

Although family occupations can readily be seen to provide opportunities for reciprocity, they may not always be symmetrical, and they almost certainly change over time (Cantor, 2000). Life course theory suggests that depending on the time of life and the particular needs of individuals, there will be an ebb and flow to reciprocity. As described above, Antonucci and Akiyama (1987) described this as the Convoy Model. A young-old individual might provide child care for grandchildren and financial support to adult children, but an individual in the oldest-old group might need care from adult children. Life events such as parental retirement (Szinovacz & Davey, 2001) or an adult child's decision to cohabit with a partner (Eggebeen, 2005) may affect opportunities for reciprocity. It would be a mistake to assume, however, that the oldest-old are not able to provide some service to their younger family members. Even elders who are quite frail may convey wisdom, comfort, or financial support to their children or grandchildren.

In modern times, a wide array of new family constellations has arisen. Some individuals have chosen to raise children outside of marriage (R.W. Johnson & Favreault, 2004), a decision that can have long-term negative consequences for financial stability. Some individuals never have children, sometimes by choice, sometimes not (Wu & Pollard, 1998). Individuals who do not have family to provide support must look to neighbors, friends, and social service agencies. Overall, they do find support, typically involving exchange within their social networks. Family also includes siblings, and elders may have positive social relationships with siblings and may be called upon to provide care (Mathews & Heidorn, 1998).

Some older adults do not have adequate support from family (Connidis, 2001). Adult children, if any, may be at an emotional or geographic distance. The older individual may live in Florida, whereas siblings and grown children live in Nebraska. Elders may be responsible for grandchildren or for their own elderly siblings. Much of the literature about aging families has provided a somewhat polarized picture of the situation of aging. On one hand is a picture of older adults with extended families, wherein a presumption is made about the availability of social and instrumental supports; on the other hand is an image of older adults living alone in situations of isolation. These are, in fact, only endpoints on a continuum. Many moderating factors related to the individual, his or her culture, societal conditions, and other factors affect the experience of aging.

Spousal Relationships and Widowhood

One of the most important social relationships in later life is that with one's spouse. The vast majority of today's cohort of elders is or has been married. Spousal relationships provide companionship and emotional and instrumental support (Szinovacz & Davey, 2004) and can be extremely rewarding in later life. Marriage is associated with better health (Schone & Weinick, 1998) and less loneliness and depression (Bookwala & Jacobs, 2004; Pinquart, 2003). Of course, not all marriages are created equal, and where long-standing problems exist, they are not likely to disappear in later life. Divorce is not unheard of late in life (Avison & Davies, 2005; Cummings, 2005) and brings its own stresses. For women, these stresses can be financial as well as emotional. In addition, some developmental changes, retirement, for example, can lead to challenges in establishing new patterns in relationships. A nonworking spouse may struggle to adjust to having a retired spouse at home and (potentially) underfoot.

Without doubt, however, the greatest challenge in the marital relationship is death of a spouse. The initial adjustment is fraught with difficulty (Williams, 2004). For both men and women, the loss of companionship and instrumental support can be devastating, at least initially. For women, the adjustment may be compounded by loss of financial resources, because in the current cohort of elders, women are unlikely to have pensions of their own (McGarry & Schoeni, 2005). During the initial adjustment, newly widowed individuals report poor health and swings in emotional well-being (Bisconti, Bergeman, & Boker, 2004). It is important for care providers to realize that the duration of the adjustment is highly variable, often taking a year or more.

Several factors predict adjustment and long-term well-being (P.S. Fry, 2001a, 2001b). Widowers have greater difficulty than widows. However, for women and men, higher socioeconomic status, religious and spiritual resources, and social resources are important in ensuring adaptation. High initial distress is associated with worse adjustment (Boerner, Wortman, & Bonanno, 2005). The quality of the marital relationship does not predict the extent of initial grief or long-term adjustment (Carr et al., 2000), reinforcing the finding that problematic relationships can be better than none for some individuals.

The choice about whether to remarry carries its own unique challenges (Davidson, 2001; Davidson, 2002). In most developed countries, women are less likely to remarry as a result of demographic realities. In addition, women are more likely to eventually adjust to being alone, and may find pleasure in a newfound freedom. Men, in contrast, are very likely to remarry relatively quickly, both because of social pressures and their own wish to have a companion and helper.

Grandparenting

As was briefly discussed above, grandparenting is a unique family role for older adults. Ninety-four percent of elders become grandparents (Szinovacz, 1998). There is no question that it is a role that has great importance in the lives of elders and that this occupation may encourage well-being (Reitzes & Mutran, 2004a). Grandparenting takes many forms (Kettmann, 2000), offering opportunities for meaningful leisure and enjoyable interaction. Grandparents may take children on outings or travel with them or may enjoy playing with them and telling stories (Bonder, 2006).

In many families, grandparenting involves providing a direct service through child-care activities. This may be infrequent, as in the case of one woman who looked after her grandchildren when they had snow days at school (Bonder, 2006). Or the grandparent may provide child care on a regular basis while adult children are at work.

The most intensive grandparenting comes in those cases where the grandparent is raising the grandchildren (Minkler & Fuller-Thomson, 2005). Well over two million grandparents in the United States are primary caregivers for grandchildren. This includes almost 10% of African American grandparents, 6% of Hispanic grandparents, and 4% of non-Hispanic White grandparents (Fields, 2003). These data suggest cultural differences in grandparenting expectations, and indeed such cultural differences have been identified (Burnette, 1999). Elders from minority or disadvantaged backgrounds are more likely to be custodial grandparents, and also to lack wide social networks that might provide support as they take on this role. On the other hand, minority families are more likely to co-reside, in which case family supports may be available (Pruchno, 1999). Surrogate parenting can increase depression in grandmothers and reduce opportunities for engagement in other meaningful occupations (Szinovacz, DeViney, & Atkinson, 1999). These effects are less pronounced in grandfathers. There is some evidence that the stresses and rewards of this kind of grandparenting are consistent across cultural groups (Pruchno & McKenney, 2002). Occupational therapy intervention may provide mechanisms for building skills for custodial grandparents whose own parenting skills may be somewhat out of date.

There is little training for custodial grandparents, and often the arrangement is the result of serious family problems such as death or disability of adult children. Custodial grandparenting carries both costs and benefits (Hayslip & Kaminski, 2005). The costs include financial demands, isolation from peers, and role overload. These problems are compensated for by the rewards, which include closeness with grandchildren and a sense of purpose.

The meaning of grandparenting varies by gender and by expectation (Somary & Stricker, 1998). In general, women are more likely to expect to have warm relationships with grandchildren and to find that the relationships meet this expectation. They find the role more satisfying overall than grandfathers. On the other hand, grandfathers feel more able to offer advice about parenting. Both grandfathers and grandmothers typically enjoy the role. The sense of self-efficacy conveyed through grandparenting also varies somewhat (King & Elder, 1998). Individuals whose own relationships with grandparents were warm, who attend church, and who have strong bonds with their adult children feel the best able to be effective grandparents. Overall, grandparenting is associated with a sense of well-being (Reitzes & Mutran, 2004a), although clearly in families already struggling with dysfunction, these relationships may be problematic as well.

Special Circumstances

One issue is what happens in the lives of gay elders who are less likely than others to have children. For these individuals, family networks include extended family and fictive kin (C. L. Johnson, 1999). As is true for other childless individuals (Koropeckyj-Cox, 1998), there is an increased risk of loneliness and depression. However, childlessness is not necessarily a cause of isolation or sadness. Perhaps a more important issue is the presence or absence of a long-term partner, as gay individuals are affected by absence or loss of a partner in much the same way as other individuals who become widowed.

Another unique concern is present in families with adult children with developmental disabilities (Decker & Hull, 2005; Evenhuis, Henderson, Beange, Lennox, & Chicoine, 2000). Elders may have ongoing responsibility for providing financial, instrumental, and emotional support for their children. They may find this to be particularly stressful if there are no extended family members they feel can be counted upon to provide support. In addition, some individuals with developmental delay start to show signs of aging, including dementia, at a younger age than is typical for others. Thus, parents who are themselves aging may have to help adult children who are dealing with the same issues (Evenhuis et al., 2000).

When Caregiving Becomes Necessary

At some point in the lives of many elders, it becomes necessary to receive support and care in managing daily life. The vast majority of this care is provided by family (C.L. Fry, 2004). This is true throughout the world (c.f., Davey et al., 2005; Lowenstein & Katz, 2000; Mahoney, Cloutterbuck, Neary, & Zahn, 2005; Sorensen & Pinquart, 2000). In fact, in the United States alone, such care has an economic value of more than $196 billion (Tennstedt, 1999). Approximately 25% of adult children are providing some care for elders. Of these, 20% have elders in co-residence; another 55% live closer than 20 minutes away. Where family is not available, fictive kin (Shippy, Cantor, & Brennan, 2004) or friends and neighbors (Barker, 2002) may step in.

An array of factors influence the experience. These include the relationship of the elder to the caregiver, such that spouses (Barrett & Lynch, 1999), sons (Campbell & Martin-Matthews, 2003), daughters (Carpenter, 2001), and children-in-law (Peters-Davis, Moss, & Pruchno, 1999) all have somewhat different characteristics. The most typical pattern is for wives and adult daughters to be at the top of the list in terms of providing care, followed by husbands, sons, and daughters-in law. Unfortunately, wives providing care may also experience greater stress in the role, perhaps because their coping styles tend to differ from those of husbands providing care (Rose-Rego, Strauss, & Smyth, 1998). Adult daughters increasingly find the caregiving role difficult, particularly if they are also in paid employment (Pavalko & Artis, 1997). It may be that women have somewhat greater expectations than men that they should be able to manage care without outside assistance (Pinquart & Sorensen, 2006).

Informal caregiving is of particular importance for occupational therapy intervention, because it is most often a new occupation that families must learn to manage. Thoughtful assistance by the therapist can reduce the stress that is so often a hallmark of this occupation (Dooley & Hinojosa, 2004; Zarit, Stephens, Townsend, & Greene, 1998) and can improve satisfaction both of the elder and the family. Elders and their families may be faced with difficult decisions about living arrangements (Bongaarts & Zimmer, 2002). There can also be significant issues about how much help is appropriate and how much is too much (Cimarolli, Reinhardt, & Horowitz, 2006). Help from an occupational therapist in evaluating the proposed environment in the context of the elder's skills can help in these decisions. In addition, an occupational therapist can help families examine realistically their own emotional and instrumental resources for providing care in alternative living arrangements. Family members may need reassurance that deciding against providing certain kinds of care does not mean they do not love the elder (Kaufman, Shim, & Russ, 2004)—allow them to be realistic in identifying their resources. These strategies for caregiving can reduce family conflict and improve decision making (Lieberman & Fisher, 1999). Discussion of strategies for assisting families is provided here.

Therapeutic Relationships

Families are complex entities, each of which has a unique set of occupational experiences together, and particular interpersonal dynamics (Connidis, 2001). Care involving families can be challenging for occupational therapists (Lawlor & Mattingly, 1998) as the multiple relationships each carry particular history and affect. To work most effectively with the family, therapists must address several issues:

- What kinds of therapeutic relationships might be developed between therapists and family members?
- What seems to be the most beneficial kind of relationship in terms of facilitating functional performance and independence in the care receiver?
- What techniques are available to the therapist to promote the best working relationship with the family member?

A therapeutic relationship is an interaction between two or more persons to promote the prevention, cure, or management of disease, ill health, and dysfunction. Hasselkus (1994) notes that therapists are expected to establish therapeutic relationships with their clients to promote optimum outcomes and that it is important to examine a number of questions:

- What type of "connection" actually promotes optimum occupational performance?
- What is the precise nature of the link between therapist and client that leads to health-promoting behaviors?
- When this connection is formed between a therapist and a family member as they try to promote health in a third person, is the nature of this therapeutic relationship different from that between therapist and patient?

Beliefs About Problems and Solutions

A therapeutic relationship can take many forms. (Table 15-3 summarizes the models described here.) Karuza, Zevon, Rabinowitz, and Brickman (1982) suggest that the form of the helping relationship depends on the participants' beliefs about who bears the responsibility for the source of the problem and for the solution. For example, according to Karuza, in the *medical model,* the client is not held responsible for either the cause of the problem or the solution. In other words, clients are seen as "victims," and the medical professional is there to minister to them. This is different from the *compensatory model,* in which the client is not held responsible for the cause of his or her problem but *is* responsible for the solution. In this model, the patient is viewed as the essential agent for change and is expected to find solutions to problems by learning new skills to overcome difficulties. The professional helper in this model takes a cooperative stance. Two other models are the *moral model* (client is responsible for both the cause and the solution) and the

enlightenment model (client is responsible for the problem but not for finding a solution). Karuza and associates hypothesize that different helping models are chosen by both the helpers and the clients to maximize their chances of bringing about what they believe to be the most desirable outcomes. They suggest that a formal assessment of a client's beliefs about the nature and origins of his or her illness be a part of program planning so that potential areas of conflicting beliefs between therapist and client can be identified and addressed.

A Power Continuum

From a different perspective, Arnstein (1971) depicted relationships as levels of participation that are determined by a continuum of power and control. This continuum ranges from full power by the professional (*manipulation*) to full power by the client (*citizen control*). For therapists, it is useful to be aware of and to reflect on the power balance in relationships with clients. If a client's participation in therapy is limited to being informed or even being consulted, this indicates an authoritarian approach to treatment and very little power on the client's part. Is such a relationship really what we want if our ultimate goal is to foster increased independent performance in activities of daily living?

In their discussion of power in the medical encounter, Bloom and Speedling (1981) state that dependence is reciprocal to power and that "the patient appears to be inherently dependent within the situation of doctor–patient exchanges" (p. 158). According to Marshall (1981), issues of the power balance between client and professional may be especially important in the relationship of *older* client to professional—again, because of stereotypes of dependency in old age and older people's lifelong patterns of deference to authority figures. Therapists must search their

---

TABLE 15-3 **Models of Therapeutic Relationships**

Medical model: The client is not held responsible for the cause or solution of a problem.
Compensatory model: The client is not held responsible for the cause but is held responsible for the solution.
Moral model: The client is responsible for both the cause and the solution of a problem.
Enlightenment model: The client is responsible for the problem but not the solution.

Source: Karuza et al. (1982).

own relationships to determine the extent of stereotyping influences and their level of comfort with different power balances.

Shared Cultures

A third concept of the therapeutic relationship is that of shared cultures. From sociology and anthropology comes a wealth of fascinating literature on illness as a cultural experience— for both the care provider and for the patient. There is a large body of literature examining the cultural factors that influence caregiving (Aranda & Knight, 1997; Connell & Gibson, 1997; Janevic & Connell, 2001; John, Hennessy, Dyeson, & Garrett, 2001). Among the cultural factors that may affect the experience are beliefs about the proper role of family in relation to elders, gender roles, and expectations about family interactions and about independence and dependence.

Kleinman's (1978; 1988) concept of explanatory models speaks to the issue of health and health care being embedded in social contexts and the corollary that, because the professional and the patient come from different social contexts, it follows that they also hold different explanations of the illness being addressed. The two explanations or perspectives often represent major discrepancies between the individuals— discrepancies in values, beliefs, and desired outcomes. Professionals' explanations tend to be derived from theoretical, scientific backgrounds, and laypeople tend to derive their explanatory models from their lives.

Models of Family Care

Beliefs about who is responsible for health problems and solutions can have a dramatic effect on the model of care used in the family caregiving situation (Hasselkus, 1994) These beliefs are the source of family attributes, including sense of commitment ("I feel like this is my responsibility"), guilt ("I should be more patient"), blame ("I think the stroke is because he smoked a lot and drank a lot of beer"), initiative ("I suggest things because the doctors don't know everything"), or resentment ("I feel forced into this and I really resent it"). Just as other health care decisions are based on individual experience, personality, and culture, caregiving will reflect these factors. Considerations become increasingly complex, however, as each family member brings his or her unique perspectives to the situation.

Therapists often transfer responsibility for solutions *to* family caregivers by teaching skills and therapy techniques to be carried on at home (Hasselkus, 1994). This transfer of responsibility is based on the assumption by the therapist that the family member also believes that he or she should be responsible for the solution. As any therapist who has worked with family members knows, this transfer process does not always go smoothly. For example, a family caregiver may continue to cling to the therapist as the source of all solutions, never gaining confidence to assume such responsibilities:

> *Caregiver:* The therapist will be through with her visits next week—I'll miss the service because then at least it (walking exercise) was done and it was done right. . . 'cuz there's lots of habits you can get into that are wrong and I wouldn't know, but she *does* know (Hasselkus, 1988a, 1988b, 1989)

Alternatively, a caregiver may accept responsibility from a therapist, but the end result is not entirely therapeutic. The therapist may unwittingly set up the care receiver for excessive care and dependence and the caregiver for excessive self-confinement, self-blame, fear of failure, and potential guilt, or the therapist may ignore the caregiver's competing responsibilities, setting her or him up for depression, exhaustion, and potential health problems.

In the example that follows, the therapist transferred responsibility for both a problem (falling) and solution (don't ever let him fall) to the family caregiver:

> *Caregiver:* The therapist said to never let him fall, so when he gets up, I get up . . . I don't ever want him to move without me being right there. Once, when I went outside to hang up clothes, I looked back in through the window and he was trying to walk to the bathroom. So now I don't even do that. . . . (Hasselkus, 1988a, 1988b, 1989)

In the transfer of caregiving responsibility from therapist to family caregiver, the family member emerges firmly in the role of second practitioner (Hasselkus, 1994). It is obvious that both the relinquishing of the role of responsibility for solutions by the therapist and the acceptance of this role by the family caregiver are complex processes that need to be approached thoughtfully and skillfully.

Cultural Explanations

If illness is a cultural experience for the person who is ill (Kleinman, 1988), it is also a cultural experience for the persons who are providing care. Both the professional and the family have explanatory models for the illness, and these explanations may not be compatible. If the therapist hopes to transfer skills and work in partnership with the family to facilitate occupational performance, then perspectives must be shared to reach mutually agreeable explanations for the illness and its treatment.

One dramatic example of an absence of cultural sharing occurred between a caregiver and a physical therapist. The physical therapist terminated her home visits with the husband (who was recovering from a stroke) because of "no improvement." The wife-caregiver stated, "She must have been trying to do the wrong thing. She was trying to repair that left arm, and that was impossible. All that I was interested in was getting him to move easier" (Hasselkus, 1994). Subsequently, the caregiver successfully attempted walking with her husband, first around the dining room table and later from his wheelchair into the bathroom. Neither caregiver nor therapist had shared with each other their own perspectives of the situation. The caregiver thought the therapist was trying to do something "impossible," and the therapist was unaware of the caregiver's priorities of "getting him to move easier." Nor did the therapist examine the absence of other family in this particular process. Two very different explanatory models were never exchanged.

Techniques for Practice

Therapeutic relationships with clients and their families are a means to facilitate functional performance best. In a partnership between the family caregiver and the professional, the therapeutic relationship illustrates compatible beliefs about the source of the problem and the solution, a sharing of power and control, and a sharing of perspectives. One caregiver described such a relationship with a nurse as she recounted her experiences of caring for her mother-in-law:

> *Caregiver:* She (the mother-in-law) was responsible for her own medicine when she first came home, but there would be times when she would either forget to take it or would be taking it too often. So between the nurse and me talking it over, she set up four packets of pills for her to take daily. . . . (Hasselkus, 1988a, 1988b, 1989)

The medication-taking system that was set up imposed a minimum of constraints on the occupational performance of both the caregiver and the care receiver, because the caregiver was free from the daily routine of medication management, and the care receiver was maximally responsible for her own pills. Such interactions are a desirable goal for all therapeutic relationships. There are specific methods by which such relationships can be established, as described in the following sections.

Ethnographic Interviewing

In health care situations, information solicited during interviews with clients and their families is expected to relate specifically to the purpose of intervention. This, by itself, can represent a significant challenge in which family concerns are to be incorporated. In some situations, the therapist may be under considerable pressure to deal with basic functional issues that will facilitate discharge, whereas clients and families may have very different priorities (Lawlor & Mattingly, 1998). The method used in interviewing and the information obtained should both incorporate a sense of the client's and the family's understanding of the illness experience (Bonder, Martin, & Miracle, 2002).

One technique for gathering information and gaining understanding of the illness experience of another person is ethnographic interviewing (Bonder et al., 2002). This is an anthropological technique that can be adapted without difficulty for use in health care. With a family caregiver, ethnographic interviewing can be used to understand the caregiver's point of view and the beliefs about the illness experience that are used to organize his or her caregiving behaviors, to help the therapist understand the family caregiver's explanatory model. Table 15-4 provides an overview of ethnographic interviewing techniques.

Ethnographic interviewing starts with very global, open-ended questions, such as "Can you start by telling me what your day is like?" or "Could we sit down and talk about what kinds of things you do during the day to take care of your husband?" As the family member starts to describe her or his day, the therapist makes note of topics that may warrant more discussion and seeks greater detail about the caregiving experience, probing into topics that have been mentioned. The therapist also pays special attention to the words that the caregiver uses to describe the situation and uses the caregiver's terms in asking further questions. The following excerpt from an ethnographic interview with a family caregiver (Hasselkus, 1994) illustrates many of these techniques:

> *Interviewer:* Maybe you could start by just telling me a little about how you and your husband spend a typical day.
>
> *Caregiver:* Well, sometimes I have to get up through the night. He kicks all the covers off, no matter how well I make the bed. That one leg is good, see, and he can kick, he can clear the bed, and he'll say, "Maw," and then I have to remake the bed, sometimes two times a night. Last night it was good, he was quiet.
>
> *Interviewer:* But usually you're up some time?
>
> *Caregiver:* Ya, I'm mostly up some time. And, well, on Monday and Tuesdays, he goes to the (adult day center). I asked them to take him for two days so I could have a little time away from him, you know? . . . then on Wednesday, I have a lady come in from the visiting nurse service and she gives him a bath . . . and then on other days, I come out and get dressed and brush my teeth and comb my hair and start breakfast, and then I get him up, bring him out here, wash him.
>
> *Interviewer:* Okay, when you say, "get him up," what does that involve?
>
> *Caregiver:* Well, I put his pants on laying down until I got them up to as far as I can go, and then I swing him off the bed and I put his stockings and shoes on and then he takes ahold of the bedpost and he holds on there while I pull up the pants and zip it and so forth. . . .

Remarkable details of everyday functional performance are evident in this brief excerpt from a 1-hour interview. Using ethnographic methods, the therapist can immediately identify several important domains of the caregiving experience—getting up at night, the day center, the visiting nurse who gives the bath, getting the client up, and the absence of other family members. The fact that the caregiver started her description of the day's activities with comments about the nighttime activity might be a clue that this is an important issue in her caregiving. The interviewer also successfully probed for more detail in her question, "when you say 'get him up,' what does that involve?" In asking this question, she also began to incorporate the caregiver's terms into the interview. This may seem to be obvious and simply common sense, but we often translate the client's language into more formalized language, perhaps without even realizing it. Being "up" at night could easily be reworded into being "disturbed" or "awakened," and getting him "up" could be reworded into getting him "out of bed." A change in the words being used to describe an experience can also change the meaning of the experience. It is best to follow the words used by the caregiver. This also indirectly reassures the caregiver that what he or she is saying and the way he or she says it is fine. Because it is the *caregiver's* perspective that we hope to understand through the interview, such reassurance is vital to reaching that goal.

For more general guidelines about conducting ethnographic interviews, see Table 15-4. Spradley (1979) has written a book, *The Ethnographic Interview,* that more precisely details types of ethnographic questions and other background information on ethnography.

Levels of Questioning

According to Payton, Ozer, and Nelson (1990), to encourage the greatest possible client participation, the therapist should start with open-ended questions, thereby enabling the person to function at the level of free choice (not unlike starting with global questions in the ethnographic interview). Then, as necessary, the therapist moves down a ladder of decreasing freedom for the client, first asking questions that offer suggestions and options from which the client can choose (multiple choice), then asking questions that offer an answer or recommendation (forced choice, concurrence), and finally asking *no* question by simply telling the client what to do (no choice). At each shift to the lower level of questioning style, the therapist should ask the client's permission by saying, for instance, "Would it be all right if I made a recommendation?" Whenever possible, the therapist should revert back to the higher level of questioning in the interview, especially at the start of a new topic (Figure 15-1).

Payton and colleagues (1990) believe that these questioning techniques will lead to maximum involvement of the client in the process of defining therapeutic concerns and goals. The further down the ladder the therapist moves in questioning techniques (toward less and less freedom or choice for the client), the more the goals will be generated by the therapist rather than the client. As these authors state, "Each therapist must develop his or her own level of tolerance for personal anxiety before intervening by 'moving down the scale' in offering suggestions and thus taking a greater role for planning than may be necessary" (p. 20). The higher the level of participation of the client in the planning process, the greater will be the client's commitment and energy available for carrying out the plan.

Identifying and Negotiating Discrepancies

The preceding sections on ethnographic interviewing and levels of questioning describe practice techniques to use in gaining understanding of both the client's and the caregiver's perspectives, or explanatory models, and in promoting the

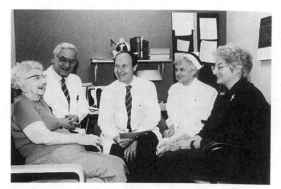

FIGURE 15-1 Clients and their caregivers should be consistently involved in the design of interventions. Here a client and her daughter meet with professional members of the health-care team. (Courtesy of the Menorah Park Nursing Home, Cleveland, Ohio, with permission.)

client's active participation in the therapeutic process. In Kleinman's (1988) model, this is the first step in the therapeutic process, and it addresses questions such as

- What do you think is wrong?
- What do you think has caused this?
- How has this affected your daily routine?
- What are your biggest fears?
- What do you think should be done?

The second step in the therapeutic process is for the therapist to explain to the caregiver the therapist's explanatory model. What does the therapist think is wrong? What does the therapist think is the cause? What does the therapist think should be done? This involves the often difficult translation of biomedical explanations into terms that are understandable to laypeople. The explanation of the therapist's perspective, if it is sensitively done, can yield for the therapist the joy of "collaborating with accurately informed patients and families who can

---

TABLE 15-4 Ethnographic Interview Techniques

1. The therapist is the *learner*; the person being interviewed is the *expert*.
2. The interview is semistructured. Start with very global questions, and then probe further based on what the person starts talking about.
3. Begin to incorporate the terms used by the client as he or she talks.
4. Repeatedly express interest in what the person is saying.
5. Be careful not to slip into the authority or expert role. Express ignorance appropriately.
6. Build in opportunities for expansion and repetition.
7. The interview should be asymmetrical with the person being interviewed doing most of the talking.

Source: Hasselkus (1990).

contribute to the therapeutic process. When it is poorly done, however, the stage is set for clinical communication to have serious problems, which can unsettle the therapeutic relationship and thereby undermine care" (Kleinman, 1988, p. 240). It is the presentation of their own perspectives and subsequent comparison to the perspectives of the caregiver that enable the therapist to identify questions and discrepancies that require further understanding.

Thus, the next step in this therapeutic process is to engage in negotiation with the client and the caregiver, actively seeking compromise in areas of differences and conflict. The therapist may assume responsibility for clarifying areas of conflict or discrepancies between views (based on the previous sharing of both explanatory models) and then lead the negotiation toward the resolution of these conflicts. The therapist must recognize and accept that resolution and compromise may be closer to the caregiver's view or it may be closer to the therapist's view—either must be possible, or it is not true negotiation. Bonder and colleagues (2002) describe this process as **mutual cultural accommodation,** a process by which all parties arrive at a compromise that preserves their most central beliefs but also supports a decision that facilitates progress.

For the therapist, there is one final step in this therapeutic process: the therapist's self-reflection on what has transpired—that is, her or his own explanatory model, the caregiver's model, the compromises, the resulting plan, and the special interests and emotions that emerged along the way (Hasselkus, 1994). As Kleinman (1988) states, such self-reflection contributes not only to the development of more therapeutic relationships but also to the therapist's own personal development.

Addressing Family Issues in the Current Health Care Environment

All too often, given current trends in health care reimbursement, the therapist is under pressure to accept a view that reflects none of these parties. Third-party payers typically require rapid termination of services and tend to assume that the family will fill the breach (Zarit,

Johansson, & Jarrott, 1998). For a variety of reasons, this may be an unrealistic assumption. Family may live far away. They may have their own families and work to tend to. They may have long-standing family tensions that interfere with the provision of required services.

Such problems are not always easily resolved, and they present significant ethical dilemmas for the practitioner. Can a client be discharged to home when family members are unable or unwilling to ensure the person's physical safety? Increasingly, negotiation with families must be complemented by negotiation with insurers about alternative services. Creative solutions must be considered, not all of which will be acceptable. For example, a family member might agree to have the client live in his or her home for a limited time, with a promise of home health care thereafter. Or the family may need to negotiate with the client about payment for services not covered by insurance. Therapists can assist families in interacting with insurers, locating alternative resources, and working toward changing unreasonable and unrealistic regulations.

On the other hand, it is easy to forget that caregiving also has benefits. Caregivers may find the role meaningful particularly when they are close to the individual (McGraw & Walker, 2004; Noonan & Tennstedt, 1997). This is particularly true when opportunities for reciprocity continue to be available (Wolff & Agree, 2004) and there are strong emotional ties between caregiver and recipient of care (McGraw & Walker, 2004).

A word about other social networks is important here. As has been discussed throughout this chapter, social interactions beyond family are highly meaningful to many individuals. In some circumstances, they provide an essential source of support when family are unwilling to do so, or when an individual has no family. Elders may struggle to build and maintain social networks as they leave jobs where social interaction was a daily part of life, as they move to new environments, or as friends of long-standing move away or die. Thus, therapists must go beyond simply looking at the family, and identify, with the client, other needs with regard to interaction. Assistance building social skills, problem solving about meeting new people, and other efforts to address social needs can be vital to successful aging.

■ Summary

Much remains to be learned about family life and social interaction in later years. The circumstances of individual older adults are complex, and their multiple relationships with family and society add to that complexity. In addition, what is understood about today's older population may not be true for older adults tomorrow, as societal and personal situations change (Velkoff et al., 2006). The relative lack of systematic understanding about older adults in the context of their families and social networks is troublesome to formal care providers and policy makers. Existing policies significantly impact services; incomplete information may contribute to misdirected rules and regulations (Moen & Forest, 1995). "At present, societal norms, institutions, and practices have not kept pace with the shifting realities of contemporary life" (p. 826). It is essential that policy be based on the best available information, and that information be expanded, enhanced, and updated as family and social circumstances change.

When health care professionals work with older adults, family issues cannot be ignored. Outcomes of treatment often reflect the effectiveness with which concerns of the whole family, not just the identified client, have been incorporated into the intervention. Therefore, interventions made by health care and social service professionals must take into account all the complex factors previously described when designing services with and for the entire family (Cantor, 2000). They must also establish effective working relationships with relevant family members. Families have considerable import in service provision for elders and represent a potential resource to reduce costs while enhancing quality of care. At the same time,

professionals must take care to remember that elders may also have important responsibilities for other family members. Families must determine how to fill the gaps caused by the older individual's illness or disability. Therapists should also remember to address goals that return the older individual to those responsibilities if they are of value to the individual and the family. Likewise, a strong extended social network can be a major source of support, especially in the absence of family.

A therapeutic relationship with a client's family can be a rich and satisfying experience for both the therapist and the family. The therapeutic relationship between therapist and family caregiver for an older person is different from that between therapist and patient. Research findings have suggested that the family caregiver tends to view himself or herself as a practitioner; it then follows that therapeutic relationships that promote partnership through sharing of control, knowledge, and cultural perspectives may best support a therapeutic alliance between therapist and family member.

The ultimate objective of occupational and physical therapy is to promote optimum performance in daily living activities. In working with families of older people in the community, an important goal is to support them in their efforts to reach, in essence, the same objective for themselves and for the person receiving the care. The relationship between therapist and family is equivalent to that between two practitioners. Our educational programs have an obligation to provide opportunities for students to experience this kind of alliance in their field practica so they may try out techniques for interviewing and negotiating care in real-life settings and clarify their own philosophies of care.

Case Study

Mrs. Jones is an 88-year-old woman whose husband died 10 years ago. Since then she has been living alone in a condominium on the second floor of a 100-unit building.
Mrs. Jones has two daughters who live within 20 minutes of her. They are both married, and each has two teenaged children. She

also has a son, an attorney, who lives at a considerable distance with his wife and three children.

Two months ago, Mrs. Jones fell on an icy sidewalk and fractured her femur. She had surgery to repair the fracture with a steel implant, and was then transferred to a nursing facility for rehabilitation. It is now time to consider discharge, because the therapists believe she has made maximal progress in their care.

Mrs. Jones wants to go back to her home; her daughters are very concerned because she is unsteady on her feet even with a walker, and she is not yet able to bathe independently or manage stairs. They are also concerned because they both work and fear that if she returns home they will be pressed into service, as she is currently far from fully independent. Her son has called the facility social worker to indicate that he expects his mother to be discharged to an assisted living facility. He has threatened legal action if his wish is not accommodated.

1. What family-related issues are evident here?

Mrs. Jones appears to value her independence, and to enjoy her previous living arrangement. It is not clear from the description what motivates her daughters. Are they concerned about their mother, or are they concerned that they might have to provide care? Or, most likely, are their motivations somewhat mixed? An added issue is the attitude of the son who lives at a distance. Family members who are not in the immediate area can have misperceptions about a situation or can feel guilty about their inability to assist. These feelings may be

expressed through unrealistic expectations about the elder, or about what is reasonable and fair to expect of those who are closer.

2. Whose values should be given precedence?

The therapist must be clear about his or her responsibility, which is most often to the elder who is receiving services. On the other hand, if family members are not comfortable with the plan, they may not participate as needed. Although it can be a challenge to do so, in ideal situations everyone reaches agreement about the plan. If this is not possible, the therapist's primary responsibility is to his or her client.

3. How might you work with the family to reach an agreement about next steps?

Family meetings can be helpful to allow everyone to express opinions. Having a skilled moderator present can ensure that participants are honest but also respectful of the feelings and needs of others. In this situation, it may be particularly important to have the son present along with the daughters, and to be sure that the precise details of Mrs. Jones' current situation and prognosis are provided. An important role for a therapist in these situations is to present information about available options and services so that Mrs. Jones and her family have the information they need to make good choices.

Review Questions

1. For elders, what kinds of occupational and emotional needs are addressed through social and family interactions?
2. Discuss the concept of reciprocity. In what ways is reciprocity important in the social interactions of elders?
3. What are some ways that elders who do not have blood relations meet family-focused occupational needs?
4. What are some important performance areas in which social and family occupations are enacted?
5. Discuss areas in which social and family interactions can be problematic in later life.
6. According to Karuza and colleagues, the form of the therapeutic relationship depends on what beliefs?
7. What is the medical model, and why is it often chosen when working with elderly clients?

continued on page 404

Review Questions (continued)

8. Describe the authoritarian model of health care and give an example. What are some of its disadvantages? Does it conflict with the goals of occupational therapy?
9. Relate the concept of responsibility for problems and solutions to the therapist–family caregiver relationship.
10. In ethnographic interviewing, the professional's use of the family caregiver's terms serves what purposes?
11. What is the difference between an illness problem list and a medical problem list?
12. According to Payton and colleagues, what type of question represents the most free choice in a client interview?
13. After the client and therapist have exchanged and shared perspectives, what is the next step in the therapeutic process?
14. How would you augment academic curricula and field practica to incorporate skills related to establishing therapeutic relationships with family members?

Web-Based Resources

www.aoa.gov/eldfam/How_To_Find/Agencies/Agencies.asp or www.n4a.org/, **Area Agencies on Aging** can be found around the United States. These organizations usually have federal and state funding, and both provide services themselves and serve as a clearinghouse for information. Accessed April 5, 2008.

www.aarp.org, **AARP.** AARP has a wealth of information both for and about families.

www.aoa.gov/prof/aoaprog/caregiver/caregiver.asp or www.aoa.gov/eldfam/eldfam.asp, **U.S. Administration on Aging.** The U.S. Administration on Aging has good information for family caregivers. Accessed April 5, 2008.

http://ethnomed.org/about/ethnoint.html, **Collecting Ethnographic Data: The Ethnographic Interview.** This website contains information about ethnographic interviewing, with an emphasis on addressing cultural factors. Accessed April 5, 2008

REFERENCES

Ajrouch, K. J., Blandon, A. Y., & Antonucci, T. C. (2005). Social networks among men and women: The effects of age and socioeconomic status. *Journal of Gerontology: Social Sciences, 60B,* S311–S317.

Akiyama, H., Antonucci, T., Takahashi, K., & Langfahl, E.S. (2003). Negative interactions in close relationships across the life span. *The Journals of Gerontology Series B: Psychological Sciences and Social Sciences, 58,* P70–P79.

Antonucci, T. C., & Akiyama, H. (1987). Social networks in adult life and a preliminary examination of the convoy model. *Journal of Gerontology, 42,* 519–527.

Aranda, M. P., & Knight, B. G. (1997). The influence of ethnicity and culture on the caregiver stress and coping process: A sociocultural review and analysis. *The Gerontologist, 37,* 342–354.

Arnstein, S. R. (1971). Eight rungs on the ladder of citizen participation. In E. S. Cahn & B. A. Passett (Eds.), *Citizen participation: Effecting community change* (pp. 69–91). New York: Praeger.

Avison, W. R., & Davies, L. (2005). Family structure, gender, and health in the context of the life course. *Journals of Gerontology: Series B, 60*(Special Issue II), 113–116.

Barker, J. C. (2002). Neighbors, friends, and other nonkin caregivers of community-living dependent elders. *Journal of Gerontology: Social Sciences, 57B,* A158–S167.

Barrett, A. E., & Lynch, S. M. (1999). Caregiving networks of elderly persons: Variation by marital status. *The Gerontologist, 39,* 695–704.

Becker, G., Beyene, Y., Newson, E., & Mayen, N. (2003). Creating continuity through mutual assistance: Intergenerational reciprocity in four ethnic groups. *Journal of Gerontology: Social Sciences, 58B,* S151–S159.

Bengtson, V., Rosenthal, C., & Burton, L. (1996). Paradoxes of families and aging. In R. H. Binstock & L. K. George (Eds.), *Handbook of aging and the social sciences* (4th ed.) (pp. 253–282). San Diego: Academic Press.

Bisconti, T. L., & Bergeman, C. S. (1999). Perceived social control as a mediator of the relationship among social support, psychological well-being, and perceived health. *The Gerontologist, 39,* 94–103.

Bisconti, T. L., Bergeman, C. S., & Boker, S. M. (2004). Emotional well-being in recently bereaved widows: A dynamical systems approach. *Journal of Gerontology: Psychological Sciences, 59B,* P158–P167.

Bloom, S., & Speedling, E. J. (1981). Strategies of power and dependence in doctor–patient exchanges. In M. Haug (Ed.), *Elderly patients and their doctors* (pp. 157–170). New York: Springer.

Boerner, K., Wortman, C. B., & Bonanno, G. A. (2005). Resilient or at risk? A 4-year study of older adults who initially showed high or low distress following conjugal loss. *Journal of Gerontology: Psychological Sciences, 60B,* P67–P73.

Bonder, B. R. (2006). Family occupations in later life. *Journal of Occupational Science, 13,* 107–116.

Bonder, B. R., Martin, L., & Miracle, A. W. (2002). *Culture in clinical care.* Thorofare, NJ: Slack.

Bongaarts, J., & Zimmer, Z. (2002). Living arrangements of older adults in the developing world: An analysis of demographic and health survey household surveys. *Journal of Gerontology: Social Sciences, 57B,* S145–S157.

Bookwala, J., & Jacobs, J. (2004). Age, marital processes, and depressed affect. *The Gerontologist, 44,* 328–338.

Brody, E. (2004). *Women in the middle: Their parent care years.* New York: Springer.

Brown, S. L., Lee, G. R., & Bulanda, J. R. (2006). Cohabitation among older adults: A national portrait. *Journal of Gerontology, 61B,* S71–S79.

Burnette, D. (1999). Social relationships of Latino grandparent caregivers: A role theory perspective. *The Gerontologist, 39,* 49–58.

Campbell, L. D., & Martin-Matthews, A. (2003). The gendered nature of men's filial care. *Journal of Gerontology: Social Sciences, 58B,* S350–S358.

Cantor, M. H. (2000). *Social care of the elderly: The effects of ethnicity, class, and culture.* New York: Springer.

Carpenter, B. D. (2001). Attachment bonds between adult daughters and their older mothers: Associations with contemporary caregiving. *Journal of Gerontology: Psychological Sciences, 56B,* P257–P266.

Carr, D., House, J. S., Kessler, R. C., Nesse, R. M., Sonnega, J., & Wortman, C. (2000). Marital quality and psychological adjustment to widowhood among older adults: A longitudinal analysis. *Journal of Gerontology: Social Sciences, 55B,* S197–S207.

Carstensen, L. L. (2001). Adult personality development. In N. J. Smelzer & P. B. Baltes (Eds.), *International encyclopedia of the social and behavioral sciences* (pp. 11290–11295). Amsterdam: Elsevier Science.

Cimarolli, V. R., Reinhardt, J. P., & Horowitz, A. (2006). Perceived overprotection: Support gone bad? *Journal of Gerontology: Social Sciences, 61B,* S18–S23.

Clarke, E. J., Preston, M., Raksin, J., & Bengtson, V. L. (1999). Types of conflicts and tensions between older parents and adult children. *The Gerontologist, 39,* 261–270.

Climo, J. (1992). *Distant parents.* New Brunswick, NJ: Rutgers University Press.

Cole, T. R. (1992). *The journey of life: A cultural history of aging in America.* Cambridge, England: Cambridge University Press.

Connell, C. M., & Gibson, G. D. (1997). Racial, ethnic, and cultural differences in dementia caregiving: Review and analysis. *The Gerontologist, 37,* 355–364.

Connidis, I. A. (2001). *Family ties and aging.* Thousand Oaks, CA: Sage.

Cummings, S. M. (2005). Widows and divorcees in later life: On their own again. *Journal of Women & Aging, 17*(1–2), 191–193.

Davey, A., & Eggebeen, D. J. (1998). Patterns of intergenerational exchange and mental health. *Journal of Gerontology: Psychological Sciences, 53B,* P86–P95.

Davey, A., Femia, E. E., Zarit, S. H., Shea, D. G., Sundström, G., Berg, S., et al. (2005). Life on the edge: Patterns of formal and informal help to older adults in the United States and Sweden. *The Journals of Gerontology Series B: Psychological Sciences and Social Sciences, 60,* S281–S288.

Davidson, K. (2001). Late life widowhood, selfishness, and new partnership choices: A gendered perspective. *Ageing and Society, 21,* 279–317.

Davidson, K. (2002). Gender differences in new partnership choices and constraints for older widows and widowers. *Ageing International, 27*(4), 43–60.

Davidson, K. (2004). "Why can't a man be more like a woman?": Marital status and social networking of older men. *Journal of Men's Studies, 13*(1), 25–43.

Decker, B., & Hull, A. H. (2005). Older adults with developmental disabilities: Encouraging participation. *OT Practice, 10*(21), CE1–CE8.

Dooley, N. R., & Hinojosa, J. (2004). Improving quality of life for persons with Alzheimer's disease and their family caregivers: Brief occupational therapy intervention. *American Journal of Occupational Therapy, 58,* 561–569.

Draper, P. (1976). Social and economic constraints on !Kung childhood. In R. B. Lee & B. I. DeVore (Eds.), *Kalahari Hunter Gatherers.* Cambridge: Harvard University Press, 200–220.

Draper, P., & Keith, J. (1992). Cultural contexts of care: Family caregiving for elderly in America and Africa. *Journal of Aging Studies, 6,* 113–133.

Eggebeen, D. (2005). Cohabitation and exchanges of support. *Social Forces, 83,* 1097–1110.

Evenhuis, H., Henderson, C. M., Beange, H., Lennox, N., & Chicoine, B. (2001). Healthy ageing—Adults with intellectual disabilities: Physical health issues. *Journal of Applied Research in Intellectual Disabilities, 14,* 175–194.

Falk, U. A., & Falk, G. (2002). *Grandparents: A new look at the supporting generation.* Amherst, NY: Prometheus Books.

Fees, B. S., Martin, P., & Poon, L. W. (1999). A model of loneliness in older adults. *Journal of Gerontology: Psychological Sciences, 54B,* P231–P239.

Fields, J. (2003). Children's living arrangements and characteristics: March, 2002. In *Current population reports* (pp. 20–547). Washington, DC: U.S. Census Bureau.

Fingerman, K. L. (1996). Sources of tension in the aging mother and adult daughter relationship. *Psychology of Aging 11,* 591–606.

Fingerman, K. L. (2000). "We had a nice little chat": Age and generational differences in mothers' and daughters' descriptions of enjoyable visits. *Journal of Gerontology: Psychological Sciences, 55B,* P95–P106.

Fingerman, K. L., & Birditt, K. S. (2003). Do age differences in close and problematic family ties reflect the pool of available relatives? *Journal of Gerontology: Psychological Sciences, 58B,* P80–P87.

Fry, C. L. (2004). Kinship and supportive environments of aging. In H. Wahl, R. J. Scheidt, & P. G. Windley (Eds.), *Annual Review of Gerontology and Geriatrics: Focus on Aging in Context: Socio-physical Environments* (pp. 313–333). New York: Springer.

Fry, P. S. (2001a). Predictors of health-related quality of life perspectives, self-esteem, and life satisfactions of older adults following spousal loss: An 18-month follow-up study of widows and widowers. *The Gerontologist, 41,* 787–798.

Fry, P. S. (2001b). The unique contribution of key existential factors to the prediction of psychological well-being of older adults following spousal loss. *The Gerontologist, 41,* 69–81.

Fuller-Thomson, E., & Minkler, M. (2001). American grandparents providing extensive child care to their grandchildren: Prevalence and profile. *The Gerontologist, 41,* 201–209.

Ganong, L., & Coleman, M. (2006). Obligations to stepparents acquired in later life: Relationship quality and acuity of needs. *Journal of Gerontology: Social Sciences, 61B,* S80–S88.

Greenberg, S. (1994). Mutuality in families: A framework for continued growth in later life. *Journal of Geriatric Psychiatry, 27,* 79–95.

Hamilton, G., Brown, S., Alonzo, T., Glover, M., Mersereau, Y., & Willson, P. (1998). Building community for the long term: An intergenerational commitment. *The Gerontologist, 39,* 235–238.

Hasselkus, B. R. (1988a). Meaning in family caregiving: Perspectives on caregiver/professional relationship. *Gerontology, 28,* 686–691.

Hasselkus, B. R. (1988b). Rehabilitation: The family caregiver's view. *Topics in Geriatric Rehabilitation, 4*(4), 60–70.

Hasselkus, B. R. (1989) The meaning of daily activity in family caregiving for the elderly. *American Journal of Occupational Therapy, 43,* 649–656.

Hasselkus, B. R. (1990). Ethnographic interviewing: A tool for practice with family caregivers for the elderly. *Occupational Therapy Practice, 2,* 9–11.

Hasselkus, B. R. (1994). Professionals and informal care givers: The therapeutic alliance. In B. R. Bonder & M. B. Wagner (Eds.), *Functional performance in older adults* (pp. 339–351). Philadelphia: F.A. Davis.

Hayslip, B., Jr., & Kaminski, P. L. (2005). Grandparents raising their grandchildren: A review of the literature and suggestions for practice. *The Gerontologist, 45,* 262–269.

Holtzman, R. E., Rebok, G. W., Saczynski, J. S., Kouzis, A. C., Doyle, K. W., & Eaton, W. W. (2004). *Journal of Gerontology: Psychological Sciences, 59B,* P278–P284.

Ingersoll-Dayton, B., Morgan, D., & Antonucci, T. (1997). The effects of positive and negative social exchanges on aging adults. *Journal of Gerontology: Social Sciences, 52B,* S190–S199.

Janevic, M. R., & Connell, C. M. (2001). Racial, ethnic, and cultural differences in the dementia caregiving experience: Recent findings. *The Gerontologist, 41,* 334–347.

John, R., Hennessy, C. H., Dyeson, T. B., & Garrett, M. D. (2001). Toward the conceptualization and measurement of caregiver burden among Pueblo Indian family caregivers. *The Gerontologist, 41,* 210–219.

Johnson, C. L. (1999). Fictive kin among oldest old African Americans in the San Francisco Bay area. *Journal of Gerontology: Social Sciences, 54B,* S368–S375.

Johnson, R. W., & Favreault, M. M. (2004). Economic status in later life among women who raised children outside of marriage. *Journal of Gerontology: Social Sciences, 59B,* S315–S323.

Karuza, J., Zevon, M. A., Rabinowitz, V. C., & Brickman, P. (1982). Attribution of responsibility by helpers and recipients. In T. A. Wills (Ed.), *Basic processes in helping relationships* pp. 107–129. New York: Academic Press.

Kaufman, S. R., Shim, J. K., & Russ, A. J. (2004). Revisiting the biomedicalization of aging: Clinical trends and ethical challenges. *The Gerontologist, 44,* 731–738.

Kettermann, S. (2000). *The 12 rules of grandparenting: A new look at traditional roles and how to break them.* New York: Facts on File.

King, V., & Elder, G. H., Jr. (1998). Perceived self-efficacy and grandparenting. *Journal of Gerontology: Social Sciences, 53B,* S249–S257.

Kleinman, A. (1978). Culture, illness and cure: Clinical lessons from anthropologic and cross-cultural research. *Annals of Internal Medicine, 88,* 251–258.

Kleinman, A. (1988). *The illness narratives.* New York: Basic Books.

Koropeckyj-Cox, T. (1998). Loneliness and depression in middle and old age: Are the childless more vulnerable? *Journal of Gerontology: Social Sciences, 53B,* S303–S312.

Krause, N. (2003). Religious meaning and subjective well-being in late life. *Journal of Gerontology: Social Sciences, 58B,* S160–S170.

Krause, N. (2006). Social relationships in late life. In R. H. Binstock & L. K. George (Eds.), *Handbook of aging and the social sciences* (6th ed.) (pp. 181–200). Burlington, MA: Elsevier.

Krause, N., & Rook, K. S. (2003). Negative interaction in late life: Issues in the stability and generalizability of conflict across relationship. *Journal of Gerontology: Psychological Sciences, 58B,* P88–P99.

Krause, N., & Shaw, B. A. (2000). Giving social support to others, socioeconomic status, and changes in self-esteem in late life. *Journal of Gerontology: Social Sciences, 55B,* S323–S333.

Lawlor, M. C., & Mattingly, C. F. (1998). The complexities embedded in family-centered care. *American Journal of Occupational Therapy, 52,* 259–267.

Legge, V., & O'Loughlin, K. (2000). The balance of benefit: A review of intergenerational transfers in Australia. *The Gerontologist, 40,* 605–611.

Lieberman, M. A., & Fisher, L. (1999). The effects of family conflict resolution and decision making on the provision of help for an elder with Alzheimer's disease. *The Gerontologist, 39,* 159–166.

Lin, K. (2005). Cultural traditions and the Scandinavian social policy model. *Social Policy Administration, 39,* 723–730.

Litwin, H. (1998). The provision of informal support by elderly people residing in assisted living facilities. *The Gerontologist, 38,* 239–246.

Litwin, H. (2001). Social network type and morale in old age. *The Gerontologist, 41,* 516-524.

Lowenstein, A., & Katz, R. (2000). Rural Arab families coping with caregiving. *Marriage & Family Review, 50*(1–2), 179–197.

Mahoney, D. F., Cloutterbuck, J., Neary, S., & Zhan, L. (2005). African American, Chinese, and Latino family caregivers' impressions of the onset and diagnosis of dementia: Cross-cultural similarities and differences. *The Gerontologist, 45,* 783–792.

Marshall, V. W. (1981). Physician characteristics and relationships with their older patients. In M. Haug (Ed.), *Elderly patients and their doctors* (pp. 94–118). New York: Springer.

Matthews, S. H., & Heidorn, J. (1998). Meeting filial responsibilities in brothers-only sibling groups. *Journal of Gerontology: Social Sciences, 53B,* S278–S286.

McGarry, K., & Schoeni, R. F. (2005). Widow(er) poverty and out-of-pocket medical expenditures near the end of life. *Journal of Gerontology: Social Sciences, 60B,* S160–S168.

McGraw, L. A., & Walker, A. J. (2004). Negotiating care: Ties between aging mothers and their caregiving daughters. *Journal of Gerontology: Social Sciences, 59B,* S324–S332.

McIntosh, B. R., & Danigelis, N. L. (1995). Race, gender, and the relevance of productive activity for elders' affect. *Journal of Gerontology Social Sciences, 50B,* S229–239.

Miller, B., & Lawton, M. P. (1997). Introduction: Finding balance in caregiver research. *The Gerontologist, 37,* 216–217.

Minkler, M., & Fuller-Thomson, E. (2005). African American grandparents raising grandchildren: A national study using the census 2000 American Community Survey. *Journal of Gerontology: Social Sciences, 60B,* S82–S92.

Moen, P., & Forest, K. B. (1995). Family policies for an aging society: Moving to the twenty-first century. *The Gerontologist, 35,* 825–830.

Musil, C. M., Warner, C. B., Zauszniewski, J. A., Jeanblanc, A. B., & Kercher, K. (2006). Grandmothers, caregiving, and family functioning. *Journal of Gerontology: Social Sciences, 61B,* S89–S98.

Noonan, A. E., & Tennstedt, S. L. (1997). Meaning in caregiving and its contribution to caregiver well-being. *The Gerontologist, 37,* 785–794.

Norgard, T. M., & Rodgers, W. L. (1997). Patterns of in-home care among elderly black and white Americans. *Journal of Gerontology: Social Science, 52B,* S93–S101.

Okun, M. A., & Keith, V. M. (1998). Effects of positive and negative social exchanges with various sources on depressive symptoms in younger and older adults. *Journal of Gerontology: Psychological Sciences, 53B,* 4–20.

Ong, F. S., & Phillips, D. (2003). Elders' quality of life and intergenerational relations: A cross national-comparison. *Hallym International Journal of Aging, 5,* 131–158.

Pavalko, E. K., & Artis, J. E. (1997). *Journal of Gerontology: Social Sciences, 52B,* S170–S179.

Payton, O. D., Ozer, M., & Nelson, C. (1990). *Patient participation in program planning: A manual for therapists.* Philadelphia: F.A. Davis.

Peters-Davis, N. D., Moss, M. S., & Pruchno, R. A. (1999). Children-in-law in caregiving families. *The Gerontologist, 39,* 66–75.

Pinquart, M. (2003). Loneliness in married, widowed, divorced and never-married older adults. *Journal of Social and Personal Relationships, 20,* 31–53.

Pinquart, M., & Sorensen, S. (2006). Gender differences in caregiver stressors, social resources, and health: An updated meta-analysis. *Journal of Gerontology: Psychological Sciences, 61B,* P33–P45.

Pruchno, R. (1999). Raising grandchildren: The experiences of black and white grandmothers. *The Gerontologist, 39,* 209–221.

Pruchno, R. A., & McKenney, D. (2002). Psychological well-being of black and white grandmothers raising grandchildren: Examination of a two-factor model. *Journal of Gerontology: Psychological Sciences, 57B,* P444–P452.

Reitzes, D. C., & Mutran, E. J. (2004a). Grandparent identity, intergenerational family identity, and well-being. *Journal of Gerontology: Social Sciences, 59B,* S213–S219.

Reitzes, D. C., & Mutran, E. J. (2004b). Grandparenthood: Factors influencing frequency of grandparent–grandchildren contact and grandparent role satisfaction. *Journal of Gerontology: Social Sciences, 59B,* S9–S18.

Rook, K. S. (1997). Positive and negative social exchanges: Weighing their effects in later life. *Journal of Gerontology: Social Sciences, 52B,* S167–S169.

Rose-Rego, S., Strauss, M. E., & Smyth, K. (1998). Differences in the perceived well-being of wives and husbands caring for persons with Alzheimer's disease. *The Gerontologist, 38,* 224–230.

Schone, B. S., & Weinick, R. M. (1998). Health-related behaviors and the benefits of marriage for elderly persons. *The Gerontologist, 38,* 618–627.

Shippy, R. A., Cantor, M. H., & Brennan, M. (2004). Social networks of aging gay men. *Journal of Men's Studies, 13*(1), 107–120.

Silverstein, M. (2006). Intergenerational family transfers in social context. In R. H. Binstock & L. K. George (Eds.), *Handbook of aging and the social sciences* (6th ed.) (pp. 165–180). Burlington, MA: Elsevier.

Silverstein, M., Conroy, S. J., Wang, H., Giarrusso, R., & Bengtson, V. L. (2002). Reciprocity in parent–child relations over the adult life course. *Journal of Gerontology: Social Sciences, 57B,* S3–S13.

Somary, K., & Stricker, G. (1998). Becoming a grandparent: A longitudinal study of expectations and early experiences as a function of sex and lineage. *The Gerontologist, 38,* 53–61.

Sorenson, S., & Pinquart, M. (2000). Preparation for future care needs by West and East German older adults. *Journal of Gerontology: Social Sciences, 55B,* S357–S367.

Spradley, J. P. (1979). *The ethnographic interview.* New York: Holt, Rinehart and Winston.

Stoller, E. P. (1998). Informal exchanges with non-kin among retired Sunbelt migrants: A case study of a Finnish American retirement community. *Journal of Gerontology: Social Sciences, 53B,* S287–S298.

Sung, K. T. (2000). Respect for elders: Myths and realities in East Asia. *Journal of Aging and Identity, 5,* 197–205.

Szinovacz, M. E. (Ed.), (1998). *Handbook on grandparenthood.* Westport, CT: Greenwood Press.

Szinovacz, M. E., & Davey, A. (2001). Retirement effects on parent–adult child contacts. *The Gerontologist, 41,* 191–200.

Szinovacz, M. E., & Davey, A. (2004). Honeymoons and joint lunches: Effects of retirement and spouse's employment on depressive symptoms. *Journal of Gerontology: Psychological Sciences, 59B,* P233–P245.

Szinovacz, M. E., DeViney, S., & Atkinson, M. P. (1999). Effects of surrogate parenting on grandparents' well-being. *Journal of Gerontology: Social Sciences, 54B,* S376–S388.

Taylor, M. G., & Lynch, S. M. (2004). Trajectories of impairment, social support, and depressive symptoms in later life. *Journal of Gerontology: Social Sciences, 59B,* S238–S246.

Tennstedt, S. (1999). *Family caregiving in an aging society.* Presented at the U.S. Administration on Aging Symposium Longevity in the New American Century, Baltimore, MD. Retrieved April 17, 2006, from www.aoa.gov/prof/research/famcare.pdf.

Unger, J. B., McAvay, G., Bruce, M. L., Berkman, L., & Seeman, T. (1999). Variation in the impact of social network characteristics on physical functioning in elderly persons: MacArthur Studies of Successful Aging. *Journal of Gerontology: Social Sciences, 54B,* S245–S251.

Usita, P. M. (2001). Interdependency in immigrant mother–daughter relationships. *Journal of Aging Studies, 15,* 183–199.

Usita, P. M., & Bleszner, R. (2002). Communication challenges and intimacy strategies of immigrant mothers and adult daughters. *Journal of Family Issues, 23,* 266–286.

van Tilberg, T. (1998). Losing and gaining in old age: Changes in personal network size and social support in a four-year longitudinal study. *Journal of Gerontology: Social Sciences, 53B,* S313–S323.

Velkoff, V. A., He, W., Sengupta, M., & DeBarros, K. A. (2006). *65+ in the United States: 2005.* Washington, DC: U.S. Census Bureau.

Weibel-Orlando, J. (2000). Grandparenting styles: Native American perspectives. In E. P. Stoller & R. C. Gibson (Eds.), *Worlds of difference* (pp. 249–251). Thousand Oaks, CA: Pine Forge Press.

Williams, N. & Torrez, D.J. (1998). Grandparenthood among Hispanics. In M. Szinovacz (Ed.), *Handbook on grandparenthood* (pp. 87-96). Westport, CT: Greenwood.

Williams, K. (2004). The transition to widowhood and the social regulation of health: Consequences for health and health risk behavior. *Journal of Gerontology: Social Sciences, 59B,* S343–S349.

Wolff, J. L., & Agree, E. M. (2004). Depression among recipients of informal care: The effects of reciprocity, respect, and adequacy of support. *Journal of Gerontology: Social Sciences, 59B,* S173–S180.

Wu, Z., & Pollard, M. S. (1998). Social support among unmarried childless elderly persons. *Journal of Gerontology: Social Sciences, 53B,* S324–S335.

Zarit, S. H., Stephens, M. A. P., Townsend, A., & Greene, R. (1998). Stress reduction for family caregivers: Effects of adult day care use. *Journal of Gerontology: Social Sciences, 53B,* S267–S277.

Zarit, S. H., Johansson, L., & Jarrott, S. E. (1998). Family caregiving: Stresses, social programs, and clinical interventions. In I. H. Nordhus, G. VandenBos, S. Berg., & P. Fromholt (Eds.), *Clinical Geropsychiatry* (pp. 345–360). Washington, DC: American Psychological Association.

CHAPTER 16

Sexuality in Late Adulthood

Andrew W. Miracle, PhD • Tina S. Miracle, EdS, LPCC

Although it is widely believed that sex no longer matters after middle age, the opposite is true, and sex often becomes more and not less important as a person grows older. Because sex is among the last pleasure-giving biological processes to deteriorate, it is potentially an enduring source of gratification at a time when these are becoming fewer and fewer, and a link to the joys of youth. These are important ingredients in the [older] person's emotional well-being.

Helen Singer Kaplan

Young love is from earth, while late love is from heaven.

Turkish proverb, cited in Hillerman (2000, p. 8)

OBJECTIVES

By the end of this chapter, readers will be able to:

1. Identify three cultural myths about sex and older adults.
2. Determine demographic factors affecting sexuality among older adults.
3. Identify the nature of the relationship between sexual activity and sexual satisfaction reported by older adults.
4. Understand how health status and health care affect the sexual activity and sexual satisfaction of older adults.
5. List common conditions and illnesses of older adults that can negatively affect sexuality.
6. Identify common prescription medications with potential sexual side effects.
7. Determine how to respond to patients' concerns about sexual issues.

Views of late-life sexuality are often based on stereotypes that sex after 50 either does not exist or that it is beset by dissatisfaction and dysfunction (Sharpe, 2004). Older women and men are seen as asexual or, if they do show an interest in sex, as "dirty old men or women." It is not only young and middle-aged but also older people themselves who are often negative about the prospects of continued sexual interest and ability. Many simply assume that the game is over. These stereotypes and misinformation lead many to ignore or take a pessimistic attitude toward late-life sexuality or make jokes about it. The fact is that we have lifelong sexual feelings, interest, activity, and capacities.

As Bob Dylan sang, "the times, they are a changing." The large number of prescriptions written for Viagra and similar medications for sexual dysfunction provide evidence that older adults are vitally concerned with sexuality. In addition, the Baby-Boom generation, the 77,702,865 Americans born between 1946 and 1965, have begun turning 60. These individuals value sexuality as an important part of life as they age. "A vast majority of mid-life to older adults shows a positive attitude toward sex. While they agree that too much emphasis is placed on sex in today's culture, they disagree that sex is only for younger people. To them, sex is enjoyable and many would be quite unhappy if they never had sex again" (AARP, 2005, p. 1).

Sex and the Elderly Population

Defining Sexuality

Sexuality includes the way we think about ourselves as sexual beings and the corresponding gender roles and behaviors, the need for intimacy, ideas about reproduction, and the feelings of excitement and pleasure that are associated with sex (Mohan & Bhugra, 2005). Sexuality also includes the entire range of sexual behaviors as well as the decision to be celibate and is an important aspect of activity and participation.

Too often, when we think of sex we think of a specific sexual act, such as **coitus,** oral sex, anal sex, or masturbation. Often, we tend to trivialize the sensuality of such intimate behaviors as kissing, holding hands, or looking into a loved one's eyes. The couple in Figure 16-1

clearly enjoys each other's company. Indeed, many Americans categorize all sexual behaviors between partners prior to penile insertion as "foreplay," a prelude to "real" sex. Many even agree that fellatio is not "having sex." Despite the distinction that is often made between caressing and fondling as "foreplay" and coitus as the "main event," many individuals find non-coital sex play pleasurable and rewarding as an end in itself—even when it does not lead to penile insertion or orgasm. This may be especially true for elderly persons or those with physical conditions that make some types of sexual activities uncomfortable, painful, difficult, or impossible.

Thus, in any discussion of sexuality in late adulthood, we need to maintain a broad definition of sexuality that will allow us to perceive existing sexual behaviors more accurately and to provide appropriate professional assistance.

Demographic Factors

Americans are now living longer than they did even a generation ago, and this trend is likely to continue (Mohan & Bhugra, 2005). There will be an increasing number of individuals who live into their 80s and beyond. Moreover, social definitions of aging are changing. In his 20s, Mick Jagger said he could not imagine performing rock and roll at age 50, but later found that it was possible to be part of both the AARP and

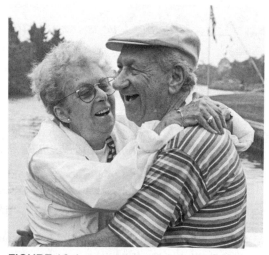

FIGURE 16-1 Couples who have been together for a long time can find pleasure in a variety of close or intimate activities. (Photo from Jeffrey M. Levine, MD. Copyright, 2007.)

MTV generations. Our ideas about how a 70-year-old should look, feel, or behave are likely to be very different when we are 20 years old than at age 40 or 60.

Unfortunately, the opportunity to develop or maintain intimate relationships is a problem for many older Americans. The groundbreaking 1994 Sex in America survey (Laumann, Gagnon, Michael, & Michaels, 1994) reported that for noninstitutionalized men and women, access to a sexual partner becomes increasingly problematic as we age. For men aged 60 to 64, the survey found that approximately 85% had a sexual partner in the past 12 months; this decreased to 45% for men 80 to 84 years old (U.S. Bureau of the Census, 1998a). The change was even more precipitous for women, who, by their very late years are very unlikely to have a sexual partner (Gott, 2005).

The demographic reality is that in the United States there are more women than men in every age category beginning at age 30 (U.S. Bureau of the Census, 1998b). Two factors help explain this situation. First, although there are more males born than females, males die naturally at a higher rate in infancy, and adult males tend to be more susceptible to certain age-related diseases, such as cardiovascular disease. Second, to a greater degree than women, men in our society traditionally have been socialized to take physical risks, fight wars, and take employment in dangerous occupations, such as mining and commercial fishing. These behaviors further decrease the number of men in society. Whatever the reasons, a woman's life expectancy exceeds a man's by as much as 6 years (U.S. Bureau of the Census, 1996). Marriage patterns in the United States also contribute to the difficulty older women have finding a spouse or partner. Despite highly publicized relationships like that of Demi Moore and Ashton Kutcher, women commonly marry men older than themselves and are more likely to survive a husband by several years.

This demographic imbalance, especially in late adulthood, makes it difficult for older heterosexual women to find a sexual partner. For those aged 75 or older, there are 1.3 women for every man in the population (U.S. Bureau of the Census, 1996). The situation for widowed women is made worse by the fact that many elderly men are married and thus not available to widowed women. Of those aged 75 or older,

66.7% of men, but only 28.8% of women, are married (U.S. Bureau of the Census, 1998b). Only half of older African Americans report having a regular sexual partner as compared to roughly two-thirds of other racial/ethnic groups.

Another demographic factor is affecting current perceptions of old age. Because baby boomers make up such a large segment of the population, they continue to have a great deal of influence on the rest of society. The "sex, drugs, and rock and roll" generation is redefining what is "old." The sexual revolutionaries of the 1960s and 1970s were exposed to the ideal of free love, and they were the first generation on "the pill." Now they are unwilling to concede that sex might end after middle age.

It should be noted that although there is relatively less research on sexuality outside the United States, existing evidence from China (Guan, 2004) and the United Kingdom (Gott, 2005) suggests that many issues with regard to sexuality in later life are universal.

Life Stage Effects

For most individuals in our society, late adulthood is a distinct life stage (Sharpe, 2004). Parents are usually deceased, and any children are adults. Given today's mobility, family members may live at some distance from one another. For many, full-time employment will have ended. Those who are employed full time may find that their responsibilities have shifted and their work is less satisfying. Many turn to hobbies and volunteer or become involved in other social activities to provide enjoyable and meaningful occupation.

Many older people find themselves alone after the death of a long-time spouse or companion. This means that the opportunities for sex, other than self stimulation, may be decreased. Nevertheless, "late life is a sexual stage of development like any other across the life span" (Sharpe, 2004, p. 199). The situation is made difficult, however, by the fact that those with whom one may be interested in exploring a sexual relationship may themselves be prisoners of the prevalent cultural stereotype.

Some contemporary retirement communities provide insight into the changing climate regarding older adults and sexuality. From Florida to California, communities where the average age is in the 70s reflect the demographics of late adulthood—increasing numbers, an imbalance of men and women, and better health and more vigor than might have been expected a decade or two ago. With their singles clubs, dance groups, social mixers, and newsletter advice columns, these communities also mirror the sexual interests and needs of their residents. They provide opportunities for meeting other people and developing relationships as part of a larger set of programs and opportunities for occupational engagement more generally.

The situation in nursing homes contrasts sharply with that in retirement communities. Adults in nursing homes tend to be treated as sexless beings by staff, and sexual activities may be actively discouraged (Sharpe, 2004). Although they may recognize the residents' rights to sexual expression, those in the nursing home industry have pragmatic concerns that often take precedence. These include a concern that patients might physically hurt themselves, a concern for what is acceptable to patients' families, as well as concerns about the possibilities of litigation. When dementia is a factor, there also is a concern about mutual consent (Ward, Vass, Aggarwal, Garfield, & Cybyk, 2005). Privacy issues are a significant concern for those wishing to sustain sexual relationships while in a nursing home. And there are significant ethical dilemmas about individuals with cognitive decline who may or may not be able to understand consent. Nursing homes have an obligation to protect those who cannot consent, but it may not always be easy to determine the wishes of the individual.

Declining health with associated decrements in performance skills can be a significant barrier to sexual fulfillment for older people. If health begins to fail, there is a resulting loss of independence that can take a heavy emotional toll. Moreover, if you are no longer able to drive, afraid to go out at night, and living on a fixed budget, you may become socially isolated. Finding and enjoying sex under such circumstances can be difficult. In addition, a decline in general health can affect sexual physiology. It may be that studies showing a decrease in sexual activity by elderly individuals are actually measuring a decline in their overall health.

In fact, older men and women report that better health for themselves and their partners is among the most important factors for improving their sexual satisfaction. Moreover, those who have a health problem that negatively affects their sexual relationships do not necessarily seek professional treatment. It is often believed that new drugs have greatly enhanced the sex lives of older adults. In reality, only a small percentage of those needing help (10% of men and 7% of women) have ever taken any medicine, hormone, or treatment to enhance sexual satisfaction. However, a majority of both men (62%) and women (59%) who have used such medications or treatments report enhanced satisfaction with their sex life, as well as improved relationships with their partners (AARP, 1999).

Gays and Lesbians in Older Adulthood

Aging can be stressful and problematic for all individuals in Western societies; however, there are no scientific data to suggest that homosexuals and heterosexuals differ in response to older adulthood. The reality is that the data on elderly homosexuals are scant. The most recent AARP sexuality study reported that only 4% of males and 1% of females reported having a same-sex partner (AARP, 2005). However, the report did not look at those who previously had a same-sex sexual relationship. Moreover, given the social changes of the past three decades, there is no reason to believe that the way current older homosexuals experience their situation will remain the same for those who are growing older during a period when attitudes toward gays and lesbians are significantly different.

What is known about the current generation of elderly gays and lesbians is summarized in this section. For those who would like additional information, Rosenfeld's (2003) volume on issues relevant to lesbian and gay elders is a good place to start. A recent study by MetLife (2006) provides insights into the views and wishes of aging gay and lesbian individuals. Many of these individuals have close partner relationships in later life, but like other elders, they worry about the prospect of outliving their partner. They also worry that health professionals will discriminate against them and will not treat their health and sexual concerns with respect. Thirty-two percent of gay men and 26% of lesbians indicated that this fear was their greatest concern about growing old. In addition, 19% reported little or no confidence that medical personnel would treat them with dignity and respect as lesbian, gay, bisexual, or transgender (LGBT) people as they age.

At the same time, there is contrast between the stereotype of unhappy old homosexuals and findings reported in the literature. For example, older gay men maintain both their interest in sex as well as their ability to function sexually (Pope & Schulz, 1991), and gay and lesbian individuals struggle with the same issues about sustaining sexual occupations later in life that characterize other populations (MetLife, 2006). It is important to remember that elders, including the transvestite shown in Figure 16-2, have as many ways of engaging in demonstrations of their personal sexual choices as do younger individuals. An attitude of acceptance is essential in working with elders, as is true in any clinical situation.

Adelman (1991) has examined the relationships of stigma, gay lifestyles, and adjustment to aging, finding that there is a significant relationship between adjustment to later life and the sequence of early gay development events. Specifically, there is a significant relationship between adjustment to later life and satisfaction with being gay; that is, high life satisfaction, low self-criticism, and few psychosomatic complaints constitute patterns of adjustment related to being "very satisfied with being gay." Those who were "less than very satisfied with being gay" attributed a perceived failing in life with respect to careers, friendships, or intimate relationships to their homosexuality. Stigma was frequently referred to as a reason for being less than very satisfied with being gay.

Sexual Attitudes and Behaviors of Older Adults

The Baby-Boom generation feels strongly that sex is for every age, not just the young. And a large majority of both men and women in their 40s and 50s see no reason that sex should not be enjoyed by singles, the divorced, and widows and widowers (National Council on Aging, 1998). Although older Americans believe that sex is emphasized too much in our society, a vast majority show a positive attitude toward sex (Table 16-1). Most adults, regardless of their age, are interested in sex, find sex satisfying, and consider sex to be an important part of their lives.

Although as we age our bodies change and we respond more slowly or differently, sex remains an important and enjoyable aspect of life for older adults. Years of sexual experience may more than compensate for any decrease in physical responsiveness. The physical changes that occur with age can provide an opportunity to revitalize lovemaking. Many older adults seize the chance to slow down and focus on intimacy, not solely on the act of coitus. They spend more time hugging and cuddling, fondling, and caressing to express their affection. In one study of adults aged 60 to 91, nearly three quarters of those who remained sexually active reported that lovemaking had become more rewarding over the years (AARP, 2005).

The cultural myth that we become less attractive and sexually appealing as we age probably goes hand in hand with the myth, too often presented in the media, that older adults are less sexual (Hilt & Lipschultz, 2005). The study conducted for the AARP and *Modern Maturity* magazine in 1999 reported that the number of people who view their partners as romantic or find them physically attractive does not decrease with age. The study found that 59% of men aged 45 to 59 gave their partners the highest possible rating for being "physically attractive." Of those men aged 75 or older, this rose to 63%. Of women aged 45 to 59 years, 52% gave their partners the highest possible rating for being "physically attractive," as did 57% of those aged 75 and older. For the same age categories, 37% of the younger men said

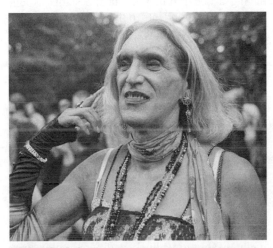

FIGURE 16-2 Elders have the same wide array of sexual orientations and behaviors as do younger individuals. (Photo from Jeffrey M. Levine, MD. Copyright, 2007.)

TABLE 16-1 **Attitudes Toward Sex After 50**

	Strongly Agree/ Agree	Neutral	Strongly Disagree/ Disagree
There is too much emphasis on sex in our society	73	19	8
Sexual activity is a critical part of a good relationship	60	28	12
Sexual activity is a pleasurable but necessary part of a good relationship	48	26	25
Sexual activity is critical to my overall quality of life	49	28	23
Sex becomes less important to people as they age	42	26	32
Sexuality is a duty to one's spouse or partner	30	35	35
I would be quite happy never having sex again	12	18	70
I do not particularly enjoy sex	10	19	71
Sex is only for young people	4	12	84

Adapted from AARP. Sexuality at Midlife and Beyond: 2004 Update to Attitudes and Behavior. Commissioned by *AARP: The Magazine.* 2005. Also available at http://assets.aarp.org/rgcenter/general/2004_sexuality.pdf

their partners were "romantic," as did 42% of the older men. For women, the percentage rose from 29% to 53% for "romantic" partners (AARP, 1999).

According to a survey sponsored by the Association of Reproductive Health Professionals (2002), 52% of men 50 to 59 were sexually active (engaged in sexual activity more than once per week), as were 26% of men 60 to 69, and 27% of men over 70. However, among women 70 and older, availability of a sex partner is relatively low. This can be particularly problematic for women who wish to sustain sexual activity, given that they can expect to spend one third of their lives after menopause (Kingsberg, 2002).

Both the 1999 and the 2005 update to the AARP/*Modern Maturity* study found that a vast majority of men and women aged 49 to over 70 report having some type of sexual activity (including kissing, hugging, sexual touching, intercourse, masturbation, and oral sex) at least once a week (see Table 16-1), and 81% reported that they always or usually had an orgasm with sex.

Not surprisingly, those older Americans who have a regular sex partner are far more likely to report having regular sexual activity (99%) than those who do not (59%). Coital frequency tends to decline with age for both men and women. Some of the change is due to increasing health problems and the loss of partners (AARP, 1999). Another study of people married for more than 50 years found that 47% had discontinued coitus and 92% reported a decline over the years (Hodson & Skeen, 1994).

The NCOA (1998) study found that 39% of respondents 60 years or older wanted to have sex more frequently than they currently do. Across all age segments (60s, 70s, and 80 years and older), older men are twice as likely as women to report wanting more-frequent sex (NCOA, 1998). Another study found that the main predictors of sexual activity for one elderly population (mean age 77.3 years) were being married, having more education, being younger, being male, and having good social networks (Matthias, Lubben, Atchison, & Schweitzer, 1997). The main predictors of sexual satisfaction for the older adult population were being sexually active, having good mental health, and having a better functional health status. About half of the respondents to the 2004 AARP study reported they were satisfied with their sex lives. According to an earlier AARP survey (1999), factors that respondents indicated might improve their sexual satisfaction included better health for themselves or their partner, less stress, and more sexual initiative from their partners.

Age-Related Physical Changes and Sexual Functioning

Certainly, older adults are more susceptible to many disabling medical conditions such as cardiac problems and arthritis, as well as normal aging changes that may make the expression of sexuality difficult as a result of changes in performance skills as well as body structures and body functions. As is shown in Table 16-2, sexual activity may diminish in frequency. In addition, the treatments used for medical conditions may hinder the older adult's sexual response. Those in late adulthood may experience a decrease in physical energy, along with increases in physical discomfort, which may affect the desire and capacity for sexual activities. One study has found that for women, age also is associated with less sexual daydreaming and more negative sexual attitudes (Purifoy, Grodsky, & Giambra, 1992). However, the need for intimacy, excitement, and pleasure continues throughout the life span, and there is nothing in the normal biology of aging that would preclude the ability for sexual activity.

Physical Changes in Men

There are several sexual changes that occur as men age, including a decrease in the production of testosterone. Consequently, the size and firmness of the testicles may decrease. There also is a reduction in sperm as men age, although unlike women, who once past menopause can no longer become pregnant, men can father children into very late life. Another common change is an increase in the size and condition of the prostate.

Men in late adulthood may notice that it takes longer to get an erection than when they were younger, and many older men need more manual or oral stimulation of the penis to produce an erection. Moreover, the erection may not be as firm or as large as it was when the man was younger (I. Goldstein, 2004). A man also may experience a longer time before ejaculating. In addition, the feeling that ejaculation is imminent may be shorter, and there is a reduction in seminal fluid. The loss of tumescence (swelling due to engorgement of blood vessels in the penis) may occur more quickly in older men. Finally, the refractory period, the amount of time it takes to achieve a subsequent erection, tends to increase with age.

As men get older, they are more likely to experience erectile dysfunction (i.e., the inability to have and maintain an erection). Traditionally, erectile dysfunction was commonly termed impotence. However, because the word "impotence" is imprecise and implies personal failure or not being "manly," the term "erectile dysfunction" is now preferred. Evidence suggests that minimal erectile dysfunction can be found in 17% of men aged 40 to 70, 25% experience moderate dysfunction, and 10%, complete dysfunction (I. Goldstein, 2004). The rate of dysfunction triples from age 40 to age 70.

The magnitude of the problem is unknown because it often goes unreported. Many men associate the inability to have an erection with loss of manhood and are embarrassed to admit they have a problem. However, in one survey, 26% of men (aged 45 and older) acknowledged having either moderate or complete erectile dysfunction (AARP, 1999).

An erection results when an aroused man's brain signals nerve cells in the penis to release nitric oxide. In turn, this produces the release of cyclic **guanosine monophosphate,** or cGMP, which is key to having an erection. The cGMP enlarges blood vessels in the penis, allowing blood to engorge the penis, thus producing an

TABLE 16-2 **Sexual Activity Engaged in at Least Once a Week in the Past Six Months**

Gender	Male			Female		
Age	50–59	60–69	Over 70	50–59	60–69	Over 70
Kissing or hugging	83	73	64	69	58	49
Sexual touching/caressing	68	67	54	57	41	27
Sexual intercourse	49	36	22	43	24	14
Self-stimulation	36	28	15	11	3	3
Oral Sex	26	15	8	10	7	2

Adapted from AARP. Sexuality at Midlife and Beyond: 2004 Update to Attitudes and Behavior. Commissioned by *AARP: The Magazine.* 2005. Also available at http://assets.aarp.org/rgcenter/general/2004_sexuality.pdf

erection. A man will continue to produce cGMP as long as he is sexually stimulated (Kolata, 1998). At the same time, however, he will produce **phosphodiesterase 5,** or PDE5, which destroys cGMP. The result is an appropriate level of engorgement. After orgasm, or when sexual stimulation ends, cGMP production ceases, PDE5 destroys any remaining cGMP, and the erection resolves.

The proportion of men who have tried potency-enhancing medicines, hormones, or other treatments has doubled since 1999. Viagra and similar medicines work by blocking the effect of PDE5 (Kolata, 1998). A man with erectile dysfunction who takes the medication may increase the effects of cGMP by slowing the impact of PDE5. The result can be an erection for a man who otherwise would not have one.

Physical Changes in Women

The common physical changes that affect women's sexuality result from lowered levels of estrogen hormones after menopause. Postmenopausal women usually experience a decrease in vaginal lubrication—which may make coitus uncomfortable—and a decrease in vaginal expansion during arousal. Nonprescription vaginal lubricants are readily available and effective for this problem.

Older women also may notice changes in the shape and flexibility of the vagina. However, these changes should not affect one's ability to enjoy sexual activity. Moreover, sensitivity of the clitoris and nipples remains unchanged with age. The sexual tension that occurs just before orgasm may be less dramatic in older women, but the constriction in the vagina and withdrawal of the clitoris under the hood is the same as in younger women. A somewhat surprising result of more men using medication for erectile dysfunction is the increased pleasure the men's use of these treatments is giving their female partners, no matter what their age—a finding that challenges the widely held belief that older women are not all that welcoming of their partner's newfound ardor (AARP, 2005).

Hormonal Changes and Sexual Response

As we age, there are accompanying changes in the levels of sex hormones, although it is not clear whether or how these may impact our sexuality. Sexual dysfunction may occur at any point of the sexual response cycle but most typically involves difficulties related to sexual arousal or to orgasm. A model proposed by Masters and Johnson (1966) consists of four phases: excitement, plateau, orgasm, and resolution. Examination of these phases in elders suggests that aging has the greatest impact on arousal (Sharpe, 2004), particularly because of changes in hormone levels. Orgasm, on the other hand, is least affected, and the refractory period is more affected in men than in women. Table 16-3 summarizes the changes described in this section.

Androgens, from the Greek word *andros* for male, circulate at the highest levels in men. The most important androgen is testosterone, which is present in both men and women. On average, men have at least 10 times more testosterone than women (Worthman, 1999). Men produce testosterone primarily in their testes, with a small additional amount produced by the adrenal glands. Testosterone levels are not constant; they fluctuate on a daily cycle and according to daily events. Research has shown that testosterone is responsive to physical, emotional, and intellectual challenges. On average, testosterone levels of U.S. males tend to go into a steady decline after age 20, and the hormone's concentration in the blood decreases by about 30% by the time a man reaches the age of 80 years (Worthman, 1999).

This pattern of hormone decline with aging, however, is not universal. For example, one cross-cultural study indicates that male subjects in Bolivia have a modest decrease in testosterone levels after age 30, with hormone levels remaining relatively stable after that time (Leary, 1992). On the other hand, testosterone in Tibetan males does not peak until the late 50s and then falls precipitously during the 60s and 70s (Worthman, Beall, & Stallings, 1997a). A study of **dihydroepiandosterone sulfate (DHEAS),** an androgen produced by the adrenal glands, also showed dramatic variations in level by age when U.S. males were compared with Bolivians and Tibetans (Worthman, Beall, & Stallings, 1997b). Neither the cause nor possible significance of this variation is known at present; however, the lack of a universal pattern suggests that environmental factors, such as nutrition and other cultural factors, may play a significant role in the regulation of these hormones.

TABLE 16-3 Normal Age-Related Changes in Sexual Response

	Women or Female	Men or Male
Arousal	Delayed lubrication Decreased Bartholin gland secretion Reduced vaginal expansion Decreased elevation of the uterus	Delayed and less firm erection Longer interval to ejaculation Less testicular elevation
Orgasm	Fewer orgasmic contractions	Shorter ejaculation time
Postorgasm	No dilation of cervical os Longer refraction period	Rapid loss of erection

Sexual desire and satisfaction may be less affected by age than arousal and ejaculation (Sharpe, 2004). That is, decreasing erectile capacity in aging men may be related to decreasing sensorineural and autonomic function; however, factors other than the frequency of and potency for sexual response are important to the overall rating of sex life. Many factors apparently contribute to this situation, including decreased health and mobility, increased incidence of disease, partner considerations, and increasing neurological dysfunction.

Women produce lesser amounts of testosterone in their ovaries and adrenal glands than men do in their testes and adrenal glands. The brain can convert testosterone into estradiol, so that the "male hormone" becomes the "female hormone." Scientists are uncertain whether testosterone has any separate effect in women other than to increase the available estrogen reaching the center of the brain that controls sexual motivation and drive.

Like testosterone, estrogens are a part of a shared male and female biology, although estrogens circulate at higher levels in women than in men. There are actually three estrogens—estrone, estradiol, and estriol—forming a closely related family. In both men and women, estrogens appear more directly necessary to staying alive than androgens. There is a great deal of controversy about the connection between blood levels of testosterone and measures of sexual desire, or libido. Moreover, some researchers have suggested measuring bioavailable testosterone rather than serum testosterone (Rowland, Greenleaf, Dorfman, & Davidson, 1993). However, the relationship of testosterone to sexuality is intriguing.

At the onset of menopause, a woman's ovaries and adrenal glands produce less testosterone and other androgens. As a result, the amount of testosterone circulating in the body is reduced by at least half. Although some women may react to this change by experiencing a noticeable drop in sexual desire, others do not. Some researchers believe women who find their sex drive diminished during menopause may respond to testosterone therapy. However, caution is suggested. There is more to libido than hormones, and a lack of sexual desire may result from any of several causes (Mohan & Bhugra, 2005).

Estrogens are produced by the testes in males and by the ovaries in females. Men make estradiol, and women make all three estrogens. Each is concentrated in a different part of the body and has its own place in the life cycle. In women, estrogens serve to maintain the condition of the vaginal lining and to produce vaginal lubrication. There is no known function for estrogen in men. However, estrogen therapy may be helpful to men as well as women. For example, researchers at Johns Hopkins University have found that a form of estrogen increased the blood flow to the heart by nearly a third in men with coronary artery disease (Blumenthal et al., 1997).

The use of hormones or other medicines (including those for erectile dysfunction) has grown tremendously. About half of former or current users of medication for a sexual problem who have a regular sex partner report that the medicine had a positive effect on their relationship with their partner. There is a lack of clear research about the benefits and risks of hormone replacement therapy, whether estrogen for women or testosterone for men or women. Therapists should encourage their clients to discuss these issues carefully with their physicians and to weigh potential advantages and disadvantages.

Effects of Disease on Sexuality

Many conditions and illnesses common among those in late adulthood can impact body systems and body functions necessary for participation in sexual activity. Moreover, some chronic conditions slowly take their toll on affected individuals' capacity to enjoy certain sexual activities (Box 16-1).

Cardiovascular Disease

Men who have vascular problems may not get enough blood flowing to the penis. In such cases, the nerves that make nitric oxide are malnourished, and erections are either absent or partial (I. Goldstein, 2004). Thus, the risk of erectile dysfunction is increased for those with vascular disease, hypertension, diabetes, and various neurological disorders. Moreover, any behavior that decreases the supply of oxygen to the penis—lack of exercise, sleep deprivation, smoking, sexual abstinence, or physical injuries—can contribute to erectile difficulties. Half the men who have undergone coronary bypass surgery have erectile problems, and many drugs used to treat heart disease interfere with blood flow, which can result in erectile dysfunction. Nerve damage from diabetes or prostate surgery can cause erectile problems, as can some hormone imbalances.

Those with diseases of the heart and cardiovascular system (which include angina, high blood pressure, heart failure, abnormal rhythms of the heart, and aortic stenosis) need to take reasonable precautions before resuming sexual activity. Usually, sexual activity is safe if the disease is mild, if it causes few symptoms, and

if blood pressure is normal. In general, if a patient can walk about 300 yards on flat surfaces or climb two flights of stairs briskly without getting chest pain or feeling breathless, sexual activity is probably safe. Those who have had a heart attack should check with their physician prior to resuming sexual activity. Use of Viagra and similar medications may be dangerous, and taking nitroglycerine with these medications is not recommended.

Cerebrovascular Accident

Cerebrovascular accident (CVA, or stroke) is the third leading cause of death in North America, yet little is known regarding sexual problems and adjustment following CVA. Several studies (Korpelainen, Nieminen, & Myllalä, 1999; Monga, 1993) suggest that cerebrovascular diseases may commonly result in sexual dysfunction, leading to a marked decrease in sexual activity. However, a Finnish study (Sjögren, Damberg, & Liliequist, 1983) found the number of patients who completely stopped having sexual intercourse after the stroke was markedly lower (33% of patients, 27% of spouses) than previously reported.

Psychological and social factors seem to exert a strong impact on sexual functioning and the quality of sexual life after stroke (Nadler, 1997). Common physical problems of those who have sustained a stroke are decreased libido and arousal, decreased vaginal lubrication, decreased incidence of orgasm, premature ejaculation or inability to ejaculate, pain, lack of satisfaction, and hypersexuality. In addition, CVA may result in sensory, motor, or cognitive deficits, spasticity, contractures, aphasia, or incontinence. Psychological changes may result in anxiety, depression, and changes in self-image or

---

BOX 16-1 Some Illnesses that May Affect Sexual Arousal or Desire

- Testosterone deficiency caused by aging, disease of the testicles, surgery or injury to the testicles, diseases of the pituitary gland, surgical removal of adrenals or ovaries
- Cardiac disease, including coronary artery disease, postcoronary recovery, high blood pressure
- Liver problems including hepatitis, cirrhosis
- Kidney problems including nephritis, renal failure, dialysis

- Pulmonary diseases
- Degenerative diseases
- Thyroid diseases
- Head injuries
- Psychomotor epilepsy
- Hypothalamic lesions
- Pituitary gland tumors
- Chronic obstructive pulmonary disease

communication. Aphasia can interfere with communication about sexuality. The site where the brain damage occurred also may affect sexuality. Kinsella and Duffy (1979) found that psychosocial factors play a crucial role in determining sexual drive, activity, and satisfaction after stroke, and their influence is even stronger than that of medical factors.

Arthritis

The pain, stiffness, fatigue, and limited ability associated with joint inflammation may interfere with sexual activity (Nadler, 1997). Several small clinical studies have shown that approximately half of arthritic men and women experience sexual problems, including fatigue, weakness, pain, and limited movement. Pain and stiffness of the hip joints were the main causes of sexual difficulty, and approximately one out of five patients reported a loss of libido or sex drive. Some arthritis drugs, especially corticosteroids, have been shown to reduce sex drive.

Sexual dysfunction in arthritic patients may be difficult to manage for several reasons. The nature of the problem may be difficult to diagnose because it often is complicated by the underlying medical condition. In addition, chronic illness places a great deal of stress on patients and their relationships. For those suffering from arthritis, it is important to find positions that avoid or reduce pain and pressure on the affected joints.

Pain management is a particular concern for individuals with arthritis, and use of appropriate pain medications may be warranted. As is true with other physical conditions, clients should be encouraged to discuss this issue with their physician to ensure that appropriate interventions are provided. Positioning and relaxation strategies can also help, and therapists will want to explore these nonmedical methods with their clients.

Chronic Obstructive Pulmonary Disease

Pulmonary diseases are not uncommon in later life. Individuals who have smoked are particularly at risk, but others may develop chronic obstructive pulmonary disease (COPD) as well. Individuals with COPD are likely to tire easily, so that sexual activity may result in excessive stress or fatigue. Someone tethered to supplemental oxygen may find that with the oxygen, activity is limited by the device, and that without it, fatigue is too great to allow for activity. Therapists can help clients explore alternatives that may reduce energy expenditure and thereby allow for sexual expression.

Other Factors Affecting Sexuality

Alcohol and Other Drugs

Alcohol and other drugs interact with the cerebral cortex, autonomic nervous system, and the neural structure of the limbic system. Drugs that affect the cerebral cortex and the limbic system interfere with motivation, judgment, and emotionality. The Massachusetts Male Aging Study (Bremner & McKinlay, 2003) found that lower amounts of alcohol intake, not smoking, and increased physical activity were related to lower rates of sexual dysfunction among men in their study. These results were also found in a study by Bacon et al. (2003), who found that physical activity greater than or equal to 2.7 hours/week was associated with lower risk for erectile dysfunction, but alcohol consumption and smoking resulted in increased risk for erectile dysfunction in men. Decreased sexual performance may provide motivation to alter these health risk behaviors.

Any substance that interferes with **vasocongestion** or **myotonia** can produce sexual problems by interfering with erection and orgasm. This can occur in men or women because the neurophysiology of orgasm is similar for both.

Excessive alcohol consumption may adversely affect sexual arousal and sexual performance at any age. However, there may be a cumulative effect on long-time heavy drinkers. Although some people report that the use of drugs and alcohol make them feel less inhibited and freer to enjoy sex, acute or chronic use of alcohol and drugs can inhibit sexual desire, performance, and satisfaction in men and women. Abuse of alcohol and drugs almost inevitably contributes to sexual problems not only directly, but also by affecting emotions and straining relationships.

Medications

As many as 400 prescription medicines are known to cause at least occasional problems with sexual desire and function. Sometimes, the problem is not with a single medication but rather may be a reaction to two or more medications taken in combination. Many medications frequently prescribed for elderly patients, including blood pressure medicine, antidepressants, and prostate-shrinkage drugs may have these side effects. Table 16-4 shows common medications with sexual side effects.

The most obvious and commonly talked about side effects are the actual physical changes, such as erectile dysfunction, changes in ejaculation and ejaculatory control, and decrease in vaginal lubrication. However, medications also can affect energy levels, emotions, and thinking.

Surgery

Many types of surgery can cause short-term sexual difficulties. Surgeries that involve sexual organs or glands may have long-term sexual effects; however, some common surgeries are often inaccurately assumed to cause inevitable sexual impairment.

Neither a hysterectomy nor a mastectomy should impair sexual functioning. If a woman seems to enjoy sexual activities less after one of these surgeries, counseling may prove helpful. It is not uncommon for women to feel less feminine or less desirable after such surgery. Ideally, postdischarge counseling should be routine for all women after such surgeries.

A prostatectomy, the surgical removal of all or part of the prostate, does not necessarily end a man's physical capacity for sexual activity. Improved surgical techniques and alternative treatments increase the likelihood that patients will continue to enjoy erections after treatment. Except for a lack of seminal fluid, the capacity for erection and orgasm after a prostatectomy should most often return to the presurgery level.

Emotional Concerns

Psychiatric illnesses, especially major depression and dementia, are frequently associated with sexual dysfunction in late life. Decreased libido is a cardinal symptom of depression. In one study it was found that more than 70% of depressed patients had a loss of sexual interest when not taking medication, and they reported that the severity of this loss of interest was worse than the other symptoms of depression (Casper et al., 1985). Depression itself can impair sexual performance, and certain antidepressants trigger sexual dysfunction. However, sexual dysfunction is a common side effect seen in patients taking antidepressants, particularly selective serotonin reuptake inhibitors (SSRIs) (Beers & Berkow, 2000). Modifications to therapy including reducing drug dosages, altering timing of drug dosages, taking drug holidays, adding an adjunctive drug, and switching to alternative antidepressants can be employed to eliminate undesirable side effects.

Alzheimer's and other dementias can have a profound effect on sexuality (Ward et al., 2005). Sometimes sexual desire increases and can result in unreasonable and exhausting demands, often at odd times or in inappropriate places. Occasionally, aggression may be shown if those needs are not met. Other individuals may lose interest in a physical relationship and may become very withdrawn. Sometimes there is a loss of inhibitions and there may be sexual advances to strangers, or other inappropriate sexual behavior such as undressing or fondling in public. Sexual advances are sometimes made because the person with dementia mistakes another person for their partner. Sometimes, an action which appears sexual (e.g., a woman lifting her skirt) may be an indication of something else, such as the need to go to the toilet.

TABLE 16-4 **Some Prescription Medications with Possible Sexual Side Effects**

Type of Drug	Trade Names	Potential Problems
Tranquilizer; antianxiety	Valium, Xanax, Ativan	Changes in libido; erection problems; delayed orgasm/ejaculation
Antidepressant	Prozac, Zoloft, Paxil, Effexor	Changes in libido, delayed orgasm/ejaculation
Antihypertensive	Clonidine, beta blockers	Erectile dysfunction, decreased libido
Ulcer medication	Tagamet	Decreased libido, erectile dysfunction

Psychosocial stresses such as the loss of a partner due to disability or death, fears of self-injury or death due to medical conditions (e.g., history of myocardial infarction, shortness of breath), or sensitivity to loss of personal appearance or control of hygiene (e.g., due to incontinence or the presence of a colostomy) can sometimes spell the end of an individual's desire for sexual activity.

Older individuals living in social isolation, suffering the threat of health problems, and coping with adjustments to physical changes associated with aging may be at especially high risk for emotional problems with consequent sexual implications. Sexuality involves a balance of emotional and physical factors: How we feel affects what we are able to do. A man who fears he may not have an erection may experience sufficient stress to prevent an erection. In fact, many aging men suffer from performance anxiety and may avoid sex rather than risk "failure" in front of a partner. On the other hand, a woman who has always associated coitus with reproduction may feel little need for sex after menopause.

Sexually Transmitted Diseases and the Elderly Population

Older men and women are at significant risk for HIV/AIDS and other sexually transmitted diseases. Not only are many older individuals sexually active, especially in retirement communities where social opportunities abound, but they may be at risk because of a lack of information. Whether you are 18 or 80, unprotected sex with a partner with an unknown sexual history carries risks. At an age when pregnancy is not a concern, many never think of using protection; the safe-sex message aimed at the younger generations is often lost on the sexually active older adult. In fact, the elderly are one sixth as likely to use condoms during intercourse as compared to those in their 20s (Gott, 2005; Goodroad, 2003).

Syphilis, genital herpes, and chlamydial infections do not appear to present any differently or to be more severe in older persons. However, elders are clearly not immune from HIV infection, and these infections appear to progress more rapidly to AIDS and death in elders as seen in Table 16-5. A report from the Centers for Disease Control (www.cdc.gov/hiv/topics/surveillance/resources/slides/epidemiology/slides/EPI-AIDS.ppt, 2005) indicates that more than 50,000 cases of AIDS have

TABLE 16-5   AIDS Cases by Age

Age	Estimated Number of AIDS Cases in 2004
50 to 54	3932
55 to 59	2079
60 to 64	996
65 and older	901

Adapted from Goodroad, B. K. (2003). HIV and AIDS in people older than 50. A continuing concern. *Journal of Gerontological Nursing, 29*(4), 18–24.

been reported among individuals older than 55. The normal aging changes in older women, such as a decrease in vaginal lubrication and thinning vaginal tissue, can put them at higher risk during unprotected sexual intercourse.

Typically, older people with HIV/AIDS are diagnosed later, experience more rapid progression of the disease, and survive a shorter period of time than those who are younger, although the observed shorter survival time may result from a delay in diagnosis, because health care professionals may not suspect HIV/AIDS among older patients (Goodroad, 2003). Symptoms of HIV infection are often nonspecific, including anorexia, weight loss, and decreased physical and cognitive function. The most common opportunistic infections in older HIV-infected patients are *Pneumocystis carinii* pneumonia, tuberculosis, *Mycobacterium avium* complex, herpes zoster, and cytomegalovirus. HIV-related dementia may be confused with Alzheimer's disease.

■ Summary

Culture and Society

There appear to be at least three cultural myths about the sexuality of older adults that are *not* true: that older adults do not have sex, that new drugs have greatly enhanced the sex lives of older adults, and that people find each other less physically attractive over time

Fewer North Americans live in generationally integrated neighborhoods. Since the birth of suburbia after World War II, there has been an increasing tendency toward age-segregated residential patterns. The popularity of retirement communities is only the most recent example of this trend, and one effect of the concentration of elderly persons in select areas is that it increases the isolation of those who either cannot or choose not to follow the trend.

Age stereotyping, sexual taboos, and lack of access to health care have an impact on sexuality in older adults. In turn, those who lack a fulfilling sexual relationship can experience an overall decrease in their general quality of life.

Relationships and Quality of Life

A fulfilling sexual relationship usually consists of physical attraction, a capacity for intimacy, and sensitivity to one's own and one's partner's needs. In addition, social attitudes and health issues may affect relationships.

The AARP/*Modern Maturity* survey (1999) found that a satisfying sexual relationship is an important component contributing to the general quality of life for many older individuals (67% of men and 57% of women). In addition, the NCOA study (1998) found that among those aged 60 and older who said they engage in sexual activity at least once a month, 79% of men and 66% of women reported that maintaining an active sex life is an important aspect of their relationship with their partner. In the AARP/*Modern Maturity* study, 92% of men and 87% of women reported that a good relationship with a spouse or partner is important to their quality of life. Moreover, 75% of men and 72% of women described their partners as "my best friend."

A majority (63%) of men and women with partners described themselves as either "extremely satisfied" or "somewhat satisfied" with their sex lives. And when all is said and done, it seems that having a mediocre sex partner is better than having no partner at all. Almost 40% of men without regular sex partners and 15% of women without regular sex partners rated their sex lives at the bottom of the satisfaction scale (AARP, 2005).

There seems little doubt that most individuals find that good interpersonal relationships with a spouse or partner, family, and friends give meaning to life, making life both pleasurable and worthwhile. The extent to which satisfying sexual activity is a necessary component of the quality of life surely varies over a wide continuum.

Implications for Health Care Providers

The preservation and enhancement of sexual activity in geriatric patients requires an understanding and sensitivity to the fact that many individuals want and intend to continue sexual activity, despite changes in physical and sexual function.

Clearly, there is a role for health professionals as advocates to represent the right of those in late adulthood to pursue sexual pleasure with other consenting adults. Providing for privacy, supporting relationships, and addressing cultural stereotypes would have positive effects on the health, self-esteem, and dignity of many elderly individuals. Medical and other health care professionals have tended to subscribe to cultural stereotypes as much as society in general. There is a need for health professionals to initiate education for change with regard to sexuality in late adulthood. After all, even young adults have a vested interest in this change, because they may expect to become older adults at some point in the future.

Despite its importance to the quality of life, when it comes to sexuality, "don't ask, don't tell" seems to be the preferred approach of most health care professionals. Although about one-fourth of older adults report seeking treatment from a medical professional for a problem related to sexual function (AARP, 2005), sexuality is typically ignored during the medical assessment of clients of any age. Cultural stereotypes about aging make it even less likely that sexuality will be discussed with older patients. If patients do bring up the subject of sex, at best they may be handed a generic informational brochure or at worst be shamed for bringing up such an "inappropriate" topic. This anxiety may be fueled by a lack of training, because few health care professionals have had formal instruction in human sexuality through the life cycle. In addition, our own sexual attitudes, values, and beliefs affect our professional responsibility to address sexuality as a legitimate health care issue. Open-minded, nonjudgmental individuals who are comfortable with their own sexuality are likely to approach the topic differently than those who believe that sexuality is limited to genital contact between married heterosexuals under a certain age.

Sexuality probably is not discussed with clients for many reasons. Health care professionals may believe that it is someone else's responsibility (H. Goldstein & Runyon, 1993). They may lack education on the subject, believe that other "more important" issues take precedence, think their clients would be embarrassed, or, more likely, would themselves feel uncomfortable. Communication with older adults and families is critical to the fulfillment of sexual health. For older couples in new relationships, it is often difficult for families to appreciate that their older relative may have a new relationship. Family meetings may help to open up communication with the couple and their loved ones.

Assessing sexual concerns can be done in the context of addressing limitations or changes in the patient's lifestyle and general health care issues. The evaluation of sexuality concerns may be done in the form of a simple checklist or as open-ended questions such as "what concerns you about your sexuality?" Another technique is to make a general statement indicating that other patients have expressed concerns about how a disability or illness affects sexuality, and to ask whether this is something that the client would like to discuss. This gives patients the opportunity to discuss any sexual concerns or to decline if they do not have any problems or do not choose to discuss them at that time or with that caregiver. Among the important considerations are the following:

- Look for possible barriers to sexuality—for example, lack of knowledge and understanding about sexuality, loss of partners, and family influence on sexual practice often present substantial barriers to sexual health among older adults.
- Privacy issues may present a substantial barrier to sexual health among older residents of long-term-care facilities. Consequently, arrangements for privacy must be made among consenting adults. These arrangements may include a resident's room or an appropriate and private common room. Patient safety while maintaining privacy should be considered by ensuring access to call lights and adaptive equipment as necessary.
- Determine the presence of any physiological changes through a health history, review of systems, and physical examination for the presence of normal and aging changes that impact sexual health.
- Address concomitant factors such as fatigue, incontinence, fear of incontinence, spasticity, pain, and hormonal issues.
- Review medications, as many of those commonly used to treat depression and hypertension among the elderly impact sexual desire and response. Potential medications should be identified by reviewing the client's medication bottles, and the client should be questioned about the potential impact of these medications on sexual health. If the medication is found to impact sexual health, alternative medications should be considered.
- The older adult should also be questioned regarding the use of alcohol, as this substance has a potential impact on sexual response. Also consider if depression may be affecting sexual health.
- Cognitively impaired older adults continue to have sexual needs and desires but may lack the capacity to make appropriate decisions regarding sexual relationships. Accurate assessment and documentation of the ability to make informed decisions regarding sexual relationships must be conducted by an interdisciplinary team. Limits must be placed on any inappropriate sexual behavior, such as public masturbation, disrobing, or making sexually explicit remarks that may be a result of dementia or other neurological conditions.
- Sexual problems resulting from chronic illnesses are prevalent among the older adult population. In many cases, these problems are treatable. For example, erectile dysfunction/impotence in older men with chronic medical illnesses is often effectively treated with new erectile agents. Physician referral for these needs should be made without hesitation.
- Occupational therapists should be aware of, and ask about, specific performance skills or body functions and body structures that contribute to sexual dysfunction. For example, an individual with arthritis might need to discuss positions that reduce pain and conserve energy.
- Should a patient present a sexual concern, the health care professional needs to assess whether it is a problem of sexual desire (e.g., decreased or hypoactive sexual desire), a problem of sexual function (e.g., erectile dysfunction), or a problem of sexual satisfaction (e.g., **anorgasmia,** premature ejaculation). Other concerns might be related to sexual self-image if the client's body, which was once a source of pleasure, is now a source of discomfort or disfigurement. In addition, there may be a relationship issue with a partner or spouse, or concerns about the loss or lack of a sexual partner.

Many professionals find the PLISSIT intervention model a helpful guide in working with sexual issues (Annon, 1976). The acronym PLISSIT stands for **P**ermission • **L**imited **I**nformation • **S**pecific **S**uggestions • **I**ntensive **T**herapy. Health care professionals should be able to provide the first two levels (PLI) of intervention, because most people simply need permission to talk about their sexual concerns in a supportive, confidential environment and be assured that their feelings are normal and acceptable. Some patients may need limited information about their specific problem and for the professional to provide accurate answers to their questions. Others, however, may require specific suggestions about how to deal with a particular problem or intensive therapy to resolve their concerns (SSIT). In such cases, the appropriate course for the health care professional may be to refer the patient to a qualified professional who is better prepared to meet the patient's needs.

Dealing with the sensitive area of sexuality also may bring up ethical considerations. Health care providers must be aware of the limits of their own comfort, knowledge, and skills, and be prepared to refer to someone better qualified to help a patient with a sexual problem.

Most codes of ethical behavior for health care professionals explicitly prohibit sexual contact between a health care provider and a client for very good reasons. Research has found that the inherent power imbalance makes a client vulnerable to exploitation and leads to negative effects for most clients who have had a sexual relationship with a health care professional (Friedman, 1997; Gabbard & Nadelson, 1995). It is imperative that professionals maintain appropriate boundaries to protect their clients from harm and protect themselves from professional or legal liability.

Boundaries are equally important if the professional is faced with a patient who makes inappropriate sexual remarks or sexual advances. Flirtatious behavior or sexual joking may be the patient's way of coping with his or her own anxiety, expressing an interest in the topic of sexuality if the topic has not been addressed directly, or "trying out" his or her sexuality (Friedman, 1997). In a firm but friendly manner, the professional can acknowledge and redirect the patient's expression of his or her needs. If a patient exhibits abusive or threatening verbal or physical sexual behavior, it should be documented and reported to a supervisor. Depending on the circumstances, psychiatric or neurological consultation may be indicated.

Health care professionals must recognize their limits and deficiencies in the area of sexuality and maintain balance and respect in what they do. Ignoring the sexual dimension may adversely affect the patient's well-being, whereas attention to this area may improve the patient's quality of life (Goldstein-Lohman & Aitken, 1995).

Case Study

Mr. Smith is a 67-year-old male who was diagnosed with Alzheimer's disease 4 years ago. Although he still lives at home with his wife, he recognizes her only intermittently. He needs help with all his self-care activities except feeding himself, and his wife feels an obligation to assist. An occupational therapist has been asked to review the home for safety, and to recommend environmental modifications to assist Mrs. Smith in providing care for Mr. Smith.

At the end of the visit, Mrs. Smith pulls the occupational therapist aside. In a somewhat halting fashion, Mrs. Smith tells the OT that her husband has recently been "bad." When the therapist inquires about what this means, it develops that Mr. Smith has been attempting to disrobe in public, and has repeatedly fondled Mrs. Smith in public. She is embarrassed and unsure how to handle this.

Questions

1. What might the occupational therapist do to respond to Mrs. Smith's concerns?
2. Given that Mr. Smith appears to want continued sexual activity with his wife, what suggestions might you make to help deal with his socially unacceptable expression of this wish?
3. How can Mrs. Smith's concerns be taken into account?

Review Questions

1. What are the major demographic factors affecting sexuality in late adulthood?
2. What is the general level of sexual activity for older men and women? How does it change through late adulthood?
3. What is the general level of sexual satisfaction for men and women in late adulthood?
4. How do health status and health care affect the sexual activity and satisfaction of older adults?
5. What are some of the diseases that can lead to erectile dysfunction? What is the primary physiological cause of erectile dysfunction?
6. How do cardiovascular diseases, stroke, and arthritis affect sexuality?
7. How does depression affect sexuality?
8. Name four prescription medications that can adversely affect sexuality, and indicate the nature of those potential side effects.
9. What are three cultural myths about sex and older adults?
10. What is the PLISSIT model?

Web-Based Resource

For helpful information about the experience of sexuality in late adulthood visit:

www.apa.org/pi/aging/sexuality.html, **The American Psychological Association Aging and Human Sexuality Resource Guide,** date connected May 23, 2007. Provides a variety of facts about sexuality in later life, along with links to other resources.

www.aarp.org/health/, **AARP (The Health Site),** date connected May 23, 2007. This site includes survey and research, as well as health care tips and information.

www.asaging.org, **American Society on Aging,** date connected May 23, 2007. A site that provides information from the Gay and Lesbian Aging Interest Network (LGAIN).

REFERENCES

AARP. (1999). *Sex—what's age got to do with it?* Retrieved April 12, 2006, from www.research.aarp.org/health/mmsexsurvey_1.html.

AARP. (2005). *Sexuality at midlife and beyond: 2004 update to attitudes and behavior.* Retrieved April 12, 2006, from http://assets.aarp.org/rgcenter/general/2004_sexuality.pdf.

Adelman, M. (1991). Stigma, gay lifestyles, and adjustment to aging: A study of later life gay men and lesbians. *Journal of Homosexuality, 20,* 7–32.

Annon, J. (1976). The PLISSIT model: A proposed conceptual scheme for the behavioral treatment of sexual problems. *Journal of Sex Education and Therapy,* 2 (Spring–Summer), 1–15.

Association of Reproductive Health Professionals. (2002). *Sexuality in middle and later life.* Retrieved April 10, 2006, from www.siecus.org/pubs/fact/fact0018.html.

Bacon, C. G., Mittleman, M. A., Kawachi, I., Giovannucci, E., Glasser, D. B., & Rimm, E. B. (2003). Sexual function in men older than 50 years of age: Results from the health professionals follow-up study. *Annals of Internal Medicine, 139,* 161–168.

Beers, M. H., & Berkow, R. (2000). *The Merck manual of geriatrics* (3rd ed.). Whitehouse Station, NJ: Merck & Co.

Blumenthal, R. S., Heldman, A. W., Brinker, J. A., Resar, J. R., Coombs, V. Y., Sloth, S. T., et al. (1997). Acute effects of conjugated estrogens on coronary blood flow response to acetylcholine in men. *American Journal of Cardiology, 80,* 1021–1022.

Bremner, W. J., & McKinlay, J. B. (2003). Age trends in the level of serum testosterone and other hormones in middle-aged men: Longitudinal results from the Massachusetts Male Aging Study. *Journal of Clinical Epidemiology and Metabolism, 872,* 589–598.

Casper, R. C., Redmond, D. E., Katz, M. M., Schaffer, C. B., Davis, J. M., & Koslow, S. H. (1985). Somatic symptoms in primary affective disorder. Presence and relationship to the classification of depression. *Archives of General Psychiatry, 42,* 1098–1104.

Centers for Disease Control. (2006). *Reported AIDS cases, by age and sex cumulative through 2005—United States and Dependent Areas.* Retrieved February 16, 2007, from www.cdc.gov/hiv/topics/surveillance/resources/slides/epidemiology/slides/EPI-AIDS.ppt.

DeLamater, J. D., & Still, M. (2005). Sexual desire in later life. *Journal of Sex Research, 42,* 138–150.

Friedman, J. D. (1997). Sexual expression: The forgotten component of ADL. *OT Practice,* (January), 20–25.

Gabbard, G. O., & Nadelson, C. (1995). Professional boundaries in the physician–patient relationship. *Journal of the American Medical Association, 273,* 1445–1495.

Goldstein, H., & Runyon, C. (1993). An occupational therapy educational module to increase sensitivity about geriatric sexuality. *Physical & Occupational Therapy in Geriatrics, 11*(2), 57–76.

Goldstein, I. (2004). Epidemiology of erectile dysfunction. *Sexuality and Disability, 22,* 113–120.

Goldstein-Lohman, H., & Aitken, M. J. (1995). Influence of education on knowledge and attitude toward older adult sexuality. *Physical & Occupational Therapy in Geriatrics, 13*(1/2), 51–62.

Goodroad, B. K. (2003). HIV and AIDS in people older than 50. A continuing concern. *Journal of Gerontological Nursing, 29*(4), 18–24.

Gott, M. (2005). Are older people at risk of sexually transmitted infections? A new look at the evidence. *Reviews in Clinical Gerontology, 14,* 5–13.

Guan, J. (2004). Correlates of spouse relationship with sexual attitude, interest, and activity among Chinese elderly. *Sexuality & Culture, 8*(1), 104–131.

Hillman, J. (2000). *Clinical perspectives on elderly sexuality.* New York: Kluwer Academic.

Hilt, M., & Lipschultz, J. H. (2005). *Mass media, an aging population, and the baby boomers.* Mahwah, NJ: Lawrence Erlbaum Associates.

Hodson, D. S., & Skeen, P. (1994). Sexuality and aging: The hammerlock of myths. *Journal of Applied Gerontology 13,* 219–235.

Kingsberg, S. A. (2002). The impact of aging on sexual function in women and their partners. *Archives of Sexual Behavior, 31,* 431–437.

Kinsella, G. H., & Duffy, F. D. (1979). Psychosocial readjustment in the spouses of aphasic patients: A comparative study of 79 subjects. *Scandinavian Journal of Rehabilitation Medicine, 11,* 129–132.

Kolata, G. (1998). FDA approves pill to overcome impotence. *The New York Times,* March 28. Accessed April 4, 2008, from www.usrf.org/breakingnews/bn_980328_viagra.html.

Korpelainen, J. T., Nieminen, P., & Myllylä, V. V. (1999). Sexual functioning among stroke patients and their spouses. *Stroke, 30,* 715–719.

Laumann, E. O., Gagnon, J. H., Michael, R. T., & Michaels, S. (1994). *The social organization of sexuality: Sexual practices in the United States.* Chicago: University of Chicago Press.

Leary, W. E. (1992, December 10). Medical panel says most sexual impotence in men can be treated without surgery. *New York Times,* D20.

Masters, W. H., & Johnson, V. E. (1966). *Human sexual response.* Boston: Little, Brown.

Matthias, R. E., Lubben, J. E., Atchison, K. A., & Schweitzer, S. (1997). Sexual activity and satisfaction among very old adults: Results from a community-dwelling Medicare population survey. *Educational Research, 37,* 6–14.

MetLife Mature Market Institute. (2006). *Out and aging: The MetLife study of lesbian and gay baby boomers.* Retrieved February 16, 2007, from www.asaging.org/networks/LGAIN/OutandAging.pdf.

Mohan, R., & Bhugra, D. (2005). Literature update: A critical review. *Sexual and Relationship Therapy, 21*(1), 115–122.

Monga, T. N. (1993). Sexuality post stroke. In R. Teasell (Ed.), *Long term consequences of stroke* (pp. 225–236). Philadelphia: Hanley & Belfus.

Nadler, R. D. (1997). Arthritis and other connective tissue diseases. In M. L. Sipski & C. J. Alexander (Eds.), *Sexual function in people with disability and chronic illness* (pp. 261–278). Gaithersburg, MD: Aspen.

National Council on Aging. (1998). *Half of older Americans report they are sexually active.* Available at www.ncoa.org/content.cfm?sectionID=105&detail=128.

Pope, M., & Schulz, R. (1991). Sexual attitudes and behavior in midlife and aging homosexual males. *Journal of Homosexuality, 20,* 169–177.

Purifoy, F. E., Grodsky, A., & Giambra, L. M. (1992). The relationship of sexual daydreaming to sexual activity, sexual drive, and sexual attitudes for women across the life-span. *Archives of Sexual Behavior, 21,* 369–385.

Rosenfeld, D. (2003). *The changing of the guard: Lesbian and gay elders, identity, and social change.* Philadelphia: Temple University Press.

Rowland, D. L., Greenleaf, W. J., Dorfman, L. J., & Davidson, J. M. (1993). Aging and sexual function in men. *Archives of Sexual Behavior, 22655,* 447–452.

Sharpe, T. H. (2004). Introduction to sexuality in late life. *The Family Journal: Counseling and Therapy for Couples and Families, 12,* 199–205.

Sjögren, K., Damberg, J.E., & Liliequist, B. (1983). Sexuality after stroke with hemiplegia, I: Aspects of sexual function. *Scandinavian Journal of Rehabilitation Medicine, 15,* 55–61.

U.S. Bureau of the Census. (1996). *Statistical abstracts of the United States, Tables 128–129.*

U.S. Bureau of the Census. (1998a). *Statistical abstracts of the United States. Table 16.*

U.S. Bureau of the Census. (1998b). *Statistical abstracts of the United States. Table 62.*

Ward, R., Vass, A. A., Aggarwal, N., Garfield, C., & Cybyk, B. (2005). A kiss is still a kiss? The construction of sexuality in dementia care. *Dementia: The International Journal of Social Research and Practice, 4*(1), 49–72.

Worthman, C. M. (1999). Faster, farther, higher: Biology and the discourses on human sexuality. In D. N. Suggs & A. W. Miracle (Eds.), *Culture, biology, and sexuality* (pp. 64–75). Athens, GA: University of Georgia Press.

Worthman, C. M., Beall, C. M., & Stallings, J. F. (1997a). Population variation in reproductive function of men. *American Journal of Physical Anthropology, 24*(Suppl.), 246–256.

Worthman, C. M., Beall, C. M., & Stallings, J. F. (1997b). Population differences in DHEAS across the lifespan: Implications for aging. *American Journal of Human Biology, 9,* 149–157.

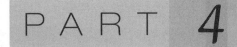

PART 4

Service Delivery

C hapters 17 through 22 in this part consider what it is that health care providers can do to assist older adults in maintaining their desired levels of activity and participation. Each of the chapters discusses a particular system in which health care is provided: the community, home health, rehabilitation, and long-term care. Type and location of service (e.g., community-based service or institutional) must be matched to the particular need. Interventions may be targeted to the individual, the social system, or the environment. Thus, following careful assessment of the individual and the environment, the care provider must decide whether to develop an intervention plan for the person, to confer with informal caregivers, or to consult with planners such as architects and policy makers.

The most helpful interventions for elders will focus on wellness, function, and life satisfaction, rather than on perfect health. It is unrealistic to expect every older adult to be "cured." It is also unnecessary, because the presence of illness does not automatically imply dysfunction.

Careful consideration must be given to the wishes of the individual. Some individuals find the possibility of being confined to a nursing home anathema. And some individuals reach a point at which they no longer perceive their lives to have adequate quality to encourage them to continue. This is often difficult for health care professionals to accept, because there is a strong societal bias toward preserving life at all costs. Similarly, there is an assumption that independence is always desirable. The Independent Living movement has given lie to that belief, holding that it is up to the individual to decide the extent and kind of independence that is optimal. An individual might choose not to dress himself of herself if this activity required a level of energy expenditure that left none for other activities that he or she defined as more gratifying.

CHAPTER 17

Evaluation of Functional Performance

Seanne Wilkins, PhD, OT Reg (Ont) • Lori Letts, PhD, OT Reg (Ont) • Julie Richardson, PhD, PT

The therapist made me feel good. She said, "Remember anything that's aged is good—wine, art, architecture, books." She made me realize that if you're aged, you're worthwhile . . . she seemed to work with [her clients'] needs, not hers . . . she was practising what they needed . . . it was what she had learned from studying people and their way of life and their whole person.

M.S. Wilkins, 1998

OBJECTIVES

By the end of this chapter, readers will be able to:

1. Outline the purposes of evaluating the functional performance of older adults.
2. Describe a philosophy of the evaluation process that is client centered and contextually based.
3. Describe a decision-making process including key questions useful in guiding the selection and implementation of assessments.
4. Identify particular issues that must be considered in the evaluation of older adults, including (a) who the client is, (b) why it is important to assess the functional performance of older adults, (c) what is the broad focus of evaluation, and (d) what general and specific factors should be considered when evaluating older adults.
5. Discuss the different evaluation methods that might be used to assess older adults, including special methodological considerations.

Health professionals perform evaluation with older adults for various purposes. The value of evaluation rests in the ability to provide information for description of **impairments, functional performance,** program planning, prediction of functional outcome, and evaluation after therapy intervention. **Evaluation** has been defined as a determination of the value of or significance of a situation through careful appraisal and study; in the rehabilitation context it is the process of gathering and interpreting data to be used as the basis for intervention with a client (American Occupational Therapy Association, 1995, 2002; Merriam-Webster Online Dictionary, n.d.). Evaluation also usually involves classification, scoring, or judgment in a quantitative or qualitative manner to enable the service provider and older adult to make sense of information related to functional performance.

Given that this text will be used internationally by both occupational therapists and physical therapists, we have decided to use terminology and models of practice that are used around the world. It is then up to the reader to apply the terminology and models of practice used in his or her own local environment when interpreting this chapter for use in his or her practice. In those cases where we have used particular terms in a specific way, these terms are highlighted in the text in bold and defined in the glossary at the end of the chapter. We also encourage readers to review some of the most helpful summaries of assessment and measurement, including Finch, Brooks, Stratford, and Mayo (2002) and Law, Baum, and Dunn (2005).

In this chapter, we discuss issues related to the meaning of evaluation with older adults; present a philosophy of a client-centered, contextual evaluation process; and outline a decision-making process to guide therapists in the evaluation process. Issues specifically related to evaluation of functional performance with older adults—including the need to identify who the client is, the need for older adults to stay engaged in purposeful activity, the promotion of a broad focus of evaluation beyond activities of daily living (ADL), and general and specific factors that may affect the evaluation process—are discussed. Finally, we focus on evaluation methods used with older adults, including **standardized** and individualized methods, qualitative and quantitative methods, the use of norms, the need for contextual evaluation, and self-report versus observation. Specific examples and quotations from seniors are used to illustrate evaluation issues.

The Meaning of Evaluation

What do we mean by evaluation? An evaluation process involves the gathering of information, using qualitative or quantitative methods, in order to assess and categorize, make appraisals, estimations, and judgments. Although evaluation is commonly considered to begin the therapy process, it is an activity that can and should occur before, during, and after a person receives rehabilitation therapy services. There are several purposes for evaluation with older adults, including screening and prevention, description, prediction, and outcome evaluation.

As persons grow older, changes in health status and an increasing prevalence of chronic diseases such as cardiovascular disease, arthritis, stroke, dementia, and Parkinson's disease may lead to increasing difficulties in performing the daily activities of self-care, household maintenance, shopping and other community activities, voluntary or work pursuits, and recreation and leisure activities. U.S. data show that limitations with activities because of chronic conditions increase with age. Among older adults 65 to 74 years old, 19.9% had difficulties with ADL, and over half (52.5%) of those 85 years and older had difficulties with ADL. Among older adults over 65 living in the community, 27.3% had difficulty performing one or more ADL, and 13.0% had difficulty with instrumental activities of daily living (IADL). In contrast, among those older adults living in institutions, 93.3% had difficulty with one or more ADL, and 76.3% had difficulty with three or more ADL (Administration on Aging, 2004). The National Health and Nutrition Examination Survey (NHANES III), designed to identify data on health status, disease, and risk factors among older adults that could be used for public health planning, provides interesting information about functional skill levels of older adults. The survey included a randomly selected group of 5000 adults over the age of 60 and described self-report data as well as data from physical examinations. For adults 60 to 69 years of age, 4% experienced difficulties in activities such as preparing meals or walking indoors. These rates of functional difficulties increased to 17% to 23% for adults over 80 years of age (Marwick, 1997). Disabled older adults living in Canada have difficulty with the following tasks: preparing meals (49%), housework (55%), heavy chores (59%), personal finances (35%), and personal care (53%) (Statistics Canada, 2002).

The compression of morbidity is increasingly viewed as the primary goal for promoting health and improving quality of life for older adults

(Fries, 1987, 2005). The theory of compression of morbidity predicts a future decrease in the number of years with severe disease and **disability** (Fried, Herdman, Kuhn, Rubin, & Turano, 1991). Active life expectancy, which can be used to evaluate compression of morbidity, is defined as the average number of years an individual at a given age will survive and remain in an active or nondisabled state. The ideal healthy population would experience long life expectancy with the effects of chronic disease compressed into a very short time before death. Aging produces changes in physical functioning and transitions through disabled states. The process of disablement is dynamic and involves varying functional states such as changes in mobility, ADL, and IADL. The onset of disability can be slow and progressive which often occurs with chronic disease or acute as occurs following a catastrophic medical event (Guralnik, Ferrucci, Balfour, Volpato, & Di Iorio, 2001). Recent work has defined the period between the onset of impairment and the onset of disability as being a stage of preclinical disability (Fried et al., 1991). Preclinical disability is a transitional state between impairment and disability which is characterized by a general decline in activity level or by limitation of ability to perform a task (using the normal method) though the individual can still accomplish the task under certain circumstances without perceived difficulty (Fried et al., 1991; Guralnik, 1996). Specifically, preclinical disability in mobility also predicts the onset of future disability (Fried, Ettinger, Lind, Newman, & Gardin, 1994). Thus, it is important for therapists to be involved in the evaluation and intervention with older adults to prevent preclinical disability that may be the result of deconditioning, and increase functional performance resulting from chronic conditions.

Because of increasing rates of difficulties with functional performance, an important role of evaluation of older adults is to screen for problems in functional performance in order to develop strategies to improve performance or prevent further deterioration in the ability to perform the activities that a person needs or wants to do. **Screening** can identify older adults who may need further evaluation or intervention, or both. It is important that screening evaluations be easy to do, take little time, and accurately identify those who require further evaluation for intervention. Examples of screening **assessments** are the Mini-Mental State Examination (Folstein, Folstein, &

McHugh, 1975), the Minimum Data Set (State University of New York at Buffalo [SUNY], 1990), IADL Screener (Fillenbaum, 1985), Functional Activities Questionnaire (Fillenbaum, 1985) the Frail Elderly Functional Assessment (Gloth, Watson, Meyer, & Pearson, 1995), and the Geriatric Depression Scale (Yesavage & Brink, 1983). There are also various measurement tools, such as the Timed "Up and Go" Test (Podsiadlo & Richardson, 1991), the Functional Reach Test (Duncan, Weiner, Chandler, & Studenski, 1990), and the Berg Balance Scale (Berg et al., 1992), that are used to screen for particular impairments associated with mobility of older adults.

Evaluations that are used for **descriptive** purposes focus on gathering information to describe characteristics of individuals and to enable differentiation between persons on the specific characteristic that is being measured (Law, 1987). This type of assessment is important to identify issues that merit intervention; to determine specific problems in the areas of impairment, activity limitation, and **participation** restriction; and to help determine the need for therapeutic services. For example, a short cognitive assessment provides information about the cognitive status of an individual and helps the person, his or her family, and the service provider decide whether there are difficulties related to cognitive status and whether intervention is warranted. Assessments used for descriptive purposes, such as the Functional Behavior Profile (Baum, Edwards, & Morrow-Howell, 1993) or the Assessment of Motor and Process Skills (Fisher, 1995), include items that have been shown to discriminate among individuals on the basis of the characteristic being assessed. The Modified Falls Efficacy Scale is an activity questionnaire that can be used to identify older adults with balance and mobility problems and reflects confidence levels and fear of falling (Hill, Schwarz, Kalogeropoulos, & Gibson, 1996). In many instances, evaluations that work well for descriptive purposes do not perform adequately in evaluating change over time after therapeutic intervention.

Assessments used for **prediction** include items related to a specific characteristic in order to forecast another trait. Examples include the Cognitive Performance Test (Allen, Earheart, & Blue, 1992) and the Tinetti Performance-Oriented Mobility Evaluation (Tinetti, 1986). The Cognitive Performance Test has been used to predict functional capacity in a range of daily activities of older adults with dementia. The Tinetti Performance-Oriented Mobility Evaluation is used to determine older adults' risk for falls. Items on a predictive measure are included if they describe the characteristic of interest and predict the trait or criterion of interest now or in the future. Table 17-1 summarizes the various uses of assessment and examples of instruments that can be used for each.

A common use for assessments is to evaluate **outcomes** or change in persons after they have received rehabilitation services. Examples include the Functional Independence Measure (FIM) (State University of New York at Buffalo [SUNY], 1990) and the Canadian Occupational Performance Measure (COPM) (Law et al., 2005). The FIM is widely used to measure the overall performance in daily living skills, providing an indicator of functional ability, and is used to evaluate the effectiveness of rehabilitation services. The COPM was designed specifically as an evaluative tool to measure clients' self-perception of change in **occupational performance** and satisfaction with performance after occupational therapy intervention. Items included on evaluative measures are those that can be demonstrated to be responsive to change in individuals when change actually occurs.

It is important for therapists to review information in the assessment manual to determine the purposes for which the assessment has been developed and validated, and to match that purpose to the given situation. For example, if an assessment that is primarily designed to describe differences between persons is used to evaluate change or outcomes after a therapeutic program, it often leads to a situation in which a clinically important change may have occurred but the evaluation is not able to measure that change. Other psychometric characteristics that therapists need to review before using an assessment include issues of **reliability, validity,** and **clinical utility** (Van Dusen & Brunt, 1997).

Evaluation Philosophy

The primary focus of occupational therapists and physical therapists working with older people is to enable older adults to maintain function. The ability to participate in important day-to-day activities gives meaning to life. Such participation evolves and changes over one's life course and is an important determinant of health and well-being (Canadian Association of Occupational Therapists, 2002; Law, Baptiste, & Mills, 1995). Our beliefs about social participation and its inherent value to people, as well as our beliefs in the ability of people to understand and make choices about their own daily activities, result in our practice being client centered. Within practice, we enter into partnerships with our clients. Client-centered practice has been defined as

> a partnership between the client and the therapist that empowers the client to engage in functional performance and fulfil his or her ... roles in a variety of environments. The client participates actively in negotiating goals, which are given priority and are at the centre of assessment, intervention and evaluation. Throughout the process the therapist listens to and respects the client's values, adapts the interventions to meet the client's needs and enables the client to make informed decisions. (Sumsion, 2000, p. 308)

TABLE 17-1 **Summary of Purpose of Assessments with Examples**

Purpose of Assessments	Examples
Screening	Mini-Mental State Examination, Minimum Data Set, IADL Screener, Functional Activities Questionnaire, Frail Elderly Functional Assessment, Geriatric Depression Scale, Timed "Up and Go" Test, Functional Reach Test, Berg Balance Scale
Descriptive	Functional Behavior Profile, Assessment of Motor and Process Skills, Modified Falls Efficacy Scale
Predictive	Cognitive Performance Test, Tinetti Performance-Oriented Mobility Evaluation
Outcome	Canadian Occupational Performance Measure, Functional Independence Measure

Part of being client centered involves listening carefully to our clients. What do they say that they want? In a seminal study of over 6000 recently hospitalized patients randomly selected from 62 hospitals across the United States, as well as 2000 of the family members or friends who served as their care partners, the Picker/Commonwealth Program for Patient-Centered Care identified seven dimensions of patient-centered care:

1. Respect for patients' values, preferences, and expressed needs
2. Coordination and integration of care
3. Information, communication, and education
4. Physical comfort
5. Emotional support and alleviation of fears and anxiety
6. Involvement of family and friends
7. Transition and continuity after discharge (Gerteis, Edgman-Levitan, Daley, & Delbanco, 1993)

Further research identified an eighth dimension as access to care (Picker Institute, n.d.).

In the case of older adults, what do they say they want as they age and require more health and social services? They clearly say that they want a voice in the development of policies and programs directed toward their care (National Advisory Council on Aging [NACA], 2000). They want the same rights and privileges guaranteed people of all ages. They realize that health and well-being require adequate income protection, universal access to health care, and the availability of a range of programs and services that support their autonomy while taking into account their individuality and cultural diversity. They want "the right to be autonomous while benefiting from interdependence and to make their own decisions even if it means 'living-at-risk'" (NACA, 2000). They see themselves as independent, capable of making their own choices and decisions. They equate independence with quality of life. Independence means being in control of one's own life and is closely tied to dignity, pride, and well-being. These beliefs are similar to those shared by therapists who practice in a client-centered way.

Some authors (Moloney & Paul, 1993) have suggested that the cohort of older people, whose values and attitudes were shaped by the Depression and World War II, embrace authority, security, and conformity and, therefore, tend to respect the medical system and comply with health professionals' recommendations. More recently, older adults are becoming more involved in directing their own care. Walker (2006) argued that this is related to the rise of consumerism and the reassertion of individualism leading to expectations for a participatory voice and more choice relative to care and services. In the experiences of the authors of this chapter, there is diversity in the ways in which older adults wish to be involved in their own care. For example, in a study of women with osteoporosis, there were a variety of ways in which participants described their interactions with health care providers, and particularly their physicians (Wilkins, 1998). One woman said *"I would suggest you go out and get the best doctor in the city and do exactly as he says."* Another woman, who suggested that she might not have been as forthright with her doctor in the past, said, *"[My doctor] wanted me to go on hormones and I said 'Okay you give me 300% guarantee that I won't get cancer again and I'll go on hormones. But otherwise forget it.'... You know that's one thing at my age I would never have said earlier."* Some women participated in what their doctors would have called "risky behaviors," such as lifting heavy items or climbing ladders while painting, but despite their doctors' warnings, they continued to participate in these valued activities. Others had discontinued taking their medications for osteoporosis or augmented their medical treatment with alternative therapies (e.g., homeopathy, naturopathy, chiropractic). As therapists, we need to be aware of the diversity among older adults and refrain from espousing stereotypical ideas about our older clients.

Among the women with osteoporosis, some had specific suggestions for health care providers. One woman described the need for health care professionals to look beyond the physical aspects of living with osteoporosis and consider the psychological and social aspects as well. When she was depressed by the death of her husband, by the need to have her hip reconstructed, and by her diagnosis of osteoporosis, her physician asked her why she was depressed, inasmuch as osteoporosis was not something from which she was going to die. This lack of recognition of the other aspects of her life left her angry and disappointed in the lack of understanding about the impact of other life events on her health. Another woman talked about the difference in approaches between her physician and physical therapist. Her physician had told her that she was old and *"all the things you shouldn't do . . . don't bend over, don't stretch, don't do this, don't do that . . . be sure you get up properly, don't slip on the rug. Do you know how restrictive that is?"* In contrast, when she had discussed this with her physical therapist, the therapist had pointed out to her how valued older things are: *"She made me feel good. She said, 'Remember anything that's aged is good— wine, art, architecture, books. She made me realize that if you're aged, you're worthwhile."* She described the therapist as someone who worked with individuals in a client-centered way: *"she seemed to work with their needs, not hers . . . she was practicing what they needed not what she'd learned from a book. It was what she had learned from studying people and their way of life and their whole person"* (Wilkins, 1998).

How do we make sure that we are meeting the individual needs of our older clients? One way to ensure that we are addressing the aspects of older adults' lives that they consider to be important is to use a model of practice or conceptual framework that considers the older adult performing activities of his or her choice within a supportive environment. Examples of such tools are the International Classification of Functioning, Disability and Health (ICF) (WHO, 2001) and Glass's (1998) Conceptual Scheme for Conjugating the Tenses of Function. These will be described in detail later in the chapter. Other models that have been developed are profession specific, such as Person-Environment-Occupation Model of Occupational Performance (Law et al., 1996). As had been described in previous chapters, the American Occupational Therapy Practice Framework (2002) incorporates many of these constructs in its guidelines for evaluation and intervention.

Why Evaluate Functional Performance in Older Adults?

Functional performance is a significant factor in the ability of older adults to participate in activities that are important to them. There is an established link between engagement in meaningful activities (function) and health and well-being. This is true for older adults as well as the rest of the population. Law, Steinwender, and

Leclair (1998) reviewed a number of studies that examined the relationships among health, well-being, and occupation. They included studies that have been conducted with older adults, with and without functional impairments. It is clear from their review that the removal of **occupation** can be detrimental to health and well-being, whereas the addition of occupation can be beneficial.

It is also well known that many older adults want to continue to participate in their community, fulfilling roles as they have always done and taking on new roles. Evaluation of functional performance can be a useful step in understanding whether functional abilities are changing and why, so that strategies can be developed to address the changes and promote optimum function. Multiple strategies can be used to address and promote functional performance. They might focus on the strengths and limitations of the person, but they can also relate to the **environment** or area of activity in which the person is engaging. It is important, then, to consider functional performance in the context in which it will be carried out (Dunn, Brown, & McGuigan, 1994). It may not be possible to change the abilities of the person, if changes are occurring as a result of a chronic progressive disease, for example. However, the activity might be maintained if the environment or task is modified.

Generally, an evaluation of functional performance can be useful to understand (1) which activities are most important to an older adult, so that priorities can be set for intervention; (2) how functional activities are balanced or changed as a person ages; and (3) how a person is actually performing so that interventions can be designed to optimize that performance.

Evaluation Realities

The evaluation philosophy described in the previous section fits the overriding goal of rehabilitation professionals to facilitate the functional performance of their clients, particularly in those areas most desired by the individual. However, realities of funding and setting also drive evaluation decisions. In the United States, most individuals receive health care paid for by a third party. This may be a government insurance plan, such as Medicaid or Medicare; a private insurance policy provided by an employer or paid for by the individual; or county- or state-funded care for indigent individuals. That third-party payer has an interest in the care provided. As a result, therapists are typically bound by reimbursement rules that dictate what can be assessed (and, as treatment progresses, what sorts of interventions will be covered). Specifics of these guidelines, which vary depending on site of care, are described in later chapters. It is important to remember, however, that the evaluation process may need to be modified to fit reimbursement guidelines. Therapists may need to promote the client's interests with the insurers, ideally providing sound economic rationale for reimbursement. As the number and scope of outcome studies and systematic reviews increases (see, for example, Bean et al., 2004; Clark et al., 1997; Gill et al., 2002, 2004; Gillespie et al., 2003; Gitlin et al., 2003; Jette et al., 1999; Steultjens et al., 2004), such arguments about the value of evaluating and intervening to address more than ADL will become easier to make.

A Conceptual Framework for Evaluation of Performance

The goal of evaluation is to ensure that the activities that older adults want to, need to, or are expected to perform are identified, and the reasons for difficulties in performance are established. The use of a conceptual framework will help therapists and older adults work together to identify the focus on evaluation and the measures to use. Various conceptual frameworks have influenced the understanding of disability over

the years (e.g., the Nagi Model, 1976; the International Classification of Impairments, Disabilities and Handicaps (ICIDH), World Health Organization [WHO], 1980). The latter was the basis for the International Classification of Functioning, Disability and Health (ICF) (WHO, 2001), described in Chapter 1, which provides standard language and a conceptual framework that can underpin the evaluation process. Consideration is given to the health condition of the individual within the body functions and structures, the activities in which he or she engages as well as participation within the various contexts that make up his or her environment.

The use of a conceptual framework depicting the interactions between the components of the ICF (WHO, 2001) enables therapists to identify attributes for evaluation and ensures that the evaluation process develops logically and focuses only on areas of evaluation that are important and meaningful to older adults and their families. Table 17-2 provides examples of how this framework is used to specify attributes for evaluation along with appropriate evaluation tools. This conceptual framework is an excellent guide to therapists and rehabilitation teams in making decisions about the specific attributes to be assessed in each clinical situation.

Glass (1998) argued that the Nagi Model (Nagi, 1976) and the ICIDH (WHO, 1980) did not go far enough to allow those working with older adults to understand disability and its complexity in later life functioning. Traditionally in aging research, measures of disability have focused on hypothetical reported functional capacity (what the older adult says he or she can do) rather than on actual performance

TABLE 17-2   Using the International Classification of Function, Disability, and Health (ICF) to Organize Evaluation

ICF Domain	Body Functions and Structures	Activities	Participation	Environmental Factors
Evaluation attribute	Body movement	Functional mobility	Participation in leisure activities	Accessibility
Evaluation	Chedoke-McMaster Stroke Assessment (Gowland et al., 1995)	Late Life Function and Disability Instrument— Function Index (Jette et al., 2002; Haley et al., 2002)	London Handicap Scale (Harwood et al., 1994)	The Housing Enabler (Iwarsson & Slaug, 2001)

in everyday life (what the older adult does do). Glass maintained that measures of capacity provide limited information and often produce disability rates that may underestimate actual levels of disability among older adults. He suggested that more focus should be given to performance rather than capacity. This resulted in the development of a "conceptual scheme for conjugating the tenses of function" (Glass, 1998, p. 103) among older adults (Figure 17-1). His conceptual scheme has three levels. The first or hypothetical level measures a person's capacity by assessing what he or she says he or she can do. Activities are not placed within a context, and self-report or proxy responses are sought in relation to the degree of difficulty or the degree of assistance required. At the second or experimental level, the person's capabilities are measured by assessing timed performance and standardized task completion in a laboratory or clinic setting or what the person could do when asked to simulate activities. The third or enacted level reflects what the person actually does in his or her home or community environment, based on self-report, proxy, or direct observations that provide measures of the frequency and duration of activities, tasks, and roles. Glass demonstrated the discrepancy between self-report and actual everyday performance through qualitative interviews with members of three sites of the EPESE survey and the MacArthur Research Network on Successful Aging. For one third of the sample, there was congruency between what they reported they did and what they actually did, one third reported poorer functioning, and one third reported higher functioning than their actual functioning. The implications of Glass' research for therapists suggest that given the complexity of aging, it is important to consider what older adults *can* do and also what they *do* do. In evaluating our interventions to determine if our clients are improving or maintaining functional performance, it is critical to measure functional outcomes that include performance rather than only ask about hypothetical functional capacity. Glass' work also reminds us of the importance of considering the context within which our clients participate as well as the importance of compensatory strategies already used to maintain activity and participation. For example,

when evaluation takes place within the client's own home or community, it is possible to observe how he or she would ordinarily manage an activity rather than how he or she performs an activity in a hospital.

A Decision-Making Process to Guide Evaluation

Making decisions about which assessments to use with older adults is a complex process. In this chapter, we outlined the importance of using assessments that are client centered and enable older adults to identify the activities in which they want to participate and difficulties

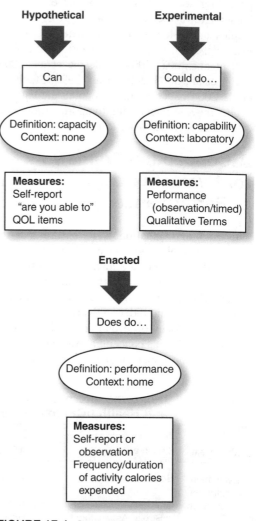

FIGURE 17-1 Conceptual scheme for conjugating the tenses of function. (From Glass, T. (1998). Conjugating the tenses of function: Discordance among hypothetical, experimental, and enacted function in older adults. The Gerontologist, 38, 101–112.)

they are having related to participation. Assessments also should meet basic psychometric criteria of clinical utility, reliability, and validity. The following key questions can be used by therapists to guide the selection and implementation of clinical evaluations:

- Do you have an evaluation method that enables the client to identify his or her functional performance issues and his or her goals for therapeutic intervention?
- What is the reason for the evaluation—to screen for problems, to describe specific performance difficulties, to predict performance, or to evaluate change or outcomes in performance after intervention?
- Is the assessment primarily for an individual client, or is it part of an evaluation protocol that is completed with all clients?
- What aspects of functional performance do you wish to assess?
- Where will the evaluation take place—in the client's home, in the community, or in the clinical setting?
- Do you have the time to conduct the assessments that are required?
- What methods of evaluation will you use—self-report, family, or **caregiver** report; service provider report; or observation of performance?
- If you require standardized assessments, do you have the budget to purchase these?
- Is the assessment that you are using reliable?
- Has the assessment you are using been validated for use with older adults?
- If you are using the measure for evaluation, is there evidence that the measure is sensitive to change?
- Have you completed any training required in order to do the assessment? If not, do you have access to the dollars required for training?
- What is the clinical utility of the assessment—amount of time to complete, cost, ease of administration and interpretation, or availability of assessment manual?
- How will you use the results of the evaluation for program or intervention planning, administrative uses, or program evaluation?
- How can the evaluation be framed to convince insurers of the value of obtaining desired information?

Issues in the Evaluation of Performance with Older Adults

Who is the Client?

For the most part, when therapists are working with adults and older adults, these clients are competent to give informed consent and to make decisions about the course of their interactions with health care providers. This situation changes with older adults who are cognitively impaired, have communication problems, have mental health problems, or are no longer deemed to be competent. Although we might discuss the client's functional abilities as well as preferences, interests, and values around function with his or her significant others, we may also wish to engage the client directly in these discussions. How do we engage in client-centered practice when the client has a cognitive impairment, has aphasia, or is depressed? Hobson (1996, 1999) addressed the issue of being client centered when the client is cognitively impaired and incompetent. She described two strategies that can allow the therapist to practice in a client-centered manner: graded decision making and advocacy.

In addressing *graded decision making,* she first clarified that there are decisions with low-risk outcomes (e.g., whether to eat one's meal in the kitchen or dining room) and those with high-risk outcomes (e.g., whether to return to living alone in one's own home). She then suggested that because modifying activities is part of the usual practice of therapists, these same skills can be applied to modifying decision making. Decisions can be graded to be less cognitively demanding. For example, the therapist might provide a list of limited options or pros, cons, and possible outcomes for a client within an environment that fosters decision making and competence. The amount of guidance and input by the therapist into decision making will depend on the client's level of cognitive impairment.

With regard to *advocacy,* Hobson (1999) argued that therapists should listen to and respect the opinions and preferences of clients, even if they are cognitively impaired and deemed incompetent. The therapist also serves as an advocate for the client, expressing the client's interests to the people who have the legal authority to make decisions on behalf of the client. Being client centered ranges from the therapist considering the client's needs to the client directing the care process (Hobson, 1999). This diversity recognizes that there are a variety of possible ways to be client centered with clients who are cognitively impaired.

There may be situations in which the client is the person providing care for the older adult who is cognitively impaired or frail. The majority of older adults living in the community who require care receive that assistance from informal caregivers, who may be spouses or partners, children, other family members, or friends (Stone, 2006). Many of those providing care may themselves be old and have chronic illnesses. There may be physical or mental strain associated with caregiving, which may result in the additional need for therapy services by the caregivers. The caregiver or care partner (Gerteis et al., 1993) may identify his or her own functional performance issues in functional mobility, self-care, productivity, and leisure.

What to Assess When Focusing on Function in Older Adults

As people age, we know that their life roles and the kinds of activities in which they participate tend to change. People may not engage in paid work as they get older (and in many countries or certain vocations, mandatory retirement policies prevent them from doing so), but many older adults engage in productive roles through volunteering. As a result of retirement, the amount of available leisure time usually increases with age. Therefore, we need to consider leisure activities as potentially significant to the client. ADL are often a focus of functional performance evaluation in older adults. Self-care is, of course, an essential component of evaluation of function, but it should not be used to the exclusion of evaluation in other areas of function, including IADL, functional and community mobility, productivity, and leisure. Functional mobility underlies many areas of performance and may be key to evaluating plan interventions to help clients meet their goals. All of these functional performance areas can be important, and together they form the balance of activities in which people participate. For an in-depth discussion of self-care, work and retirement, and leisure, refer to Chapters 11, 12, and 13 respectively.

There are a number of functional performance evaluations that can be used with older adults that address a broad range of functional areas of performance. Some examples follow to assess the following:

- Lower extremity performance: the Short Physical Performance Battery (Guralnik, Ferrucci, Simonsick, Salive, & Wallace, 1995), including balance tests, repeated chair stands, and an 8-meter walk
- Exercise capacity and tolerance: the Two and Six Minute Walk (Butland, Pang, Gross, Woodcock, & Geddes, 1982) and the Long Distance Corridor Walk (Simonsick, Montgomery, Newman, Bauer, & Harris, 2003)
- Functional mobility: the Environmental Analysis of Mobility Questionnaire (EAMQ), Shumway-Cooke and colleagues (2002, 2005) reporting the frequency of encounter and avoidance of 24 features of the physical environment, grouped into eight dimensions
- A person's usual or actual performance of mobility: The Life Space Diary (May, Nayak, & Issacs, 1985)—the environment in which a person expects to move within a day, for example, is divided into concentric zones and persons record over 24-hour periods areas in which they have moved during the day; Stavley, Owsley, Sloane, and Ball (1999) developed a questionnaire version of this approach—the Life-Space Questionnaire (LSQ) consists of nine questions that ask whether respondents have been to each of the regions of their environment within the past 3 days
- Performance difficulties in self-care, productivity, and leisure areas: the Canadian Occupational Performance Measure (Law et al., 2005)
- Roles that are important sources of activity for older adults: the Role Checklist (Oakley, Keilhofner, Barris, & Reichler, 1986) or the Activity Card Sort (Baum & Edwards, 1995); leisure and social activities are incorporated into these instruments
- ADLs and IADLs: the Kitchen Task Assessment (Baum & Edwards, 1993), Arnadottir OT-ADL Neurobehavioral Evaluation (A-ONE) (Arnadottir, 1990), the Physical Self-Maintenance Scale, and the Instrumental ADL Scale (Lawton & Brody, 1969), the Functional Autonomy Measurement System (Hebert, Carrier, & Bilodeau, 1988), and the

Assessment of Living Skills and Resources (Williams et al., 1991)

- Multiple domains of physical functions using observed performance of tasks: the Physical Performance Test (Reuben & Siu, 1990)
- Home safety: the Safety Evaluation of Function and the Environment for Rehabilitation—Health Outcome Measurement and Evaluation (SAFER-HOME v3) (Chiu & Oliver, 2006; Chiu et al., 2006) focuses on the person's ability to manage functional activities safely within the home environment

Although this is not a comprehensive listing of functional assessments available for use with older adults, it provides evidence of the vast array of instruments available that address functional mobility, self-care, productivity, and leisure.

Specific Issues Related to Evaluation of Functional Performance

A number of factors are unique to evaluating functional performance with older adults, such as considerations of how changes in lower extremity function or sensory and motor systems might influence outcomes of functional performance evaluations, and how the presence of chronic conditions may need to be considered. There also are a number of factors that need to be considered in any evaluation of functional performance that are equally important when evaluating function with older adults. These issues will be discussed in this section.

Changes in Lower Extremity Function
There is strong evidence that changes in lower extremity function are the hallmark for the onset of disability with aging. However, assessment using performance measures as part of routine functional assessment of lower extremity function is more likely to include walking speed assessment rather than functional limitations (e.g., stooping, kneeling, crouching, pushing objects, climbing stairs, and transferring) as an indicator of mobility. These latter items are from the Nagi (1976) assessment and the Rosow-Breslau Scale (Rosow & Breslau, 1966). This level of functioning is sometimes obtained in surveys through self-report but rarely assessed through performance. Performance of these activities would indicate changes in functioning which would identify persons who are experiencing changes in lower extremity functioning and who might be prevented from making the transition to disability. The relationship between impairments, such as muscle strength, range of movement, pain, and flexibility, to functional limitation items and lower extremity functioning needs to be considered. The final issue that needs to be addressed in lower extremity performance is what is usual performance and how does the individual perform within his or her environment (Glass, 1998)?

Interventions targeted at prevention of functional limitations should focus on screening for changes in lower extremity functioning. Analyses of data from the Longitudinal Study on Aging (LSOA) found that age, walking activities, and musculoskeletal problems have a greater influence on lower body functional limitations than on IADL. Lower body disability predicted lower body and upper body disability 3 years later, whereas, upper body disability only predicted future upper body disability (Lawrence & Jette, 1996). A further cross-sectional study that examined the relationship between impairments and different types of disability in 207 community-dwelling volunteers found that mobility disability rather than upper or lower extremity strength predicted overall disability, basic physical disability, ADL, or IADL (Jette, Assmann, Rooks, Harris, & Crawford, 1998). Data from the Asset and Health Dynamics among the Oldest Old (AHEAD) Study used to assess the structure of Health Status in 6470 community-dwelling adults, 70 years and older, showed that lower body limitations were the most important factor in how older persons perceived their health when compared to basic ADL, IADL, and predicted future health status (Stump, Clark, Johnson, & Wolinsky, 1997). Finally, in a large cohort study of older community-dwelling persons with the lowest scores and intermediate scores on performance tests at baseline (walk one-half mile, climb stairs, ADL), were at increased risk of disability, RR = 4.2 – 4.9 and RR = 1.6 – 1.8 at 4 years compared to persons with highest performance scores (Guralnik et al., 1995). For therapists, then, this implies that although it may be important to evaluate both upper and lower body disability, lower body functioning may be more predictive of future activity and participation limitations.

It is well documented that poor lower extremity function predicts subsequent disability. There is also evidence that gait speed alone accurately predicted onset of incident disability almost as well as a battery of lower extremity performance tests (Guralnik et al., 2000). Therefore, it is worth considering using walking speed and gait assessments as an evaluation of current abilities and to predict future physical functioning. An index of ambulatory mobility-related physiological limitations (MOBLI), which has information about self-reported walking difficulty, walking speed, time to complete five chair stands, and peak expiratory flow, has established evidence of responsiveness and predictive validity over a 4-year period with evidence of a **dose response** relationship. The predictive validity of this index was similar to self-reported mobility (Melzer, Lan, & Guralnik, 2003). If emphasis is on prevention of decline, therapists may want to consider adopting this index as one of the assessments to screen for potential decline.

Changes to Sensory and Motor Systems with Usual Aging

Sensory loss occurs often as a part of the process of usual aging. Sensory loss includes changes in vision (e.g., presbyopia), hearing, and touch, all of which can influence functional performance. At the same time, there are changes in motor performance that can be detected. Balance and coordination may not be as efficient in older adults as in younger adults. There may also be differences in the speed or quality of performance. Despite these differences at the level of sensory and motor skills, these changes do not necessarily result in significant changes in the level of functional performance needed to perform daily roles. It is important to keep in mind that for many older adults, their functional performance abilities continue to be adequate for them to participate in daily activities. They may not experience functional changes in their performance as a result of sensory or motor system changes. Chapters 4 and 6 provide further descriptions of tools that assess motor and sensory function.

When evaluating functional performance, however, it is important to consider that changes in sensory or motor systems may, in fact, be the cause of difficulties with performance, particularly when standardized tests are being used. For tests that have norms for comparison, the normative sample should include a group of older adults, so that usual aging changes will occur in the normative sample as they may in the client group.

During evaluation, it may also be useful to set up the evaluation environment in such a way as to limit the extent to which sensory changes cause difficulties in performance of functional activities. When evaluating older adults, it is useful to ensure that

- Lighting is adequate in the environment
- All materials presented to the person, especially written materials, should be in print that is large and a contrasting color with the background, so that they can easily be read.
- The environment should have minimal background noise to enable the client to focus on the evaluation and any interaction with the assessor.
- The assessor should face the client, and verbal communications should be clear, allowing the client to hear what is said optimally and at the same time see the face of the assessor and pick up any nonverbal communication as well.

Depending on what is being assessed, consideration should also be given to performance expectations on the basis of the following:

- The client's familiarity with the environment: An older person may perform a meal preparation task quite easily in his or her own home but may have more difficulties with finding items or remembering where they are in a different setting. Depending on where the person will actually be performing the task, this is an important consideration.
- The client's familiarity with the task: Tasks such as dressing and toileting that have been done frequently by a person are more familiar than others and may be performed with greater ease.

All of these factors may influence the functional performance of an older person in evaluation and should be considered when the person's performance is being assessed.

When evaluating older adults, it is important to avoid stereotypes related to expectations for performance. Older adults may well be able to accommodate aging changes in ways to enable them to maintain their function. It may be most useful to consider which activities are of most importance to a client, and then examine the quality and speed of functional performance.

Aging with a Chronic Disability or Illness

Often when conducting a functional performance evaluation with an older adult, the client may have one or more chronic illnesses or disabilities that should be taken into account. It is important to consider what problems people have experienced in the past, so that current difficulties can be placed in the context of past difficulties. It is also useful to explore how past difficulties were addressed, because people have vast experience in developing individually adaptive techniques to deal with their personal challenges.

When evaluating someone who has a chronic condition, it is useful to also be clear about the purpose of the examining function. Is the goal to describe how the person is performing at one point in time (i.e., now) or to get a sense of how the chronic condition is changing with time, or responding to intervention? The expectations of the client's performance or ability to change or improve may be modified based on his or her status and previous problems.

Other Important Factors to Consider in any Evaluation of Functional Performance

There are a number of factors related to functional evaluation that are important to consider with any person. They are no less important when conducting evaluations of functional performance with older adults. They include the following:

Literacy Level. Particularly if the evaluation requires any kind of written language or numeric work, it is important to ensure that the client is able to read and understand the materials.

Language Spoken. In addition to the significance of written words in functional evaluations, if the client's first language is different than that of the evaluation setting, difficulties in performance may be related more to comprehension of instructions than to actual performance problems.

Cultural Background. Not only language but also cultural expectations and norms may influence performance. People in some cultures may not approach functional activities such as meal preparation or dressing in the manner expected in a functional evaluation. These factors need to be considered when selecting and administering evaluations. Two evaluations that consider the cultural relevance of daily activities are the

Assessment of Motor and Process Skills (AMPS) (Fisher, 1995; Fisher, Liu, Velozo, & Pan, 1992) and the Structured Observational Test of Function (SOTOF) (Laver, 1996; Laver & Powell, 1995).

Personal Factors. Such factors as the mood, motivation, education, and cognition of the person may influence his or her abilities to perform in a functional evaluation. Ideally, the client should understand why the evaluation is being conducted and agree to the process as it unfolds. This will help ensure that the performance observed is at an optimum for the person.

Economic Resources. Depending on the coverage the older adult has for health and rehabilitation services, evaluations by therapists may or may not be covered by the public sector (e.g., Medicare, Medicaid). The lack of financial resources may also limit access to community-based services.

Evaluation Methods

A range of evaluation methods can be used to gather information about functional performance in older adults. Such methods can be quantitative or qualitative in nature. Evaluations may focus on gathering information in either a standardized or individualized fashion.

Quantitative evaluations allow service providers to gather structured, scoreable information about a specific attribute. Such assessments are usually standardized so they have an underlying theory, specific administration instructions, a set number of items, and detailed information about how the evaluation is scored and the results interpreted. The advantage of quantitative, standardized evaluations is that they help ensure that the evaluation is done in a reliable manner and that the same information is collected and can be used for group analysis to provide information for evaluation of programs. It is important to note here that using standardized assessments often entails special training. Any modification of a standardized assessment will invalidate the norms and reliability and validity of the measure.

Individualized evaluations have become more popular in the past few years as an alternative to standardized evaluation. Individualized evaluations can assess attributes for which no standardized measures exist, may be more responsive to small changes in function over time, and may reflect more accurately client-centered goals (Russell, King, Palisano, & Law, 1995). Examples of individualized evaluations used with older adults include the Canadian Occupational Performance Measure (Law et al., 2005), the Patient Specific Function Scale (Stratford, Gill, Westaway, & Binkley, 1995), goal attainment scaling (Ottenbacher & Cusick, 1990, 1993), and the use of behavioral objectives (O'Neill & Harris, 1982). Individualized evaluations provide specific information about the client's goals for therapy intervention and are efficient evaluation methods to use. As with standardized evaluations, it is important that individualized evaluations be used in a systematic way in order to ensure their clinical utility. There is also some controversy about the aggregation of data from individualized evaluations because calculating an average score over a group of people may lose meaning as compared with the individualized results.

Evaluation can also be accomplished using *qualitative* or *naturalistic evaluation methods* such as narrative interviews, participant observation, or review of print or visual materials. Such approaches are ideally suited to the professions of occupational therapy and physical therapy with our interest in function and life experiences and our skill in human interaction. Issues related to the use of these methods include the time that data collection and thematic analysis can take, along with the need for increased training for most therapists in order to be able to interpret qualitative data dependably. However, this approach to evaluation does offer a unique, in-depth appraisal of the functional performance of a person within his or her environment and can serve as the basis for the development of a function-based intervention plan.

Screening for functional performance difficulties is a special use of evaluation methods. In screening situations, the purpose of doing an evaluation is to identify persons who have a higher probability of a functional performance difficulty in the specific area. For example, one might use a balance evaluation to screen for older adults who have a higher probability of balance difficulties that could potentially lead to a greater incidence of falls. It is important to consider the amount of time that screening evaluations will take, the accuracy with which the screening evaluation identifies a problem, and the availability of services to address these problems.

The accuracy of screening evaluations is determined by calculating the sensitivity and specificity of the screening tool (Sackett, Haynes, Guyatt, & Tugwell, 1991). The *sensitivity* of a screening assessment reflects the true positive rate of the evaluation—that is, the number of persons with positive screening results compared with the total number of persons with the attribute of interest. In the case of a balance evaluation, this would be the number of persons with a balance problem identified on the screening test compared with the total number of persons in the sample who had balance problems as confirmed by a gold standard test. In contrast, the *specificity* of a screening evaluation is the true negative rate of the evaluation for the number of persons with negative test results compared with the total number of persons who do not have the attribute of interest. In our balance assessment, this would be the number of persons without a balance problem on the screening test compared with the total number of persons in the sample who did not have balance problems as confirmed by a gold standard test. A screening evaluation that provides high sensitivity and specificity results in improved screening accuracy and minimizes the number of persons who are falsely identified as having difficulties when they do not or as not having difficulties when they do. Riddle and Stratford (1999) used the Berg Balance Test to illustrate the validity of different scores to predict falling.

Many standardized measures have been developed using normative data. The collection of normative data or norms is usually done by administering the evaluation to a reference population of "normal" persons. From these data, the normal distribution is calculated to include 95% of the sample in the two standard deviations above or below the mean. When using an evaluation with normative data, the therapist is able to compare the performance of a person with the norm to determine whether performance is significantly above or below normal and warrants intervention or further evaluation. Normative data are particularly useful for evaluations used for descriptive and screening purposes. The Short Physical Performance Battery (Guralnik et al., 1995) is an example of an evaluation that has established norms. However, there are potential difficulties with the use of normative evaluations with older adults. Many evaluations have been developed and standardized using adults across a wide age range. Normative data that have been collected across such a range should not be used to make decisions about persons in a narrow part of that age range. Many evaluations used with older adults do not have normative data for that specific population. Therefore, interpretation of the evaluation results is not accurate if normative data for adults are used. Another difficulty arises related to the use of the word *normal* to mean lifestyles or habits that are culturally desirable. The use of evaluation data on functional performance to make statements or decisions about intervention based on social desirability is not consistent with a client-centered evaluation philosophy.

Evaluations of functional performance in older adults can be completed through direct observation or subjective report from the person or caregiver, or both. Evaluation through direct observation yields information about the actual performance or what a person does do in a particular context. In contrast, evaluation based on self-report may be more subjective and yield information about what a person says he or she can do as well as what he or she may actually do or not do. It is obviously easier and more efficient to gather evaluation information via self-report. Moreover, self-report, particularly when the evaluation is done in the clinical environment, can provide a more accurate reflection of what the person does within the environment in which he or she lives. Often, self-report provides the therapist with significant information about the desires and needs of the person.

However, there are controversies about the use of self-report with older adults (McDowell & Newell, 1996), because the information can be biased. McDowell and Newell have stated that "subjective ratings of health blended [an] estimate of the severity of the health problem with a personal tendency to exaggerate or conceal the problem—a bias that varies among people and over time" (p. 25). For example, persons receiving services may exaggerate their difficulties on a first encounter to ensure that services are received, and subsequently diminish their difficulties after rehabilitation is finished (Streiner & Norman, 2003). A particular concern in rehabilitation can occur when an older adult has experienced a relatively sudden change in health or disability status, or both. In this situation, a self-report evaluation of functional performance may be inaccurate because the person does not know what he or she is capable of performing since the change in functional status (Glass, 1998).

Self-report evaluations are very useful for gathering information on how a person perceives his or her performance. When using self-report evaluations as a substitute for direct observation, the results are likely to be more valid when the person has no cognitive impairment and when the evaluation is focused on simple performance activities such as daily self-care. High levels of agreement have been found between self-report and observational evaluations for basic self-care activities (Kivela, 1984; Shinar et al, 1987). Bedard, Molloy, Guyatt, and Standish (1998) compared self-administered and interview-administered evaluations of ADL, sleep problems, and dysfunctional behavior conducted with caregivers of older adults with dementia. The results indicated intraclass correlation coefficients from 0.71 to 0.89 between the two evaluation methods, suggesting that self-administered evaluations by caregivers are valid.

The validity of evaluation results is influenced by the environment in which the evaluation takes place. Research that has compared the use of the same evaluation in different environments has found that evaluation results are affected by the evaluation environment (Nygard, Bernspang, Fisher, & Winblad, 1993; Park, Fisher, & Velozo, 1993). If evaluations are based on direct observation of performance of the task and that task is performed in an unfamiliar environment, it is probable that the results of the evaluation will not be valid. If possible, observational evaluations should be conducted in environments that are familiar to the person or, at least, after the person has had sufficient time to familiarize himself or herself with the environment.

■ Summary

In summary, we have discussed a philosophy of client-centered evaluation, and we have provided a conceptual framework for the evaluation of performance as well as a decision-making process to guide evaluation of older adults. We have focused on issues that must be considered during the evaluation of older adults and have considered the types of evaluation methods used with older adults. The following section provides two evaluation examples that will illustrate some of the key points discussed earlier in this chapter.

Case Study

Janet Fuller is a 62-year-old woman who was diagnosed with osteoporosis 2 years ago during her yearly medical examination with her family physician. She was referred to the osteoporosis clinic at a major teaching hospital. During appointments at the clinic, her diagnosis was confirmed. She has been given medication and has been counseled on changes she should make to her life in order to avoid fractures.

Mrs. Fuller is married and has two adult children who live in the same city. She and her husband live in an apartment in the city and have a country home a 3-hour drive away. Mrs. Fuller worked as a librarian but retired at 50 years of age to accompany her husband on business trips. When not traveling, they spend 4 days a week in the city and spend 3 days in the country. Mrs. Fuller manages both homes herself, although she has found that she often has back pain after doing household activities.

Mrs. Fuller volunteers at her local hospital, delivers meals-on-wheels once a week, and is on the board of a local women's shelter. She enjoys outdoor sports, including golf and skiing, although she has given up downhill skiing since being diagnosed with osteoporosis. She also plays the piano but finds that she is not able to do so for long periods of time as she has in the past:

I don't downhill ski. That's the one thing that I don't do any more. And even sitting playing the piano, you have to sit upright. I can't play for very long. I'm just too tired. And really I think to say, "Well, I can't play the piano as long as I did." I think that is frivolous. And I don't think, if that's all it interferes [with] or the fact that I can't downhill ski, those things are frivolous. They shouldn't be important and so therefore that's why I don't consider that. If I'm crippled and I can't get up in the morning or like I see people who are so bent over, their bones are so brittle and I haven't had any fractures. What can I complain about? (Wilkins, 1998, p. 156)

Questions

1. How could you explore areas of occupational performance in more detail?
2. What is your impression of Mrs. Fuller's functional performance?
3. What other issues are important to assess in this situation?
4. What could be done to help Mrs. Fuller to maintain her activities and prevent further problems with her osteoporosis?
5. What client factors may be important in ensuring Mrs. Fuller's safety?

Review Questions

Using the scenarios about Mrs. Fuller, consider the following questions:

1. Why would you be evaluating Mrs. Fuller?
2. How would you use the ICF model to consider your evaluation of Mrs. Fuller?
3. How would you use Glass' conceptual scheme to inform your evaluation of Mrs. Fuller?
4. How would you select the specific assessments for Mrs. Fuller?
5. What particular issues would you consider to be important in your evaluation of Mrs. Fuller?
6. How would you ensure that you are client centered in your approach to Mrs. Fuller?
7. What evaluation methods would you consider in your evaluation of functional performance for Mrs. Fuller?

Web-Based Resources

For helpful information about the experience of the evaluation of function performance, visit:

www.bu.edu/hdr/products/llfdi/index.html, **Boston University (n.d.) Late-Life Function and Disability Index (LLDFI),** date connected September 4, 2007. This site describes an instrument that is used with community-residing elders. The instrument has both a function dimension and a separate disability dimension.

www.enabler.nu, **The Enabler Web Site,** date connected September 4, 2007 (S. Iwarsson and B. Slaug. [2001, 2006]. *The Enabler Web Site: Providing tools for professional assessments of accessibility problems in the environment.*). An instrument designed to evaluate homes and community environments, with a specific emphasis on accessibility. Includes references, related research projects, and multiple links.

www.canchild.ca/portals/0/outcomes/pdf/measguid.pdf, **The CanChild Centre for Childhood Research, McMaster University, Hamilton, Ontario,** date connected September 4, 2007. Defines themes found in the M.Eaasrate.PDF that follows. This also provides an extensive rating form useful in evaluation instruments to be used for assessment.

REFERENCES

Administration on Aging, U.S. Department of Health and Human Services. (2004). *A profile of older Americans: 2004.* Retrieved April 17, 2006, from www.aoa.gov/prof/Statistics/profile/2004/2004profile.doc.

Allen, C. K., Earheart, C. A., & Blue, T. (1992). *Occupational therapy treatment goals for the physically and cognitively disabled.* Rockville, MD: American Occupational Therapy Association.

American Occupational Therapy Association (AOTA). (1995). Clarification of the use of terms assessment and evaluation. *American Journal of Occupational Therapy, 49,* 1072–1073.

American Occupational Therapy Association (AOTA). (2002). Occupational therapy practice framework: Domain and process. *American Journal of Occupational Therapy, 56,* 609–639.

Arnadottir, G. (1990). *The brain and behavior: Assessing cortical dysfunction through activities of daily living.* St Louis: C.V. Mosby.

Baum, C., & Edwards, D. (1993). Cognitive performance in senile dementia of the Alzheimer's type: The Kitchen Task Assessment. *American Journal of Occupational Therapy, 47,* 431–436.

Baum, C., & Edwards, D. (1995). *The Activity Card Sort.* St. Louis, MO: Occupational Therapy Program, Washington University.

Baum, C., Edwards, D., & Morrow-Howell, N. (1993). Identification and measurement of productive behaviors in senile dementia of the Alzheimer's type. *The Gerontologist, 33,* 403–408.

Bean, J. F., Herman, S., Kiely, D. K., Leveille, S. G., Fielding, R. A., & Frontera, W. R. (2004). Increased velocity exercise specific study exploring the effect on leg, balance and mobility in community-dwelling older women. *Journal of the American Geriatrics Society, 52,* 799–804.

Bedard, M., Molloy, D. W., Guyatt, G. H., & Standish, T. (1998). Self-administered and interviewer-administered instruments in dementia research. *Clinical Gerontologist, 19,* 25–35.

Berg, K. O., Wood-Dauphinee, S., Williams, J., & Maki, B. (1992). Measuring balance in the elderly: Validation of an instrument. *Canadian Journal of Public Health, 83,* S7–S11.

Butland, R. J., Pang, J., Gross, E. R., Woodcock, A. A., & Geddes, D. M. (1982). Two-, six-, 12-minute walking test in respiratory disease. *British Medical Journal, 284,* 1607–1608.

Canadian Association of Occupational Therapists (CAOT). (2002). *Enabling occupation: An occupational therapy perspective* (rev ed.). Ottawa, Ontario, Canada: CAOT Publications ACE.

Chiu, T., & Oliver, R. (2006). Factor analysis and construct validity of the SAFER-HOME. *OTJR: Occupation, Participation and Health, 26,* 132–142.

Chiu, T., Oliver, R., Ascott, P., Choo, L. C., Davis, T., Gaya, A., et al. (2006). *Safety assessment of function and the environment for rehabilitation—Health outcome measurement and evaluation (SAFER-HOME) version 3 manual.* Toronto, Ontario, Canada: COTA Health.

Clark, F., Azen, S. P., Zemke, R., Jackson, J., Carlson, M., Mandel, D., et al. (1997). Occupational therapy for independent-living older adults: A randomized controlled trial. *Journal of the American Medical Association, 278,* 1321–1326.

Duncan, P., Weiner, D., Chandler, J., & Studenski, S. (1990). Functional reach: A new clinical measure of balance. *Journals of Gerontology, 45,* M192–M197.

Dunn, W., Brown, C., & McGuigan, A. (1994). The ecology of human performance: A framework for considering the effect of context. *American Journal of Occupational Therapy, 48,* 595–607.

Fillenbaum, G. (1985). Screening the elderly: A brief instrumental activities of daily living measure. *Journal of the American Geriatrics Society, 33,* 698–706.

Finch, E., Brooks, D., Stratford, P., & Mayo, N. (2002). *Physical rehabilitation outcomes measures. A guide to enhanced clinical decision-making.* Hamilton, Ontario, Canada: B.C. Decker.

Fisher, A. G. (1995). *Assessment of motor and process skills.* Ft. Collins, CO: Third Star Press.

Fisher, A. G., Liu, Y., Velozo, C. A., & Pan, A. W. (1992). Cross-cultural assessment of process skills. *American Journal of Occupational Therapy, 46,* 876–885.

Folstein, M. F., Folstein, S. C., & McHugh, P. (1975). Mini-Mental State: A practical method for grading the cognitive state of patients for the clinician. *Journal of Psychiatric Research, 12,* 189–198.

Fried, L. P., Ettinger, W., Lind, B., Newman, A. B., & Gardin, J. (1994). Physical disability in older adults: A physiological approach. *Journal of Clinical Epidemiology, 47,* 747–760.

Fried, L. P., Herdman, S., Kuhn, K. E., Rubin, G., & Turano K. (1991). Preclinical disability: Hypotheses about the bottom of the iceberg. *Journal of Aging and Health, 3,* 285–300.

Fries, J. (1987). An introduction to the compression of morbidity. *Gerontologica Perspecta,* 5–19.

Fries, J. (2005). The compression of morbidity. *The Milbank Quarterly, 83,* 801–823.

Gerteis, M., Edgman-Levitan, S., Daley, J., & Delbanco, T. (Eds.). (1993). *Through the patient's eyes: Understanding and promoting patient-centered care.* San Francisco: Jossey-Bass.

Gill, T. M., Baker, D. I., Gottschalk, M., Peduzzi, P. N., Allore, H., & Byers, A. (2002). A program to prevent functional decline of physically frail, elderly persons who live at home. *New England Journal of Medicine, 347,* 1068–1074.

Gill, T. M., Baker, D. I., Gottschalk, M., Peduzzi, P. N., Allore, H., & VanNess, P. H. (2004). A prehabilitation program for the prevention of functional decline. *Archives of Physical Medicine & Rehabilitation, 85,* 1043–1049.

Gillespie, L. D., Gillespie, W. J., Robertson, M. C., Lamb, S. E., Cumming, R. G., & Rowe, B. H. (2003). Interventions for preventing falls in elderly people. *The Cochrane Database of Systematic Reviews 2003,* Issue 4, Art. No.: CD000340. DOI: 10.1002/14651858. CD000340.

Gitlin, L., Winter, L., Corcoran, M., Dennis, M. P., Schinfeld, S., & Hauck, W. (2003). Effects of the home environmental skill-building program on the caregiver–care recipient dyad: 6-month outcomes from the Philadelphia REACH Initiative. *The Gerontologist, 43,* 532–546.

Glass, T. (1998). Conjugating the tenses of function: Discordance among hypothetical, experimental, and enacted function in older adults. *The Gerontologist, 38,* 101–112.

Gloth, F., Watson, J., Meyer, J., & Pearson, J. (1995). Reliability and validity of the Frail Elderly Functional Assessment Questionnaire. *American Journal of Physical Medicine & Rehabilitation, 74,* 45–53.

Gowland, C., Stratford, P., Ward, M., Moreland, J., Torresin, W., Van Hullenaar, S., et al. (1995). *The Chedoke-McMaster Stroke Evaluation Manual.* Hamilton, Ontario, Canada: Chedoke-McMaster Hospitals.

Guralnik, J. M. (1996). Assessing the impact of comorbidity in the older population. *Annals of Epidemiology, 6,* 376–380.

Guralnik, J. M., Ferrucci, L., Balfour, J. L., Volpato, S., & Di Iorio, A. (2001). Progressive versus catastrophic loss of the ability to walk: Implications for the prevention of mobility loss. *Journal of the American Geriatrics Society, 49,* 1463–1470.

Guralnik, J. M., Ferrucci, L., Simonsick, E. M., Salive, M. E., & Wallace, R. B. (1995). Lower-extremity function in persons over the age of 70 years as a predictor of subsequent disability. *New England Journal of Medicine, 332,* 556–561.

Guralnik, J. M., Pieper, C. F., Leveille, S. G., Markides, K. S., Ostir, G. V. S., Berkman, S., et al. (2000). Lower extremity function and subsequent disability: Consistency across studies, predictive models, and value of gait speed alone compared with the Short Physical Performance Battery. *Journals of Gerontology, 55A,* M221–M231.

Harwood, R. H., Rogers, A., Dickinson, E., & Ebrahim, S. (1994). Measuring handicap: The London Handicap Scale, a new outcome measure for chronic disease. *Quality in Health Care 3,* 11–16.

Hebert, R., Carrier, R., & Bilodeau, A. (1988). The functional autonomy measurement system (SMAF): Description and validation of an instrument for the measurement of handicaps. *Age and Ageing, 17,* 293–302.

Hill, K. D., Schwarz, J. A., Kalogeropoulos, A. J., & Gibson, S. J. (1996). Fear of falls revisited. *Archives of Physical Medicine & Rehabilitation, 77,* 1025–1029.

Hobson, S. (1996). Being client-centred when the client is cognitively impaired. *Canadian Journal of Occupational Therapy, 63,* 133–137.

Hobson, S. (1999). Using a client-centred approach with persons with cognitive impairment. In T. Sumsion (Ed.), *Client-centred practice in occupational therapy: A guide to implementation* (pp. 51–60). New York: Churchill Livingstone.

Iwarsson, S., & Slaug, B. (2001). *Housing Enabler: An instrument for assessing and analysing accessibility problems in housing.* Nävlinge and Staffanstorp, Sweden: Veten and Skapen HB, Slaug Data Management AB.

Jette, A., Assmann, S., Rooks, D., Harris, B., & Crawford S. (1998). Interrelationships among disablement concepts. *Journals of Gerontology. Series A: Biological Sciences and Medical Sciences, 53,* 863–871.

Jette, A. M., Haley, S. M., Coster, W. J., Kooyoomijian, J. T., Levenson, S., Heeren, T., et al. (2002). Late Life Function and Disability Instrument—Development and evaluation of the function component. *Journals of Gerontology. Series A:Biological Sciences and Medical Sciences, 57*(4), M217–M222.

Jette, A., Lachman, M., Giorgetti, M. M., Assman, S. F., Harric, B. A., Levenson, C., et al. (1999). Exercise— It's never too late: The strong-for-life program. *American Journal of Public Health, 89,* 66–72.

Kivela, S. L. (1984). Measuring disability—Do self-ratings and service provider ratings compare? *Journal of Chronic Disease, 37,* 27–36.

Laver, A. (1996). The occupational therapy intervention process: Occupational therapy assessment and evaluation of older clients. In K. O. Larson, R. Stevens-Ratchford, L. Pedretti, & J. Crabtree (Eds.), *ROTE: The role of OT with the elderly* (pp. 507–537). Bethesda, MD: American Occupational Therapy Association.

Laver, A., & Powell, G. (1995). *The Structured Observational Test of Function (SOTOF).* Berkshire, UK: NFER-NELSON.

Law, M. (1987). Criteria for the evaluation of measurement instruments. *Canadian Journal of Occupational Therapy, 54,* 121–127.

Law, M., Baptiste, S., Carswell, A., McColl, M., Polatajko, H., & Pollock, N. (2005). *Canadian Occupational Performance Measure* (4th ed.). Ottawa, Ontario, Canada: CAOT Publications ACE.

Law, M., Baptiste, S., & Mills, J. (1995). Client-centred practice: What does it mean and does it make a difference? *Canadian Journal of Occupational Therapy, 62,* 250–257.

Law, M., Baum, C., & Dunn, W. (2005). *Measuring occupational performance: Supporting best practice in occupational therapy* (2nd ed.). Thorofare, NJ: SLACK.

Law, M., Cooper, B., Strong, S., Stewart, D., Rigby, P., & Letts, L. (1996). The Person-Environment-Occupation Model: A transactive approach to occupational performance. *Canadian Journal of Occupational Therapy, 63,* 9–23.

Law, M., Steinwender, S., & Leclair, L. (1998). Occupation, health and well-being. *Canadian Journal of Occupational Therapy, 65,* 81–91.

Lawrence, R., & Jette, A. (1996). Disentangling the disablement process. *Journals of Gerontology: Social Sciences, 51B,* S173–S182.

Lawton, M. P., & Brody, E. M. (1969). Assessment of older people: Self-maintaining and instrumental activities of daily living. *The Gerontologist, 9,* 179–186.

Marwick, C. (1997). NHANES III health data relevant for aging nation. *Journal of the American Medical Association, 277,* 100–102.

May, D., Nayak, U. S., & Isaacs, B. (1985). The life-space diary: A measure of mobility in old people at home. *International Rehabilitation Medicine, 7,* 182–186.

McDowell, I., & Newell, C. (1996). *Measuring health: A guide to rating scales and questionnaires* (2nd ed.). Oxford, UK: Oxford University Press.

Melzer, D., Lan, T. Y., & Guralnik, J. M. (2003). The predictive validity for mortality of the index of mobility-related limitation—Results from the EPESE study. *Age & Ageing, 32,* 619–625.

Merriam-Webster Online Dictionary. (n.d.). Retrieved April 17, 2006, from www.m-w.com/netdict.htm.

Moloney, T., & Paul, B. (1993). Rebuilding public trust and confidence. In M. Gerteis, S. Edgman-Levitan, J. Daley, & T. Delbanco (Eds.), *Through the patient's eyes: Understanding and promoting patient-centered care* (pp. 280–298). San Francisco: Jossey-Bass.

Nagi, S. (1976). An epidemiology of disability among adults in the United States. *Milbank Quarterly, 54,* 439–468.

National Advisory Council on Aging (NACA). (2000). *The NACA position on enhancing the Canadian health care system* (Cat. No. H-71-2/2-21-2000). Ottawa, Ontario, Canada: Minister of Supply and Services Canada.

Nygard, L., Bernspang, B., Fisher, A. G., & Winblad, B. (1993). Comparing motor and process ability in home versus clinical settings with persons with suspected dementia. *American Journal of Occupational Therapy, 48,* 689–696.

Oakley, F., Keilhofner, G., Barris, R., & Reichler, R. K. (1986). The Role Checklist: Development and empirical assessment of reliability. *Occupational Therapy Journal of Research, 6,* 157–170.

O'Neill, D. L., & Harris, S. R. (1982). Developing goals and objectives for handicapped children. *Physical Therapy, 62,* 295–298.

Ottenbacher, K. J., & Cusick, A. (1990). Goal attainment scaling as a method of clinical service evaluation. *American Journal of Occupational Therapy, 44,* 519–525.

Ottenbacher, K. J., & Cusick, A. (1993). Discriminative versus evaluative assessment: Some observations on goal attainment scaling. *American Journal of Occupational Therapy, 47,* 349–354.

Park, S., Fisher, A. G., & Velozo, C. A. (1993). Using the Assessment of Motor and Process Skills to compare performance between home and clinical settings. *American Journal of Occupational Therapy, 48,* 519–525.

Picker Institute. (n.d.). *Our mission, our values.* Retrieved April 17, 2006, from www.pickerinstitute.org.

Podsiadlo, D., & Richardson, S. (1991). The timed "up and go": A test of basic functional mobility. *Journal of the American Geriatrics Society, 39,* 142–148.

Reuben, D. B., & Siu, A. L. (1990). An objective measure of physical function of elderly outpatients: The Physical Performance Test. *Journal of the American Geriatrics Society, 38,* 1105–1112.

Riddle, D. L., & Stratford, P. (1999). Interpreting validity indexes for diagnostic tests—An illustration using the Berg Balance Test. *Physical Therapy, 79,* 939–948.

Rosow, I., & Breslau, N. A. (1966). A Guttman Health Scale for the Aged. *Journal of Gerontology, 21,* 556–559.

Russell, D., King, G., Palisano, R., & Law, M. (1995). *Measuring individualized outcomes.* Hamilton, Ontario, Canada: Neurodevelopmental Clinical Research Unit, McMaster University.

Sackett, D. L., Haynes, R. B., Guyatt, G. H., & Tugwell, P. (1991). *Clinical epidemiology: A basic science for clinical medicine* (2nd ed.). Boston: Little, Brown.

Shinar, D., Gross, C. R., Bronstein, K. S., Licata-Gehr, E. E., Eden, D. T., Cabrera, A. R., et al. (1987). Reliability of the activities of daily living scale and its use in telephone interview. *Archives of Physical Medicine and Rehabilitation, 68,* 723–728.

Shumway-Cook, A., Patla, A., Stewart, A., Ferrucci, L., Ciol, M., & Guralnik, J. (2002). Environmental demands associated with community mobility in older adults with and without mobility disabilities. *Physical Therapy, 82,* 670–681.

Shumway-Cook, A., Patla, A., Stewart, A., Ferrucci, L., Ciol, M., & Guralnik, J. (2005). Assessing environmentally determined mobility disability: Self-report versus observed community mobility. *Journal of the American Geriatrics Society, 53,* 700–704.

Simonsick, E., Montgomery, P., Newman, A., Bauer, D., & Harris, T. B. (2003). Measuring fitness in healthy older adults: The Health ABC Long Distance Corridor Walk. *The American Geriatrics Society, 49,* 1544–1548.

State University of New York at Buffalo (SUNY). (1990). *Guide for the uniform data set for medical rehabilitation (Adult FIM)* (Version 4.0). Buffalo, NY: Author.

Statistics Canada. (2002, May). Disability-free life expectancy at age 65, by sex, Canada, provinces, territories, health regions and peer groups. *Health Indicators* (Catalogue no. 82-221-XIE), 1–6.

Stavley, B., Owsley, C., Sloane, M., & Ball, K. (1999). The Life Space Questionnaire: A measure of the extent of mobility of older adults. *Journal of Applied Gerontology, 18,* 460–479.

Steultjens, E. M. J., Dekker, J., Bouter, L. M., Jellema, S., Bakker, E. B., & van den Ende, C. H. M. (2004). Occupational therapy for community dwelling elderly people: A systematic review. *Age and Aging, 33,* 453–460.

Stone, R. (2006). Emerging issues in long-term care. In R. Binstock & L. George (Eds.), *Handbook of aging and the social sciences* (6th ed., pp. 397–418). Thousand Oaks, CA: Sage.

Stratford, P., Gill, C., Westaway, M., & Binkley, J. (1995). Assessing disability and change on individual patients: A report of a patient specific measure. *Physiotherapy Canada, 47,* 258–263.

Streiner, D. L., & Norman, G. R. (2003). *Health measurement scales: A practical guide to their development and use* (3rd ed.). Oxford, UK: Oxford University Press.

Stump, T. E., Clark, D. O., Johnson, R. J., & Wolinsky, F. D. (1997). The structure of health status among Hispanic, African American, and white older adults. *Journals of Gerontology: Social Sciences 52B*(Special Issue), 49–60.

Sumsion, T. (2000). A revised occupational therapy definition of client-centred practice. *British Journal of Occupational Therapy, 63,* 304–309.

Tinetti, M. (1986). Performance-oriented assessment of mobility patterns in elderly patients. *Journal of the American Geriatrics Society, 34,* 119–126.

Van Dusen, J., & Brunt, D. (1997). *Assessment in occupational therapy and physical therapy.* Philadelphia: W.B. Saunders.

Walker, A. (2006). Aging and politics: An international perspective. In R. Binstock & L. George (Eds.), *Handbook of aging and the social sciences* (6th ed., pp. 339–359). Thousand Oaks, CA: Sage.

Wilkins, M. S. (1998). *Aging, chronic illness and self-concept: A study of older women with osteoporosis.* Unpublished doctoral dissertation, University of Toronto, Toronto, Ontario, Canada.

Williams, J. H., Drinka, T. J. K., Greenberg, J. R., Farrell-Holtan, J., Euhardy, R., & Schram, M. (1991). Development and testing of the Assessment of Living Skills and Resources (ALSAR) in elderly community-dwelling veterans. *The Gerontologist, 31,* 84–91.

World Health Organization. (1980). *International classification of impairment, disability and handicap.* Geneva: Author.

World Health Organization. (1998). *ICIDH-2: International classification of impairment, activities and participation—Beta 1 version.* Geneva: Author.

World Health Organization. (2001). *International classification of functioning, disability and health (ICF).* Geneva: Author.

Yesavage, J. A., & Brink, T. L. (1983). Development and validation of a geriatric screening scale: A preliminary report. *Journal of Psychiatric Research, 17,* 37–49.

CHAPTER 18

Health Promotion and Wellness

Marjorie E. Scaffa, PhD, OTR/L, FAOTA • Bette R. Bonder, PhD, OTR/L, FAOTA

Something remains for us to do or dare;
Even the oldest tree some fruit may bear;
For age is opportunity no less Than youth
itself, though in another dress

Longfellow, 1858

OBJECTIVES

By the end of this chapter, the reader will be able to:

1. Describe the health status of older adults in terms of demographic trends.
2. Define the concept of wellness.
3. Describe the specific factors that have been associated with promoting wellness in older adults.
4. Apply the Transtheoretical Model to health behavior change.
5. Discuss health behavior change strategies that are appropriate for elders.
6. Describe the process of health promotion program development.
7. Identify specific interventions and programs that have been developed to promote wellness.

Between 2000 and 2030, the number of Americans over age 65 will have doubled; that means that one of every five persons in the United States will be an older adult (Centers for Disease Control and Prevention [CDC], 2004). Although currently, older persons make up just over 12% of the population, they account for one-third of health care dollars spent (CDC, 2004). Chronic disease is a common occurrence in this age group and includes, in order of prevalence, the following conditions: arthritis, heart disease, hearing impairment, high blood pressure, orthopedic impairment, and cataracts.

However, the vast majority of older adults maintain functional ability well into later life. Good health and function during later life can be attributed to many factors. Environmental factors such as exposure to toxic substances play a role in the experience of aging. Genetics also play a role. However, there is growing evidence that genetics contribute less to successful aging than was generally thought. The majority of factors that promote good health and function in later life are within the control of the individual. Good nutrition, exercise, and avoidance of harmful substances like tobacco are positive lifestyle habits that can help the older adult maintain wellness. In addition, the presence of a good social support system, a sense of spiritual fulfillment, positive personal coping mechanisms, and a satisfying array of occupations contribute to what has come to be called "successful aging."

Successful aging refers to a combination of "avoidance of disease and disability, maintenance of cognitive and physical function, and sustained engagement with life" (Rowe & Kahn, 1998, p. 39). As was noted in Chapter 1, critics of this conceptualization note that while it may not be possible to avoid disease and disability, it is possible to maintain engagement with life. Kane (2003) has elaborated his views, noting that the potential to age successfully with a disability is enhanced if health care shifts from a focus on cure to a focus on care, which requires preventing the transition from disease or disability to dysfunction. Minkler and Fadem (2002) stress an ecological approach that emphasizes environmental accommodations and policy change to enhance the health and well-being of older adults.

The health and well-being of older adults is a national priority and will remain so for the foreseeable future as the baby boomer generation ages. The federal government has a particular interest in health promotion programming, as evidenced by *Healthy People 2010* (U.S. Department of Health and Human Services [USDHHS], 2000). Many of the objectives identified in *Healthy People 2010* have direct relevance to elders. A sampling of objectives directed at older adults of interest to therapy professionals are listed in Table 18-1. Now in the planning stages, Healthy People 2020 (USDHHS, 2008) will undoubtedly contain at least as many objectives that relate to aging.

TABLE 18-1 Selected *Healthy People 2010* Objectives Related to Older Adults

Objective Number	Description
1-15	Increase the proportion of persons with long-term care needs who have access to the continuum of long-term care services
1-16	Reduce the proportion of nursing home residents with a current diagnosis of pressure ulcers
2-9	Reduce the proportion of adults with osteoporosis
2-10	Reduce the proportion of adults who are hospitalized for vertebral fractures associated with osteoporosis
5-1	Increase the proportion of persons with diabetes who receive formal diabetes education
5-2	Prevent diabetes
5-9	Reduce the frequency of foot ulcers in persons with diabetes
5-10	Reduce the rate of lower extremity amputations in persons with diabetes
5-17	Increase the proportion of adults with diabetes who perform self-blood-glucose-monitoring at least once daily
7-12	Increase the proportion of older adults who have participated during the preceding year in at least one health promotion activity
10-5	Increase the proportion of consumers who follow key food safety practices
15-1	Reduce hospitalization for nonfatal head injuries
15-15	Reduce deaths caused by motor vehicle crashes
15-16	Reduce pedestrian deaths on public roads
15-25	Reduce residential fire deaths
15-27	Reduce deaths from falls
15-28	Reduce hip fractures among older adults
17-3	Increase the proportion of primary care providers, pharmacists and other health care professionals who routinely review with their patients aged 65 years and older and patients with chronic illnesses or disabilities all new prescribed and over-the-counter medications
18-4	Increase the number of states, territories and the District of Columbia with an operational mental health plan that addresses mental health crisis interventions, ongoing screening, and treatment services for elderly persons
19-1	Increase the proportion of adults who are at a healthy weight

19-2	Reduce the proportion of adults who are obese
22-1	Reduce the proportion of adults who engage in no leisure-time physical activity
22-2	Increase the proportion of adults who engage regularly, preferably daily, in moderate physical activity for at least 30 minutes per day
22-4	Increase the proportion of adults who perform physical activities that enhance and maintain muscular strength and endurance
22-5	Increase the proportion of adults who perform physical activities that enhance and maintain flexibility
22-14	Increase the proportion of trips made by walking
27-1	Reduce tobacco use by adults
27-5	Increase smoking cessation attempts by adult smokers
28-10	Increase vision rehabilitation
28-13	Increase access by persons who have hearing impairments to hearing rehabilitation services and adaptive devices, including hearing aids, cochlear implants, or tactile or other assistive or augmentative devices

Source: U.S. Department of Health and Human Services, Public Health Service: *Healthy People 2010*. Retrieved September 30, 2006 from www.health.gov/healthypeople.

This chapter focuses largely on the situation in the United States. Many developed nations, including in particular those like Canada and Sweden that enjoy national health insurance, have more advanced programs of wellness and health promotion, having recognized that such interventions can reduce health care expenditures. On the other hand, some developing nations do not as yet have the resources to provide these kinds of interventions. In some settings, nongovernmental organizations (NGOs) attempt to provide at least some population-based health promotion interventions, and occupational therapists are increasingly involved in these efforts.

This chapter discusses the factors that impact the health and well-being of elders, health behavior change strategies, and the design of health promotion interventions that facilitate successful aging.

Defining Wellness and Health Promotion

The factors listed earlier contribute to a state that has been termed *wellness*. Wellness is not the same as good health. In fact, it is possible to be well while having several medical diseases. Rather, **wellness** is the individual's perception of physical and psychological well-being characterized by adequate physical capacity for accomplishment of desired activities, coupled with overall satisfaction with one's life situation (Gallup, 1999). Clearly, this is a state that can be reached by many individuals, even those

with significant physical limitations. In the *Occupational Therapy Practice Framework: Domain and Process (Framework)*, wellness is considered one of the potential outcomes of occupational therapy interventions (American Occupational Therapy Association [AOTA], 2002).

Absence of disease is not a prerequisite for wellness. This is an important point, because absolute good health is unlikely for older individuals. Treas (1995) notes that the majority of older adults report at least one chronic condition. Arthritis is by far the most common, affecting almost half of the elderly population. Nevertheless, older individuals with such conditions can and most often do identify themselves as well. One of the most effective ways to intervene with older adults is to focus on promotion of wellness, rather than on remediation of dysfunction. Preventing problems before they occur enhances quality of life for the older adult. At the same time, this strategy has the potential to reduce overall health care costs by reducing or delaying the need for expensive, high-tech interventions.

Wellness is the desired outcome, and health promotion and prevention are processes to facilitate the achievement of that objective. The *Framework* identifies health promotion and disability prevention as appropriate occupational therapy intervention strategies to facilitate health and well-being (AOTA, 2002). **Health promotion** is defined as "an intervention approach that does not assume a disability is present or that any factors would interfere with performance. This approach is designed to provide enriched contextual and activity experiences that will enhance performance for all persons in the natural contexts of life" (AOTA, 2002, p. 627). **Prevention** approaches in occupational therapy focus on individuals at-risk for occupational performance problems and are designed to promote healthy lifestyles and "prevent the occurrence or evolution of barriers to performance in context" (AOTA, 2002, p. 627). **Preventive occupation** is the "application of occupational science in the prevention of disease and disability and the promotion of health and wellbeing of individuals and communities through meaningful engagement in occupations" (Scaffa, 2001, p. 44). The use of occupation in health promotion and prevention is the unique contribution of occupational therapy to public health.

Factors That Promote Wellness

A number of factors have been identified as central to wellness and successful aging. Among factors suggested by research are genetics, physical activity, nutritional habits, social participation and social support, occupational engagement, mental health, and spirituality (Rowe & Kahn, 1998). Each of these factors will be considered individually, although in reality they operate synergistically to impact health positively or negatively.

Genetics

There is no question that one's genetic heritage influences the aging process. The main impact of genetic factors on later life has to do with predisposition to potentially disabling or fatal diseases. It is now clear that type II diabetes, Alzheimer's disease (AD), heart disease, and a number of cancers have a genetic component. In some of these diseases, the genetic component is clear and compelling. For example, individuals with the gene for Huntington's disease have a 100% probability of developing the disorder. For other diseases, however, the influence of genetics is less clear. In the case of AD, for example, several genetic anomalies have been identified in families with a high incidence of the disease. The current thinking is that there are two forms of early-onset AD, sporadic, which has no genetic component, and familial, which does (National Institute on Aging [NIA], 2004).

The familial form of early-onset AD is thought to carry a 50/50 genetic risk of developing the disorder. However, for late-onset AD, genetic factors have been identified in some families, but the likelihood of developing the disorder is much less predictable.

With the exception of diseases that will be expressed regardless of health habits (e.g., Huntington's disease), it is possible to reduce the risk of genetic disorders by half or more (Finch, 1990). The interventions described in the next section are highly appropriate for individuals whose genetic characteristics would put them at high risk for disabling conditions. Thus, genetics is not destiny, but only a form of predisposition that can, in many instances, be moderated.

Physical Activity

Substantial evidence exists demonstrating that regular exercise or physical activity is a powerful health promotion strategy (Centers for Disease Control [CDC], 2001; Miller et al., 2000). Regular physical activity has been linked to improved cardiovascular function, enhanced pulmonary function, increased strength and flexibility, enhanced memory, and improved mood. Enhanced strength, flexibility, coordination, balance, and movement velocity reduce the risk of falls in the elderly. Reducing the likelihood of falls also lessens the risk of negative consequences of falls, including fractures and death. Further, individuals who fear falls often limit other activities, which contributes to a downward spiral in quality of life. Thus, interventions to reduce fall risk can dramatically improve overall quality of life. For individuals who have risk factors predisposing them to disease and disability, regular physical activity can prevent or minimize a whole array of disorders. Among them are heart disease, osteoporosis, arthritis, diabetes, hypertension, and cerebrovascular disease.

According to the World Health Organization (n.d.), there are many physiological and psychological benefits of physical activity. A list of these benefits can be found in Box 18-1.

Individuals who exercise regularly have more energy and are better able to focus on cognitive tasks. Physical activity also promotes the body's production of endorphins, which are naturally occurring opioid-like substances, which produces a general sense of well-being.

Physiological Benefits of Physical Activity

- Regulation of glucose levels
- Stimulation of adrenaline and noradrenaline
- Improved sleep
- Enhanced aerobic and cardiovascular capacity
- Increased muscle strength
- Enhanced flexibility
- Improved balance and coordination
- Improved regulation of movement velocity

PSYCHOLOGICAL BENEFITS OF PHYSICAL ACTIVITY

- Relaxation
- Reduced stress and anxiety
- Enhanced mood state
- General well-being
- Improved mental health
- Improved cognition
- Enhanced skill acquisition

(American Council on Exercise, 1998.)

Some fitness experts claim that a person must exercise for a specific duration and number of times to reduce the risk of certain diseases. However, any level of physical activity has health benefits (CDC, 2001). Common occupations such as walking the dog, gardening, and cleaning the house can improve fitness. There are a number of good exercise guidelines for older adults. Although their recommendations vary somewhat, all suggest that elders engage in three different kinds of exercise: aerobic, strengthening, and flexibility. Suggested aerobic activities include walking, jogging, swimming, and biking. Activities performed around the house like cleaning and gardening also may also have aerobic effects. Although the typical recommendation is for 30 or more minutes of sustained aerobic exercise, there is growing evidence that even brief periods of physical activity are helpful. For people whose mobility is limited, aerobic exercise may be structured to be done while in a swimming pool or while sitting in a chair.

Strengthening exercises are helpful in building bone mass or reducing bone mass loss. They are also useful in building or maintaining muscle mass. Both are important to mobility and to fall prevention. Strength training should involve all major muscle groups and should be done against resistance. Even limited movement against relatively light resistance or against gravity has some positive impact. As with aerobic training, strength training can be readily adapted for individuals who have physical limitations.

Flexibility training includes gentle stretching, and a relatively small amount of stretching is sufficient to obtain significant benefits. Bouncing can reduce the effectiveness of the muscle stretch and therefore should be avoided. Stretching can be done in bed, in a chair, or on the floor.

Physical activity is a wellness intervention with potential benefits for all older adults, including those with significant disease or disability (American College of Sports Medicine, 1997). Its positive effects apply regardless of the baseline from which intervention is begun. However, exercise programs for older adults must be planned with careful attention to any preexisting conditions. Increases must be gradual and monitoring done with care, especially for individuals with cardiac disease. Warm-ups and cool-downs must be done consistently to avoid injury. In addition, the interaction among multiple medical conditions should be considered. For example, an individual may have both arthritis and osteoporosis. The recommendation for osteoporosis is weight-bearing exercise to maintain bone mass or reduce bone loss. However, such exercise may be especially hard on arthritic knee and hip joints. In such situations, therapists must carefully assess risks and benefits. Referring clients to an Arthritis Foundation exercise group (Arthritis Foundation, 2007 [www.arthritis.org/conditions/exercise/default.asp]) can ensure that they learn appropriate strategies for engaging in walking, yoga, and other weight-bearing exercise that can strengthen bones while avoiding further injury to joints.

Perhaps the greatest challenge is motivating elders to start and continue physical activity and exercise programs. Several strategies may be of value. For example, there is a definite benefit to social exercise. Walking with a group will provide social interaction that may be as rewarding as the exercise. Mall walking is an example of a modification that some elders find motivating, particularly if the walk is followed by a cup of tea with friends. Another strategy recommended by some fitness experts is goal-setting, monitoring, and appropriate rewards for program adherence. Probably the most useful motivation strategy is identification of physical activities that the individual enjoys. There is compelling evidence that individuals are most likely to continue those activities that they find personally meaningful or enjoyable.

Whereas one person may enjoy jogging, another may prefer square dancing, gardening, or tai chi. Cultural factors influence preferred forms of exercise and should be considered in planning. For example, in some cultures, women are not comfortable with the idea of wearing a bathing suit, particularly in the presence of men. For such women, no matter how well planned the program, pool exercises are not likely to be effective. If an individual cannot easily get out to shop or cannot afford acceptable footwear, this inability to purchase the appropriate equipment, such as tennis shoes, can be a barrier to safely participating in physical activities. The most accessible physical activities are those that require little to no special equipment and can be done in a variety of settings. Because the evidence is so convincing that any physical activity is beneficial, its form is a secondary consideration.

Nutrition

Throughout the life span, good nutrition is essential for health. Nutrition has an impact on normal growth and development, preservation of health, healing, and recovery from illness. According to Chernoff (2001), "Building muscle strength, developing antibodies to potential invading microorganisms, maintaining immune function, preserving cellular integrity, healing wounds, and experiencing a general sense of wellbeing and an active lifestyle are all dependent on maintaining nutritional health" (p. 43).

Like physical activity, proper nutrition is important for health maintenance in the older adult. Older adults are more at risk than younger individuals for poor nutrition. The older person's sense of taste may diminish, making food less enjoyable, or the individual may be on a low-salt or other restricted diet that makes food less appealing. Some elders who have lost significant others may not eat well when alone. Perhaps they have reduced incomes, which leads them to economize on food. If they are obese, their physicians may recommend weight loss without providing accompanying nutritional information. Because older adults require fewer calories, weight loss diets can lead to excessive restriction with accompanying malnutrition. At the same time, their ability to absorb needed nutrients may diminish, leading to a need for greater amounts of various nutrients in the diet.

General nutritional recommendations for older adults include reducing calories by about 10% by age 75, maintaining fat intake at 30% or less of diet, and eating a wide array of fruits, vegetables, and whole-grain foods (American Academy of Family Physicians, American Dietetic Association, National Council on the Aging, Inc., n.d.). As with other health recommendations, it is important to remember that chronic health conditions can alter recommendations. Older adults need slightly more protein than younger individuals. This is not typically a problem, but for individuals on limited budgets or who have difficulty chewing meat, protein deficiency may be a real concern. There are many alternative sources of protein, but not all older adults know that eating beans, nuts, and cheeses can fulfill this requirement. Similarly, a varied diet can supply all the needed vitamins and minerals, but older adults may have difficulty absorbing them. Vitamin supplementation may be beneficial but limited to those individuals with economic means to purchase the supplements.

In addition, it may be difficult in later life to maintain adequate hydration. Older adults may avoid drinking because they find that they experience urinary frequency that can be challenging for individuals with various mobility limitations. They may also experience less sensation of thirst. Although this loss of sensation may be problematic in daily life, it becomes a crucial issue in elders who develop flu or other infectious diseases. Dehydration can cause serious problems if it is not corrected (Reichel, 1995).

Sugars are less well metabolized by older adults and can contribute to widely fluctuating levels of blood sugar. Salt may cause fluid retention, which can be hazardous for individuals with high blood pressure. Alcohol is problematic when used to excess. Excessive alcohol use is associated with a high rate of injuries and deaths, as well as liver disease, ischemic heart disease, cardiomyopathy, and hemorrhagic stroke (Mukamal et al., 2003). Light alcohol use (two to seven drinks weekly) in healthy individuals may be of some health benefit, including a mild reduction in risk for heart disease (Mukamal et al., 2003). At-risk drinking is defined as more than one drink per day or seven drinks per week for women, and as more than two drinks per day or 14 per week for men (Dawson, Grant, & Li, 2005). For older adults who may be taking an array of prescription medications, alcohol can have greater potential danger than for younger individuals. In addition, it may be less well metabolized, increasing its effects and duration.

Although specific dietary advice is best left to dieticians and other nutritional experts, all health care professionals should be alert to the effects of malnutrition, dehydration, and excessive alcohol consumption. An important role for occupational therapists is in ensuring that the individual is capable of obtaining needed nutrition and is motivated to do so. The Practice Framework (AOTA, 2002) reflects the potential complexity of associated tasks and skills, including getting to a grocery store, shopping for food, making good food choices, preparing meals, and eating them. Sometimes, specific skill training is warranted. In other instances, motivation is the most important factor requiring attention. Finding social occasions for eating, identifying community-dining opportunities at senior centers, and so forth, are often vital interventions focused on ensuring adequate nutrition. The cultural aspects of eating may also provide clues to improved nutrition. For example, lunches at a senior center in a mostly Hispanic neighborhood should be planned to include foods that are preferred by individuals of that culture.

Social Participation and Social Support

Social participation, an area of occupation, is essential to successful aging. **Social participation** is defined as "activities associated with organized patterns of behavior that are characteristic and expected for an individual interacting with others within a given social context" (AOTA, 2002, p. 621). Elders who have social networks experience less dysfunction than those who are isolated. Individuals with higher levels of perceived social environment make fewer visits to the hospital (Bosworth & Schaie, 1997) and have lower mortality rates (Bennett, 2002; Sugisawa, Liang, & Liu, 1994). However, research is unclear about the particulars of this phenomenon, such as the

types, frequency, and duration of interactions that produce optimal benefit.

Older adults derive satisfaction from a sense of connectedness with others, past, present, and future (Bonder & Martin, 2000). This sense of connectedness is strongly associated with a sense of well-being. A study of the experiences of elders on a Kibbutz in Israel confirmed that the sense of social inclusion and involvement is a strong predictor of well-being (Levitan, 1999). The positive benefits of such support also extend to individuals with serious illness, as demonstrated by the evidence of increased longevity and well-being among terminally ill cancer patients who are involved in support groups (DeVries et al., 1997). Not all older adults have a ready source of social interaction. Friends and spouses die or move. Adult children, if any, may move away.

The implications for health care providers are clear. Wellness programs must involve opportunities for meaningful and supportive social interaction. Such interaction can readily be provided at the same time as other interventions. Group physical activity provides benefits that exercise in isolation cannot; similarly, groups emphasizing nutrition are likely to have benefits beyond improved diet. Furthermore, they are more likely to result in improved nutrition because of the importance of peer support in making behavioral changes.

Intergenerational activities are particularly valued by many elders. Older adults tend, on the whole, to prefer engagement with individuals of all ages and to find satisfaction in sharing their experiences and wisdom with younger individuals. Programs such as foster grandparents are popular for this reason, because they offer intergenerational experiences for elders who may not have grandchildren or whose grandchildren may be at a distance.

Among individuals who are socially isolated, interaction with pets can provide a substitute for human interaction (Park, 1999). The research literature has explored benefits of pets for community-residing individuals as well as those in institutions, and benefits have been found in all settings. In addition, for elders who are isolated because of their living arrangements (e.g., those in rural settings) or because of mobility problems, the telephone and computer offer opportunities for interaction. Many elders report particularly enjoying the Internet as a way to make contact around the world (Bass, Mcciendon, Brennan, & McCarthy, 1998).

Occupational Engagement

Rehabilitation personnel have long recognized the value of meaningful occupation, and its health benefits (Carlson et al., 1998). In fact, older adults often evaluate their lives in terms of their ability to accomplish meaningful activities. Elderly persons are likely to say that they want their lives prolonged only so long as they are capable of engaging in activities important to them (Ditto et al., 1996).

Identification of meaningful occupations is a highly individual matter. Although there are common themes that can be identified, elderly persons express those themes through individualized activity patterns and choices. For example, connection with others is a common theme. This theme may be expressed through babysitting for grandchildren, volunteering in a school, tending to a sick neighbor, or countless other ways. The goal for intervention is to ensure that the individual continues to find meaning in their everyday activities. This may require lifestyle redesign (Jackson, Carlson, Mandel, Zemke, & Clark, 1998), learning new activities, altering the pattern of activities, or modifying choices. Sometimes the environment must be adapted to support or facilitate occupation.

Menec (2003) studied the relationship between ordinary, everyday activities and indicators of successful aging, such as function, well-being, and mortality. Activity, in general, was found to be positively related to happiness, and activity level corresponded to improved function and reduced mortality. In addition, participation in social and productive activity appeared to delay functional decline. Solitary activity, such as reading the newspaper, writing letters, and listening to music, is also important to successful aging and was associated with the psychosocial domain of happiness.

Care must be taken to assess the individual's wishes and desires accurately. Being busy is not necessarily the desired outcome of activity. In fact, some older adults may prefer time for quiet reflection and be concerned that others will perceive this as withdrawal or isolation. Care providers must gather information carefully and be overt about their reasons for inquiring. Cultural differences about preferences must be taken into account. Therapists must clarify that their responsibility is to ensure good quality of life for the elder.

Mental Health

Depression is the most frequently occurring mental health problem in the elderly and is often precipitated by significant life stressors including death of a spouse, social isolation, loss of meaningful occupational roles, multiple illnesses, and forced moves from familiar environments (Glass, 2006). As discussed in Chapter 10, depression is quite common in later life, although it must be distinguished from grief reactions that are also common among elders. Suicide is a significant risk among the elderly. Although they make up only 20% of the population, adults over age 60 account for 40% of all suicide deaths. White males over the age of 80 are particularly vulnerable, with suicide rates nearly six times the national average for the U.S. population (Kinsella & Velkoff, 2001). Unfortunately, older adults are unlikely to seek help for depression from a health professional. Although depression is not part of the normal aging process, its symptoms are often overlooked in the elderly, particularly when they coincide with other medical conditions. As a result, depression is often untreated or undertreated in this population.

Risk factors for major depressive disorder (MDD) include family history of depression, personal history of depression, and history of mental trauma, chronic illnesses, and chronic pain. Marital status also has an effect: higher rates are found in unmarried males, widows, widowers, and separated and divorced individuals (Quan & Gitlin, 2004). Nearly 25% of older adults experiencing a cerebrovascular accident (CVA) suffer depression that meets diagnostic criteria for MDD (National Institute of Mental Health [NIMH], 2007). Although symptoms of depression are common immediately after the loss of a spouse, one-sixth of widows and widowers continue to experience MDD at the end of one year (NIMH, 2007).

By 2020, the WHO estimates that MDD will be second only to heart disease in terms of disability experienced by sufferers (Quan & Gitlin, 2004). Depression has adverse effects on adherence to medical regimens and health habits as well, including poor diet, increased alcohol consumption and smoking, and sedentary lifestyle. The direct physiological effects of MDD, along with maladaptive behaviors, help explain the association with increased morbidity and mortality. Older persons with symptoms of depression have approximately 50% higher health care costs than their nondepressed peers (NIMH, 2007). Presenting complaints for depression in the elderly often include physical symptoms such as sleep disturbances, gastrointestinal problems, headaches, fatigue, and appetite and weight changes.

Because depression is so common, therapists must be alert to signs and ready to provide appropriate interventions and referral to other professionals. Strategies that occupational therapists can provide include opportunities for expression of emotion and assistance in developing coping strategies.

Perceived Control and Coping Strategies

A person's psychological characteristics can have a considerable influence on physical health. Among the factors associated with good health are perceived control, a sense of self-efficacy, and effective problem-solving coping strategies.

Individuals who experience a sense of control over their circumstances (**perceived control**) perceive their health as better, and their lives as more satisfying. Such individuals place more importance on good health, perhaps leading them to engage in more positive behaviors. Regardless of the reasons, perceived control is associated with lower rates of hospitalization and reduced mortality (Menec & Chipperfield, 1997). Interventions focused on enhancing perceived control can improve health for older adults. For example, research in nursing homes suggests that individuals who are provided with personal choice over diet, clothing, and activities maintain better health and feel more satisfied with their situations (McCabe, Walker, & Clark, 1997). Similarly, it is likely that individuals residing in the community will also benefit from opportunities to exert control over their situations. In situations in which family members are exercising undue influence, for example, it may be helpful to support the elder in making important life decisions.

Self-efficacy, a belief that one can organize and execute courses of action needed to achieve a desired goal or succeed at desired undertakings, also influences health status. Unlike perceived control, self-efficacy relates more to psychological assessment of health than to physical health. In other words, individuals with a strong sense of self-efficacy are more likely to perceive themselves as functional, regardless of their actual physical status. This factor, in turn, has a positive impact on mental health and improves quality of life (Blazer, 2002). Self-efficacy is enhanced through experiences of success, particularly success in overcoming difficulties. The elderly person may need to be provided with direct opportunities to affirm their abilities. In fact, many elders seek opportunities for creative expression of their observations of the world, some of them in public arenas where they can receive positive feedback (Bonder & Martin, 2000).

Both perceived control and self-efficacy are associated with choice of coping response. Coping responses have been categorized as being either problem solving or emotional. Inadequate coping can lead to stress, depression, anger, and anxiety, all of which have been associated with physical disease. **Problem-solving coping strategies,** such as information seeking and other behavioral and cognitive actions, have been found most effective in promoting both a sense of well-being and physical health. Emotional coping responses, particularly those that are passive, when used solely are associated with poor health outcomes.

There is evidence that coping strategies can be taught. Folkman and Lazarus (1991) suggest that teaching a combination of cognitive problem solving with positive reappraisal can lead to an improved emotional state. This suggests that individuals can learn to adopt a cognitive problem-solving approach to health-related concerns, thereby enhancing the state of their health. Unutzer (2006) found that elders with depression who participated in a four- to eight-session series of behavioral interventions designed to improve problem-solving abilities demonstrated less-frequent thoughts of suicide than those who received standard care for at least up to 12 months. Thus, health care providers can support both physical and emotional well-being by ensuring that elders have adequate control over their own lives, by supporting their self-efficacy, and by ensuring that they have effective, health-promoting problem-solving strategies.

Spirituality

It has long been observed that individuals seem to become more focused on spiritual concerns in later life. Reasons for this renewed interest are hypothesized to relate to the imminence of death and a renewed focus on life's greater meanings. **Spirituality** involves the development of an "internalized personal relation with the sacred or transcendent that is not bound by race, ethnicity, economics, or class and promotes wellness and welfare of self and others" (Crowther, Parker, Larimore, Achenbaum, & Koenig, 2002, p. 614). It is important to note that the expression of spirituality varies widely from individual to individual. For example, among Mexican Americans, elders who attended church experienced greater life satisfaction and less depression than those who did not (Levin, Markides, & Ray, 1996).

For some, participation in traditional religious services may be the activity of choice. Others find spiritual expression in creative arts, in communing with nature, or with meditation. The variety of ways to express spirituality is probably as vast as the range of individuals. A careful meta-analysis of research on the relationship of spirituality to health found "a positive relationship between religious beliefs, behaviors, and mental or physical health" (Koenig, 1994, p. xv). The overwhelming evidence supports the value of spirituality in promoting well-being in later life.

In spite of these findings, health care professionals are likely to overlook the power of spirituality in their interactions with their clients. Nevertheless, as Moberg (1996) notes, "the religious commitments and connections of older people provide rich opportunities for enhancing therapy and services to improve their wellbeing" (p. 267). Forcing religion or spirituality on older adults is likely to be counterproductive, but offering opportunities for voluntary expression can promote satisfaction with life and help them cope with whatever their current situation may be. Health care professionals can support their clients by eliciting such expressions, and by listening carefully and supporting them. Attendance at religious ceremonies may be a motivating factor that health care professionals can use to encourage elders to participate in other kinds of wellness programs. For example, a physical therapist might find a client more willing to work on ambulation if the identified goal is the ability to walk to the sanctuary from the parking lot at church.

Health Behavior Change

Obviously, to be beneficial, the factors listed earlier must be given careful consideration and personal behavior altered. This is not a simple matter. It is well established that access to information, by itself, is not sufficient to lead to change. An individual may well be aware, for example, that smoking is bad for one's health but not choose to stop. Or an individual may know that exercise is a positive health habit but exercise sporadically or not at all. Likewise, making a decision to undertake behavior change is also not sufficient, as we witness the number of New Year's resolutions that have fallen by the wayside before the end of January. A number of theories exist that attempt to describe how health behavior change occurs. For the purposes of this chapter, the Transtheoretical (or Stages of Change) Model will be described as an example and applied to health behavior change.

Transtheoretical Model (TTM)

This model suggests that individuals' health behavior change can be conceptualized as occurring in five stages: precontemplation, contemplation, preparation, action, and maintenance (Table 18-2). During each stage, specific interventions have the potential to encourage movement to the next stage. In the contemplation stage, weighing of pros and cons of the new behavior may provide a basis for movement to preparation. The model has been tested in an array of programs, including mammography and smoking cessation, and has provided valuable insight into health behavior change (Prochaska, Redding, & Evers, 2002).

The ultimate motivation for change may be highly personal. For example, one individual explained that he smoked his last cigarette on the day his father died of lung cancer. Knowing for years that it was harmful to his health was insufficient motivation; seeing the impact of lung cancer on someone he loved was a powerful motivator. In the development of wellness programs, identifying such motivation for change is an important factor. Health promotion programs based on appropriate theoretical models

TABLE 18-2 The Transtheoretical Model

Stage	Behaviors	Intervention to Move to Next Phase
Precontemplation	Individual becomes aware of issue	Information, advertising, public awareness campaigns
Contemplation	Individual considers implications of issue for himself or herself, considers behavior change	Information, health screening, consumer or client education
Preparation	Individual decides to make change, develops plan	Health information, resource exploration, client education
Action	Individual implements plan	Reward system, social support, behavior modification program
Maintenance	New behavior becomes habit	Reward system, social support, behavioral evaluation

ensure the best possible outcomes. Combining the TTM with evidence-based health behavior change strategies can enhance the effectiveness of health promotion and wellness programs for older adults.

Application of The TTM

The TTM can be applied to a variety of health issues older persons face. One example might be for fall prevention. Consider an elderly woman with osteoarthritis and resultant pain in both knees. She has sustained two falls in the past 6 months. As her osteoarthritis progressed, she became more and more sedentary which increased her risk of falls due to diminished muscle strength and balance. Her daughter has encouraged her to join an exercise class to improve her physical fitness, but the mother declines. The mother is in the precontemplation stage. After visiting her physician, she was sent to an occupational therapist for a home evaluation for fall prevention. The occupational therapist facilitated movement from the precontemplation stage to contemplation by suggesting a variety of physical activities that would improve strength and balance that might be more enjoyable than an exercise class. The suggestion that seemed of most interest was tai chi, so the occupational therapist showed the client some basic tai chi moves and encouraged her to imitate them. The older woman stated that she liked this activity but was not inclined to take a course with other people. She preferred to exercise alone, so the occupational therapist recommended using a tai chi videotape.

On the client's next trip to the shopping mall with her daughter, she purchased a videotape and thus moved into the preparation stage. She also acquired some new, comfortable "exercise" clothes to wear as she practiced the tai chi moves. It was then easy for her to begin the action phase, and she practiced with the video twice a week with her daughter's encouragement. Over a short period of time, the woman noticed she was sleeping better, she was more stable on her feet, and she had less pain. These reinforcers helped her to move into the maintenance stage. A strength of this model is its circular nature, whereby individuals can enter the change cycle at any point, and repeated attempts to change and maintain health behaviors are possible.

Strategies for Health Behavior Change

There are many evidence-based approaches to health behavior change. Three strategies that have particular relevance for elders will be discussed here. These include enhancing health literacy, chronic disease self-management, and lifestyle redesign.

Health Literacy

Healthy People 2010 defines **health literacy** as the "degree to which individuals have the capacity to obtain, process, and understand basic health information and services needed to make appropriate health decisions" (USD-HHS, 2000, Chapter 11, Health Communication). According to the Institute of Medicine's (IOM) report titled *Health literacy: A prescription to end confusion,* nearly half of adults in the United States have difficulty comprehending, responding to, and appropriately acting on health information (IOM, 2004). The national emphasis on health literacy is based, in part, on research that demonstrates a relationship between health literacy and health outcomes (USDHHS, 2000).

According to Osborne (2005), "health literacy is a shared responsibility in which patients and providers each must communicate in ways the other can understand" (p. 2). In addition, health literacy does not simply apply to written information; it includes all forms of communication between health care providers, patients, families, and caregivers. Because low health literacy limits a person's understanding of their health conditions, they are more likely to report poor health and have higher rates of hospitalization (USDHHS, 2000).

Services to enhance health literacy among the elderly may include

* Individualized health counseling
* Health education group sessions on a variety of topics
* Referral to self-help and support groups
* Preparation of individuals to participate in health care interactions with providers

Chronic Disease Self-Management

A significant percentage of elderly persons over 70 years of age have at least one of the following chronic diseases or conditions: arthritis, cancer, cerebrovascular accident, diabetes mellitus, heart disease, hypertension, or respiratory disease (Chodosh et al., 2005). As a result of rising health care costs, patient self-management of chronic disease is being increasingly emphasized. There are varying definitions in the literature, but essentially, **chronic disease self-management** involves individuals and families actively participating in the health care process, self-monitoring symptoms or physiological processes, making informed decisions about their health, and managing the impact of the disease on their daily life. The purpose of chronic disease self-management programs is to enable individuals to prevent complications and control and manage their health conditions (Chodosh et al., 2005).

Therapists have knowledge of chronic diseases and their effects on daily life functioning which would enable them to develop chronic disease self-management programs in health care and community settings, train persons with chronic diseases to instruct and lead groups, and evaluate the outcomes. The research available supports the efficacy of generic chronic disease self-management programs and their cost-effectiveness for persons with multiple comorbidities (Centers for Disease Control and Prevention [CDC], 2006). Effective chronic disease self-management programs generally share the following characteristics: tailoring, group setting, feedback, psychological emphasis, and offered by medical care providers. Programs tailored to the specific needs and circumstances of the individual, offered by medical care providers, and conducted in group settings appear to be more beneficial than standard programs offered to individuals by non-health-care personnel. Routine review and feedback and attention to the person's psychosocial concerns also appear to be important determinants of effectiveness (Chodosh et al., 2005).

Lifestyle Redesign

The Lifestyle Redesign concept emerged from the landmark study by Clark et al. (1997) that compared the outcomes of an occupational therapy preventive intervention for elders living in the community with a social activities program led by nonprofessionals, and a group that received no intervention. The elders receiving the occupational therapy program had better outcomes than either of the other two groups, and the results were maintained at a 6-month follow-up. The occupational therapy group demonstrated greater gains in physical and social functioning, mental health, and life satisfaction. The outcomes for the social activities group were similar to those who received no treatment at all (Clark et al., 1997).

Lifestyle Redesign focuses on educating older adults about the importance of occupation to enhance physical, mental, emotional, social, and spiritual health and on preparing them to be reflective about their occupational choices. The combination, of knowledge of the health benefits of occupation and the skills to be reflective, permits the person to "construct daily routines in a manner that would optimize their health and psychosocial wellbeing" and to participate in a process of lifestyle redesign (Jackson et al., 1998, p. 329).

Many of the health problems experienced by older persons are lifestyle related and have multiple occupation-linked determinants. Positive health behavior changes can only be sustained if they are embedded in the occupations of a person's daily life. Lifestyle redesign principles include the following:

- Occupation is essential for human life.
- Occupation can create visions of new possibilities and potential life changes.
- Occupation has an effect on physical and mental health and life order and routines.
- Occupational therapy can be used for prevention and health promotion (Mandel, Jackson, Zemke, Nelson, & Clark, 1999).

Designing and Funding Programming

Health promotion programming is somewhat different from other forms of intervention in a number of respects. First, it is often population based. This means that, rather than focusing on the design of an intervention plan for an individual, programming is designed to address problems identified through epidemiological data. For example, a health promotion program might incorporate physical activity, not because an individual has been identified as needing an exercise program, but rather because it is established that lack of physical activity is a general problem in a particular population. Some wellness programs are completely invisible to the service population, as in the case of environmental modifications that support function but are implemented in the original planning of a building as opposed to retrofitting it for a specific individual.

Second, health promotion programs are often implemented outside of traditional health care settings. Programs for the elderly may be offered in a range of community settings, such as assisted living facilities, senior centers, faith-based organizations, libraries, homes, workplaces, adult day care centers, and community housing apartments. Health promotion services can be provided by a variety of health professionals, including physicians, nurses, therapists, health educators, and public health professionals.

Third, because health promotion interventions often occur outside the traditional medical setting, mechanisms for funding are also different. In some instances, interventions to enhance wellness are funded by health care insurers. A cardiac rehabilitation program, including exercise, diet, stress management, and smoking cessation interventions, might be funded for an individual who has just had coronary bypass surgery. In many instances, however, particularly for those interventions perceived as less "medical," funding must come from other sources. Sometimes the source is direct payment from the individual. Elders or their families may be willing to pay directly for home safety surveys, for example, or may pay to come to a lecture series focused on prevention and health promotion topics.

Another source of funding is government agencies. For example, the Older Americans Act includes funding for nutrition and other wellness programming at senior centers nationwide. Federal funding is directed first to programs that address the objectives identified in *Healthy People 2010*; state and local offices on aging also fund health promotion programs. These are likely to include health screening, nutrition programs, and vaccination programs. They are less likely to include social support, occupational interventions, and education about coping strategies.

Funding for less medically focused programming may come from industry or from local foundations. For example, some businesses now fund preretirement seminars for prospective retirees, focused on financial planning, health practices, and time usage. Foundations and other charitable institutions may support health-specific programming.

Finally, the emphasis of wellness programming is on prevention and health promotion rather than remediation. The goal of wellness programs is to enhance function and reduce the incidence of disease, rather than to rehabilitate or cure.

These differences make it somewhat difficult to document the effectiveness of health promotion programming. Outcomes, like the interventions, may best be documented based on broad, population-based benefits. Overall reductions in hospitalization rates, illness, morbidity, and increases in self-reported health and well-being are all markers that health promotion programs are valuable.

Program Development

The development of health promotion programs follows a similar process regardless of the health problem targeted. Upon reflection, the program development process appears remarkably similar to the evaluation and intervention processes occupational therapists use everyday. However, the terminology for describing the processes is different. The program development process is depicted in Figure 18-1.

The process starts with preplanning or exploration, where the problem, resources, barriers, goals, and target population are identified. This is comparable to the chart review in clinical practice. The next step is **needs assessment,** or data gathering and analysis. In the needs assessment, data are collected and analyzed in order to determine priorities and formulate an action plan. This step is comparable to client evaluation. The intended population should be carefully identified and health risks for that population clarified. Depending on the ethnic background of the service population, health risks may differ. African Americans are at higher risk for high blood pressure but lower risk for osteoporosis than their white counterparts.

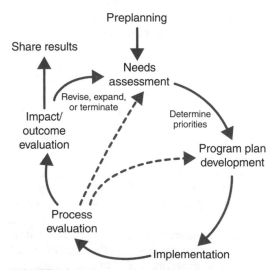

FIGURE 18-1 The cycle of program development. (From M. E. Scaffa, *Occupational therapy in community-based practice settings,* 2001, Figure 6-1, Philadelphia, F.A. Davis.)

After priorities are established, a plan is developed, including the establishment of goals and objectives, intervention strategies, procedures, and timelines. This step is comparable to intervention planning with clients. The planning process should identify specific components of the program, as well as the environment in which they will occur. Ideally, the environment enhances the effectiveness of the program. Funding must be considered in conjunction with program planning. As noted earlier, an array of funding possibilities must be explored. Although some programs respond to specific funding initiatives (e.g., announced health priorities of a state department of health), many require somewhat creative funding mechanisms.

Then the health promotion program is implemented in the same way therapy interventions are implemented, based on the treatment plan and the client's goals and objectives. The health promotion program should take into account the characteristics of the service neighborhood. For example, although social support is an intervention that would be of value in almost any wellness program, in some communities, it will be more effective if it is planned around church activities. In other neighborhoods, a lecture series might be more likely to attract participants. The time frame is also important. Some individuals prefer evening programs, whereas others go out only during the day. Individuals must be made aware of the program, enrolled, and, if necessary, provided with transportation. Wellness programs require good public relations efforts to publicize them in ways that will be noticed. Information in newsletters that are widely read, notices in community newspapers, announcements at senior centers and churches, brochures provided to physicians and to social service agencies, and posts on popular Web pages are all mechanisms to consider.

The next step in the program development process is **program evaluation.** Evaluation consists of monitoring the program's process, impact, and outcomes to determine its effectiveness. This parallels the client reevaluation process in therapy. Outcome evaluation should be a prominent consideration during the planning process. Effective evaluation involves careful data collection throughout the program development process. The first step is identifying desired outcomes (e.g., smoking cessation, more positive health and function). Once outcomes have been identified, specific data-collection mechanisms can be identified (e.g., interview, questionnaire, standardized instrument).

Examples of Wellness Programs

Effective community-based health promotion programs have certain characteristics in common. These may be considered "best practices" and include the following:

- Tailoring the program to a specific population within a particular context
- Involving program participants in the planning, implementation, and evaluation of the program
- Integrating efforts aimed at changing individuals, environments (physical and social), communities, and policies
- Linking participants' concerns about health to broader life concerns
- Using existing resources within the community
- Incorporating the strengths of participants and their social networks
- Building community capacity for health
- Preparing participants to become self-advocates and managers of their own health (Scaffa, 2001)

A few health promotion programs for older adults that incorporate aspects of these best practices will be described briefly as examples. These include the Health Enhancement Program, OASIS Institute's Health Stages, and Designing a Life of Wellness Program.

The *Health Enhancement Program* developed by the University of Washington provides participants with a health self-evaluation. Participants are referred from various local sources and evaluated by a nurse and a social worker. In addition, a university-based geriatrician is affiliated with the program. The nurse helps participants identify personal health goals, and every 6 months the health program is updated for the participant and the referring physician. Each participant is assigned a health mentor. The health mentor is "a trained community-based volunteer who may accompany the participant to exercise classes, provide weekly calls and support, or engage in other activities supporting the participant in reaching health goals" (Centers for Disease Control and Prevention [CDC], 2004, Phase 2, Senior Wellness Project, p. 1). Program fees are on a sliding scale based on income, and the health department funds a nurse at each of five sites and interpreters as needed. Analysis of program outcome data indicated a 72% decrease in length of hospital stay and a 38% reduction in hospitalization rates (CDC, 2004).

Health Stages is the health promotion component of the OASIS Institute, a national nonprofit educational organization designed to enrich the lives of older adults. The OASIS Institute is sponsored by Federated Department Stores and BJC Health Care. The Health Stages program is provided in 26 cities and consists of the following three components: (1) a state-of-the-art curriculum, (2) an implementation model that is tailored to meet the needs and interests of local participants, and (3) a comprehensive evaluation plan. Health Stages focuses on seven areas: physical activity, nutrition, mental wellness, memory, sensory health, disease management, and general health promotion. The program promotes successful aging by enabling participants to set personal goals and develop health management skills. Health Stages is based on the TTM and provides a variety of learning opportunities for people at different stages of readiness to make health ehavior changes. Curricular offerings are categorized by goal: awareness, knowledge, skill building, or maintenance of behavior change (OASIS Institute, 2006).

Designing a Life of Wellness Program is an occupation-based health promotion program developed by Matuska, Giles-Heinz, Flinn, Neighbor, and Bass-Haugen (2003). Sixty-five older adults (ages 70 to 92 years) from three senior apartment complexes and individuals living in the community participated in the program. The program consisted of weekly 1-hour educational classes over a period of 6 months. Occupational therapy faculty members and students on their Level II fieldwork experience conducted the educational sessions. The program emphasized the importance of engagement in meaningful occupations as a means of enhancing quality of life and was designed to remove personal and environmental barriers to social participation. Results from the pilot study, using pretest and posttest scores of the SF-36 Health Survey, indicated significantly enhanced vitality, social functioning, and mental health. In addition, the number of participants who communicated with family, friends, or support persons at least three times a week increased from 47% to 56%; and participation in social or community activities rose from 47% to 66%. Eighty-seven percent of participants rated their overall satisfaction with the program as good or excellent. This study provides additional evidence of the benefits of occupation-based health promotion programs for the elderly.

■ Summary

The AOTA (2001) official document on the role of occupational therapy in prevention and health promotion emphasizes the importance of providing services for individuals, groups, organizations, and communities. Health promotion services may aim to reduce health risk factors, increase protective factors, or a combination of both. Occupational therapists are uniquely trained to identify and remediate the risk factors for occupational dysfunction, which include occupational imbalance, occupational alienation, and occupational deprivation (Wilcock, 1998).

The potential for occupation-based health promotion interventions for the elderly is great, and there is considerable evidence that at least some programs have significant positive impact. Although much remains to be learned about health promotion programs for the elderly, they offer opportunities for the reframing of health care as focused on wellness as opposed to illness. Opportunities for allied health practitioners in such programs are limited only by the creativity of the practitioner in meeting the needs of the community.

Case Study

Mrs. Allen is a 78-year-old woman who was recently widowed. She lives in a small bungalow in a close-in suburb of a medium-sized city. Before her husband died, they had settled into a relatively traditional division of labor. She handled shopping, food preparation, laundry, and housecleaning, while he paid the bills, did outside maintenance of the house, and drove. Mrs. Allen never learned to drive. As a couple, they enjoyed playing bridge with friends. They frequently went to the movies, and they walked each evening. Each Sunday they attended the local Lutheran Church together; the church is less than a mile from Mrs. Allen's home.

Mrs. Allen's daughter is concerned because her mother now seems at loose ends. On a recent visit, the daughter found little food in the refrigerator, and her mother had not left home for almost a week. She has asked you to provide an occupational therapy consultation to help her decide how to best assist her mother.

Questions

1. How would you go about assessing the situation?
2. What occupational issues do you feel are most salient?
3. How might you recommend Mrs. Allen and her daughter address these issues?

Review Questions

1. What factors most strongly influence wellness and successful aging for older adults?
2. How do cultural characteristics of the target population influence programs being planned?
3. In what ways might it be important to use a theoretical model to guide program planning?
4. How might environmental design promote wellness?

Web-Based Resources

For helpful information about the experience of Health Promotion and Wellness, visit:

Websites and Resources on Aging

Website Name	Website Address
Ageline	http://www.research.aarp.og/ageline/
American Society on Aging	http://www.asaging.org
Gerontological Society of America	http://geron.org
AARP	http://www.aarp.org
National Association of Area Agencies on Aging	http://www.n4a.org
World Health Organization	http://www.who.org
National Caucus and Center on Black Aged	http://www.ncbablackaged.org
Robert Wood Johnson Foundation	http://www.rwjf.org
National Institute on Aging	http://nih.gov/nia/
US Administration on Aging	http://www.aoa.gov

Other Websites for Manuals and Content Specific Information on Successful Aging

Website Address

http://www.asaging.org/cdc/
http://www.ncoa.org/content.cfm?sectionID=99&detail=99
http://www.agingstats.gov/chartbook2000/default.htm
https://www.ncoa.org/Downloads/healthy_living.pdf.pdf

Note: Websites and addresses change frequently.

REFERENCES

American Academy of Family Physicians, The American Dietetic Association, National Council on the Aging, Inc. (n.d.). *Nutrition interventions manual for professionals caring for older Americans.* Retrieved January 26, 2007, from www.eatright.org/ada/files/NSIOlderAmericansComplete1.pdf.

American Council on Exercise: Exercise for Older Adults. (1998). *Human kinetics.* Champaign, IL: Author.

American Occupational Therapy Association (AOTA). (2001). Occupational therapy in the promotion of health and the prevention of disease and disability statement. *American Journal of Occupational Therapy, 55*(6), 656–660.

American Occupational Therapy Association (AOTA). (2002). *Occupational therapy practice framework: Domain and process.* Bethesda: Author.

Arthritis Foundation. (2007). *Exercise and arthritis.* Retrieved January 26, 2007, from www.arthritis.org/conditions/exercise/default.asp.

Bass, D. M., McClendon, M. J., Brennan, P. F., & McCarthy, C. (1998). The buffering effect of a computer support network on caregiver strain. *Journal of Aging and Health, 10,* 20–43.

Bennett, K. M. (2002). Low level social engagement as a precursor of mortality among people in later life. *Age and Ageing, 31,* 165–168.

Blazer, D. G. (2002). Self-efficacy and depression in late life: A primary prevention proposal. *Aging & Mental Health, 6*(4), 315–324.

Bonder, B. R., & Martin, L. (2000). Personal meanings of occupation for women in later life. *Women and Aging, 4*(12), 177–193

Bosworth, H. B., & Schaie, K. W. (1997). The relationship of social environment, social networks, and health outcomes in the Seattle longitudinal study: Two analytical approaches. *Journal of Gerontology: Psychological Sciences, 52B,* P197–P205.

Carlson, M., Clark, F., & Young, B. (1998). Practical contributions of occupational science to the art of successful aging. How to sculpt a meaningful life in older adulthood. *Journal of Occupational Science: Australia, 5,* 107–118.

Centers for Disease Control and Prevention. (2001). Increasing physical activity. A report on recommendations of the Task Force on Community Preventive Services. *MMWR. Recommendations and Reports, 50*(RR-18), 1–16.

Centers for Disease Control and Prevention. (2004). *Live well, live long: Health promotion and disease prevention for older adults.* Retrieved August 16, 2006, from www.asaging.org/cdc/module1/phase1/phase1_2b.ctm.

Centers for Disease Control and Prevention. (2006). *CDC Funded Science: Comparisons of the outcomes of the arthritis self help course and the chronic disease self management program among people with arthritis.* Retrieved January 8, 2007, from www.cdc.gov/arthritis/funded_science/projects/arthritis-self-help-course-chronic-disease-self-management-program-unc.htm.

Chernoff, R. (2001). Nutrition and health promotion in older adults. *Journals of Gerontology Series A: Biological Sciences and Medical Sciences, 56,* 47–53.

Chodosh, J., Morton, S. C., Mojica, W., Maglione, M., Suttorp, M. J., Hilton, L., et al. (2005). Meta-analysis: Chronic disease self-management programs for older adults. *Annals of Internal Medicine, 143,* 427–438.

Clark, F., Azen, S. P., Zemke, R., Jackson, J., Carlson, M., Mandel, D., et al. (1997). Occupational therapy for independent-living older adults: A randomized controlled trial. *Journal of the American Medical Association, 278,* 1321–1326.

Crowther, M., Parker, M., Larimore, W., Achenbaum, A., & Koenig, H. (2002). Rowe and Kahn's model of successful aging revisited: Spirituality the missing construct. *The Gerontologist, 42*(5), 613–620.

Dawson, D. A., Grant, B. F., & Li, T. (2005). Quantifying the risks associated with exceeding recommended drinking limits. *Alcoholism: Clinical & Experimental Research, 29,* 902–908.

De Vries, M. J., Schilder, J. N., Mulder, C. L., Vrancken, A. M. E., Remie, M. E., & Garssen, B. (1997). Phase II study of psychotherapeutic intervention in advanced cancer. *Psycho-Oncology, 6,* 129–137.

Ditto, P. H., Druley, J. A., Moore, K. A., Danks, J. H., & Smucker, W. D. (1996). Fates worse than death: The role of valued life activities in health-state evaluations. *Health Psychology, 15,* 332–343.

Finch, C. E. (1990). *Longevity, senescence and the genome.* Chicago: University of Chicago Press.

Folkman, S., & Lazarus, R. S. (1991). Coping and emotion. In A. Monat & R. S. Lazarus (Eds.), *Stress and coping: An anthology* (3rd ed., pp. 207–227). New York: Columbia University Press.

Gallup, J. W. (1999). *Wellness centers: A guide for the design professional.* New York: Wiley.

Glass, T. A. (2006). Social engagement and depressive symptoms in late life: Longitudinal findings. *Journal of Aging & Health, 18,* 604–628.

Institute of Medicine. (2004). *Health literacy: A prescription to end confusion.* Washington, DC: National Academies Press.

Jackson, J., Carlson, M., Mandel, D., Zemke, R., & Clark, F. (1998). Occupation in lifestyle redesign: The well elderly study occupational therapy program. *American Journal of Occupational Therapy, 53*(5), 326–336.

Kane, R. L. (2003). The contribution of geriatric health services research to successful aging. *Annals of Internal Medicine, 139*(5), 460–462.

Kinsella, K., & Velkoff, V. A. (2001). *An aging world: 2001.* Washington, DC: U.S. Census Bureau publication P95/01-1.

Koenig, H. G. (1994). *Aging and God: Spiritual pathways to mental health in midlife and later years.* Binghamton, NY: Haworth Pastoral Press.

Levin, J. S., Markides, K. S., & Ray, L. A. (1996). Religious attendance and psychological wellbeing in Mexican

Americans: A panel analysis of three-generations data. *The Gerontologist, 36,* 454–463.

Levitan, U. (1999). Contribution of social arrangements to the attainment of successful aging—The experience of the Israeli kibbutz. *Journal of Gerontology: Psychological Sciences, 54B,* P205–P213.

Mandel, D., Jackson, J. M., Zemke, R., Nelson, L., & Clark, F. A. (1999). *Lifestyle redesign: Implementing the well elderly program.* Bethesda, MD: American Occupational Therapy Association.

Matuska, K., Giles-Heinz, A., Flinn, N., Neighbor, M., & Bass-Haugen, J. (2003). Outcomes of a pilot occupational therapy wellness program for older adults. *American Journal of Occupational Therapy, 57,* 220–224.

McCabe, B. W. Walker, S. N., & Clark, K. A. (1997). Health promotion in long term care facilities. *Journal of Nursing Science, 2,* 153–167.

Menec, V. H. (2003). The relation between everyday activities and successful aging: A 6-year longitudinal study. *Journals of Gerontology Series B: Psychological and Social Sciences, 58,* S74–S82.

Menec, V. H., & Chipperfield, J. G. (1997). The interactive effect of perceived control and functional status on health and mortality among young-old and old-old adults. *Journal of Gerontology: Psychological Sciences, 52B,* P118–P126.

Miller, M. E., Rejeski, W. J., Reboussin, B. A., Ten Have, T. R., & Ettinger, W. H. (2000). Physical activity, functional limitations, and disability in older adults. *Journal of the American Geriatrics Society, 48,* 1264–1272.

Minkler, M., & Fadem, P. (2002). "Successful aging": A disability perspective. *Journal of Disability Policy Studies, 12,* 229–235.

Moberg, D. O. (1996). Religion in gerontology: From benign neglect to belated respect. *The Gerontologist, 36,* 264–266.

Mukamal, K. J., Conigrave, K. M., Mittleman, M. A., Camargo, C. A., Stampfer, M. J., Willett, W. C., et al. (2003). Roles of drinking pattern and type of alcohol consumed in coronary heart disease in men. *New England Journal of Medicine, 348*(2), 109–118.

National Institute on Aging. (2004). *Alzheimer's disease genetics fact sheet.* U.S. Department of Health and Human Services, NIH publication No. 03-3431.

National Institute of Mental Health. (2007). *Older adults: Depression and suicide facts.* Retrieved September 7, 2007, from www.nimh.nih.gov/publicat/elderlydepsuicide.cfm.

OASIS Institute. (2006). *Health Stages.* Retrieved January 8, 2007, from www.oasisnet.org/learn/ health.htm.

Osborne, H. (2005). *Health literacy from A to Z: Practical ways to communicate your health message.* Boston: Jones and Bartlett.

Park, K. (1999). Pets bring therapeutic benefits to nursing homes. *Balance, 3,* 18–20.

Prochaska, J. O., Redding, C. A., & Evers, K. (2002). The transtheoretical model and stages of change. In K. Glanz, B. K. Rimer, & F. M. Lewis (Eds.), *Health behavior and health education: Theory, research, and practice* (3rd ed., pp. 99–120). San Francisco, CA: Jossey-Bass.

Quan, M., & Gitlin, M. (2004). *Get a life! Recognition and management of depression from diagnosis to remission.* California Academy of Family Physicians. Retrieved September 7, 2007, from www.familydocs.org/assets/Publications/Monographs/CAFP_Depression.pdf.

Reichel, W. (1995). *Care of the elderly: Clinical aspects of aging* (4th ed.). Baltimore: Williams & Wilkins.

Rowe, J. W., & Kahn, R. L. (1998). *Successful aging.* New York: Pantheon Books.

Scaffa, M. E. (2001). *Occupational therapy in community-based practice settings.* Philadelphia: F.A. Davis.

Seeman, T. E., Unger, J. B., McAvay, G., Mendes de Leon, C.F.M. (1999). Self-efficacy beliefs and perceived declines in functional ability: MacArthur studies of successful aging. *Journal of Gerontology: Psychological Sciences, 54B,* P214–P222.

Sugisawa, H., Liang, J., & Liu, X. (1994). Social networks, social support, and mortality among older people in Japan. *Journal of Gerontology: Social Sciences, 49,* S3–S13.

Treas, J. (1995). *Older Americans in the 1990s and beyond.* Washington, DC: Population Reference Bureau.

Unutzer, J. (2006). Reducing suicidal ideation in depressed older primary care patients. *Journal of the American Geriatric Society, 54*(10), 1550–1556.

U.S. Department of Health and Human Services, Public Health Service. (2000). *Healthy People 2010.* Retrieved September 30, 2006, from www.health.gov/healthypeople.

U.S. Department of Health and Human Services (2008). Healthy People 2020 retrieved June 21, 2008 (from www.healthypeople.gov/HP2020/.

Wilcock, A. A. (1998). *An occupational perspective of health.* Thorofare, NJ: Slack.

CHAPTER 19

Community-based Services

Georgia J. Anetzberger, PhD, ACSW

I find that the "winding down" process of life isn't much different than the "growing up" process: New experiences everyday and problems to be solved. We had lots of help in growing up and we have lots of help in winding down.

Richard Kauffman, retired musician and settlement house worker, at age 88

OBJECTIVES

By the end of this chapter, readers will be able to:

1. Discuss factors that influence the use of services.
2. Identify levels of service barriers.
3. Describe resources that link individuals with available community services.
4. List the various resources available for older adults to remain active through work, learning, volunteerism, or social and recreational experiences.
5. Explain the nature of adult protective services.
6. Identify housing options that exist for older adults.

Nearly all older adults want to remain in the community and out of institutions (Pynoos & Golant, 1996; Wagnild, 2001). Most believe that they will be able to remain in their current homes until they die (AARP, 2003). It is not so much that medical and nursing facilities are seen as uncaring or unsafe. Rather, community dwelling carries with it a sense of familiarity, individual identity, personal control, and freedom. As adults age, remaining in the community becomes more challenging. Impairments and social losses can serve to compromise well-being and independence. Facing these challenges usually means confronting the need for services. Much help comes from family and friends (Levine et al., 2000; National Alliance for Caregiving & American Association of Retired Persons, 1997; Thompson, 2004). The rest is available from organizations or housing options in the community. Many of these community-based services are described here; others are considered in the remaining chapters.

Discussion in this chapter focuses on recent growth in community-based services before identifying various ways to classify them, selecting a functional approach for the subsequent organization of chapter contents. Service utilization and barriers to service use are explored, with special attention given to ethnicity and sexual orientation as potential group-level service barriers. Identifying community-based services can be difficult without the help of linkage resources, which connect individuals with available services. This chapter describes these and then discusses various community-based services in terms of their provision of something to do, someone to care, and someplace to live. Throughout, case examples act to introduce these service classifications as well as to illustrate the use of select services. In addition, where appropriate, models of community-based services found in other countries, but currently not in the United States, are introduced, because the origins of many services now common here were in Great Britain or elsewhere.

Service Growth

Community-based services have grown significantly during the past few decades. For example, the number of adult day centers increased 1233% between 1978 and 1997, and the number of home care agencies increased 89% from 1991 to 1999 (National Council on Aging, 1997; Office of Strategic Planning & Health Care Financing Administration, 1999). Service growth has been fueled by many factors, including growth of the elderly population and decline of available informal caregivers, as family size, structure, and mobility changed. In addition, public policy propelled growth, bolstered by old age interest groups, considered to be among the nation's most powerful lobbies (Day, 1998; Binstock, 2005). Federal legislation, like the Older Americans Act, Title XX of the Social Security Act, and Medicaid waivers, provided funding for community-based services and encouraged more organizations to become senior service providers. In addition, the 1999 U.S. Supreme Court decision on *Olmstead v. L.C.* gave priority to community-based services by recognizing the general responsibility of states to serve people with disabilities in the community if they are eligible and do not oppose receiving services there. The ruling is widely seen as a stimulus for changing the long-term care balance from institutional to community-based care (Velgouse, 2000).

Service Classifications

There are numerous ways to classify community-based services. Three of the more common are as follows:

- Along a **continuum of care**
- By location
- According to function

Continuum of Care

Continuum of care describes the system of services that supports the well-being of older adults at every stage of functioning. It is typically presented in linear fashion. Older adults without service needs are at one end (independence), and those requiring total care or assistance are at the other end (dependence). Community-based services fall all along the continuum of care. For example, transportation ranges from driving a car oneself to being transported by ambulance. In between these extremes are such options as community response transport and escort services. Housing, too, ranges from living in one's own home or apartment to residing in a nursing facility, with congregate care and assisted living found midway in this continuum. The extent and type of services required by older people primarily reflect their physical and mental health. Those who are well and able need no or very few services. Those who are ill and disabled may need many and varied services.

In selecting services along the continuum of care, three considerations must be kept in mind. First, older adults usually require a comprehensive assessment in order to determine specific service needs. Comprehensive assessments explore an individual's physical, intellectual, emotional, social, financial, and environmental status. They evaluate level of functioning, particularly with respect to the individual's ability to perform tasks, like bathing, and fulfill social roles, such as being a spouse (Miller, 2004). Comprehensive assessments often involve an interdisciplinary team of professionals, minimally including a physician, nurse, and social worker. They also are available in most communities in hospital, clinic, or agency settings. Second, it is essential that older adults receive the level and type of services required to address their needs. Too much help can foster dependency or helplessness (Cimarolli, Reinhardt, & Horowitz, 2006; Thompson & Sobolew-Shubin, 1993). Too little help can risk health and safety (Dong, 2005; O'Brien, Thibault, Turner, & Laird-Fick, 1999). Third, service needs may change over time, making ongoing reassessment necessary. Older adults do not necessarily follow the continuum of care linearly. Most do not experience a consistent and gradual decline in functional capacity over time from independence to dependence. Rather, they move into and out of various states of independence and dependence based upon health, performance skills, personal factors, and circumstances.

Walter illustrates this dynamic quality of well-being and service need after his recent discharge from a hospital following a stroke. At home alone, he was assisted by his daughter who lived nearby as well as by community-based agencies which provided home care, housekeeping, chore, and home-delivered meal services. An occupational therapist came to do a home safety evaluation, and worked with Walter to develop energy conservation strategies in the home. A physical therapist developed a home exercise plan to help Walter regain strength and maintain mobility. As his recovery and rehabilitation progressed, his need for these services disappeared. Eventually Walter only required transportation, so he contacted the local office on aging to arrange a minivan to take him to doctor appointments.

Location

Community-based services can be classified by their location, in which case three types are usually presented: in-home care, outside-of-the-home assistance, and housing modifications or options. In-home care represents services provided in the homes of older adults. They include homemaking, chore services, and home-delivered meals. They are appropriate when older adults need help to maintain themselves at home but do not require around-the-clock care or supervision. Outside-of-the-home assistance is available for those able to travel to a service site where often group activities are highlighted. They include adult day care, congregate meals, and **senior centers.** Finally, housing modifications or options represent changes in residence

or living arrangements which address functional limitations on the part of older adults. Modifications represent alterations to an existing home so that it is more accessible to an individual with deficits. Examples include ramps at entrances, grab bars for tubs, and electric openers for garage doors. Housing options are the range of residences available to older adults which offer services or other accommodations to meet their specific needs. They include assisted living, board and care, and accessory apartments.

Function

The last classification presented here considers the general function of community-based services and will be used to describe available resources in the remainder of the chapter. This approach focuses on ways in which services meet the basic needs of older people. Accordingly, community-based services offer

- Something to do (performance areas)
- Someone to care (social and interpersonal context)
- Someplace to live (environmental context)

Service Utilization

Most older adults do not use community-based services even when they are readily available and needed (Black & Mindell, 1996; Krout, 1983; Mitchell, 1995). Older adults prefer help from family, friends, and neighbors (Cantor, 1991; Tennstedt, Harrow, & Crawford, 1996). Assistance from the informal care network, as it is called, usually reflects a history of reciprocity and is easier to arrange, longer-term, free, and based on emotional bonds. In contrast, community-based services from the formal care network tend to be shorter term and require payment. They can seem hard to locate and overly structured and impersonal. In 1984, the National Center for Health Statistics, in studying service utilization by persons age 65 and older found that only 20% used one or more community-based services during the preceding year. However, where recipients are well organized, service utilization tended to be higher. There is evidence that increasingly, older adults are receiving assistance from the combination of formal and informal care networks (Liu, Manton, & Aragon, 2000). In part this may stem from growing awareness of community-based services, particularly among family caregivers, who often facilitate care arrangement and monitoring for elderly relatives.

Community-based service utilization is lower in the United States than in Europe, Canada, or even some Asian countries (Eaton, 2005; Lassey, Lassey, & Jinks, 1997). For example, in comparing patterns of formal and informal help to older adults in the United States and Sweden, Davey et al. (2005) found formal service use was higher in Sweden and informal use was lower. Sweden provides health and long-term care to all citizens based on need. Consequently, 43% of persons over age 80 receive home care, often supplemented by such other community-based services as housekeeping and shopping (Johansson, 1991). Core cultural values differentiate countries generous in publicly supported services for older adults from countries that are not. Sweden, like most other European countries, Canada, and Japan emphasize solidarity, community, equity, and dignity, values missing or deemphasized in the United States (Brown, 2003).

Occupational therapists in many developed countries provide community-based services (Hearle, Prince, & Rees, 2005). In Canada, community-based therapy services are widespread, although a shift to increased assessment and less intervention has been described (Hollis, Madill, Darrah, Warren, & Rivard, 2006). In the United Kingdom, and elsewhere in Europe, the emphasis in community-based occupational therapy intervention is on maintaining both independence and meaningful occupations (Hearle et al., 2005). Community-based occupational therapy can be challenging in unfamiliar environments, particularly in developing countries (Bourke-Taylor & Hudson, 2005). Because most therapists tend to be educated in Western countries, careful identification of local values and beliefs is essential to effective intervention.

Research on the use of services by older adults suggests the importance played by three sets of characteristics (Anderson, 1995; Anderson & Aday, 1978): (1) need characteristics, like self-rated health, number of illnesses, and disabling conditions; (2) predisposing characteristics, such as age, gender, and race or ethnicity; and (3) enabling characteristics, including education, income, and residence with another person.

Although there is some variability among research findings, in general they suggest the following patterns about the use of community-based services by older adults:

1. Need characteristics are most likely to influence use (Coulton & Frost, 1982).
2. Health conditions and physical disabilities are the primary need characteristics that determine whether or not and to what extent services are used (Bass, Looman, & Ehrlich, 1992; Johnson & Wolinsky, 1996).
3. The older the person the greater the likelihood of service use because of increased frailty and impairment (Diwan & Coulton, 1994; Short & Leon, 1990).
4. Women use services more than men, because they are more likely to live longer and be widowed (Stone, Cafferata, & Sangl, 1987).
5. Racial and other minorities receive fewer services than do nonminorities, a subject that will be discussed in more detail later in this chapter (Greene & Monahan, 1984; National Alliance for Caregiving & American Association of Retired Persons, 1997; Norgard & Rodgers, 1997).
6. High- and low-income older adults are more likely to use community-based services than are middle-income older adults—persons with high incomes because they can pay for the services, and persons with low incomes because the services are funded by government sources (Stommel, Collins, & Given, 1994).
7. Older people who live with other persons or have available, willing informal care delay use or are less likely to rely exclusively on community-based services (Deimling, Bass, Townsend, & Noelker, 1989; Horowitz, 1977).
8. Older adults who live in rural areas are less likely to use services than those who live in urban areas for reasons that include differences in help orientations and accessibility of care (Spense, 1992).

Service Barriers

Barriers can exist which inhibit use of specific services or community-based service in general. D.E. Biegel and Farkas (1989) suggest three levels of service barriers: system, agency, and individual. Applied to programs for older adults (D.E. Biegel, Farkas, & Wadsworth, 1992), they can be distinguished in the following manner:

- System-level barriers are political, economic, and social forces that influence policy development, such as the cost of transportation or lack of linkage between formal and informal care.
- Agency-level barriers are structures, staffing, funding, and procedures within organizations that affect service delivery, such as difficulty in recruiting and retaining paraprofessional staff or the complications of having multiple funding sources to support adult day care operations.
- Individual-level barriers are personal attitudes or behaviors toward services, such as the perception of formal assistance as "welfare" and "charity" or discomfort with group recreational activities because of shyness or fear of strangers.

These three levels of barriers provide understanding about why some older adults refuse or fail to use existing community-based services. However, to capture fully the reasons that exist, a fourth conceptual barrier must be added—group-level barriers. Group-level barriers are inhibitors to service use that relate to membership in or identity with a larger social entity. Although there are a wide range of groups that can influence service use, two will be discussed briefly to illustrate the concept: ethnicity and sexual orientation.

Ethnicity

Older adults who are members of ethnic minorities tend to use community-based services less frequently than nonminority elders (Harbert & Ginsberg, 1990; Johnson & Tripp-Reimer, 2001; U.S. Department of Health and Human Services, 1990). For example, Hispanic elders are more likely than Anglo elders to turn to families for support rather than use community-based services (Aguilera, 1992). Despite the growth of this population within the United States, there is evidence that their participation in most Older Americans Act programs has declined. Cited reasons for lack of participation include absence of bilingual or bicultural staff, locating services outside of ethnic communities, and perception by ethnic minorities that they are not welcome in the programs (Hyde & Torres-Gil, 1991; U.S. Administration on Aging, 2000).

Reliance of Hispanic elders on family for assistance reflects a cultural tradition that underscores respect for older adults and obligates family members to collaborate for mutual support. According to one Puerto Rican elder, "The people who brought those children into the world must be loved no matter what they say. The children must respect them, be considerate with them, and love them forever" (Anetzberger, Korbin, & Tomita, 1996, p. 203. In fact, ethnic minority elders who need care are more likely than nonminority elders to receive it from family members. Nearly three in ten Hispanic households provide assistance to chronically ill relatives or friends compared to one in four Anglo households (National Alliance for Caregiving & American Association of Retired Persons, 1997).

Asian American elders also tend to underutilize community-based services. Reasons given include social alienation, culturally inappropriate services, preference for informal care, and Asian values (Lee, 1987; Young, McCormick, & Vitaliano, 2002). Moon and Williams (1993) suggest that norms of shame and face-saving keep many Korean American elders from using services like mental health counseling. More specifically, the problem of mental illness can disgrace families. Therefore, they may attempt to conceal afflicted members from the public by avoiding formal services. Similarly, Korean traditions emphasize family care and respect for elders. This means that acts like elder abuse remain hidden and help is not sought because of the associated stigma (Kim, Kim, Lee, & Kwon, 2003; Levande, Herrick, & Sung, 2000).

The organization of community-based services can create additional barriers for Asian American elders. Agencies may offer services that have no linguistic equivalent. For example, because there are no Korean words for hospice or case management, it is not surprising that when surveyed, Korean elders find these service concepts incomprehensible. Similarly, in Asian culture it is common for clients to give gifts to professionals, like physicians and attorneys, as gestures of reciprocity (Cho, 1998). Refusing the gifts insults the giver. However, accepting gifts violates standards of ethical practice for most American professionals. Finally, programs may fail to take into account the dietary or religious traditions that have been integral to the lives of many Asian American elders. Foods like fried chicken, mashed potatoes, and apple pie are popular at congregate meal sites frequented by elders of European descent; they are not popular among Korean Americans. Moreover, the celebration of Christian holidays like Easter or Christmas at senior centers has little meaning to persons who are Buddhist.

Sexual Orientation

Like ethnic minorities, older gays and lesbians are underserved by traditional community-based agencies (Behney, 1995; Goldschmidt, 1998). Part of the reason rests with perceptions on the part of older gays and lesbians themselves. Having lived through the McCarthy era and possible police harassment in bars and social gatherings, many have a distrust of authority (Almvig, 1982; Kimmel, 1978). Others may be concerned about discrimination from service providers (Connolly, 2002; McFarland & Sanders, 2003). Still others may feel that heterosexual participants at senior centers and congregate meal sites have little understanding of the implications of alternative lifestyles, such as the need for supportive counseling following the death of a beloved partner or close friend and "family member."

Likewise, staff at some agencies are heterosexist, if not sometimes homophobic; that is, they have an irrational fear of gays and lesbians (Hartman & Laird, 1998; Metz, 1997). The origin of this prejudice undoubtedly is complex and may include religious interpretations as well as discomfort with sexuality as a general topic, long a taboo in American culture. The result, however, is set of stereotypes and discriminatory practices which sometimes keep community-based services from being extended to older gays and lesbians (Anetzberger, Ishler, Mostade, & Blair, 2004). Having spent many years in program management, the author of this chapter has personally encountered stereotyping and discriminatory behavior on the part of staff or community contacts. For example, a home care aide refused to provide an older lesbian a bath, because the service seemed "too intimate." A social worker refused to visit the home of an older gay man, because he believed that contracting AIDS was a possibility. A mayor would not allow the municipal office of aging to publicize its senior center as a meeting place for older gays and lesbians out of fear that local citizens would consider the act "too gay-friendly" and not reelect her to public office. Finally, a nursing home administrator surveyed on policies to enable sexual expression by residents, including gays and lesbians, replied, "We don't have that problem here."

It is estimated that there are as many as two million gay and lesbian elders (Cahill, South, & Spade, 2000). Not only are many invisible to community-based service providers, they are invisible within the gay community as well, with its historic emphasis on youth and vitality along with recent practice of openness and "coming out" (Lee, 1989). This invisibility isolates older gays and lesbians, providing them with few options for support anywhere when personal and peer resources erode (Kochman, 1997). Sometimes estranged from relatives and often lacking adult children, traditional sources of informal care further may be lacking, placing older gays and lesbians in a position to manage on their own despite need. To the extent that they are able to succeed under these circumstances probably reflects a lifetime of self-reliance as the primary social option and crisis mastery as the only means for survival (Berger, 1996; Jones & Nystrom, 2002).

Linkage

Most communities have a variety of services for older adults. Moreover, many types of services have multiple providers in any locale. The "catch" is to find those most appropriate based upon need, eligibility, and preference considerations. Several resources exist which help to connect individuals with available services. Outreach by professionals can help elders learn about their options (Figure 19-1).

Each has its own method of linkage and inherent limitations. The mostly common linkage forms are information and referral, case management, outreach, service guides, and educational programs. These linkage forms are described and some of their limitations identified in Table 19-1.

In addition to local linkages, national ones have evolved to accommodate the needs of families living at a distance from elderly members and service providers advocating for older adults about to relocate. Many of these national linkages are accessible through the Internet. For those wishing to speak with a professional, the Eldercare Locator offers access to the information and referral networks of state

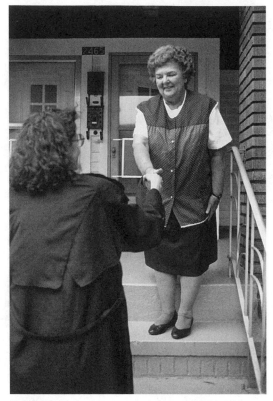

FIGURE 19-1 Outreach by professionals helps older adults learn about available community services. (Courtesy of The Benjamin Rose Institute, Cleveland, Ohio.)

and local area agencies on aging. Available weekdays 9:00 a.m. to 8:00 p.m. by calling 1-800-677-1116, this service is sponsored by the Administration on Aging and administered by the National Association of Area Agencies on Aging and National Association of State Units on Aging.

Something to Do

Martha was sixty-eight years old and widowed three times. When her last husband died of cancer, she vowed never to marry again. Death had not left Martha without financial resources. It did, however, leave her lonely and unoccupied. She had no close friends with whom to talk, eat meals, shop, or take trips. Having reasonably good health and adult children busy with their careers and families, Martha felt anxious to find meaningful activity and human connections at this stage of life.

An array of community-based services has evolved since the mid-1960s providing Martha with numerous opportunities to remain active and to stay connected. Categorically they can be divided by primary function or performance area:

- Working
- Learning

TABLE 19-1 Linkage Forms Connecting Individuals with Services

Form	Description	Arrangement
Information and referral	Resources that link older adults to services and services to each other, usually through telephone contact or internet access	Stand-alone service or as a component of other services offered by an organization like a community center
Case management	Use of human service professional to arrange and monitor a comprehensive package of services	Health or social service agency function or available from a professional social worker or nurse in private practice
Outreach	Actions taken by service providers to reach individual older adults and encourage their use of available services	Community or senior center or office on aging function
Service guides	Lists of available services, often arranged by locale or function	Provided by government agencies, planning organizations, or private entrepreneurs
Educational programs	Lectures, workshops, demonstrations, and fairs highlighting available services	Offered by health and social service organizations, colleges and universities, and the mass media

- Giving
- Experiencing

Each area will be examined briefly with respect to use by older adults, available options, and public policy connections.

Working

Under the federal Age Discrimination in Employment Act (ADEA), persons become "older workers" beginning at age 40. Most adults remain active in the labor force until their early 60s. Workers age 55 and above make up 15.6% of the total labor force in the United States, those age 65 and above 3.2%. Four out of five persons age 55 to 64 and one-fourth of those age 65 to 74 are employed. The rate drops to 9.0% among persons age 75 and older. Men are more likely to be employed than women in each of these age groups (Toossi, 2005). Among ethnic populations, Hispanic men are more likely to work in old age than white men, and black elderly women are more likely to be employed than their white counterparts, often because of a lack of financial security for retirement due to historic employment disparities (Hudson, 2002; U.S. Department of Labor, 2002).

The labor force is aging. The growth rate of workers age 55 and above is projected to be more than four times that of the overall working population between 2004 and 2014. Indeed, those age 55 and above represent the fastest-growing segment of the labor force. In 2000, there were 18 million of these older workers. By 2015 their number is expected to increase to more than 31 million, largely due to the aging of the baby boomers and the trend to delay full retirement. Surveys suggest that eight of ten baby boomers plan to continue working after age 65, at least part time. Since 1987 there has been a 40% increase in the number of persons 65 and over who are working or trying to find a job. In 2015 workers age 55 and above will make up 20% of the labor force, including increasing numbers in managerial and supervisory positions because of their experience and skills (AARP, 1998; Federal Interagency Forum on Aging-Related Statistics, 2004; Grant, 2003; Toossi, 2005; U.S. General Accounting Office, 2001). There are several forces driving elder workers to stay working or to return to work. These include white-collar workers finding little distinction between their avocations and vocations; rise in

defined contribution plans, which serve as an incentive to remaining on the job; broader reach of the ADEA to cover occupations previously not covered, such as academic faculty; and inadequate retirement savings (Grant, 2006).

Thirty-six percent of persons age 60 to 69 and 72% of those age 70 or older who are employed work part time (less than 35 hours weekly). In comparison to younger workers, they are more likely to be self-employed or in sales or service occupations (National Academy on an Aging Society, 2000). Older workers tend to earn less following any job loss or separation ("Older workers are less likely to find jobs comparable to ones lost," 2003). On the other hand, they also enjoy the lowest unemployment rate and have outpaced the rest of the work force in job gains during the 1990s (Quadagno & Hardy, 1996). Older adults work for various reasons, including income to maintain an adequate living standard, enjoyment, and activity to occupy time. In addition, within American culture, to be an adult means to work. Work is a central value and key to self-identity and esteem.

However, among older adults who are not currently in the labor force, only 2% want to be employed. The reasons older adults give for not working are many, including illness, disability, other responsibilities, adequacy of retirement income, desire to spend time with family, or belief that they will be unable to obtain a job (LaRock, 2002; U.S. House Select Committee on Aging, 1992).

Once unemployed, older adults typically have a harder time finding employment than do younger adults. Age discrimination in employment is the major cause, and it is both pervasive and persistent. Harris polls in the 1970s, 1980s, and 1990s indicate that the vast majority of Americans believe that most employers discriminate against older workers in hiring, retention, and promotion practices (U.S. Senate Special Committee on Aging, 1993). In support of this perception is the fact that the third leading type of employment discrimination charge filed with the U.S. Equal Employment Opportunity Commission each year concerns age. In 2004 there were 17,837 such charges filed (U.S. Equal Employment Opportunity Commission, n.d.). Age discrimination complaints also are on the increase, jumping 41% from 1999 to 2002, compared to only a 2% increase for other types of discrimination complaints during the same period (Harris, 2003). Some employers see older workers as "over the hill" and "dead wood." They hold myths about older workers that actually have no basis in reality—for example, that older workers are unproductive, inflexible, frequently absent, or accident prone. Other employers are recognizing that they need older workers as much as increasingly older people want to work (J. Biegel, 2001). As a result, corporate America is beginning to make changes to accommodate an aging workforce. For example, in 2005, 40% of employers allowed staff to work from home, an increase of 20% from 2000, and 75% offered flexible hours, a 17% increase from 1995 (Dychtwald & Kadlec, 2005).

The federal government supports several programs for older adults. The two most important of which are described here:

• Senior Community Services Employment Program (SCSEP): Established as a demonstration project in 1969, SCSEP is authorized under Title V of the Older Americans Act and administered by the U.S. Department of Labor. It is the only federally funded employment program for low-income older persons. Grants are awarded to national organizations, like AARP and the National Caucus and Center on Black Aged, as well as to state and territorial agencies, principally state units on aging. These groups recruit and place older adults in part-time, subsidized minimum-wage community-service jobs in the public and voluntary sectors. Eligible individuals must be at least 55 years of age, unemployed, and with incomes of no more than 125% of poverty level. Priority is given to persons over age 60 and veterans or their spouses. Each year more than 100,000 program participants receive training and over 20,000 are placed with employers. The goal of participation is to move into unsubsidized employment. Almost one quarter of program participants do.

• Age Discrimination in Employment Act (ADEA): ADEA promotes employment based on ability rather than age and protects workers age 40 and above from arbitrary age discrimination in employment. Enacted in 1967 and expanded in subsequent amendments, ADEA covers nearly all workers except for a few occupations, like public safety officers.

Delegates at the 2005 White House Conference on Aging gave priority to public and private initiatives for enhancing employment opportunities in later life. Of 15 top-ranked resolutions, two dealt with efforts to strengthen labor force conditions for older workers by (1) promoting incentives to continue working and improving employment training and retraining programs, and (2) removing barriers to the retention and hiring of older workers, including age discrimination. The private sector also has developed various employment programs to accommodate the needs of older workers. Illustrations of these programs are found in Table 19-2. For greater elaboration on issues of work and retirement, see Chapter 13.

TABLE 19-2 Private Sector Employment Programs for Older Workers

Job modifications	Job sharing, flex time schedules, and reduced work weeks are found at numerous companies, including Borders, Walgreen's, Stouffer Foods, and Polaroid
Job redesign	Xerox allows unionized older workers to bid on lower stress positions with pay adjustments, and Monsanto gives older workers special projects for completion on a flexible schedule so long as they pass on their technical expertise to younger workers in the process
Work training	General Electric offers a technical renewal program to company aerospace engineers to help keep them abreast of the latest scientific advances
Job enhancements	Aerospace Corporation allows senior employees to take unpaid leaves of absence for up to 3 months each year in order to pursue their own interests
Rehiring retirees	Many companies are bringing retirees back as consultants or independent contractors

Learning

A second option for Martha is to return to school. The intent may not be to train for reentry into the labor force. Rather, Martha can pursue adult education for personal growth, to advance a hobby, for socialization, or to learn a skill. People have a capacity to learn throughout their lives (Schaie, 1994). Many older adults want to participate in a learning process and become actively engaged in that process when it is interesting, relevant, and recognizes the experience they bring to the education context.

The concept of **lifelong education** originated in the 1930s and has evolved over the years. By definition, it implies a cradle-to-grave approach to education and recognizes that adults of any age can be learners (Manheimer, Snodgrass, & Moskow-McKenzie, 1995). Federal programs like the National Endowment for the Arts funded demonstration projects at institutions of higher learning as a national goal, but without public funding, in 1976. Since these beginnings, the federal Office of Vocational and Adult Education has helped adults acquire basic literacy skills, and the Administration on Aging has encouraged **area agencies on aging** to collect and disseminate information on local colleges and universities that offer tuition-free education to older adults. Area agencies on aging also sponsor various educational programs for older adults on topics ranging from Medicare prescription drug coverage to advance directives and other legal concerns.

One way to classify the various educational opportunities that exist for older adults is where they are located. Accordingly, there are three primary locations:

- Institutions
- Community
- Home

The options available in each locale will be discussed briefly.

Institutions

The majority of states provide statutory authority for public universities to offer tuition waiver programs for older adults. Requirements vary, but few enroll. In contrast, many older adults attend the educational programs specifically established for them at community colleges. Over one fourth of all community or junior colleges offer such programs, the most popular of which are taught in person, during multiple sessions, in group settings, and without credit (Ventura-Merkel, 1991).

Annually, 170,000 older adults attend Elderhostel. Elderhostel is a nonprofit organization that combines education, travel, and adventure at almost 2000 participating institutions nationwide, usually on college campuses. It is generally regarded as the world's largest educational travel organization for persons age 55 and over. For several hundred dollars, participants enjoy a five- to six-night stay, take noncredit courses, and engage in a number of organized activities. The best part for passionate learners, there are no homework assignments, exams, or grades. Elderhostel also offers international programs in nearly 90 countries. Stays and costs are more than their domestic counterparts.

Community

An increasing number of agencies and organizations in the community offer educational programs aimed at older adults. They include hospitals, senior centers, libraries, civic associations, and religious institutions. Senior centers, for example, routinely offer them in conjunction with congregate meals, often focusing on available community resources and health promotion activities. Some businesses have even become involved in providing education programs. For example, Federated Department Stores and the May Department Stores Company Foundation sponsor OASIS (Older Adult Services and Information), which holds courses in 26 cities and serves 350,000 annually. OASIS was started in 1982 as a public–private partnership providing lifelong learning and service opportunities to adults age 50 and over. Sponsors, often health care organizations or retail establishments, may offer financial support for educational sessions focused on the arts, humanities, wellness, and technology.

Home

Learning experiences at home have grown as a result of computer and communication technology. Once largely confined to bookmobiles and tapes distributed by sight centers, the options have expanded in recent years to include cable television courses, Internet information sharing, and correspondence study. The emergence of home-based learning as an option greatly enhances the ability of impaired older adults to augment their knowledge and skills. It also provides self-directed learners with more avenues to pursue individual study. The website www.lifelonglearning.com lists various online schools, courses, and degrees that may interest older adults.

Giving

Volunteerism would provide Martha with constructive use of her time and the opportunity to contribute her talent in a meaningful way to the community. Twenty-four percent of persons age 65 years and over spend an average of 88 hours per year helping others (Wilhelm, 2004). Some older adults volunteer informally by providing assistance to family and friends. Others do it formally through public or nonprofit organizations. The proportion of older adults among American volunteers has increased in recent decades (Independent Sector, 1998). Currently over 16 million adults age 55 and over volunteer (Wilhelm, 2004). Across the life span, volunteerism increases with age. Although the highest probability of doing volunteer work occurs in middle age, older volunteers invest more hours than do younger ones (Gallagher, 1994).

The motivations to volunteer for older adults differ from those of younger adults. Younger adults tend to volunteer for status, material reward, or career advancement. Older adults volunteer for personal growth, religious belief, or productive use of time (Kovacs & Black, 1999). In addition, the character of volunteerism among older adults varies demographically. Men tend to volunteer for altruistic reasons and women for socialization. Blacks and other racial minorities are more likely than whites to volunteer informally or within religious organizations (Fischer & Schaffer, 1993). Individuals who volunteered earlier in life are more likely to continue at an older age than those who have never had this experience. Finally, persons with higher incomes and education volunteer more than those with less income and education (Peters-Davis, Burant, & Brauschweig, 2001). Volunteerism promotes the well-being of older adults. Various studies show that formal volunteerism improves self-reported health, decreases functional dependency, lowers depression levels, and even improves mortality rates (Adler, 2004; Lum & Lightfoot, 2005; Musick, Herzog, & House, 1999; Van Willigen, 2000). Volunteering in later life also has been shown to provide role identity, give purpose to life, and increase life satisfaction (Greenfield & Marks, 2004; Morrow-Howell, Hinterlong, Rozario, & Tang, 2003).

Volunteer opportunities for older adults are many and diverse, although few charitable organizations have taken advantage of the growing interest in volunteerism among older people (Berkshire, 2005). Those that have offer opportunities that range from serving as docents at museums and zoos to staffing blood banks for the Red Cross to handling the registration line at congregate meal programs. Many volunteer experiences are intergenerational in nature. For example, older adults are found in elementary and secondary schools helping students learn to read or mentoring certain skills. They also provide care to young children and call those who are home alone after school to see how they are doing and offer companionship.

Four of the most important volunteer programs for older adults were established by the federal government in the 1960s and 1970s. Currently, most are administered by the Corporation for National and Community Service's Senior Corps.:

• Retired Senior and Volunteer Program (RSVP): Begun as a demonstration project by the Community Service Society of New York in 1965, RSVP has grown to become the largest federally funded volunteer association in the United States, with more than 750 projects in 50 states deploying nearly one-half million volunteers to 63,000 public and nonprofit community agencies and providing them with 78 million service hours annually. RSVP volunteers serve in a variety of settings without compensation, except on-duty insurance and perhaps program-related expenses. Participation is not restricted by income or minimum time commitment requirements. RSVP sponsors are responsible for developing and managing projects within federal guidelines. The government provides up to 70% of the project's budget; the rest comes from such local sources as individual donations, foundations, and in-kind support.

- Foster Grandparents Program: The purpose of the Foster Grandparents Program is to provide low-income older adults with the opportunity to assist children having special needs. At the same time volunteers receive limited financial compensation and derive social meaning in service of others. Foster Grandparents work 4 hours daily in such settings as day care centers, pediatric departments of hospitals, and homes for children with mental retardation or developmental disabilities. From 21 demonstration projects in 1965 the Foster Grandparents Program has grown to over 340 projects today with about 32,500 volunteers. Collectively they serve 263,600 children annually. Eighty-five percent are 12 years old or younger, and 68% have learning, developmental, or emotional disabilities.
- Senior Companion Program: Established in 1973 and modeled after the Foster Grandparents Program, the Senior Companion Program is based on the concept of low-income older adults helping their frail and impaired counterparts with socialization and other kinds of assistance. In exchange for their efforts, Senior Companions receive a small stipend, some program-related expenses, on-duty insurance, training, and an annual physical examination. There are 227 Senior Companion Program projects. They are found in all states and employ approximately 16,500 volunteers to serve 57,700 clients at 3700 stations annually (Figure 19-2). The typical client is over age 75 with self-care and chronic health disabilities.
- Service Corps of Retired Executives (SCORE): SCORE is a nonprofit association dedicated to entrepreneurial education. It places retired executives in small businesses in order to foster their growth and success. Volunteers range from former company presidents to physicians. Services are provided by more than 10,500 retired executives each year in 389 chapters and 800 branches. These volunteers offer advice, mentoring, counseling, and workshops to approximately 300,000 entrepreneurs annually. SCORE originated in 1964 and is a resource partner with the Small Business Administration. Its services extend from helping those starting businesses for the first time to those whose businesses are failing.

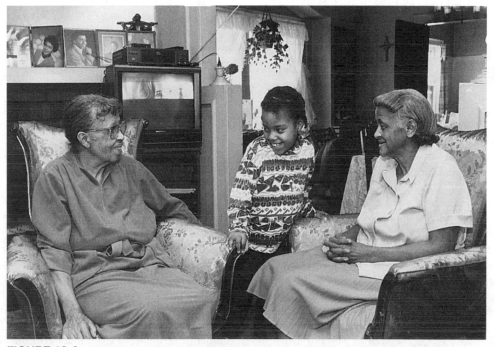

FIGURE 19-2 Senior companions offer friendly visiting and socialization to homebound older adults. (Courtesy of the Benjamin Rose Institute, Cleveland, Ohio.)

Experiencing

Each community offers an array of social and recreational options intended to provide older adults like Martha with interpersonal contact, stimulation, and activity. They include

• Senior centers
• Congregate meal programs
• Adult day services

Community-based services that offer older adults experiences exist for varied reasons. Senior centers serve as community focal points, providing opportunities for older adults to come together for services and programs "which enhance their dignity, support their independence and encourage their involvement in and with the community" (National Institute of Senior Centers, 1978, p. 18). Congregate meal programs offer lunches in group settings in order to improve the nutrition of older adults. At the same time, these programs typically provide nutrition education and information on benefits or other services available locally. Finally, adult day services offer socialization to reduce the isolation of older adults with disabilities along with a variety of services that have health maintenance or restoration as their goal. Moreover, adult day services evolved to address the respite needs of caregivers as much as the dependency of older adults with impairments that limit their ability to self-care.

Senior Centers

The first senior center in the United States was the Williams Hodson Community Center in New York City, established in 1943 by the municipal department of welfare. It was followed in 1947 by the formation of senior centers in San Francisco and Philadelphia with voluntary sector auspices. Although the number of senior centers grew during the 1950s and 1960s, the most significant increase happened during the 1970s with amendments to the Older Americans Act under which senior centers became community focal points and received special consideration in the receipt of funding to support the development and delivery of a range of services. According to the U.S. Administration on Aging (2001), there are about 11,300 centers across the country. Three-fourths of these are considered multipurpose, meaning they represent community facilities for the organization and deliver a broad spectrum of services for older adults.

Older Americans Act funding stagnated beginning in the early 1980s. In addition, some research and certain respected gerontologists began questioning the usefulness of senior centers as a service concept. For example, in a literature review of research on senior centers, Ralston (1987) concluded that the results were mixed. Programs and services at senior centers expanded over a 20-year period. However, few were evaluated for effectiveness. Quality issues frequently arose, as senior centers undertook ambitious programming that reflected the high expectations that policy makers and practitioners had for these organizations.

More older adults (about 15% of the population age 65 and above) avail themselves of senior centers than any other type of community-based service (Gelfand, 1993). However, Atchley (2000) argues that this small percentage hardly suggests senior centers represent community focal points for recreation and education, as delineated in the Older Americans Act. Part of the problem may be access barriers, such as transportation and disability. Part, too, may be the image of senior centers and the changing interests of older people. The National Council on Aging (1995) recognized these issues in its publication *Senior Centers in America: A Blueprint for the Future*. Since then, some states have taken on the challenge of revitalizing their senior centers. In preparation, for example, the Ohio Department of Aging (2002) undertook a comprehensive assessment of the state's more than 325 senior centers and their services. It then identified priorities for providing quality services that would appeal to aging baby boomers, benchmarked against recommendations contained in the *Blueprint*.

Various models for senior centers have been proposed. In general, they distinguish senior centers based upon physical facilities, activities and services location, or participants. A study of senior centers, using a nationally representative sample, found that most senior centers are located in separate buildings, limiting operations because of space problems. Two-thirds are units of other agencies. Less than one-fifth of program funding comes from the federal government; most comes from local government or private sources. The typical center has 100 daily and 1850 annual participants. The largest number of participants are age 65 to 74 and fairly active. Eleven activities and sixteen services usually are offered at a senior center. The most frequent areas of programming relate to education, recreation, health, nutrition, information, and access (Krout, 1994). Other research suggests that in comparison to nonparticipants, senior center participants tend to be older, have lower incomes, are less likely to be employed, and are less likely to own their own homes. They also tend to have more social contacts, enjoy better mental health, experience fewer daily living limitations, and have more links to other services (Calsyn, Burger, & Roades, 1996; Calsyn & Winter, 1999). The personal characteristics of participants also influence the experience and perceived benefits of senior center activities (Turner, 2004).

Recent trends have been identified in program development. For instance, more senior centers are offering home-delivered meals and intergenerational programming (Ohio Department of Aging, 2002; Wacker & Blanding, 1994). However, senior center programming is basically of two types: recreation and education, or services. Recreation and education may include arts, crafts, dance, movies, fitness activities, music, and trips. Services may include counseling, information and referral, employment services, meals, legal assistance, friendly visiting, telephone reassurance, transportation, health screening, and outreach.

Congregate Meals Programs

The impetus for a federally supported meals program grew out a 1956 national study on food consumption and dietary levels among Americans, which showed that six to eight million older adults had deficient diets. To address this problem, demonstration projects were funded to design appropriate delivery of nutrition services in settings that facilitated peer social interaction (Cain, 1977).

What began as 32 pilots has evolved to 4000 congregate meal programs nationwide, supported through Older Americans Act funding (U.S. Administration on Aging, 2003a). The purpose of these programs has been to

provide older Americans, particularly those with low income, low cost, nutritionally sound meals served in strategically located centers ... where they can obtain better social

and rehabilitative services. Besides promoting better health among the older segment of population through improved nutrition, such a program is aimed at reducing the isolation of old age, offering older Americans an opportunity to live their remaining years in dignity. (*Federal Register,* 1972, p. 16845)

By law, Older Americans Act congregate meals programs must provide at least one hot meal five days each week in a group setting. For fiscal year 2006, 385.3 million federal dollars were appropriated for congregate meals, more than for any other program area under the U.S. Administration on Aging. Combined with money for home-delivered meals, 43% of agency funds target the nutrition needs of older adults (U.S. Administration on Aging, 2006). The continued importance of these meals programs lies in the fact that an estimated 1.6 to 2 million older adults report not having enough to eat or enough of the right kinds of food. Nonetheless, many older people in need of nutrition assistance and eligible for publicly supported programs do not participate in them. Reasons include the following: participation compromises independence or is seen as carrying the stigma of charity; awareness of the programs is lacking; and the food is unappealing or unsuited for special diets (U.S. General Accounting Office, 2000). Users of congregate meals tend to have lower incomes, poorer health, and greater isolation than older adults in general. Perhaps not surprisingly, when asked why they participate in these programs, the most common replies relate to obtaining an affordable meal, supplementing their diet, social interaction and stimulation, and community involvement (Wacker, 1992; Wellman & Kamp, 2004). More specifically, a recent study of Older Americans Act Title III service recipients found that the majority of congregate meal users lived alone or were age 75 and above and were poor or near poor. Forty-three percent were at high and 25% moderate nutritional risk. Fifty-eight percent received one-half or more of their daily food intake from the congregate meal, and 11% did not always have enough money or food stamps to buy food (Bauer, 2003).

Adult Day Services

Adult day services are designed for older adults with long-term care needs. They offer an array of health, social, and support services in a protective setting during any portion of the day, but less than 24 hours. The intent of adult day services is to enable chronically ill adults to remain at home by providing services to program participants and respite for their nonworking informal caregivers or surrogate care for their working ones (Nadash, 2003). The concept of adult day services was imported from Great Britain. The first center in the United States opened in 1947 as part of the Menninger Clinic. Growth of adult day services was slow until the 1980s. In 1979 there were only 200 centers nationwide. Today there are over 3500 serving 150,000 daily at an average cost of $56. Seventy-eight percent of centers are non-profit operations, and 74% are affiliated with larger organizations, such as social service agencies or skilled nursing facilities (National Adult Day Services Association, 2006). Most centers are located in urban areas, leaving many rural older adults without adult day services as an option. Partners in Caregiving (2003) estimates that more than 5400 additional centers are needed, including nearly 4000 in urban parts of the country. A variety of adult day services models have been identified:

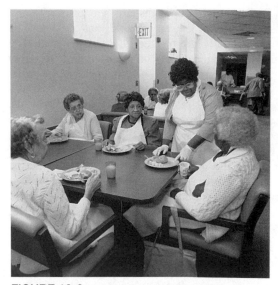

FIGURE 19-3 Adult day services benefit functionally impaired adults through structured programming in a protected setting. (Courtesy of the Benjamin Rose Institute, Cleveland, Ohio.)

- Medical: usually under the auspice of hospitals or nursing homes and emphasizing rehabilitative and health services
- Social: typically affiliated with social service agencies and stressing recreation, nutrition, and functional maintenance
- Special purpose: targeting older adults with specific problems such as dementia or mental illness, and concentrating on disease-specific interventions and participant safety

In surveys of dementia-specific centers, 25% were medical models, 17% social models, and the remaining combined medical and social services (Cox & Reifler, 1994; Reifler, Henry, Sherril, Asbury, & Bodford, 1992).

Adult day services are funded through multiple sources, including Medicaid, Older Americans Act, Social Services Block Grant, United Way, local government, and private dollars. The majority of centers provide the following types of services: activities, exercise, meals, social services, transportation, education, personal care, nursing services, rehabilitative therapy, medication management, and medical care ("Top ADC services, activities are identified," 2001) (Figure 19-3).

Centers generally operate weekdays for eight or more hours daily. They typically serve 25 participants a day using both paid staff and volunteers. In addition to the center director, the most common staff positions are activities director, nurse, aide, driver, and social worker ("Straight from our survey. How do you measure up?," 2001). The typical center user is a 76-year-old female, living with another person (usually an adult child or spouse), and both functionally and cognitively impaired (Reifler, Henry, & Cox, 1995). Consumer satisfaction for adult day services tends to be high from both participants and their caregivers (Baumgarten, Lebel, LaPrise, LeClerc, & Quinn, 2002; Jarrott, Zarit, Parris-Stephens, Townsend, & Greene, 1999). However, adult day services have not been shown to broadly affect health or mental status for participants (Gaugler & Zarit, 2001).

Someone to Care

Ruth was eighty-one years old and had multiple health problems, including a heart condition, emphysema, and arthritis. She took several medications and regularly visited her physician, with transportation and assistance from her nephew, Jim. In spite of efforts to stay well and active, Ruth was less and less able to do routine tasks, and traveling outside the home was becoming a formidable challenge. Ruth's poor health rendered her increasingly homebound, isolated, and depressed. But even more worrisome was the behavior of Jim, her only living relative. Recently unemployed and exhibiting drinking problems, Jim expected financial help from Ruth, something she could not afford to do with less than $800 income each month. At times Jim became insistent, occasionally threatening Ruth, once with a kitchen knife, if she did not give him money. Jim also stole Ruth's credit card, running up about $4000 in debt before the bank became suspicious. In addition, because Jim had taken so much of her money, Ruth had fallen behind in her rent and utility bills. Now faced with eviction from her apartment of 15 years, Ruth was afraid for the future.

A variety of supportive services exist which, simply speaking, suggest that "someone cares" for older adults like Ruth. Collectively these services have three intents: regular contact or emotional support, guidance, and protection. A number of supportive services are identified in Table 19-3. They are described and the primary problems they impact and their typical arrangements are discussed. One service, however, requires separate attention because of its importance in addressing the problem of elder abuse.

Adult Protective Services

Ruth could have benefited from any one of the supportive services described in this section. Friendly visiting would have offered regular contact with volunteers from the local senior center. Telephone reassurance would alert someone to check on her well-being if she failed to answer the prearranged call. An emergency response device would enable Ruth to get immediate assistance in the event of a fall. Financial management would have helped with payment of daily bills and dealing with creditors. Legal services may be able to forestall the eviction. Finally, counseling, especially that offered in the home, might help to alleviate Ruth's emotional problems of anxiety and depression. However, even if all of the above

TABLE 19-3 Supportive Services for Older Adults

Service	Description	Types of Problems Addressed	Arrangements
Friendly visiting	Regular companionship and activity	Homebound person with few social contacts who is lonely	Function of a senior center, office on aging, or religious institution
Telephone reassurance	Prearranged calls to check need for help	Homebound person with chronic health problems and few social contacts who is at risk	Function of a senior center, office on aging, or religious institution
Emergency response systems	Devices to alert response centers that help is needed	Persons with health conditions that may require immediate attention and an inability to obtain it through other means of contact	Monthly fee service of private businesses or health care organizations
Financial management	Assistance with daily money matters, including bill payment	Person who because of physical or cognitive limitations cannot manage household finances	Function of an accounting firm, social service agency, or attorney
Legal services	Consultation or assistance in legal matters	Person requiring advocacy or representation about eligibility in government programs, like Medicare and Social Security, or help with wills, probate, and housing issues	Function of legal services corporation agencies, legal hotlines, or elder law attorneys in private practice
Counseling	Treatment for emotional or addiction problems	Person expressing anxiety or depression due to recent trauma or loss or person with substance abuse problems	Activity of community mental health centers, social services agencies, substance abuse treatment centers, and professionals in private practice

supportive services were offered, Ruth still would need help because of Jim. As a victim of psychological abuse and financial exploitation, Ruth requires adult protective service intervention.

Adult protective services represent a constellation of services and potential use of legal authority to address situations where adults are harmed or at risk of harm (Byers, Hendricks & Wiese, 1993; Collins, 1982). According to the National Adult Protective Services Association, adult protective services are "those services provided to older people and people with disabilities who are in danger of being mistreated or neglected, are unable to protect themselves, and have no one to assist them" (Teaster, Dugar, Mendiondo, & Otto, 2005, p. 9). Begun in the late 1960s, adult protective services are the primary means for preventing and treating elder abuse broadly defined. In every state adult protective services operates through legal mandate, typically requiring public departments of social services or aging to receive and investigate reports of suspicion that adults have been subject to abuse and neglect because of the actions of other persons or themselves (Anonymous, 2002). In addition to report receipt and investigation, adult protective services involves three other activities:

1. **Assessment** of client status and service need
2. Provision and coordination of services to correct the harm or prevent further harm
3. Obtainment of legal intervention, if indicated, in the form of surrogate decision-making authority for mentally incapacitated adults or criminal penalty for the abuse perpetrator (Anetzberger, 2002)

Adult protective services are primarily funded through the Social Services Block Grant (formerly Title XX of the Social Security Act) as well as state and local government funds. Evaluative research has not shown the effectiveness of adult protective services in alleviating elder abuse (Fulmer & Anetzberger, 1995). Indeed, there is widespread frustration with this intervention mode. Part of the frustration may be based upon unrealistic expectations, because adult protective services agencies are unable to select cases and routinely receive those that other agencies cannot handle (Quinn & Tomita, 1997). Part, too, may reflect the increase in elder abuse reporting at a time of dwindling government funding for adult

protective services, leaving those who do this work hard-pressed to even fulfill legal requirements, never mind providing adequate services and follow-up to prevent the reoccurrence of elder abuse (Otto & Bell, 2003). Finally, some elder abuse situations cannot be satisfactorily resolved, because older adults are choosing to live at risk and have the mental capacity and constitutional right to make this decision. For more information about elder abuse and strategies for protecting elders, see Chapter 25.

Someplace to Live

Tom and Mary had lived in their current home for 53 years, enough time to raise three daughters and retire from two jobs. It had served them well. Structurally sound and nestled in an older suburb of a large metropolitan area, the house had readily adapted to their changing needs.

This was no longer the case. During the past year Tom suffered a stroke and Mary fell and broke a hip. Now mobility impaired and needing help with lifting and strenuous tasks, two stories became impossible for Tom and Mary to navigate. Maintaining the large house and yard were a strain, and covering the cost of regular help became difficult in the face of mounting medical bills. In addition, the neighborhood was beginning to change. Nearby friends had moved away or died, and crime became a concern, as several properties converted from owner-occupied to rental. For the first time Tom and Mary thought about leaving. It might be possible to remain in their current residence with some of the accommodations identified in Table 19-4 along with home care and supportive services. However, Tom and Mary preferred moving, especially to a housing arrangement with available services and people with whom to socialize.

Ninety-five percent of older Americans live in community settings: only 5% reside in nursing homes or other institutions. Seventy-seven percent own their own homes, including those of advanced old age (i.e., 67% of those 85 and older) (Pynoos & Golant, 1996). Among older adults in community settings, just 5% live in planned housing of various types, such as those that offer supportive services to residents.

TABLE 19-4 **Creating More Supportive Housing in Later Life**

Name	Description
Home modification	Adaptations made to a residence to accommodate a person's changing physical needs, such as adding grab bars for tubs, lever handles on doors, and ramps at entrances
Home weatherization programs	Assistance available to those who meet income eligibility guidelines to improve energy conservation in a residence by such measures as adding insulation or caulking windows
Home matching services	Programs that link people who have housing space with individuals seeking housing, providing the homeowner with added income, companionship, or help with chores
Homestead exemption	Government programs that offer reductions in property taxes for income-eligible older or disabled homeowners
Utility or energy assistance	Various programs available for low-income persons to manage the costs of heating, cooling, and other utilities through direct assistance, credits, deferred payments, or discounts
Home equity conversion	Reverse mortgages that turn the equity value of a house into a source of income without the need to sell or move, with the loan usually paid to the homeowner in the form of monthly checks to meet expenses or purchase services, and loan repayment with the sale of the house when the owner dies or moves
Home maintenance and repair	Programs that provide such minor repairs and maintenance as replacement of broken windows and new plastering, usually for income-eligible persons in order to keep homes in good condition or to meet established housing codes
Rental assistance	Federal and state programs for income-eligible persons, enabling them to live in privately owned housing and pay an established percentage of their home for rent, with the local housing authority administering the program, paying the difference up to the amount established as fair market value

Of the approximately 22 million households headed by older adults, 80% are owners and 20% are renters (U.S. Administration on Aging, 2003b). Fifty-four percent of noninstitutionalized older adults live with spouses, and 30% reside alone (Federal Interagency Forum on Aging-Related Statistics, 2004). Four in ten older adults have remained in their current home for over 20 years, and eight in ten wish to stay there and never move (AARP, 2003). Older Americans change residence at less than one-half the rate of the rest of the population, and when they move, the vast majority remain in their original county, typically to be near adult children or other family members who play an important role in their lives (Haas & Serow, 2002).

There is a wide range of housing options for Tom and Mary to explore. Indeed, there has been a boom in senior housing in recent years that is unlikely to slow anytime soon. It is propelled by several factors, including growth in households age 75 and older, likelihood of impairments with advancing age, growing acceptance of such housing options as assisted living, shrinkage of available caregivers, and continuing increases in long-term care costs.

The major types of housing options available to older adults are identified and described in Table 19-5. Obviously, not every housing option is appropriate for every older adult. A number of factors must be examined in selecting housing options or living arrangements, including impairment status, financial resources, social needs, personal preferences, and long-range considerations. In addition, because the meaning of "home" is so important and individual, especially to older adults, housing relocation should involve sufficient planning and preparation to help insure a positive transition and subsequent adjustment in the new dwelling.

TABLE 19-5 Housing Options for Older Adults

Name	Description
Single-room occupancy (SRO)	Low-cost lodging typical in inner-city hotels or rooming houses with simple furnishings, no kitchen, and shared bathroom facilities
Public housing	Government-subsidized housing complexes for income-eligible persons, including high-rise apartments and town houses
ECHO housing	Elder cottage housing opportunity—small, free-standing, removable dwelling located near a single-family home, usually to provide independent residence for an elderly parent close to the house of an adult child
Accessory apartment	Independent living quarters within a single-family home that includes a private sleeping area, kitchen, bathroom, and sometimes a separate entrance
Shared housing	A group of unrelated persons residing together, sharing common space, and pooling resources for household maintenance, sometimes with staff support and often under the sponsorship of a voluntary organization or government agency
Congregate living	A private apartment in a planned retirement setting, with limited services and at least one meal daily provided in the rental fee, for persons who need minimal assistance and require no continuous supervision, personal care, or nursing
Board and care	Residences that for a monthly rental fee offer a protected environment, meals, and personal care to unrelated persons who cannot live alone due to physical or mental impairments
Assisted living	Unit within a planned residential setting that provides three daily meals, supervision, personal care, health services, transportation, and social activities for persons requiring regular help but not continuous medical or skilled nursing care
Continuous care retirement community	A planned residential arrangement that provides a range of housing options from independent housing to nursing care as well as various supportive services and recreational programs through long-term contract in one location

Implications for Occupational Therapy

Occupational therapists have an important role to play in community-based care (Scaffa, 2001). As is true in other care sites, the primary emphasis is on sustaining and enhancing function in those performance areas that are most valued by the individual. Among the strategies that can be employed are

1. Performance skills: Provision of education regarding safety and community resources can enhance ability to undertake values roles and to maintain self-care (Painter & Elliott, 2004)
2. Enhanced contexts: Safety evaluations and identification of support services and resources can enhance performance and enable elders to remain in the community if they desire

3. Expanded or sustained quality of life: Assisting elders in the community to identify meaningful occupations can greatly enhance quality of life, as those to which they are accustomed either diminish because of normal life-course events or reduced capacity

In fact, it can be (and has been) argued that the community is the most natural site for occupational therapy interventions because of its focus on performance of everyday occupations (Scaffa, 2001). There are a wide array of available services, but elders are frequently confused by the lack of coordination. Occupational therapists can undertake the kind of comprehensive review of occupational performance that identifies areas of current or potential functional problems and can assist in developing strategies for sustaining performance for the longest possible period.

■ Summary

An aging society has increasing need for services that promote the well-being and self-sufficiency of older adult members. Assistance not provided by family and friends is sought from formal care providers and housing options. A vast array of community-based services has evolved in recent decades to offer older adults something to do, someone to care, and someplace to live. In addition, linkage resources have emerged to connect individuals with services and services with each other.

It has been suggested that the last 30 years represent a period of unprecedented model building and experimentation in service delivery to older adults. Certainly, vast sums of public and private dollars were used to fund this effort, and many scholars or practitioners were willing innovators. Unfortunately, evaluation of the resulting programming has mixed findings. Rarely has there been shown clear direction for future growth. Even more problematic is the fact that the baby boomers have decidedly different interests than their predecessors and are likely to have very different needs in their old age. For example, this generation of older adults participated in senior centers, the next is more likely to prefer spiritual and holistic health centers. This generation has been subjected to intervention by adult protective services when there was likelihood of abuse or neglect; the next is more likely to use legal action to protect their right to privacy and against unwanted intrusion by outside agencies.

In the decades ahead, some community-based services will remain. Those that do will have demonstrated success at meeting essential need and ability to transcend the idiosyncrasies of individual generations. Other community-based services will change and adapt to new generations, and still others will be replaced by more relevant service and housing options.

In this sense, the chapter ends appropriately with a quotation from *The Tibetan Book of Living and Dying,* "I ask myself often: 'Why is that everything changes?' And one answer comes back to me: That is how life is" (Rinpoche, 1992, p.25).

Case Study

Marge is 69-years-old and lives alone in her apartment of many years. She never married. An only child, her parents died more than a decade ago. Until retiring last year, Marge worked as a sales clerk at the local department store. Arthritis had made it difficult to stand long periods of time, and diminished hearing had made it hard to grasp what the customers said. Still, Marge hated to retire. Although she earned little pay, she always enjoyed the work and being around people all day. Now she found herself lonely and depressed, with little useful or interesting to do. In addition, meager Social Security benefits left Marge with barely enough money to cover the rent, food, and other essentials.

Questions

1. What seem to be Marge's concerns?
2. What additional information is required to assess her needs?
3. Which community-based services might be helpful in this situation?

Review Questions

1. What is the continuum of care?
2. What influences the use of service by older adults?
3. Identify four levels of service barriers. What measures can be taken to overcome these barriers?
4. Which community resources are designed to link individuals with available services? Where are the limitations of each?
5. Which federally supported programs provide work and volunteer opportunities for older adults?
6. Illustrate learning options that have evolved for older adults in each of the following locations: institutions, community, and home.
7. Contrast senior centers and adult day services.
8. What is the purpose of adult protective services?
9. List supportive services for older adults that offer regular contact, emotional assistance, or guidance.
10. What changes can older adults make in their current living arrangements to make them more handicap accessible, in better condition, or more affordable?
11. Identify various housing options that exist for older adults. What is their availability and use locally?
12. Describe roles for occupational therapists in providing care in the community.

Web-Based Resources

For helpful information about the experience of community-based services visit:

www.aarp.org, **AARP,** date connected June 4, 2007. AARP has an array of links and information items for consumers and their families. AARP is the largest self-help and advocacy organization for older adults in the United States.

www.aoa.dhhs.gov, **U.S. Administration on Aging,** date connected June 4, 2007. The U.S. Administration on Aging site includes a vast array of information and resources both for professionals and consumers. It provides information about available services, sources of payment, and other critical concerns, as well as numerous links to other sites.

www.eldercare.gov, **Eldercare Locator,** date connected June 4, 2007. A government-sponsored site that provides valuable information for individuals and professionals seeking services.

REFERENCES

AARP. (1998). *America's changing work force: Statistics in brief.* Washington, DC: Author.

AARP. (2003, May). *These four walls ... Americans 45+ talk about home and community.* Washington, DC: Author.

Adler, R. P. (2004, July–August). The volunteer factor. *Aging Today, 5,* 10.

Aguilera, E. (1992). *Meeting the needs of Hispanic elderly: Hispanic service providers' perspectives.* Washington, DC: National Council of La Raza.

Almvig, C. (1982). *The invisible minority: Aging and lesbianism.* New York: Utica College of Syracuse University.

Anderson, R. (1995). Revisiting the behavioral model and access to medical care: Does it matter? *Journal of Health and Social Behavior, 36*(1), 1–10.

Anderson, R., & Aday, L. (1978). Access to medical care in the U.S.: Realized and potential. *Medical Care, 16,* 533–546.

Anetzberger, G. J. (2002). Adult protective services. In D. J. Ekerdt (Ed.), *Encyclopedia of aging.* New York: Macmillan Reference USA.

Anetzberger, G. J., Ishler, K. J., Mostade, J., & Blair, M. (2004). Gray and gay: A community dialogue on the issues and concerns of older gays and lesbians. *Journal of Gay & Lesbian Social Services, 17*(1), 23–45.

Anetzberger, G. J., Korbin, J. E., & Tomita, S. K. (1996). Defining elder mistreatment in four ethnic groups across two generations. *Journal of Cross-Cultural Gerontology, 11,* 187–212.

Anonymous. (2002). Protecting older Americans: A history of federal action on elder abuse, neglect, and exploitation. *Journal of Elder Abuse & Neglect, 14*(2/3), 9–31.

Atchley, R. C. (2000). *Social forces and aging: An introduction to social gerontology* (9th ed.). Belmont, CA: Wadsworth Thomson.

Bass, D. M., Looman, W. J., & Ehrlich, P. (1992). Predicting the volume of health and social services: Integrating cognitive impairment into the modified Anderson framework. *The Gerontologist, 32,* 33–43.

Bauer, C. (2003). *Highlights from the pilot study: First national survey of Older Americans Act Title III service recipients—Paper no. 2.* Retrieved November 11, 2004, from www.gpra.net/surveys/2ndhighlights.pdf.

Baumgarten, M., Lebel, P., LaPrise, H., LeClerc, C., & Quinn, C. (2002). Adult day care for the frail elderly: Outcomes, satisfaction, and cost. *Journal of Aging and Health, 14*(2), 237–259.

Behney, R. (1994, Winter). The aging network's response to gay and lesbian issues. *Outword: Newsletter of the Lesbian and Gay Aging Issues Network,* p. 2.

Behney, R. (1995, September/October). Research: Gauging the aging network's response.*Aging Today,* p. 8.

Berger, R. M. (1996). *Gay and gray: The older homosexual man* (2nd ed.). New York: Harrington Park Press.

Berkshire, J. C. (2005, June 6). Tapping older volunteers. *Chronicle of Philanthropy.* Available at: http://www.philanthropy.com/free/articles/v17/i17/17004201.htm. Accessed April 6, 2008.

Biegel, D. E., & Farkas, K. J. (1989). *Mental health and the elderly: Service delivery issues.* Cleveland, OH: Western Reserve Geriatric Education Center.

Biegel, D. E., Farkas, K. J., & Wadsworth, N. (1992). Social service programs for older adults and their families: Service use and barriers. In P. K. H. Kim (Ed.), *Services to the aging and aged: Public policies and programs* (pp. 141–178). New York: Garland Press.

Biegel, J. (2001, July–August). Business, labor explore growing need for older workers. *Aging Today,* p. 13.

Binstock, R. H. (2005). The contemporary politics of old age policies. In R. B. Hudson (Ed.), *The new politics of old age policy* (pp. 265–293). Baltimore, MD: Johns Hopkins University Press.

Black, J., & Mindell, M. (1996). A model for community-based mental health services for older adults: Innovative social work practice. *Journal of Gerontological Social Work, 26*(3/4), 113–127.

Bourke-Taylor, H., & Hudson, D. (2005). Cultural differences: The experience of establishing an occupational therapy service in a developing community. *Australian Occupational Therapy Journal, 52,* 188–193.

Brown, L. D. (2003). Comparing health systems in four countries: Lessons for the United States. *American Journal of Public Health, 93*(1), 52–56.

Byers, B., Hendricks, J. E., & Wiese, D. (1993). An overview of adult protective services. In B. Byers & J. E. Hendricks (Eds.), *Adult protective services: Research and practice* (pp. 3–31). Springfield, IL: Charles C Thomas.

Cahill, S., South, K., & Spade, J. (2000). *Outing age: Public policy issues affecting gay, lesbian, bisexual, and transgendered elders.* New York: Policy Institute of the National Gay and Lesbian Taskforce.

Cain, L. (1977). Evaluative research and nutrition programs for the elderly. In J. E. O'Brien & G. F. Streib (Eds.) *Evaluative research on social programs for the elderly* (DHEW Publication No. 77-20120). Washington, DC: U.S. Government Printing Office.

Calsyn, R. J., Burger, G. K., & Roades, L. A. (1996). Cross-validation of differences between users and non-users of senior centers. *Journal of Social Service Research, 21*(3), 39–56.

Calsyn, R. J., & Winter, J. P. (1999). Who attends senior centers? *Journal of Social Service Research, 26*(2), 53–69.

Cantor, M. H. (1991). Family and community: Changing roles in an aging society. *The Gerontologist, 31,* 337–346.

Cho, P. J. (1998). Awareness and utilization: A comment. *The Gerontologist, 38,* 317–319.

Cimarolli, V. R., Reinhardt, J. P., & Horowitz, A. (2006). Perceived overprotection: Support gone bad? *Journal of Gerontology: Social Sciences, 61B*(1), 518–523.

Collins, M. (1982). *Improving protective services for older Americans: A national guide series. Social worker role.* Portland, ME: University of Southern Maine.

Connolly, L. (2002). Long-term care issues for LGBT older adults. *Healthcare and Aging, 9*(3), 5.

Coulton, C., & Frost, A. K. (1982). Use of social and health services by the elderly. *Journal of Health and Social Behavior. 23,* 330–339.

Cox, N. J., & Reifler, B. V. (1994). Dementia care and respite services program. *Alzheimer's Disease and Associated Disorders, 8*(3), 113–121.

Davey, A., Femia, E. E., Zarit, S. H., Shea, D. G., Sundstrom, G., Berg, S., et al. (2005). Life on the edge: Patterns of formal and informal help to older adults in the United States and Sweden. *Journal of Gerontology: Social Sciences, 60B*(5), S281–S288.

Day, C. L. (1998). Old age interest groups in the 1990s: Coalition, competition, strategy. In J. S. Steckenrider & T. M. Parrott (Eds.), *New direction in old-age policies* (pp. 131–150). Albany: State University of New York.

Deimling, G. T., Bass, D. M., Townsend, A. L., & Noelker, L. S. (1989). Care-related stress: A comparison of spouse and adult child caregivers in shared and separate households. *Journal of Aging and Health, 1,* 67–82.

Diwan, S., & Coulton, C. (1994). Period effects on the mix of formal and informal home care used by urban elderly. *Journal of Applied Gerontology, 13*(3), 316–330.

Dong, X. (2005). Medical implications of elder abuse and neglect. *Clinics in Geriatric Medicare, 21,* 293–313.

Dychtwald, K., & Kadlec, D. (2005). *The power years.* Hoboken, NJ: John Wiley & Sons.

Eaton, S. C. (2005). Eldercare in the United States: Inadequate, inequitable but not a lost cause. *Feminist Economics, 11*(2), 37–51.

Federal Interagency Forum on Aging-Related Statistics. (2004). *Older Americans 2004: Key indicators of well-being.* Hyattsville, MD: National Center for Health

Statistics. *Federal Register* (1972, August 19). *37*(162), 16845.

Fischer, L. R., & Schaffer, K. B. (1993). *Older volunteers: A guide to research and practice.* Newbury Park, CA: Sage.

Fulmer, T., & Anetzberger, G. J. (1995). *Knowledge about family violence interventions in the field of elder abuse: Background paper for the Committee of the National Research Council and Institute of Medicine.* Unpublished manuscript.

Gallagher, S. K. (1994). Doing their share: Comparing patterns of help given by older and younger adults. *Journal of Marriage and the Family, 56,* 567–580.

Gaugler, J. E., & Zarit, S. H. (2001). The effectiveness of adult day services for disabled older people. *Journal of Aging & Social Policy, 12*(2), 23–47.

Gelfand, D. E. (1993). *The aging network: Programs and services* (4th ed.). New York: Springer.

Goldschmidt, J. (1998). *Policy issues facing GLBT seniors: An overview of the issues.* Washington DC: Policy Institute.

Grant, A. (2003, September 2). Americans working longer or working after retirement. *Plain Dealer,* pp. C1, C3.

Grant, A. (2006, February 8). Work pushing away retirement. *Plain Dealer,* pp. C1, C5.

Greene, V. L., & Monahan, D. (1984). Comparative utilization of community-based long-term care services by Hispanic and Anglo elderly in a case management system. *Journal of Gerontology, 39,* 730–735.

Greenfield, E. A., & Marks, N. F. (2004). Formal volunteering as a protective factor for older adults' psychological well-being. *Journal of Gerontology: Social Sciences, 59B*(5), S258–S264.

Haas III, W. H., & Serow, W. J. (2002). The baby boom, amenity retirement migration and retirement communities: Will the golden age of retirement continue? *Research on Aging, 24*(1), 150–164.

Harbert, A. S., & Ginsberg, L. H. (1990). *Human services for older adults: Concepts and skills* (2nd ed.). Columbia, SC: University of South Carolina Press.

Harris, D. (2003, July–August). Simple justice: The inside story of the biggest age bias in U.S. history. *AARP Magazine,* pp. 64–70.

Hartman, A., & Laird, J. (1998). Moral and ethical issues in working with lesbians and gay men. *Families in Society: The Journal of Contemporary Human Services, 79,* 263–276.

Hearle, P., Prince, J., & Rees, V. (2005). An exploration of the relationship between place of residence, balance of occupation and self-concept in older adults as reflected in life narratives. *Quality in Ageing, 6*(4), 24–33.

Hollis, V., Madill, H., Darrah, J., Warren, S., & Rivard, A. (2006). Canadian therapists' experiences of community-based rehabilitation services. *International Journal of Therapy and Rehabilitation, 13*(1), 7–14.

Horowitz, A. (1977). Social networks and pathways to psychiatric treatment. *Social Forces, 56,* 86–105.

Hudson, R. B. (2002). *People of color and the challenge of retirement security.* Public Policy & Aging Research Brief. Washington, DC: National Academy on an Aging Society.

Hyde, J. C., & Torres-Gil, F. (1991). Ethnic minority elders and the Older Americans Act: How have they fared? *Generations, 15*(3), 57–61.

Independent Sector. (1998). *America's senior volunteers.* Washington, DC: Author.

Jarrott, S. E., Zarit, S. H., Parris-Stephens, M. A., Townsend, A., & Greene, R. (1999). Caregiver satisfaction with adult day service programs. *American Journal of Alzheimer's Disease, 14*(4), 233–244.

Johansson, L. (1991). Elderly care policy, formal and informal care: The Swedish case. *Health Policy, 18*(3), 231–242.

Johnson, R. A., & Tripp-Reimer, T. (2001). Aging, ethnicity, & social support: A review—part 1. *Journal of Gerontological Nursing, 27*(6), 15–21.

Johnson, R. J., & Wolinsky, F. D. (1996). Use of community-based long-term care services by older adults. *Journal of Aging and Health, 8,* 512–537.

Jones, T. C., & Nystrom, N. M. (2002). Looking back...looking forward: Addressing the lives of lesbians 55 and older. *Journal of Women & Aging, 14*(3/4), 59–76.

Kim, K., Kim, H., Lee, M., & Kwon, J. (2003). *Comprehensive study for the elderly welfare policy in Seoul: Survey and policy recommendations.* Seoul Development Institute.

Kimmel, D. C. (1978). Adult development and aging: A gay perspective. *Journal of Social Issues, 34,* 113–130.

Kochman, A. (1997). Gay and lesbian elderly: Historical overview and implications for social work practice. *Journal of Gay & Lesbian Social Services, 6*(1), 1–10.

Kovacs, P. J., & Black, B. (1999). Volunteerism and older adults: Implications for social work practice. *Journal of Gerontological Social Work, 32*(4), 25–39.

Krout, J. (1983). Knowledge and use of services by the elderly: A critical review of the literature. *International Journal of Aging and Human Development, 17,* 153–167.

Krout, J. A. (1994). Changes in senior center participant characteristics during the 1980s. *Journal of Gerontological Social Work, 22*(1/2), 41–60.

LaRock, S. (2002, January–February). Lengthening work-life of boomers may be exaggerated. *Aging Today,* pp. 7–8.

Lassey, M. L., Lassey, W. R., & Jinks, M. J. (1997). *Health care systems around the world: Characteristics, issues, reforms.* Upper Saddle River, NJ: Prentice Hall.

Lee, J. (1987). Asian American elderly: A neglected minority group. *Ethnicity and Gerontological Social Work, 9,* 103–117.

Lee, J. A. (1989). Invisible men: Canada's aging homosexuals. Can they be assimilated into Canada's "liberated" gay communities? *Canadian Journal on Aging, 8*(1), 79–97.

Levande, D. I., Herrick, J. M., & Sung, K. T. (2000). Eldercare in the United States and South Korea: Balancing family and community support. *Journal of Family Issues, 21,* 632–651.

Levine, C., Kuberis, A. N., Gould, D. A., Navaie-Waliser, M., Feldman, P. H., & Dorelan, K. (2000). *A survey of family caregivers in New York City: Findings and implications for the health care system.* New York: United Hospital Fund.

Liu, K., Manton, K. G., & Aragon, C. (2000). Changes in home care use by disabled elderly persons: 1982–1994. *Journal of Gerontology: Social Sciences, 55B*(4), S245–S253.

Lum, T. Y., & Lightfoot, E. (2005). The effects of volunteering on the physical and mental health of older people. *Research on Aging, 27*(1), 31–55.

McFarland, P., & Sanders, S. (2003). A pilot study about the needs of older gays and lesbians: What social workers need to know. *Journal of Gerontological Social Work, 40*(3), 67–80.

Manheimer, R., Snodgrass, D., & Moskow-McKenzie, D. (1995). *Older adult education: A guide to research, programs, and policies.* Westport, CT: Greenwood.

Metz, P. (1997). Staff development for working with lesbian and gay elders. *Journal of Gay & Lesbian Social Services, 6*(1), 35–45.

Miller, C. A. (2004). *Nursing for wellness in older adults: Theory and practice* (4th ed.). Philadelphia: Lippincott Williams & Wilkins.

Mitchell, J. (1995). Service awareness and use among older North Carolinians. *The Journal of Applied Gerontology, 14*(2), 193–209.

Moon, A., & Williams, O. (1993). Perceptions of elder abuse and help-seeking patterns among African American, Caucasian American, and Korean American elderly women. *The Gerontologist, 33,* 386–395.

Morrow-Howell, N., Hinterlong, J., Rozario, P. A., & Tang, F. (2003). Effects of volunteering on the well-being of older adults. *Journal of Gerontology: Social Sciences, 58B*(3), S137–S145.

Musick, M. A., Herzog, A. R., & House, J. S. (1999). Volunteering and mortality among older adults: Findings from a national sample. *Journal of Gerontology: Social Sciences, 54B*(3), S173–S180.

Nadash, P. (2003, August). Adult day centers: Everything you wanted to know but were afraid to ask! *CARING Magazine,* pp. 6–8.

National Academy on an Aging Society. (2000, August). *How financially secure are young retirees and older workers?* Washington, DC: Author.

National Adult Day Services Association. (2006). *Facts and stats.* Retrieved April 6, 2008, from http://www.nadsa.org/adsfacts/default.asp

National Alliance for Caregiving & American Association of Retired Persons. (1997). *Family caregiving in the U.S.: Findings from a national survey.* Washington, DC: American Association of Retired Persons.

National Center for Health Statistics. (1984). *Health interview survey, Supplement on aging, Analysis of long term care data bases.* Unpublished report.

National Council on Aging. (1995). *Senior centers in America: A blueprint for the future.* Washington, DC: Author.

National Council on Aging. (1997, August 20). Centers offering adult services have nearly doubled since 1989 as demand mushrooms (Press release). Washington, DC: Author.

National Institute of Senior Centers. (1978). *Senior center standards: Guidelines for practice.* Washington, DC: National Council on the Aging.

Norgard, T. M., & Rodgers, W. L. (1997). Patterns of in-home care among elderly black and white Americans. *Journals of Gerontology: Social Sciences, 52B,* 93–101.

O'Brien, J. G., Thibault, J. M., Turner, L. C., & Laird-Fick, H. S. (1999). Self-neglect: An overview. *Journal of Elder Abuse & Neglect, 11*(2), 1–19.

Office of Strategic Planning and Health Care Financing Administration. (1999). *A profile of Medicare home health chartbook.* Washington, DC: Health Care Financing Administration.

Ohio Department of Aging. (2002). *Senior centers: Ohio's blueprint for the future.* Columbus: Author.

Older workers are less likely to find jobs comparable to ones lost. (2003, June 9). *Plain Dealer,* pp. E1, E3.

Otto, J., & Bell, J. B. (2003). *Problems facing adult protective services programs and the resources needed to resolve them.* Denver, CO: National Association of Adult Protective Services Administrators.

Painter, J., & Elliott, S. (2004). Meeting community-dwelling older adults' needs through community education programs. *Physical & Occupational Therapy in Geriatrics, 22*(4), 53–66.

Partners in Caregiving. (2003). *The role of adult day service: National trends.* Princeton, NJ: The Robert Wood Johnson Foundation.

Peters-Davis, N. D., Burant, C. J., & Braunschweig, H. M. (2001). Factors associated with volunteer behavior among community dwelling older persons. *Activities, Adaptation, & Aging, 26*(2), 29–44.

Pynoss, J., & Golant, S. (1996). Housing and living arrangements for the elderly. In R. H. Binstock & L. K. George (Eds.), *Handbook of aging and the social sciences* (4th ed., pp. 303–324). San Diego, CA: Academic Press.

Quadagno, J., & Hardy, M. (1996). Work and retirement. In R. H. Binstock & L. K. George (Eds.), *Handbook of aging and the social sciences* (4th ed., pp. 325–345). San Diego: Academic Press.

Quinn, M. J., & Tomita, S. K. (1997). *Elder abuse and neglect: Causes, diagnosis, and intervention strategies* (2nd ed.). New York: Springer.

Ralston, P. A. (1987). Senior center research: Policy from knowledge? In E. F. Borgatta & R. J. V. Montgomery (Eds.), *Critical issues in aging policy: Linking research and values* (pp. 199–234). Newbury Park, CA: Sage.

Reifler, B., Henry, R. S., & Cox, N. (1995). *Adult day services in America.* Wake Forest, NC: Robert Wood Johnson Partners in Caregiving, The Dementia Services Program.

Reifler, B. V., Henry, R. S., Sherrill, K. A., Asbury, C. H., & Bodford, J. S. (1992). A national demonstration program on dementia day centers and respite services: An interim report. *Behavioral Health & Aging, 2,* 199–205.

Rinpoche, S. (1992). *The Tibetan book of living and dying.* San Francisco: Harper.

Scaffa, M. E. (2001). *Occupational therapy in community-based practice settings.* Philadelphia, PA: F.A. Davis.

Schaie, K. W. (1994) The course of adult intellectual development. *American Psychologist, 49*(4), 304–313.

Short, P., & Leon, J. (1990). *Use of home and community services by persons ages 65 and older with functional difficulties.* DHHS Publication No. 90-3466, National Medical Expenditure Research Findings 5. Rockville, MD: Public Health Service.

Spense, S. A. (1992). Use of community-based social services by older rural and urban blacks: An exploratory study. *Human Services in the Rural Environment, 15*(4), 16–19.

Stommel, M., Collins, C. E., & Given, B. A. (1994). The cost of family contributions to the care of persons with dementia. *The Gerontologist, 34,* 199–205.

Stone, R., Cafferata, G., & Sangl, J. (1987). Caregivers of the frail elderly: A national profile. *The Gerontologist, 27,* 616–626.

Straight from our survey: How do you measure up? (2001, June). *Adult Day Services Letter,* pp. 1–3.

Teaster, P. B., Dugar, T. A., Mendiondo, M. S., & Otto, J. M. (2005, September). *The 2004 survey of state adult protective services: Abuse of vulnerable adults of all ages.* Washington, DC: National Center on Elder Abuse.

Tennstedt, S., Harrow, B., & Crawford, S. (1996). Informal care vs. formal services: Changes in patterns of care over time. *Journal of Aging & Social Policy, 7*(3/4), 71–92.

Thompson, L. (2004). *Long-term care: Support for family caregivers* (Issue brief). Washington, DC: Georgetown University, Long-Term Care Financing Project.

Thompson, S. C., & Sobolew-Shubin, A. (1993). Perceptions of overprotection in ill adults. *Journal of Applied Social Psychology, 23,* 85–97.

Toossi, M. (2005). Labor force projections to 2014: Retiring boomers. *Monthly Labor Review, 128*(11), 25–44.

Top ADC services, activities are identified. (2001, October). *Elderly Health Services Letter,* pp. 5–7.

Turner, K. W. (2004). Senior citizens centers: What they offer, who participates, what they gain. *Journal of Gerontological Social Work, 43*(1), 37–47.

U.S. Administration on Aging. (2000, May). *Culturally competent service delivery: An overview.* Washington, DC: Author.

U.S. Administration on Aging. (2001). *Senior centers: fact sheet.* Washington, DC: Author.

U.S. Administration on Aging. (2003a, August 27). *Elderly nutrition program: Fact sheet.* Washington, DC: Author.

U.S. Administration on Aging. (2003b). *A profile of older Americans: 2003.* Washington, DC: Author.

U.S. Administration on Aging. (2006). *Budget.* Retrieved February 13, 2006, from www.aoa.gov/ABOUT/legbudg/current_budg/docs/FY_2007_Presidents_Budget.pdf.

U.S. Department of Health and Human Services. (1990). *National health interview survey, longitudinal study of aging, 70 years and over, 1984–1989.* Hyattsville, MD: U.S. Department of Health and Human Services, National Center for Health Statistics.

U.S. Department of Labor, Bureau of Labor Statistics. (2002, January). *Employment and earnings.* Washington, DC: U.S. Government Printing Office.

U.S. Equal Employment Opportunity Commission. (n.d.). *Types of complaints: Age.* Retrieved February 7, 2006, from www.eeoc.gov/types/age.html.

U.S. General Accounting Office. (2000). *Food assistance: Options for improving nutrition for older Americans* (Publication No. RCED-00-238). Washington, DC: Author.

U.S. General Accounting Office. (2001). *Older workers: Demographic trends pose challenges for employers and workers.* Washington, DC: Author.

U.S. House Select Committee on Aging. (1992). *Older workers in the labor market* (Committee Publication No. 102–839). Washington, DC: U.S. Government Printing Office.

U.S. Senate Special Committee on Aging. (1993). *Developments in aging, 1992,* Vol. 1. Washington, DC: U.S. Government Printing Office.

Van Willigen, M. (2000). Differential benefits of volunteering across the life course. *Journal of Gerontology: Social Sciences, 55B*(5), S308–S318.

Velgouse, L. (2000). *The Olmstead decision: Responses and impact* (An AAHSA technical assistance brief). Washington, DC: American Association of Homes and Services for the Aging.

Ventura-Merkel, C. (1991). Community colleges in an aging society. In W. A. Heil & L. N. Marks (Eds.) *Resourceful aging: Today and tomorrow* (Vol. 5, pp. 47–51). Washington, DC: American Association of Retired Persons.

Wacker, R. R. (1992). *What do you think? An evaluation of the Weld County senior nutrition program.* Greeley, CO: University of Northern Colorado.

Wacker, R. R., & Blanding, C. (1994). *Comprehensive leisure and aging study: Final report.* Washington, DC: National Recreation and Park Association.

Wagnild, G. (2001). Growing old at home. *Journal of Housing for the Elderly, 14*(1/2), 71–84.

Wellman, N. S., & Kamp, B. (2004). Federal food and nutrition assistance programs for older people. *Generations, 28*(3), 78–85.

Wilhelm, I. (2004, January 8). Stepping up to serve charity: Number of Americans who volunteer is on rise. *Chronicle of Philanthropy,* pp. 43–44.

Young, H. M., McCormick, W. M., & Vitaliano, P. P. (2002). Attitudes toward community-based service among Japanese American families. *The Gerontologist, 42,* 814–825.

CHAPTER 20

Home Health Care

Ben J. Atchison

*I*t *is no longer necessary to speak of the value of occupational*
therapy and try to prove what it can do and
what it has done in the home; we have
seen this and we know its value.

E. Collins, Archives of Occupational
Therapy, 1921, p. 3.

OBJECTIVES

By the end of this chapter, readers will be able to:

1. Describe the events that led to the rapid growth in home-health-care utilization.
2. List the home-health-care services provided for Medicare beneficiaries.
3. List the criteria used by Medicare to determine eligibility for home-health-care services.
4. List the most common diagnostic groups treated in home health care.
5. List the core competencies required to practice in the home-health-care setting and give examples of each.
6. Describe the efforts by the Centers for Medicare and Medicaid Services to develop quality outcome measures in home-health-care services.
7. Describe the OASIS data set and how it is used in home health care to identify outcomes of intervention.

Health care providers, including occupational therapists, have long extolled the benefits of providing home-based therapy. As early as 1925, Sullivan described the positive effects of occupational therapy in her account of a case involving a 35-year-old man with polio (Sullivan, 1925). This patient, a person who had supported himself and his family by begging, was referred to occupational therapy so he could be provided with meaningful activity and skill training. In a home-based program, she taught this client the art of chair caning, a skill that enabled him to make chairs that he sold to retailers in his community (Jackson, 1992). Other accounts published in the early occupational therapy literature recognized the value of providing care in the home (Collins, 1921; Strange, 1926; Sullivan, 1925). Belief in the value of home-based care is now well established in many rehabilitation professions.

In its early history, development of self-employability for homebound clients was often the focus of occupational therapy intervention. Today, the emphasis of the services provided by occupational therapists is to promote engagement and participation in all areas of occupational performance and ultimately to decrease the need for continuous care—a paradigm that is also driven by health care economics.

History of Home Health Care

Although this chapter is focused on home health care services for older adults in the United States, it is valuable to recognize that there are many efforts around the globe, some of them predating those in the United States, and some that are much more extensive and encompassing. In Sweden, Denmark, the Netherlands, and Great Britain, long-term care systems include home-based care designed to optimize quality of care, ensure more efficient delivery of services, and control or lower costs. Initiatives in these countries have aimed to develop care management techniques to better target appropriate services to each elderly client and have provided incentives for different types of care providers to coordinate their work, resulting in improved service delivery and greater client satisfaction. In addition, their policies have discouraged the building of additional nursing homes and instead supported the development and expansion of a range of housing alternatives for the older adult population.

Unlike the United States, greater responsibility is placed on local governments in Europe for delivering long-term care services, bringing those services closer to those who need them (Coleman, 1995). This is similar to Canada, where there is no centralized agency to regulate home health care. In fact, some provinces do not require a physician's referral. Each locality is responsible for providing its older adults with home-based care. In Australia, varied programs provide home-based health care including the Home and Community Care Program that provides traditional domestic and personal care services, the Extended Aged Care Package that includes services for people who need a higher level of care, and the Community Aged Care Packages that include those who need a high level of community and home care.

In 1995, following a study of long-term care services (including home care) in Germany, Sweden, and Holland, Poland reformed its health care system to include multilevel systems that included creation of agencies that provide care in the home (May, Onarcan, Olechowski, & Myron, 2004). In Japan, all citizens 40 years and older with an income must pay long-term care insurance (LTCI) premiums, and those who are identified as having a disability are eligible to receive these benefits with no restrictions based on income or family situation. The program covers 90% of the cost of institutional or community-based care. The idea of long-term care provided by the government is a significant variation from traditional family-based care as it moves toward the socialization of care of the elderly, and the integration of medical care and welfare services. In fact, there is criticism in Japan that this system totally neglects the family situation. It is therefore important to assess the new system to determine whether the family caregiving situation still has an impact on service use (Nanako, Kazue, & Eiji, 2002).

In the United States, employment of occupational and other therapists in the home-health-care industry was slow to develop. From the early 1880s to the mid 1960s, voluntary organizations such as the Visiting Nurses Association and governmental agencies (e.g., public health nurses) were focused on the delivery of home-based nursing services to indigent populations (Youngstrom, 1997). In 1965, the enactment of the Medicare Acts (Title XVIII of the Social Security Act) and Medicaid (Title XIX of the Social Security Act), resulted in the inclusion of home-health-care services as part of the overall health care program for older adult and indigent populations (Levit, 1996). This legislation resulted in a rapid growth of home-care utilization with the total number of agencies providing home health expanding from 1100 in 1963 to approximately 8100 Medicare-certified agencies in 2005, serving approximately 2.4 million persons across the United States. Medicare funds an estimated 85% to 90% of the total cost of home health agency services amounting to a total of $8,700,000,000 (Moyle, 2005, p. 1).

Services Provided by Home-Health-Care Agencies

Home health care is a benefit covered under Part A of Medicare and is intended to provide intermittent, medically necessary care that is considered "skilled." Nursing, physical therapy, occupational therapy, and speech-language therapy are included in the category of "skilled" services. Services must be ordered by a physician and may include part-time assistance with personal care provided by a certified nursing assistant (CNA). In order to receive in-home services, the person must meet criteria for **homebound status.** Homebound status is defined as being unable to leave one's home unassisted. To be homebound means that leaving home takes considerable and taxing effort. However, this does not exclude participation in short, nonmedical outings to a hairdresser or religious services (Moyle, 2005, p. 2). Additionally, attending an adult day care program does not negate homebound status. This is a recent compromise in the strict definition that resulted from a demonstration project initiated by the Centers for Medicare and Medicaid Services (CMS). That program provides an opportunity for home health agencies to partner with medical adult day care facilities to provide medical adult day care services to Medicare beneficiaries as a substitute for a portion of home health services that would otherwise be provided in the home (Kinsella, 2005). The rationale for this change is that adult day treatment can enhance quality of life, reducing health consequences of depression that might increase health care costs. Medicare is testing, with a very small test group, a program where selected home health agencies can provide adult day health care instead of home health services. If successful, the program will offer a new dimension in Medicare home care (*Medical News Today,* 2005). In addition, under the new definition, Medicare will allow and pay for home visits from doctors who specialize in homebound elderly patients. Limited office visits are also allowed under the new definition. More recently, Medicare is paying for home telehealth visits through a home telehealth computer workstation. Telehealth is being used with some success to provide home care in rural areas where it would be difficult to arrange the personal visit from a home-health-care agency (Kinsella, 2005).

Of reimbursable services, the most frequently utilized professional discipline in home health is nursing, which serves as gatekeeper for the provision of other services. The second most often utilized service is physical therapy, followed by social work services, occupational therapy, and speech-language services (U.S. Census Bureau, 2006). The discrepancy between the number of physical therapy visits and occupational therapy (double the amount) is of concern and suggests a lack of awareness and understanding by nurses about the services provided. Because nurses typically seek physician approval for services, it is essential that there be a clear understanding of the value of all services to ensure that all appropriate and necessary care is provided. It should also be noted here that home health aides provide many essential home health services, particularly those focused on immediate care (for example, help with bathing or with light housekeeping tasks), while the individual gains strength and skill through therapeutic interventions.

Home Care Patient Population

The majority of people receiving home-health-care services are Medicare beneficiaries, with a very small number being under the age of 65. Seventy-three percent (73%) are over the age of 75, most (68%) are women, and 76% are Caucasian. The most common health disorders requiring home health intervention, in order of frequency, are as follows (U.S. Census Bureau, 2006):

- Cardiovascular 34%
- Injuries and poisoning 17%
- Musculoskeletal and connective tissue 16%
- Respiratory diseases 12%
- Endocrine, nutritional metabolic, and immune disorders 12%
- Cancers and tumors 8%
- Nervous system and sensory 2%

Ninety-four percent of home care recipients live in a private or semiprivate residence. The vast majority of adults in the United States who receive long-term care at home get all their care from unpaid family and friends, mostly wives and adult daughters. It is estimated that 75% of older adults who receive home care depend on family members or other unpaid help for assistance (Thompson, 2004). There are 22 million households with at least one member who provides unpaid assistance to a person older than 50 years of age living in that home (National Alliance for Caregiving, 2004). The number of unpaid, informal caregivers is much larger when care is provided for an elder not co-residing is taken into account. Given these data, it is critical that the rehabilitation program plans be both client and family centered. Recognition of potential caregiver burnout as well as overall safety issues for the client must be standard elements of the team plan of care. The concept of "caring for the caregiver" has been given increasing attention in home care. Opacich (1997) calls for occupational therapists to be cautious about placing excessive burden on family members and suggests that realistic expectations, plans, and supports be provided for patients and caregivers.

Payment for Home-Health-Care Services

Approximately 90% of all formal or paid home health agency care is paid for by Medicare or Medicaid if eligibility criteria are met (Moyle, 2005, p. 7). Prior to 1997, home care agencies could bill for services provided for each episode of service, through a **retrospective payment system.** This changed dramatically with the passage of The Balanced Budget Act (BBA) of 1997, which mandated a prospective payment system (PPS) for Medicare home health services.

Under **prospective payment,** Medicare pays home health agencies (HHAs) a predesignated base payment that varies with the health condition and care needs of the beneficiary. Additionally, there is consideration of the geographic differences in wages for agencies across the country. These considerations for the health condition and service needs of the beneficiary contribute to the **case-mix adjustment** (CMS, 2006b). The home health PPS will provide agencies with payments for each 60-day **episode of care** for each beneficiary. Episode of care is the label given by Medicare to a unit of time for which services are authorized when a request for payment is made. If a beneficiary is still eligible for care after the end of the first episode, a second episode can begin. At the time of this publication, there are no limits to the number of episodes a beneficiary can receive as long as he or she continues to meet eligibility requirements. Payment for each episode is adjusted to reflect the beneficiary's health condition and needs, and a special outlier provision exists to ensure appropriate payment for those beneficiaries who have the most expensive care needs.

The Prospective Payment System (PPS)

Discussed below are the six major features of the PPS system that must be understood by any professional who is employed by a HHA, as each one has direct implications for how one practices in this environment (CMS, 2006b).

Payment for the 60-Day Episode

Each beneficiary who is eligible for home care services is certified for a 60-day episode of care. HHAs receive 50% of the estimated base payment for the full 60 days when the initial claim for services is received by Medicare. As previously described, this estimate is based upon the patient's condition and care needs, referred to as the case-mix assignment. At the end of the 60-day certification period (or at discharge), after the physician signs all subsequent supplemental orders, the agency will submit a detailed bill to the intermediary that lists all of the services provided (by visit, in 15-minute increments). On receipt of this end-of-episode bill, the intermediary will pay the agency the other half of the Home Health Resource Group (HHRG) payment (CMS, 2006b; Siebert, 2000).

If, at the end of this episode of care, a person continues to have need for services and is eligible, another 60-day episode can be initiated. The average length of service provided is 41.5 days. Often, a person continues to need supervision or care after Medicare has determined that services are no longer medically necessary. At that point, some other source of payment, perhaps through private pay, will be required (Moyle, 2005). It is worth noting that in families that have the resources to do so, private payment may well be forthcoming. Clearly, this raises ethical concerns about those individuals who cannot afford to pay.

Case-Mix Adjustment

Following a physician order or prescription or a home health plan of care, the HHA conducts an initial evaluation visit to assess the patient's condition and determine the need for skilled nursing care, rehabilitation services, medical social services, and home health aide services. The assessment must be done for each individual episode of care. Only a nurse, physical therapist, or speech-language therapist can open a case or conduct this initial assessment. Even though occupational therapists cannot conduct this assessment, they may provide stand-alone service once a case is opened.

The instrument used for the initial assessment required by Medicare since July of 1999 is known as the Outcome and Assessment Information Set (OASIS). OASIS was developed by the Center for Health Services Research (CHSR) at the University of Colorado specifically for the home health setting. CMS funded the research program (which was co-funded by the Robert Wood Johnson Foundation) to develop a system of outcome measures for home health care. OASIS was developed and refined over a 10-year period of clinical and empirical research.

The OASIS items encompass sociodemographic, environmental, support system, health status, and functional status factors as well as the need for rehabilitative services (physical, speech-language pathology, or occupational therapy) and are used to determine the case-mix adjustment to the standard payment rate. Eighty case-mix groups, or Home Health Resource Groups (HHRG), are derived from these items which result in patient classification. Each HHRG includes three dimensions: the clinical dimension (continuing medical problems), the functional status dimension (ability to care for personal needs), and the services utilization dimension, which includes the projected need for therapy. These items determine the HHRG that will be submitted to Medicare, along with the home health plan of care and certification of eligibility signed by the physician.

Outlier Payments—Paying More for the Care of the Costliest Beneficiaries

Additional payments are made to the 60-day case-mix adjusted episode payments for beneficiaries who incur unusually large costs. These outlier payments are made for the 60-day episode in which the cost is more than the amount allotted for the case-mix group. Outlier costs are calculated for each episode by applying standard per-visit amounts to the number of visits by discipline (skilled nursing visits, or physical, speech-language pathology, occupational therapy, or home health aide services) reported, and coverage is based on OASIS data that recognize an unusually complex case.

Adjustment for Beneficiaries Whose Condition Only Requires a Few Days of Care During the 60-Day Episode

Medicare provides a low-utilization payment adjustment for beneficiaries whose episodes consist of four or fewer visits. These episodes will be paid the standardized, service-specific per-visit amount multiplied by the number of visits actually provided during the episode. Savings from reduced episode payments are redistributed to all episodes paid under the PPS so that if a plan required more visits than initially determined, a payment adjustment is made.

Adjustments for Significant Changes in a Condition

When a beneficiary experiences a significant change in condition during the 60-day episode that is not envisioned in the original physician's plan of care and original case-mix assignment, a significant change in condition (SCIC) adjustment can occur. A SCIC adjustment requires that a new payment amount be determined. The SCIC payment adjustment occurs within a given 60-day episode.

Adjustments Made When the Beneficiary Changes a HHA

If the beneficiary wishes to transfer to another HHA or if he or she is discharged and readmitted to the same HHA during the 60-day episode of care, there is a partial episode payment (PEP) adjustment and a new episode clock is initiated. The PEP will provide a simplified approach to the episode definition that takes into account key intervening health events in a patient's care. The PEP allows the 60-day episode clock to end and a new clock to begin if a beneficiary transfers to another HHA or is discharged but returns because of a decline in his or her condition to the same HHA within the 60-day episode. When a new 60-day episode begins, a new plan of care and a new assessment are necessary. As can be seen in this discussion, payment regulations are complex. Therapists must be aware of the rules, though, so that their intervention will be covered. It is important to be aware, too, that the regulations change frequently, meaning that home health therapists must expect to keep up. One reason for both the complexity and the change is an effort to control costs.

Strategies to Create Evidence-Based Practice in Home Health Care

The continuing escalation of health care costs has resulted in a mandate by all third-party reimbursement agents, particularly the federal government, to install systems of accountability for all health care providers, including home health agencies. A recent survey of medical and health care literature documents that home care is more cost-effective than institutional care. Studies published in the *Journal of the American Geriatrics Society, Health Care Financing Review,* and other journals illustrate the value of home care. For example, one study demonstrated that home intervention can minimize fall risk and improve life quality for elders, and that these improvements are sustained over time (Gitlin et al., 2006). In June of 2005, the American Association for Homecare called on Congress to consider these studies and others and to support policy that emphasizes greater use of home care. U.S. Department of Health and Human Services Secretary Michael Leavitt has described home-based care "radically more efficient" for Medicaid recipients, and the studies that are emerging do support that this principle is the same for Medicare.

The CMS principal quality improvement priority for the home health setting is to reduce avoidable acute care hospitalizations. To that end, CMS has identified key strategies to provide quality outcomes in home health care. Thus far, these strategies have been effective in establishing clear goals for home health agencies so that optimal outcome-based services can be provided for the home-health-care client and family.

Measure and Report Performance

CMS seeks to identify opportunities for improvement and track progress. This is being accomplished by measures of clinical outcomes derived from the OASIS data that help identify best practices, and patient and staff evaluations. The creation of comparative outcome data reports seeks to improve agency performance by way of public reports of quality, pay for performance, and health care organization accreditation. The specific quality measures that are listed on the public website include measures of improvement in getting around, patients' self-care abilities, reduced shortness of breath, patient medical emergencies, and long-term outcomes. Box 20-1 shows the specific factors included.

This information allows a consumer (including referral sources) to determine the quality of a home-health-care agency and thus motivates the agency to acquire the best ratings possible. Table 20-1 provides a sample of three of these measures in terms of the method of measure and the clinical significance as developed by CMS (2006a).

Adopt Health Information Technology

For both accuracy and efficiency, CMS has promoted the use of technology systems to generate measures of reporting outcomes. The

---

BOX 20-1 Quality Measures in Home Health

Improvement in getting around:
- Percentage of patients who get better at walking or moving around
- Percentage of patients who get better at getting in and out of bed
- Percentage of patients who have less pain when moving around

Patient's activities of daily living:
- Percentage of patients whose bladder control improves
- Percentage of patients who get better at bathing
- Percentage of patients who get better at taking their medicines correctly (by mouth)

- Percentage of patients who are short of breath less often

Long-term outcomes
- Percentage of patients who stay at home after an episode of home health care ends

Patient medical emergencies:
- Percentage of patients who had to be admitted to the hospital
- Percentage of patients who need urgent, unplanned medical care

TABLE 20-1 Sample Outcomes Publicly Reported from the OASIS Data Sets

OASIS Measure	Description of Measure	Clinical Significance
Improvement in bathing	Percentage of patients who get better at bathing	Being able to stay clean and healthy and to remain independent at home
Improvement in transfers	Percentage of patients who get better at getting in and out of bed	Being able to get in and out of bed is necessary before a person can do many things for himself or herself, like getting dressed or getting to the toilet, and to remain independent at home
Improvement in ambulation/ locomotion	Percentage of patients who get better at walking and moving around in a wheelchair safely	Many patients who get home care are recovering from an injury or illness and may need help from a person or equipment; getting better at walking or moving around in a wheelchair may be a sign of improvement

implementation of electronic health record systems combined with electronic physician prescription and orders will enable home health agencies to procure the necessary physician approval without an inordinate amount of extra paperwork and time typically required.

Redesign Care Processes

CMS emphasizes person-centered care that is safe and efficient with a fundamental design that addresses the quality outcomes emphasized in Table 20-1. Agencies are expected to provide proven tools and processes using a systematic flow-based design for care management, patient self-management, and scheduling.

Transform Organizational Culture

Senior leadership engage staff to support quality improvement goals and to provide resources for achievement. These strategies focus on empowering leaders and staff to identify quality issues, make changes to improve processes, and assess performance. Creating a person-centered work environment with management support for open communication and teamwork may facilitate improvement in care.

To support this work, CMS has funded Quality Improvement Organizations (QIOs) in every state, territory, and the District of Columbia to work directly with HHAs and other providers to improve care for Medicare beneficiaries. QIOs educate and support home health agencies in adopting more effective, person-centered processes, designing efficient systems, and

implementing organizational cultures of quality. These strategies are designed to accelerate the rate of quality improvement and result in improved patient outcomes for Medicare beneficiaries who receive home-health-care services (CMS, 2006a).

Occupational Therapy in Home Health Care

Occupational therapy is a qualifying service listed by Medicare. In this chapter thus far, the essential policies regarding beneficiary eligibility status and payment requirements have been briefly presented. Understandably, most professionals prefer to leave policy details to administrators and policy analysts. However, it is obvious that these policies have a direct impact on the delivery of services, occupational therapy among them, including the essential components that Medicare has mandated as part of plans of care. Prior to the prospective payment system and the advent of the OASIS documentation system, when activities of daily living (ADL) or instrumental activities of daily living (IADL) problems were identified, the home health aide typically addressed these concerns. There was not an emphasis on client participation in care, but rather on doing *for* the person or on the *delivery* of care (Siebert, 2000).

With the initiation of Outcome and Outcome-Based Quality Improvement (OBQI) reports, generated by the analysis of data from the OASIS, home health agencies are sharply focused on outcomes of care as measured by client factors and have developed plans to identify and implement methods to achieve not so much an effective process of care, but more a definitive product of care. There are 41 outcome measures currently calculated from OASIS data, and 10 outcomes have been identified as being Medicare priorities in the Home Health Setting published by the CMS. Of these outcomes, most have direct implications for the occupational therapist because they focus on client performance (Siebert, 2005). There is a clear link between these outcomes and the potential impact that occupational therapy has on facilitating each one. It is a challenge as well as an opportunity for occupational therapists to be active team players in enabling the patient to achieve these outcomes, while simultaneously documenting the value of home health agencies for individuals and for society.

Occupational therapy's emphasis on performance is now embraced in agency-wide care practices as a result of the emphasis placed by CMS on functional outcomes. Siebert (2005) states that "assessment and intervention strategies that are routine to occupational therapists are strategies that can contribute to agency-wide care practices that enhance client outcomes" (p. 3). She also suggests that occupational therapy practitioners can play an active role in facilitating best-care practices by being involved as a member of the OBQI team. Occupational therapy practitioners also may become involved in training staff to implement practices derived from occupational therapy strategies. Siebert also notes that "many practices that are routine to occupational therapy practitioners (and may even be considered "common sense") are actually valuable contributions to the toolbox of best care practices that agencies are beginning to develop" (p. 3).

One example of this is the development of fall prevention programs. Occupational therapists play an instrumental role in creating effective team-oriented educational programs to prevent in-home falls among the elderly (Gitlin et al., 2006). A meta-analysis conducted by Steultjens et al. (2004) to determine the effectiveness of home care services provided by occupational therapy in the Netherlands indicated that prescription of assistive devices and safety instruction as part of a home hazards assessment increased functional ability and decreased the incidence of falls. Other reports support the effectiveness of the inclusion of occupational therapy as part of a multidisciplinary theme in the prevention of in-home falls (Gitlin et al., 2006; Hornbrook et al., 1994; Toto, 2006; Weinstein & Booth, 2006).

Core Competencies of Occupational Therapy Practice in Home Health Care

The practitioner who works in home health care requires a variety of critical thinking, interpersonal, and clinical and technical competencies. In a series of interviews with expert occupational therapist practitioners in home health care, several core competencies were identified (Atchison, 2003) (Box 20-2). Although this research focused on the perceptions of expert occupational therapists, the findings are also relevant to physical therapists and speech pathologists. A discussion of the meaning of each of these themes follows.

Cultural Competence

One of the most enriching aspects of home health care is the opportunity to become immersed in the contextual aspects of the client's occupational performance. The cultural aspect of the home is one of the most significant themes that expert practitioners have identified as unique and powerful in home care. Cultural competence has also been identified by the Joint Commission on Accreditation of Health Care Organizations (JCAHO) as a critical standard of care. To achieve cultural competence, the first step is to recognize that cultural sensitivity and a belief in ethnorelativism is an essential aspect

---

BOX 20-2 Core Competencies

- Cultural competence
- Creating advocacy: discovering and using resources
- Context sensitivity
- Ethical practice
- Situation analysis
- Conflict management
- Flexibility

of "best practice." **Ethnorelativism** is the belief that all cultures are equally valid and deserving of respect (Tripp-Reimer, 1985). Every client and family has values, beliefs, and rituals that must be considered when planning and providing care. A suggested cultural assessment checklist is described later in this chapter in the section on assessment (Lipson, 1985 as found in Narayan, 1997).

Developing cultural competence can be both a challenge and an enriching experience. The therapist enters the home of a client and begins to learn about the beliefs, values, customs, and attitudes of that person. With repeated experiences of encountering the cultural space of others and then reflecting on those experiences, the therapist becomes more aware of his or her own cultural assumptions (McGruder, 1998). To become culturally sensitive, a person needs to be aware of his or her own values and be willing to explore the values of others in a nonjudgmental way. Bonder, Martin, and Miracle (2001) suggest use of an inquiry-based approach to cultural competence that makes use of ethnographic strategies including respectful questioning to secure necessary information about culturally relevant factors in assessment and intervention.

Creating Advocacy: Discovering and Using Resources

Experts have described the role of advocate in several ways. One occupational therapist in the Atchison study described the process of "creating streams of advocacy" (n.p.) which involves not only therapist-centered advocacy for the client in order to ensure best practice but also advocacy by the client for himself or herself, advocacy by the family for the client, and advocacy by the other health care team members. Advocacy emerges from a genuine sense of commitment and caring for the identified needs of others. Effective advocacy requires knowledge of needed resources and professional commitment to ensure that needed resources are accessible to the client and family. It involves giving family members choice and voice. Effective advocacy also involves having knowledge of the multiple resources in the community and providing this information to family members and clients. These resources include information necessary for economic, emotional, and physical well-being, as well as ensuring the client's safety needs. For example, knowing about the most appropriate technologies for ensuring optimal and safe occupational performance is an essential competency for home-health-care therapists.

In addition to advocacy for the client and family, the need to advocate for the benefits of rehabilitation is necessary for survival in a health care system in which there is a continuing trend toward service reduction. It is increasingly important that the therapist advocate for the role they have historically practiced. That role is centered on assisting clients to resume safe and optimal occupational performance in as independent a way as they prefer, as opposed to a focus on the medical model of restorative, curative practices. "Function" is of major interest to third-party payers. Consequently, all professionals who provide home care are now articulating the importance of focusing on functional outcomes. In addition, providers are increasingly required to validate the effectiveness of their interventions.

Context Sensitivity

To maximize performance, it is best to provide intervention in the actual setting where the person carries out his or her occupational roles. In home health care, the therapist is able to observe and work with an individual in the physical space, social, and cultural context in which he or she must function. Dunn (1994) described the influence of context on performance by noting that a person does not exist in a vacuum; the physical environment as well as social, cultural, and temporal factors all influence behavior.

The home is a source of self-identity and is a place of meaning for a client. It is where important events occur, and it is the place where people have their most important and meaningful objects (Rockwell-Dyla, 1997). "Home" is more than a physical structure in which a person engages in ADL or receives health care, just as *care* is more than the provision of discrete services.

Therapist sensitivity to the extrinsic clues during the initial observation in the client's home is fundamental to competent care. The ability to analyze cultural nuances that affect the client's well-being is an important competency for all therapists who work in home health care. The therapist must make a transition from the traditional medical model of practice, in which the client is a passive recipient of therapy, to the consumer-centered model. In the consumer-centered model, the client is an active participant in the program and is considered a partner in planning and carrying out the intervention program. This naturally allows the client to choose priorities from the point of view of the context in which occupational performance will take place. Specific suggestions for the implementation of this model in the evaluation process are described in the "Evaluation: Occupational Profile and Analysis of Occupation" section, below.

Ethical Practice

Opacich (1997) describes the moral obligations to clients, caregivers, society, professional associates, agencies, and payers that occupational therapists have in providing home care. All therapists, regardless of their profession, have an obligation to develop and maintain competence, particularly in the home-care environment, where minimal supervision is available. In terms of obligations to clients, Opacich (1997) notes that the duty of the therapist is to "preserve the dignity of home-care patients and promote the quality of life" (p. 432). The burdens imposed on clients and caregivers need to be considered, because not all families are able to meet adequately the demands of using high-tech equipment or the daily physical and emotional toll that caregiving demands. The home-health-care team has an obligation to establish cooperation to ensure the best interests of the client. Opacich further notes that "trust is predicated on mutual respect and shared commitment, rather than on competition for recognition or market dominance (p. 435). Finally, she suggests that therapists try to influence policy and practices in the home-care agencies for which they work, as well as in the overall health system, in order to allow them to provide the care to which "they are philosophically and ethically committed" (p. 433).

Situation Analysis

One of the most commonly identified core competencies by occupational therapists is the ability to use activity analysis (Atchison, 2003). In a clinic setting, the performance of the client is completed in what could be described as a context-free environment. For example, when teaching a person with hemiplegia how to prepare a meal, the occupational therapy clinic has the necessary space to move around adequately,

the proper adaptive equipment and tools, and the individual guidance of the therapist. In the home, the client performs this activity with the added stress of family dynamics, constrained space, and an environment not designed for persons with disabilities. Assessment of occupational performance requires an analysis of the physical requirements of a task as well as an analysis of the situational elements that affect performance. The therapist working with the client in the home does not have to worry about whether the client will transfer skills from the clinic to the home environment.

Other disciplines find similar advantages and disadvantages to care in the home. For example, a physical therapist in a clinic setting has access to an array of equipment designed to facilitate strength and endurance development, and to protect clients as they practice mobility skills. At home, there is no equipment, meaning the therapist must design interventions using everyday materials (e.g., cans for weight training). In addition, the home may not only lack specific safety devices for functional mobility but actually present significant barriers (e.g., loose rugs, piles of paper). Although the home environment presents added problems in designing intervention, it provides a much clearer picture of what the client must actually be able to do.

Conflict Management

In the home setting, the social dynamics that impact on the well-being of the client take center stage. The attitudes, beliefs, and behaviors of other family members are important to the success of the intervention plan that the therapist and the client have developed cooperatively. For example, it is common for the client to want to resume meal preparation, while the spouse believes this will be unsafe. In this situation, the therapist needs to consider the spouse's concerns and weigh them against the client's insistence on resuming the activity. It is also common for the client to share the concerns about family members' reactions to their illness or disability. It is important to listen to the client and allow the freedom to express concerns, fears, and perhaps even anger with respect to the family's reactions. The next step is to work with the care team to identify a strategy to manage these conflicts.

More serious, life-threatening conflicts emerge in the case of client neglect or emotional and physical abuse by family members. It is not uncommon for therapists to encounter a situation in which the spouse, child, or even hired caregiver is harming the client through negative communication or threats, or even by withholding necessary care. In these cases, the therapist must be aware of the policies and procedures that the agency has in place to report such incidents to local protective services for further investigation. In most cases, the social worker manages these issues and provides team leadership in development of a team plan. Chapter 25 provides a detailed discussion of elder abuse.

Flexibility

In the consumer-oriented model of home care, the client controls scheduling of appointments and can challenge the provision of care. If the therapist wants to schedule a client in the early morning but the family believes that an early visit is too disruptive, the therapist—not the client—will be required to reconsider the visit plan. Flexibility in scheduling requires managing unexpected changes or disruptions. On arriving at the home, the therapist may encounter an important visitor in the home who has dropped by to see the client when he or she is scheduled for therapy. Another health care member may be there at the same time, or traffic and weather conditions may disrupt the therapist's timely arrival at a client's home on a given day.

In all of these cases, the therapist needs to manage the incident with a simple, common-sense approach. A phone call ahead of the scheduled visit to confirm that the appointed time is acceptable is helpful. If a therapist cannot provide a precise appointment time because of traffic, weather, or delays at earlier appointments, the client can be advised of that. Most families and clients can accept the need for flexible scheduling if the reasons are explained. When scheduling clients for therapy, it is also important to consider intervals between other services provided so the client is not overwhelmed. Therapy sessions should not all be scheduled back to back on the same day, and the clients' natural ebb and flow of energy levels also need to be considered. Teaching the client to bathe at an hour that is far from his or her ordinary time can be disruptive to the natural rhythm of the patient's ADL. Demanding that the client begin activities at an early hour is inappropriate as well. It is also important that

clients' wishes for scheduling are observed as much as possible so that no visit is scheduled during mealtime or during a favorite television program (Robinet, 1997).

The Occupational Therapy Process in Home Health Care

In this section, a discussion of evaluation, program planning, documentation, and discharge planning unique to the home-care setting is presented. Application of Medicare requirements are included in this discussion because the majority of home-care clients are Medicare beneficiaries, and it is important that the regulations and procedures required by this program are adhered to.

Preliminary Procedures

Although referrals for therapy services can come from a variety of sources, agencies require a physician's prescription to initiate services. Occupational therapists cannot be the first service to provide an initial visit because Medicare Part A regulations require that a "skilled service" such as nursing, physical therapy, or speech pathology be involved in a case before occupational therapy can be initiated. Because occupational therapy is often a secondary service, it is essential that a checklist be provided to the case manager so that an appropriate referral can be made. Johnson suggests that the referral checklist include two questions (Johnson, 1997):

1. What are the tasks the client must need to do?
2. Does the client want to do these tasks?

Evaluation: Occupational Profile and Analysis of Occupation

Although the OASIS data set has been the key tool for determining outcomes of home health care services as well as strengthening the team approach to client evaluation, it is not a stand-alone instrument for discipline-specific assessment. The occupational therapist contributes to the OASIS data set by completing an occupational profile and analysis of occupation. This is accomplished through a process that incorporates the therapist's theoretical beliefs about occupational performance and addresses the client's ability to engage and participate in activities of everyday life that are valued and meaningful to him or her in the context of the home.

Following development of an occupational profile, the occupational therapist works with the client to determine the performance skills necessary to participate in occupations. As described in the Practice Framework (American Occupational Therapy Association [AOTA], 2002), these skills include motor, process, and communication/interaction skills. In addition, an assessment of performance patterns should examine habits, routines, and roles related to the client's occupation. Habits are specific automatic behaviors; routines are established sequences of occupations or activities to provide a structure for daily life; and roles are comprised of behaviors that have been determined by the person's sociocultural sphere of influence for which there is an accepted code of norms (AOTA, 2002).

On receipt of a referral, the therapist initiates the evaluation and begins with an interview that allows the client to describe important occupations. This approach requires that the therapist listen to what the client perceives as priority issues. A useful assessment tool that may be used by occupational therapists for this purpose is the Canadian Occupational Performance Measure (COPM). The COPM is designed to elicit information from the client about his or her perception of current level of performance in terms of essential or highly valued occupations. The use of this measure sets the tone for both an occupation and client-centered practice approach in home health care (Law et al., 1990).

As noted earlier, it is important to assess cultural factors through a client-centered approach. Box 20-3 (Narayan, 1997) provides a checklist to consider in the development of a therapeutic relationship.

BOX 20-3 Cultural Assessment Checklist

- Patient-identified cultural/ethnic group
- Religion
- Cultural etiquette and social customs:
  - What is the typical greeting used?
    Is a handshake appropriate?
    Are shoes removed before entering the home?
  - Social customs before "business"
    What are social exchanges?
    Is it considered an insult to refuse a refreshment?
- Nonverbal patterns of communication
  - Is eye contact considered polite or rude?
  - What does a soft voice or loud voice mean in this culture?
  - Is personal space wider or narrower than in American culture?
  - What do smiles, nods, and hand gestures mean?
  - Is touch valued? When, where, and by whom can a client be touched?
- Client's expectations of problem
  - Diagnosis
    What do you call this illness?
    How would you describe this problem?
  - Onset
    When did the problem start?
    What started the problem?
  - Cause
    What caused the problem?
    What might other people think is wrong with you?

- Course
  How does the illness work?
  What does the illness do to you?
  What do you fear most about this problem?
  - Treatment
    How have you treated the problem so far?
    What treatment should you receive?
    Who in your family or community can help you?
  - Prognosis
    How long will the problem last?
    Is it serious?
  - Expectations
    What are you hoping the therapists will do for you when they come?
- Pain assessment
  - What is the cultural response to pain? Is it stoic? Is it expressive?
  - What is the patient's perception of pain response?
  - When did you last have pain?
  - What did you do to relieve it?
- Psychosocial assessment
  - Who is the decision maker in the family?
  - What are the characteristics of the sick role in the client's culture?
  - Are there language barriers?
  - What are the resources available from the client's cultural community?

Source: Narayan, M. (1997). Cultural assessment in home health care. *Home Health Care Nurse,* 15, 10.

An assessment of client factors specifically associated with the diagnosis that the client presents with is necessary. Client factors include body structures and functions related to physical, cognitive, and psychosocial factors that support the ability to engage and participate in occupations.

The occupational therapist must then conduct an analysis of activity demands of the activities that the client needs to accomplish. Activity demands refer to the objects, space, social demands, sequencing or timing, required actions, and required underlying body functions and body structure needed to carry out the activity (AOTA, 2002).

Documentation

Accurate, relevant, and thorough documentation is a critical component of effective delivery of services in home care. It is, in fact, the thread that all home-care agencies see as critical to survival. This is fact: "If it's not written down, it didn't happen." Without explicit, accurate, thorough, and clearly written accounts of care, agencies are not reimbursed for their services.

McGuire (1997) analyzed the coverage guidelines as set forth by Medicare and developed a set of principles that help assure practitioners that their documentation effectively meets these requirements. In summary, documentation should provide the six elements shown in Box 20-4.

Focus on Function

McGuire (1997) suggests that documentation focus on the client's prior level of function. Again, clients should be asked to identify meaningful activities that they feel they need to be able to do again. In reporting goals, it is important to be aware that a focus on the performance

BOX 20-4   **Elements of Documentation**

A focus on function
• A focus on underlying causes
• A focus on progress
• A focus on safety
• A statement of expectations for progress
• An explanation of slow progress or lack of progress

components (e.g., strength, range of motion, balance) should be addressed only if improvements in these areas will have a major impact on functional outcomes. In summarizing the client's goal, the language in the documentation must emphasize performance areas. It is appropriate to describe the need to improve sitting balance, for example, to enable the client to safely use a tub transfer bench and bathe himself. In cases in which it is not expected that the client will make gains in performance but there is risk of regression from current performance level, a functional maintenance program is appropriate. Periodic reevaluation of the maintenance program is reasonable, according to Medicare guidelines, but the goals must be clearly written in order to justify the need for this level of programming.

Focus on Underlying Causes

Occupational therapy is considered necessary when the severity of the physical/emotional/perceptual/cognitive disability requires complex and sophisticated knowledge to identify current and potential capabilities. This requires that the therapist have a firm grasp of the impact of various medical conditions on function in order to know what components need to be analyzed. For example, the problems associated with Parkinson's disease and subsequent difficulties related to feeding will need to be articulated—for example, "swallowing deficits associated with dysphagia interfere with safe, efficient eating behaviors." It is necessary to report specifically the observed factors that interfere with function and the level at which that interference occurs.

Focus on Progress

The OASIS B-1 is the document used at the time of recertification or other follow-up evaluation, such as a transfer from home-health-care status to skilled nursing care or to another HHA. It is expected as part of the comprehensive assessment. Each item is an explicit behavioral statement of the client's functional status and incorporates concepts from self-care assessments traditionally used by occupational therapists. As noted earlier, CMS continues to refine the OASIS data set. It is required of HHAs as a way to report client progress. OASIS data form the basis for evidence about the efficacy and quality of care provided by an individual agency and contribute to aggregate data about the effectiveness of home care in general.

Focus on Safety

Problems with safety include high probability of falling, lack of environmental safety awareness, swallowing difficulties, abnormal aggressive/destructive behavior, severe pain, loss of skin sensation, progressive joint contracture, and joint protection/preservation requiring skilled occupational therapy intervention to protect the patient from further medical complication. The role of occupational therapy is recognized in addressing these concerns, and it is important that the issue of safety and prevention be assessed on a regular basis and be clearly documented by all members of the home health care team.

State Expectations for Progress

For therapy services to be covered, documentation must clearly cite the therapist's professional assessment that progress is imminent and that continued improvement is expected and will be significant. This requires that the therapist clearly identify level of assistance if the client is not progressing quickly from one level to the next. For example, a client may need "maximal assistance" to perform a self-care task, but the patient is now able to perform the task without verbal reminders. This indicates progress within a level, and reporting this change can be an indicator that there is continued expectation for improvement.

Explanation of Slow Progress or Lack of Progress

It is common for home-care clients to have setbacks because of changes in their medical condition or situational crises. Therapists may encounter a client and family member who are not able to learn certain steps of a task because of perceptual cognitive impairments or other learning difficulties. Medicare guidelines allow a reasonable amount of time for the therapist to provide effective training. However, the therapist must clearly cite the various difficulties that confound the person's ability to perform a given task. These could include lack of memory required in task sequencing or difficulty with motor planning. It is recognized that if training is taking place, there will need to be a reasonable amount of teaching sessions to achieve the goal.

Intervention

After evaluating the client to determine his or her priorities, as well as those of the family, the therapist works with the client and family to establish a theoretically based intervention plan. The goals of the intervention should be documented in terms of performance areas as described in the *Practice Framework* (AOTA, 2002), because these most closely fit the concept of function as described in Medicare guidelines. It is appropriate to use client-factor terms to describe the focus of a specific intervention, but it is necessary to frame these in relation to performance. Use of the *Practice Framework* terminology is recommended to promote standard use of language in occupational therapy practice. The therapist must consider whether the intervention selected is reasonable and necessary and whether or not progress can realistically be expected. The most important question for the therapist to ask is whether the therapeutic approach is likely to promote change in functional performance.

Holm, Rogers, and Stone (1997) suggest that intervention by therapists in home care falls into three broad categories:

- *Remediation/restoration:* Used to establish new skills, restoring deficits in performance components
- *Compensation through use of adapted methods:* Assistive devices or environmental changes
- *Education:* Providing information about the effects of a given pathological condition and its consequences, preventive approaches to limit the effects of pathology, and specific procedures to restore or compensate

Box 20-5 provides some suggestions of questions to guide therapists in deciding the most appropriate intervention approach. Box 20-6 provides a quick summary of assessment and intervention strategies.

The modern health care system has adopted standards that highlight efficiency, productivity, and measurable outcomes of service. One important aspect of home health care is the potential for overlap among disciplines. Because a client may not be eligible for all the possible services reimbursed by Medicare, the nurse, physical therapist, or occupational therapist may need to address some aspect of care not typically associated with his or her practice. Obviously, this must be done with great caution so that the professional does not exceed his or her scope of practice or expertise. However, all professionals should recognize the potential need to appropriately identify the whole spectrum of client needs, to know which he or she can effectively address, and to know when referral must be made.

Regardless of economic constraints, the responsibility of the home-care agency is to provide the client with appropriate and necessary

---

BOX 20-5   Questions to Determine an Appropriate Intervention Approach for a Specific Task Disability

REMEDIATION
Would there be a change in safe performance in a reasonable amount of time if the program plan used
• Sensory re-education
• Visual perception
• Passive range of motion
• Active assistive, active, or resistive exercises for strengthening?
• Continuous passive motion?
• Inhibitory or facilitory treatment?
• Prosthetic training?
• Desensitization program?
• Postural stability exercises?
• Weight-shifting exercises?
• Balance exercises?
• Cognitive retraining? Habit training?

COMPENSATION
Would there be a change in safe performance, in a reasonable amount of time if

• The client used an alternate method to perform the task?
• Objects were adapted to make them safer and less difficult for the client to use?
• Assistive technology was provided?
• Environmental changes was made, including physical and human?

EDUCATION
Would there be a change in a safe performance in a reasonable amount of time if clients and caregivers
• Had their priorities considered?
• Demonstrated knowledge of interventions taught to them?
• Were given clear, written instructions?
• Were provided with graphic examples of interventions taught to them?

BOX 20-6   General Suggestions for Assessment and Intervention

SUGGESTIONS FOR ASSESSMENT
• The occupational therapist in home health care must be fluent in the use of the Outcome and Assessment Information Set (OASIS). The entire document has been made available by the Center for Health Services Research for download at no cost at this website: www.cms.hhs.gov/apps/hha/oasisdat.asp#B
• The Canadian Occupational Performance Measure (4th ed.) (COPM) is an excellent tool for client-centered, occupation-based assessment and is available at this website www.caot.ca

SUGGESTIONS FOR INTERVENTION
• In home health care, the emphasis of occupational therapy intervention will be to enable the client to participate in occupation. This will

occur through selection of activities that are meaningful and relevant to the client and that will enable safe, productive activities in the context of the home.
• The COPM and the OASIS form the baseline for client-centered intervention objectives. Success in meeting objectives is in large part based on the effectiveness of the occupational therapist in creating a collaborative relationship with the client and the caregivers.
• Fall prevention programs have been cited in the literature the most with regards to effectiveness of including an occupational therapist on the home-health-care team. Many protocols for assessment and education are available on AOTA's website. Also check the references in this article related to that topic.

care to ensure safety in the home. It is the responsibility of the home-care agency and each of its employees to use resources in both an efficient and an appropriate manner. Careful case management has become a critical tool for all home-care agencies. Social workers and therapists must recognize the importance of being highly visible and active participants of the team. The team must carefully evaluate the client's needs, determine an intervention plan that can be justified, and effectively communicate the rationale for that choice to the case manager.

better opportunity to demonstrate the relevance of the services of the rehabilitation team. A major paradigm shift has occurred in home care, from a medical model that has focused on pathology and long-term-care approach to one that increasingly embraces the potential of a client- or consumer-centered approach and emphasizes the importance of functional outcomes. This shift provides a wonderful opportunity for occupational therapy to expand its role (Barnes & Frock, 2003) and to enhance quality of life for elders and their families.

■ Summary

At no other time in the evolution of the home-health-care industry has there been given a

Case Study

Luisa is a 58-year-old homemaker who lives with her husband, Jorge, 60, and their 23-year-old son, James, who is attending college full time. They live in a Hispanic community in the Detroit area and have strong ties to their neighborhood community.

Luisa is diagnosed with rheumatoid arthritis. She has experienced significant hip joint pain in the last 3 years. Her pain was severe enough that it restricted not only her work in the home but also the ordinary ADL. Her pain has not been relieved by anti-inflammatory drugs. Recently, she has had to use a cane and has experienced significant stiffness of the hip. She decided to consult an orthopedic surgeon after talking with her general practitioner. X-ray studies indicated significant deterioration of the hip joint and associated cartilaginous destruction. She was advised that joint hip arthroplasty was the only means of affording pain relief and a chance for increased mobility. Following the surgery, she was treated with antibiotics to prevent infection. A catheter was applied because difficulty with urination is a side effect of anesthesia. It was removed 2 days after her operation.

To prevent the common complication of blood clots in her lower extremities,

compression stocking sleeves were applied as well as elastic hose, and she was instructed to complete simple ankle range-of-motion exercises to prevent clotting. Generally, the surgery was believed to have been successful, and Luisa was discharged 7 days after surgery to be cared for in the home. The discharge coordinator set up home-care services to begin the same day Luisa arrived home.

Luisa was discharged at 9 a.m. and came home by ambulance because she could not safely enter her home otherwise. She was scheduled for a follow-up appointment with her surgeon in 3 weeks to have her staples removed. The durable medical equipment services department of the hospital was contacted to ensure that a hospital bed was available in the home to be used during Luisa's recovery.

Nursing

The registered nurse arrived at 12 p.m. to open the case and determine the care plan. Luisa's entire family was present for the initial visit. The nurse reviewed the operation procedure as it related to the need for particular follow-up care now that Luisa was home. In general, the nursing care plan included monitoring of surgical healing, pain control, nutritional intake (especially adequate fluids), coughing, and deep-breathing exercises to prevent respiratory complications. Luisa complained of back discomfort, which is typically caused by the general postsurgical condition of the hip area and by the extended lack of movement required before, during, and after surgery. She was instructed to change her position periodically to help relieve discomfort and prevent skin breakdown. The nurse pointed out to the family the need for vigilance in providing support to Luisa as she went through her recovery period, which was estimated by her surgeon to last 6 weeks. Because patients recovering from hip replacement surgery are susceptible to dislocation, the nurse reviewed critical positioning issues that Luisa and the family needed to follow for the next 6 weeks. Luisa was cautioned against sitting up in bed, because this position can cause the artificial humeral head to dislocate from the acetabulum. She was instructed to restrict the elevation of the hospital bed to no more than 70 degrees until she was more stable. In addition, Luisa was instructed to use two to three pillows between her legs and to avoid adduction and rotation of the hips that would occur especially by crossing her legs in bed. Luisa was instructed to continue wearing elastic stockings until her return appointment to her physician. Luisa was also instructed to keep the incision clean and dry and to be alert for certain warning signs. She was advised to call her physician immediately if she noticed any swelling, increased pain, drainage from the incision site, redness around the incision, or fever.

The nurse continued to monitor Luisa's vital signs for the presence of infection such as strep throat or pneumonia. Luisa would not be able to shower until after her staples were removed, and bathing was contraindicated until total healing occurred. A certified nursing assistant (CNA) was ordered to provide daily bed baths and to assist with hygiene and grooming care needs. In addition, referrals were made for physical and occupational therapy evaluation and follow-up. The nurse indicated that she would be making daily visits for the first week and then would taper the frequency of her visits to three times per week, barring any complications. Even though she left a copy of written instructions with Luisa, she "quizzed" Luisa and the family members as to the instructions she had provided to ensure that they understood the importance of following all the necessary steps.

Physical Therapy

During the first 4 days in the hospital after her surgery, Luisa worked with a physical therapist to begin walking, going up and down stairs, getting in and out of bed, and performing range-of-motion and strength exercises of the hip. She was advised that a home-care therapist would assist her in continuing appropriate exercises, which were to be completed daily at home. The next day after Luisa's arrival home, a physical therapist initiated a program of home exercises that he taught the family as well to ensure proper follow-through. These included specific active exercises for hip and knee flexion, internal and external rotation, abduction, strengthening exercises for quadriceps setting, gluteal setting, isometric hip abduction, straight leg raising, and hip extension. Diagrams of these exercises were provided to Luisa, and the family was asked to review each one to assure that they could coach Luisa through the active exercise program. Visits were scheduled three times weekly, with discharge likely in 1 month, if progress was made in terms of mobility and strength.

Occupational Therapy

The occupational therapist was called in to emphasize functional issues that would allow Luisa to be as independent as possible in her home. Luisa was depressed because she could not resume her home management activities and felt anxious about "the men" having to perform meal preparation and cleanup, as well as all the other home management activities. Jorge and James both were not adept at these activities because they had relied on Luisa to take care of all of these areas. In addition, they had to coach Luisa along in her recovery and were beginning to complain about all the multiple tasks involved in their caregiving.

continued on page 510

Questions

1. Based on what you've learned from the evaluation above, and from the other disciplines, how might the OT proceed with evaluation?

The evaluation by the occupational therapist focused on ADL, with an emphasis on specific precautions that needed to be followed during all activities.

2. What client factor interventions might the occupational therapist recommend? Specific suggestions regarding positioning included "Dos and Do Nots" for hip positioning, such as

- DO NOT move your operated hip toward your chest (flexion) any more than a right angle. This is 90 degrees.
- DO grasp chair arms to help you rise safely to standing position. Place extra pillows or cushions in your chair so that you do not bend your hip more than 90 degrees.
- DO NOT sit on chairs without arms.
- DO use a chair with arms. Place your operated leg in front and your uninvolved leg well under.
- DO NOT sit low on a toilet or chair.
- DO use a long-handled reacher to pull up sheets or blankets or do as directed by the therapist.
- DO NOT try to put on your own shoes or stockings in the usual way. By doing this improperly you could bend or cross your operated leg too far.

- DO NOT cross your operated leg across the midline of your body (in toward your other leg).
- DO NOT lie down without a pillow between legs.
- DO keep a pillow between your legs when you roll onto your "good" side. This is to keep your operated leg from crossing the midline.

3. What equipment might help the client?

Equipment that would prevent the hip from being raised more than 90 degrees during toileting was ordered, as was a long-handled reacher, an extended bath brush so the patient could wash her feet, and a handheld shower that she could use after removal of her staples and after obtaining authorization by her physician to sit on a shower bench for showers.

4. What family factors might be important, and how can they be addressed?

Jorge and James were the primary caregivers even though Jorge worked full time and James attended school full time. A meeting with the nurse and the family allowed discussion of how Luisa's daily care needs would be met. It was decided that James would provide needed care during the day because most of his classes were in the evening, and that Jorge would be available each evening after work.

Review Questions

1. What are some advantages of home health care for functional rehabilitation and for health maintenance?
2. Who are the main recipients of home health services, and how are those services paid for?
3. Given the kind of funding available, what are some important limitations with regard to the kinds of occupational therapy goals and interventions that can be provided?
4. Why is it important to document performance change in home health interventions?
5. What unique ethical issues are important in home health care?

Web-Based Resources

For helpful information about the experience of home health care, visit:

www.cms.hhs.gov/apps/hha/all.pdf, **The Outcome and Assessment Information Set (OASIS),** date connected March 16, 2007. This site is the intellectual property of the Center for Health Services Research, Denver, Colorado, but is made available for free to individual use for assessment purposes.

www.cms.hhs.gov/center/hha.asp, **Centers for Medicare and Medicaid Services Home Health Center page,** date connected March 16, 2007. An array of resources focused on reimbursement and regulations for home health care.

www.nahc.org, **The National Association for Home Care,** date connected March 16, 2007. The primary professional organization and best source of current information on home-health-care policy and practice.

www.independenceinc.org/ability.html, **The Giant Disability Resource Page,** date connected March 16, 2007. This site maintains a comprehensive directory of links to disability-related and assistive technology sites.

www.aota.org (follow the link to the Wilma West Library), **The Special Interest Section for Home and Community Health Special Interest Section Quarterly (HHSIS), American Occupational Therapy Association,** date connected March 16, 2007. An excellent resource for home-care practice, including references, links, and other resources. If you are a member of AOTA, you can access the online archive of past issues.

REFERENCES

American Occupational Therapy Association (AOTA). (2002). Occupational therapy practice framework: Domain and process. *American Journal of Occupational Therapy, 56,* 609–639.

Atchison, B. (2003). Identification of competencies of community based practice as identified by expert occupational therapists. Unpublished raw data.

Barnes, P. A., & Frock, A. H. (2003). The expanded role for rehabilitation in home care. *Home Health Care Management & Practice, 15,* 305–313.

Bonder, B. R., Martin, L., & Miracle, A. W. (2001). *Culture in clinical care.* Thorofare, NJ: SLACK.

Centers for Medicare and Medicaid Services. (2006a). *Home health compare.* Retrieved May 28, 2006, from Center for Medicare and Medicaid Services, U.S. Department of Health and Human Services Access www.medicare.gov/HHCompare/Home.asp?dest= NavIHomeIAboutIOverview#TabTop.)

Centers for Medicare and Medicaid Services. (2006b). *Home health PPS: An overview.* Retrieved May 3, 2006, from CMS Website via Office of Clinical Standards and Quality Access www.cms.hhs.gov/ HomeHealthPPS/.

Coleman, B. (1995). European models of long-term care in the home and community. *International Journal of Health Services, 25*(3), 455–474.

Collins, E. (1921). Occupational therapy for the homebound. *Archives of Occupational Therapy, 1,* 33.

Dunn, W. (1994). The ecology of human performance: A framework for considering the effect of context. *American Journal of Occupational Therapy, 48,* 595–607.

Gitlin, L. N., Winter, L., Dennis, M. P., Corcoran, M., Schinfeld, S., & Hauck, W. W. (2006). A randomized trial of a multicomponent home intervention to reduce functional difficulties in older adults. *Journal of the American Geriatrics Society, 54,* 809–816.

Holm, M., Rogers, J., & Stone, M. (1997). Referral, evaluation, and intervention (module 4, p. 1). In M. Steinhauer & M. J. Youngstrom (Eds.), *Occupational therapy in home health: Preparing for best practice.* Bethesda, MD: American Occupational Therapy Association.

Hornbrook, M. C., Stevens, V. J., Wingfield, D. J., Hollis, J. F., Greenlick, M. R., & Ory, M. G. (1994). Preventing falls among community-dwelling older persons: Results from a randomized trial. *The Gerontologist, 34*(1), 16–23.

Jackson, B. (1992). Home based occupational therapy: Then and now. *American Journal of Occupational Therapy, 46,* 84–85.

Johnson, K. (1997). Screening tool for occupational therapy referrals. *Home and Community Special Interest Section Quarterly, 3,* 1–2, as cited in M. Holm, Referral, evaluation, and intervention (module 4, p. 1). In M. Steinhauer & M. J. Youngstrom, (Eds.), *Occupational therapy in home health: Preparing for best practice.* Bethesda, MD: American Occupational Therapy Association.

Kinsella, A. (2005). *About home telehealth. Guide to long term planning.* Retrieved April 29, 1996, from *Medical News* website. Access www.longtermcarelink.net/ eldercare/home_telehealth.htm#is.

Law, M., Baptiste, S., McColl, M., Opzoomer, A., Polatajko, H., & Pollock, N. (1990). The Canadian Occupational Performance Measure: An outcome measure for occupational therapy. *Canadian Journal of Occupational Therapy, 57,* 82–87.

Levit, K. (1996). National health expenditures. *Health Care Financing Review Fall, 13,* 175–214.

Lipson, J., & Meleis, A. (1985). Culturally appropriate care: The case of immigrants. *Topics in Clinical Nursing, 7,* 46–48.

May, V., Onarcan, M., Olechowski, C., and Myron, C. (2004). International perspectives on the role of home care and hospice in aging and long term care. *Caring, 23,* 1.

McGruder, J. (1998). Culture and other forms of human diversity in occupational therapy. In M. Neisdadt & E. Crapeau (Eds.), *Willard and Spackman's occupational therapy* (3rd ed., pp. 386–407). New York: JB Lippincott.

McGuire, M. (1997). Documenting progress in home health care. *American Journal of Occupational Therapy, 51,* 436–445.

Medical News Today. (2005). *CMS announces Medicare demonstration for day care services under the home health benefit.* Retrieved April 13, 2006, from www.medicalnewstoday.com/medicalnews.php?newsid= 26606Centers for Health Services Research.

Moyle, N. (2005). *Using professional home care services. Guide to long term care planning.* Retrieved April 6, 2008, from http://www.longtermcarelink.net/ eldercare/personal_care_home_care.htm

Nanako, T., Kazue, Y., & Eiji, Y. (2002). Use of home health services covered by new public long-term care insurance in Japan: Impact of the presence and kinship of family caregivers. *International Journal for Quality in Health Care, 14,* 295–303.

Narayan, M. (1997). Cultural assessment in home healthcare. *Home Healthcare Nurse 15,* 663–672.

National Alliance for Caregiving and American Association of Retired Persons. (2004). *Caregiving in the U.S.* (pp. 18–20). Washington, DC: Author.

Opacich, K. (1997). Moral tensions and obligations of occupational therapy practitioners providing home care. *American Journal of Occupational Therapy, 51,* 430–439.

Robinet, R. (1997). Professional responsibilities in the home care setting. In M. Steinhauer & M. J. Youngstrom (Eds.), *Occupational therapy in home health: Preparing for best practice* (module 2, p. 1). Bethesda, MD: American Occupational Therapy Association.

Rockwell-Dyla, L. (1997). The meaning of home: Establishing a frame of reference for occupational therapy in home health care. In M. Steinhauer & M. J. Youngstrom (Eds.), *Occupational therapy in home health: Preparing for best practice.* Bethesda, MD: American Occupational Therapy Association.

Siebert, C. (2000, March). An overview of the proposed prospective payment system for home health care. *Home & Community Health Special Interest Section Quarterly, 7,* 3–4.

Siebert, C. (2005, September). Home health outcomes and quality improvement. *Home & Community Health Special Interest Section Quarterly, 12*(3), 3–4.

Steultjens, E., Dekker, J., Bouter, L., Jellema, S., Bakker, E., & van den Ende, C. (2004). Occupational therapy for community dwelling elderly people: A systematic review. *Age and Aging, 33,* 453–460.

Strange, B. (1926). Work among the homebound. *Occupational Therapy and Rehabilitation, 5,* 55.

Sullivan, S. (1925). Work for crippled and disabled persons: Cleveland's experience. *Occupational Therapy and Rehabilitation, 4,* 101.

Thompson, L. (2004). *Long-term care: Support for family caregivers. Long-term financing project.* Washington DC: Georgetown University Press.

Toto, P. (2006). Success through teamwork in the home health setting: The role of occupational therapy. *Home Health Care Management and Practice, 19,* 31–37.

Tripp-Reimer, T. (1985). Cultural assessment. In J. Bellack & P. Bamford (Eds.), *Nursing assessment* (p. 265). North Scituate, *MA: Duxbury Press.*

U.S. Census Bureau. (2006). *Statistical abstract of the United States. Health and nutrition.* Retrieved May 29, 2006, from U.S. Census Bureau website via Administrative and Customer Services Division Statistical Compendia Branch www.longtermcarelink.net/ eldercare/ personal_care_home_care.htm.

Weinstein, M., and Booth, J. (2006). Preventing falls in older adults: A multifactorial approach. *Home Health Care Management and Practice, 19,* 45–50.

Youngstrom, M. J (1997). Occupational therapy in the health setting: An introduction. In M. Steinhauer & M. J. Youngstrom (Eds.), *Occupational therapy in home health: Preparing for best practice.* Bethesda: MD: American Occupational Therapy Association.

CHAPTER 21

Rehabilitation

Vanina Dal Bello-Haas, PhD, PT • Joyce Tryssenaar, PhD, OT Reg (Ont)

Dreams are renewable. No matter what our age or condition, there are still untapped possibilities within us and new beauty waiting to be born.

Dale E. Turner, Retrieved March, 16, 2006, from
www.bestinspiration.com/quotes-1/of/Dale_E._Turner.htm

In his 87th year of life, the great Michelangelo Buonarotti (1475–1564) was believed to have said, "Ancora Imparo" ("Still, I am learning")

Retrieved April 5, 2006, from
http://en.thinkexist.com/quotes/michelangelo/3.html

OBJECTIVES

By the end of this chapter, the reader will be able to:

1. Relate the demographics of disability in the older adult to the extent of problems that may be encountered during rehabilitation.
2. Outline the unique aspects of rehabilitation as they relate to the older adult.
3. Discuss the different team approaches to the rehabilitation of the older adult and the complementary relationship between occupational therapy and physical therapy.
4. Define comprehensive assessment as it relates to rehabilitation of the older adult.
5. Review common assessment tools and interventions used in older adult rehabilitation settings.
6. Discuss the personal and environmental factors that may enhance or impede the rehabilitation process.
7. Describe the various delivery systems in which rehabilitation of the older adult can take place and the related reimbursement issues.
8. Consider the psychological impacts of trauma and illness on the rehabilitation process.
9. Be aware of rehabilitation issues for older adults with preexisting conditions.

There are many definitions of rehabilitation, rather than one universally accepted definition, and some consider rehabilitation too complex to define (Sinclair & Dickinson, 1998). Rehabilitation is typically considered a *continuous process* aimed at enabling people to maximize, restore, and maintain their optimal physical, sensory, intellectual, psychological, and social functional levels (Figure 21-1). Through a client-focused partnership, usually involving several health care professionals and including family and caregivers whenever possible, rehabilitation provides people with the tools they need to attain the highest possible level of independence and self-determination. Rehabilitation includes providing for and restoring activity limitations and participation restrictions, relearning previous skills, and learning how to adapt to different circumstances in order to compensate for the loss or absence of a function or for a functional limitation (adapted from WHO, 2006).

Rehabilitation can be carried out in a variety of settings, and the scope, types, and intensity of services provided, the type of patients served, and the overall philosophy and focus of the program offered within each setting can vary. Thus, rehabilitation will involve a variety of health care professionals working across a number of health- and social-care sectors. The key to successful rehabilitation of the older adult involves the accurate identification of problems and needs, an understanding of the relationship between identified problems to impaired body functions and structures, activity limitations and participation restrictions, and the influence of personal and environment factors that may positively or negatively influence rehabilitation interventions and overall outcomes. Successful rehabilitation of the older adult requires

1. A broad perspective
2. Accurate identification and management of medical, social, and psychological problems, in addition to occupational performance and physical functioning issues
3. A thorough understanding of the differences between "normal aging" and pathological changes
4. An understanding of how these "normal aging" and pathological changes interact with the disablement process (Box 21-1)

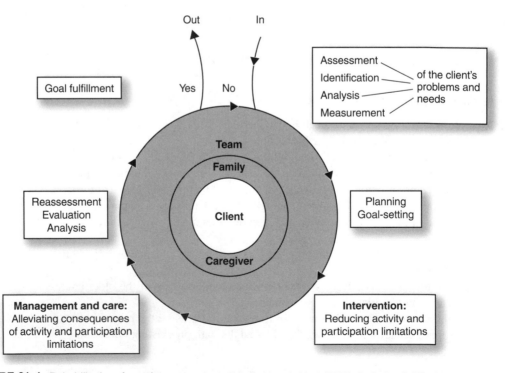

FIGURE 21-1 Rehabilitation: A continuous process. (Adapted from Lokk, J. (1999), Geriatric rehabilitation revisited. *Aging: Clinical and Experimental Research, 11*(6), 353–361.)

BOX 21-1 **As You Read the Chapter Think about How the Major Concepts, Issues, and Settings are Relevant to Uncle Alphonse.**

My Uncle Alphonse . . .

When we were little he always had candies in his pocket and would take us for ice cream. He always played lots of games, card games, sports, board games as long and as often as we all wanted to play . . .

When I was older he was interested in what I wanted to do when I grew up, who my boyfriend was, and what I did for fun. He had the biggest laugh. My mother says he also has a bad temper when they were growing up but I never saw it . . .

When I was 14 he married Sophia who was fashion model and very cool and a few years later he had babies of his own but he was still interested in our lives and what we were doing.

He was an importer/exporter; he traveled all over the world. He loved work, he said, and he loved play, and he loved people, he loved his nieces and nephews and his own children, and God. He lived a big life. He had lots of strong opinions but could laugh at himself too.

He danced at my wedding, toasted the bride, and later spoiled my own children as he had spoiled me. He took up water skiing and golf and bird watching. He said he wanted to live life to the fullest each and every day.

When he was 67 he fell off his roof and hurt his back. With his back injury he experienced significant pain and disability for the first time in his life. The loss affected all areas of his life and his health and resulted in grieving and depression. He focussed his life on a search for a cure. He tried acupuncture, and cold packs, and drugs, and prayer, and massage, and psychotherapy, and naturopathy, and finally he tried surgery in the hope that he would have less pain and a better quality of life. Tragically the surgery resulted in permanent lower limb paralysis and my Uncle Alphonse had to go to rehabilitation to learn to live independently again . . .

Disability Demographics

Almost 75% of older adults aged 60 and over have at least one chronic illness and about 50% have at least two chronic illnesses (Calkins, Boult, Wagner, & Pacalaet, 1999). Chronic conditions may lead to severe and immediate impairments, as well as progressive activity limitations that slowly decrease the ability of the older adult to care for himself or herself (Fried & Guralnik, 1997). In 1997, more than half of the older population (54.5%) reported having at least one disability of some type (physical or nonphysical), and over a third (37.7%) reported at least one severe disability. Although some of these disabilities may be relatively minor, they may be limiting enough to cause older people to require assistance to attend to their personal needs. For example, about 14.3% of people age 65 and over require assistance with bathing, dressing, preparing meals, or shopping (Banthin & Cohen, 1999). Limitations with activities because of chronic conditions increase with age as do the number of disabilities (Figure 21-2), with disabilities affecting most of the very old. Almost 75% of those aged 80 and over report at least one disability, and over half (57.6%) of

those aged 80 and over had one or more severe disabilities. Over a third (34.9%) of these individuals reported needing assistance as a result of their disability (Administration on Aging, 2005). An orderly progression of disability has been reported in older adults aged 75 and older, with self-care activities dependent on lower extremity function being lost before activities that are dependent on upper extremity function (Jagger, Arthur, Spiers, & Clarke, 2001; Spector & Fleishman, 1998). For example, Jagger and colleagues (2001) found that bathing was the first activity of daily living (ADL) with which older adults had difficulty, followed by general mobility, toileting, dressing, transfer from bed, transfer from chair, and feeding. There is a strong association between disability status and reported health status. For example, among those 65 and older with a severe disability, 68% reported their health as fair or poor. In those who reported no disability, only 10.5% reported their health as fair or poor (Administration on Aging, 2005). The association between age and prevalence of disability is not absolute. It is important to note that although people tend to develop chronic conditions as they age, growing old does not have to necessarily mean becoming

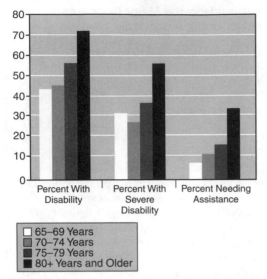

FIGURE 21-2 Percent of older people with disabilities, by age. Limitations with activities due to chronic conditions increase with age, as do the number of disabilities. (Adapted from Administration on Aging. (2005). *A profile of older Americans: 2005.* Retrieved October 23, 2007 from www.aoa.gov/PROF/Statistics/profile/2005/16.asp.)

disabled. Most older adults are independent and able to function on their own or with minimal assistance, and recent data suggest that the amount of time elderly people can expect to live without disability is increasing. Disability among older people appears to be declining in France, Belgium, Taiwan, Italy, the Netherlands, and Switzerland, but in other countries, such as Australia, Canada, and Britain, no substantial decline in disability rates is apparent; however, there is also no consistent evidence that disability rates are rising (Administration on Aging, 2005).

Psychological Consequences of Disabling Events

Many older adults seen for rehabilitation are adjusting to real and perceived losses from the sequelae of disabling events—traumas, conditions, and illnesses. These losses range from those sustained at the impairment level, such as range of motion, balance, strength, endurance to intrapersonal losses, such as the loss of a sense of self, loss of valued roles, loss of relationships, and loss of power leading to activity limitations. Finally, the older adult who faces disabling

events can experience losses affecting participation such as the disengagement from prior meaningful activities like volunteer work, the loss of living independently, and financial losses.

Loss is defined as irrevocable and can be any valued object—a loved person, a job, status, home, a cherished possession, and health—whereas grief is our response to loss and often includes the loss of the future as we expect it (Bruce & Schultz, 2001). Losses can be sudden, gradual, anticipated, temporary, or permanent. The concept of nonfinite loss has been developed by Bruce and Schultz to describe loss that is contingent on development and time and involves a process of realization that occurs over an individual's life span. Other authors use the term "chronic sorrow" (Lindgren, Burke, Hainsworth, & Eakes, 1992) to capture the essence of ongoing loss and grief usually associated with chronic conditions across the life span. Many older individuals also experience loss because of the deaths of friends and family members in their age group.

Spaniol, Gagne, and Koehler (1999) state that trauma and illness can have a number of devastating impacts on the lives of people who experience them, as well as on the lives of their caregivers. These include a loss of sense of self, the loss of connectedness that results from stigma and discrimination, loss of power from the loss of one's sense of agency and the loss of belief in oneself, and the loss of valued roles. Although Spaniol et al. are basing their work on the experiences of persons with mental illness, it is evident that these losses can also be experienced by an individual who has had a physical illness or trauma. For example, a person with a stroke may feel the loss of physical and cognitive competence (loss of sense of self), may feel isolated and different because he or she now uses a wheelchair (the loss of connectedness that results from stigma and discrimination), may experience a loss of power (loss of independence in self-care), and have lost valued roles (driving, social activities).

Drench (2006) identifies five important factors for therapists in working with loss and grief issues:

1. The importance of dialogue and relationship for healing and transformation. A busy therapist may not feel he or she has the time to spend talking about grief if that is what the individual requires, but it is essential for transformation to occur.

2. A focus on process as opposed to outcome.
3. The importance of the process of life review. Older adults often wish to review their lives, and loss may bring the need for life review to the forefront.
4. Confrontation of the nature of absence and emptiness.
5. Being present to what is experienced rather than the need for change.

Some essential therapy skills and tasks include communication about the loss and grief which may involve listening and reflecting, being present, and allowing grieving. Touching (as appropriate) and other physical means (tissues, cups of tea, etc.) of comforting are also important. Providing a hope-charged environment and making available opportunities to engage in meaningful occupations can be a means of reworking expectations and creating resilience within the person. All of the above strategies are dependent on what the client wants, but it is the therapist's responsibility to assess and support the individual in his or her experienced loss and resulting grief.

Aging with a Preexisting Disability

Chapter 17 identifies the importance of considering chronic disabilities or illnesses in evaluation. The prevalence of persons aging with preexisting disabilities is increasing rapidly as medical interventions allow individuals to not only survive but to live longer. Rehabilitation can be a very different process for the therapist when working with someone who has had numerous experiences with rehabilitation. Positive previous experiences allow caregivers to work in a collegial relationship with the client (i.e., the client has developed some expertise in managing his or her condition and is open to the rehabilitation experience and the therapist respects his or her expertise). Negative prior experiences may challenge the therapist to process these experiences before moving forward and to be sensitive to how these past experiences may affect current and future rehabilitation.

Issues for Persons with Intellectual Disability

Although children born with Down Syndrome in the 1930s were not expected to live beyond childhood, studies in the 1980s reported life expectancy of approximately 55 years, and that can be expected to increase (Adlin, 1993). Sutton (1997) suggests that within the next 20 years, the number of people with developmental disabilities over the age of 55 is expected to increase by 87%. Living longer means that these individuals will face the same age-related health concerns as the general population (Delorme, 1999). Some potential challenges in rehabilitation for persons with intellectual disability include negative experiences with institutions in their childhood, lack of supportive relationships, and limited services and programs. Salvatori, Tremblay, and Tryssenaar (2003) found age-related health issues facing both older adults and their aging parents contributed to increased caregiver burden and the need for permanency planning.

Issues for Persons with Serious Mental Illness

According to Cohen et al. (2000), older persons with schizophrenia generally received very little service and support from the mental health system except for medication; they received less than adequate health care, had increased levels of depression and decreased cognitive function; and their social networks were smaller than their age peers. There is some evidence that older clients receive less help from both formal and informal systems and are less optimistic about the future than are younger clients (Horwitz & Uttaro, 1998). Bartels, Levine, and Shea (1999) emphasize that optimal services for older persons with serious mental illness require close collaboration of primary medical care and mental health services; that older persons with serious mental illness typify the most complex, vulnerable, resource-poor, and high-risk long-term-care patients.

Rehabilitation practitioners need to be aware that among those individuals with mental illnesses, there may also be physical health problems that become part of the aging process. In a qualitative study of family members of individuals aging with serious mental illness (Tryssenaar & Tremblay, 2002), one participant reported "My husband has been classified as a mild schizophrenic, but he also had a major stroke 2½ years ago, so he now has both a physical disability and a mental disability" (p. 260). This study also found that participants reported ongoing concerns that physical health needs were not considered with a prior mental illness diagnosis. The inadequate physical health of persons with serious mental illness has also been documented in the nursing literature (Byrne, Isaacs, & Voorberg, 1991). Having a mental illness does not rule out having a physical condition in later life.

Issues for Persons with Physical Disabilities

There are common health problems related to aging with physical disabilities such as spinal cord injury, post-polio syndrome, and multiple sclerosis. These include various musculoskeletal problems, declining energy and strength, osteoporosis, and stress. Exploring these common health problems, while keeping in mind the natural processes of aging, is part of the challenge for therapists working in rehabilitation. Recognition of the individual's expertise in living with his or her preexisting condition must be considered in rehabilitation.

What Makes Older Adult Rehabilitation Unique?

Rehabilitation of the older adult presents several unique aspects for therapists. The older adult client frequently presents with multiple diagnoses or pathologies in combination with the processes of normal aging. The interaction between conditions and normal aging may exacerbate impairments and limitations and may affect the response to some rehabilitation interventions. Although specific diseases can cause specific types of disability (Fried, Ettinger, Lind, Newman, & Gardin, 1994; Fried & Guralnik, 1997), some diseases seem to interact in a unique, synergistic manner with one another, producing greater activity limitations and participation restrictions over what might be expected from either condition alone (Verbrugge, Lepkowski & Imanaka, 1989; Verbrugge, Lepkowski, & Konkol, 1991). Thus, many of the occupational performance or functional problems experienced by an older adult are the result of interactions between decreased physiologic reserve, an acute or chronic illness, and the environment in which the person resides. As the numbers of diseases increase, there is increasing risk of problems with activities of daily living (ADL) (Mor et al., 1989; Verbrugge et al., 1989), instrumental ADL (IADL) (Mor et al., 1989;

Verbrugge et al., 1989), and mobility (Campbell et al., 1994; Guralnik et al., 1993; Verbrugge et al., 1989; Verbrugge et al., 1991).

Chronologic age is not always a reflection of physiologic age. There is a great deal of heterogeneity and variability in overall presentation and functional limitations in older adults, secondary to differences in decline in the physiologic systems, such as cognition, neuromuscular (e.g., strength), cardiovascular, sensory (e.g., vision), and other physical functions (see Chapters 4, 5, 6, and 7). Older people age at different rates from one another, and within each older person, organ systems age at different rates. Differences among and within individuals need to be taken into account when planning rehabilitation programs. There is also evidence that the course of disability does not necessarily progress in a uniform manner among older people. Some older adults may have several impairments without any activity or participation limitations, and in others, activity and participation limitations are the sum effect of several different impairments. For example, Laura is 75 years old. She has osteoporosis and decreased physical mobility and has had a stroke limiting the use of her dominant hand and arm. Using a variety of compensatory techniques and adaptive devices, she continues to garden, play cards, and do the majority of her usual activities. On the other hand, Elgin, who is 65, has impaired vision and hearing and early cognitive impairments, and he does not feel able to participate in many of his usual activities even with the provision of adaptations and compensatory strategies.

The incidence of a catastrophic event precipitating activity and participation limitations is less likely for an older adult (Figures 21-3 and 21-4). Although many older adults become disabled by an acute illness such as a major stroke, fractured neck of the femur, or pneumonia, a slowly progressive pattern of disability because of worsening of chronic conditions such as arthritis or diabetes, often occurs with age. Older adults are more likely to experience progressive disability as opposed to catastrophic disability, and thus, they may be more likely to need rehabilitation intermittently over a number of years. Rates of progressive disability increase with age and are greatest for those age 85 and older (Guralnik, Ferrucci, Balfour, Volpato, & DiIorio, 2001).

Biological factors may have important effects on the development of **frailty** (Fried et al., 2001).

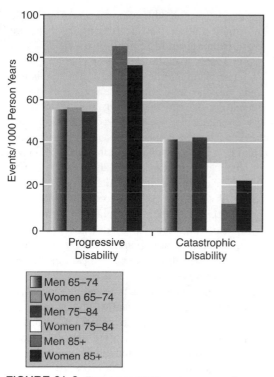

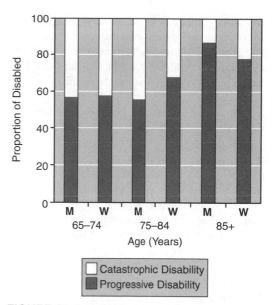

FIGURE 21-4 Proportion of progressive and catastrophic disability according to age and gender. (Adapted from Guralnik, J. M., Ferrucci, L., Balfour, J. L., Volpato, S., & DiIorio, A. (2001). Progressive versus catastrophic loss of the ability to walk: Implications for the prevention of mobility loss. *Journal of the American Geriatrics Society, 49,* 1463–1470.)

FIGURE 21-3 Rates per 1000 person-years of progressive and catastrophic disability, according to age and gender. (Adapted from Guralnik, J. M., Ferrucci, L., Balfour, J. L., Volpato, S., & DiIorio, A. (2001). Progressive versus catastrophic loss of the ability to walk: Implications for the prevention of mobility loss. *Journal of the American Geriatrics Society, 49,* 1463–1470.)

Frailty is considered an age-related loss of physiologic reserve; thus, even minor stressors can result in disproportionate functional consequences, and potentially, on the ability of frail, older adults to respond to rehabilitation. Depression and cognitive impairment, both of which are associated with poor functional outcomes, are common in older rehabilitation clients (Wells, Seabrook, Stolee, Borrie, & Knoefel, 2003a). Financial resources may be more limited in older adults, and caregivers (often older adults) may also have some decline in function themselves. Thus, the abilities of the person providing care also need to be assessed and considered as they relate to the rehabilitation management plan.

Management may not be directed to traditionally thought of vocational or educational outcomes, and at times rehabilitation may be more focused toward prevention of further decline, rather than restoration. Healthy aging over a life-course is important. Because of the higher incidence of chronic diseases in older adults,

overall rehabilitation management should take into account interventions aimed at chronic disease management and disease prevention and promotion of health and wellness, so that older adults can learn to live with their condition and become actively involved in its management. Regardless of these unique features, there are basic principles of rehabilitation for older adults that need to be kept in mind (Box 21-2).

The Rehabilitation Team

The most important member and key member of the team is the client. Rehabilitation is maximized when a comprehensive and holistic approach, with input from the family and caregivers and a variety of skilled professionals, is utilized. Evidence highlights the importance of eliciting family and patient input when setting goals. Studies have found agreement on goals between older patients, family members, and the health care team to be poor overall, and lack of agreement between family members and the health care team has been noted, regardless of setting (Bogardus et al., 2001; Glazier, Schuman, Keltz, Vally, & Glazier, 2004; Rockwood, Graham, & Fay, 2002). Although there was agreement in some goal categories, there was substantial disagreement about areas of main concern and priority. In addition, patients and caregivers tended to identify more goals, especially in the areas of medical care, psychosocial issues, spirituality, future planning (Glazier et al., 2004), and related to leisure, social interaction, behavior, and function (Rockwood et al., 2002). Explicit goal setting is a central component in the rehabilitation of older adults. Goals should be informed by careful evaluation of the client and precede all rehabilitation interventions. A rehabilitation goal is a precise statement and should be constructed so that its achievement is unambiguous (Box 21-3).

Teams may be **multidisciplinary** (MD), **interdisciplinary** (ID), or **transdisciplinary** (TD), and although the terms are often used interchangeably, they each have a specific meaning. MD teams are discipline oriented, with each team member responsible for his or her own unique scope of practice, and the team's outcome is the sum of each team member's efforts. In ID teams, team members are involved in problem solving beyond the scope of their own discipline. The whole team identifies goals for the client; once identified, each team member then works toward goal attainment within their scope of practice. Within TD teams, one team member is chosen to be the primary leader or therapist depending on the specific needs of the client. The leader is responsible for care delivery regardless of his or her discipline, and other team members contribute information and recommendations, necessitating cross-training and flexibility of health care professionals (Latella, 2000).

The number of health care professionals who make up the rehabilitation team varies greatly depending on the care setting and the needs of the client, but typically includes a geriatrician (a physician who specializes in geriatric medicine) or a physiatrist (a physician who specializes in physical medicine and rehabilitation), a nurse or a geriatric nurse practitioner, a social worker (SW), physical therapist (PT), occupational therapist (OT), and support personnel. In some countries, team members have specialized skills or specialist certification. For example, in the United Kingdom, geriatricians may have specialized skills in stroke or orthogeriatric rehabilitation, and in the United States (US), physical therapists may be Geriatric Certified Specialists (GCS) and occupational therapists may be Board Certified in Gerontology. Other health professionals, such as psychologists, speech-language pathologists (SLPs), audiologists, nutritionists, recreational and respiratory therapists, and pharmacists are also frequently part of a team that may evaluate and manage care for the older adult (Figure 21-5). An Irish study found that individual health care professionals often failed to see the patient's situation as a whole; rather each team member approached the patient from the vantage point of

---

BOX 21-2 Basic Principles of Rehabilitation for Older Adults

- Use client-centered focus—set realistic, individualized goals
- Include caregivers and family members whenever possible
- Use a team approach
- Address primary impairments, activity and participation limitations

- Prevent secondary impairments, activity and participation limitations
- Address health promotion and wellness needs
- Emphasize optimal functional independence
- Consider interclient variability
- Consider how personal and environmental factors may influence overall management and outcomes

---

BOX 21-3 Essential Components of Rehabilitation Goals

- Meaningful—appropriate to circumstances of the client and the problems identified
- Individualized
- Mutually Agreed Upon—negotiated between client, family, caregivers, and the rehabilitation team

- Clearly communicated
- Realistic—challenging, but achievable
- Measurable

their respective special skills and emphasized that particular angle. There were low levels of detection by professions of some disabilities outside their traditional areas of responsibility, highlighting the fact that no one member is as good at detecting disability as the team working as a whole (Cunningham et al., 1996).

Although some older adults requiring rehabilitation do not present with complex needs, usually the majority of clients seen in this practice area do have multifaceted issues. Interdisciplinary teams are an essential component of practice in the rehabilitation of older adults in part because no one person or discipline can have expertise in all the areas of specialty knowledge needed for the most effective care of clients with complex disorders (Perkins & Tryssenaar, 1994). An interdisciplinary approach is particularly recommended when dealing with specific client populations with chronic and complex conditions (Runciman, 1989), and with clients who traditionally have difficulty dealing with the health care system (Bachrach, 1989). Sommer, Silagy, and

Rose (1986) suggest a team approach can also be a means of improving treatment efficiency and meeting the health needs of the community. Although each individual profession makes a unique contribution to rehabilitation, "it must be acknowledged that it is the sum of individual team members' contributions and team collaboration that makes the greatest positive difference in client care outcomes" (OANPHSS, 2000, p. 9). Implicit in this belief is the premise that individuals from different health care backgrounds must be working as an effective team.

Effective teamwork requires that members bring their respective specialized knowledge and skills to the situation, recognize and appreciate the contribution of each individual member, take part in decision making, and assume responsibility for their own decisions and team decisions. Good communication among team members greatly enhances the effectiveness of the overall management plan delivery, and cooperation and coordination among team members should be seamless. A method found to promote coordination of

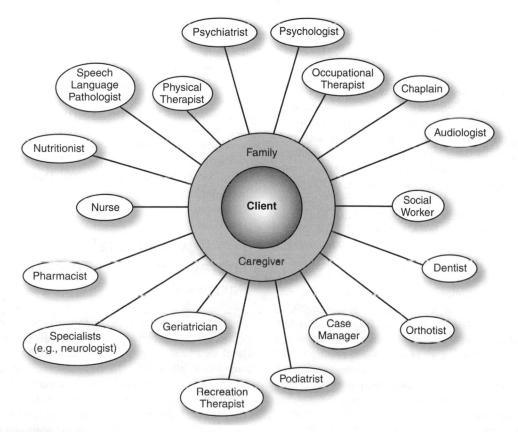

FIGURE 21-5 The rehabilitation team.

rehabilitation teams is shared documentation, weekly summary sheets on which treatment goals and expected client progress are recorded. Rates of discharge to home were increased through the use of shared documentation, and it is thought that the process requires team building and shared ownership, both of which may lead to the improved outcomes (Rosenberg et al., 1986). Although coordination of effort between rehabilitation team members may be difficult to achieve, evidence suggests a comprehensive rehabilitation team positively influences outcomes for older adults (Boult et al., 2001; Cohen et al., 2002; Landefeld, Palmer, Kresevic, Fortinsky, & Kowal, 1995; Reuben et al., 1995; Stuck et al., 1995).

Coordinating the Rehabilitation Team

Case Management

The term **case management** was first used in North America in the 1950s for the provision of care to community-residing clients with psychiatric problems. By the 1980s, case management was embraced as a strategy, along with managed care by American health maintenance organizations (HMOs), to both contain and manage the spiraling costs associated with caring for older adults. Revisions of Medicaid reimbursement rules required case management to be in place for reimbursement of home care in the mid-1990s. In the United Kingdom, case management was adopted in the early 1990s as "care management" in response to national changes to public provision of community care. Models of case management for older adults have also been reported in Australia, Canada, Italy, and Sweden (Bernabei et al., 1998; Hebert, Durand, Dubuc, & Tourigny, 2003; Hokenstad & Johansson, 1996; Lim, Lambert, & Gray, 2003).

Case management is based on the assumption that people with complex health problems need assistance in using the health care system effectively and efficiently. Older adults often use multiple health care providers and require varied social services to help them live independently. During the course of rehabilitation, many clients will require services from several health care professionals. In order to ensure that the correct interventions are applied in the correct order, and that complications, delays, and duplications are avoided, a large number of decisions will have to be coordinated. This means that decisions must be made in full awareness of many other client care issues, such client preferences, postdischarge resources in the client's home, availability of family and caregivers, community resources, and so forth. Case management assumes that no single health professional involved in the care of a client can be sure to take into account all of these issues, in addition to considering how a client's own values and life situations may affect their choices and priorities for care.

The case management approach appoints an individual or a small team, who may or may not also be responsible for the direct provision of hands-on care, to take responsibility for guiding the client through this complex process in the most efficient, effective, and acceptable way. **Case managers** facilitate communication between health care providers and ensure that services are not duplicated, while required services are provided. Thus, case management offers a practical, one-step approach to helping clients coordinate their care. There is no widely agreed model of case management. However, different models employ nurses, nurse practitioners, social workers, or other health care professionals, such as occupational or physical therapists, to be case managers. Studies in the United Kingdom, Italy, and the United States have found positive benefits to using a case management approach for older adults, including decreased levels of institutional care, high levels of client satisfaction, less functional decline, and lower levels of hospital admission rates (Bernabei et al., 1998; Knapp et al., 1992; Marshall, Long, Voss, Demma, & Skerl, 1999).

The Occupational Therapy/Physical Therapy Partnership

The unique partnership between the professions of occupational therapy and physical therapy developed from the growth of rehabilitation medicine after World War II. At that time, Seidel (1998) indicates the rehabilitation movement was oriented toward helping individuals with chronic illnesses and conditions to live productive lives and initiated the use of the treatment team made up of professionals trained in rehabilitation.

Treischmann (1987) suggests that the field of rehabilitation pioneered the multidisciplinary approach to treatment.

Current clinical practice resonates with themes of collaboration, ranging from merely knowing what the other profession does to being able to share tasks interprofessionally. Given expectations by regulatory professional bodies and the present sharing of expertise at a clinical level, it becomes critical to educate rehabilitation therapists for future interdisciplinary practice. Because of the shared bodies of knowledge between occupational and physical therapy, interdisciplinary education with these two professions has been tried in a variety of situations. For example, in Canada, as early as 1935, LeVesconte envisioned a shared core curriculum combining occupational with physical therapy. Joint curricula in physical and occupational therapy graduating combined trained professionals began in the 1940s but were gradually phased out across Canada by 1983, although many rehabilitation programs continue interdisciplinary courses between the professions (Tryssenaar, Perkins, & Brett, 1996). Saarinen and Salvatori (1994) argue that there are many advantages to joint education, including strengthened communication between the professions and an educational reflection of future health care practice. A survey by Tryssenaar, Perkins, and Brett (1996) exploring interdisciplinary educational activities in entry-level curricula reflects many of the trends indicated in the literature: interdisciplinary education is regularly included, valued at multiple institutional levels, is being maintained or expanded, and is integrated into regular curriculum. The shared history of the professions, the common bodies of knowledge, and the focus on rehabilitation grounded in ongoing entry-level and continuing education experiences anchor the occupational therapy and physical therapy partnership (Figures 21-6).

Delivery Systems

Rehabilitation can be carried out in a variety of settings, such as in a hospital, an outpatient clinic, in the client's home, or in other settings in the community. However, settings are characterized internationally by wide variation in availability, type, level, scope, and content of care provided. For example, in the United Kingdom,

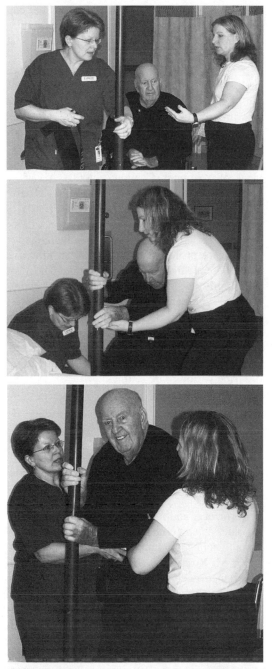

FIGURE 21-6 Physical and occupational therapists often co-treat to achieve a client's rehabilitation goals. (Courtesy of the Geriatric Day Hospital, specialized Geriatric Services, Saskatoon Health Region, Saskatoon, Saskatchewan, with permission.)

rehabilitation services can be classified under an umbrella term "intermediate care." Intermediate care is a range of services designed to facilitate transition from hospital to home and from medical independence to functional independence

(Steiner, 1997), and models of service can include community assessment and rehabilitation teams, "hospital at home," "hospice at home," rapid response teams, and nurse-led units (Lees, 2004). Scope of services within each setting can vary from community to community, with larger metropolitan communities offering more specialized services compared to rural community settings, and intensity of services can range from 1 to 8 hours a day and 1 to 3 days per week of treatment to 7 days per week of treatment (Capilouto, 2000). A variety of external factors, including reimbursement, can affect rehabilitation care differentially across settings (McCue & Thompson, 1995; Mitchell & Scott, 1992). Thus, the challenge for health care professionals is to deliver effective and efficient care regardless of setting. The most thoroughly studied aspect of older adult rehabilitation is the care setting, and better outcomes have consistently been shown for older clients treated in specialized units (Cohen et al,. 2002; Stuck, Siu, Wieland, Adams, & Rubenstein, 1993). Chapters 18, 19, 20, and 22 further describe various care settings.

Acute Care

Many older adults become disabled by an acute illness such as a stroke, fractured neck or femur, or pneumonia and require emergency hospital admission for medical care. Acute hospitalization is often associated with a decrease in occupational performance, and research has found up to 50% of older hospitalized patients experience functional decline (Bergman et al., 1997; Hebert, 1997; M. Rosenberg & Moore, 1997), one-third experience declines in their ability to perform ADLs, and only half of these individuals returned to their preadmission level of function 3 months following discharge (Sager et al., 1996). In the acute care setting, medical stabilization and determination of a medical diagnosis is the priority, and management may include surgery, medication, and initiation of therapies. Due to cost factors, older adults requiring longer-term rehabilitation are usually referred to other settings/facilities for management. Thus, a typical route of entry to rehabilitation is through an acute-care, community-based hospital. Because length of stay is often short, the role of the therapist in the acute-care setting is often to assist in the identification of appropriate discharge plans, and

planning for discharge usually begins at the initial therapy visit. In the United States, billing fees are prospectively based on preestablished rates, **prospective payment service (PPS)** that involve the type and amount of intervention required for a specific diagnostic-related group (DRG).

Transitional Care Facilities and Units

Transitional care facilities and units provide intermediate care or post-acute care. In the United States, skilled nursing facilities (SNFs), subacute units, or transitional care units are the most commonly described settings, however they vary in the degrees of services provided. Medicare-certified SNF units may be located in free-standing nursing homes or in hospitals, although hospital units are commonly referred to as subacute, swing bed, transitional care, or restorative care units. Clients cannot access SNF units directly without a hospital stay. Need for rehabilitation is a major criterion that qualifies an individual for SNF, and although clients in SNF settings must receive daily rehabilitation skilled services such as PT, OT, or SLT, no time requirement for that therapy is imposed. Clients must demonstrate measurable progress during the duration of the stay, and thorough documentation is essential to demonstrate the need for continued care. Over the past decade, with Medicare's shift to a PPS for skilled nursing facilities and encouragement of incentives for HMOs to provide care under contract with Medicare, there has been a decrease in the duration and intensity of therapy provided to patients in SNFs.

Rehabilitation Units

Characteristically, **geriatric rehabilitation units** (GRUs) are distinct units housed within community hospitals, free-standing rehabilitation hospitals, or long-term care facilities and are staffed by multidisciplinary teams specializing in the management of the medical, social, physical, psychological, and economic well-being of older adults. The philosophy of GRUs emphasizes both the physical and emotional elements of client care (Hoenig, Nusbaum, & Brummel-Smith, 1997). **Geriatric assessment units (GAUs)** and GRUs have many similarities, as both provide rehabilitation with an interdisciplinary team trained in the care of the elderly, with attention to medical, psychosocial, and functional issues. Management plans are established and reviewed in regular team meetings with therapeutic and rehabilitative teams. However in a GAU, there tends to be more emphasis on medical treatment and evaluation, and rehabilitation goals are usually short term. Within a GRU, there is a greater emphasis on longer-term rehabilitation and achieving maximal function (Wells, Seabrook, Stolee, Borrie, & Knoefel, 2003b).

In the United States, for clients to be admitted to a rehabilitation unit, they must be medically stable and able to tolerate at least 3 hours of intervention a day, 5 or 6 days a week. As with transitional care facilities, clients must demonstrate measurable progress during the duration of the stay, and thorough documentation is essential to demonstrate the need for continued care. Once clients have maximized their rehabilitation potential, they may be discharged home, and if returning home is not feasible, then a long-term-care facility is the typical discharge placement. Discharge to a long-term-care facility can be predicted by the presence of medical complications, lower functional status at discharge from the acute facility, and severity of impaired gait status. In long-term care, individuals may participate in less-intense therapy programs and may later be transferred to a rehabilitation unit. As described in Chapter 22, rehabilitation units may often be located in long-term care facilities.

Day Hospital Care/Adult Day Care Facilities

The first day hospital (UK term) for older adults was opened in the United Kingdom in 1952 (Farndale, 1961) and developed rapidly in the 1960s as an important component of older adult-care provision designed to augment inpatient services. The model has since been widely applied in New Zealand, Australia, Canada, the United States, and several European countries. Day hospitals have served several functions, including assessment, rehabilitation, maintenance, provision of medical, nursing, and social services, and respite care (Brocklehurst & Tucker, 1980); however, rehabilitation and maintenance tend to be the main focus of most day hospitals, and rehabilitation has been regarded as the most important function (Brocklehurst, 1995).

Adult day care (U.S. term) programs offer an alternative to institutionalization for newly or chronically disabled adults who cannot stay alone during the day, but who do not need 24-hour inpatient care. Designed to promote maximum independence, clients usually attend on a scheduled basis, and services may include nursing, counseling, social services, restorative services, medical and health care monitoring, medication administration, well-balanced meals, and transportation to and from the facility, exercise programs, field trips, recreational activities, in addition to occupational, physical, and speech therapy. Day hospitals can also provide respite services for family members and caregivers. The Program of All-Inclusive Care for the Elderly (PACE), described in Chapter 18, is a U.S. federally supported project designed to increase the availability of day care programs, as an alternative to institutionalization. A variety of services are provided, including distribution of prescription drugs, physician services, rehabilitation services, personal care, socialization and leisure activities, hospitalization, and nursing home care. Additionally, case management, extended home care, and respite care may be provided.

Day services have been found to decrease primary-caregiver stress and improve psychological function (Zarit, Stephens, Townsend, & Greene, 1998), and evidence suggests day hospital care appears to be an effective outpatient service for older people, but no more effective and possibly more expensive than other forms of comprehensive care for older adults (Forster, Langhorn & Young, 1999).

Home Health/Domiciliary Care

Home health care is provided in the client's residence and is recognized as an increasingly important alternative to hospitalization or care in a nursing home for older adults who do not need 24-hour professional supervision. Many older adults find it possible to remain at home for the entire duration of rehabilitation or at least to shorten their hospital stay with the provision of home health care. Interestingly, studies have found that relatively modest levels of home care therapy are associated with benefits (Gladman, Forster, & Young, 1995). A variety of health services can be provided in a home-health-care program, and it has been found that older adults receiving rehabilitation in their home (compared to hospital) took more initiative in expressing and determining their own goals (von Koch, Wottrich, & Holmvist, 1998).

In the United States, older adults qualify for home health care based on the need for "home confinement," as certified by a physician, and the need for skilled nursing or therapy, including OT and PT. The physician is required to recertify the continued need for skilled care, and the criteria for skilled therapy service are the same as those for SNF.

Outpatient Care/Ambulatory Care

Outpatient rehabilitation can be provided in a number of settings, including hospitals, free-standing clinics, private practices, and in **comprehensive outpatient rehabilitation facilities (CORFs).** CORFs offer a more comprehensive array of services than typical outpatient rehabilitation settings and utilize interdisciplinary team goals (Capilouto, 2000). Use of interdisciplinary teams in outpatient settings has been shown to improve functional outcomes and increase patient satisfaction with care. Toseland and colleagues (1996) compared frail older patients assigned to outpatient geriatric assessment and management with patients receiving usual outpatient primary care. The patients receiving team assessment and management reported higher satisfaction with the services. Outpatient rehabilitation requires that evaluation effectively select those individuals who have potential for improvement (Rodriguez & Goldberg, 1993), and a description of various community agencies can be found in Chapter 19.

Respite Care

The provision of short-term, periodic relief to families caring for dependent older adults offers tremendous potential for maintaining individuals in a familiar and least restrictive environment. Respite care services can vary in time from part of a day to several weeks and can be offered by hospitals, religious and nonreligious affiliated programs, nursing homes, in day service programs, home health care, or through volunteer service.

Palliative Care

The World Health Organization defines **palliative care** as ". . . the active total care of patients whose disease is not responsive to curative treatment. Control of pain, of other symptoms, and of psychological, social and spiritual problems is paramount. The goal of palliative care is achievement of the best possible quality of life for patients and their families" (The World Health Organization Expert Committee, 1990, p. 11). Rehabilitation in the context of palliative care does not aim to reverse the terminal illness, but rather helps restore the individual to optimal functioning and well-being, within the limits imposed by the disease process. Hospice care is an approach to caring for terminally ill individuals that stresses palliation. The emphasis of hospice care is on keeping the client at home with family and friends as long as possible, and pain and symptom control are a major focus. Although the vast majority of hospice services are provided in the individual's home, hospices may be located as a part of a hospital, nursing home, SNF, or home health agency. In the United States, hospices must meet specific federal requirements and be separately certified and approved for Medicare participation, and individuals are usually admitted if they have a prognosis of 6 months or less to live. See Chapter 26 for more information on terminal illness and palliative care.

Evaluation

Chapter 17 provides extensive detail regarding the purposes of assessing older adults, a philosophy of client-centered and contextually based assessment, issues specific to older adults when considering assessment, and different methods used to assess older adults. Within a rehabilitation context, a standardized and comprehensive assessment is important to ensure the systematic evaluation of the older adult, the identification of relevant problems requiring further investigation and treatment, the facilitation of care planning, and collection of data to allow quality improvement and research to be conducted (Royal College of Physicians and British Geriatrics Society, 1992).

Although a systematic screening assessment is useful to identify potential problems that may be modified, findings of screening assessments indicate the need for further evaluation and assist in directing a more comprehensive assessment. In rehabilitation settings, a **comprehensive geriatric assessment (CGA)** tends to be the norm and is often viewed as an approach designed to improve the health of the older adult and defines care for this client population (Rubenstein, 2004). Many older adults who require rehabilitation have several conditions of varying severity. Thus, identifying the components impacting on function and occupational performance problems and developing an individualized management plan can be challenging. Since its development in the United Kingdom, CGA has been introduced and adopted in many other countries and is conducted in a variety of settings, such as hospital, home, and nursing homes, and with varying program types and levels of intensity, such as hospital **geriatric evaluation units (GEUs),** geriatric assessment units (GAUs) or **geriatric evaluation and management services (GEMs), acute care for the elderly units (ACE),** hospital consultation teams, outpatient brief screening assessment programs, or intensive in-home assessment and case management programs (Rubenstein, 2004).

Comprehensive geriatric assessment is a multidimensional, interdisciplinary process that is used to determine an elderly person's medical, psychosocial, functional, and environmental needs resources and problems, and is linked with an overall plan for management and follow-up. CGA helps health care professionals determine and prioritize problems, develop long- and short-term plans of care, and implement rehabilitation strategies that optimize management, improve function and outcomes, prevent further deterioration, optimize living location, decrease unnecessary health care resources and service use, arrange long-term case management, and prolong survival of older adults. CGA has a number of major measurable dimensions, usually grouped into the domains of (1) physical health (e.g., traditional history and physical examination, medical assessment, nutritional assessment, medication review, laboratory data, disease-specific severity indicators, and preventive health practices); (2) functional status (e.g., ADL, IADL, and other functional status as mobility and quality of life); (3) psychological health (mainly cognitive and affective status), and, (4) socioenvironmental parameters (e.g., social networks and supports, economics, and environmental safety, adequacy, and needs) (Rubenstein, 2004).

Stuck and colleagues have reported that there is evidence regarding the effectiveness of comprehensive assessment of older adults carried out by a multidisciplinary team. In a meta-analysis of 28 controlled trials (8 in the United Kingdom, 15 in North America, 3 in Sweden, 1 in Denmark, and 1 in Australia) of comprehensive assessment of older persons in a hospital inpatient unit, comprehensive assessment resulted in improved cognitive and physical function, decreased mortality, decreased subsequent readmissions, and increased numbers of people living at home (Stuck et al., 1993).

Assessment Instruments

Rehabilitation outcomes for older adults not only should measure individuals' performance in functioning domains, but should also evaluate the extent to which older adults participate in valued life activities. There are numerous widely known and widely used standardized tools that can be used to assess the older adult in a rehabilitation setting. In the United States, some assessments are mandatory, such as the Long-Term Care Minimum Data Set, for clients admitted to certain settings (see Chapter 22 for more information). One must keep in mind that although assessment tools are important for data collection, relying too heavily on numeric scores can oversimplify a situation and shift attention away from the individual and his or her abilities within the context of his or her particular situation (Gudmundsson & Carnes, 1996). Some commonly used assessment instruments are described below.

ADL and IADL are carefully documented in a CGA and in the older adult rehabilitation setting. The Barthel Index assesses the level of independence or dependence for 10 activities of daily living using an ordinal scale. It is quick and easy to use and has been well researched (Mahoney & Barthel, 1965). The main disadvantages of the Barthel Index are that it can be insensitive to change (patients may improve or deteriorate without a change in score) and it has a low "ceiling" (patients may have a maximum score but still be restricted). The Katz ADL scale assesses a client's ability to function in six areas using a three-point scale and can be completed by the patient or caregiver (Katz, 1983). It is brief, reliable, and valid but is not very sensitive to change. The IADL Scale examines eight areas of self-performance including the ability to use a telephone, shop, prepare food, complete housework, do laundry, utilize public transportation, administer medication, and handle financial responsibilities (Lawton & Brody, 1969) and has proven to be valid and reliable in the older population. The Functional Independence Measure (FIM®) (Research Foundation of the State University of New York, 1987) assesses functional status in six domains including self-care, sphincter control, mobility, locomotion, communication, and social cognition. The tool has 18 items and each is rated on a seven-point scale ranging from completely dependent (1) to completely independent (7). Total FIM scores can range from 18 for complete dependency in all areas of functional ability to 126 for independence in all measures. The validity and reliability of the FIM have been extensively reported (Kidd & Yoshida, 1995; Reker, O'Donnell, & Hamilton, 1998; Research Foundation of the State University of New York, 1987).

Tests of specific function are also commonly used. Assessment of gait and balance is one example. The timed up and go (TUG) test involves timing a client as he or she rises from a chair, walks 3 meters, turns around, walks back to the chair, and sits down (Podsiadlo & Richardson, 1991). The TUG has good inter- and intra-rater reliability and validity, and time taken to complete the test is strongly correlated to level of functional mobility (Podsiadlo & Richardson, 1991; Rockwood, Awalt, Carver, & MacKnight, 2000). The Berg Balance Scale (BBS) is a 14-item battery consisting of everyday life balance and mobility activities. The items are graded on a scale of 0 to 4, giving a total of 56 points, with higher scores representing better performance. The BBS has good test–retest, inter- and intra-rater reliability, and has been validated for use in older adults (Berg, Maki, Williams, Holliday, & Wood-Dauphinee, 1992; Berg, Wood-Dauphinee, Williams, & Gayton, 1989; Berg, Wood-Dauphinee, Williams, & Maki, 1992).

Assessing cognitive status and the presence of depression are essential as part of a CGA. The best-known measure of cognition is the Mini-Mental Status Exam (MMSE) (Folstein, Folstein, & McHugh, 1975). The MMSE was developed as a brief tool for the examination of cognitive impairment in older adults and is also used for screening dementia. It has been extensively validated, is easy to administer, and has been standardized (Molloy, Alemayehu, & Roberts, 1991). There are several assessment tools that are used to assess symptoms of depression, including the Geriatric Depression Scale (GDS) (Yesavage et al., 1983), the Hamilton Depression Rating Scale (Hamilton, 1960), the Beck Depression Inventory (Beck, 1967), and the Beck Depression Inventory–Fast Screen (Beck, Guth, Steer, & Ball, 1997). The GDS is commonly used, and there are 5-point, 15-point, and 30-point versions available. The Beck Depression Inventory–Fast Screen was developed to permit more rapid detection of depression in the primary care setting for individuals with medical diagnoses (Beck, Guth, Steer, & Ball, 1997; Steer, Cavalieri, Douglas, & Beck, 1999). See Chapters 9 and 10 for further discussion of cognitive and depression assessment tools.

The Medical Outcomes Study 36-item Short Form (SF-36) is a multidimensional generic quality-of-life measure (Ware & Sherbourne, 1992) that is widely used to measure health status in older adults. It consists of 36 items in eight subscales: physical functioning, limitations due to physical health problems (role, physical), bodily pain, general health, vitality, social functioning, limitations due to emotional health problems (role, emotional), and mental health. Subscores are transformed to a scale of 0 to 100, with higher scores representing better health status.

Personal and Environmental Factors to Consider

Assisting older adult clients in reaching their goals and optimizing service delivery within the current constraints of the health care system requires an understanding of the factors that facilitate or impede the rehabilitation process. Most rehabilitation studies have focused on demographic variables, mental status, mood, and functional status on admission as predictors of rehabilitation outcomes. Age (Mossey, Mutran, Knott, & Craik, 1989), evidence of social support (Cummings et al., 1988; Magaziner, Simonsick, Kashner, Hebel, & Kenzora, 1990), admission function (Resnick & Daly, 1998), and interruptions in the rehabilitation process (Heinemann, Linacre, Wright, Hamilton, & Granger, 1994) have been found to be statistically significant predictors of function following rehabilitation. Specifically, those that are younger, have better function on admission, are able to complete their rehabilitation course without interruptions due to acute illness, surgery, or financial problems, and are more likely to have higher function at discharge from a rehabilitation program. In addition, cognitive status and depression have been found to be significantly correlated with lower levels of functional ability at the time of discharge from rehabilitation (Harris, O'Hara, & Harper, 1995; Resnick & Daly, 1998). It is important to note that most study findings are mixed, and jointly the above predictor variables only account for a small portion of the variance (Patrick, Knoefel, Gaskowski, & Rexroth, 2001).

Personal Factors that May Impact Rehabilitation

Age

Age is a factor believed to affect rehabilitation outcomes, but research findings suggest that clients should not be excluded from rehabilitation by age alone, and that regardless of age, older adults can benefit from rehabilitation. Some studies have found age to influence rehabilitation outcomes, and others have shown that age does not predict length of stay (LOS) or functional improvements (Rondinelli, Murphy, Wilson, & Miller, 1991). Adults 75 years old or older showed worse admission and discharge function than younger individuals; however, they were still able to demonstrate improvements in functional gain (Diamond, Felsenthal, Macciocchi, Butler, & Lally-Cassady, 1996; Falconer, Naughton, Strasser, & Sinacore, 1994). In studies that controlled for medical comorbidities, age alone did not explain rehabilitation outcomes (Patrick et al., 2001). People 80 years old or older were observed to have a longer length of stay (LOS) and were less likely to be discharged to home after rehabilitation in Sweden, in contrast to a shorter LOS reported in the United States (Ceder, Thorngren, & Wallden, 1980; Falconer et al., 1994), a discrepancy that might be related to differences in the health care systems in those countries.

Frailty

A more important factor that may determine rehabilitation outcomes is frailty. The interplay of frailty, dependence, and disability has been noted, and it is generally agreed that frailty is a pathological state that leads to physical impairments, functional limitations, and disability (Leveille, Fried, McMullen, & Guralnik, 2004). Thus, frailty implies a diminished capacity to perform ADL (Brown, Renwick, & Raphael, 1995). The term *frailty* is widely used clinically and in research settings, yet there is no one definition (Markle-Reid & Browne, 2003). The combination of inactivity and weight loss often characterizes frailty (Chin et al., 1999), although many other factors have been associated with the condition. Frailty has been characterized as a multisystem or multidimensional impairment that results in instability, a decline in physical function, and an increased risk for adverse outcomes (Bortz, 2002; Fried, Ferrucci, Darer, Williamson, & Anderson, 2004; Markle-Reid & Browne, 2003; Rockwood, Hogan, & MacKnight, 2000). It encompasses deterioration in multiple organ systems, including musculoskeletal, cardiovascular, metabolic, and immunologic systems, which results from and contributes to declining physical function (Bortz, 2002).

Motivation

Poor rehabilitation outcomes are often attributed to the lack of motivation on the part of the client (Stoedefalke, 1985). *"When people say that someone is not motivated, they usually mean that they do not understand why that person is acting a certain way, that they do not condone his or her actions, or that his or her actions go against sociocultural norms"* (Kemp, 1988, p. 42). Motivation has been found to be important in older adults' recovery from disabling events (Geelen & Soons, 1996; Resnick, 1998a) and in older adults' continued performance of functional activities (Resnick, 1998b, 1999). There are numerous theories of motivation which try to explain why people behave as they do, what sustains and directs a person's attention, and what arouses and instigates behavior, gives direction or purposes to behavior, continues to allow behavior to persist, or leads one to choose or prefer a particular behavior. Motivation should not be confused with **adherence,** the extent to which a client follows a health care professional's advice or recommendations.

One theory used to explain why people behave the way they do is the theory of self-efficacy (Bandura, 1977, 1986). Self-efficacy refers to the state of belief of one's ability(ies), which in turn will affect one's belief about future accomplishments. In other words, personal evaluations of one's own performance capabilities on a particular task or activity will affect one's motivation to perform that task and will influence the outcome expectations related to the task or activity. A very interesting qualitative study used semistructured interviews to examine how self-efficacy and outcome expectations are strengthened and how these expectations influenced motivation and behavior in 77 older adults (55 females, 22 males) in a rehabilitation program (Resnick, 2002). Some of the key findings of this study and sample strategies for addressing key areas are summarized in Table 21-1.

Depression

Depression in older adults is common, is associated with functional disability, tends to be undertreated, and can be a significant barrier to rehabilitation. The incidence of depression in geriatric inpatient rehabilitation settings has been estimated to range from 20% to 63% (Fitz & Teri, 1994; Galynker et al., 2000). Whether or not there is a correlation of depression with function at admission or discharge from rehabilitation remains to be elucidated (Fitz & Teri, 1994;

Harris, Mion, Patterson, & Frengley, 1988; Johnson, Kramer, Lin, Kowalsky, & Steiner, 2000; Resnick & Daly, 1998). For example, depression has not been found to be associated with functional gain (Gillen, Tennen, McKee, Gernert-Dott, & Affleck, 2001; Harris, Mion, Patterson, & Frengley, 1988) but was related to lower **rehabilitation efficiency,** the amount of functional gains per day of service, and longer LOS (Galynker et al., 2000). The limited number of studies and wide variability in study designs, populations, and settings preclude conclusions about the effects of depression on rehabilitation outcomes in elders. However, the therapist must not ignore the possibility of undiagnosed depression being present prior to or during the rehabilitation experience.

Cognitive Status

Older adults with cognitive impairments often have problems with being admitted to or reimbursed for rehabilitation services (Department of Health & Human Services, 2001), most

---

TABLE 21-1 Personal Expectation and Self-Efficacy Factors that Affect Motivation and Strategies that can be Used to Motivate the Older Adult in Rehabilitation

Personal Expectations Themes		Strategies
Specific beliefs about ability (*self-efficacy*)	" I just do it (walk). I just go ahead and do it. I believed I could do it, so I just go on and do it." " I was just scared and frightened on the stairs, and just don't think I can do it. Maybe after I get home, but right now, I can't even think about the stairs."	Explore and determine a client's belief by asking: "If you _____, what are you afraid might happen?"; "When you think of _____, what do you think of?";
Specific beliefs about outcomes (*outcome expectations*)	"I was sure the therapy would help, but I didn't think that I could do it. I gave it a try and I learned that I could do it. You can do a lot if you just try." "No matter how hard you try and how much therapy you get at 93, there is a limit to what you can get out of it. At 93, I just don't expect to get stronger."	"Why don't you want to _____? Assist with reinterpretation of signs and symptoms (cognitive restructuring) Allow client to verbally express emotional factors and beliefs associated with activities
General beliefs about outcomes (*general outcome expectations*)	"I realize it is just going to take some time for this thing to heal up. It won't be too long before I will start to get around again. Once it heals I will be able to walk."	Explain to client what he or she can expect

Information that Influenced Efficacy Beliefs		Strategies
Role models	"When there are other people exposed to the same thing as you are, it does motivate you as you know that you are not in it alone." "I saw the other people in therapy and was doing the same things as them. It didn't affect me. I kept my mind on what I was doing."	Treat client in group settings Introduce client to someone who has successfully completed rehabilitation Introduce client to someone who has similar problems
Verbal encouragement	"The encouragement helped me believe that I could do it. She said, 'you are not going to have any trouble with the steps. We are going to make it easy!' And I didn't have any trouble at all with those steps. Her telling me I could do it helped a lot." "Encouraging me along helped a lot. Oh, just try it one time. You know. Like lifting my leg. I thought I'd never get that done but I figured she wouldn't tell me to do it if I couldn't so I gave it a try."	Use positive verbal and nonverbal communication Design activities that are challenging, but reasonable in terms of the client's capabilities
Progress	"When I saw the improvements I was making, that helped me keep going and helped me do a little bit more. Since the exercises in therapy helped, when I got back to the room I would sit here and try to do the exercises some more to help me."	Inform client of positive objective findings Remind client of capabilities Break skills into very small, manageable tasks; ensure each small task is successfully completed
Past experiences	"I have had other experiences with rehab and I have made it before, so that kind of helped."	Remind client of past successes
Spiritually	"Nobody knows but I said to myself, 'God, if it be your will help me make it to the top of the stairs and I will try and help myself down.'"	Respect client's spiritual needs Listen to and support expressions of spirituality
Physical sensations	"Today I feel crummy and I don't think I can make it through the therapy today. Not today. I am just too tired." "The pain stopped me. I just couldn't push over the pain. The therapists were wonderful. If I could, I would get up, but the pain stops me." "The pain was there but I worked through it. I knew the therapist was trying to help me, and I knew I had to do the therapy to get stronger."	Identify and decrease any physical discomfort associated with an activity (e.g., coordinate treatment sessions with pain medication)
Social supports	"I could not have done it without my family. They were here to help me, and help pass the time." "My family helped me to get the things ready to go home. I think they also gave me moral support."	Encourage family member and caregiver participation in rehabilitation
Individualized care	"She (the therapist) found out that I wasn't feeling well yesterday. She came to get me when I was lying on the bed and I needed to get my shoes on or something. Anyhow, she told me that she had someone	Ensure treatment environment is perceived as sensitive to the client's individual needs Provide opportunities for the client to have some choice and control over activities

continued on page 532

TABLE 21-1 **Personal Expectation and Self-Efficacy Factors that Affect Motivation and Strategies that can be Used to Motivate the Older Adult in Rehabilitation** (continued)

Information that Influenced Efficacy Beliefs		Strategies
	else she could take and she would come back and get me. She told me to get some rest. I did a lot better after resting. I felt that she was concerned about how I felt. That made a lot of difference."	
Personality	"I got that determination and willpower. They used to tell me I was awful strong. What you can do yourself you shouldn't ask other people to do."	Recognize and respect differences among clients
	"I just made up my mind I was going to do it. I guess that is just the way I am. When I set my mind to something I am just going to do it. I am going to get this much done or that much done. I have done hard work all my life."	Realize you cannot change someone's personality or who a person is; you can only change how you respond to someone
		Work with client's individual strengths
Goals	"I want to get better to be able to take care of myself like I could before."	Explore what is important to the client; what the client wants and why
	"I want to be able to drive my car."	
	"I like to be able to go to the mall and have lunch."	Help client set appropriate and attainable goals that have meaning to him or her
	"When I first came in I had a goal, but I wasn't happy with it. I just wanted to stay put and forget about everything."	Set short-term and long-term goals

Personal Expectations Themes. Data from Resnick, B. (2002). Geriatric rehabilitation: The influence of efficacy beliefs and motivation, *Rehabilitation Nursing*, 27 (4), 152–159.

likely due to evidence that suggests the odds of successful rehabilitation outcomes in those with cognitive impairments to be lower than those without dementia. People with dementia are capable of learning through implicit pathways (Dick et al., 1996; Eslinger & Damasio, 1986; Zanetti et al., 1997), can acquire motor skills normally (Bondi & Kaszniak, 1991; Hirono et al., 1996), and can retain such skills for a period of time (Dick, Nielson, Beth, Shankle, & Cotman, 1995; Mochizuki-Kawai et al., 2004). Even those with moderate to severe dementia can show improvements in motor learning and maintain improvements for over a month (Dick et al., 1996).

Although severity of cognitive impairment has been found to be related to higher mortality and less successful return to independent living, the evidence related to cognitive impairment and positive rehabilitation outcomes is equivocal. For example, some studies have found cognitive impairment not to be associated with rehabilitation efficiency or daily functional gains (Gillen et al., 2001), and others have found cognitive impairment to be associated with worse rehabilitation efficiency (Heruti, Lusky, Barell, Ohry, & Adunsky, 1999; Zwecker et al., 2002).

Comorbidities

As discussed previously, many older adults have one or more chronic conditions. Physical and psychologic comorbidities have been shown to contribute to poorer functional gain, lower rehabilitation efficiency, longer LOS, and higher rates of institutionalization in inpatient rehabilitation settings only when five or more medical comorbidities were present (Ceder et al., 1980; Patrick et al., 2001; Rodriguez & Goldberg,

1993). Primary rehabilitation diagnoses tend to influence the effects of medical comorbidities on rehabilitation outcomes (Patrick et al., 2001).

Environmental Factors that May Impact Rehabilitation

Family Members and Caregivers

Family members and caregivers are an integral part of the care team. They know the older adult and can often provide additional information about the older person's perspectives, habits, behaviors, and needs; can provide emotional and instrumental support; and can facilitate adherence to treatment recommendations. Conflicts may arise if the goals of the older adult and family and caregivers differ. Full-time care of an aging spouse or relative can be stressful, and often the spouse also has a chronic illness or disability (Brown, McWilliam, & Mai, 1997). Some caregivers are also part of the sandwich generation, a generation of people who are caring for their aging parents while supporting their own children. Williams (2004) identifies these individuals as often dealing with the conflicting demands of raising children and caring for aging parents or other relatives.

If the family member is the older person's chief caregiver, he or she may be depressed, anxious, and need support services as well. Psychological and physical health problems are common in caregivers (Canwath & Johnson, 1987; Wade, Leigh-Smith, & Hewer, 1986), caregiver burden can be high, and burnout can and does occur. Research related to caregiving has found that many family caregivers report loss or curtailment of employment, and feelings of anger, apprehension, guilt, and social alienation (Biegel, Milligan, Putman, & Song, 1994; Braithwaite, 1992; Zarit, Zarit, & Rosenberg, 1990). The underprovision of adaptive devices and equipment has led some caregivers to improvise with potentially dangerous home-made gadgets designed to assist with transfers, toileting, and self-care (Brown & Mulley, 1997a). Deficiencies in caregiver training about safe handling skills and consequent risk of injury (Brown & Mulley, 1997b) are also areas of concern. Thus, in addition to the older client's needs, caregivers' needs require special attention and assessment, and it is important to provide caregivers the resources they need.

Living Arrangements

Whether an activity limitation becomes a participation restriction or not depends on the physical and social environments a person inhabits. For some older adults, there is an increased likelihood of living alone, with limited support systems. The effects of living arrangement on rehabilitation outcomes have not been sufficiently researched and the evidence is unclear. For example, some have reported that living alone was associated with longer inpatient length of stay and less likelihood for being discharged to home (Ceder et al., 1980), but others have disputed these findings (MacNeill, Lichtenberg, & LaBuda, 2000). Therefore, the effect, if any, of living arrangement on rehabilitation outcomes in older adults remains unclear. Regardless, because activity and environment cannot be separated, the way in which the older person's home or discharge environment is designed with respect to safety, accessibility, security, and support of functional performance needs to be considered. Assessment and adaptation of the home environment are essential components of overall rehabilitation management and allow the older adult to age in place.

Therapist–Client Interaction

Young (1996) describes rehabilitation management as being hard or soft (Figure 21-7). Hard interventions are those that are more observable, objective, and can be costed, such as hands-on treatment or direct management of client problems. Soft interventions are those that are not always easily evident or recognizable, but are equally, if not more, important and involve great skill. These skills are the therapeutic skills related to interpersonal communication and encompass the development of a relationship and trust, all of which embody the therapist–client interaction. The therapist acts as a facilitator, assisting the older client to make the most appropriate decisions regarding care. Effective communication skills, a nonjudgmental attitude, respect for the client's wishes and priorities, allowing time for the client to express his or her fears and concerns, and being supportive and encouraging are key aspects of being able to establish an effective therapeutic relationship.

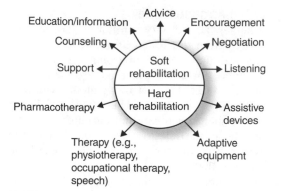

FIGURE 21-7 Hard and soft rehabilitation. (Adapted from Young, J. (1996). Rehabilitation and older people. *British Medical Journal, 313,* 677–681.)

Rehabilitation Reimbursement and Management Issues in the United States

Unlike most other industrialized countries, the United States does not have a single unified system of health care. Health care for older adults is funded by a combination of Medicare, Medicaid, private insurance, or out-of-pocket expenditures. Health care facilities offering rehabilitation services are subject to a plethora of standards and regulations by which they are expected to operate. Standards vary according to the setting in which services are delivered (Capilouto, 2000; Table 21-2) and level and scope of services are often driven by reimbursement

regulations that are subject to change. Reimbursement for rehabilitation services has undergone dramatic change. The Balanced Budget Act (BBA) of 1997 created a prospective payment system (PPS) for all postacute rehabilitation, in order to reduce Medicare expenditures. Resultant rehabilitation practice has been heavily influenced by reimbursement rules, with little empirical research on optimal management, and complex, rapidly changing guidelines and regulations complicate efforts to ensure continuity of care.

Medicare

Medicare is the largest payer of health care services in the United States and is the dominant form of insurance for persons over 65 years of age. Part A Medicare, the hospital insurance, provides for hospital, short-stay skilled nursing facility care, home health, and hospice care. Part B Medicare (Supplementary Medical Insurance) provides coverage for out-patient services, office visits to therapists, and durable medical equipment needs. Medicare payment for reasonable costs for therapy services, including occupational and physical therapy, are continuously updated, and complex regulations include rules about eligibility, dual services, plan of treatment, progress notes, levels of assistance; and documentation of evaluation. Therapists should continuously monitor Medicare reimbursement regulations because revisions occur on a regular basis. It is important for therapists to understand the rules defining skilled and nonskilled services, as

---

TABLE 21-2 Standards for Rehabilitation Services and Settings

Licensure	Set by individual states and directed by state governments
Certification	Examines standards related to facility, fire safety, cleanliness, equipment, personnel
	Federally mandated
	Allows facility to receive payment from Medicare and Medicaid programs
	Specific directives related to care e.g., maintenance of medical records, physician involvement in planning and delivery of care *Joint Commission on Accreditation of Health Care Organizations (JCAHO)*
Accreditation	Performance standards for structure, organization and processes of a wide range of facilities, including those offering rehabilitation services
	Commission on Accreditation of Rehabilitation Facilities (CARF)
	Examines programmatic regulations and provider commitment to quality improvement, in addition to performance standards e.g., personnel qualifications, medical record maintenance, client rights, client education and training

Data from: Capilouto, G.J. (2000). Rehabilitation settings. In: S. Kumar, *Multidisciplinary Approach to Rehabilitation,* pp. 1–26. Butterworth-Heinemann, Boston.

billing Medicare for the provision of nonskilled services is considered fraud.

Managed Care

Since the 1990s, focus has been on persuading Medicare beneficiaries to enroll in managed care programs. Managed care organizations (MCOs) are varied, but all integrate the delivery and financial mechanisms of health care services, by controlling access to health care services and by creating payment mechanisms that encourage efficiency. An HMO is a form of managed care, and HMOs participating in the Medicare program are required to provide a full range of benefits, including post-acute benefits. Bureaucracy of some MCOs may result in lapse of time from referral to treatment, impacting outcomes and further complicating efforts to ensure continuity of care.

Rehabilitation for Older Adults—The Evidence

There is general consensus regarding the benefits of rehabilitation, including preventative rehabilitation for older adults. Although the cost-effectiveness of some kinds of interventions continues to be debated, studies have found rehabilitation for older adults is frequently associated with improved functional abilities and decreased nursing home placement, even for individuals with severe disability or advanced age (Evans, Connis, Hendricks, & Haselkorn, 1995; Harris et al., 1995; Liem, Chernoff, & Carter, 1986; Penington, 1992; Reutter-Bernays & Rentsch, 1993). As discussed in Chapters 6 and 8, research has determined exercise is important for maximizing physical function and for reducing falls (American Geriatrics Society, British Geriatrics Society, and American Academy of Orthopedic Surgeons Panel on Falls Prevention, 2001; Chandler & Hadley, 1996, Feder, Cryer,

Donovan, & Carter, 2000; Province et al., 1995; Schnelle, MacRae, Ouslander, Simmons, & Nitta, 1995). Rehabilitation positively affects physical impairments and functional abilities, especially for older adults with arthritis, general deconditioning, and older adults postamputation, joint replacement, or stroke (Harris et al., 1995; Liem et al., 1986; Wilkinson, Buhrkuhl, & Sainsbury, 1997). Even individuals with cognitive impairments benefit from rehabilitation through improved functional performance and an increase in discharge rates to home (Goldstein, Strasser, Woodard, & Roberts, 1997; Hamman, 1997).

■ Summary

This chapter reviews a broad range of issues essential to the rehabilitation of older adults. Understanding the demographics of older adult disability and the unique aspects of rehabilitation for this population group sets the scene for practice in this area. Rehabilitation to improve or maintain functional and occupational performance can be effective for many older adults. Effective management and care begin with evaluation that includes screening, comprehensive assessment, and careful selection of assessment instruments, regardless of setting. To assist clients, continuity of care can be better facilitated if therapists have a practical understanding of rehabilitation delivery systems, reimbursement issues, practice management concerns, and the unique aspects of rehabilitation in older adults. Personal and environmental factors should not necessarily rule out whether or not an older person can participate in rehabilitation, but need to be carefully considered during the evaluation process and when planning interventions and deciding on the appropriate rehabilitation setting. The evidence strongly suggests that rehabilitation is beneficial for a variety of diagnostic conditions that affect older persons.

C a s e   S t u d y

Mr. King is a 68-year-old man with a grade 4 glioblastoma. He has a rapid-onset dense left hemiplegia and is being seen by home care nursing, physical therapy, and occupational therapy under the palliative care program. In June, a craniotomy was done to debulk the tumor. After surgery he discharged himself, against medical recommendations that he stay for inpatient rehabilitation.

continued on page 536

Case Study (continued)

On his arrival home, you received an urgent request from your colleagues to clarify his new mobility/transfer status for the Home Support Workers (HSW). On your arrival, it was clear the family were hoping for intensive in-home rehabilitation, and in fact expected Mr. King to walk again. Examination revealed grade 1 to 2 strength in scattered leg muscles and a flaccid left arm. Mr. King was unable to sit unsupported. Standing pivot transfers were maximum lift × 2, so you recommended use of the mechanical lift be resumed. These findings were essentially unchanged from Mr. King's preoperative status. You explain to the family that you could not provide intensive rehabilitation, but that you could teach the HSWs range of motion and facilitation exercises, and that you could see him weekly at best, with ongoing reevaluation.

Over the succeeding 3 months, you have seen Mr. King eight times and there has been no motor or sensory recovery. There have been very small functional gains—Mr. King is now able to roll to his weak side in bed using the bedrail. Mr. King has variable wheelchair sitting tolerance (10 to 60 minutes). Last week, Mrs. King asked you about admission to a rehabilitation facility to capitalize on these gains. You told her you did not feel Mr. King was likely to be accepted. The King's planned to approach their physician with the request. You sent the physician a letter describing your clinical findings. You have not yet heard back from the family or the doctor.

Questions

1. Tell the story from the person's perspective—the therapist, the client, and the wife/family member. Give each story a title.
2. What else do you need to know?
3. What advice would you like to give this circle of care?
4. Is the scenario describing rehabilitation? If yes, why? If not, why not?

Review Questions

1. In your own words, describe rehabilitation.
2. What are the unique features of rehabilitation for older adults?
3. What is the difference between a multidisciplinary team, an interdisciplinary team, and a transdisciplinary team?
4. What are the benefits of using a team approach in older adult rehabilitation?
5. Why is it important to use a comprehensive approach when assessing an older adult?
6. Discuss at least five strategies that may be beneficial in motivating an older adult.
7. Compare and contrast the various rehabilitation settings.
8. Consider the following two client cases and answer the following questions:
   a. What personal and environmental factors may influence rehabilitation for Mr. Williams and Mrs. Peters?
   b. Describe the potential continuum of rehabilitation settings for Mr. Williams and Mrs. Peters.

Client #1: Mr. Williams

Mr. Williams is a 77-year-old man who retired from teaching at age 65. He remains active in an informal group of retired teachers who meet weekly for breakfast. This group also organizes a monthly dinner or special event to which spouses and guests are invited. He has been an avid reader and sports fan throughout his life and maintains participation in retirement. His wife is also a retired teacher and participates in some of these activities. They own their own home and continue to manicure the landscaped yard they developed over 30 years in this location. Their three children are all self-supporting and live out of state.

Mr. Williams had been in relatively good health during retirement. He has experienced an intermittent need for medication adjustments for his hypertension. Over the past 1 to 2 years, he has rested a bit more often, but generally has maintained participation in his activities. Two days ago he was admitted to the hospital via the emergency department. He was diagnosed with a stroke affecting his left side.

Client #2: Mrs. Peters

Mrs. Peters is a 63-year-old woman who had total hip replacement surgery because of progressively increasing pain, ADL restrictions, and functional mobility problems resulting from osteoarthritis. She deliberated for several months before deciding to have the surgery. Mrs. Peters is a financial planner and has a busy practice with several clients who depend on her service. She is active in gardening and enjoys attending the activities of her grandchildren with her husband. The surgery was routine.

Web-Based Resources

For helpful information about the experience of rehabilitation visit:

www.cms.hhs.gov/default.asp, **Centers for Medicare and Medicaid Services (U.S. Department of Health and Human Services),** date connected October 23, 2007. This site contains information on Medicare services, coverage, and reimbursement.

www.carf.org, **Commission on Accreditation of Rehabilitation Facilities,** date connected October 23, 2007. Numerous resources, including free online publications for consumers, providers, payers, and surveyors. It is an independent not-for-profit organization that conducts an in-depth review of the quality of services offered by rehabilitation service providers and grants or denies accreditation dependent on whether the provider meets national standards of consumer-focused, state-of–the-art performance.

www.phac-aspc.gc.ca/seniors-aines/index_pages/publications_e.htm, **Public Health Agency of Canada, Division of Aging and Seniors,** date connected October 23, 2007. Numerous sources of reliable information about aging and Canadian seniors, for health care professionals and older adults.

www.dh.gov.uk/PolicyAndGuidance/HealthAndSocialCareTopics/OlderPeoplesServices/fs/en, **National Service Framework for Older People (UK Department of Health),** date connected October 23, 2007. This website provides numerous resources and Web links for health care providers and older adults.

www.ncoa.org, **National Council on the Aging (NCOA),** date connected October 23, 2007. This site is a national network of senior centers, area agencies on aging, adult day service centers, faith-based service organizations, senior housing facilities, employment services, consumer groups and leaders from academia, business, and labor. The website provides advocacy, program and research information, in addition to numerous publications for older adults and health care professionals.

www.udsmr.org, **Uniform Data System for Medical Rehabilitation,** date connected October 23, 2007. This is the official website for the FIM® system. Provides ordering and training information.

REFERENCES

Adlin, M. (1993). Health care issues. In E. Sutton, A. Factor, B. Hawkins, T. Heller, & G. Seltzer (Eds.), *Older adults with developmental disabilities: Optimizing choice and change* (pp. 49–60). Baltimore, MD: Paul Brookes.

Administration on Aging. (2005). *A profile of older Americans: 2005.* Retrieved March 23, 2006, from www.aoa.gov/PROF/Statistics/profile/2005/16.asp.

American Geriatrics Society, British Geriatrics Society, and American Academy of Orthopedic Surgeons Panel on Falls Prevention. (2001). Guideline for the prevention of falls in older persons. *Journal of the American Geriatrics Society, 49,* 664–672.

Bachrach, L. L. (1989). The legacy of model programs. *Hospital and Community Psychiatry, 40*(3), 234–235.

Bandura, A. (1977). Self-efficacy: Toward a unifying theory of behavioral change. *Psychological Review, 84,* 191–215.

Bandura, A. (1986). *Social foundations of thought and actions: A social cognitive theory.* Englewood Cliffs, NJ: Prentice Hall.

Banthin, J. S., & Cohen, J. W. (1999). *Changes in the Medicaid community population: 1987–96.* MEPS Research Findings No. 9. AHCPR Pub. No. 99-0042. Rockville, MD: Agency for Health Care Policy and Research.

Bartels, S. J., Levine, K. J., & Shea, D. (1999). Community-based long-term care for older persons with severe and persistent mental illness in an era of managed care. *Psychiatric Services, 50*(9), 1189–1197.

Beck, A. T. (1967). *Depression: Clinical and experimental theoretical aspects.* New York: Harper & Row.

Beck, A. T., Guth, D., Steer, R. A., & Ball, R. (1997). Screening for major depressive disorders in medical inpatients with the Beck Depression Inventory for Primary Care. *Behavior Research and Therapy, 35,* 785–791.

Berg, K., Maki, B., Williams, J. I., Holliday, P., & Wood-Dauphinee, S. (1992). A comparison of clinical and laboratory measures of postural balance in an elderly population. *Archives of Physical Medicine and Rehabilitation, 73,* 1073–1083.

Berg, K., Wood-Dauphinee, S., Williams, J. I., & Gayton, D. (1989). Measuring balance in the elderly: Preliminary development of an instrument. *Physiotherapy Canada, 41,* 304–311.

Berg, K. O., Wood-Dauphinee, S. L., Williams, J. I., & Maki, B. (1992). Measuring balance in the elderly: Validation of an instrument. *Canadian Journal of Public Health, 83,* S7–S11.

Bergman, H., Beland, F., Lebel, P., Contanriopoulos, A., Tousignant, P., Brunelle, Y., et al. (1997). Care for Canada's frail elderly population: Fragmentation or integration? *Journal of Canadian Medical Association, 157,* 1116–1121.

Bernabei, R., Landi, F., Gambassi, G., Sgadari, A., Zuccala, G., Mor, V., et al. (1998). Randomised trial of impact of model of integrated care and case management

for older people living in the community. *British Medical Journal, 316*(7141), 1348–1351.

Biegel, D. E., Milligan, S. E., Putman, P. L., & Song, L. Y. (1994). Predictors of burden among lower socioeconomic status caregivers of persons with chronic mental illness. *Community Mental Health Journal, 30*(5), 473–494.

Bogardus, S. T., Bradley, E. H., Williams, C. S., Maciejewski, P. K., van Doorn, C., & Inouye, S. (2001). Goals for the care of frail older adults: Do caregivers and clinicians agree? *American Journal of Medicine, 110,* 97–102.

Bondi, M. W., & Kaszniak, A. W. (1991). Implicit and explicit memory in Alzheimer's disease and Parkinson's disease. *Journal of Clinical Experimental Neuropsychology, 13,* 339–358.

Bortz, W. M., II. (2002). A conceptual framework of frailty: A review. *Journals of Gerontology Series A: Biological Sciences and Medical Sciences, 57,* M283–M288.

Boult, C., Boult, L. B., Morishita, L., Dowd, B., Kane, R. L., & Urdangarin, C. F. (2001). A randomized clinical trial of outpatient geriatric evaluation and management. *Journal of the American Geriatrics Society, 49,* 351–359.

Braithwaite, V. (1992). Caregiving burden: Making the concept scientifically useful and policy relevant. *Research on Aging, 14*(1), 3–27.

Brocklehurst, J. (1995). Geriatric day hospitals. *Age and Ageing, 24*(2), 89–90.

Brocklehurst, J. C., & Tucker, J. (1980). *Progress in geriatric day care.* London: King's Fund.

Brown, A. R., & Mulley, G. P. (1997a). Do it yourself: Home made aids for disabled elderly people. *Disability and Rehabilitation, 19,* 20–25.

Brown, A. R., & Mulley, G. P. (1997b). Injuries sustained by caregivers of disabled elderly people. *Ageing, 26,* 21–23.

Brown, J. B., McWilliam, C. L., & Mai, V. (1997). Barriers and facilitators to seniors' independence. *Canadian Family Physician, 43,* 469–475.

Brown, I., Renwick, R., & Raphael, D. (1995) Frailty: Constructing a common meaning, definition, and conceptual framework. *International Journal of Rehabilitation Research, 18,* 93–102.

Bruce, E. J., & Schultz, C. L. (2001). *Non-finite loss and grief: A psychoeducational approach.* Baltimore, MD: Paul H. Brookes.

Byrne, C., Isaacs, S., & Voorberg, N. (1991). Assessment of the physical health needs of people with chronic mental illness: One focus for health promotion. *Canada's Mental Health,* March, pp. 7–12.

Calkins, E., Boult, C., Wagner, E., & Pacalaet, J. T. (1999). *New ways to care for older people. Building systems based on evidence.* New York: Springer.

Campbell, A. J., Busby, W. J., Robertson, M. C., Lum, C. L., Langlois, J. A., & Morgan, F. C. (1994). Disease, impairment, disability and social handicap: A community based study of people aged 70 years and over. *Disability Rehabilitation, 16,*72–79.

Canwath, T. C. M., & Johnson, D. A. W. (1987). Psychiatric morbidity among spouses of stroke. *British Medical Journal, 294,* 409–411.

Capilouto, G. J. (2000). Rehabilitation settings. In S. Kumar (Ed.), *Multidisciplinary approach to rehabilitation* (pp. 1–26). Boston: Butterworth-Heinemann.

Ceder, L., Thorngren, K., & Wallden, B. (1980). Prognostic indicators and early home rehabilitation in elderly patients with hip fracture. *Clinical Orthopedics and Related Research, 152,* 173–185.

Chandler, J., & Hadley, E. (1996). Exercise to improve physiologic and functional performance in old age. *Clinics in Geriatric Medicine, 1*(4), 761–784.

Chin, A., Paw, M. J., Dekker, J. M., Feskens, E. J., Schouten, E. G., & Kromhout, D. (1999). How to select a frail elderly population? A comparison of three working definitions.*Journal of Clinical Epidemiology, 52,* 1015–1021.

Cohen, C. I., Cohen, G. D., Blank, K., Gaitz, C., Katz, I. R., Leuchter, A., et al. (2000). Directions for research and policy on schizophrenia and older adults: Summary of the GAP committee report. *Psychiatric Services, 5*(3), 299–302.

Cohen, H. J., Feussner, J. R., Weinberger, M., Carnes, M., Hamdy, R. C., Hsieh, F., et al. (2002). A controlled trial of inpatient and outpatient geriatric evaluation and management. *New England Journal of Medicine, 346,* 905–912.

Cummings, S., Phillips, S., Wheat, M., Black, D., Goosby, E., Wlodarczyk, D., et al. (1988). Recovery of function after hip fracture: The role of social support. *Journal of the American Geriatrics Society, 36,* 801–806.

Cunningham, C., Horgan, F., Keane, N., Connolly, P., Mannion, A., & O'Neil, D. (1996). Detection of disability by different members of an interdisciplinary team. *Clinical Rehabilitation, 10,* 247–254.

Delorme, M. (1999). Aging and people with developmental disabilities. In I. Brown & M. Percy (Eds.), *Developmental disabilities in Ontario* (pp. 189–195). Toronto, Ontario, Canada: Front Porch.

Department of Health & Human Services, Centers for Medicare & Medicaid Services (CMS). (2001). *Program memorandum intermediaries/carriers.* Transmittal AB-01-135. Retrieved June 26, 2008 from www.cms.hhs.gov/transmittals/downloads/AB-01-135.pdf

Diamond, P. T., Felsenthal, G., Macciocchi, S. N., Butler, D. H., & Lally-Cassady, D. (1996). Effect of cognitive impairment on rehabilitation outcome. *American Journal of Physical Medicine & Rehabilitation, 75*(1), 40–43.

Dick, M. B., Nielson, K. A., Beth, R. E., Shankle, W. R., & Cotman, C. W. (1995). Acquisition and long-term retention of a fine motor skill in Alzheimer disease. *Brain and Cognition, 29,* 294–306.

Dick, M. R., Shankle, R. W., Beth, R. E., Dick-Muehlke, C., Cotman, C. W., & Kean, M. (1996). Acquisition and long-term retention of a gross motor skill in Alzheimer's disease patients under constant and varied practice conditions. *Journal of Gerontology, Series B, Psychological Sciences and Social Sciences, 51*(B),103–111.

Drench, M. E. (2006). *Loss, grief, and adjustment: A primer for physical therapy, Parts 1 & 2.* APTA Continuing Education Series: American Physical Therapy Association. Retrieved April 10, 2006, from www.apta.org/AM/ Template.cfm?Section= Home&TEMPLATE=/CM/ContentDisplay. cfm&CONTENTID=28430.

Eslinger, P. J., & Damasio, A. R. (1986). Preserved motor learning in Alzheimer disease: Implications for anatomy and behaviour. *Journal of Neuroscience, 6,* 3006–3009.

Evans, R., Connis, R., Hendricks, R., & Haselkorn, J. (1995). Multidisciplinary rehabilitation versus medical care: A meta-analysis. *Social Science and Medicine, 40*(12), 1699–1706.

Falconer, J., Naughton, B. J., Strasser, D. C., & Sinacore, J. M. (1994). Stroke inpatient rehabilitation: A comparison across age groups. *Journal of the American Geriatrics Society, 42,* 39–44.

Farndale, J. (1961). *The day hospital movement in Great Britain.* Oxford: Pergamon Press.

Feder, G., Cryer, C., Donovan, S., & Carter, Y. (2000). Guidelines for the prevention of falls in people over 65. The Guidelines' Development Group. *British Medical Journal, 321*(7267), 1007–1011.

Fitz, A. G., & Teri, L. (1994). Depression, cognition, and functional ability in patients with Alzheimer's disease. *Journal of the American Geriatrics Society, 42,* 186–191.

Folstein, M. F., Folstein, S. E., & McHugh, P. R. (1975). "Mini-mental state." A practical method for grading the cognitive state of patients for the clinician. *Journal of Psychiatric Research, 12,* 189–198.

Forster, A., Langhorn, P., & Young, J. (1999). Systematic review and meta-analysis of day hospital care for older people. *British Medical Journal, 318,* 837–841.

Fried, L. P., Ettinger, W. H., Lind, B., Newman, A. B., & Gardin, J. (1994). Physical disability in older adults: A physiological approach. *Journal of Clinical Epidemiology, 47,* 747–760.

Fried, L. P., Ferrucci, L., Darer, J., Williamson, J. D., & Anderson, G. (2004). Untangling the concepts of disability, frailty, and comorbidity: Implications for improved targeting and care. *Journals of Gerontology Series A: Biological Sciences and Medical Sciences, 59,* 255–263.

Fried, L. P., & Guralnik, J. M. (1997). Disability in older adults: Evidence regarding significance, etiology, and risk. *Journal of the American Geriatrics Society, 45*(1), 92–100.

Fried, L. P., Tangen, C. M., Walston, J., Newman, A. B., Hirsch, C., Gottdiener, J., et al. (2001). Frailty in older adults: Evidence for a phenotype. *The Journals of Gerontology, Series A: Biological Sciences and Medical Sciences, 56,* M146–M156.

Galynker, I., Cohen, L., Salvit, C., Miner, C., Phillips, E., Focseneanu, M., et al. (2000). Psychiatric symptom severity and length of stay on an intensive rehabilitation unit. *Psychosomatics, 41*(2), 114–120.

Geelen, R., & Soons, P. (1996). Rehabilitation: An "everyday" motivation model. *Patient Education and Counseling, 28,* 69–77.

Gillen, R., Tennen, H., McKee, T. E., Gernert-Dott, P., & Affleck, G. (2001). Depressive symptoms and history of depression predict rehabilitation efficiency in stroke patients. *Archive of Physical Medicine and Rehabilitation, 82,* 1645–1649.

Gladman, J., Forster, A., & Young, J. (1995). Hospital and home-based rehabilitation after discharge from hospital for stroke patients: Analysis of two trials. *Age and Aging, 24,* 49–53.

Glazier, S. R., Schuman, J., & Keltz, E., Vally, A., & Glazier, R. H. (2004). Taking the next steps in goal ascertainment: A prospective study of patient team, and family perspectives using a comprehensive standardized menu in a geriatric assessment and treatment unit. *Journal of the American Geriatric Society, 52,* 284–289.

Goldstein, F. C., Strasser, D. C., Woodard, J. L., & Roberts, V. J. (1997). Functional outcome of cognitively impaired hip fracture patients on a geriatric rehabilitation. *Journal of the American Geriatric Society, 49,* 35–42.

Gudmundsson, A., & Carnes, M. (1996). Geriatric assessment: Making it work in primary care practice. *Geriatrics, 51*(3), 53–57.

Guralnik, J. M., Ferrucci, L., Balfour, J. L., Volpato, S., & DiIorio, A. (2001). Progressive versus catastrophic loss of the ability to walk: Implications for the prevention of mobility loss. *Journal of the American Geriatric Society, 49,* 1463–1470.

Guralnik, J. M., LaCroix, A. Z., Abbott, R. D., Berkman, L. F., Satterfield, S., Evans, D. A., et al. (1993). Maintaining mobility in late life: Demographic characteristics and chronic conditions. *American Journal of Epidemiology, 137,* 845–857.

Hamilton, M. (1960). Rating scale for depression. *Journal of Neurology, Neurosurgery and Psychiatry, 23,* 56–61.

Hamman, R. J. (1997). Rehabilitation following hip fracture in patients with Alzheimer's disease and related disorders. *American Journal of Alzheimer's Disease, 12,* 209–211.

Harris, R. E., O'Hara, P. A., & Harper, D. W. (1995). Functional status of geriatric rehabilitation patients: A one year follow-up study. *Journal of the American Geriatrics Society, 43*(1), 51–55.

Harris, R. E., Mion, L. C., Patterson, M. B., & Frengley, J. D. (1988). Severe illness in older patients: The association between depressive disorders and functional dependency during the recovery phase. *Journal of American Geriatrics Society, 36,* 890–896.

Hebert, R. (1997). Functional decline in old age. *Journal of Canadian Medical Association 157,* 1037–1045.

Hebert, R., Durand, P. J., Dubuc, N., & Tourigny, A. (2003). Frail elderly patients. A new model for integrated service delivery. *Canadian Family Physician, 49,* 992–997.

Heinemann, A. W. W., Linacre, J. M., Wright, B. D., Hamilton, B. B., & Granger, C. (1994). Prediction of rehabilitation outcomes with disability measures.

Archives of Physical Medicine and Rehabilitation, 75, 133–143.

Heruti, R. J., Lusky, A., Barell, V., Ohry, A., & Adunsky, A. (1999). Cognitive status at admission: Does it affect the rehabilitation outcome of elderly patients with hip fracture? *Archives of Physical Medicine and Rehabilitation, 80,* 432–436.

Hirono, N., Yamadori, A., Mori, E., Yamashita, H., Takatsuki, Y., & Tokimasa, A. (1996). Tactile perceptual skill learning and motor skill learning in Alzheimer's disease. *Behavioral Neurology, 9,* 11–16.

Hoenig, H., Nusbaum, N., & Brummel-Smith, K. (1997). Geriatric rehabilitation: State of the art. *Journal of American Geriatric Society, 45,* 1371–1381.

Hokenstad, M. C., & Johansson, L. (1996). Eldercare in Sweden: Issues in service provision and case management. *Journal of Case Management, 5,* 137–141.

Horwitz, A. V., & Uttaro, T. (1998). Age and mental health services. *Community Mental Health Journal, 34*(3), 275–287.

Jagger, C., Arthur, A. J., Spiers, N. A., & Clarke, M. (2001). Patterns of onset of disability in activities of daily living with age. *Journal of American Geriatric Society, 49,* 404–409.

Johnson, M. F., Kramer, A. M., Lin, M. K., Kowalsky, J. C., & Steiner, J. F. (2000). Outcomes for older persons receiving rehabilitation for medical and surgical conditions compared with hip fracture and stroke. *Journal of the American Geriatrics Society, 4,* 1389–1397.

Katz, S. (1983). Assessing self-maintenance: Activities of daily living, mobility, and instrumental activities of daily living. *Journal of the American Geriatrics Society, 31*(12), 721–727.

Kemp, B. J. (1988). Motivation, rehabilitation, and aging: A conceptual model. *Topics in Geriatric Rehabilitation, 3*(3), 41–51.

Kidd, T., & Yoshida, K. (1995). Critical review of disability measures: Conceptual developments. *Physiotherapy Canada, 47,* 108–119.

Knapp, M., Cambridge, P., Thomson, C., Beecham, J., Allen, C. A., & Darton, R. (1992). *Care in the community: Challenge and demonstration.* Canterbury: University of Kent: Personal and Social Services Research Unit.

Landefeld, C. S., Palmer, R. M., Kresevic, D. M., Fortinsky, R. H., & Kowal, J. (1995). A randomized trial of care in a hospital medical unit especially designed to improve the functional outcomes of acutely ill older patients. *New England Journal of Medicine, 332,* 1338–1344.

Latella, D. (2000). Team work in rehabilitation. In S. Kumar (Ed.), *Multidisciplinary approach to rehabilitation* (pp. 27–42). Boston: Butterworth-Heinemann.

Lawton, M. P., & Brody, E. M. (1969). Assessment of older people: Self-maintaining and instrumental activities of daily living. *The Gerontologist, 9*(3), 179–186.

Lees, L. (2004). Spotlight on intermediate care: A deeper analysis. In S. Wade (Ed.), *Intermediate care of older people* (pp. 19–35). London: Whurr.

Leveille, S. G., Fried, L. P., McMullen, W., & Guralnik, J. M. (2004). Advancing the taxonomy of disability in older adults. *The Journals of Gerontology, Series A: Biological Sciences and Medical Sciences, 59*(1), 86–93.

LeVesconte, H. P. (1935). Expanding fields of occupational therapy. *The Canadian Journal of Occupational Therapy, 3,* 4–12. (Reprinted in *The Canadian Journal of Occupational Therapy, 53* [Commemorative Issue], 9–15, 1986.)

Liem, P., Chernoff, R., & Carter, W. J. (1986). Geriatric rehabilitation unit: A 3 year outcome evaluation. *Journal of Gerontology, 14*(1), 44–50.

Lim, W. K., Lambert, S. F., & Gray, L. C. (2003). Effectiveness of case management and post-acute services in older people after hospital discharge. *Medical Journal of Australia, 178,* 262–266.

Lindgren, C. L., Burke, M. L., Hainsworth, M. A., & Eakes, G. G. (1992). Chronic sorrow: A lifespan concept. *Scholarly Inquiry in Nursing Practice, 6*(1), 27–40.

MacNeill, S., Lichtenberg, P. A., & LaBuda, J. (2000). Factors affecting return to living alone after medical rehabilitation: A cross-validation study. *Rehabilitation Psychology, 45*(4), 356–364.

Magaziner, J., Simonsick, E. M., Kashner, T. M., Hebel, J. R., & Kenzora, J. E. (1990). Predictors of functional recovery one year following hospital discharge for hip fracture: A prospective study. *Journal of Gerontology, 45,* M101–M107.

Mahoney, F. I., & Barthel, D. (1965). Functional evaluation: The Barthel Index. *Maryland State Medical Journal, 14,* 56–61.

Markle-Reid, M., & Browne, G. (2003). Conceptualizations of frailty in relation to older adults. *Journal of Advanced Nursing, 44,* 58–68.

Marshall, B. S., Long, M. J., Voss, J., Demma, K., & Skerl, K. P. (1999). Case management of the elderly in a health maintenance organization: The implications for program administration under managed care. *Journal of Healthcare Management, 44,* 477–491.

McCue, M. J., & Thompson, J. M. (1995). The ownership difference in relative performance of rehabilitation specialty hospitals. *Archives of Physical Medicine and Rehabilitation, 76,* 413–418.

Mitchell, J. M., & Scott, E. (1992). Physician ownership of physical therapy services: Effects on charges, utilization, profits, and service characteristics. *Journal of the American Medical Association, 268,* 2055–2059.

Mochizuki-Kawai, H., Kawamura, M., Hasegawa, Y., Mochizuki, S., Oeda, R., Yamanaka, K., et al. (2004). Deficits in long-term retention of learned motor skills in patients with cortical or subcortical degeneration. *Neuropsychologia, 42,* 1858–1863.

Molloy, D. W., Alemayehu, E., & Roberts, R. (1991). A Standardized Mini-Mental State Examination (SMMSE): Its reliability compared to the traditional Mini-Mental State Examination (MMSE). *American Journal of Psychiatry, 148,* 102–105.

Mor, V., Murphy, J., Masterson-Allen, S., Willey, C., Razmpour, A., Jackson, M. E., et al. (1989). Risk of functional decline among well elders. *Journal of Clinical Epidemiology, 42,* 895–904.

Mossey, J., Mutran, E., Knott, K., & Craik, R. (1989). Determinants of recovery 12 months after hip fracture: The importance of psychosocial factors. *American Journal of Public Health, 79,* 279–286.

Ontario Association of Non-profit Homes and Services for Seniors. (2000, February). *The professional care team in long term care: A discussion paper.* Retrieved May 20, 2006, from www.oanhss.org/StaticContent/StaticPages/about/PositionPapers/pp2.pdf.

Patrick, L., Knoefel, F., Gaskowski, P., & Rexroth, D. (2001). Medical comorbidity and rehabilitation efficiency in geriatric inpatients. *Journal of the American Geriatrics Society, 49*(11), 1471–1478.

Penington, G. (1992). Benefits of rehabilitation in the presence of advanced age or severe disability. *Medical Journal of Australia, 157*(10), 665–666.

Perkins, J., & Tryssenaar, J. (1994). Making interdisciplinary education effective for rehabilitation students. *Journal of Allied Health, Summer,* 143–151.

Podsiadlo, D., & Richardson, S. (1991). The timed "Up & Go": A test of basic functional mobility for frail elderly persons. *Journal of the American Geriatrics Society, 9,* 142–148.

Province, M. A., Hadley, E. C., Hornbrook, M. C., Lipsitz, L. A., Miller, J. P., Mulrow, C. D., et al. (1995). The effects of exercise on falls in elderly patients. A preplanned meta-analysis of the FICSIT trials. Frailty and injuries: Cooperative studies of intervention techniques. *Journal of the American Medical Association, 273,* 1341–1347.

Reker, D., O'Donnell, J., & Hamilton, B. (1998). Stroke rehabilitation outcome variation in Veterans Affairs rehabilitation units: Accounting for case-mix. *Archives in Physical Medicine and Rehabilitation, 70,* 751–757.

Research Foundation of the State University of New York. (1987). *Guide for the use of the uniform data set for medical rehabilitation.* Buffalo, NY: Author.

Resnick, B. (1998a). Efficacy beliefs in geriatric rehabilitation. *Journal of Gerontological Nursing, 24*(7), 34–44.

Resnick, B. (1998b). Functional performance of older adults in a long-term care setting. *Clinical Nursing Research, 7,* 230–246.

Resnick, B. (1999). Motivation to perform activities in daily living in the institutionalized older adult: Can a leopard change its spots? *Journal of Advanced Nursing, 29,* 792–799.

Resnick, B. (2002). Geriatric rehabilitation: The influence of efficacy beliefs and motivation. *Rehabilitation Nursing, 27*(4), 152–159.

Resnick, B., & Daly, M. P. (1998). Predictors of functional ability in geriatric rehabilitation patients. *Rehabilitation Nursing, 23,* 21–29.

Reuben, D. B., Borok, G. M., Wolde-Tsadik, G., Ershoff, D. H., Fishman, L. K., Ambrosini, V. L., et al. (1995). A randomized trial of comprehensive geriatric assessment in the care of hospitalized patients. *New England Journal of Medicine, 332,* 1345–1350.

Reutter-Bernays, D., & Rentsch, H. P. (1993). Rehabilitation of the elderly patient with stroke: An analysis of short-term and long-term results. *Disability and Rehabilitation, 15,* 90–95.

Rockwood, K., Awalt, E., Carver, D., & MacKnight, C. (2000). Feasibility and measurement properties of the Functional Reach and the Timed Up and Go Tests in the Canadian Study of Health and Aging. *Journal of Gerontology, 55A*(2), M70–M73.

Rockwood, K., Graham, J. E., & Fay, S. (2002). Goal setting and attainment in Alzheimer's disease patients treated with donepezil. *Journal of Neurology, Neurosurgery, and Psychiatry, 73,* 500–507.

Rockwood, K., Hogan, D. B., & MacKnight, C. (2000). Conceptualisation and measurement of frailty in elderly people. *Drugs & Aging, 17,* 295–302.

Rodriguez, G. S., & Goldberg, B. (1993). Rehabilitation in the outpatient setting. *Clinical Geriatric Medicine, 9,* 873–881.

Rondinelli, D. R. D., Murphy, J. R., Wilson, D. H., & Miller, C. C. (1991). Predictors of functional outcome and resource utilization in inpatient rehabilitation. *Archives of Physical Medicine and Rehabilitation, 72,* 447–453.

Rosenberg, M., & Moore, E. (1997). The health of Canada's elderly population: Current status and future implications. *Journal of the Canadian Medical Association, 157,* 1025–1032.

Rosenberg, W., Parkes, J., Jenkins, A., Denham, M. J., Royston, J. P., Sullens, C. M., et al. (1986). Making a rehabilitation hospital for the elderly work. *Health Trends, 18,* 66–72.

Royal College of Physicians and British Geriatrics Society. (1992). *Standardized assessment scales for elderly people.* London: Royal College of Physicians.

Rubenstein, L. Z. (2004). Comprehensive geriatric assessment: From miracle to reality *The Journals of Gerontology, Series A: Biological Sciences and Medical Sciences, 59*(5), 473–478.

Runciman, P. (1989). Health assessment of the elderly at home: The case for shared learning. *Journal of Advanced Nursing, 14,* 111–119.

Saarinen, H., & Salvatori, P. (1994). Educating occupational therapists and physiotherapists for the year 2000: What, no anatomy course? *Physiotherapy Canada, 46,* 81–86.

Sager, M., Franke, T., Inouye, S. K., Landefeld, C. S., Morgan, T. M., & Rudberg, M. A. (1996). Functional outcomes of acute medical illness and hospitalization in older adults. *Journal of the American Geriatrics Society, 48,* 1545–1552.

Salvatori, P., Tremblay, M., & Tryssenaar, J. (2003). Living and aging with a developmental disability: Perspectives of individuals, family members and service providers. *Journal of Developmental Disabilities, 10*(1), 1–19.

Schnelle, J. F., MacRae, P. G., Ouslander, J. G., Simmons, S. F., & Nitta, M. (1995). Functional incidental training, mobility performance, and incontinence care with nursing home residents. *Journal of the American Geriatrics Society, 43*(12), 1356–1362.

Seidel, A. C. (1998). Theories derived from rehabilitation perspectives. In M. Neistadt & E. B. Crepeau (Eds.), *Willard and Spackman's occupational therapy* (pp. 536–538). Philadelphia: Lippincott-Raven.

Sinclair, A., & Dickson, E. (1998). *Effective practice in rehabilitation: The evidence of systematic reviews.* London: King's Fund.

Sommer, S. J., Silagy, C. A., & Rose, A. T. (1986). The teaching of interdisciplinary education. *Medical Journal of Australia, 157*(1), 31, 34, 36–37.

Spaniol, L., Gagne, C., & Koehler, M. (1999). *The recovery framework in rehabilitation: Concepts and practices from the field of serious mental illness.* Paper presented at the International Association of Psychosocial Rehabilitation Services, PSR—Bridges to Recovery Conference, Minneapolis, MN.

Spector, W. D., & Fleishman, J. A. (1998). Combining activities of daily living with instrumental activities of daily living to measure functional disability. *Journals of Gerontology, Series B: Psychological Sciences & Social Sciences, 53*(1), S46–S57.

Steer, R., Cavalieri, T., Douglas, I., & Beck, A. (1999). Use of the Beck Depression Inventory for Primary Care for major depression disorders. *General Hospital and Psychiatry, 21,* 106–111.

Steiner, A. (1997). *Intermediate care: A conceptual framework and review of the literature.* London: King's Fund.

Stoedefalke, K. G. (1985). Motivating and sustaining the older adult in an exercise program. *Topics in Geriatric Rehabilitation, 1,* 78–83.

Stuck, A. E., Aronow, H. U., Steiner, A., Alessi, C. A., Bula, C. J., Gold, M. N., et al. (1995). A trial of annual in-home comprehensive geriatric assessments for elderly people living in the community. *New England Journal of Medicine, 333,* 1184–1189.

Stuck, A. E., Siu, A. L., Wieland, G. D., Adams, J., & Rubenstein, L. Z. (1993). Comprehensive geriatric assessment: A meta-analysis of controlled trials. *Lancet, 342,* 1032–1036.

Sutton, E. (1997). Enriching later life experiences for people with developmental disabilities. *Activities, Adaptation, & Aging, 21*(3), 65–69.

Toseland, R. W., O'Donnell, J. C., Engelhardt, J. B., Hendler, S. A., Richie, J. T., & Jue, D. (1996). Outpatient geriatric evaluation and management: Results of a randomized trial. *Medical Care, 34,* 624–640.

Treischmann, R. B. (1987). *Aging with a disability.* New York: Demos.

Tryssenaar, J., Perkins, J., & Brett, L. (1996). Undergraduate interdisciplinary education: Are we educating for future practice? *Canadian Journal of Occupational Therapy, 63*(4), 245–251.

Tryssenaar, J., & Tremblay, M. (2002). Aging with a serious mental disability in rural northern Ontario: Family members' experiences. *Psychiatric Rehabilitation Journal, 25*(3), 255–264.

Verbrugge, L. M., Lepkowski, J. M., & Imanaka, Y. (1989). Comorbidity and its impact on disability. *Milbank Quarterly, 67,* 450–484.

Verbrugge, L. M., Lepkowski, J. M., & Konkol, L. L. (1991). Levels of disability among U.S. adults with arthritis. *Journal of Geriatrics Society Science, 46,* S71–S83.

von Koch, L., Wottrich, A. W., & Homqvist, L. W. (1998). Rehabilitation in the home versus the hospital: The importance of context. *Disability and Rehabilitation, 10,* 367–372.

Wade, D. T., Leigh-Smith, J., & Hewer, R. L. (1986). Effects of living with and looking after survivors of stroke. *British Medical Journal, 293,* 418–420.

Ware, J. E., & Sherbourne, C. D. (1992). The MOS 36-item short form health survey (SF-36): Conceptual framework and item selection. *Medical Care, 30,* 473–483.

Wells, J. L., Seabrook, J. A., Stolee, P., Borrie, M. J., & Knoefel, F. (2003a). State of the art in geriatric rehabilitation. Part I: Review of frailty and comprehensive geriatric assessment. *Archives of Physical Medicine and Rehabilitation, 84,* 890–897.

Wells, J. L., Seabrook, J. A., Stolee, P., Borrie, M. J., & Knoefel, F. (2003b). State of the art in geriatric rehabilitation: Part II. Clinical challenges. *Archives of Physical Medicine and Rehabilitation, 84,* 898–903.

Wilkinson, T., Buhrkuhl, D., & Sainsbury, R. (1997). Assessing and restoring function in elderly people— More than rehabilitation. *Clinical Rehabilitation, 11*(4), 321–328.

Williams, C. (2004). The sandwich generation. *Perspectives on Labour and Income, 5*(9), Statistics Canada (Catalogue no. 75-001-XIE). Retrieved November 8, 2006, from www.statcan.ca/Daily/English/040928/d040928b.htm.

The World Health Organization. (2006). Retrieved March 23, 2006, from www.who.int/disabilities/care/en/.

The World Health Organization Expert Committee. (1990). *Cancer pain relief and palliative care.* Geneva: Author.

Yesavage, J. A., Brink, T. L., Rose, T. L., Lum, O., Huang, V., Adey, M. B., et al. (1983). Development and validation of a geriatric depression screening scale: A preliminary report. *Journal of Psychiatric Research, 17,* 37–49.

Young, J. (1996). Rehabilitation and older people. *British Medical Journal, 313,* 677–681.

Zanetti, O., Binetti, G., Magni, E., Rozzini, L., Bianchetti, A., & Trabucchi, M. (1997). Procedural memory stimulation in Alzheimer's disease: Impact of a training programme. *Acta Neurologica Scandinavica, 95,* 152–157.

Zarit, S. H., Stephens, M. A., Townsend, A., & Greene, R. (1998). Stress reduction for the family caregivers: Effects of adult care use. *Journal of Gerontology Series B: Psychological Sciences and Social Sciences, 53*(5), S267–S277.

Zarit, S. H., Zarit, J. M., & Rosenberg, T. S. (1990). A special treatment unit for Alzheimer's disease: Medical, behavioral, and environmental features. *Clinical Gerontologist, 9*(3–4), 47–63.

Zwecker, M., Levenkrohn, S., Fleisig, Y., Zeilig, G., Ohry, A., & Adunsky, A. (2002). Mini-Mental State Examination, cognitive FIM Instrument, and the Loewenstein Occupational Therapy Cognitive Assessment: Relation to functional outcome of stroke patients. *Archives of Physical Medicine and Rehabilitation, 83,* 342–345.

ACKNOWLEDGMENTS

"My Uncle Alphonse" is based on the experiences of a family member of the second author. The scenarios of Mr. King and Mr. Schultz are based on actual real-life patient scenarios, were originally developed from the clinical experience of two students in the postprofessional MSc (Rehabilitation Science) program at McMaster University, and have been modified and used with their permission.

Special thanks to Tasha Thornhill and Liz Scott for their assistance with this chapter.

CHAPTER 22

Long-Term Care

Ruth E. Plautz • Cameron J. Camp

*Meaning and meaningful activities, then, are our goals, our purpose
and our challenge. What we bring or do not bring is all these
individuals we serve will Cameron J. Camp or will not have.*

Ann M. Rancourt, 1991

*If a lifetime … follows a path, there is a need for a leader. In the
progressive phase where the path leads upward to greater skill,
the leader is a teacher; in the regressive phase when tasks need
simplifying the leader is a caregiver or therapist.*

Barbara B. Dreher, 1997

OBJECTIVES

By the end of this chapter, readers will be able to:

1. Name and describe critical legislation that created the "modern" nursing home.
2. Describe the types of residents typically found in long-term-care settings today.
3. Describe the occupational performance of residents in long-term care.
4. Discuss the utility of applying principles of occupational therapy to occupational performance in long-term-care settings.
5. Discuss the need to integrate occupational performance tasks within an interdisciplinary framework.
6. Discuss reimbursement and regulatory issues involved with delivering occupational therapy and activities services to residents in long-term care.
7. Describe the major components of Kitwood's model of the factors that influence the manifestation of dementia.
8. Describe the parallels between Montessori-based activities and occupational therapy.
9. Discuss methods of infusing principles of occupational therapy into the daily routine of long-term residents within the context of current and future reimbursement and management systems.
10. Give examples of the influence of culture on the formulation of appropriate occupational performance tasks.

In this chapter, we will discuss occupational performance in long-term-care settings. We will begin by describing how the nursing home industry has been changed by federal regulations in the past 25 years. We will then describe typical nursing home residents. This will be followed by a discussion of the role of occupational performance within the nursing home setting. In particular, we will focus on how interventions to enhance performance skills are implemented, regulated, and reimbursed.

In the next section of the chapter, we will specify some recent innovative trends in activities implemented in long-term care, including a discussion of how to use activities as interventions/mechanisms for rehabilitation in long-term care. We will conclude with a summary and a depiction of challenges still facing implementation of occupational therapy and activities programming in long-term care. Throughout the chapter, we will attempt to illustrate and inform various points of discussion through use of examples culled from our experience working with long-term care residents at Menorah Park Center for Senior Living.

The chapter focuses on long-term care in the United States. Because of the wide range of types of long-term care, and the centrality of specific government and third-party payer regulations, it is beyond the scope of a single chapter to cover long-term care around the globe. In some countries, long-term-care facilities are rare either because economic circumstances make it impossible to afford such care, or because families feel strongly about providing care themselves. In other countries, an array of long-term-care options may provide alternative models worthy of consideration for implementation in the United States. Certainly, as the population ages worldwide, options for ensuring adequate care for elders at the end of their lives will become increasingly important.

Evolution of the "Modern" Nursing Home

The nursing home industry in the United States has been in a state of change since 1965, when the health entitlement programs Medicare and Medicaid were created. These programs provided financial resources for nursing home care and served as the impetus for tremendous growth in the nursing home industry. The population of elderly adults in nursing homes in the United States increased by 55% from 1970 to 1980, and by another 29% from 1980 to 1990 (Aronson, 1999). In 2005, approximately 1.5 million persons over age 65 lived in nursing homes (National Center for Health Statistics, 2005). However, the increase in number of beds available for older adults in these facilities did not result in an increase in quality of care for residents.

Historically, an older adult living in a nursing home was characterized as disheveled, sleeping in a wheelchair in a slumped position, and not socially engaged with the environment. This individual was thought to be almost totally dependent in activities of daily living and incapable of decision making. The environment was perceived as custodial rather than restorative, and older adults dreaded the thought of nursing home institutionalization.

Fifteen years after the entitlement programs were enacted, *Unloving care,* was published (Vladeck, 1980). This was the first systematic evaluation of nursing homes and nursing home policy. Its findings revealed that nursing homes were places where nurses spent little time in direct patient care and physicians seldom visited, and residents were physically and chemically restrained. Residents' rights were limited, the environment often smelled of urine or disinfectant, and there were few if any meaningful activities made available to residents. Such was the general result of entitlement programs for older adults. It wasn't until 1986 and the Institute of Medicine report, *Improving quality of care in nursing homes* and the Omnibus Budget Reconciliation Act (OBRA) of 1987, that the nursing home of the 1960s began to change (Institute of Medicine, 1986; OBRA, 1991). This occurred through creation and enforcement of regulations emphasizing consistent quality of care, quality of life, residents' rights, and development of a standardized assessment tool, called the Resident Assessment Instrument (RAI), which included the **minimum data set (MDS)** (Hawes, Morris, et al., 1997; Hawes, Phillips, et al., 1997; Mor et al., 1997; Phillips et al., 1997). Nursing homes now were being held accountable for adhering to national standards of care.

MDS and RAPs

The MDS is assessed for each resident upon admission to a facility. It also is administered when there is a change in a resident's status (e.g., when a resident must be hospitalized). Even without a change in status, the MDS is assessed on a quarterly basis for all residents of skilled nursing facilities. (Alternative forms of this assessment tool are in development for other forms of long-term care, such as assisted living facilities.)

The MDS is a survey, with most items rated on a "present or absent" or on a Likert scale. For example, in Section N of the MDS, involving "Activity Pursuits," there is a list of activity preferences (e.g., Crafts/arts, Helping Others, Reading/writing, Spiritual/religious activities). Each activity preference is scored as to whether or not it is a preference of the resident. Another item in Section N assesses the average time that the resident is involved in activities ("0" = most—more than 2/3 of time; "1" = some—from 1/3 to 2/3 of time; "2" = little—less than 1/3 of time; "3" = none). Section T of the MDS involves "Therapy Supplement for Medicare PPS." Items assess the amount of recreational therapy provided over the last 7 days, as well as the amount of physician-ordered therapies such as occupational therapy, physical therapy, or speech pathology services.

It is important to know that the MDS was designed to be an initial assessment to screen for residents' problems and also for abilities and preferences. When particular patterns of MDS items scores are obtained, this sets off a triggering mechanism that should lead to additional information gathering. Such triggers within the MDS set in motion the use of resident assessment protocols (RAPs). There are 18 RAP areas in the current version (2.0) of the MDS. These RAP areas are listed in Box 22-1. (Readers should be aware that version 3.0 of the MDS will probably be implemented in the near future, if not by the time this book goes to press.)

After examining what items triggered a RAP for a resident, a care plan is developed by an interdisciplinary team. Note that some triggers focus on rehabilitation potential, as would be the case if a resident expressed an interest in demonstrating increased independence. All RAP areas potentially could benefit from interventions with input from rehabilitation staff. However, areas such as ADL Functional/ Rehabilitation Potential, Activities, Cognitive Loss, Communication, and Behavioral Symptoms are especially salient areas where rehabilitation professionals could provide meaningful

> **BOX 22-1 RAPs Categories of the MDS**
>
> 1. Delirium
> 2. Cognitive loss
> 3. Visual function
> 4. Communication
> 5. ADL functional/rehabilitation potential
> 6. Urinary incontinence and indwelling catheter
> 7. Psychological well-being
> 8. Mood state
> 9. Behavioral symptoms
> 10. Activities
> 11. Falls
> 12. Nutritional status
> 13. Feeding tubes
> 14. Dehydration/fluid maintenance
> 15. Oral/dental care
> 16. Pressure ulcers
> 17. Psychotropic drug use
> 18. Physical restraints

input in care plan development, implementation, and evaluation.

A Change in Perception

The new legislation focused on changing society's perception of the aging process and stereotypes regarding older adults. In the nursing home industry, a change began occurring in the basic philosophy regarding the type of care to be delivered. Warehousing older adults in facilities no longer matched the intent of the new legislation, and society needed to be educated about the potentials and abilities of older adults, even as they lived out their last years in nursing care facilities.

OBRA legislation focused on a wellness philosophy embracing the concept that the older adult possesses numerous capabilities or abilities and should be treated with dignity and respect. OBRA developed new standards of care as well as new survey and enforcement procedures. It was necessary to develop objective standards to ensure consistent delivery of adequate care. The survey process became oriented toward functional outcomes, objectively assessing issues such as the prevalence of weight loss, staff training standards, and competency of staff, while subjectively assessing quality of life issues such as privacy and resident satisfaction. Lack of adherence to the legislated standards created immediate sanctions, such as fines, for facilities that were out of compliance. The new standards of care challenged nursing home administrators and caregivers to change their paradigm for care delivery and begin redefining the concept of long-term care and its organizational structure.

The Omnibus Budget Reconciliation Act of 1987—"OBRA '87"—was developed in a less medically complex environment than what exists at present. Today, nursing homes are not necessarily just an environment for non-hospital-based interventions focusing on chronic care and not cure. Rather, nursing homes provide various levels of care from posthospital **subacute care** to specialized pavilions such as ventilators, wound care, AIDS, and hospice care. There is actually a blurring of the definition of a "traditional" nursing home. In general, however, nursing home care can be thought of as falling into three main categories: skilled, which provides high-level medical care immediately following a hospitalization (this includes subacute and some ventilator care); rehabilitative, which includes stays of several weeks to several months during which time the individual is expected to improve and, probably, to return to a less-restrictive environment; and true long-term care, in which the *home* aspect of nursing home care is most prominent. There are also residential alternatives such as assisted living and community resources such as adult day centers that provide less-restricted care.

There are innovative, nontraditional, stand-alone models of care such as the Wellspring Program and the Eden Alternative. These models focus on using 24 hours a day as potential time for engagement in the various areas of **occupation** such as social participation or instrumental activities of daily living. The Wellspring Program, a model for residents with memory loss, is designed to foster a self-regulating series of behavior-based feedback loops among the resident, staff, and family members. This approach fosters independence and spontaneity creating activities for the moment. The Eden Alternative attempts to redesign the experience of aging and limitations by utilizing animals, plants, and children to transform the nursing home environment into habitats where individuals enjoy living. They continually ask, "What is best for the resident?" The resident remains the central focus at all times, ensuring that each day reflects the natural rhythms of life and freedom of choice.

Other factors that affect the current model of nursing homes are the introduction of long-term-care insurance (dictating the amount of money that will be paid for care, not necessarily based on the client's medical needs) and shortened length of stay in acute-care settings. Therefore, the nursing home of tomorrow will be challenged to create a niche within the continuum of care, perhaps creating specialized services, or forming alliances with other specialty providers and developing strategies about how to successfully operate within a restricted reimbursement environment.

In 2003, the majority of nursing homes (65%) were owned by for-profit companies, 28% were operated by nonprofit entities, and the remainder were government owned, such as Veterans Administration facilities. The primary payer source for the vast majority of nursing home residents, 65% to 70%, was Medicaid, but only 10% to 15% were covered by Medicare, with the rest covered by private or other payer sources (Centers for Medicare and Medicaid Services [CMS], 2005). Because the yearly cost of staying in a nursing home is more than $74,000, most residents must rely on entitlement programs such as Medicare and Medicaid to pay (Kaiser Foundation, 2006). Therefore, nursing homes must adhere to legislated standards of care to remain certified. OBRA '87 made adherence to national standards a requisite for facilities to maintain certification in the entitlement programs. This provided the incentive to change from the custodial model of the 1960s to the current restorative model of nursing home care.

Nursing home care improved after the inception of OBRA. For example, use of physical restraints decreased from 40% in 1989 to 20% in 1993 according to data collected by the Health Care Financing Administration. There was also a decrease in chemical restraints. In addition, changes have been noted in the areas of residents' rights and improved outcomes in the areas of dehydration, falls, pressure ulcers, and malnutrition (Hawes, Morris, et al., 1997; Hawes, Phillips, et al., 1997; Mor et al., 1997; Phillips et al., 1997).

However, today's nursing home resident is sicker, more cognitively impaired, and physically dependent, with an increased need for intensive medical, skilled nursing, and rehabilitative services than in the past. The majority of nursing home residents are female (72%) and have no spouse (60% are widowed) (American Geriatric Society [AGS] Foundation, 2005). Because women generally outlive men and have marital partners their own age or older, they are less likely than men to have a caregiver at home should they become disabled. Therefore, men are less likely to enter nursing homes than women. Today, almost half of all persons living in nursing homes are 85 years of age or older (AGS Foundation, 2005). Because disabilities increase in frequency with age, most nursing home residents are disabled. Of those residents aged 65 and older, when admitted to a nursing home, 75% need assistance with three or more activities of daily living (ADL) such as bathing (96%), dressing (88%), and toileting (82%). A majority of these residents (55%) are bladder incontinent, and 45% are bowel incontinent (American Health Care Association [AHCA], 2005). More than a third have difficulty with hearing or seeing (AGS Foundation, 2005). Although the vast majority of nursing home residents aged 65 and older receive various forms of medical care, only 19% receive rehabilitation. With regard to pharmacology, 64% receive psychoactive medication, compared to 24.5% receiving pain medication and 8% receiving antibiotics (AHCA, 2005). As the population continues to age, it is projected that the nursing home of tomorrow will focus increasingly on chronic illness, not age-specific dysfunction.

OBRA '87 Philosophy and Occupational Therapy

There has been a change in practice patterns of occupational therapists in nursing home environments. Occupational therapy services, along with the other rehabilitative services, focus on functional problems as their primary concern (Fried & Guralnik, 1997). The current pattern of nursing home intervention by occupational therapists is to emphasize performance skills such as range of motion, strength, and coordination, with the expectation of functional physical gains within a limited time period. Treatment standards and definitions are controlled by federal and state legislation and by Medicare and Medicaid. That is not to say that there are not other opportunities for occupational therapists to treat older adults.

However, federal and state legislation and reimbursement policies along with changes in facility policies have forced therapists to treat specific impairments, not the whole person. Change in performance skills is measured by the assistance needed in performance areas such as self-feeding or grooming rather than in a person's acceptance of his or her altered roles and redesigned performance patterns.

The theoretical basis of occupational therapy is that purposeful occupation enhances an individual's quality of life by providing meaning and direction, and that a relationship exists between occupation and health (Iwarsson, Isacsson, Persson, & Schersten, 1998; Zimmer-Branum & Nelson, 1995). The model of human occupation describes positive adaptation as the ability to function effectively during each stage of the life cycle (Nelson, 1988). Occupational therapists embrace the concept that activity contains within itself curative properties that will affect function when appropriately planned and executed (Nelson & Peterson, 1989; Trombly, 1995). Therapists have been trained to promote holistic, client-centered occupational-centered practice, and promote prevention while working as part of a health care team.

It is also recognized that each individual has a unique perception of purposefulness. Older adults living in an institutionalized environment have lost many of their life roles and routines, decreasing their opportunities to maintain a positive sense of self-worth. In addition, the roles available to older adults in long-term-care settings generally are not perceived to be productive by either society or older adults themselves. It should be noted that the type of activity presented to an older adult is as significant as the presence or absence of participation opportunities, and that engagement or participation style may vary with age of residents or type of engagement (e.g., observational versus active physical involvement). Institutionalized elderly adults who take advantage of the opportunity to participate in available activities tend to be more active physically, cognitively, and socially than those who choose not to participate (Duellman, Barris, & Kielhofner, 1986).

Occupational therapy has an important role in the prospective payment system and is reimbursed through indication of the number of days and total number of minutes the resident was treated. However, the reimbursement tool has been designed to pay for dependency, not independence.

An example of this is seen in the **prospective payment system (PPS)** regulations requiring nursing staff to evaluate and implement restorative nursing programming for long-term-care residents. In restorative nursing programs, nursing staff must implement and monitor the effects of interventions to maintain or improve level of functioning in long-term-care residents. Even though occupational therapists should be able to assist nursing staff in creating restorative nursing programs, the role of rehabilitation staff within such programs has remained consultative in nature. A more collaborative approach emphasizes that once a resident has maximized his or her skills through reimbursable occupational, physical, and speech therapy, nursing staff reinforces the learned skill. New models for interaction and cooperation between disciplines need to be developed within long-term-care environments so that residents can most fully benefit under the PPS reimbursement system.

It is not surprising that there is a dearth of information in occupational therapy literature on the development of areas of occupation for residents in nursing homes who do not exhibit acute medical problems or are not capable of recovering "normal" levels of performance. Therapy is usually discontinued when the resident has reached his or her maximum potential and there is variable follow-up by support personnel to maintain outcomes of the therapy intervention. What happens when rehabilitation or restoration of skills of the institutionalized older adult is not a likely goal? It is necessary to raise the question of what is realistic, achievable, and desired outcomes for the frail elderly in institutions (Hirdes & Carpenter, 1997). Typically, these individuals decline in functional abilities. This may partially be the result of reimbursement policies, because occupational therapy services are most frequently reimbursed only when significant functional progress is expected and demonstrated.

To some extent, this situation arises because of the view that occupational therapy is a form of rehabilitation, and that rehabilitation implies restoration to normal life through training (see Wilson, 1997, for a discussion of contrasting views of what does or does not constitute rehabilitation). However, it is useful to look at the World Health Organization's (WHO, 1986, 2001) definition of rehabilitation:

> Rehabilitation includes all measures aimed at reducing the impact of disability for an individual, enabling him or her to achieve independence, social integration, a better quality of life and self-actualization. Rehabilitation includes not only the training of disabled people but also interventions in the general systems of society, adaptations of the environment and protection of human rights. Protection of human rights is an obligation.

Wilson (1989) defined cognitive rehabilitation as "... any intervention strategy or technique which intends to enable clients or patients, and their families, to live with, manage, by-pass, reduce, or come to terms with cognitive deficits precipitated by injury to the brain." Engagement in occupation can be rehabilitative if it enables residents in long-term care to reduce or better live with deficits. To the extent that the therapeutic use of occupations and activities enables residents to maintain skills, retain useful habits and roles, and bypass or manage deficits, engagement in occupations are rehabilitative.

Statistics indicate that the older adult population, especially the old-old (85 years of age and older), is the most rapidly increasing portion of the older adult population.

People age 65 have at least a 40% risk of entering a nursing home at some point in their lives (American Association of Homes and Services for the Aging [AAHSA], 2006). Age is a substantial risk factor for entering a nursing home, with 1.4% of persons who are 65 to 74 years of age living in nursing homes, and 20% of persons age 85 and older living in these facilities. Additional risk factors for nursing home placement include low income, low levels of social activity, functional or mental difficulties, and poor family support (especially if there is a lack of a spouse and children) (AGS Foundation, 2005). Nearly half of the residents in long-term care are experiencing some form of dementia. The number of therapists necessary to care for the institutionalized older adult population will increase in the coming years (Jacelon, 1995). There are questions regarding how therapists will be utilized in long-term care in the future, particularly in light of the current managed cost environment and the implementation of the PPS. The long-term-care provider is under tremendous pressure from third-party payers to pursue the most economical approach to providing services. Will therapists focus on short-term acute problems, or will they be able to utilize their theoretical knowledge base to support activities programming or engagement in occupation?

OBRA '87 mandates that "Nursing homes must care for residents in such a manner and in such an environment as will promote maintenance of enhancement of the quality of life of each resident." For occupational therapists, the mandate from OBRA parallels their original philosophical basis for therapeutic interventions—focusing on a holistic approach to a person's abilities rather than their disabilities, enhancing functional independence, encouraging choice and decision making, and promoting previous lifestyle pursuits.

Occupational therapists have historically been responsible for the development and delivery of **purposeful activity** to enhance independence, maximize functional abilities, and improve the quality of life of institutionalized elders (Baum & Edwards, 1995; Fidler, 1981; Clark & Larson, 1993; Nelson, 1988, 1997). The concept of quality of life and the focus on successful aging are naturally embodied within occupational therapy theory (Bissell, 1981; Breines, 1984; Nelson, 1988, 1997). Therapists have been trained to treat the whole person and to foster an environment supportive of life and living, rather than death and dying. This is done by enabling older adults to continue an autonomous, meaningful existence in spite of chronic disabilities, less than optimal living situations, learned helplessness, as well as social, emotional, and financial losses (Jackson, 1996).

The OBRA '87 legislation provides owners and operators of long-term-care facilities latitude in the implementation of the regulations. For example, the federal OBRA laws mandate that for ongoing activities, "The facility must provide for an ongoing program of activities designed to meet, in accordance with the comprehensive assessment, the interests and the physical, mental and psychosocial well-being of each resident" (OBRA, 1991, Tag number F248).

According to the federal regulations, the activities program must be directed by a qualified professional who

1. Is a qualified therapeutic recreation specialist or an activities professional who—
   a. Is licensed or registered, if applicable, by the state in which practicing; and
   b. Is eligible for certification as a therapeutic recreation specialist or as an activities professional by a recognized accrediting body on or after October 1, 1990; or
2. Has 2 years of experience in a social or recreational program within the last 5 years, one of which was full time in a patient activities program in a health care setting; or
3. Is a qualified occupational therapist or occupational therapist assistant; or
4. Has completed a training course approved by the state (OBRA, 1991).

The regulations suggest that different types of personnel are equally capable of fulfilling the intent of the law. As a result, it is logical to expect long-term-care residential facilities to opt for the least-expensive provider. Generally, facilities do not understand the complexity of developing intervention approaches around the concepts of work, play, leisure, and previous life roles while accommodating or remediating physical and cognitive limitations. Because occupation-based interventions focused on quality of life are not government mandated or reimbursed, most owners and operators will continue to focus on cost rather than effectiveness of activities programming and decide to provide activities directed by the least-expensive qualified professional.

Occupational Performance in Long-Term Care

Whether treatment planning for specific medical deficits or for occupational engagement in an occupational therapy context, all facets of an individual must be considered. A comprehensive occupational profile will describe a person's routine, habits, values, and interests. The connectedness elders have with their rich lifetime experiences and past relationships, as well as their physical, emotional, social, and cognitive abilities, should be taken into account. The goal of an effective activities program, under the direction of an occupational therapist, is to focus on goal- and process-directed, purposeful tasks that capitalize on a person's abilities and growth potential—not busywork (Breines, 1984). A nonreimbursable occupation-based program can be viewed as an ongoing, long-term approach to the maintenance and enhancement of functional abilities, and thus a preventative health program rather than a short-term solution to a specific deficit.

Occupational therapists have the skills to develop and adapt activities programs that are goal and process directed, that create a sense of competence and fulfillment, and that are based on an individual's abilities rather than disabilities (Hinojosa, Sabari, Rosenfeld, & Shapiro, 1983). According to Hinojosa and Kramer (1997), "goal directed" does not always require a physical product or an outcome but does involve active engagement that meets personal goals or needs. Within the context of an activities program, a resident can practice skills learned in the functional occupational therapy program (Dutton, 1989). Intervention is based on a wellness model rather than a medical model. Clark and her colleagues (1997) demonstrated that preventive health programs based on occupational therapy theory were capable of decreasing health risks for community-dwelling older adults, but socially based activities programs did not affect the general well-being of the participating individuals. Therefore, it might be hypothesized that occupational therapy using ongoing activities as the basis for preventive care could have a similar effect on the health and well-being of institutionalized older adults.

As appropriate interventions are identified for the institutionalized elderly, one must consider various deficits that an older adult may present, including those who are aging with a preexisting disability such as polio. Deficits may include physical, cognitive, and social changes, redefined relationships, sensory impairments, changes in life roles and self-esteem, and many others. Attention must be given to the individual's health needs and health improvements without sacrificing the residential, social environment.

Occupational performance is the ability to carry out activities of daily living. Occupational performance is the accomplishment of the selected activity or occupation resulting from the dynamic transaction among the client, the context, and the activity. Improving or enabling skills and patterns in occupational performance leads to engagement in occupations or activities

(Law, Polatajko, Baptiste, & Townsend, 1997). **General activities programs** are defined as "events or tasks designed to provide incentive and opportunity to engage in continuing life experiences and hence, to satisfy interests and meet general activity needs. General activities programs focus on enjoyment, stimulation and repetition of present skills" (Crepeau, 1986). *Occupational therapy* is defined as the "application of occupation or goal-directed activity to achieve optimum function, to prevent dysfunction, and to promote health" (p. 5). The term *occupation,* as used in occupational therapy, refers to "Occupation is everything people do to occupy themselves ... enjoying life ... and contributing to the social and economic fabric of their communities" (p. 3).

Goals for occupational performance programs can focus on a wide variety of target areas, including promoting change in intrapersonal skills (appropriately tolerating frustration, developing realistic expectations of self); promoting change in communication skills; demonstrating appropriate impulse control; actively listening; promoting change with cognitive and task performance skills (organizing own tasks, self-correcting task errors); promoting change in independent living skills (effectively managing time, using appropriate safety judgment, and developing a sense of emotional well-being); and promoting maintenance or improvement of physical skills (dexterity for self-care independence, ability to produce a legal signature). Occupational performance programs have as many diverse goals as the therapists possess creativity.

Steultjens et al. (2004) conducted a systematic review on the effects of research involving the use of occupational therapy with older adults living independently in the community. They concluded that there was strong evidence for the efficacy of advising on assistive devices, some evidence for the training of skills in decreasing incidence of falls in at-risk elderly clients, and some evidence for the efficacy of occupational therapy on functional ability, social participation, and quality of life. These areas should become commonly targeted for persons with dementia living in skilled nursing facilities, as well.

To accommodate cognitive loss that accompanies dementia, therapists rely more heavily on the use of external cues. Memory books and other cuing systems can be very helpful in assisting persons with dementia to reach therapeutic goals (Bourgeois, 2007). This is especially true when combined with other procedures such as errorless learning (Camp, 2006a; Wilson, Baddeley, Evans, & Shiel, 1994), teaching task-specific routines or self-monitoring related to executive dysfunction (Sohlberg & Mateer, 2001), or spaced-retrieval, which is described in more detail later in this chapter.

As of June 2006, CMS guidelines and regulations regarding activities provided to residents of skilled nursing facilities changed. There is now a renewed emphasis on insuring that activities match the individual resident's personal interests, age, gender, and level of cognitive functioning. One target area for surveyors following these guidelines is to determine whether facility staff other than those in activity departments are involved with activity programming. Camp, Breedlove, Malone, Skrajner, and McGowan (2007) have described areas being targeted for more intense scrutiny by surveyors, and provided an extensive list of recommendations on how to address these issues using Montessori-based activities, which we will describe in more detail later in this chapter.

Interdisciplinary Teams in Long-Term Care

Given the wide variety of needs of long-term-care residents, a variety of professionals are required to meet these needs. As a result, professionals creating occupational performance programs for long-term-care residents must work as part of an interdisciplinary team. Members of the interdisciplinary team must work in collaboration and partnership with one another, advocating for the rights of the resident and never losing sight of the resident's needs. The composition of the long-term-care interdisciplinary team is dependent upon the size of the organization, its staffing patterns (e.g., whether most staff are contractual versus employees), and the needs of the residents. Long-term-care residents and organizations benefit from having a comprehensive team of skilled health care professionals holistically evaluating and treating residents based on their physical, cognitive, and psychosocial needs. Members of the team will bring their unique specialties and perspectives to the decision-making process. The interdisciplinary team is typically composed of a variety of specialists such as nurses, nurse assistants, physicians, social workers, and therapists from various disciplines—art therapy, (Figure 22-1A and 22-1B), audiology, music therapy, occupational therapy, physical therapy, and speech/language pathology, nutritionists, and recreational specialists. Of course, the most important members of the team are the resident and family members or significant others, who should be involved whenever possible to assist in establishing goals and making informed decisions. Based on the assessments of all the team members, a comprehensive, personalized plan of care is developed, outlining all aspects of care delivery for a resident. The plan of care should reflect individualized cognitive and physical problems, goals, and intervention strategies and

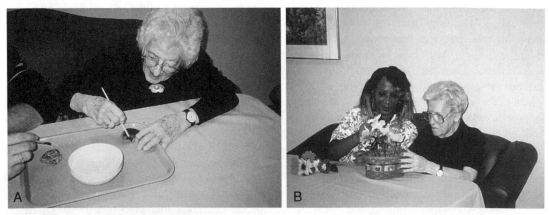

FIGURE 22-1 (A) Rock painting emphasizes focused concentration, fine motor skills, and range of motion. (B) Flower arranging emphasizes fine and gross motor skills, aesthetic appreciation, color identification, and care of the environment. (Courtesy of Myers Research Institute, Menorah Park Center for the Aging, Beachwood, Ohio, with permission.)

identify which disciplines will be responsible for providing the intervention. Interdisciplinary meetings for each resident are held at least quarterly or more frequently if and when there is a change in medical status, whether it is improvement or decline. The team is charged with the responsibility to creatively develop a plan of intervention that will maximize an individual's abilities and focus on successful interactions while maintaining the resident's dignity and feelings of self-worth.

Staff attitudes and communication are the most significant determinants of whether an interdisciplinary team will be successful or not. Staff members must focus on the needs of the client and set aside individual differences and potential competitiveness among disciplines. This may be especially challenging in this era of managed care and changes within the government entitlement programs. Considering staffing patterns for long-term care, it will be critical for all care providers to work cooperatively to create and maintain environments that support and maintain optimal programming for residents. Professionals must view themselves as having the potential and responsibility of maintaining interventions initiated by persons outside their own discipline.

It is quite possible for an interdisciplinary rehabilitation team to be very successful at creating an occupational performance project while maintaining the integrity of their individual disciplines. For example, at Menorah Park Center for Senior Living in Beachwood, Ohio, an interdisciplinary team was developed to create a quilt describing significant personal life events of a number of residents in the long-term-care facility (Figure 22-2). This was a collaborative effort of staff from art therapy, music therapy, occupational therapy, and speech/language pathology. The goals of the task included providing an avenue for reminiscing; increasing feelings of accomplishment; enhancing clients' satisfaction and reaffirming their value in society; enabling individuals to make a unique contribution to a whole that was far more than the sum of its parts; providing a way for residents to be as independent as possible during a creative process; and finally, providing a forum to connect with families, careers, hobbies, and past life experiences. In this case, the occupational therapist was an equal member of the interdisciplinary team, and each discipline focused on its area of expertise with the resident.

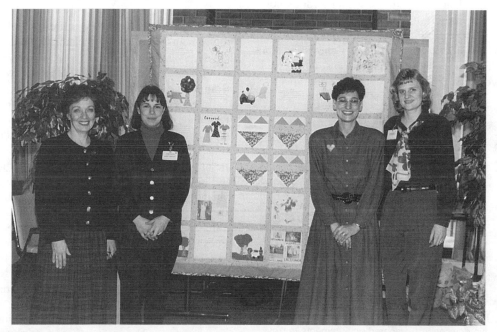

FIGURE 22-2 The memory quilt was developed by an interdisciplinary team from rehabilitation services in collaboration with residents in long-term care. (Courtesy of Myers Research Institute, Menorah Park Center for the Aging, Beachwood, Ohio, with permission.)

Therapies and Total Environment

Along with the expertise and attitude of the staff, the general environment of an organization can and should support the delivery of a quality occupational performance program, and the environment must be supportive of a variety of activities. Each of the residents has an array of previous life skills that can be incorporated into programming. It is a mistake to believe that rehabilitation can occur only within a traditional clinic setting focusing on tabletop tasks and therapy materials. We must look beyond the obvious and utilize the total living environment as an element in occupational performance treatment planning.

The **therapeutic environment** can be anything from the resident's room to the facility at large. At Menorah Park, for example, the treatment environment includes a horticulture area; an in-house nature center; in-house pets; therapeutic and recreational swimming facilities; work trial areas in a snack shop, gift shop, or reception area; an on-site child care facility for volunteer experiences; available technology such as environmental controls, aids for the visually impaired, Internet access, and computer learning modules; vehicles for exploring and integrating into the community at large; a specific place for worship and meditation; a resident bank and beauty shop, exterior garden spaces with putting greens, and raised flower beds (Figure 22-3); an ice cream parlor;

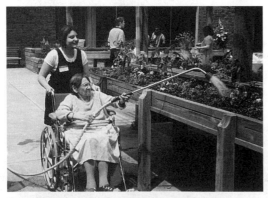

FIGURE 22-3 Wheelchair gardening. The use of assistive devices and prepared environments makes outdoor gardening accessible to residents. (Courtesy of Myers Research Institute, Menorah Park Center for the Aging, Beachwood, Ohio, with permission.)

an auditorium used for entertainment, evenings of formal dining with visiting family members, and dances, and so on. It is the responsibility of the therapist to look outside of the traditional box and utilize the environment in treatment planning. Some facilities may have limited environmental resources, but even an outdoor picnic table, a courtyard with flowerbeds, or an activity space can be therapeutically valuable. The interdisciplinary team must be committed to being creative in utilizing the existing environment to achieve goals, always remembering that the facility is actually an individual's home and not a sterile clinic environment.

Regulatory and Reimbursement Issues

Therapists must become accustomed to constructively dealing with the continual changes within the regulatory world while not losing sight of the residents' needs. The regulatory changes are often mandated by the various payer sources rather than through the legislative process. It will always be necessary to work within the framework of regulations governing long-term care such as the PPS. Therapists may consider the regulatory world as encouraging evaluation of current methods of conducting business and providing care. Often, regulatory requirements will raise questions about care delivery systems and challenge an organization to problem-solve effective solutions within resource constraints.

In general, administrators must evaluate how to provide quality occupational performance-based programming, while meeting regulatory standards, with the least-expensive intervention. The area of reimbursement is constantly changing, sometimes resulting in a greater emphasis on managing cost than managing care, though it is important to note that containing costs and providing quality care do not have to be opposing forces (Phillips, Hawes, & Fries, 1994). The attitudes of the various payer sources, whether traditional Medicare or managed care, affect the scope of service provided and at what cost. There are several state providers of Medicaid services that focus on therapy services and provide an incentive to increase therapy involvement to improve the functional abilities of long-term-care residents. But in general, therapy-based services are paid for by third-party payers with an emphasis on achieving specific goals rather than preventing deterioration or decline.

Innovative Trends

As a result of these factors, innovation and creativity are required to assure that the principles and philosophy of occupational therapy will be part of engagement for long-term-care residents. An example of this is the Occupational Performance Clinic at Menorah Park. This model clinic utilizes the skills of an occupational therapist to evaluate the physical, cognitive, and psychosocial abilities of residents on various units who express the interest and capability to benefit from extended participation in activities away from their unit. Additional staff includes OT assistants and, of course, the support of the other rehabilitation disciplines. Each resident has an individualized plan of care, with individualized clinic activities integrated within the care plan. Each plan focuses on utilizing a resident's physical and cognitive abilities, and adaptive techniques and equipment as necessary. The tasks access previous life experiences such as homemaking and clerical skills and may also involve community outreach projects. The clinic serves approximately 30 clients each day, with 45 total residents in the program. The occupational therapist also develops engagement plans to export to other caregivers, including family members, so that residents can continue to benefit from exposure to appropriate tasks during nonclinic hours. The goals of the Occupational Performance Clinic are accomplished within the constraints of reimbursement, with corresponding documentation requirements and the need to adhere to facility productivity standards.

Collaboration with Research

Another example of the search for innovative ways to deliver services is seen in the collaborations at Menorah Park between the Rehabilitation Department and the Myers Research Institute. The research institute is a division of Menorah Park and focuses on applied research in the areas of public policy and psychosocial interventions affecting long-term-care residents. With regard to psychosocial interventions, researchers are committed to working with care delivery staff to insure that treatments created by research staff can be effectively implemented within the real-world context of long-term-care facilities.

An example of this trend is seen in the development of a memory intervention for persons with dementia called **spaced retrieval (SR).** SR involves giving persons with memory deficits practice at successfully remembering information over increasingly long periods of time, and it has been shown to enable persons with a variety of different dementing conditions to retain new information across clinically meaningful (i.e., days, weeks, or months) periods of time (Camp, 1999, 2006a; Camp et al., 2000; Camp & Foss, 1997; Camp, Foss, O'Hanlon, & Stevens, 1996; Camp, Foss, Stevens, Reichard, McKitrick, & O'Hanlon, 1993; Camp & Mattern, 1999; Camp & McKitrick, 1992).

In a collaborative effort between speech-language pathologists and research staff at Menorah Park, SR has been developed into an intervention for persons with dementia that can be implemented by therapists from a number of different disciplines, including occupational, physical, music and art therapy, as well as speech-language pathology, within the contexts of regular therapy sessions (Brush & Camp, 1998a, 1998b; 1999; Bourgeois et al., 2003). Thus, SR can enable clients in long-term care to accomplish additional therapy goals within the same time frame as regular therapy sessions, enabling therapists to accomplish more within the context of the number of therapy sessions imposed by PPS.

Within the contexts of interventions for dementia in general, and the creation of therapeutic activities in particular, research staff have been heavily influenced by the work of Tom Kitwood. Kitwood (1996, 1997) proposed a model for describing the development and manifestation of dementia. He compares his approach against what he refers to as the "standard paradigm" for describing the cause of dementia:

$$X \Rightarrow \text{neuropathic change} \rightarrow \text{dementia}$$

In this linear model, the X refers to factors such as genetic causes, vascular disease, and so forth, that may lead to progressive, neuropathic change. This, in turn, leads to progressive dementia. Interventions from the standpoint of a medical model, such as is seen in clinical trials of drugs, focus on finding ways to influence the

X in this model. Drugs are designed to eliminate or otherwise influence *X*. For those who focus on genetic determinants of dementia, an eventual hope is that gene therapy or interventions designed to modify harmful genetic processes can be found to influence *X* in this model.

Kitwood discusses three significant problems with this model. First, even though correlations between measures of dementia and indices of the extent of neuropathology are statistically significant, they are often quite weak. Second, some individuals show a more rapid degeneration in short periods of time than could be attributed to rate of nervous tissue degeneration. Third, dementia can become stable for long periods of time or even display partial recovery of function. These problems are viewed as resulting from difficulties in relating aspects of mind versus brain.

As an alternative conceptualization, Kitwood proposed this model:

$$D = P + B + H + NI + SP$$

Dementia (D) in any particular individual is manifested through the combined effects of five key factors. Three of these, personality (P), biography (B) or personal life history, and neurological impairment (NI), are relatively outside the control of current interventions and are viewed as fixed. These factors vary across individuals and account for variability in how persons react to their conditions, adhere to medication regimens, and so forth. Physical health (H) also plays a key role in the manifestation of dementia (e.g., whether the person has a healthy diet, high blood pressure, etc.), along with affecting opportunities for maintaining competence and the ability to interact with the social and physical environment. The fifth factor is a person's social psychology (SP), which surrounds the individual and critically influences the way in which dementia is manifested to or interpreted by society. Kitwood states that everything should be done to promote the highest level of physical health in persons with dementia, but he suggests that the social psychology of dementia should be the focus of intervention for occupational persons working with dementia.

These factors in the overall model are described as interacting in this manner: "In a very general way, then, the symptomatic presentation of dementia in any individual arises from a complex interaction between all five factors, while the progression of the illness depends primarily on the interplay between NI and SP ..." (Kitwood, 1997, p. 274). For example, a husband with dementia living in long-term care may have a wife who visits often, reads to him, and provides social and cognitive stimulation on a regular basis. He suddenly loses his wife's support due to her death (change in SP). Though NI may remain at a steady state, manifestation of dementia can rapidly progress if the level of facilitation previously provided by his wife is no longer available to him.

Although neurological impairment cannot be reversed, it is useful to focus on abilities that are spared or less impaired over the course of dementia as the basis for improving the social psychological environment within long-term care. For example, Squire (1992, 1994) has described a number of abilities, such as priming, classical conditioning, and skills and habits, which might serve as the basis for interventions for persons with dementia (Camp, 1999, 2006b; Camp & Foss, 1997; Camp et al., 1993, 1996; Camp & Mattern, 1999; Camp & McKitrick, 1992; Camp & Nasser, 2003; Kitwood, 1997; Squire, 1992, 1994). Camp and his colleagues used this approach to create an intergenerational program in which individuals with dementia living on an Alzheimer's Disease Special Care Unit served as teachers and mentors for preschool children using Montessori teaching materials and lessons as the basis for the program (Camp et al., 1997), as well as in an adult day health center (Camp, Orsulic-Jeras, Lee, & Judge, 2004). Montessori-based activities and materials employ many principles found in occupational therapy and have goals similar to those found in occupational therapy. These include breaking down tasks into their simplest components; providing feedback and high probability of success; providing structure and order; giving practice and repetition within the context of completing tasks; using everyday materials; attempting to increase independence and self-esteem; focusing on the circumvention of deficits; using adaptive or assistive devices; attempting to increase range of motion, motor skills, use of tools, grip strength, eye–hand coordination, and self-care capacities; and providing meaningful activity and meaningful social roles (Auer, Sclan, Yaffee, & Reisberg, 1994; Camp, 1999, 2006b; Camp et al., 2006;

Joltin, Camp, Noble, & Antenucci, 2005). In addition, there is evidence that Montessori-based activities are based on forms of learning in Squire's model described earlier that are relatively preserved in dementia (Camp, 1999, 2006b; Camp & Brush, 1999).

Residents in the program were trained to complete and demonstrate Montessori-based activities to preschool children from the child care center that serves employees of Menorah Park (Figure 22-4). Residents with dementia were able to display high levels of competence doing this. Most importantly, even though disengagement from their social psychological environment was a common occurrence on the unit as evidenced by observational data, disengagement was not seen when these residents were fulfilling the roles of teacher and mentor to children. This pilot study was expanded into a 3-year project involving both residents in long-term care and adult day care clients with dementia (Camp et al., 2004).

In another study funded by the national Alzheimer's Association, Montessori-based activities have been given directly to persons with moderate to advanced dementia. Using this approach is based on the idea that there may be a developmental progression to the loss of abilities in dementia, roughly following a "first-in, last-out" model of cognitive deterioration labeled by Reisberg (1986; Reisberg et al., 2002) as "retrogenesis" (see also Auer et al., 1994; Barinaga, 1998; Camp, 1999; Nolen, 1988; Sclan, Foster, Reisberg, Franssen, & Welkowitz, 1990; Thornbury, 1992; Vance, Camp, Kabacoff, & Greenwalt, 1996).

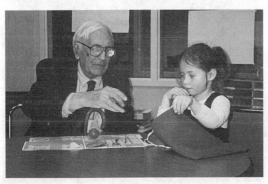

FIGURE 22-4 Intergenerational programming for dementia. Montessori-based activities provide the structure and guidance to allow persons with dementia to serve as mentors to preschool children. (Courtesy of Myers Research Institute, Menorah Park Center for the Aging, Beachwood, Ohio, with permission.)

Working in conjunction with occupational therapists at Menorah Park and with Montessori teachers, activities were developed by research staff and provided to persons on a number of long-term-care units who were at various stages of dementia. Both group and individual activities incorporating Montessori teaching principles (and occupational therapy approaches) were created (Box 22-2). Initial results, based on observational data, indicate that persons with dementia displayed significantly higher levels of active engagement during Montessori programming than in standard activities programming (Camp, 1999, 2006b). What has been especially interesting in this study is that research staff trained activities therapists, social workers, nurse assistants, and volunteers to implement some of these activities effectively in the course of their usual caregiving routines (Camp & Brush, 1999; Camp & Nasser, 2003; Orsulic & Judge, 1998; Schneider, Diggs, Orsulic, & Camp, 1999). This approach parallels that taken by staff within the Therapeutic Activities Clinic; that is, they search for ways to enable activities based on occupational therapy principles to be made available to residents on their units when occupational therapists may not be available there (Figure 22-5A and 22-5B).

Additionally, researchers at the Myers Research Institute have taken this approach a step farther, training clients and residents with early- to moderate-stage dementia to serve the role of small group activity leader for groups of persons with more advanced dementia (Camp & Skrajner, 2004; Camp, Skrajner, & Kelly, 2005). In these cases, the small group activities involved an activity developed to resemble bingo for persons who could no longer take part in that game, and a reading/discussion group activity designed for persons with dementia (Camp, 1999).

In a similar fashion, research staff have been working to develop an assessment tool for persons with advanced dementia, called the **Myers-Menorah Park/Montessori-based Assessment System (MMP/MAS).** As described in more detail elsewhere (Camp et al., 1999), the MMP/MAS is composed of a set of seven **Montessori-based activities.** It is designed to be administered by an occupational or recreational therapist charged with creating activities programming for persons with dementia, and yields information more relevant to this purpose than more standard assessments of cognitive assessment in late-stage dementia.

BOX 22-2 **Key Montessori-Based Dementia Programming® Principles for Working with Persons with Dementia**

- Invite clients to participate in an activity.
- Offer choice to the clients about what activity to pursue, when possible.
- Sit in a closed circle/square to increase participation.
- Talk less. Demonstrate more. Let the client learn what to do by observation.
- Match your speed to their speed.
- Use visual hints/external cues/templates whenever possible.
- Give the clients something to hold/manipulate.
- Work from the simple to the complex.
- Ask clients at the end of an activity, "Did you enjoy this?" or "Would you like to do this again?"
- Think THEIR SUCCESS! If the client is not succeeding, ask yourself how the procedures and materials should be modified to accommodate the strengths and weaknesses of the client to enable the client to succeed.

©2006 Myers Research Institute. Used with permission.

An example of the types of information that the MMP/MAS might yield is shown in Appendix 1 on pages 565–567, along with programming suggestions and goals based on MMP/MAS results (Fig. 22-6A and 22-6B).

This is another example of an attempt to infuse principles of occupational therapy into long-term-care settings. Of course, the administration and interpretation of Montessori-based activities or an instrument such as the MMP/MAS might be most effectively accom-plished by persons with training in occupational therapy. However, current reimbursement regulations reduce contact between long-term-care residents and occupational therapists. As a result, although the long-term solution of this dilemma is the

restructuring of the present regulatory and reimbursement system for occupational therapists providing services to persons with dementia, in the short term it is important that residents have access to activities that embody principles of occupational therapy. For this reason, a version of the MMP/MAS is now being developed as an assessment tool for restorative nursing programs in long-term-care settings. In so doing, it is possible to sensitize caregivers and administrators to the benefits that can be derived for long-term-care residents (and their caregiving staff) when more purposeful activities are made available. In addition, we hope to encourage activities staff, nursing assistants, volunteers, and others who use such activities to become more cognizant of the

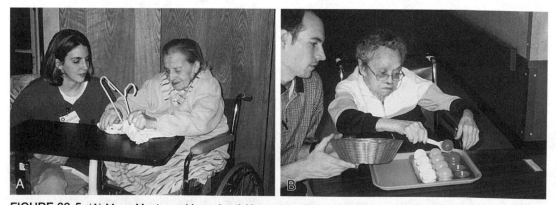

FIGURE 22-5 (A) Many Montessori-based activities emphasize practice in activities of daily living, such as hanging up clothing, which are similar to activities utilized by occupational therapists. (B) Practice in using tools to transfer large objects will be followed by activities transferring small, solid objects, and then transferring liquids. Skills required for self-care, such as eating soup, can be practiced and refined through the use of programmatic sets of activities. (Courtesy of Myers Research Institute, Menorah Park Center for the Aging, Beachwood, Ohio, with permission.)

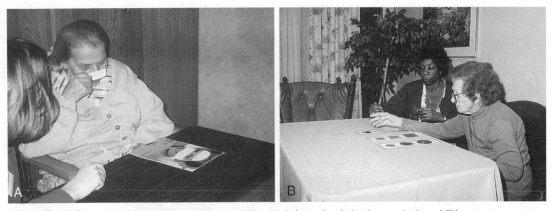

FIGURE 22-6 (A) Cognitive stimulation, motor skills, whole/part discrimination, and other abilities are practiced in such tasks as face puzzles. Such puzzles can include faces of family members, staff, or famous persons familiar to residents. (B) Shapes are sorted by size and type. This is a preliminary assessment of matching and discrimination ability. (Courtesy of Myers Research Institute, Menorah Park Center for the Aging, Beachwood, Ohio, with permission.)

rehabilitation potential of residents and, in turn, to become important referral sources for occupational therapists.

Cross-Cultural Issues

As discussed in other chapters, it is important to be sensitive to cross-cultural issues when creating activities related to occupational performance. To date, manuals and other materials created by the Myers Research Institute in collaboration with the rehabilitation staff of Menorah Park Center for Senior Living have been translated into Japanese, Mandarin, Korean, Spanish, and French. In addition, we are actively working to have these materials translated into other languages. However, we have found that it is important to translate specific tasks into a culture, as well. For example, tasks that involve use of spoons or forks in Western cultures must involve transfer using chopsticks in Eastern cultures.

A task in our first *Manual for Montessori-Based Dementia Programming*® (Camp, 1999) involves using a slotted spoon to scoop objects hidden in a tub filled with rice. When the object (i.e., "buried treasure") has been found and scooped up, the spoon is gently shaken to sift out the rice through the slots in the spoon. The object is then placed on a mat inside of one of several circles. When all of the circles have an object inside, the client knows that all of the objects have been found. In Japan, we had to substitute lentils or some other substance less

familiar to older Japanese. We were told that older Japanese would view the use of rice in this way as something close to sacrilegious, because these persons had lived through times when rice was scarce and each grain was important to sustain life. A visiting researcher from India suggested that in her culture the activity would involve putting rocks inside of the tub of rice, and that sifting out the rocks would be similar to an activity of daily living. Even at Menorah Park, an Orthodox Jewish facility, cultural issues impact this activity. During the feast of Passover, we cannot use this activity with residents, because their religious beliefs mean that they should not touch a grain at this time, even it if will not be eaten.

■ Summary

Occupational therapists must objectively prove to regulators and reimbursement sources that activities-based programs designed and implemented by occupational therapists versus generalists, provide positive, objective, and sustained functional outcomes. Positive clinical outcomes will be the most important factor in determining the future of occupational therapists and activity-based programming. In the future, the long-term-care industry is expecting to admit more frail older adults with multiple medical diagnoses. Many long-term-care facilities may maintain their focus on provision of health care needs from the medical model, but truly progressive organizations will attempt to meet these needs whenever possible without sacrificing the psychosocial needs of the resident.

The resident of the future will present with chronic disease and pose conflicting goals for the organization. The resident will desire safety, autonomy, and excellent medical services but may be unwilling or unable to pay for the services. To meet the needs of residents and deliver services within long-term-care settings, therapists must be creative and innovative when approaching the subject of activities programming and be able to demonstrate tangible benefits of such programming for both residents and staff.

An individual's age should not be the determinant of whether a person should or should not participate and benefit from a therapeutic activities program. But will third-party payers understand the significance of quality-based activities programs for the frail older adult and be willing to reimburse therapists for their skills? There is recent evidence that this indeed may be happening. As of June 2006, regulations from the Center for Medicare and Medicaid Services have begun to emphasize the need for high-quality, age-, gender-, and stage-of-dementia-appropriate activities programming. This may well portend a renewed interest in providing truly therapeutic activities for long-term-care residents. If so, the skills and knowledge of occupational therapists may become more salient to facilities seeking to comply with regulatory imperatives.

Case Study

Mrs. Johnson is an 87-year-old African American widow, currently residing in a nursing home. She lived alone in her own home until 2 years ago, when her five adult children became concerned about her memory and her ability to manage daily tasks. Mrs. Johnson has had arthritis for at least the past 10 years; it causes her moderate pain most days. She also has diabetes, which she developed at age 50. She requires both diet management and medication to manage this condition.

However, the main concern about her condition is her rapidly developing dementia. Her children noticed about 4 years ago that her recent memory was deteriorating. They decided that she needed nursing home care following an incident in which one of the children came for a visit and found an empty pot sitting on the stove over an open flame.

The children and grandchildren remain involved with Mrs. Johnson and are frequent visitors. However, staff members want to ensure that she remains as functional as possible and have noted that recently she's been relatively withdrawn and less involved with activities. In addition, they are concerned about her arthritis and the limitations it imposes on her daily function. They have referred her to OT for an evaluation of her condition and suggestions about a care plan.

Questions

1. In order to adequately develop a treatment plan for Mrs. Johnson, what additional information should the OT seek?
2. Mrs. Johnson's children report that she used to sing in the church choir, and that prior to entering the nursing home, she was very involved in the church sisterhood. They also report that she used to be a very good bridge player, and had a regular game with three longtime friends. How might this information be helpful to the occupational therapist?
3. What aspects of a comprehensive occupational profile are missing? What other activities might help maintain Mrs. Johnson's quality of life?
4. How might these services be provided given that goals focused on "leisure" are not reimbursable?
5. What cultural factors are apparent in Mrs. Johnson's situation?

Review Questions

1. How did enforcement of OBRA '87 influence nursing home standards of care?
2. Discuss the implications of OBRA '87 legislation on activities programming in long-term-care facilities.
3. What factors influence the role of occupational therapists in long-term-care settings?
4. Does rehabilitation mean restoration to previous levels of functioning?
5. Under OBRA regulations, what constitutes a "qualified professional" who can direct activities programming in long-term care?
6. Describe the different kinds of goals that might be set for occupational performance programming.
7. Discuss the use of interdisciplinary teams for creating occupational-performance-based plans of care for persons with dementia.
8. What is the therapeutic environment?
9. Describe Kitwood's model of dementia. How does it relate to activities programming?
10. How are Montessori-based activities similar to occupational therapy practices?
11. What are some examples of how cultural issues can influence creation of occupational activities in long-term-care settings?

Web-Based Resources

For helpful information about the experience of long-term care visit:

www.myersresearch.org, **The Myers Research Institute,** date connected September 20, 2007. Provides a listing of resources (print and electronic) available through the Institute, describes current research and staff, and provides additional information about Montessori-based intervention.

www.ahca.org, **American Health Care Association,** date connected September 20, 2007. An advocacy group for long-term care. Includes information about current efforts, the advocacy process, and links to other resources.

www.aahsa.org, **American Association of Homes and Services for the Aging,** date last connected September 20, 2007. Many resources for individuals working in nursing home settings. Includes references, links, and general information.

www.healthinaging.org/agingintheknow/, **American Geriatrics Society Foundation for Health in Aging,** date connected September 20, 2007. Feature articles about the aging process, information about how to get information from health care providers. Primarily focused on consumers.

www.cms.hhs.gov, **Centers for Medicaid and Medicare Services of the U.S. Department of Health and Human Services,** date connected September 20, 2007. A comprehensive and authoritative resource for information about the complex rules and policies governing these two government programs. Use of a website is essential because the rules change frequently.

www.wellspringis.org, **Wellspring,** date connected September 20, 2007. An organization of independent, not-for-profit institutions serving older adults. Includes resources for program planning and links to other resources.

www.edenalt.com/about/htm, **The Eden Alternative,** date last connected September 20, 2007. A well-known organization that advocates focusing on strengths of elders, rather than a deficit model. Discusses this philosophy and provides resources.

REFERENCES

Allen, C. K. (1993). Position paper: Purposeful activity. *The American Journal of Occupational Therapy, 47,* 1081–1085.

American Association of Homes and Services for the Aging (AAHSA). (2006). *Aging services in America: The facts.* Retrieved from www.aahsa.org/aging_services/default.asp. Accessed April 8, 2008.

American Geriatric Society (AGS) Foundation. (2005). *Aging in the know.* Retrieved from www.healthinaging.org/agingintheknow/. Accessed April 8, 2008.

American Health Care Association (AHCA). (2005). *The state long-term health care sector 2004: Characteristics, utilization, and government funding.* Retrieved from www.ahca.org/research/statestatsrpt_20050328_final.pdf. Accessed April 8, 2008.

American Occupational Therapy Association, Inc. (1977). AOTA representative assembly: Minutes. *The American Journal of Occupational Therapy, 31,* 599–604.

American Occupational Therapy Association, Inc. (1996). *AOTA member data surveys.* The American Occupational Therapy Association, Inc. 1995–96.

Aronson, M. K. (1999). Chronic pain and behavioral symptoms in the nursing home setting. *Dimensions, 6*(1), 5–6.

Auer, S. R., Sclan, S. G., Yaffee, R. A., & Reisberg, B. (1994). The neglected half of Alzheimer's disease: Cognitive and functional concomitants of severe dementia. *Journal of the American Geriatrics Society, 42,* 1266–1272.

Barinaga, M. (1998). Alzheimer's treatments that work now. *Science, 282,*1030–1032.

Baum, C., & Edwards, D. (1995). Position paper: Occupational performance: Occupational therapy's definition of function. *The American Journal of Occupational Therapy, 49,* 1019–1020.

Bissell, J. C. (1981). The use of crafts in occupational therapy for the physically disabled. *The American Journal of Occupational Therapy, 35,* 369–374.

Bourgeois, M. S. (2007). *Memory books and other graphic cuing systems.* Baltimore: Health Professions Press.

Bourgeois, M. S., Camp, C. J., Rose, M., White, B., Malone, M., Carr, J., et al.. (2003). A comparison of training strategies to enhance use of external aids by persons with dementia. *Journal of Communication Disorders, 36,* 361–379.

Breines, E. (1984). An attempt to define purposeful activity. *The American Journal of Occupational Therapy, 38,* 543–544.

Brush, J. A., & Camp, C. J. (1998a). Using spaced retrieval as an intervention during speech-language therapy. *Clinical Gerontologist, 19,* 51–64.

Brush, J. A., & Camp, C. J. (1998b). Using spaced retrieval to treat dysphagia in a long-term care resident with dementia. *Clinical Gerontologist, 19*(2), 96–99.

Brush, J. A., & Camp, C. J. (1999). *A therapy technique for improving memory: Spaced retrieval.* Beachwood, OH: Menorah Park Center for Senior Living.

Camp, C. J. (1999). Memory interventions for normal and pathological older adults. In R. Schulz, M. P. Lawton,
& G. Maddox (Eds.), *Annual review of gerontology and geriatrics* (Vol. 18, pp. 155–189). New York: Springer.

Camp, C. J. (2006a). Spaced retrieval: A case study in dissemination of a cognitive intervention for persons with dementia. In D. Koltai Attix & Kathleen A. Welsch-Bohmner (Eds.), *Geriatric neuropsychological assessment and intervention* (pp. 275–292). New York: The Guilford Press.

Camp, C. J. (2006b). Montessori-Based Dementia Programmings™ in long-term care: A case study of disseminating an intervention for persons with dementia. In R. C. Intrieri & L. Hyer (Eds.), *Clinical applied gerontological interventions in long-term care* (pp. 295–314). New York: Springer.

Camp, C. J., Bird, M. J., & Cherry, K. E. (2000). Retrieval strategies as a rehabilitation aid for cognitive loss in pathological aging. In R. D. Hill, L. Bäckman, & A. S. Neely (Eds.), *Cognitive rehabilitation in old age* (pp. 224–248). New York: Oxford University Press.

Camp, C. J., Breedlove, J., Malone, M. L., Skrajner, M. J., & McGowan, A. (2007). Adjusting Activities to Meet CMS Guidelines Using Montessori-Based Dementia Programming(r). *Activity Director's Quarterly, 8*(1), 34–46.

Camp, C. J., & Brush, J. A. (1999). *Montessori-based interventions for persons with dementia.* Teleconference presented at the National Center for Neurogenic and Communication Disorders, University of Arizona, Tucson, February.

Camp, C. J., & Foss, J. W. (1997). Designing ecologically valid memory interventions for persons with dementia. In D. G. Payne & F. G. Conrad (Eds.), *Intersections in basic and applied memory research* (pp. 311–325). Mahwah, NJ: Lawrence Erlbaum & Associates.

Camp, C. J., Foss, J. W., O'Hanlon, A. M., & Stevens, A. B. (1996). Memory interventions for persons with dementia. *Applied Cognitive Psychology, 10,* 193–210.

Camp, C. J., Foss, J. W., Stevens, A. B., Reichard, C. C., McKitrick, L. A., & O'Hanlon, A. M. (1993). Memory training in normal and demented populations: The E-I-E-I-O model. *Experimental Aging Research, 19,* 277–290.

Camp, C. J., Judge, K. S., Bye, C. A., Fox, K. M., Bowden, J., Bell, M., et al. (1997). An intergenerational program for persons with dementia using Montessori methods. *The Gerontologist, 37,* 688–692.

Camp, C. J., Koss, E., & Judge, K. S. (1999). Cognitive assessment in late stage dementia. In P. A. Lichtenberg (Ed.), *Handbook of assessment in clinical gerontology* (pp. 442–467). New York: John Wiley & Sons.

Camp, C. J., & Mattern, J. M. (1999). Innovations in managing Alzheimer's disease. In D. E. Biegel & A. Blum (Eds.), *Innovations in practice and service delivery across the lifespan* (pp. 276–294). New York: Oxford University Press.

Camp, C. J., & McKitrick, L. A. (1992). Memory interventions in DAT populations: Methodological and theoretical issues. In R. L. West & J. D. Sinnott (Eds.), *Everyday memory and aging: Current research and methodology* (pp. 155–172). New York: Springer-Verlag.

Camp, C. J., & Nasser, E. H. (2003). Nonpharmacological aspects of agitation and behavioral disorders in dementia: Assessment, intervention, and challenges to providing care. In P. A. Lichtenberg, D. L. Murman, & A. M. Mellow (Eds.), *Handbook of dementia: Psychological, neurological, and psychiatric perspectives* (pp. 359–401). New York: John Wiley & Sons.

Camp, C. J., Orsulic-Jeras, S., Lee, M. M., & Judge, K. S. (2004). Effects of a Montessori-based intergenerational program on engagement and affect for adult day care clients with dementia. In M. L. Wykle, P. J. Whitehouse, & D. L. Morris (Eds.), *Successful aging through the life span: Intergenerational issues in health.* (pp. 159–176). New York: Springer.

Camp, C. J., Schneider, N., Orsulic-Jeras, S., Mattern, J., McGowan, A., Antenucci, V. M., et al. (2006). *Montessori-based activities for persons with dementia* (Vol. 2). Beachwood, OH: Menorah Park Center for Senior Living.

Camp, C. J., & Skrajner, M. J. (2004). Resident-assisted Montessori programming (RAMP): Training persons with dementia to serve as group activity leaders. *The Gerontologist, 44,* 426–431.

Camp, C. J., Skrajner, M. J., & Kelly, M. (2005). Early stage dementia client as group leader. *Clinical Gerontologist, 28*(4), 81–85.

Centers for Medicare and Medicaid Services (CMS). (2005). *Health care industry market update.* (cited in www.ahca.org/research/cms_market_update_030520.pdf).

Clark, F., Azen, S. P., Zemke, R., Jackson, J., Carlson, M., Mandel, D., et al. (1997). Occupational therapy for independent-living older adults. *Journal of the American Medical Association, 278,* 1321–1326.

Clark, F. & Larson, E.A.. (1993). Developing an academic discipline: The science of occupation. In H. Hopkins & H. Smith (Eds.), *Willard and Spackman's occupational therapy* (8th ed., pp. 44–57). Philadelphia: J. B. Lippincott.

Crepeau, E. L. (1986). *Activity programming for the elderly.* Boston: Little, Brown & Co.

Dreher, B. B. (1997). Montessori and Alzheimer's: A partnership that works. *American Journal of Alzheimer's Disease, 12,* 138–140.

Duellman, M. K., Barris, R., & Kielhofner, G. (1986). Organized activity and the adaptive status of nursing home residents. *The American Journal of Occupational Therapy, 40,* 618–622.

Dutton, R. (1989). Guidelines for using both activity and exercise. *The American Journal of Occupational Therapy, 43,* 573–580.

Fidler, G. S. (1981). From crafts to competence. *The American Journal of Occupational Therapy, 35,* 567–573.

Fried, L. P., & Guralnik, J. M. (1997). Disability in older adults: Evidence regarding significance, etiology and risk. *Journal of American Geriatric Society, 45*(1), 92–100.

Hawes, C., Morris, J. N., Phillips, C. D., Fries, B., Murphy, K., & Mor, V. (1997). Development of the nursing home resident assessment instrument in the USA. *Age and Ageing, 26*(Suppl. 2), 19–25.

Hawes, C., Phillips, C., Morris, J., Mor, V., Fries, B., Steele-Freidlob, E., et al. (1997). The impact of OBRA-87 and the RAI on indicators of process quality in nursing homes. *Journal of the American Geriatric Society, 45*(8), 977–985.

Hinojosa, J., & Kramer, P. (1997). Statement-fundamental concepts of occupational therapy: Occupation, purposeful activity, and function. *The American Journal of Occupational Therapy, 51,* 864–866.

Hinojosa, J., Sabari, J., Rosenfeld, M. S., & Shapiro, D. (1983). Purposeful activities. *The American Journal of Occupational Therapy, 37,* 805–806.

Hirdes, J. P., & Carpenter, G. I. (1997). Health outcomes among the frail elderly in communities and institutions: Use of the Minimum Data Set (MDS) to create effective linkages between research and policy. *Canadian Public Policy (23sl),* pp. 53–69.

Institute of Medicine. (1986). *Improving the quality of care in nursing homes.* Washington, DC: National Academy Press.

Iwarsson, S., Isacsson, A., Persson, D., & Schersten, B. (1998). Occupational and survival: A 25 year follow-up study of an aging population. *The American Journal of Occupational Therapy, 5,* 65–70.

Jacelon, C. S. (1995). The effect of living in a nursing home on socialization in elderly people. *Journal of Advanced Nursing, 22,* 539–546.

Jackson, J. (1996). Living a meaningful existence in old age. In R. Zemke & F. Clark (Eds.), *Occupational science: The evolving discipline* (pp. 339–361). Philadelphia: F.A. Davis.

Joltin, A., Camp, C. J., Noble, B. H., & Antenucci, V. M. (2005). *A different visit: Activities for caregivers and their loved ones with memory impairment.* Beachwood, OH: Menorah Park Center for Senior Living.

Kaiser Foundation. (2006). Financing Long Term Care. http://www.kaiseredu.org/tutorials/longtermcare/longtermcare.html. Accessed April 8, 2008.

Kitwood, T. (1996). A dialectical framework for dementia. In R. T. Woods (Ed.), *Handbook of the clinical psychology of aging* (pp. 267–282). Chichester, UK: Wiley.

Kitwood, T. (1997). *Dementia reconsidered.* Buckingham, UK: Open University Press.

Law, M., Polatajko, H., Baptiste, W., & Townsend, E. (1997). Core concepts of occupational therapy. In E. Townsend (Ed.), *Enabling occupation: An occupational therapy perspective* (pp. 29–56). Ottawa, Ontario, Canada: Canadian Association of Occupational Therapists.

Mor, V., Intrator, O., Hiris, J., Fries, B., Phillips, C., Hawes, C., et al. (1997). Impact of the MDS on changes in nursing home discharge rates and destinations. *Journal of the American Geriatrics Society, 45*(8), 1002–1010.

National Center for Health Statistics. (2005). *Health, United States, 2005, with chartbook on trends in the health of Americans.* Hyattsville, MD: National Center for Health Statistics.

Nelson, D. L. (1988). Occupation: Form and performance. *The American Journal of Occupational Therapy 42,* 633–641.

Nelson, D. L. (1997). Eleanor Clark Slagle lecture, 1997: Why the profession of occupational therapy will flourish in the 21st century. *The American Journal of Occupational Therapy, 51,* 11–24.

Nelson, D. L., & Peterson, C. Q. (1989). Enhancing therapeutic exercise through purposeful activity: A theoretic analysis. *Geriatric Rehabilitation, 4*(4), 12–22.

Nolen, N. R. (1988). Functional skill regression in late-stage dementias. *The American Journal of Occupational Therapy, 42,* 666–669.

Omnibus Budget Reconciliation Act (OBRA) of 1987. (1991, October). *The Federal Register, 56* (48), 865.

Orsulic, S., & Judge, K. (1998). *Implementation of Montessori-based activities for dementia by long-term care and adult day care staff.* Paper presented at the annual meeting of the Gerontological Society of America, Philadelphia, PA, November.

Pedretti, L. W., & Pasquinelli, S. (1996). *Occupational therapy practice skills for physical dysfunction* (4th ed.). Philadelphia: Mosley-Year Book.

Phillips, C. D., Hawes, C., & Fries, B. (1994). High costs of restraints. *Provider, 20*(2), 33–34.

Phillips, C., Morris, J., Hawes, C., Mor, V., Fries, B., Murphy, K., et al. (1997). The impact of the RAI on ADL's, continence, communication, cognition, and psychosocial wellbeing. *Journal of the American Geriatrics Society, 45*(8), 986–993.

Rancourt, A. M. (1991). Programming quality services for older adults in long-term care facilities. *Activities, Adaptation, & Aging, 15,* 1–11.

Reilly, M. (1962). Occupational therapy can be one of the great ideas of the 20th century medicine. *The American Journal of Occupational Therapy, 16,* 1–9.

Reisberg, B. (1986). Dementia: A systematic approach to identifying reversible cues. *Geriatrics, 4,* 30–46.

Reisberg, B., Franssen, E. H., Souren, L. E. M., Auer, S. R., & Akram, I. (2002). Evidence and mechanisms of retrogenesis in Alzheimer's and other dementias: Management and treatment import. *American Journal of Alzheimer's Disease® and Other Dementias, 17*(4), 202–212.

Schneider, N. M., Diggs, S., Orsulic, S., & Camp, C. J. (1999). N.A.s teaching Montessori activities. *Journal of Nurse Assistants, 26* (March), 13–15.

Sclan, S. G., Foster, J. R., Reisberg, B., Franssen, E., & Welkowitz, J. (1990). Application of Piagetian measures of cognition in severe Alzheimer's Disease. *Psychiatric Journal of the University of Ottawa, 15*(4), 221–226.

Sohlberg, M. M., & Mateer, C. A. (2001). *Cognitive rehabilitation.* New York: Guilford Press.

Squire, L. R. (1992). Memory and the hippocampus: A synthesis from findings with rats, monkeys, and humans. *Psychological Review, 99,* 195–231.

Squire, L. R. (1994). Declarative and nondeclarative memory: Multiple brain system supporting learning and memory. In D. L. Schacter & E. Tulving (Eds.), *Memory systems 1994* (pp. 203–232). Cambridge, MA: The MIT Press.

Steultjens, E. M. J., Dekker, J., Bouter, L. M., Jellema, S., Bakker, E. B., & van den Ende, C. H. M. (2004). Occupational therapy for community dwelling elderly people: A systematic review. *Age and Ageing, 33,* 453–460.

Thornbury, J. M. (1992). Cognitive performance on Piagetian tasks by Alzheimer's disease patients. *Research on Nursing and Health, 15,* 11–18.

Trombly, C. A. (1995). Eleanor Clarke Slagle lecture, 1995: Occupation: Purposefulness and meaningfulness as therapeutic mechanism. *The American Journal of Occupational Therapy, 49,* 960–972.

Vance, D., Camp, C. J., Kabacoff, M., & Greenwalt, L. (1996). Montessori methods: Innovative interventions for adults with Alzheimer's disease. *Montessori Life, 8,* 10–12.

Vladeck, B. C. (1980). *Unloving care.* New York: Basic Books.

Wilson, B. A. (1989). Models of cognitive rehabilitation. In R. L. Woods & P. Eames (Eds.), *Models of brain injury rehabilitation* (pp. 117–141). London: Chapman & Hall.

Wilson, B. A. (1997). Cognitive rehabilitation: How it is and how it might be. *Journal of the International Neuropsychological Society, 3,* 487–496.

Wilson, B. A., Baddeley, A., Evans, J., & Shiel, A. (1994). Errorless learning in the rehabilitation of memory impaired people. *Neuropsychological Rehabilitation, 4,* 307–326.

World Health Organization (WHO). (1986). *Optimum care of disabled people.* Report of a WHO meeting, Turku, Finland, 1986.

World Health Organization (WHO). (2001). *ICF: International Classification of Functioning, Disability and Health.* (http:/www3.who.int/icf/icftemplate.cfm).

Yerxa, E. J. (1980). Occupational therapy's role in creating a future climate of caring. *The American Journal of Occupational Therapy, 34,* 529–534.

Zimmer-Branum, S., & Nelson, D. L. (1995). Occupationally embedded exercise versus rote exercise: A choice between occupational forms by elderly nursing home residents. *The American Journal of Occupational Therapy, 49,* 397–402.

ACKNOWLEDGMENT

Preparation of this manuscript was supported, in part, by grant # R01 AG021508-01A1 from the National Institute on Aging and grant # R21 MH063395-01A2 from the National Institute of Mental Health to the second author.

Appendix 1

Myers-Menorah Park/Montessori-Based Assessment System (MMP/MAS)

Coding Sheet for Montessori Activities

Resident: B.

Examiner: T.P.

Date: 5/18/98 (completed)

Directions:

Demonstrate each activity under standard procedures. If the resident is able to perform the activity under standard procedures, then only "able to complete task under standard procedures" is checked. If the resident is unable to perform the activity under standard procedures, then "unable to complete task under standard procedures" is checked. Also, any component of the task that was completed correctly is checked. Additional subjective notes regarding the resident's motor, cognitive, sensory, and social skills are noted for every task, and an overall global assessment is made pertaining to suitable programming for the resident.

Background Information:

Hidden Coin Search:

___ Able to complete task under standard procedures.
_X_ Unable to complete task under standard procedures.
___ Able to find coins (7).
___ Able to count number of coins (1–7).
___ Able to place coins on stars.
_X_ Able to place coins back into corn.

- Resident was able to follow the example of the examiner and put hands into the corn, find them, and hand them to the examiner.

She was also able to hide coins in the corn when they were handed back. She did not respond to prompts to count, or to place the coins on stars on the tray. She did not respond to comments about colors of the coins. She did, however, talk the whole time using short phrases or sentences and show pleasure.

Golf-ball Scooping:

___ Able to complete task under standard procedures.
_X_ Unable to complete task under standard procedures.
_X_ Able to identify colors (white, *yellow,* orange).
___ Able to match colors correctly (between golf balls and colored wells).
___ Able to use large/small scoop independently.
___ Able to use scoop with assistance of using hands.
_X_ Able to transfer golf balls using only hands.
___ Able to transfer golf balls back into the container.

- Resident referred to the yellow color of golf balls as "gold" and repeatedly used the phrase "gold star." This may have been a carryover from the hidden coins activity. She was able to transfer golf balls by hand into wells in the muffin tin but did not match by color. She did not attempt to use the scoop, but did show pleasure through smiling during the entire activity.

Living/not-living Picture Sort:

___ Able to complete task under standard procedures.
_X_ Unable to complete task under standard procedures.
_X_ Able to read labels.
_X_ Able to identify the pictures.
(some) Able to decide if picture is living or not living.
(some) Able to place pictures under correct label.
___ Able to put pictures and labels back into Ziploc bag.

- Correctly named cows, zebras, car, and bear. Gave the correct color of the car (red) and cows. Did not identify the record player or butterfly. Smiled when she saw ice cream cone but did not identify. Correctly categorized car and tractor and could place some pictures under correct labels with prompting.

Happy/not-happy Picture Sort:

___ Able to complete task under standard procedures.

X Unable to complete task under standard procedures.

X Able to read labels.

X* Able to identify the pictures. [* about half, with redirection and assistance]

X Able to decide if the picture is happy or not happy. [* about half, able to comment on some]

X* Able to place pictures under correct label. [*with direction]

___ Able to put pictures and labels back into Ziploc bag.

• Resident was able to comment on the pictures and correctly able to judge if they were "happy" or "not happy" for about half of the pictures. She needed redirection to help her keep focused and on task. She was enthusiastic when photos led to talking about her family.

Liquid Seriation:

___ Able to complete task under standard procedures.

X Unable to complete task under standard procedures.

___ Able to distinguish between large and small.

___ Able to seriate using concrete operations (i.e., able to compare and contrast different sizes by physically manipulating them).

___ Able to seriate using formal operations (i.e., able to compare and contrast different sizes by mentally manipulating them).

• Resident was able to place the test tubes in the holes, though not in any order. She named the color of the liquid (black) and of the tip of the tube (blue).

Pom-pom with Tweezers:

___ Able to complete task under standard procedures.

X Unable to complete task under standard procedures.

X Able to identify colors.

X Able to use *large*/small tweezers to transfer pom-poms.

X Able to use hands to transfer pom-poms.

___ Able to match pom-poms to correct colored wells.

___ Able to transfer pom-poms back into container.

• Resident was able to transfer pom-poms using large tweezers but not the small ones. She could not match the color of pom-pom to the corresponding color of well in the ice cube tray. She named all colors of pom-poms appropriately, except for white. She enjoyed talking about the colors. She started to put the pom-poms back into the bowl, but then asked examiner to finish for her. Resident did not respond to attempts to get her to count the pom-poms.

Shape Sorting:

___ Able to complete task under standard procedures.

X Unable to complete task under standard procedures.

___ Able to identify the shapes correctly (triangle, square, and circle).

___ Able to identify the sizes correctly (small, medium, and large).

X Able to match the shapes according to size.

___ Able to pick out correct shape and size.

• Resident was able to work with only one shape (square, circle, triangle) at a time. She was able to match small, medium, and large circles to their corresponding outlines but did not complete corresponding matching on the other shapes. She needed frequent redirection to stay focused. She would often stop the task to start telling stories about her family, which may have been a carryover from the happy/not happy sorting activity.

Overall Assessment

• **COGNITIVE:** B. is very verbal, responds well to multistep commands, and has a long attention span. B. is able to count and make some category decisions, with the help of provided verbal descriptions. B. enjoys discussing the activity with T.P. and at times begins verbalizing off of the topic. However, this can be easily redirected.

- **MOTOR:** B. has limited motor capabilities, because her hands act as her eyes. It would be difficult for her to use the scoop for golfball scoop because she uses both of her hands to feel her surroundings. B. is able to transfer using her hands. The smaller tools are difficult for B. to manipulate; the larger ones are more adaptable. B. has no visible motor problems, such as tremors or paralysis.
- **SENSORY:** B. has no apparent tactile or auditory problems. B. is completely blind. However, B. compensates well by using her hands. Tactile stimulation is extremely important for B. B. enjoys feeling things, such as the corn in hidden coin search and the softness of the pom-poms.
- **SOCIAL:** B. is very socially appropriate while participating in the Montessori activities. She is very attentive and willing to participate while in programming. B. comments that the activities are very enjoyable.

Programming Suggestions and Goals

Sensory activities, focusing on auditory and tactile stimulation, should be incorporated into programming for B. Activities such as sound cylinders, seashell matching, and thermic tablets would be beneficial. Motor activities utilizing her hands, such as hidden coin search, cylinder blocks, geometric shapes, and transferring activities, would be most beneficial and promote the most engagement for this resident. Picture and word-sorting activities are also good activities for B. to engage in cognitively, with some assistance. These activities will help promote verbalization and expression of remaining cognitive abilities. Goals for B. include tapping into remaining cognitive abilities (despite vision problems), use of fine motor skills, and increased decision making.

Myers-Menorah Park/Montessori-Based Assessment System (MMP/MAS). (©1998 Myers Research Institute & Menorah Park Center for the Aging.)

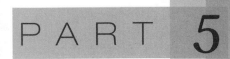

PART 5

Context

O lder adults have both unique and universal circumstances. All of us deal on a regular basis with the implications of a multicultural society, and other countries have similar cultural issues. For older adults, cultural factors like those discussed in Chapter 23 may be of particular salience either because they are immigrants or because older adults are likely to be more traditional than younger individuals. Professional cultures of the care providers they encounter can have significant impact on the outcomes of care, as values and beliefs can diverge in important ways. There is compelling evidence that health disparities are marked in later life, with individuals from disadvantaged minority groups struggling economically and functionally (Whitfield, 2004).

Technological advances, as explored in Chapter 24, have done more than prolong life. They have provided a wide range of methods for making life more satisfying and helping individuals accomplish what they need and want to do. Some professionals are tempted to assume that older adults do not relate well to "high-technology" interventions. Although this may be true for some, it is equally true that many elderly individuals respond extremely well to new technologies and find them enjoyable and gratifying. In addition, emphasis on **universal design** that enhances environments for everyone has improved and simplified some technologies that might previously have increased rather than reduced environmental barriers. In circumstances in which new technologies are not well accepted, it may be due to the manner in which they are introduced, not to the technologies themselves.

Elder abuse has been an increasing area of concern in gerontology. Abuse is not new, but attention is only recently being paid to the ways in which older adults can suffer from neglect or from direct injury. Financial abuse is also rampant. All professionals must attend to signs that elders are being abused and must help take steps to ameliorate problems both by reporting suspected abuse and by educating the public about elder abuse and its terrible toll. Chapter 25 describes the problem as well as the responsibilities of health-care practitioners in addressing it.

And finally, later life can be a time of great pleasure and satisfaction, but it ends for all of us. As Chapter 26 suggests, working with individuals who are dying and their families is an area of growing interest. Palliative and hospice care can help make the end of life as satisfying as possible for the individual and for family members. It is also incumbent on professionals to recognize when there is hope and when an individual is giving up prematurely, perhaps because of depression. This is not an easy distinction, but an important one. One 95-year-old woman, who described herself as being in good health, except, of course, for macular degeneration, high blood pressure, and arthritis, complained that she had buried all her friends and had no desire to go on. When she suffered a mild stroke, from which someone in her physical condition would most typically have recovered, she stated that she was ready to be with her friends, stopped eating, and died 3 weeks later. This is not the inevitable outcome of such a series of losses, and most older adults choose to find ways to cope. However, it is important for care providers to be aware of the potential for such downward spirals. It is also important for care providers to recognize situations in which palliative care is appropriate and to help families accept the inevitable.

In working with older adults, health-care professionals must consider all of the special circumstances that characterize the aging process. In doing so, they can help ensure that the later stages of life are satisfying to the individual, the family, and the broader community. This is a challenge to the professional, but one that carries considerable potential benefit for all.

Whitfield, K. E. (Ed.). (2004). *Closing the gap: Improving the health of minority elders in the new millennium.* Washington, DC: Gerontological Society of America.

CHAPTER 23

Culture and Aging

Bette R. Bonder, PhD, OTR/L, FAOTA

M uch of what we call culture and civilization consists in efforts people have made, generally against over whelming odds, to create a sense of purpose for themselves and their descendants.

Mihaly Csikszentmihalyi, 1990, p. 215

OBJECTIVES

By the end of this chapter, readers will be able to:

1. Define culture.
2. Describe the characteristics of culture.
3. Discuss the ways in which culture interacts with individual personality and experience to create unique expressions of culture.
4. Discuss the ways in which culture influences the experience of aging.
5. Discuss the concept of health disparities and the ways in which culture contributes to these disparities.
6. Describe strategies for effectively incorporating culture into intervention planning and implementation, including the concepts of culture-specific knowledge, scientific-mindedness, and dynamic sizing skills.
7. Describe characteristics of specific cultures, including those based on racial, ethnic, and religious identities, as well as cultures based on disability, sexual orientation, and profession.
8. Discuss the implications of culture for service use.
9. Describe the way cultures interact based on individual experience, to result in the emergence of culture in specific interactions.
10. Discuss strategies for generating hypotheses about the impact of culture on assessment and treatment with individuals.
11. Describe skills that facilitate dynamic sizing.
12. Describe strategies for self-evaluation that enhance increased cultural competency.

As was briefly discussed in Chapter 1, **culture** has profound import in the experience of aging. The rapid global growth of the older population, the increasing mobility of populations from one country to another, and historical trends in migration have all contributed to the growing need to understand culture and to incorporate cultural values, beliefs, and preferences in health care interventions.

Both the International Classification of Function (ICF) (World Health Organization, 2001) and the American Occupational Therapy Association (AOTA) Practice Framework (2002) list culture as a contextual factor—that is, a factor that affects health and function but exerts its influence on the individual from the environment rather than the reverse. This is something of an oversimplification as we shall see in this chapter, but having culture clearly identified as a factor in development across the life span and in provision of health care is a major step forward in addressing its centrality to human occupation.

Demographic trends are a good indicator of some important cultural issues in aging. In the United States, the population is growing both older and more diverse. U.S. Census Bureau projections (2001) suggest that the white population in the United States will grow by 81% by 2030; for African Americans it will grow by 131%; for American Indians, Eskimos, and Aleuts, 145%; Asian and Pacific Islanders, 285%; and Hispanics, 328%. As noted in Chapter 1, the age pyramid is shifting toward aging in all countries. Many of the developed countries, as is true for the United States, are also experiencing increased immigration (Organisation for Economic Co-operation and Development, 2004) so that their aging populations are increasingly diverse. And world-wide, the proportion of the population that is older is growing rapidly (United Nations Division for Social Policy and Development, 2006). Culture influences public policies that affect the experience of aging, dealing with such issues as access to health care and social services, pension and other financial support, and perceptions about appropriate roles for older adults (Walker, 2006).

Culture may affect individuals' expectations about what old age will be like, their plans and goals for this period of their lives, their values and attitudes about being older and about health care, and their motivations for engaging in or withdrawing from occupations. Many aspects of culture can be exaggerated in later life. For example, the current cohort of elders is more likely than their offspring to be first-generation immigrants and to have retained more aspects of their home countries. This may influence such traits as emotional inhibition, leaving some groups of elders less equipped to express emotional concerns in later life (Consedine, Magai, Cohen, & Gillespie, 2002). A particularly important issue is their retention of the language of their native country. Elders may not learn the new language, or may be less fluent than subsequent generations. They may also retain traditional beliefs about health and health care and be more likely to use traditional healing methods.

Culture affects not only roles but also values and interpretations of the aging experience. For example, in the United States, *generativity,* productive engagement in the lives of others or in the society, is viewed as important in later life as a way to establish a sense of continuity. Generativity is less valued in cultures where there is a strong belief in the afterlife or spirit life (Alexander, Rubinstein, Goodman, & Laborsky, 1991), and roles tend to be somewhat vague. By contrast, "in the West, and in the United States in particular, the self rests within the individual, and within a larger ethos of individualism" (Rubenstein & De Medeiros, 2004, p. 61).

Even perceptions of what constitutes a "good" old age vary. In the United States, being vital and active is considered important, while in Ireland, the time to relax and have freedom from work is more valued (Fry et al., 1997). In the United States, older minority women are at greater risk for health problems because of income, poor education, housing, malnutrition, and barriers to health care (Hopper, 1993). In some cultures, though, older women are particularly valued for their wisdom, or have important ongoing functions as decision makers for health issues for the whole family.

As noted in Chapters 1 and 3, care must be taken in describing "successful aging," as different cultural groups may have different perspectives of what this means (Fox, 2005). In Greece, subjective quality of life was associated with positive affect and ability to adapt to old age (Efklides, Kalaitzidou, & Chankin, 2003). Among older Chinese, functional status and productive involvement status were associated with successful aging (Chou & Chi, 2002). Frequent contact with friends was especially important in China. These are subtle differences, but they are potentially important in thinking about OT intervention.

There are some common beliefs across cultures with regard to aging. Most notably, almost all cultures make a distinction between frail and able elders, and this distinction accounts for much of the difference in the aging experience (Draper & Harpending, 1994). There are many common elements of subjective well-being across cultures (Diener & Suh, 1998). Commonality across cultures in terms of correlates of successful aging include physical functioning and performance (Andrews, Clark, & Luszcz, 2002) and positive affect (Diener & Suh). At the same time, cultural differences cannot be ignored. So, for example, it may be important to know that for Jewish Israelis, life satisfaction was predicted most strongly by health status, but for Arab Israelis, social visitation was more important (Litwin, 1995).

There is no way to present all the cultural differences that affect the experience of aging; however, examination of a number of cultural groups provides instructive information regarding factors that may be common across cultures and factors that are unique to specific groups. It is noteworthy that even in cultures that appear to the outsider to be relatively similar, dramatic differences may exist. Likewise, there are commonalities across cultures, even those that appear quite different.

with preferences, with contextual factors that support or impede performance, or with other cultural variables. In examining the various performance areas, it is important to keep in mind that culture is not static. So, for example, in the Asia-Pacific region, a new image of a more active elder is emerging (Phillips, 2000). This means that in addition to having a fundamental knowledge of occupations in individual cultures, it is also helpful to have some sense of world events that are likely to play some role in altering cultures.

An interesting and helpful example of the impact of culture on the experience of aging has been presented by Draper and her colleagues (Brooks & Draper, 1998; Draper & Harpending, 1994). They studied two groups found in Africa, the !Kung and the Herero. The !Kung, a tribe in Botswana, sustain a traditional lifestyle that has not been greatly influenced by Western cultural norms. The !Kung live by a combination of food-producing and food-gathering–hunting techniques, and are extremely poor. In contrast, the Herero are pastoralists who live in Namibia and Botswana (Figure 23-1). Both the !Kung and Herero have had low to moderate fertility, and older adults are not scarce. Despite close similarity in the numbers of available children, the two societies make very different use of the potential labor pool represented by children. The

Culture and Occupation

Culture affects every area of occupation, as well as the underlying and contextual factors associated with performance. Because of the many interacting factors that can influence a particular individual's values, beliefs, and behaviors, it is not reasonable to assume that a care provider can know everything about every culture. The discussion that follows is designed to provide an overview of some of the considerations that should be taken into account when working with elders. It is followed by a discussion of strategies for attending to culture in the intervention process.

Performance in Areas of Occupation

Every area of occupation is influenced to some extent by culture. The impact may have to do

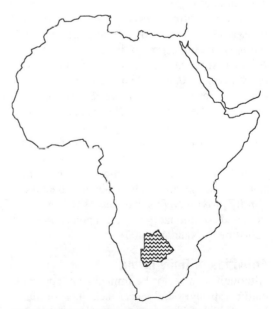

FIGURE 23-1 This map shows the location of the !Kung and Herero groups in Africa.

work performance of old people in the two societies varies accordingly.

Although the social environment of aging in simple societies may be desirable and generally superior to that of aging in complex industrial societies, the physical environment does not permit older adults to cushion themselves against the physical losses of aging. In !Kung society, everyone who is neither very young nor very old performs the same chores, although with varying degrees of vigor, depending on age, health, and to some extent, gender. Old people remain physically active as long as possible. They derive self-esteem from the belief that they are "able to take care of themselves." In Herero society, elders in their 60s and 70s undertake only light tasks, but with age, more of the work is accomplished with the help of others, especially children. The !Kung cannot count on this type of help.

In a comparison of !Kung and Herero, outward signs of the value of old people are most prominent among the Herero, but among the !Kung, the old are also given at least some respect and support. Herero elders can assume that material and social resources will be provided. Among the !Kung, older people enjoy no special status, privileges, or authority as a matter of custom. Some elders are well provided for, but when this occurs, it is the result of having successful adult children with whom the elder is on good terms rather than on a more general cultural sense of obligation to elders.

Culture affects occupation in developed nations as well. So, for example, as compared with other ethnic groups in the United States, African Americans have more difficulties with daily tasks (Sloan & Wang, 2005) and higher disability rates (Kelley-Moore & Ferraro, 2004; Mendes de Leon, Barnes, Bienias, Skarupski, & Evans, 2005). And immigration brings new complexity to the equation, as demonstrated by the fact that Asian Indian immigrants to the United States have encountered social, emotional, and spiritual obstacles to adaptation. Family proximity, positive reasons for immigration, and commonality of values predict positive adjustment (Nandan, 2005).

Activities of Daily Living

Although it may not be immediately apparent, culture strongly influences activities of daily living (ADL). This category includes dressing (sari or slacks?), eating (fork or chopsticks?), hygiene (bath or shower?), mobility (sitting on a chair or on the floor?), and other basic self-care functions. Among the important factors to consider is the particular set of cultural standards for competence (Rubenstein & de Medieros, 2004). Two individuals with identical ability to perform self-care tasks as viewed by an observer may perceive their own competence quite differently.

Among the observations about function among different groups in the United States, more than half of Native Americans aged 75 and older experience at least one significant ADL limitation; the number increases to more than 70% of those over 85 (Ludtke, McDonald, & Allery, 2002). Because the number of elders in these groups is growing rapidly, the number with significant ADL limitation is likewise expected to grow rapidly. Interestingly, although African Americans have been reported to have greater functional limitations overall, some research also finds they have somewhat less loss of ADL function than whites as they aged (Sloan & Wang, 2005).

Instrumental Activities of Daily Living

Instrumental activities of daily living (IADL) function is strongly mediated by gender role expectations in particular cultures. In Hong Kong, women are unlikely to learn to manage their finances, and they are at high risk for poverty in later life (Lee, 2003). Among elders in Berlin, women are very likely to spend a great deal of time on household activities, although those who lived with a partner had more time for leisure activities (Klumb & Baltes, 1999). Community mobility can be a problem for women who have never learned to drive if they live in cities without good public transportation. Men can also be disadvantaged by these gender expectations, because in some cultures they may never have learned to cook or to maintain a home.

Certainly culture plays a role in IADL choices. Food preferences and cooking styles are clear examples. Making a stir-fry requires different skills and abilities than roasting a turkey. Money management varies by cultures. For example, the Muslim religion generally proscribes taking loans from banks (*Nida'ul Islam Magazine,* 1995). Informal lending structures have arisen in these communities to fill the void; they mean that interventions emphasizing money management must be modified to suit these kinds of arrangements.

Lest one think that culture is something that happens to others, consider the kinds of cultural influences on IADL performance in mainstream U.S. culture. Typically, men handle house repairs and maintenance of the yard, and women cook and keep the interior of the home clean. Elders who choose to dress for comfort rather than for style sometimes find themselves disparaged by younger individuals.

Education

Education has a profound influence on the experience of aging. There is considerable evidence that individuals who are well educated have a more positive experience of aging (Kinsella & Phillips, 2005). The reasons are not clear—it may be that better-educated individuals have better access to health information, or that they are more likely to have the financial resources to afford healthy food and good health care, or it may be that they have more access to meaningful occupations.

Once again, differences in gender roles can affect educational attainment. In Asian countries, older women are more likely than men to be illiterate (Knodel, Ofstedal, & Hermalin, 2002). In the United States, by contrast, in African American communities, women are much more likely than men to have attended college (Babco, 2001).

Work

Because culture affects education, it is reasonable to assume it also influences participation in work. Research evidence confirms that this is so. In the United States, for example, African American women have longer paid work histories than other women but have less income from social security because their work is more likely to be in low-paid jobs (Carstensen, 2001). In the Asia-Pacific region, there is an array of work activities, including rural semisubsistence, which conveys no retirement benefits so that many elders continue to work, and corporate work, which historically had good benefits that enabled retirement (Phillips, 2000). However, as is true in the United States, retirement benefits are being cut in many parts of the world. As a result of the loss of benefits, labor force participation has changed in Asia, so that older men are increasingly likely to be working, and among older women, rates of participation are lower, but increasing (Knodel, Ofstedal, & Hermalin, 2002).

It is important to remember that for elders, "work" may be too restrictive a construct. As noted in Chapter 13 the concept of "productive occupation" is important. Elders may well engage in occupations like child care or volunteer activities that have economic value but that do not come with a paycheck. In less-developed countries, there is an expectation that everyone who is able will make a contribution to the survival of the economic unit, usually the family.

Leisure and Play

As regards leisure and play, there are substantial differences across countries and cultures. One particular issue is whether the particular group has opportunities for retirement. In less-developed locations, and in agrarian cultures, individuals may be expected to make economic contributions until they are too frail to do so, and work may extend throughout the day and evening. The !Kung, described by Draper and her colleagues (Brooks & Draper, 1998; Draper, 1976; Draper & Harpending, 1994), and the Maya (Bonder, Bazyk, Reilly, & Toyota, 2005) are examples of cultures in which occupations undertaken purely for purposes of leisure are very rare. Although women in Guatemala certainly describe engagement in pleasurable activities, they must often find this pleasure in the course of productive occupations.

Leisure occupations fill a number of needs for elders, as noted in Chapter 12. An important issue related to culture is the opportunity for occupations to reinforce cultural values and beliefs. So, for example, for older Korean Americans, well-chosen leisure activities can facilitate a sense of "Koreanness" and a sense of security in an unfamiliar country (Kim, Kleiber, & Kropf, 2001).

At the same time, culture influences the particular leisure occupations chosen by elders. Older Spanish women are less likely than men to engage in physical activity; this results in poorer health-related quality of life for women (Guallar-Castillion, Sendino, Banegas, Lopez-Garcia, & Rodriguez-Artalejo, 2005). In the United States, these differences are related not only to culture but to socioeconomic circumstances. It has been noted that differences in education and health status account for almost all racial/ethnic differences in leisure-time physical activity (He & Baker, 2005).

Social Participation

One of the most consistent findings in the research about occupations of elders as they contribute to life satisfaction is the importance of social participation. The nature of that participation, the kinds of social networks that are available to elders, and the frequency of contact are all mediated by culture. So, for example, for African Americans, sense of community, sense of accomplishment in spite of adversity, spiritual connection, and social activity are correlates of positive aging (Terry-Cox, 2003). However, research suggests that African Americans have smaller social networks and lower levels of social engagement than whites (Barnes, Mendes de Leon, Bienias, & Evans, 2004). However, some African Americans find most of their social support through their families (Figure 23-2) and churches. The findings about social occupations are consistent for many

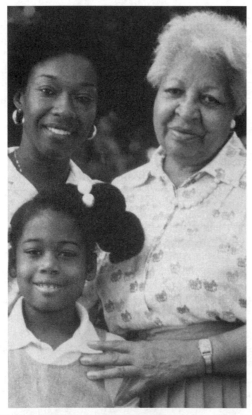

FIGURE 23-2 Family relationships are highly valued by African American elders. (From Memory and Aging. The Alzheimer's Association, Chicago, 1991, with permission.)

cultures. So, for example, socially active Japanese elders are more active in other ways as well. They have more hobbies and stay physically active, and are healthier than those who are not as socially connected (Ohno et al., 2000).

Performance Skills

Although less frequently reported than its impact on performance areas, culture has interesting interaction with performance skills. It is noteworthy that culture can affect human factors typically associated with biological processes.

Motor Skills

Even though there is not a large body of research on this point, evidence suggests that motor skills are developed consistent with the occupation demands in particular cultures. Observations of Mayan weavers (Bonder, 2001) showed that over the course of a lifetime of this activity, they were able to sit on the ground, either with legs extended or with knees flexed, or to kneel on the ground, for long periods of time. Other culturally mediated occupations may be associated with similar development of particular motor skills, or absence of those not needed.

Process Skills

There is a growing literature focused on the ways in which cultural factors influence cognition (e.g., Park, Nisbett, & Hedden, 1999). African Americans score lower on tests of cognitive function (Sloan & Wang, 2005). In particular, culture shapes reasoning and categorization (Atran, Medin, & Ross, 2006). East Asians tend to process information in a holistic, contextual fashion, and Europeans process information in an analytical fashion (Park et al., 1999). This has been attributed to the nature of Asian languages, which tend to be pictographic, thereby encouraging holistic perception of the world.

Interestingly, there is some evidence that Japanese Americans who speak Japanese have some protection against Alzheimer's disease (Graves, Rajaram, Bowen, McCormick, McCurry, & Larson, 1999). Culture affects many aspects of Alzheimer's disease, including not only prevalence, but also diagnosis and intervention strategies (Manly & Espino, 2004). Further, more acculturated African Americans (that is, those who had greater exposure to the majority culture) had better performance on neuropsychological testing (Manly, Byrd, Touradji, & Stern, 2004), perhaps associated with higher levels of education. Over time, African Americans show somewhat less deterioration in cognitive function than whites (Sloan & Wang, 2005).

Communication/Interaction Skills

Elders, particularly older immigrants, often struggle in terms of communication. The literature makes it clear that young children learn new languages most readily, and that language acquisition ability diminishes with age. This is a significant issue, as learning the language of the new country may be an important factor in establishing social networks, accomplishing important daily tasks, and becoming comfortable in new surroundings. So, for example, strong English-language skills predicted ability to live independently or serve as head of household for older Mexican immigrants. This difference is less evident in communities where the primary language is Spanish (Burr & Mutchler, 2003). Elderly Spanish-speakers are less likely than younger individuals to be proficient in English (Mutchler & Brallier, 1999).

Performance Patterns

As can be seen from the discussion above, occupational choices made by elders are culturally mediated (He & Baker, 2005). Patterns of engagement are likewise influenced by culture. As one example, older African Americans are less likely than whites to participate in social organizations or job-related organizations (Miner & Tolnay, 1998) but are more likely to be actively engaged in their churches (Rasheed & Rasheed, 2003). Another example can be seen in Figure 23-3 where Mayan women use a traditional method for carrying supplies from the market to their homes along cobblestone streets that would make it difficult to maneuver wheeled carts more typically found in the United States.

Habits and Routines

For elders, well-established habits can support function as physical capacity diminishes. The ability to complete self-care activities without conscious thought, for example, can conserve energy for other valued occupations. Even when capacity is significantly reduced, long-standing habits can support occupation. For example, Camp, Bird, and Cherry (2000) examined therapeutic effects of activities that draw on **procedural memory** in working with elders with Alzheimer's disease. They found that

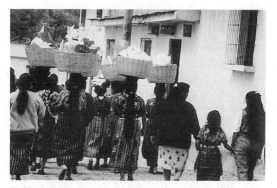

FIGURE 23-3 In some cultures, as is true for these Mayan women in the highlands of Guatemala, performance patterns may be based on age-old routines as well as environmental factors.

elders could participate in both self-care and leisure occupations more effectively when long-term habits were incorporated.

Unfortunately, not all habits are positive. In countries like the United States, where elders from some minority groups may have experienced significant discrimination throughout their lives, there can be long-term consequences for behavior and for quality of life (Dixon & Richard, 2003). These individuals may be suspicious of formal care providers and may have established habits that lead them to avoid services that might be able to support their function. Expectations about the probability of discrimination or about the absence of resources have been shown to result in stressful fears for African American elders (Weitzman, Dunigan, Hawkins, Weitzman, & Lefkoff, 2001).

Roles

In Western countries, where retirement is a life-course expectation, roles for elders are less clearly defined than for others. The lack of clear role expectations can be both a positive and a negative reality. In the positive sense, elders may feel more freedom than others to self-identify important roles. In the negative sense, elders may experience a certain amount of anxiety with regard to identity. In developing countries, and in some ethnic or religious groups, there are clear roles for elders; these enable them to retain a sense of self and of self-esteem. Grandparenting among Native Americans includes the highly valued role of "cultural conservator" (Weibel-Orlando, 2001). In these cultures, old age represents "an important time of life when a number of milestones have been attained" (Gardiner & Kosmitzki, 2005, p. 97). In Arab communities, elders are looked to as advisors, perceived as having wisdom born of experience (EthnoMed, 1996). This is also true in Brazil, Colombia, Japan, China, and many other collectivist societies, in which elderly people are revered and given high social status.

Gender expectations are apparent in the roles ascribed to elders (Cochran, Brown, & McGregor, 1999). For African American and white older women, roles include grandparenting, providing care, and volunteering, all of which are activities that can reduce depression. AIDS in Africa may force grandparents to take on custodial roles for grandchildren. In the United States, multiple roles are associated with lower rates of depressive symptoms (Cochran et al., 1999; Gallo, Cooper-Patrick, & Lesikar, 1998), which might suggest that providing care for grandchildren might have some positive consequences; this is less clear in other countries (especially Africa) where grandparents are frequently pressed into service. Marriage, employment, and total number of social roles were the most powerful predictors of depression for both African American and white women, but employment was more important in reducing depression in African American women (Cochran et al., 1999).

A dilemma in terms of roles is the impact of cultural change. Immigration can adversely affect roles as traditions are lost. Among Asian immigrants to the United States, respect for the knowledge of elders is diminished because it does not apply in the new environment (Carstensen, 2001). For Japanese-American elderly individuals, acculturation of subsequent generations changes sense of filial responsibility (Yamaguchi & Silverstein, 2003). However, reduced valuing of filial responsibility seems to increase affectional ties. In these situations, all generations continued to feel satisfied with their relationships.

Changing roles result from other societal factors, too. China's one-child policy and other causes of low fertility will have profound consequences for the notion of filial piety there (Phillips, 2000). In addition, younger people are less likely to believe that their parents should live with them (Hsu, Lew-Ting, & Wu, 2001). Although perceptions of elders are more positive in Chinese culture than in the United States (Zhang, Hummert, & Garstka, 2002), coresidence with adult children is diminishing because adult daughters no longer believe as strongly in allowing

this and are often in the workforce and therefore less available to provide care (Zimmer, 2005). In Ghana, diminished availability of family support because of changes in occupations of younger individuals and because of the loss of adult children to AIDS, there is a growing normative expectation of self-reliance (Aboderin, 2004).

Context

Occupations do not occur in a vacuum. The environment in which occupations are undertaken has strong influence on what they are and how they are enacted.

Cultural

As can be seen from the discussion so far, cultural context is a major factor in occupational choice. Beliefs about the role of family, independence and dependence, and proper societal supports can influence basic decisions, including residence and support networks. So, for example, in most countries in the Asia-Pacific region, aging is regarded primarily as a family concern. Changes in the ability of families to care for elders have generated considerable discussion and concern in this region (Phillips, 2000).

Culture affects sources of meaning derived from occupations. A study of young-old and older-old Israeli Jews and Arabs found that family and communal values were ranked high for all four groups, but higher for Arabs. Autonomy and independence and interpersonal relationships were ranked high by all, but were higher for older-old Jews. Communal activity was high overall, but higher for Arabs. Attainment of tranquility was very important for all, and highest for Jewish older adults, and self-development was lower for Arabs. Leisure activities with others were of medium-high significance, with differences between genders as well as cultures (less important to Arab women, and more important for men in all groups, more important for older Jewish women than younger Jewish women). Having good relationships was important, but less so for the older than the younger women in both groups (Bar-Tur, Savaya, & Prager, 2001). This is but one example of the differences in cultural values in late life.

Physical

An important aspect of the physical environment, and one that has received considerable attention in the research literature, is residential choice. In particular, decisions about whether to stay in the home, to migrate, or to live with adult children is associated with cultural values. It is, however, sometimes hard to discern whether the decision to live with family is the result of preference or economic considerations. "Although Hispanic, black, and Asian Americans are more likely than Caucasian Americans to live in extended family households, living arrangements are often determined more by economic need than by desire" (Carstensen, 2001, p. 267).

Many elders want to remain in their own homes. This choice certainly supports performance habits and can meet important psychological needs. "'Home' is known and individually appropriated through personal use, routines, and local meanings" (Rubenstein & de Medeiros, 2004, p. 62). In some cultures, this is an expected choice that is supported by family members and through publicly funded social services. In others, it is expected that elders will remain in the home.

Other aspects of culturally mediated physical environments affect the experience of aging. "Many Asian urban and rural areas offer an environment that is in effect hostile to older people" (Phillips, 2000, p. 25) including dense traffic, uneven surfaces, and wide roads. Individuals in wheelchairs, with unsteady gait, or with poor balance are at risk trying to manage damaged pubic walkways, but in developing countries, upgrades to provide adequate access may not be at the top of the list of priorities for spending on public health.

In recognition of the importance of the physical environment, immigrant families may choose to have elders return to their country of origin. Eritrean refugees believe that their elders will be more comfortable in more familiar surroundings (Ethnomed, 1996), and some Puerto Rican elders living in the mainland United States may decide to return to Puerto Rico for the same reason.

Social

The nature and reciprocity of social networks is culturally mediated (Ferraro & Su, 1999). Families are clearly at the center of those networks, but as families change, so does the character of their engagement with elders. In Japan there is a "dual structure" for familial caregiving, one modern and one traditional. Japanese elders who are in traditional families report high levels

of well-being. Those in modern families are similar to Japanese Americans in terms of worries about the future. However, this is somewhat ameliorated in Japanese Americans because they perceive themselves as having other options for care (Iwamoto, Rogers, & Gall, 2003). Studies in Hong Kong have had similar findings (Lee & Hong-kin, 2005; Ng, Phillips, & Lee, 2002). There is concern that changes in the valuing of filial piety will have significant consequences for elders.

In other countries, acculturation of younger generation has led to some dissatisfaction among elders. This has been reported for Chinese New Zealanders, who report a gap in expectations between younger and older individuals about reverence for the elderly. New Zealanders of European descent did not share the expectation and were therefore not disappointed by their children's attitudes toward them (S. B. Gee, Liu, & Ng, 2002).

Overall, widows or widowers living alone may be at highest risk for isolation (Williams, 2001), although it is impossible to generalize from living arrangements to quality of life (E. M. Gee, 2000). What is well established, though, is that social networks influence quality of life in later life, and that cultural expectations about appropriate roles affect the extent to which elders are able to establish and maintain satisfying networks.

Personal

In several chapters in this book, the concept of cohort has been discussed. Cohort experiences differ for various cultural groups (Dixon & Richard, 2003). So, for example, the current cohort of African American elders in the United States has experienced significant discrimination throughout life. Those experiences reflect both context and personal interpretation of external events. It is inevitable that they will have profound impact on occupation, and, as a result, on other circumstances of life. Although some of the consequences may be negative, greater poverty and poorer health, for example, there can also be positive consequences, in terms of such factors as strong social networks (Angel & Angel, 2006).

Spiritual

The spiritual context for occupation can have profound implications for quality of life. East Asian countries are influenced by Confucianism, Buddhism, Islam, and, to a lesser extent, Christianity (Phillips, 2000). Cultural characteristics that result include a strong value placed on family and societal harmony. Native American elders indicate that those who pray frequently and perceive their faith as important to them tend to have better mental health, regardless of their living situation or their age (Meisenhelder & Chandler, 2000). Overall, elders are more tolerant of religious difference as they age, and they attempt to find meaningful practices from a variety of traditions. Religious individuals, those who engage in formal, structured involvement with religious organizations, are more likely to benefit from social networks; spiritual individuals, those who focus on the presence of a higher power, rather than on formal religious participation, benefit from personal growth (McFadden, Brennan, & Hicks Patrick, 2003).

Conventional wisdom suggests that for African Americans, the church substitutes for formal social service agencies (Trinitapoli, 2005). Trinitapoli suggests that churches are much less likely to provide instrumental support than has been assumed, although their spiritual benefits may be substantial.

It is important to note that spirituality is not always equivalent with religion. Some individuals self-describe as highly spiritual in the sense that they believe in a higher power, a purpose or meaning greater than their self-interest. They may or may not enact those beliefs through traditional religious worship, and they may choose to express their spirituality through creative endeavors, through meditation, or through service to others. A qualitative study of older adults (Bonder, 2000) described how two women, both self-described as spiritual, enacted this value. One attended services regularly, participated in church-sponsored study groups, and was an active volunteer in community-service activities sponsored by the church. Another never attended services, but was active in choreographing dance performances held at her church that expressed her spiritual side. Another participant in the study, whose responses were not reported in the paper cited here, indicated that she felt her spirituality most profoundly when gardening, because the connection with nature seemed to her to reflect a higher and greater power.

Temporal

Cultural groups often have particular perceptions about time and its importance in life. So, for example, Native Americans in the United States tend to be aware of time more in terms of changes in the natural world than in terms of hour of the day (Alvord & Van Pelt, 1999). This results in a tendency to disregard the clock, with an accompanying tendency to be "late" for appointments that can be frustrating for those who focus more on the importance of being "prompt." And in some Hispanic cultures, a relaxed attitude toward time is also prominent. This can be a source of conflict with health care providers whose work is often strongly regulated by expectations for productivity.

Activity Demands

Objects Used and Their Properties

In my study of weaving in Guatemala and in the United States, I described the differences in the looms used by weavers (Bonder, 2001). Mayan women in Guatemala typically engage in back-strap weaving, in which the loom is constructed of sticks and the warp of the fabric, with the weaver providing the tension for the warp and thus serving as a part of the loom. Women in the United States who were weavers are more likely to use floor or table looms with more complicated mechanisms to provide tension. The weaver sits on a bench and is not, physically, a part of the loom. Likewise, Mayan women in Guatemala often make tortillas by grinding the corn, gathering wood, forming the tortillas by hand, and cooking them on a wood-burning stove (Bonder, Martin, & Miracle, 2002), while in the United States, tortillas are most often purchased ready-made at the store. Clearly, the objects used to weave and to cook are quite different in these two cultures and impact the extent to which elders will be able to maintain valued occupations.

Space Demands

Cultures differ with regard to perceptions about appropriate locations and spaces for work, prayer, and other occupations. Likewise, living arrangements differ among cultural groups such that the living space for elders may vary greatly. Because elders living alone, regardless of race or ethnicity, have more difficulty with daily tasks (Waite & Hughes, 1999), living arrangements can have dramatic consequences for occupational performance.

Social Demands

Societal expectations can either support or impede performance. In places where retirement is publicly supported and expected, elders who might prefer to continue in paid employment may experience unpleasant pressure to leave work. Likewise, pressure to stay "busy" can be difficult for elders who might prefer more placid and reflective lives (Ekerdt, 1986). Cultures like that of the United States that place particular value on youth may leave elders feeling marginalized.

A particular challenge for elders can be the experience of immigration. Elderly Russian immigrants to Israel reported that the experience was difficult but ultimately positive. They did not learn the language because they stayed in Russian immigrant communities; they reported difficulty finding housing, inadequate income, and weakening of ties with their younger family members (Remennick, 2003). Older Somali immigrants in London did best when they had family support. Those who did not perceived lower life satisfaction and were more likely to be depressed. They also experienced more disability and loneliness (Silveira & Alleback, 2001).

Required Body Functions/Required Body Structures

Because culture mediates the way in which particular occupations are undertaken, the required body functions and structures will also vary. Some older Mayan weavers struggle because of developing limitations in joint mobility or vision (Bonder, 2001). Because they had learned to weave in a particular fashion, these limitations led them to conclude that they could no longer weave. Simple adaptations to the occupation might have allowed them to move weft through warp, but in their view, this was no longer weaving. For these women, good vision, flexible limbs, and endurance for particular postural positions were essential to accomplish the task.

Client Factors

Body Functions/Body Structures

For individuals of all ages, stress is associated with negative affect and emotion inhibition. However stress-response illnesses emerge in different patterns in different cultural groups.

One study found that negative affect was disproportionately associated with arthritis in Eastern Europeans (as compared with European Americans), and the effect of negative affect on sleep disorders was less for Caribbean Africans than African Americans (Consedine et al., 2002).

Because the nature of particular occupations differs depending on culture, the needed body structures also differ. In addition, body structures develop differently across the life span depending on the occupations undertaken. Mayan weavers have considerable joint mobility in their lower extremities but also report high rates of "*artritis*" (joint pain) as a consequence of long years of sitting on the floor.

Culture and The Intervention Process

There is now a large literature describing differences in use of health care services (Smedley, Stith, & Nelson, 2003). Many cultural factors are associated with health care utilization (Dunlop, Manheim, Song, & Chang, 2002). In the United States, Hispanic women are less likely than other women or men to use nursing home care, and disabled African Americans are less likely to use services than other groups (White, 2000). Underrepresented minorities tend to have poor access to mental health services (Abramson, Trejo, & Lai, 2002). Native Americans have substantially worse health and poorer access to adequate care (John, 2004), a finding that is consistent with the circumstances of indigenous populations in many countries (cf., Ranzijn & Bin-Sallik, 2001).

History plays a role in service utilization. A study of all-Black towns in Oklahoma demonstrated that historical racism has led elders to use parallel or alternative services as opposed to formal health care systems (McAuley, 1998). And, of course, most health care providers in the United States are familiar with the chilling effect of the Tuskegee Syphilis Study on perceptions about the formal health care system among African Americans (Cargill, 2005). Health disparities are diminishing somewhat for elders in Medicare, possibly because of increased attention to the problem (Trivedi, Zaslavsky, Schneider, & Ayanian, 2005), but the United States has a long way to go before elders from all cultural groups receive satisfactory and equitable care.

Differences in service use also appear across international lines. Elders in Sweden make greater use of formal services, particularly focused on ADLs, and those in the United States make greater use of informal services (Shea et al., 2003). Foreign-born elders were at higher risk of poor emotional health than native-born counterparts (Angel, Buckley, & Sakamoto, 2001).

Interacting Demographic Factors as They Affect Intervention Planning

Many factors are associated with culture, and it is not always clear what is cause and what is effect (McCallum & Shadbolt, 1989). Numerous methodological problems plague research: differences in education, income, and social network patterns may be the variables that really contribute to differing situations. Markides and Lee (1990) found that education was a good predictor of well-being for older adults regardless of cultural background. A similar finding has been reported for African Americans (Manly et al., 2004). McCallum and Shadbolt (1989) noted that elderly Mexican Americans seem to rely primarily on families for support, whereas white individuals rely more on friends. Differences in support networks may be the result of cultural differences, or they may be the result of other factors, such as immigrant status. It is unclear whether cultural differences persist into old age, as "double jeopardy," or whether the experience of aging serves as the great leveler (Markides & Black, 1996). Because aging leads to increasing individual differences, cultural and societal factors may diminish in importance.

Some cultural differences are reflected in the kinds of health conditions seen by care providers. For example, African American individuals have lower life expectancy than white individuals until they reach the age of 75 years. They have higher rates of high blood pressure, with resultant kidney problems and cardiovascular accidents (Smedley et al., 2003). In addition, they have higher rates of cardiovascular disease, some cancers, and diabetes. After age 75, the life expectancy for African Americans is greater than for any other group (Manton & Stallard, 1997). They have greater bone density than white people, possibly reducing risk of injury secondary to osteoporosis. In addition, it may be that African Americans who survive into late life have already demonstrated unusual

hardiness. Asian individuals have lower risk of some cancers and cardiovascular disease. These differences may be biological rather than cultural, meaning that greater attention to differences among ethnic groups may yield important information about disease prevention.

Because the number of immigrants worldwide is likely to remain high (Gelfand & Yee, 1991), therapists will need to remember that culture can serve both to enhance the experience of later life and to make it more problematic. The opportunity to establish a clear identity is helpful; the associated tendency to remain apart from others can be detrimental (Gelfand & Yee, 1991.

To complicate matters further, people have more than one culture (Bonder et al., 2002). Our discussion so far has been primarily about ethnicity, however, we have also noted that there are distinct gay and lesbian cultures. There are also age-associated cultures (think about high school students, or elders in retirement communities). Disability groups and professions have distinct cultures, too. So it is likely that each client will have a unique set of interacting cultural values that must be discerned before intervention can be planned effectively.

Although there are clear cultural differences among groups, there are also many similarities (Mahoney, Cloutterbuck, Neary, & Zhan, 2005; Yang, McCrae, & Costa, 1998). Adult children of individuals from Chinese, African American, and Latino groups, when identifying onset of Alzheimer's disease reported similar reactions. In all three groups, there was a delay in seeking care because their initial impression was that forgetfulness was a normal part of aging. African Americans tended to label this "old timer's disease," Chinese used the term *"hu tu,"* and Latinos used the phrase *"el loco."* All tended to normalize symptoms, and all looked to family first for advice. For most cultural groups, life satisfaction does not decline with age (Diener & Suh, 1998), although elders tend to experience lower levels of control across groups (Shaw & Krause, 2001).

Sokolovsky (1997, p. xxv) suggested six key factors to bear in mind regarding culture and aging:

1. A single cultural system may provide successful solutions for some problems of aging and fail at others.
2. Not all non-Western, nonindustrial societies provide a better milieu for aging.

3. Social change does not automatically reduce the quality of life of the elderly.

4. A single cultural system may offer different opportunities for successful aging based on gender, class, or rural or urban variation.

5. The potential security and quality of life of the aged is maximized when both community and kin provide roles.

6. There are no "geriatric utopias."

Behaviors

Culturally mediated behavioral choices can affect the ability of older adults to age well and to cope with the inevitable challenges that occur with age. Among studies examining these interactions, research has found that African American elders show determination, perseverance, and tenacity even when seriously ill. This has been attributed to the fact that racism shaped their responses such that independence, spirituality, and survival were highly valued (Becker & Newsom, 2005).

Willingness to comply with treatment is also culturally mediated. Concern about side effects of antidepressant medication led African American and Latino elders to fail to follow instructions. This was attributed to forgetfulness (Latino) or intentional dissatisfaction with the medications (both) (Ayalon, Arean & Alvidrez, 2005). Native Americans tend to be less assimilated and to view psychiatric (and other) disorders as a result of spiritual imbalances and disharmony (Abramson et al., 2002).

Gay and lesbian elders have unique needs for service provision (Beeler, Rawls, Herdt, & Cohler, 1999) and make decisions about health behaviors based on their experience of acceptance or rejection. Cohort differences affect their needs because subsequent generations have experienced increasingly more social acceptance (Herdt & de Vries, 2003). Many gay and lesbian individuals construct fictive kin networks and turn to these friends and partners for support (Shippy, Cantor, & Brennan, 2004).

There are cultural differences in use of alternative health care. Blacks and Hispanics use fewer dietary supplements than whites, but more personal practice of complementary medicine (Ness, Cirillo, Weir, Nisly, & Wallace, 2005). Elderly Koreans who have chronic conditions such as arthritis, and who have insurance and are not depressed are most likely to use traditional Korean healers (Pourat, Lubben, Wallace, & Moon, 1999).

Cultural Competency

Growing recognition of the cultural aspects of occupation and health has led to growing attention to ensuring that care providers are **culturally competent.** Cultural competence is "a set of congruent behaviors, attitudes, and policies that come together in a system, agency, or among professionals that enables effective work in cross-cultural situations" (U.S. Department of Health and Human Services Office of the Secretary, 2000, p. 80865). The evidence is limited about the extent to which cultural competence actually affects outcomes of care, but it appears that, at a minimum, it increases client satisfaction. Thus, "clinicians will need immediate answers on how to appropriately assess, diagnose, and treat patients from various racial and ethnic groups in order to provide culturally competent care for all patients" (Faison & Mintzer, 2005, p. 541).

It is impossible to know everything about every group. This is true in part because cultural background interacts with personality and experience to create unique expression in every individual. Further, there are so many cultures, and they are evolving in so many ways, that what is true for one small group at one point in time may not be true later or in other communities with the "same" cultural profile. As a case in point, the experiences of Soviet Jews, many of whom are from Ukraine, differ significantly from those of the larger Ukranian population, most of whom observe the Russian Orthodox faith (EthnoMed, 1996). Likewise, in countries with indigenous populations, each group may have its own unique characteristics, mediated by history, location, and many other factors (Ranzijn & Bin-Sallik, 2001).

All these factors affect the intervention process at every stage. It is, therefore, important that practitioners have the needed knowledge, attitude, and skills to recognize and respond to the cultural beliefs and values of the client. There is a growing body of literature to suggest that ethnographic strategies, those used by qualitative researchers in the social sciences, can provide helpful guidance in building cultural competence (cf., Bonder et al., 2002). As was described in Chapter 15, ethnographic interviewing is a strategy for eliciting important information through the use of open-ended questions and careful observation.

Evaluation

The first step in any effective intervention is a thoughtful evaluation. To acquire the needed information, therapists must build rapport with clients. Such simple matters as greetings, names, and the environment in which evaluation occurs can greatly affect success in acquiring information and incorporating it into an intervention plan. As is true at every phase of intervention, it is useful to have a fund of knowledge about clients' cultures. So, for example, knowing that, as a rule, individuals from Arab Muslim backgrounds might be uncomfortable being touched by someone of the opposite gender, or that African American elders most often prefer to be called by their last names as a sign of respect would provide the practitioner with a place to begin an encounter. However, as should be clear by now, these culturally mediated preferences are also influenced by personal preference and experience. Thus, the best strategy might be to ask, "How would you like to be addressed?" or "Is it all right if we shake hands?" Asking the question helps avoid uncomfortable errors and typically conveys a sense of respect for, and genuine interest in, the preferences of the individual.

Occupational Profile

By now it should also be clear that occupational profiles will be influenced by cultural factors. It is not enough to ask a client whether he or she can manage his or her own meals. It is important to know of what the meals consist, who cooks, and how cooking is accomplished. Because the typical goal of occupational therapy intervention is to facilitate accomplishment of what the individual needs and wants to do, it is important to grasp the precise nature of the occupation, not just its category.

Analysis of Occupational Performance

The occupational profile should guide the analysis of performance. If an elder prefers traditional methods of Thai cooking, she may sit on the floor to do much of the preparation. This requires a different degree of flexibility and endurance than standing at a kitchen counter. Donning a *hijab* involves different movement patterns than donning slacks.

If standardized instruments are used, it is important to know how they have been developed, and whether they have taken cultural factors into account (Fernandez-Ballesteros et al.,

2004; Shulman & Feinstein, 2003). Some instruments used in occupational therapy, such as the Assessment of Motor and Process Skills (AMPS) (Goldman & Fisher, 1997) and the Canadian Occupational Performance Measure (COPM) (Law et al., 2005), have been examined extensively with regard to their applicability across cultures, but for other instruments this may not have been addressed. However, specific items and the constructs on which they have been based may not cross cultures. Keep in mind that this is true not just for populations from other countries, but also for cultural groups within national boundaries.

Intervention

The acceptability of various kinds of intervention has a clear cultural component. Even where the individual might be willing to go for care is culturally mediated. For example, in the United States, African Americans are less likely than whites to use nursing homes. They substitute paid home care, informal care, or they do without assistance (Wallace, Levy-Storms, Kington, & Andersen, 1998). In any case, intervention planning and implementation will be effective largely to the extent that individual preferences are addressed. And doing so involves understanding individual cultural values, personal experiences, and personality.

Intervention Plan

If evaluation has been successful, the intervention plan can be designed based on the specifics of the individual's situation. Both goals and modalities are influenced by culture. So, for example, if the care provider and client are in agreement that building physical endurance is an important goal to facilitate playing with grandchildren, the provider will need to recognize that suggesting swimming at the local community pool is unlikely to be an acceptable mechanism for doing this if the client is a Muslim woman who would find this immodest.

Intervention Implementation

In working with older adults, it is not unusual to involve the family or other sources of informal support. In some instances, the care provider must mediate differing expectations about the roles and contributions of different family members. In the case of an East Indian immigrant to the United States, the elder might expect, based on cultural norms, that his or her adult children (particularly daughters) would provide care. The elder might demonstrate a wish for dependency that is unacceptable in Western cultures. If the adult children have acculturated to mainstream U.S. culture, they may live at a distance, have full-time jobs, and have developed attitudes more consistent with Western views of the importance of independence and self-sufficiency. As discussed in Chapter 15, this can lead to serious family conflict and may leave the elder feeling depressed and abandoned.

Intervention Review

In some cultures, it is considered rude to directly challenge an authority figure. In such a situation, the care provider may believe that the client is in agreement with an intervention plan and then be surprised and disappointed when the plan is not implemented by the individual. This "noncompliance" suggests that the process of negotiating intervention has not been successful, and a return to the plan to revisit the client's preferences would be in order.

Outcomes

There is limited systematic evidence as yet that incorporating culture into care improves objective outcomes. On the other hand, there is substantial evidence that clients are more satisfied with such care (Fortier & Bishop, 2003). Occupational therapists recognize the importance of client-centered care—that is, care that identifies the client's goals and helps him or her to reach them. Because culture is inextricably linked to occupational choice and occupational performance, it is reasonable to assume that it must be understood and incorporated into intervention.

Developing cultural competency is an ongoing, lifelong process that requires a commitment to continued learning and to self-evaluation and reflection. As a follow-up to each encounter, a therapist would do well to review the process, and to identify those aspects of the encounter that seemed satisfactory and those that did not. The therapist can ask the client for input and suggestions. Many clients appreciate being queried and take this as a sign of the therapist's serious intent to be responsive and helpful.

It is inevitable that from time to time the therapist will make a misstep. It may be that the therapist's fund of culture-specific knowledge was misapplied, or that the therapist did not know an important fact about a particular culture. Even if the therapist has accurate and comprehensive knowledge about the culture, the client's individual experiences may influence his or her reactions. And, of course, because everyone has many cultures (ethnicity, religion, professional culture, age-associated culture, etc.), it may not be possible to determine accurately which cultural values dominate in the therapeutic encounter. In these cases, a sincere apology and a request for clarification and suggestions can go a long way toward remedying the situation (Bonder et al., 2002).

Case Study

Mrs. P* is 62 years old and an immigrant to the United States from Iran. She has lived in the United States for the past three decades. She visits her remaining family in Iran. She and her immediate family (three sons), all of whom moved to the United States together, are *Shia* Muslims but are not particularly observant. Mrs. P. reads the *Qur'an* from time to time but does not fast during Ramadan or wear the *hijab* other than during her visits to Iran. Her sons do not identify themselves as Muslim.

Mrs. P's behavior is not what would stereotypically be expected of a Muslim woman. She is strong and independent and had a relationship with her late husband based on equality. However, her command of English is not good; her sons speak Farsi with her. Unlike her, her sons have not integrated into the Iranian community in their new city, but she is proud of the fact that they have all completed graduate degrees.

Mrs. P's most important occupation, as she describes it, is looking after her only granddaughter twice a week. She very much wants to be able to continue this occupation. At present, she is very healthy, and she is concerned about remaining so in order to be able to continue this occupation.

continued on page 586

Case Study (continued)

Other than this, Mrs. P's occupations are somewhat limited. She visits with friends in the Iranian community, and used to enjoy travel. However, she worries now about travel because of her single status and because of fears about discrimination or racial profiling. She also worries about crime in her neighborhood, so she tends not to go out alone. Her sons do not believe the neighborhood to be particularly dangerous and worry about her isolation. They have urged her to start dating, but because of cultural norms, she is unwilling to do so.

Questions

1. What do you see in this description that might contribute to successful aging?
2. What do you note as factors discussed in this chapter that might affect Mrs. P's experience of growing older?
3. Do you see any particular risk factors in this description of Mrs. P?

This case study is loosely based on one that appears in Salari (2002).

Review Questions

1. In what ways does culture affect occupational performance, patterns, and choices?
2. How are process and motor skills affected by culture?
3. Discuss ways in which activity demands are affected by culture.
4. What is meant by cultural competence?
5. How does culture influence the various steps in the intervention process?

Web-Based Resources

For helpful information about the experience of culture and aging, visit:

www.csis.org/gai, **Center for Strategic and International Studies,** date connected September 20, 2007. This site describes the Global Aging Initiative, established in 1999. The site includes many links to information about specific countries and their experiences with changing demographics.

www.aginginstride.org, **Aging in Stride,** date connected September 20, 2007. This site includes a great deal of information that is useful in working directly with clients. It provides consumer-friendly advice about physical safety, aging in place, senior living options, health issues, choosing a nursing home, financial concerns, death and dying, and social networks.

www.nethealthinc.com/cultural, **Western Reserve Geriatric Education Center,** date connected September 20, 2007. Access an instructional program focused on building cultural competence in working with older adults.

REFERENCES

Aboderin, I. (2004). Decline in material family support for older people in urban Ghana, Africa: Understanding processes and causes of change. *Journal of Gerontology: Social Sciences, 59B,* S128–S137.

Abramson, T. A., Trejo, L., & Lai, D. W. L. (2002). Culture and mental health: Providing appropriate services for a diverse older population. *Generations, 26*(1), 21–27.

Alexander, B. B., Rubinstein, R. L., Goodman, M., & Laborsky, M. (1991). Generativity in cultural context: The self, death and immortality as experienced by older American women. *Aging and Society, 11,* 417–442.

Alvord, L. A., & Van Pelt, E. C. (1999). *The scalpel and the sliver bear: The first Navajo woman surgeon combines Western medicine and traditional healing.* New York: Bantam.

American Occupational Therapy Association. (2002). Occupational therapy practice framework: Domain and process. *American Journal of Occupational Therapy, 56,* 609–639.

Andrews, G., Clark, M., & Luszcz, M. (2002). Successful aging in the Australian Longitudinal Study of Aging: Applying the Mac Arthur model cross-nationally. *Journal of Social Issues, 58,* 749–765.

Angel, R. J., & Angel, J. L. (2006). Diversity and aging in the United States. In R. H. Binstock & L. K. George (Eds.), *Handbook of aging and the social sciences* (6th ed., pp. 94–106). Burlington, MA: Academic Press.

Angel, J. L., Buckley, C. J., & Sakamoto, A. (2001). Duration or disadvantage? Exploring nativity, ethnicity, and health in midlife. *Journal of Gerontology: Social Sciences, 56B,* S275–S284.

Atran, S., Medin, D., & Ross, N. (2006). Evolution and devolution of knowledge. *Psychological Review, 111,* 960–983.

Ayalon, L., Arean, P. A., & Alvidrez, J. (2005). Adherence to antidepressant medications in black and Latino elderly patients. *American Journal of Geriatric Psychiatry, 13,* 572–580.

Babco, E. L. (2001). *Under-represented minorities in engineering: A progress report.* Washington, DC: The American Association for the Advancement of Science.

Bar-Tur, L., Savaya, R., & Prager, E. (2001). Sources of meaning in life for young and old Israeli Jews and Arabs. *Journal of Aging Studies, 15,* 253–269.

Barnes, L. L., Mendes de Leon, C. F., Bienias, J. L., & Evans, D. A. (2004). A longitudinal study of black-white differences in social resources. *Journal of Gerontology: Social Sciences, 59B,* S146–S153.

Becker, G., & Newsom, E. (2005). Resilience in the face of serious illness among chronically ill African Americans in later life. *Journal of Gerontology: Social Sciences, 60B,* S214–S223.

Beeler, J. A., Rawls, T. W., Herdt, G., & Cohler, B. J. (1999). The needs of older lesbians and gay men in Chicago. *Journal of Gay & Lesbian Social Services, 9*(1), 31–49.

Bonder, B. (2001). Culture and occupation: A comparison of weaving in two traditions. *Canadian Journal of Occupational Therapy, 65,* 310–319.

Bonder, B. R., Bazyk, S., Reilly, B., & Toyota, J. (2005). Women's work in Guatemala. *Work, 24*(10), 3–10.

Bonder, B. R., & Martin, L. (2000). Personal meanings of occupation for women in later life. Two women compared. *Women and Aging, 12,* 177–193.

Bonder, B. R., Martin, L., & Miracle, A. W. (2002). *Culture in clinical care.* Thorofare, NJ: SLACK.

Brooks, A. S., & Draper, P. (1998). Anthropological perspectives on aging. In R. O. Selig & M. R. London (Eds.), *Anthropology explored: The best of Smithsonian AnthroNotes* (pp. 286–297). Washington, DC: Smithsonian Institution Press.

Burr, J. A., & Mutchler, J. E. (2003). English language skills, ethnic concentration, and household composition: Older Mexican immigrants. *Journal of Gerontology, Social Sciences, 58B,* S83–S92.

Camp, C. J., Bird, M. J., & Cherry, K. E. (2000). Retrieval strategies as a rehabilitation aid for cognitive loss in pathological aging. In T. D. Hill, L. Backman, & A. S. Neely (Eds.), *Cognitive rehabilitation in old age* (pp. 224–248). New York: Oxford University Press.

Cargill, V. (2005). HIV/AIDS: A minority health issue *Medical Clinics of North America, 89,* 895–912.

Carstensen, L. L. (2001). Selectivity theory: Social activity in life-span context. In A. J. Walker, M. M. Manoogian-O'Dell, L. A. McGraw, & D. L. G. White (Eds.) *Families in later life: Connections and transitions* (pp. 265–275). Thousand Oaks, CA: Pine Forge Press.

Chou, K., & Chi, I. (2002). Successful aging among the young-old, old-old, and oldest-old Chinese. *International Journal of Aging and Human Development, 54,* 1–14.

Cochran, D. L., Brown, D. R., & McGregor, K. C. (1999). Racial differences in the multiple social roles of older women: Implications for depressive symptoms. *The Gerontologist, 39,* 465–472.

Consedine, N. S., Magai, C., Cohen, C. I., & Gillespie, M. (2002). Ethnic variation in the impact of negative affect and emotion inhibition on the health of older adults. *Journal of Gerontology: Psychological Sciences, 57B,* P396–P408.

Diener, E., & Suh, E. (1998). Age and subjective self-being: An international analysis. *Annual Review of Gerontology & Geriatrics, 17,* 304–324.

Dixon, C. G., & Richard, M. (2003). Contemporary issues facing aging Americans: Implications for rehabilitation and mental health counseling. *Journal of Rehabilitation, 69*(2), 5–12.

Draper, P. (1976). Social and economic constraints on !Kung childhood. In R. B. Lee & B. L. DeVore (Eds.), *Kalahari hunter gatherers* (pp. 199–217). Cambridge: Harvard University Press.

Draper, P., & Harpending, H. (1994). Cultural considerations in the experience of aging: Two African cultures. In B. R. Bonder & M. B. Wagner (Eds.), *Functional performance in older adults* (pp. 15–27). Philadelphia: F.A. Davis.

Dunlop, D. D., Manheim, L. M., Song, J., & Chang, R. W. (2002). Gender and ethnic/racial disparities in health care utilization among older adults. *Journal of Gerontology: Social Sciences, 57B,* S221–S233.

Efklides, A., Kalaitzidou, M., & Chankin, G. (2003). Subjective quality of life in old age in Greece: The effect of demographic factors, emotional state, and adaptation to aging. *European Psychologist, 8*(3), 178–191.

Ekerdt, D. J. (1986). The busy ethic: Moral continuity between work and retirement. *The Gerontologist, 27,* 239–244.

EthnoMed: Voices of the Community. (1996). Retrieved February 22, 2006, from http://ethnomed.org/ethnomet/voices.html/.

Faison, W. E., & Mintzer, J. E. (2005). Editorial: The growing, ethnically diverse aging population: Is our field advancing with it? *American Journal of Geriatric Psychiatry, 23,* 541–544.

Fernandez-Ballesteros, R., Zamarron, M. D., Rudinger, G., Schroots, J. J. F., Hekkinnen, E., Drusini, A., et al. (2004). Assessing competence: The European Survey on Aging Protocol (ESAP). *Gerontology, 50,* 330–347.

Ferraro, K. F., & Su, Y. (1999). Financial strain, social relations, and psychological distress among older people: A cross-cultural analysis. *Journal of Gerontology: Social Sciences, 54B,* S3–S15.

Fortier, J. P., & Bishop, D. (2003). *Setting the agenda for research on cultural competence in health care: Final report,* (Edited by C. Brach.) Rockville, MD: U.S. Department of Health and Human Services Office of Minority Health and Agency for Healthcare Research and Quality.

Fox, N. J. (2005). Cultures of ageing in Thailand and Australia (What can an ageing body do?). *Sociology, 39,* 481–498.

Fry, C. L., Dickerson-Putman, J., Draper, P., Ikels, C., Keith, J., Glascock, A. P., et al. (1997). Culture and the meaning of a good old age. In J. Sokolovsky (Ed.), *The cultural context of aging: Worldwide perspectives* (2nd ed., pp. 99–137). Westport, CT: Bergin & Garvey.

Gallo, J. J., Cooper-Patrick, L., & Lesikar, S. (1998). Depressive symptoms of whites and African Americans aged 60 years and older. *Journal of Gerontology: Psychological Sciences, 57B,* P277–P286.

Gardiner, H. W., & Kosmitzki, C. (2005). *Lives across cultures: Cross-cultural human development* (3rd ed.). Boston: Allyn & Bacon.

Gee, E. M. (2000). Living arrangements and quality of life among Chinese Canadian elders. *Social Indicators Research, 51,* 309–329.

Gee, S. B., Liu, J. H., & Ng, S. H. (2002). The veneration gap: Generational dissonance and well-being among Chinese and European parents. *Hallym International Journal of Aging, 4,* 45–65.

Gelfand, D., & Yee, B. W. K. (1991). Trends and forces: Influence of immigration, migration, and acculturation on the fabric of aging in America. *Generations, 15*(Fall/Winter), 7–10.

Goldman, S. L., & Fisher, A. G. (1997). Cross-cultural validation of the Assessment of Motor and Process Skills (AMPS). *British Journal of Occupational Therapy, 60,* 77–85.

Graves, A. B., Rajaram, L., Bowen, J. D., McCormick, W. C., McCurry, S. M., & Larson, E. B. (1999). Cognitive decline and Japanese culture in a cohort of older Japanese Americans in King County, WA: The *Kame* project. *Journal of Gerontology: Social Sciences, 54B,* S154–S161.

Guallar-Castillion, P., Sendino, A. R., Banegas, J. R., Lopez-Garcia, E., & Rodriguez-Artalejo, F. (2005). Differences in quality of life between women and men in the older population of Spain. *Social Science & Medicine, 60,* 1229–1240.

Hahn, R. A. (1995). *Sickness and healing: An anthropological perspective.* New Haven, CT: Yale University Press.

He, X. Z., & Baker, D. W. (2005). Differences in leisure-time, household, and work-related physical activity by race, ethnicity, and education. *Journal of General Internal Medicine, 20,* 259–266.

Herdt, G., & deVries, B. (2003). *Gay and lesbian aging: A research agenda for the 21st century.* New York: Springer.

Hopper, S. V. (1993). Ethnicity and the health of older women. *Clinical Geriatric Medicine, 9,* 231–259.

Hsu, H., Lew-Ting, C., & Wu, S. (2003). Age, period, and cohort effects on the attitude toward supporting parents in Taiwan. *The Gerontologist, 41,* 742–750.

Iwamoto, K., Rogers, A., & Gall, J. (2003). Cultural influences on life satisfaction: A comparative study of Japanese and Japanese American elderly. *Hallym International Journal of Aging, 5,* 19–39.

John, R. (2004). Health status and health disparities among American Indian elders. In K. E. Whitfield (Ed.), *Full-color aging: Closing the gap: Improving the health of minority elders in the new millennium* (pp. 27–44). Washington, DC: Gerontological Society of America.

Kelley-Moore, J. A., & Ferraro, K. F. (2004). The black/white disability gap: Persistent inequality in later life? *Journal of Gerontology: Social Sciences, 59B,* S34–S43.

Kim, E., Kleiber, D. A., & Kropf, N. (2001). Leisure activity, ethnic preservation, and cultural integration of older Korean Americans. In N. G. Choi (Ed.), *Social work practice with the Asian American elderly.* (pp. 107–130). New York: Haworth Press.

Kinsella, K., & Phillips, D. R. (2005). *Global aging: The challenge of success.* Washington, DC: Population Reference Bureau.

Klumb, P. L., & Baltes, M. M. (1999). Time use of old and very old Berliners: Productive and consumptive activities as functions of resources. *Journal of Gerontology: Social Sciences, 54B,* S271–S278.

Knodel, J., Ofstedal, M. B., & Hermalin, A. I. (2002). The demographic, socioeconomic, and cultural context of the four study countries. In A. I. Hermalin (Ed.), *The well-being of the elderly in Asia: A four-country comparative study* (pp. 25–63). Ann Arbor: The University of Michigan Press.

Law, M., Baptiste, S., Carswell, A., McColl, M. A., Polatajko, H., & Pollock, N. (2005). *Canadian Occupational Performance Measure.* Toronto: Canadian Association for Occupational Therapy.

Lee, W. K. M. (2003). Women and retirement planning: Towards the "feminization of poverty" in an aging Hong Kong. *Journal of Women & Aging, 15*(1/2), 31–53.

Lee, W. K. M., & Hong-kin, K. (2005). Older women and family care in Hong Kong: Differences in filial expectation and practices. *Journal of Women & Aging, 17*(1/2), 129–150.

Litwin, H. (1995). *Uprooted in old age: Soviet Jews and their social networks in Israel.* Westport, CT: Greenwood Press.

Ludtke, R., McDonald, L., & Allery, A. (2002). *Long term care and health needs of America's Native American elders.* National Resource Center on Native American Aging, Center for Rural Health, University of North Dakota School of Medicine and Health Sciences, July.

Mahoney, D. F., Cloutterbuck, J., Neary, S., & Zhan, L. (2004). African American, Chinese, and Latino family caregivers' impressions of the onset and diagnosis of dementia: Cross-cultural similarities and differences. *The Gerontologist, 45,* 783–792.

Manly, J. J., Byrd, D. A., Touradji, P., & Stern, Y. (2004). Acculturation, reading level, and neuropsychological test performance among African American elders. *Applied Neuropsychology, 11,* 37–46.

Manly, J. J., & Espino, D. V. (2004). Cultural influences on dementia recognition and management. *Clinical Geriatric Medicine, 20,* 93–119.

Manton, K. G., & Stallard, E. (1997). Health differences among racial and ethnic groups. In L. G. Martin & B. J. Soldo (Eds.), *Racial and ethnic differences in the health of older Americans* (pp. 43–104). Washington, DC: National Academy of Sciences.

Markides, K. S., & Black, S. A. (1996). Race, ethnicity, and aging: The impact of inequality. In R. H. Binstock & L. K. George (Eds.), *Handbook of aging and the social sciences* (4th ed., pp. 153–170). San Diego, CA: Academic Press.

Markides, K. S., & Lee, D. J. (1990). Predictors of wellbeing and functioning in older Mexican Americans and Anglos: An eight-year follow-up. *Journal of Gerontology: Social Sciences, 45*(Suppl.), S69–S73.

McAuley, W. J. (1998). Historical and contextual correlates of parallel services for elders in African American communities. *The Gerontologist, 38,* 445–455.

McCallum, J., & Shadbolt, B. (1989). Ethnicity and stress among older Australians. *Journal of Gerontology: Social Sciences, 44*(Suppl.), S89–S96.

McDonald, J., Quandt, S. A., Arcury, T. A., Bell, R. A., & Vitolins, M. Z. (2000). Nutritional self-management strategies of rural widowers. *The Gerontologist, 40,* 480–491.

McFadden, S. H., Brennan, M., & Hicks Patrick, J. (2003). Charting a course for 21st century studies of late life religiousness and spirituality. In S. H. McFadden, M. Brennan, & J. Hicks Patrick (Eds.), *New directions in the study of late life religiousness and spirituality* (pp. 1–10). New York: Haworth Pastoral Press, Haworth Press.

Meisenhelder, J. B., & Chandler, E. N. (2000). Faith, prayer, and health outcomes in elderly Native Americans. *Clinical Nursing Research, 9,* 191–203.

Mendes de Leon, C. F., Barnes, L. L., Bienias, J. L., Skarupski, K. A., & Evans, D. A. (2005). Racial disparities in disability: Recent evidence for self-reported and performance-based disability measures in a population-based study of older adults. *Journal of Gerontology: Social Sciences, 60B,* S263–S271.

Miner, S., & Tolnay, S. (1998). Barriers to voluntary organization membership: An examination of race and cohort differences. *Journal of Gerontology: Social Sciences, 53B,* S241–S248.

Mutchler, J. E., & Brallier, S. (1999). English language proficiency among older Hispanics in the United States. *The Gerontologist, 39,* 310–319.

Nandan, M. (2005). Adaptation to American culture: Voices of Asian Indian immigrants. *Journal of Gerontological Social Work, 44,* 175–203.

Ness, J., Cirillo, D. J., Weir, D. R., Nisly, N. L., & Wallace, R. B. (2005). Use of complementary medicine in older Americans: Results from the health and retirement study. *The Gerontologist, 45,* 516–524.

Ng, A., Phillips, D., & Lee, W. K. M. (2002). Persistence and challenges to filial piety and informational support of older persons in a modern Chinese society: A case study in Tuen Mun, Hong Kong. *Journal of Aging Studies, 16,* 135–153.

Nida'ul Islam Magazine. (1995). *Principles of Islamic banking.* Retrieved April 20, 2006, from www.usc.edu/dept/MSA/economics/nbank1.html.

Ohno, Y., Aoki, R., Tamakoshi, A., Kawamura, T., Wakai, K., Hashimoto, S., et al. (2000). Successful aging and social activity in older Japanese adults. *Journal of Aging and Physical Activity, 8,* 129–139.

Organisation for Economic Co-operation and Development (OECD). (2004). *Trends in international migration 2004.* Paris: Author.

Park, D. C., Nisbett, R., & Hedden, T. (1999). Aging, culture, and cognition. *Journal of Gerontology: Psychological Sciences, 54B,* P75–P84.

Phillips, D. R. (2000). Ageing in the Asia-Pacific region: Issues, policies and contexts. In D. R. Phillips (Ed.), *Aging in the Asia-Pacific region: Issues, policies and future trends* (pp. 1–34), London: Routledge.

Pourat, N., Lubben, J., Wallace, S. P., & Moon, A. (1999). Predictors of use of traditional Korean healers among elderly Koreans in Los Angeles. *The Gerontologist, 39,* 711–719.

Ranzijn, R., & Bin-Sallik, M. A. (2001). The health and well-being of Aboriginal elders. *National Conference of Australian Psychological Society,* Adelaide.

Rasheed, M. N., & Rasheed, J. M. (2003). Rural African American older adults and the Black helping tradition. *Journal of Gerontological Social Work, 41*(1/2), 137–150.

Remennick, L. (2003). Retired and making a fresh start: Older Russian immigrants discuss their adjustment in Israel. *International Migration, 41*(5), 153–175.

Rubenstein, R. L., & de Medeiros, K. (2004). Ecology and the aging self. In H. Wahl, R. J. Scheidt, & P. G. Windley (Eds.), *Annual review of gerontology and geriatrics* (pp. 59–84). New York: Springer.

Salari, S. (2002). Invisible in aging research; Arab Americans, Middle Eastern immigrants, and Muslims in the United States. *The Gerontologist, 42,* 580–588.

Shaw, B. A., & Krause, N. (2001). Exploring race variations in aging and personal control. *Journal of Gerontology: Social Sciences, 56B,* S119–S124.

Shea, D., Davey, A., Femia, E. E., Zarit, S. H., Sundstrom, G., Berg, S., et al. (2003). Exploring assistance in Sweden and the United States. *The Gerontologist, 43,* 712–721.

Shippy, R. A., Cantor, M. H., & Brennan, M. (2004). Social networks of aging gay men. *Journal of Men's Studies, 13*(1), 107–120.

Shulman, K., & Feinstein, A. (2003). *Quick cognitive screening for clinicians.* London: Martin Dunitz, Taylor and Francis Group.

Silveira, E., & Alleback, P. (2001). Migration, ageing and mental health: An ethnographic study on perceptions of life satisfaction, anxiety and depression in older Somali men in east London. *International Journal of Social Welfare, 10,* 309–320.

Sloan, F. A., & Wang, J. (2005). Disparities among older adults in measures of cognitive function by race or ethnicity. *Journal of Gerontology: Psychological Sciences, 60B,* P242–P250.

Smedley, B. D., Stith, A. Y., & Nelson, A. R. (2003). *Unequal treatment: Confronting racial and ethnic disparities in healthcare.* Washington, DC: Institute of Medicine.

Sokolovsky, J. (1997). Starting points: A global cross-cultural view of aging. In J. Sokolovsky (Ed.), *The cultural context of aging: Worldwide perspectives* (2nd ed, pp. xiii–xxxi). Westport, CT: Bergin & Garvey.

Terry-Cox, L. P. W. (2003). Factors that contribute to positive aging in African-Americans. *Dissertation Abstracts International Section A: Humanities and Social Sciences, 64*(1–A), 75.

Trinitapoli, J. (2005). Congregation-based services for the elders. *Research on Aging, 27,* 241–264.

Trivedi, A. M., Zaslavsky, A. M., Schneider, E. C., & Ayanian, J. Z. (2005). Trends in the quality of care and racial disparities in Medicare managed care. *New England Journal of Medicine, 353,* 692–700.

United Nations Division for Social Policy and Development. (2006). *The ageing of the world's population.* Retrieved April 10, 2008, from http://www.un.org/esa/population/publications/ageing/ageing2006.htm

U.S. Census Bureau. (2001). Introduction. In *An aging world: 2001* (pp. i–iv). Washington, DC: Author.

U.S. Department of Health and Human Services Office of the Secretary. (2000). National standards on culturally and linguistically appropriate services (CLAS) in health care. *Federal Register, 65*(247), 80865–80879.

Waite, L. J., & Hughes, M. E. (1999). At risk on the cusp of old age: Living arrangements and functional status among black, white and Hispanic adults. *Journal of Gerontology: Social Sciences, 54B,* S136–S144.

Walker, A. (2006). Aging and politics: An international perspective. In R. H. Binstock & L. K. George (Eds.), *Handbook of aging and the social sciences* (6th ed., pp. 339–358). Burlington, MA: Academic Press.

Wallace, S. P., Levy-Storms, L., Kington, R. S., & Andersen, R. M. (1998). The persistence of race and ethnicity in the use of long-term care. *Journal of Gerontology: Social Sciences, 53B,* S104–S112.

Weibel-Orlando, J. (2001). Grandparenting styles: Native American perspectives. In A. J. Walker, M. Manoogian-O'Dell, L. A. McGraw, & D. L. G. White (Eds.), *Families in later life: Connections and transitions* (pp. 139–145). Thousand Oaks, CA: Pine Forge Press.

Weitzman, P. F., Dunigan, R., Hawkins, R., Weitzman, E. A., & Levkoff, S. E. (2001). Everyday conflict and stress among older African American woman: Findings from a focus group study and pilot training program. *Journal of Ethnic & Cultural Diversity in Social Work, 10*(2), 27–44.

White, S. I. (2000). Racial patterns in disabled elderly persons' use of medical services. *Journal of Gerontology: Social Sciences, 55B,* S76–S89.

Williams, N. (2001). Elderly Mexican American men: Work and family patterns. In A. J. Walker, M. Manoogian-O'Dell, L. A. McGraw, & D. L. G. White (Eds.), *Families in later life: Connections and transitions* (pp. 202–207). Thousand Oaks, CA: Pine Forge Press.

World Health Organization (WHO). (2001). International classification of functioning, disability, and health (ICF). Geneva, Switzerland: Author.

Yamaguchi, M., & Silverstein, M. (2003). The impact of acculturation and ethnic identity on the intergenerational relations and psychological well-being of Japanese-American elderly in a retirement residence. *Hallym International Journal of Aging, 5*(1), 1–17.

Yang, J., McCrae, R. R., & Costa, P. T. (1998). Adult age differences in personality traits in the United States and the People's Republic of China. *Journal of Gerontology: Psychological Sciences, 53B,* P375–P383.

Zhang, Y. B., Hummert, M. L., & Garstka, T. (2002). Stereotype traits of older adults generated by young, middle aged, and older Chinese participants. *Hallym International Journal of Aging, 4,* 119–140.

Zimmer, Z. (2005). Health and living arrangement transitions among China's oldest-old. *Research on Aging, 27,* 526–555.

CHAPTER 24

Products and Technology

William C. Mann • Eric E. Hicks

*O*ld age deprives the intelligent man only of qualities
useless to wisdom.

Joubert, Pensées, 1842

OBJECTIVES

By the end of this chapter, readers will be able to:

1. Describe the three ways the built environment can be adapted or modified to benefit people with disabilities.
2. Differentiate between accessible design, adaptable design, transgenerational design, and universal design.
3. Define and describe assistive technology.
4. Differentiate between high-tech and low-tech devices.
5. Describe the devices used for individuals with mobility impairments, including environmental control devices and mobility aids.
6. Describe the devices that may be helpful to individuals with visual impairments.
7. Describe devices that may be helpful to individuals with hearing deficits.
8. Describe how the World Health Organization's International Classification of Functioning (ICF) model and Occupational Therapy Practice Framework (AOTA, 2002) can be used to determine the types of devices that may be helpful to a particular individual.
9. Discuss the limitations in the usefulness of technological devices.

Introduction

This chapter provides an overview of how the built environment can be adapted or modified to increase or maintain functional performance for older individuals with disabilities. This is followed by a discussion of how the World Health Organization (WHO) International Classification of Functioning (ICF) model and culture can impact the appropriate provision of assistive devices. Then, we describe some common **assistive technology devices** used to compensate for various age-related problems (i.e., mobility, vision, hearing, and cognition) and conclude with a brief discussion of important issues related to technology and older adults. An appendix at the end of the chapter lists resources on assistive technology for older adults.

Aging and Functional Performance

Recent data suggest that most people over 64 years old are living longer and healthier lives compared to the same age group 10 years ago (Administration on Aging, 2004; Freedman et al., 2004; He, Sengupta, Velkoff, and DeBarros, 2005). However, with advancing age come two major challenges that impact functional performance. The first is a gradual decline that can result in decrements in hearing, vision, mobility, and cognitive processes. The second is the probability that one or more chronic diseases, such as arthritis, macular degeneration, heart disease, or Alzheimer's disease will result in additional disabilities. Figure 24-1 shows a continuum along which individuals may be located as their level of age-associated decline increases and their number of chronic conditions increases.

Demographic factors, such as age, gender, race, health, living arrangements, and social support, which have been discussed previously in this volume, contribute to both limitations in functional performance and diversity or heterogeneity of the older population in the United States (He et al., 2005). While facing chronic conditions and age-related functional impairments, Schafer (2000) found that 9 out of 10 seniors 64 and older prefer to live at home. Because most housing and communities are not typically designed to meet the needs and preferences of seniors as they age, various solutions are being implemented in homes and communities to assist older persons in "aging in place"—remaining in their homes as long and as independently as possible.

The Built Environment and Functional Performance

> Almost everything we do in life is affected by what has been built around us. Our ability to receive an education, find housing, attend a church or synagogue, shop, bank, recreate, travel, and earn a living are all affected by the built environment. Yet for almost 200 years, our schools, courts, houses, churches and synagogues, stores, banks, theaters, restaurants, public transit systems, and overall workplaces were built with the able-bodied population in mind. Access to these buildings, facilities, and services was only a dream shared by millions of individuals with disabilities. (Peterson, 1998, p. 15)

The concept of designing products and the built environment for people with disabilities did not emerge until the 1960s when the American National Standards Institute (ANSI) established Standard A117.1, *"Making Buildings Accessible to and Usable by the Physically Handicapped."* These standards were followed, over the years, by legislation (e.g., Americans with Disabilities Act and Fair Housing Amendment Act) that increased the rights of people with disabilities to access all public buildings and public and private housing (Kose, 1998; Peterson, 1998; Vanderheiden, 1998). Although these laws improved the

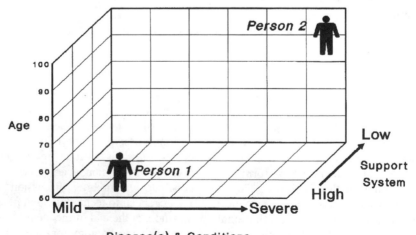

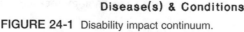

FIGURE 24-1 Disability impact continuum.

opportunities and independence afforded to those with disabilities, they have not adequately addressed the needs of older adults which in some ways are different from the needs of younger people with disabilities (Kose, 1998). Older adults often experience simultaneous decline in several abilities (i.e., vision, mobility, and hearing) which cannot be addressed solely by removing certain environmental barriers.

Three different approaches can be taken to ensure effective interaction with the environment:

1. Change the individual
2. Change the environment
3. Provide individuals with tools they can use (Vanderheiden, 1998)

Each approach is seen as equally important and necessary to "function effectively in the various environments and situations they encounter on a daily basis" (Vanderheiden, 1998, p. 31). Each area is briefly discussed in the following sections.

Change the Individual

This approach addresses the methods used to enhance the physical, psychological, and social abilities of the individual for accessing and using the environment (Vanderheiden, 1998). These methods include the following interventions: surgery, therapy, training, education, and teaching of compensatory strategies and adaptive techniques. One advantage of this approach is that it improves the innate abilities, skills, and strategies that individuals "carry" with them.

Change the Environment

In many cases, the impact of disability on functional performance can be overcome or reduced through the design of the places we live, work, play, and worship. This is often referred to as accessible design, defined as "design that meets prescribed code requirements for use by people with disabilities" (Story, 1998, p. 4). Accessible design is often achieved by providing separate design features for specific disabilities, such as paddle blade handles on large lowered sinks in public restrooms for those with mobility impairments. These solutions can be costly because they are added onto existing designs or new construction at the end of the design process. They can be stigmatizing because they draw attention to the

individuals who have to use these features (e.g., ramps next to entrances with stairs). There are three subsets of design that fall under the broad category of accessible design. These are adaptable design, transgenerational design, and universal design. Even though all are considered to be subsets of accessible design, designs may incorporate features from one, two, or all of these subsets. A height-adjustable stovetop, for instance, is an accessible design feature within an environment that incorporates features of both the adaptable and universal design subsets but not the transgenerational design subset because the feature was not specifically made to accommodate all of the changes a person might experience as they age.

Adaptable Design

Adaptable design involves making modifications to a standard design for the use by a particular individual with a disability, like adding large grips to kitchen utensils to help someone with rheumatoid arthritis (Story, 1998). Similar to accessible design, these features sometimes appear added onto a product or environmental space which may result in the design being stigmatizing and expensive.

Transgenerational, or Life-Span, Design

Transgenerational, or life-span, design considers the changes individuals experience as they age (Story, 1998). This type of design does not address the full range of possibilities that can affect individuals throughout their lifetime, such as congenital conditions, injury, illness, gender, cultural background, and literacy level. Grab bars in a bathroom might help both young children and elders but are not specific to particular kinds of conditions.

Universal Design

Universal design is defined as "the design of products and environments that can be used and experienced by people of all ages and abilities, to the greatest extent possible, without adaptation" (Story, 1998, p. 4). This is the most inclusive and least stigmatizing of the three types of designs because it benefits everyone—young and old, men and women, children and older adults, small people and large people. Furthermore, universal design solutions are fully integrated into the environmental design before the process begins in order to accommodate a wide range of the populations. The goal of universal design is to minimize the amount of adaptation needed by the individual and maximize the individual's natural inclusion into all daily activities. There has been widespread attention to "smarthouse" designs that incorporate microchip-controlled lights, heating, and appliances, as a mechanism for improving home management for everyone.

The Center for Universal Design (1997) in Raleigh, North Carolina, established seven principles that can be used to guide the design process, evaluate existing and new designs, and teach what universal design encompasses. These principles are as follows:

1. Principle one: Equitable use—The design is useful and marketable to people with diverse abilities.
2. Principle two: Flexibility in use—The design accommodates a wide range of individual preferences and abilities.
3. Principle three: Simple and intuitive use—Use of the design is easy to understand, regardless of the user's experience, knowledge, language skills, or current concentration level.
4. Principle four: Perceptible information—The design communicates necessary information effectively to the user, regardless of ambient conditions or the user's sensory abilities.
5. Principle five: Tolerance for error—The design minimizes hazards and the adverse consequences of accidental or unintended actions.
6. Principle six: Low physical effort—The design can be used efficiently and comfortably and with a minimum amount of fatigue.
7. Principle seven: Size and space for approach and use—Appropriate size and space is provided for approach, reach, manipulation, and use regardless of the user's body size, posture, or mobility. (n.p.)

There are several advantages of universal design, including reduced need for assistive technology, decreased cost of a device, increased availability of usable designs, increased longevity and reliability and ease-of-repair, increased inclusion of people with disabilities into society, reduced social stigmatism, and decreased amount of personal assistance needed by people with disabilities (Story, 1998). Universal design offers people with disabilities many advantages, but it will not fully replace the need for interventions to enhance the individual's abilities, or the need to provide individuals with tools, or assistive technology. Thus, for some individuals and for some activities, there will always be a need for devices and personal assistance.

Provide Individuals with Tools

Humans are "tool users," and with the exception of chimpanzees who use sticks to dig up insects, and sea otters who use rocks to break clam shells, no other species use objects, or tools, to enhance task performance. Our tools range in complexity from spoons to space shuttles and from can openers to computers. Tools that are used to strengthen, compensate, or provide a better match between a person's abilities and the demands of the environment are called assistive technologies, adaptive devices, or assistive devices. Specifically, **assistive technology device** is defined by the Technology Related Assistance for Individuals with Disabilities Act of 1988 (1994) *as any item, piece of equipment, or product system, whether acquired commercially off the shelf, modified or customized, that is used to increase, maintain, or improve functional capabilities of individuals with disabilities. (n.p.)* This broad definition includes **low-tech devices** (i.e., those traditionally used by therapists, such as button hooks and reachers) and **high-tech devices** (which often involve microprocessors and include computer hardware and software, such as voice output and screen magnification software for persons with low vision, and environmental control units).

Two advantages of assistive technology are that they can be custom selected and fitted to meet the needs of a particular individual, and they can be specifically adapted to meet the needs of the individual and the constraints of the environment in which they will be used (Vanderheiden, 1998). Several disadvantages of assistive technology devices are the cost, lack of consumer awareness of products, social stigma regarding use of assistive technology, and that assistive technology advancements cannot keep up with the rate at which mainstream technology is advancing.

Aging in Place

Three areas that should be addressed when helping older adults "age in place" include interventions at the person level, changes to the environment, and provision of assistive devices. All areas should be taken into consideration when working with a client. Mann, Ottenbacher, Fraas, Tomita, and Granger (1999) demonstrated this point by investigating the effectiveness of assistive technology and home modifications in reducing the rate of declined functional status for physically frail older persons living at home. Furthermore, this study documented the cost-effectiveness of an intensive approach to the provision of assistive technology and home modifications. Individuals who receive all the assistive devices and home modifications they need spend less time in hospitals and nursing homes, and average costs associated with institutional care are significantly less. These findings provide strong support for a thorough approach to functional and home evaluation, followed by procurement of needed devices and home modifications, with appropriate training and follow-up. The remainder of this chapter focuses on assistive technology.

Assessing the Need for Assistive Technology

The heterogeneity of those 64 and older makes it difficult to predict a person's level of functional performance and need for assistive technology (He et al., 2005; Schafer, 2000). For example, one person may experience only the effects of the normal aging process, such as decreased hearing and vision, but another person may have several medical conditions or age-related diseases that can significantly impact independence. The WHO's ICF (2001) model, as discussed previously in this book, provides practitioners with a systematic way to assess and select appropriate assistive technology devices to accommodate the needs of their clients (Jette, Haley, & Kooyoomjian, 2003; Perenboom, & Chorus, 2003; Ustun, Chatterji, Kostansjek, & Bickenbach, 2003). The ICF model not only depicts the person and his or her performance of tasks or activities in a state of health rather than disability, but it also delineates and conceptualizes functional performance into three classification levels—body structure/function, activity, and participation—prior to adding in disease or disorder. Any resulting impact caused by disease, disorder, condition, and personal and environmental factors on one or more classification levels is viewed as unique to the individual and is not always in a direct one-to-one relationship. Thus, the ICF model can be used as a guide for the provision of medical and therapeutic intervention, including evaluating

and selecting assistive technology, at each classification level for a particular individual given their health or disability, as well as environmental and personal factors.

Assistive technology evaluation, provision, training, and follow-up is guided by the environmental factors component of the ICF model. Specifically, the environmental factors component constitutes the physical, social, and attitudinal environment in which people live and includes five areas:

1. Products and technology
2. Natural environment and human-made changes to environment
3. Support and relationships
4. Attitudes
5. Services, systems, and policies (Schneidert, Hurst, Miller, & Ustun, 2003)

According to the ICF, assistive technology would be included under the area of **products and technology**—"natural or human made products or systems of products, equipment, and technology in an individual's immediate environment, that are gathered, created, produced or manufactured" (p. 591). Selecting and providing appropriate assistive technology devices for a person depends on the number and type of classification levels affected by that person's disease, condition, or disorder. Devices used to compensate for impairments at the body structure/function level include hearing aids, pacemakers, and prosthetics. Technology solutions at the activity level can be low tech or high tech. Some low-tech solutions are utensils with built-up or weighted handles, reachers, and sock aids. Several high-tech examples include environmental control units and specialized computer hardware or software. Assistive technology used to compensate for limitations in participation often overlap with the devices recommended for the body structure/function and activity levels. For example, a person with a mobility impairment may use a powered wheelchair to compensate for an inability to walk as well as to accomplish specific tasks or actions, such as cleaning the kitchen. In short, the more classification levels impacted by a disease, condition, or disorder will determine the amount and type of assistive technology devices needed to function independently.

Many chronic diseases affect hearing, vision, cognition, and movement. Assistive technology is available for people with hearing, vision, memory, communication, and movement impairments. The overview of assistive technology in the next section focuses primarily on high-tech devices, assuming that the reader is familiar with the range of low-tech devices that have been available for many years. It is important to point out that high-tech is not synonymous with complicated. In fact, high-tech devices may be easier to use than traditional devices designed for the same purpose. That is, they may be "smarter" and save the user steps. A good example of this is the Beyond™ Smart Microwave Oven that features a built-in scanner that reads the bar code label on the food package and automatically sets the time and temperature controls for the correct cooking of the food product. The electronics for this oven are complex, but the process of cooking is simplified for the user; if the user has a visual or cognitive impairment, independent cooking may be possible only with such a device. The Beyond Smart Microwave Oven will have a much broader market than older persons with cognitive and visual impairments and could be considered a universally designed product.

Assistive Technology for Older Adults

There are over 20,000 products listed in *Abledata,* a computerized database of assistive devices. In discussing products that might be useful for older adults, this section will cover the following categories of assistive devices: devices for persons with movement impairments (including walking aids, environmental control devices, and robots) and those with vision, hearing, cognitive, and communication limitations. It is important to keep in mind that older adults often have more than one chronic condition and resultant impairments and may benefit from devices in several categories. Multiple impairments may also require modification of devices.

Devices for Persons with Mobility or Motor Impairments

Walking Aids and Wheelchairs
Walking aids are among the most common of all assistive devices. The cane, second only to eyeglasses in popularity and numbers, is also one of the oldest assistive devices. Persons experiencing some loss of balance may decide on their own to purchase a cane. For those with more serious gait impairments, perhaps as a result of stroke or Parkinson's disease, a variety of canes and walkers are available to make mobility easier and safer. Walker types vary in design and functionality. They range from regular walkers and canes to ones with built-in seats that allow a person to sit and rest when tired.

Wheelchairs offer another option for independent mobility, as well as making assisted mobility possible. Advances in wheelchairs have led to lighter, more comfortable designs. Depending on the needs of the person who will use the wheelchair, therapists must make recommendations involving cushions, armrests, wheels, tires, hand rims, and power. Therapists also make recommendations for wheelchair accessories including transfer boards, lapboards and trays, safety belts, clothing guards, and bags and pockets. Several references provide detailed information on wheelchairs, useful for therapists working with older adults who may need a wheelchair (Cooper, 1998; Giannini, 1998).

Environmental Control Units
Environmental control devices are designed primarily for persons with physical disabilities, although they often benefit people with cognitive or visual impairments as well. For older adults, whether living at home or in a nursing home, an environmental control device can increase ability to operate almost any device that runs on electricity: radios, computers, phone, lights, and security systems, to name just a few. Handheld remote controls for televisions could be considered an environmental control device, one that reaches a much broader market than people with impairments. Originally, handheld remotes were designed for young people with excellent fine motor control, excellent vision, and a love for "bells and whistles" because of the small size of the buttons, the small print on or under each button, and the various complicated features. However, there are several handheld remotes now that incorporate universal design features like larger buttons, more room between buttons, more simplified layouts, and easy-to-read print.

Haataja and Saarnio (1990) identified five components that make up an environmental control device:

1. A switch that provides the user a means to operate the device

2. A control device that provides a means for transmitting commands, through sound waves, infrared light, or hard-wired connections
3. A target device such as a lamp or radio that is actually turned on or off
4. Connections such as the sensors that pick up the infrared light signal
5. A feedback device that lets the user know the status of the system

One recent study employed a cross-sectional design with 15 experienced users of electronic aids to investigate the impact of continued use of a device and to identify the functions the device assists with or performs for an individual (Ripat, 2006). Device use was found to make participants feel more competent. Their well-being was stable over a long period compared with new users of electronic devices. Furthermore, participants noted that environmental control units were used to perform the following functions: increase and maintain independence, control devices for entertainment, and communicate basic needs.

An X-10 environmental control device is pictured in Figure 24-2. Environmental control devices range in price from $24 to approximately $10,000, and their functions vary from simple on–off of one or a few appliances to computer-based control of the total home environment, the computer, and telecommunications. A table listing different environmental control units, a brief description of each, the manufacturer, and the cost is available from Abledata. In helping a person select an environmental control device, Dickey and Shealey (1987) offer several questions to consider: Will the system be difficult (how difficult) to operate? How reliable and durable is the system? How will the system be installed? How easy is it to install? How portable is the system, especially if it will need to be moved? Who is the manufacturer, and will the manufacturer be in business when support or repair is required? Are the features of the device appropriate for the intended user? How much training will be required to ensure that the user will be successful with its operation?

Robots

Environmental control devices "operate" on the electrical environment. An environmental control device could be used to operate a mechanical device such as a lift (Figure 24-3), but the combination of electronics and mechanical functions falls into the area of robotics. Robots have been developed to assist people with performing industrial, military, personal, and medical tasks (Davenport, 2005). Personal robot research and development has lagged behind the advances made with industrial robots because personal robots have to "operate in a semiautonomous to autonomous state in changing

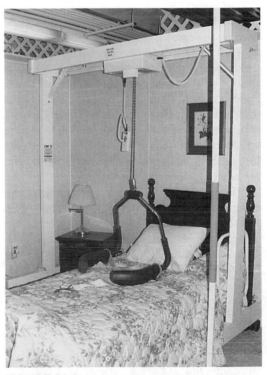

FIGURE 24-3 Overhead lift operated by remote control device.

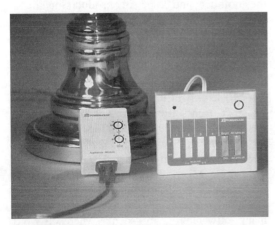

FIGURE 24-2 An X-10 environmental control device system.

environments while industrial robots function in fixed environments" (p. 76). However, development of personal robots is expected to increase in the near future due to less-expensive robotic components, recent advances in power consumption, and better sensor technology. Current personal robot use and development is in the following areas: mobility devices, exoskeletons, powered wheelchairs, entertainment, household assistance, and monitoring.

Devices for Persons with Vision Impairments

Vision loss is common among older persons. In fact, age-related vision loss and blindness affect 5.5 million noninstitutionalized Americans who are 55 years and older (American Foundation for the Blind [AFB], 2006). Additionally, about 1.8 million noninstitutionalized older adults state they have difficulty performing basic activities of daily living (ADL), like bathing, reading, and dressing, due to a severe visual impairment (Desai, Pratt, Lentzner, & Robinson, 2001). Visual loss may be caused by diabetic retinopathy, cataracts, glaucoma, and macular degeneration, as well as normal aging. A discussion of visual loss can be found in Chapter 5.

Vision loss among the elderly is associated with a decrease in outdoor mobility. A recent study of 404 older adults determined that vision significantly affects the performance of activities of daily living outside the home (Wahl, Heyl, & Schilling, 2002). They also found that vision impairment affected a participant's ability to engage in outdoor activities. Those who participated in outdoor activities reported a higher level of life satisfaction than those who did not engage in outdoor activities.

Eyeglasses are the most common assistive device, and they are typically provided by an optometrist. For individuals who require other devices or devices that provide stronger magnification, occupational therapists often participate in providing assistive devices. The following are some basic guidelines for assisting persons with visual impairments who do not necessarily require an assistive device:

1. In speaking with a person with a visual impairment, do not increase your speaking volume unless the person also has a hearing impairment. Be sure to tell the person who you are. Tell the person when you are leaving.
2. Ask the person if assistance is needed; do not wait to be asked.
3. Allow the person to hold your arm and follow a few steps behind when guiding a person with a severe vision loss.
4. When providing assistance with setting up activities, provide larger images when possible. For example, you can set the enlargement feature on a photocopy machine to increase the size of print or pictures.
5. Position the person closer to the objects involved in the task.
6. Increase the amount and intensity of light, but at the same time reduce glare.
7. Provide contrasting colors (e.g., dark objects on a light surface). This may require placing a cloth on the table for activities (AFB, 2006, n.p.).

There are a wide variety of low-cost, simple assistive devices for persons with visual impairments. These include magnifying glasses, pens that write with a bold line, and writing guides. Materials prepared in large print are available in many bookstores and libraries. Banks can print checks with large characters, and games can be bought with enlarged boards. Most electronics stores carry phones with large buttons and large numbers. Thermometers, clocks, watches, and blood sugar monitors are all available with either large-print or voice-output features. Figure 24-4 pictures a thermostat with enlarged numbers and marks.

Today, various hardware and software solutions and video-based technology have increased the number and type of products available for persons with visual impairments. The features offered by these devices make them very appropriate for older adults. These products are categorized by the features they offer.

Screen Enlargement Software

There are many software programs that magnify the image on the computer screen, making it possible for a person with low vision to read what is on the screen. Prices range from under $100 to $600. All of the current Microsoft operating systems provide free limited magnification of the computer screen through its accessibility options. There are also many software programs, such as Microsoft Word, Microsoft Excel, and WordPerfect, which have free limited character enlargement features by increasing the viewing size of the page. These free built-in features found in Microsoft Windows and Office applications are also another example of universal design. A list of screen enlargement software can be obtained from Abledata.

Closed Circuit Televisions (CCTVs)

These devices increase the size of any written material or picture. The systems include a monitor, anywhere from 14 to 26 inches, and a viewing table where the book or other materials are placed. Some viewing tables are automated and can be controlled with a foot pedal. For older adults with visual impairments, a CCTV could make the difference in being able to read the newspaper and books. In fact, one study found that reading was one of the two activities that visually impaired older participants missed doing most (Mann, Hurren, Kuruza, & Bentley, 1993). Figure 24-5 illustrates a stand-alone print enlargement system.

Braille Output Devices

Most of us are familiar with braille printed on heavy paper. Software is available that, together with a braille printer, permits braille printing of text produced on a computer with a word processor. "Refreshable braille displays" attach to the computer and use tiny pins that move up and down to produce braille characters that represent a portion of the computer screen. Various refreshable braille display models exist and are available in 20-, 40-, and 80-character-long strings. Although a smaller percentage of visually impaired persons are now learning braille, a significant portion of older adults who have been blind since youth are benefiting from these computer-based braille output devices. However, those who acquire vision loss later in life often have difficulty learning to read braille due to sensory loss in the fingers. Figure 24-6 shows a refreshable braille display.

Screen Reading Software

Screen reading software can be added to a computer which will allow the words on the computer monitor to be read out loud through the computer speakers. This allows a person to navigate the computer desktop, access files and documents, and use various word processing, scheduling, and spreadsheet software. Existing files can be read to the visually impaired person. Together with an optical character recognition system (described in the following section), which takes text that is

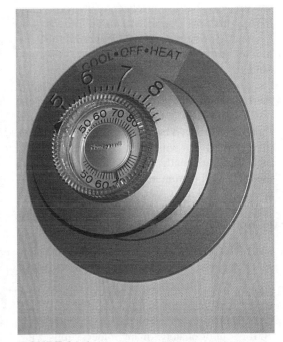

FIGURE 24-4 Thermostat with large numbers.

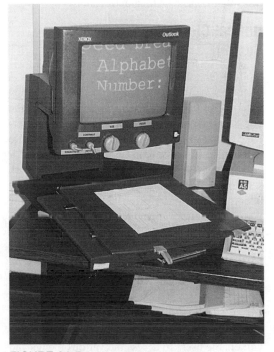

FIGURE 24-5 Print enlargement system.

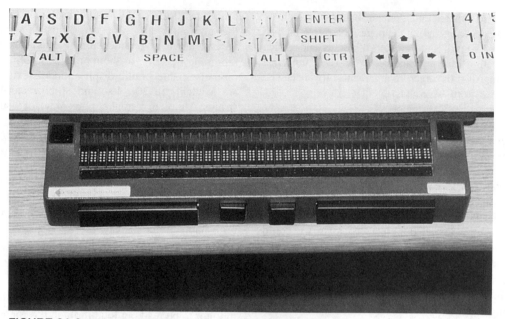

FIGURE 24-6 Refreshable braille display on the navigator.

already printed and converts it into a computer file, virtually any printed material becomes available to the person with a visual impairment. For older adults with severe vision loss, a talking computer may make it possible to continue working, leisure reading, and carrying out household tasks that require writing and reading.

Optical Character Recognition System

Optical character recognition systems use a computer scanner that is similar to a photocopy machine in that you place a printed page on the copying surface to get a second copy. The difference is that the scanner produces a computer file that can be saved or read (with screen reading or enlargement software). Computer systems with screen reading capabilities and a scanner have become much more affordable in the past few years, and they provide virtually complete access to printed materials.

Mobile Devices

Recent technological advances have made the development of mobile devices for people with visual impairments possible. Cell phones can be programmed with voice-output software that will enable users to access the various menus and dialing features of their phone. Personal digital assistants (PDAs) have been developed to provide the same functionality and programs for people with visual impairments as off-the-shelf PDAs provide to those without visual impairments. These PDAs have various input (standard or braille keyboard) and output (refreshable braille display or audio) methods. A global positioning system can also be attached to many of these PDAs, making it possible for a person who is visually impaired to navigate around the community. Development of portable CCTVs and optical character recognition (OCR) scanners has improved access to printed materials in the home and community and has reduced the reliance on the larger desktop models of the same products. These mobile devices have provided those with visual impairments an increased independence and freedom in both the home and community environments that was unheard of even 5 years ago.

Devices for Persons with Hearing Impairments

Hearing impairment is common among older adults: One out of three persons over age 65 have some hearing impairment; this increases to almost one out of two persons over age 85 (Desai et al., 2001). Unfortunately, many older adults view hearing loss as a normal part of aging and do nothing about it. Hearing loss can impact on communication, which in turn can result in isolation and depression (Capella-McDonnall, 2005). Hearing loss affects health and safety in other ways, such as not being able to understand instructions for taking medications or not being able to hear fire alarms. Causes and types of hearing loss are discussed in Chapter 5.

The first step in addressing hearing impairment is to seek medical advice. Surgery is employed for some types of hearing loss; age should not be the determinant in considering a surgical approach (Capella-McDonnall, 2005). A relatively new surgical procedure, developed for profoundly deaf persons, involves implanting electrodes that bypass damaged hair cells surrounding the cochlea. Although a cochlear implant can enable a person to hear sounds, the procedure has not yet been developed to the point that a person is able to discriminate speech. Cochlear implants are a promising new technology, but most older adults do not have the type of profound hearing loss that would require this procedure.

Approximately 174 in 1000 people over 64 experience tinnitus (U.S. Public Health Service, 1995). There is no cure for tinnitus, but "maskers" are sometimes used to provide a more acceptable sound than that produced by the tinnitus. Hearing aids are often used to offset the effect of the hearing loss that can accompany tinnitus. Surgery is sometimes employed to reduce tinnitus, as are drugs, relaxation techniques, and biofeedback (Desai et al., 2001).

Hearing Aids

There are many assistive devices for people with hearing impairments, the most common of which is the hearing aid, typically prescribed by an audiologist. Therapists encounter many older adults who use hearing aids but because of fine motor or vision impairment, have difficulty replacing batteries, positioning the device, or adjusting the controls. Working with older adults, the therapist often establishes a goal of improved fine motor performance that can lead to independence in use of the hearing aid. The therapist might also assist a person in finding "tools" for working the controls or replacing the batteries more easily.

Assistive Listening Devices

When hearing aids do not provide adequate sound amplification, *assistive listening devices* (ALDs) may be used. ALDs include microphones for the person speaking, amplifiers to capture the

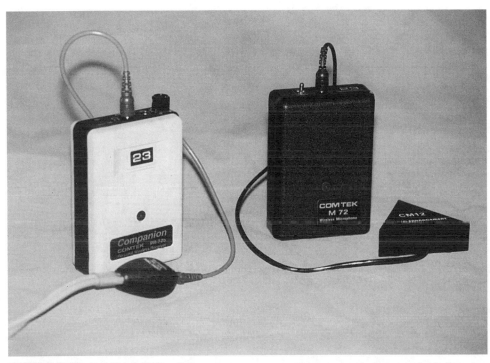

FIGURE 24-7 Assistive listening device.

sounds, and, for the person with the hearing loss, a headset or ear receiver. ALD systems are hard-wired or use either FM radio waves or infrared signals. Many churches, schools, and theaters have ALD systems, usually FM and infrared systems. The hard-wired system is more often used in a home. Figure 24-7 illustrates an assistive listening device.

Telecommunication Devices

Telecommunication devices for the deaf (TDDs) are actually small microprocessor-based devices that have a screen, keyboard, and modem. With a TDD at both ends of a telephone line, messages can be typed in and read at each end. Relay services are available in every state so that a person with a hearing impairment can type in a message to an operator, who in turn provides the final receiver with the spoken message. TDDs are now available in public places such as airports. Figure 24-8 provides a picture of a TDD.

Amplification Devices

Electronics and phone stores carry phones that offer amplified sound and devices that can be added to an existing phone to provide

amplification. Closed-captioned television provides text at the bottom of the screen on televisions equipped with a special decoding device. All new televisions with a screen greater than 13 inches now have this feature installed in the factory. Other devices include smoke detectors that provide a visual alert such as a flashing light or vibration. A number of these low-cost devices can make it possible for older adults with hearing loss to continue their involvement in important life roles.

Devices for Persons with Cognitive Impairments

Personal Digital Assistants (PDAs)

Memory loss can occur with a number of diseases associated with aging. One low-tech solution to memory impairment is to write notes on paper and post them in appropriate places. An alternative, high-tech solution is to use a PDA. A number of these are available for under $500. The alarm can be used to provide a reminder for taking medications. Many digital wristwatches now offer similar features. One recent study reported the effectiveness of use of an electronic memory

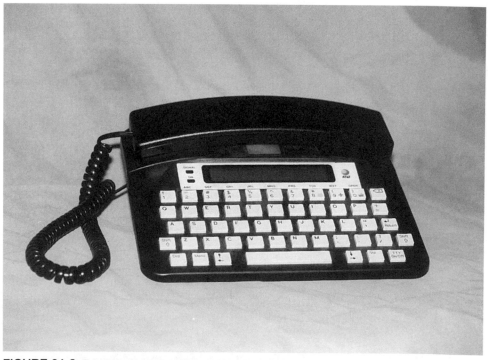

FIGURE 24-8 Telecommunication device for the deaf (TDD).

device by persons with Alzheimer's disease. In this study, participants made significantly more statements of fact and fewer ambiguous utterances. In addition, participants showed more initiative in conversations (Bourgeoris, 1990). However, caution must be exercised in recommending these devices, as some may be too complex for someone to operate even in the early stages of Alzheimer's disease.

Other Devices

Other helpful devices include automatic turn-off switches for stove burners, automatic timers for lights, movement-sensitive light switches that turn lamps on when a person enters a room, and security systems that can sound an alarm when someone attempts to open a secured door.

Determining Assistive Technology Needs Using the ICF and Practice Framework

The *World Health Organization's International Classification of Functioning (ICF)* (2001) and the *Occupational Therapy Practice Framework* (AOTA, 2002) can guide the practitioner throughout the assistive technology process from assessment to follow-up. Specifically, the ICF model provides the underlying foundation of the process by giving the practitioner a picture of the client in a healthy and an unhealthy state at various levels of functioning and contextual factors. The Practice Framework delineates the procedures to follow during each step of the process. A practitioner uses the ICF model to gain an understanding of a person's "typical" functional performance and contextual factors without a disease, disorder, or condition, and, in turn, uses this information to determine the client's functional needs, abilities, limitations, and impact of various contextual factors. The first level of the ICF model—the body structure/function level—is where the practitioner assesses the client's previous physiological and anatomical integrity and the changes that occurred at this level due to a disease, condition, or disorder. The second and third levels of the ICF model—the activity and participation levels— consist of obtaining the client's prior level of functioning at these levels, and then evaluating the client's activity limitations and participation

restrictions caused by a condition, disease, or disorder. Environmental factors are deemed as facilitators if they positively impact one's functional performance, or hindrances and limitations if they negatively affect a person's functional performance (Arthanat, Nochajski, & Stone, 2004). Personal factors, such as age, gender, fitness, coping abilities, and social background, are also important in determining how the person will react to intervention. Thus, the ICF model provides the practitioner with a framework for gathering necessary information about the client—needs, abilities, and limitations—before and after the onset of a disease, condition, or disorder.

According to the Practice Framework (AOTA, 2002), any occupational therapy evaluation, including the assistive technology assessment, begins with constructing an occupational profile of the client. After an occupational profile is gathered, the practitioner analyzes the client's occupation performance. This includes evaluating the person's performance skills (e.g., motor and process skills), performance patterns (e.g., habits and roles), and performance in areas of occupation (i.e., ADLs and instrumental activities of daily living [IADLs]). Impairments, limitations, restrictions, and barriers in any of these areas are explored to determine which therapeutic strategy or combination of strategies—therapeutic intervention, compensatory techniques, assistive technology, or environmental modifications— would give the client the most independent level of functional performance. Assistive technology should be selected when the other strategies are not adequate or sufficient in helping the client achieve his or her full functional potential, and for energy conservation, joint protection, or to reduce repetitive motion. An outcome assessment is performed after assistive technology provision and training to determine whether or not the technology was successful in helping the client reach the desired goals. The following section will explore the appropriate application of technology for people given the number and type of classification levels affected by that person's disease, condition, or disorder.

Person 1 is a community-dwelling older male who enjoys golfing, meeting with his friends to play cards, reading the newspaper, and doing crossword puzzles. He has recently developed an age-related eye condition called presbyopia that affects the accommodative power of his intraocular lens causing decreased visual acuity at near distances. He has noticed increased difficulty reading the newspaper, filling out crossword puzzles, and reading road signs when driving. He does not have any difficulty performing any other ADLs or IADLs. According to the ICF model, the condition, presbyopia, directly affects the body structure/function level, and indirectly affects the other levels as noted by only minor activity limitations and participation restrictions mentioned above. Although this is not a typical client seen for occupational therapy services, this client does represent a person on the high functioning end of the continuum; that is, the client has a condition that affects one level on the ICF model with minimal effects to the other, and only requires low-tech assistive technology (i.e., eyeglasses) to remediate these limitations and restrictions.

Person 2 is an older female with mild dementia who resides with her daughter's family. Prior to developing dementia she lived independently and had no difficulty performing her ADLs and IADLs. Currently, she is beginning to have difficulty remembering to take her medications and to turn off the stove after cooking. Occasionally, she also gets confused when performing certain self-care and home management tasks, as well as getting disoriented when walking in the neighborhood. Her family is concerned for her safety because she is home alone while they are working or going to school. In this case, the condition affects the body/structure level of the ICF model, as well as the activity and participation levels. The client appears to have many positive environmental factors (e.g., good social support network), but also several negative environmental factors that endanger her safety (e.g., stove burners without automatic shutoff). Interventions cannot be implemented at the body structure/function level to alleviate problems in the other two levels. Because the evaluation results show no other impairments except for memory and cognitive-processing skills, intervention focuses on environmental modifications, compensatory strategies, and family education. An outcome assessment performed by the therapist concludes that the goals relating to the patient's safety and medication management have not been fully met. Thus, the occupational therapist begins to explore assistive technology options with the client and her family, taking into account her strengths, limitations, and acceptability of the device. The client, her family, and the therapist decide on the following devices: burners with automatic shutoffs, electronic pill organizer and reminder, an electronic notebook that provides audible reminders, and a bracelet locator for when she gets disoriented (www.abledata.com/abledata.cfm?pageid=19327&ksectionid=19327). A follow-up evaluation found that with the intervention and assistive technology, the client successfully met her goals and will be able to continue to live with her family members.

Issues Relating to Use of Assistive Technology with Older Adults

Repair and maintenance of assistive devices are important concerns. What are the costs, will it be available when needed, and how long will it take? Lack of repair and maintenance can be dangerous and fail to provide the optimal amount of assistance. A study of 227 adults with various disabilities found that 29.3% of all devices were abandoned (Phillips & Zhao, 1993). Furthermore, this study found that device abandonment was significantly related to one of four factors:

1. Lack of consideration of user opinion in selection
2. Easy device procurement
3. Poor device performance
4. Change in user needs or priorities

In recommending assistive devices, first it is important to give the client options of different assistive technology devices and work with vendors to allow the client to try equipment out before making the purchase, especially with more expensive devices. After determining which device the client prefers, the therapist should help the client in identifying funding for the device. Last, the therapist should provide training in the use of the device, and leave instructions regarding repair and maintenance, either with the device user or with a caregiver. Locating service providers capable of offering quality assistive technology services is often difficult not only for the older consumer but for other service providers who make referrals. There is also some fragmentation of services as a result of specialization. Experts in vision, hearing, and cognitive disabilities may not be capable of working with the complex interweave of factors that often are present in an older person. Occupational therapists are often the most knowledgeable about assistive technology services and either make an intervention or refer the client to another provider. One source of information on service providers is the lead agency in each state under the Technology Related Assistance for Individuals with Disabilities Act. The Society for the Advancement of Rehabilitative and Assistive Technology (RESNA) in Washington, DC, provides technical assistance to the states and could be contacted for information on your state's lead agency.

Funding is another problem with assistive devices and the services required for successful use. Even though many devices are low in cost and can be covered by the user, many other devices are expensive and not affordable to all who need them. The national trend is for less public funding for health care and for greater out-of-pocket funding: The findings demonstrate the startling and accelerating growth in the elderly's out-of-pocket costs for health care. In fact, the elderly's out-of-pocket health expenditures have grown much faster than Medicare and Medicaid program costs (Crystal, Johnson, Harman, Sambamoorthi, & Kumar, 2000). Assistive devices help people maintain or regain independence and, thus, can reduce overall health care costs. However, access to assistive devices is often blocked, restricted, or limited because third-party payers do not cover them.

Acceptability of the device to the individual is a crucial factor. The person's needs and wishes must be considered. Some people may find the devices unacceptable cosmetically, and some may resist being "dependent" on these devices. Further, "high tech" is intimidating to some older adults. It may be possible to address this factor in a training program for the use of a certain device, but it is also possible that the device will still be left in a closet to collect dust or, worse, that it will get in the way and make function more difficult.

Although there are problems related to assistive technology and environmental interventions, these tools offer great potential for helping older adults maintain independence and lead satisfying lives. Occupational and physical therapists as well as other service providers often play an important role in identifying the appropriate technology, in training older persons in how to use it, and in providing follow-up support. Audiologists deal with devices related to hearing, and physical therapists, mobility devices. Opticians or optometrists may be knowledgeable about vision aides. Social workers are vital in identifying sources of financing for all these devices and services.

Case Study

Mrs. Jones is a 78-year-old female who had a right cerebrovascular accident (CVA) and left hemiplegia several years ago and uses a manual wheelchair for all of her mobility needs. She lives alone in the community but has family members who live next door and come and check on her at least once a day. She also has home health nurses come by once a week to check on her and nursing assistants that come by three times a week to assist her with bathing, dressing, and light house chores. Recently, the client has reported increased difficulty moving around her house and operating appliances.

Questions

1. What is the first step for an occupational therapist?
2. Based on this assessment, how would you evaluate her difficulties at each level of the ICF? What environmental factors might affect her performance?
3. What kinds of occupational therapy intervention might be most helpful?

Review Questions

1. What is the difference between high-tech and low-tech assistive devices? What makes universal design important to all older adults—that is, including those who have only minimal functional limitations? Mrs. A is a 67-year-old widow with mild arthritis and mild presbycusis. How might environmental control devices assist her in maintaining independence in her apartment?
2. Mr. Y is in the early stages of macular degeneration. What assistive devices might a therapist consider to help him as his vision declines?
3. A therapist has provided an environmental control device for Ms. D. On a home visit, she notes that the device is sitting on the table, collecting dust. What are the possible reasons that Ms. D might not use the device, and what could the therapist do?

Web-Based Resources

For helpful information about the experience of products and technology, visit:

Product Reports (2003–2005).

www.aarp.org, **American Association of Retired Persons (AARP),** date connected July 16, 2007. Developed for AARP members, each of these reports provides overviews of the device type and comparative information. Several reports are planned, but those currently available include "Wheelchairs," "Hearing Aids," and "Personal Alerting Devices."

www.phhp.ufl.edu/centers/rerc.htm, **Rehabilitation Engineering Research Center on Aging,** date connected July 16, 2007. A series of training material for professionals and information on products for consumers, including videos, slides, booklets, training guides, and case studies.

www.RESNA.org, *Assistive Technology* **(journal), published by RESNA Press,** date connected July 16, 2007. This quarterly journal is the official publication of RESNA, The Society for the Advancement of Rehabilitative and Assistive Technology.

www.abledata.com, **Abledata,** date connected July 16, 2007. This site includes a large number of products that can be helpful to individuals with physical disabilities and for older adults.

Resources

Smart technology for aging, disability, and independence: The state of the science (2005). published by Wiley Interscience, Hoboken, NJ. This 379-page text covers assistive technology devices for various disabilities and contains a unit on assistive technology information.

Technology and Disability, IOS Press, 5795-G Burke Centre Parkway, VA 22015. This journal communicates knowledge about the field of assistive technology devices and services, within the context of the lives of end users—persons with disabilities and their family members. Although the topics are technical in nature, the articles are written for a broad comprehension despite the reader's education or training. Its contents cover research and development efforts, education and training programs, service and policy activities, and consumer experiences. The journal publishes original research papers, review articles, case studies, program descriptions, Letters to the editors, and commentaries. Suggestions for thematic issues and proposed manuscripts are welcomed.

REFERENCES

Administration on Aging. (2004). *A profile of older Americans: 2004* (Department of Health and Human Services Publication). Washington, DC: Author.

American Foundation for the Blind. (2006). *Quick fact and figures on blindness and low vision.* Retrieved April 10, 2008 from www.afb.org/Section.asp?SectionID = 42&DocumentID=1374.

American Occupational Therapy Association. (2002). Occupational therapy practice framework: Domain and process. *American Journal of Occupational Therapy, 56,* 609–639.

Arthanat, S., Nochajski, S. M., & Stone, J. (2004). The international classification of functioning, disability and health and its application to cognitive disorders. *Disability and Rehabilitation, 26*(4), 235–245.

Bourgeoris, M. (1990). Enhancing conversation skills in patients with Alzheimer's disease using a prosthetic memory aid. *Journal of Applied Behavior Analysis, 23*(1), 29–42.

Capella-McDonnall, M. E. (2005). The effects of single and dual sensory loss on symptoms of depression in the elderly. *International Journal of Geriatric Psychiatry, 20*(9), 855–861.

Center for Universal Design. (1997). The principles of universal design (Version 2.0). Raleigh, NC: North Carolina State University. Retrieved April 10, 2008 from http://www.design.ncsu.edu/cud/about_ud/udprinciplestext.htm.

Cooper, R. A. (1998). *Wheelchair selection and configuration.* New York: Demos Medical.

Crystal, S., Johnson, R. W., Harman, J., Sambamoorthi, U., & Kumar, R. (2000). Out-of-pocket health care costs among older Americans. *The Journals of Gerontology. Series B, Psychological Sciences and Social Sciences, 55*(1), 551–562.

Davenport, R. (2005). Robotics. In W. Mann (Ed.), *Smart technology for aging, Disability, and independence: The state of the science* (pp. 67–109). Hoboken, NJ: Wiley-Interscience.

Desai, M., Pratt, L. A., Lentzner, H., & Robinson, K. N. (2001). Trends in vision and hearing among older Americans. *Aging Trends, 2,* 1–8.

Dickey, R., & Shealey, S. (1987). Using technology to control the environment. *American Journal of Occupational Therapy, 41,* 717–721.

Edwards, N. I., & Jones, D. A. (1998). Ownership and use of assistive devices amongst older people in the community. *Age and Ageing, 27,* 463–468.

Freedman, V. A., Crimmins, E., Schoeni, R. F., Spillman, B. C., Aykan, H., Kramarow, E., et al. (2004). Resolving inconsistencies in trends in old-age disability: Report from a technical working group. *Demography, 41*(3), 417–441.

Giannini, M. J. (1998). *Choosing a wheelchair system.* Baltimore, MD: Department of Veterans Affairs.

Haataja, S., and Saarnio, I. (1990). An evaluation procedure for environmental control systems. In

J. J. Presperin (Ed.), Proceedings of the 13th Annual RESNA Conference (pp. 177–178). Washington, D.C.: RESNA, 1990.

He, W., Sengupta, M., Velkoff, V. A., & DeBarros, K. A. (2005). 65+ in the United States: 2005 (U.S. Census Bureau Publication No. P23-209). Washington, DC: U.S. Government Printing Office.

Jette, A. M., Haley, S. M., & Kooyoomjian, J. T. (2003). Are the ICF activity and participation dimensions distinct? *Journal of Rehabilitation Medicine, 35,* 145–149.

Kose, S. (1998). Form barrier-free to universal design: An international perspective. *Assistive Technology, 10*(1), 44–50.

Mann, W. C., Hurren, D., Charvat, B., & Tomita, M. R. (1998). Problems with wheelchairs experienced by frail elders. *Technology and Disability, 5,* 101–111.

Mann, W., Hurren, D., Kuruza, J., & Bentley, D. (1993). Needs of home-based older visually impaired persons for assistive devices. *Journal of Visual Impairment and Blindness, 87*(4), 106–110.

Mann, W., and Lane, J. (1991). *Assistive technology for persons with disabilities: The role of occupational therapy.* Rockville, MD: American Occupational Therapy Association.

Mann, W., Ottenbacher, K., Fraas, L., Tomita, M., & Granger, C. (1999). Effectiveness of assistive technology and environmental interventions in maintaining independence and reducing home care costs for the frail elderly: A randomized trial. *Archives of Family Medicine, 8,* 210–217.

Perenboom, R. J. M., & Chorus, A. M. J. (2003). Measuring participation according to the International Classification of Functioning, Disability and Health (ICF). *Disability and Rehabilitation, 25*(11–12), 577–587.

Peterson, W. (1998). Public policy affecting universal design. *Assistive Technology, 10*(1), 13–20.

Phillips, B., & Zhao, H. (1993). Predictors of assistive technology abandonment. *Assistive Technology, 5*(1), 36–45.

Ripat, J. (2006). Function and impact of electronic aids to daily living for experienced users. *Technology and Disability, 18*(2), 79–87.

Schafer, R. (2000). *Housing America's seniors.* Cambridge, MA: Harvard University.

Schneidert, M., Hurst, R., Miller, J., & Ustun, B. (2003). The role of environment in the International Classification of Functioning, Disability and Health (ICF). *Disability and Rehabilitation, 25*(11–12), 588–595.

Story, M. F. (1998). Maximizing usability: The principles of universal design. *Assistive Technology, 10*(1), 4–12.

Technology Related Assistance for Individuals with Disabilities Act of 1988 as Amended in 1994. Retrieved April 10, 2008 from http://www.handinet.org/tech_act.htm.

United States Public Health Service. (1995). Prevalence of selected chronic conditions, United States, 1990–1992. Advanced Data from Vital and Health Statistics, No. 194 (DHHS Pub No (PHS) 88-1250). Hyattsville, MD.

Ustun, T. B., Chatterji, S., Kostansjek, N., & Bickenbach, J. (2003). WHO's ICF and functional status information in health records. *Health Care Financing Review, 24*(3), 77–88.

Vanderheiden, G. C. (1998). Universal design and assistive technology in communication and information technologies: Alternatives or complements? *Assistive Technology, 10*(1), 29–36.

Wahl, H., Heyl, V., & Schilling, O. (2002). The role of vision impairment for the outdoor activity and life satisfaction of older adults: A multi-faceted view. *Visual Impairment Research, 4*(3), 143–160.

World Health Organization. (2001). *International Classification of Function.* Geneva: Author. Retrieved February 26, 2006, from www3.who.int/icf.

CHAPTER 25

Elder Abuse

Georgia J. Anetzberger, PhD, ACSW

. . .Our society must address the abuse of the elderly and disabled persons as a critical social problem. The lessons learned in responding to the needs of those individuals may serve as guideposts for advancing the quality of life for all older adults and their families.

Rosalie S. Wolf, PhD (1927–2001),
Founder of the National Committee for
the Prevention of Elder Abuse

OBJECTIVES

By the end of this chapter, readers will be able to:

1. Delineate various forms of elder abuse.
2. Provide an historical account of elder abuse awareness.
3. Discuss the prevalence, incidence, and reporting of this problem.
4. Distinguish between examples, signs, and risk factors for elder abuse.
5. Describe the role of various service systems in preventing and treating elder abuse.
6. Give the benefits of multidisciplinary teams in problem intervention.

The National Center on Elder Abuse offers almost daily listings of headlines on elder abuse. They are compiled from newspapers nationwide and posted on the Center's listserve. The listserve is used by more than one thousand subscribers—all professionals actively involved in research, education, public policy, program planning, or service delivery on behalf of abused elders.

Anyone perusing these headlines cannot help but be struck by the frequency of elder abuse, its potentially severe effects, and the occurrence of the problem in all parts of the country and in both urban and rural settings. The headlines dispel common myths about the problem—that it is rare, not serious, and mostly an issue for older people who live in big cities.

A sample of these newspaper headlines follows:

- 71-year-old's emaciated body described
- Nursing home failed to protect alleged rape victims
- Daughter charged with neglecting impaired mom
- Health aide says she stole $250,000 from two elderly sisters
- Woman accused of stealing from grand-mother; suspect charged with exploitation of an endangered adult

- Former nursing assistant accused of beating patient
- Man sentenced to 10 to 25 years for stabbing mom
- 83-year-old woman found in condemned home
- Brothers kept mom's body in storage; police say duo cashed her checks
- 81-year-old goes on trial for killing his wife

Examining the Problem of Elder Abuse

Definitions and Forms

Elder abuse has no universally accepted definitions and forms, although advocates have emphasized the need for them over the past two decades (National Center on Elder Abuse, 2001; National Research Council, 2003; Stein, 1991; University of New Hampshire, 1986; U.S. Department of Health and Human Services, 1992; Watson, 1995). Standardized definitions and forms are important for comparison of research results and state reporting statistics. Without them, generalizations are impossible.

There are several reasons for the lack of uniform elder abuse definitions and forms, including

- There has been no federal funding incentive to standardize definitions in state law, as occurred with child abuse.
- Opinions vary on how broad the meaning of elder abuse should be. For example, should self-abuse and self-neglect be included as **elder abuse forms,** or should their lack of perpetrator (other than the victim) preclude this?
- Some believe that only intentional acts constitute elder abuse; others would include passive acts as well, such as benign neglect.
- There is disagreement on whether or not vulnerability on the part of the victim due to frailty, disability, or some other factor is a prerequisite for elder abuse.
- A range of opinion exists on the degree to which consequences, frequency, severity, or duration are considerations in defining elder abuse.

There have been several efforts to standardize definitions and forms for elder abuse. Notable research efforts were undertaken by Johnson (1986), Hudson (1991), and the National Research Council (2003). Johnson's definitions and forms of elder mistreatment include four sequential stages that conceptualize the problem, identify its behavioral manifestations, specify measurable observations, and distinguish cause from act. They are derived from her synthesis and analysis of the literature on elder abuse at the time. In contrast, Hudson's definitions and forms reflect a three-round Delphi survey of elder abuse experts. They have five levels and eleven definitions, beginning with general forms of violence perpetrated against elder adults (Level I) and ending with specific types of abusive or neglectful behaviors (Level V). Finally, the National Research Council's definitions of elder mistreatment were developed for scientific purposes by a panel of health and legal academics and elder abuse experts. The Council elected to use the term "elder mistreatment" over "abuse" and "neglect," because it perceived the latter terms to have legal connotations based upon state statutes.

Similarly, there have been efforts to derive uniform public policy elder abuse definitions and forms. Early related activity is evident in legislation introduced into the U.S. House of Representatives by Mary Rose Oakar and Claude Pepper, titled the Prevention, Identification, and Treatment of Elder Abuse Act of 1981 (HR 7551). With only minor modifications, its definitions of abuse, neglect, and exploitation were eventually incorporated into the United States Code, under Title 42, Chapter 35, Subchapter I. Later the National Center on Elder Abuse defined seven elder abuse forms based upon its 1995 analysis of existing federal and state statutes (Anonymous, 2002). Nonetheless, individual state definitions and forms vary widely. Current federal legislation before the U.S. Senate, the Elder Justice Act of 2006 (S 2010), would support comprehensive description and comparative analysis of state elder abuse laws toward greater uniformity for improved understanding and practice regarding the problem (Box 25-1).

Historical and Cultural Dimensions

Elder abuse is not a new phenomenon. There is evidence of its existence centuries ago. More recent is recognition of elder abuse as a health and social problem. In the United States this first surfaced in the 1950s, but it was not until the 1980s that elder abuse "came of age" as a

Box 25-1   Elder Abuse Definitions and Forms

RESEARCH

Johnson (1986)

- Stage 1: A state of self- or other-inflicted suffering unnecessary to the maintenance of the quality of life of the older person.
- Stage 2: Identified as one or more behavioral manifestations categorized as physical, psychological, sociological, or legal circumstances.
- Stage 3: Measured by determining the intensity and density of the behavioral manifestations.
- Stage 4: Treated on the basis of whether the cause is the result of passive neglect, active neglect, passive abuse, or active abuse (p. 180).

Hudson (1991)

- Level I: Violence involving elder adults
  - Self-mistreatment
  - Elder mistreatment
  - Crime by stranger
- Level II: Relationship between victim and perpetrator
  - By person in personal/social relationship
  - By person in professional/business relationship
- Level III: How the destructive behavior is carried out
  - Neglect
  - Abuse
- Level IV: Purpose motivating the destructive behavior
  - Intentional
  - Unintentional
- Level V: The specific type of destructive behavior
  - Physical
  - Psychological
  - Social
  - Financial

Note: Levels move from general to specific. Everything from Level II through Level V relates to elder mistreatment. Elder mistreatment is defined as destructive behavior that is directed toward an older adult, occurs within the context of a relationship connoting trust and is of sufficient intensity or frequency to produce harmful physical, psychological, social, or financial effects of unnecessary suffering, injury, pain, loss, or violation of human rights and power quality of life for the older adult (p. 14).

NATIONAL RESEARCH COUNCIL (2003)

Mistreatment is defined as intentional actions that cause harm or create a serious risk of harm, whether or not intended, to a vulnerable elder by a caregiver or other person who stands in a trust relationship to the elder, or failure by a caregiver to satisfy the elder's basic needs or to protect the elder from harm.

- Caregiver. A person who bears or has assumed responsibility for providing care or living assistance to an adult in need of such care or assistance.
- Harm. Injuries or unmet basic needs attributable to acts or omissions by others.
- Trust relationship. A caregiving relationship or other familial, social, or professional relationship where a person bears or has assumed responsibility for protecting the interests of the older person or where expectations of care or protection arise by law or social convention.
- Vulnerability. Financial, physical, or emotional dependence on others or impaired capacity for self-care or self-protection (p. 39).

PUBLIC POLICY

42 United States Code 35, Subchapter I, §3002

- Abuse is the willful (a) infliction of injury, unreasonable confinement, intimidation, or cruel punishment with resulting physical harm, pain, or mental anguish; or (b) deprivation by a person, including a caregiver of goods or services that are necessary to avoid physical harm, mental anguish, or mental illness (13).
- Neglect is (a) the failure to provide for oneself the goods or services that are necessary to avoid physical harm, mental anguish, or mental illness; or (b) the failure of a caregiver to provide the goods or services (37).
- Exploitation is the illegal or improper act or process of an individual, including a caregiver, using the resources of an older individual for monetary or personal benefit, profit, or gain (26).

National Center on Elder Abuse (2006)

- Physical abuse: Use of physical force that may result in bodily injury, physical pain, or impairment.
- Sexual abuse: Non-consensual sexual contact of any kind with an elderly person.
- Emotional abuse: Infliction of anguish, pain, or distress through verbal or nonverbal acts.
- Financial/material exploitation: Illegal or improper use of an elder's funds, property, or assets.
- Neglect: Refusal, or failure to fulfill any part of a person's obligations or duties to an elderly person
- Abandonment: Desertion on an elderly person by an individual who has physical custody of the elder or by a person who has assumed responsibility for providing care to the elder.
- Self-Neglect: Behaviors of an elderly person that threaten the elder's health or safety.

major concern of older Americans. However, elder abuse is not confined to a single locale. Rather, it is a global problem, found in both developed and developing countries.

Colonial America

There are numerous accounts during colonial America where family conflict had negative consequence for older members (Fischer, 1978; Stearns, 1986). For example, adult children sometimes scorned their parents for controlling family property. Dependent elders might be cast out when families lacked the money or will to provide care. Older women were the usual targets in witch hunts and occasionally put to death when they were seen as burdening family resources or threatening access to property desired by younger kin.

Elder abuse roused little public interest during early America, partly because age was generally exalted. In addition, relatively few people even reached old age, and family matters usually remained family, not community, concerns. In fact, it was not until the mid-twentieth century that elder abuse engendered public attention.

Early Awareness

The 1950s represented a time of contradictions for older Americans. On the one hand, their numbers increased as penicillin and other drugs meant survival from infectious disease. Public benefit expansion enabled more older people to live on their own. The deinstitutionalization movement emptied mental hospitals and other such settings of older residents, who might better manage in the community. On the other hand, over one-third of older Americans were impoverished (Federal Interagency Forum on Aging-Related Statistics, 2004). Job opportunities were limited due to ageism in the workplace (Achenbaum, 1978). Postwar prosperity found younger families highly mobile, searching for better jobs and lifestyles. This often meant leaving older kin behind. Elders who were frail or impaired, especially those with mental disabilities, and living alone became of particular concern in urban communities. It was feared that they might be subjected to neglect or exploitation without nearby family who could offer assistance and oversight (American Public Welfare Association, 1962: O'Neill, 1965).

Cities like Chicago, Houston, San Diego, and Cleveland sought to remedy this emerging problem through the creation of protective services.

According to Cleveland community planner Mildred Barry (1963, p. 4), speaking at the Arden House Seminar on Protective Services for Older People in Harrison, New York, this type of intervention focused on persons characterized by "aberrant behavior...which manifested itself in ways detrimental to health and safety of self and others ... [and a] combination of problems which seemed to call for different types of professional help..."

What began as individual community initiatives expanded in the 1960s and early 1970s into national dialogues and demonstration projects aimed at delineating the elements of protective services, determining its clientele, and assessing its outcomes (Blenkner, Bloom, Nielson, & Weber, 1974; Horowitz & Estes, 1971; U.S. Senate Special Committee on Aging, 1977). Despite disappointing program evaluation results, adult protective services spread nationwide during the 1970s through professional embrace and available funding. The funding came from the 1974 enactment of Title XX of the Social Security Act. Under it, adult protective services was identified as a universal service, making the protection of adults "found in circumstances and situations which are considered to be harmful or dangerous" (Burr, 1982, p. 2) a government agency concern, which it has remained ever since.

Growing Interest

Public awareness about the broad spectrum of elder abuse forms took root by the late 1970s. It started with scholarly publications by American and British physicians focused on physical abuse and self-neglect or self-abuse. The former was variously labeled "battered old person syndrome" (Butler, 1975) and "granny battering" (Baker, 1975; Burston, 1975). The latter was termed a "Diogenes syndrome" (Clark, Mankikar, & Gray, 1975) or described as "self-injurious behavior" (Kastenbaum & Mishara, 1971). Awareness expanded with four pioneering studies on elder abuse forms and victim/perpetration characteristics. They were conducted in Ohio (Lau & Kosberg, 1979), Maryland (Block & Sinnott, 1979), Massachusetts (O'Malley, Segars, Perez, Mitchell, & Knuepfel, 1979), and Michigan (Douglass, Hickey, & Noel, 1980). The investigators were typically social scientists or practitioners. In contrast, the earliest Congressional testimony on elder abuse came from a family violence expert. Suzanne Steinmetz (1978) was invited to speak before the U.S. House Science and Technology Committee on overlooked aspects of this problem. Along with battered husbands and sibling abuse, she discussed battered parents.

Call to Action
The above publications, studies, and testimony set the stage for public and professional action regarding elder abuse in the following decade. They also provided the impetus for an elder abuse agenda in health care, adult protective services, and domestic violence programming, all **service systems** with strong interest in the problem today. During the 1980s, activity to understand and address elder abuse traversed multiple formats. The end result was that by the early 1990s, elder abuse was regarded as a major social problem confronting older Americans, an important aspect of family violence, a public health concern, and a crime deserving of law enforcement attention. Evidence of all this is found in the following illustrative events:

- Older Americans Act reauthorization with new provisions for elder abuse prevention and service coordination
- Family Violence Prevention and Services Act amendment identifying older people as a potential targeted group for funding
- Adult protective services or elder abuse **reporting** law passage by the majority of states
- Declaration by U.S. Surgeon General Louis Sullivan that elder abuse is public health and criminal justice issue at a workshop on family violence
- Publication of the *Journal of Elder Abuse & Neglect* by Haworth Press, the first scholarly journal exclusively focused on the topic
- Establishment of the Clearinghouse on Abuse and Neglect of the Elderly (CANE) at the University of Delaware, currently holding the nation's largest collection of elder abuse publications and providing individually designed annotated bibliographies and literature searches
- Formation of the National Committee for the Prevention of Elder Abuse, the only national multidisciplinary professional association focused on elder abuse research, education, and public policy advocacy
- Creation of numerous local elder abuse networks, including the Ohio Coalition for Adult Protective Services and Cleveland's Consortium Against Adult Abuse, considered to be the oldest state and community elder abuse networks in the country

Recent Trends
During the last 15 years, the field of elder abuse has witnessed better research, broader focus, and heightened cultural perspective. Early research on elder abuse often was criticized for its weak theory, poor design and measures, and lack of control groups (National Research Council, 2003; Stein, 1991; University of New Hampshire, 1986). Although problems remain, the field has benefited from the demand for improved study methods, expanded funding opportunities, and entry of skilled new investigators. The demand was articulated through a series of forums to enhance research on elder abuse and establish national research agendas that would respond to the needs of policy makers and practitioners. These forums were sponsored by the University of New Hampshire in 1986, National Aging Resource Center on Elder Abuse in 1990, National Institute of Aging in 1991, and National Research Council in 1994–1997 and 2002. The first major funding initiatives geared exclusively to elder abuse research occurred in 2005 through the National Institute on Justice and National Institute on Aging. They served to heighten interest in the subject among many investigators new to the field and to provide support for inquiry into aspects of elder abuse not studied or only inadequately studied in the past.

Elder abuse research has assumed broader focus in recent years, examining such topics as sexual assault, battered older women, and mistreatment in residential care settings (e.g., Burgess, Dowdell, & Prentky, 2000; Fisher & Regan, 2006; Jogerst, Daly, & Hartz, 2005; Mouton et al., 2004; Teaster & Roberto, 2004). In addition, a growing number of investigators have explored variation in recognition, meaning, and response to elder abuse among cultural groups in the United States (Box 25-2). Finally, elder abuse in an international context has captured the attention of researchers and practitioners alike, spurred on by importance given the problem at the Second World Assembly on Aging (United Nations Economic and Social Council, 2002) and activities initiated by the International Network for the Prevention of Elder Abuse. These latter activities include a world environmental scan of elder abuse awareness and interventions as well as declaration of

Box 25-2 **Select Research on Elder Abuse Among Minority Older Americans**

MULTIPLE GROUPS

• African Americans or Caucasian Americans were less likely than Korean American older women to view a situation as abusive and to seek help for it, usually because of a reluctance to reveal "family shame" to others and a fear of creating conflict among family members (Moon & Williams, 1993).

• A study of four ethnic groups found that European American, African American, Puerto Rican, and Japanese American elders were similar in terms of the importance that they placed on psychological abuse and psychological neglect as the "worst things" that family members could do to older persons (Anetzberger, Korbin, & Tomita, 1996).

• Studies of within-group differences among two Native American and five Caucasian American groups in North Carolina found contrasts with regard to the boundaries of what constitutes elder abuse (Hudson, Armachain, Beasley, & Carlson, 1998; Hudson et al., 2000).

AFRICAN AMERICANS

• Domestic violence is high among African American families, and has been found to continue as partners age (Griffin, Williams, & Reed, 1998).

• In a study of reported elder abuse cases in Wisconsin, African American victims were more likely than other ethnic groups to be younger, experience a life-threatening form of maltreatment, and use protective services offered (Longes, 1992).

• Younger African American respondents were more likely than older ones to regard verbal abuse as a mild form of elder mistreatment. Both groups considered physical abuse an extreme form (Tauriac & Scruggs, 2006).

ASIAN AMERICANS

• A sample of 100 Korean American elders identified 46 known elder abuse cases, with financial abuse and psychological abuse comprising over half. Physical abuse and sexual abuse were rarely mentioned, perhaps in part because of the shame and stigma attached to them (Chang & Moon, 1997).

• Japanese American elders regard silence and avoidance as extreme forms of punishment and as emotionally devastating as physical abuse (Tomita, 1994).

• A study of Vietnamese American elderly women found emotional and verbal abuse fairly common and physical abuse nonexistent, with the incidence of mistreatment increasing when older people became frail and could no longer baby sit for grandchildren or provide other assistance in the households that they shared with adult children (Le, 1997).

LATINOS

• Strong family ties and respect for elders in Hispanic culture are thought to minimize the incidence of elder abuse and may reduce the reporting of the problem as well (Montoya, 1997).

• A study of Mexican Americans in Detroit, Michigan, and Carson City, Nevada found that both groups were most likely to talk to family members if an elderly neighbor was being abused by her or his family, but those in Detroit were more willing to contact authorities about the situation than those in Carson City (Sanchez, 1999).

• A Puerto Rican study of domestic violence in later life revealed that nearly all elderly women respondents condemned violence in a marriage. However, one-third of the respondents also believed that men could be violent when women were unfaithful and half argued that women should preserve the child's father no matter what (Baba, Colon, & Cruz, 1996).

NATIVE AMERICANS

• In two studies of elder abuse among Navajos, defining exploitation represented a form of cultural conflict, with older people feeling that they should share their incomes with other family members as a matter of responsibility and service providers considering it financial abuse (Brown, Fernandez, & Griffith, 1990).

• Investigation of two geographically distinct Plains Indian reservations discovered that elder abuse was more common in the reservation with the higher unemployment and substance abuse rates and little potential income from the land (Krassen Maxwell & Maxwell, 1992).

• A retrospective medical record review of 550 Indians and Alaskan Natives age 50 and over served by the Seattle Indian Health Board revealed that 10% definitely or probably had been physically abused (Buchwald et al., 2000).

the first World Elder Abuse Awareness Day, held on June 15, 2006.

Elder abuse has been documented in many countries (Kosberg & Garcia, 1995; Malley-Morrison, Nolido, & Chawla, 2006; Ockleford et al., 2003). Frequency rates vary, depending on problem definition and methods, but include 15% for Greece (Pitsiou-Darrough & Spinellis, 1995), 5% to 8% for Holland (Comijs, Penninx, Knipscheer, & VanTilberg, 1999), 8% for Denmark and Sweden (Tornstam, 1989), and 0.6% for Western Australia (Boldy et al., 2005). Elder abuse also is thought to be on the rise globally, largely due to such variables as modernization, economic difficulties, elder dependency, and societal violence.

Understanding Elder Abuse

Prevalence and Incidence

Unlike other aspects of family violence, there has never been a national **prevalence** study on elder abuse conducted in the United States. There-fore, our knowledge regarding the scope of the problem is based upon local, often limited, studies along with estimates using international sources. Collectively, the American investigations suggest a prevalence rate of 1% to 10% (Block & Sinnott, 1979; Gioglio & Blakemore, 1983: Lau & Kosberg, 1979; McLaughlin, Nickell, & Gill, 1980; Pillemer & Finkelhor, 1988). Applying these figures to the current population age 65 and older indicates a range of 360,000 to 3.6 million older American elder abuse victims. Other esti-mates have been suggested by Congress. In 1990 the U.S. House Select Committee on Aging (1990) offered a 1 to 2 million range. A decade later, when introducing the Elder Justice Act, Senator John Breaux stated that between 500,000 and 5 million older Americans were abused annually (Anonymous, 2002).

The best-regarded American prevalence study was undertaken in the metropolitan Boston area using telephone interview methods. Pillemer and Finkelhor (1988) surveyed a random sample of 2020 elderly households with inquiries about three elder abuse forms. The results revealed an overall prevalence rate of 3.2%, with 2.2% of the sample experiencing physical abuse, 1.1% verbal aggression, and 0.4% neglect. Often comparable research in Canada, Great Britain, Finland, and the Netherlands suggests prevalence rates of 4% to 6%, with financial abuse and verbal aggression the most common elder abuse forms (Comjis, Pot, Smit, Bouter, & Jonker, 1998; Kivela, Kongas-Saviaro, Kesti, Pahkala, & Ijas, 1992; Ogg & Bennett, 1992; Podnieks, 1992).

The National Center on Elder Abuse (1998) in collaboration with Westat, Inc., conducted a national elder abuse **incidence** study to uncover the number of new domestic cases occurring in 1996. Gathering data from adult protective service agencies and sentinels (i.e., specially trained personnel in community agencies serving the elderly) in a representative sample of 20 counties in 15 states, researchers estimated the incidence rate that year at 551,011. Self-neglect was the most common form, followed in order by neglect, psychological abuse, exploitation, and physical abuse.

Reporting

The national elder abuse incidence study found that only 21% of the cases were reported to and later substantiated by adult protective services. Adult protective services is the lead agency for receiving and investigating reports of domestic, and sometimes institutional, elder abuse nation-wide. A one in six reporting rate was estimated 15 years earlier in a landmark Congressional report, *Elder Abuse (An Examination of the Hidden Problem)* (U.S. House Select Commit-tee on Aging, 1981) and reduced to one in eight in the follow-up report a decade later (U.S. House Select Committee on Aging, 1990). Pillemer and Finklehor's (1988) prevalence data suggest an even lower rate; just 1 in 14 situa-tions ever get reported to authorities.

All American states and territories have enacted laws authorizing adult protective services in elder abuse situations (American Bar Associa-tion Commission on Law and Aging, 2005). With rare exception, these laws require reporting of the problem minimally by select categories of health and social service professionals (Tatara, 1995). Those professionals most likely to be identified as mandatory reporters include physicians, nurses, mental health practitioners, and social workers (Moskowitz, 1998). Originally, mandatory report-ing was regarded as important for case finding and referral (Regan, 1990; Zborowsky, 1985). There is evidence, however, that it may be less effective than professional training and public awareness

(Fredriksen, 1989; U.S. General Accounting Office, 1991; Wolf, Godkin, & Pillemer, 1986; Wolf & Li, 1999). In addition, mandatory reporting is highly controversial, with critics claiming that it is ageist, can inappropriately label people as perpetrators, and is irresponsible without adequate funding for adult protective services (Callahan, 1988; Capezuti, Brush, & Lawson, 1997; Faulkner, 1982; Macolini, 1995).

Low elder abuse reporting rates offer confirmation that mandatory reporting laws alone do not guarantee professional referral of the problem. The literature cites numerous reasons for this (Anetzberger, 1993; Balaswamy, 1993; Coyne, Petenza, & Berbig, 1996; Daniels, Baumhover, & Clark-Daniels, 1989; Fulmer & O'Malley, 1987; Gilbert, 1986; Meagher, 1993; Thobaben, 1989):

- Lack of confidence in the referral agency
- Professional confidentiality
- Fear of eroding rapport established with clients
- Lack of awareness about reporting requirements or processes
- Fear of litigation
- Belief in the sanctity of families
- Fear of reprisal by the victim or perpetrator
- Inadequate evidence that elder abuse occurred
- Belief that reporting violates the elder's rights of autonomy and self-determination
- Desire to avoid possible court involvement
- Belief that reporting will not make any positive difference
- Concern about possible reprisal against the victim
- Belief that the situation will be reported by someone else

Still, the number of elder abuse reports has grown. It increased 150% in the decade 1986–1996, from 117,000 to 293,000 (Tatara, 1996; Tatara & Kuzmeskus, 1997). More recent compilations indicate that adult protective services nationwide received almost 566,000 reports of elder and vulnerable adult abuse in 2004, up 20% from 2000 (Teaster, Dugar, Mendiondo, & Otto, 2005; Teaster, 2003). In 2004 the most commonly reported elder abuse form was self-neglect (29%), followed by caregiver neglect (26%), financial exploitation (19%), psychological abuse (12%), and physical abuse (12%). Sexual abuse represented less than 1% of all reports. Among states providing data on race, the vast majority of victims age 60 and over were Caucasians (77%) followed by African Americans (21%). American Indians, Alaskan Natives, Asians, Native Hawaiians, and Pacific Islanders each represented less than 1% of all reports.

Theoretical Underpinnings

A variety of theories have been suggested to explain elder abuse. The first proposals may have been offered by Jordan Kosberg (1979) at the 32nd Annual Scientific Meeting of the Gerontological Society of America. Among the theories that he identified as potentially relevant to elder abuse were

- Psychopathology: Elder abuse is perpetrated by those who exhibit abnormal or deviant behavior, such as mental illness or substance abuse.
- Life crisis: Elder abuse occurs when perpetrators experience an excessive number or magnitude of life-changing events, which result in exhaustion, inability to adjust, or loss of control.
- Intergenerational conflict: Abuse results from conflict between elderly relatives and their family members over scarce resources.

A few years later, Phillips (1986) suggested that the three most popular theories to explain elder abuse were

- Situational: As stress increases for perpetrators, so does the likelihood of abuse directed at vulnerable elders seen to be associated with the stress.
- Social exchange: Abused elders are more powerless, dependent, and vulnerable than their perpetrators; consequently, they have fewer options to maintaining interaction than do the perpetrators.
- Symbolic interaction: Elder abuse occurs in social interactions between victims and perpetrators where there exist discrepancies between behaviors and role expectations.

Phillips also identified the strengths and limitations of each theory, often using her own research for support, before concluding that we simply do not have sufficient knowledge to explain elder abuse or predict its occurrence. That was over 20 years ago. Not much has changed. Certainly more theories have been proposed. Like the earlier ones, they often are borrowed from other aspects of family violence. For instance, in addition to situational theory, child abuse offered role theory and functionalism.

In all of these, elder abuse is thought to stem from inadequate caregiving. In addition to social exchange theory, partner abuse provided conflict theory and feminist theory. In these, elder abuse is believed to be the result of inequities in power and control.

Although no theory has been rigorously tested, some have received support from empirical study. These include psychopathology (Anetzberger, Korbin, & Austin, 1994; Greenberg, McKibben, & Raymond, 1990; Paveza et al., 1992; Pillemer & Finlehor, 1989; Reay & Browne, 2001; Wolf, Godkin, & Pillemer, 1984), situational (Lachs, Berkman, Fulmer, & Horwitz, 1994; Phillips, 1983; Wolf, Godkin, & Pillemer, 1984), and symbolic interaction (Steinmetz, 1988). However, none of the theories borrowed from child abuse and partner abuse considers the impact of the aging process. None alone seems sufficient for explaining elder abuse across all variation of forms, settings, and perpetrators.

There have been efforts to combine or collapse theories in order to produce an overarching perspective on elder abuse as a problem. For example, Ansello's (1996) environmental press model incorporates situational, vulnerability, and social exchange theories. Using housing the elderly as a launching pad, Carp (2000) proposes an ecological model that recognizes both victim and perpetrator needs in the context of available resources. Last, the National Research Council's (2003) transactional model links the social embeddedness and individual-level factors of victim and perpetrator within a sociocultural context that considers status inequity, relationship type, and power and exchange dynamics. Like their simpler predecessors, these theoretical models have not been subjected to rigorous testing.

Examples, Signs, and Risk Factors

Three concepts are key to decision making in identifying, referring, and treating elder abuse situations. Each concept is unique in the degree it evidences elder abuse and the level of attention that should be directed at the problem. "Examples" are illustrations of elder abuse. They have been observed or reported by reputable sources. Among the three concepts, examples provide the highest evidence that elder abuse exists and requires attention. Examples of elder abuse include watching an adult son slap and demean

his elderly mother as well as listening to a bedbound elderly husband report that his wife refuses to give him more than two glasses of water daily as punishment for his incontinence.

"Signs" are the consequences of elder abuse examples. They offer less assurance that the problem has occurred and intervention is needed. This is because signs can be caused by phenomena other than elder abuse. However, the existence of signs should raise suspicion of elder abuse, and suspicion is a sufficient standard for reporting the problem under most state laws. Signs of elder abuse include bruises, depression, and dehydration, following our previous examples. More exploration is required to know for certain, because bruises can happen from a fall, depression from personal loss, and dehydration from acute illness.

Finally, "risk factors" indicate the possibility of elder abuse. They represent characteristics of victims, perpetrators, or environments found through research to be associated with the problem. Risk factors are commonly accepted conditions that are linked with theory presumed to explain elder abuse. Nonetheless, like signs, they can be associated with phenomena other than elder abuse. Elder abuse risk factors include alcoholism or caregiver stress on the part of the perpetrator, which may be risk factors for depression as well.

The literature on elder abuse frequently fails to differentiate examples, signs, and risk factors for elder abuse. This is a problem for both research and practice. In empirical study, failure to differentiate can compromise attempts to unravel problem causation. Risk factors are important in this regard, but signs are not. In practice, failure to differentiate can lead to confusion over whether or not to report the problem. Most state reporting laws require referral of any known or suspected instances of elder abuse. This means reporting upon awareness of examples or signs, but not risk factors.

Screening or Assessment Instruments for Elder Abuse Detection

Detecting elder abuse examples, signs, and risk factors is enhanced through the use of **screening or assessment instruments.** Such tools are important for

1. Assuming that clues to case identification are not missed

2. Organizing information collected about abuse victims and their circumstances
3. Systematically documenting data for court proceedings or research purposes

There are many elder abuse screening or assessment instruments. Some are specialized, geared to particular professional disciplines, clinical settings, or abuse forms. Others have general application for practitioners in contact with either community-dwelling older adults or those in institutional settings. Formats for the tools also vary, from checklists to narrative guidelines. Finally, some screening or assessment instruments are relatively simple, examining only a few areas of detection. Others are complex, considering many areas and layering inquiry. However, no elder abuse screening or assessment instrument has universal acceptance, and few have been tested for reliability and validity. In addition, some clinical settings elect to employ multiple detection phases, with a different instrument used for each phase, in recognition of the demands placed on practitioner time and potential negative consequence of mistakes in case detection. In these instances, a prescreen typically is used to detect situations of potential elder abuse within large vulnerable populations, followed by a screen to narrow detection to situations of probable abuse that warrant investigation.

Brief descriptions of select elder abuse screening or assessment instruments are given in Table 25-1. A set of three screening tools is provided in Figures 25-1, 25-2, and 25-3. It is unique among available instruments in clearly differentiating examples, signs, and risk factors for elder abuse. The tool set was developed and tested by staff at the Benjamin Rose Institute in Cleveland. The process was collaborative, involving national and local adult protective service and domestic violence experts as well as Ohio service providers from diverse systems, including law enforcement, health care, and aging networks. Each specific tool provides a list of the more common examples, signs, or risk factors for elder abuse emerging from the research literature and clinical experience. However, all possibilities are not given.

The tool set was created at the request of and with funding from Ohio public officials in order to improve the detection and referral of elder abuse cases in the state. After local distribution, the tools were incorporated into the state training curriculum for adult protective services. The tools also were broadly disseminated through a special issue of the *Journal of Elder Abuse & Neglect* (Anetzberger, 2001a, 2001b; Bass, Anetzberger, Ejaz, & Nagpaul, 2001) and represent "one of only a few instruments that state agencies use that its developers have studied" (Fulmer, Guadagno, Dyer, & Connolly, 2004, p. 300).

Signs

The signs of elder abuse can be physical, behavioral, psychological, or social in nature (Anetzberger, 1997). Physical signs range from injuries to death. Those most commonly seen in hospital emergency departments are bruises, lacerations, head trauma, and fractures (Jones, 1990). Research suggests that elder abuse victims die two to three times sooner than nonvictims (Lachs, Williams, O'Brien, Pillemer, & Charlson, 1998). Behavioral signs include anger, helplessness, and suicidal actions. Osgood and Manetta (2000–2001), for example, found that older women with a history of psychiatric hospitalization and either suicidal ideation or attempt were more likely to have been physically or sexually abused at some time. Psychological signs include fear, anxiety, and depression. Depression in particular has been found associated with elder abuse in comparison group studies of victims (Harris, 1996; Phillips, 1983; Pillemer & Prescott, 1989). Finally, social signs include limited contacts and withdrawal. Pillemer (1986) found that elder abuse victims were more likely than nonvictims to have fewer social contacts. In a study of older women in long-term abusive relationships, Zink, Regan, Jacobson, and Pabst (2003) found that victims' shame and embarrassment caused them to withdraw and develop internal barriers to seeking help.

Risk Factors

Risk factors have greater power for predicting elder abuse when found in combination or complex interaction. In addition, those risk factors that are characteristic of the perpetrator tend to be more predictive of abuse occurrence than those that are characteristic of either the victim or environment (Lachs & Pillemer, 1995; Reis & Nahmiash, 1998). Although many risk factors have been proposed, only a handful have been validated by substantial evidence (National Research Council, 2003).

TABLE 25-1 Description of Select Elder Abuse Screening or Assessment Instruments

Instrument	Reference	Description
Conflict Tactics Scale	Straus, 1979	The original 19-item self-report focuses on examples of physical and psychological abuse. It is not specific to elder abuse but has been used in research studies and clinical settings to determine whether or not individuals have been subjected to domestic assault or threat.
H.A.L.F.	Ferguson & Beck, 1983	The 37-item tool assesses various elder abuse forms in the context of family dynamics, across the broad domains of health, attitudes toward aging, living arrangements, and finances. Using a Likert-type scale, clinicians indicate the frequency of occurrence for specific elder abuse examples, signs, or risk factors.
Hwalek-Sengstock Elder Abuse Screening Test Revised	Hwalek & Sengstock, 1986	The 15-item screen explores likely or possible physical, psychological, or financial abuse using broad assessment categories. It is used with the community-dwelling older adult as respondent.
Indicators of Abuse Screen	Reis & Nahmiash, 1998	The 28-item instrument screens for physical abuse, psychological abuse, and neglect by assessing both the caregiver and older adult in the home. It has application for case identification by practitioners in health and social service agencies.
Elder Assessment Instrument Revised	Fulmer, Paveza, Abraham, & Fairchild, 2000	The 35 items cover most elder abuse forms and reflect established theory and reporting law. The instrument uses the caregiver as respondent to identify persons most at risk of abuse.
Occupational Therapy Elder Abuse Checklist	Lafata & Helfrich, 2001	The checklist has two comparable versions: elders who live alone, and those who live with others. Questions address several domains: health issues, caregiver attitudes, financial issues, support systems for caregiver and client, and safety issues. The intent is to complete a thorough evaluation and uncover possible elder abuse.

continued on page 620

TABLE 25-1 **Description of Select Elder Abuse Screening or Assessment Instruments** (continued)

Instrument	Reference	Description
Nursing Home Abuse Prevention Checklist	National Association of State Units on Aging, 2005	This is a lengthy checklist that considers three board categories of risk factors for elder abuse in nursing homes: facility, resident, and relationship. The tool can apply to specific nursing home or most of those in a state or region. A Likert-type scale is used to rate degree of risk.

The most important risk factors for victims are reduced functional capacity and problem behaviors (Anetzberger, 1987; Comijs, Pot, Smit, & Jonker, 1998; Lachs, Williams, O'Brien, Hurst, & Horwitz, 1997; Wolf & Pillemer, 1989). Reduced functional capacity can render victims dependent on abusers, unable to leave abusive situations, or unaware that help is needed. Problem behaviors on the part of victims may include being aggressive, demanding, or complaining. They can spark anger and resentment in perpetrators, which may ignite abusive actions. A considerable body of research links dementia and elder abuse (Compton, Flanagan, & Gregg, 1997; Cooney & Mortimer, 1995; Dyer, Pavlik, Murphy, & Hyman, 2000; Homer, & Gilleard, 1990; Steinmetz, 1988). Dementia also may result in both reduced functional capacity and problem behaviors. As a consequence, it should not be surprising that various studies suggest that family members who provide care for persons with dementia are up to three times more likely to physically abuse the care recipient as those who care for relatives without dementia (Coyne, Reichman, & Berbig, 1993; Paveza et al., 1992; Pillemer & Suitor, 1992).

Among various proposed perpetrator risk factors, pathology and dependency receive the most support from empirical investigation. Pathology includes alcoholism, mental illness, and emotional distress. Research suggests that more than nonabusers, abusers tend to be self- or other-identified as having an alcohol problem and to drink regularly (Anetzberger, Korbin, & Austin, 1994; Bristowe & Collins, 1989; Greenberg, McKibben, & Raymond,

1990; Homer & Gilleard, 1990). In addition, perpetrators are more likely to have a diagnosed mental illness and to have spent time in a psychiatric hospital (Anetzberger, 1987; Paveza et al., 1992; Pillemer & Finkelhor, 1989; Reis & Nahmiash, 1998; Wolf & Pillemer, 1989). Perpetrator dependence on the victim usually takes the form of finances or housing (Anetzberger, 1987; Greenberg, McKibben, & Raymond, 1990; Pillemer & Finkelhor, 1989; Wolf & Pillemer, 1989). It may result from unemployment or underemployment, mental disorders, greed, or selfishness.

Other risk factors suggested for the perpetrator have less substantiation through research. However, some have been traditionally popular explanations for elder abuse, especially caregiver stress (Douglas, Hickey, & Noel, 1980; Steinmetz, 1988; Steinmetz & Amsden, 1983). This is probably due to its universal appeal and analogy with child abuse, making the problem of elder abuse more understandable and its resolution more amenable using existing social services.

The environmental risk factors best supported by research are shared living arrangements and social isolation. Typically the victim and perpetrator reside together (Anetzberger, 1987; Wolf & Pillemer, 1989). Such close proximity can produce tension and conflict, and sometimes even violence. Elder abuse victims and perpetrators also tend to feel alone and to have low levels of social support (Compton et al., 1997; Lachs et al., 1994; Phillips, 1983; Wolf & Pillemer, 1989). The isolation may be self-imposed due to deviance or estrangement, or it may result from conditions like poor health, disability, or forced confinement.

Name of Client _____ Case Number _____

The victim or reliable party reports, or you directly observe the following acts of domestic violence, abuse, neglect, or exploitation. (This list is not exhaustive but contains some examples.) A single check indicates the perceived presence of domestic violence or elder abuse.

	(check)
Examples of Physical Abuse	
• Hit, pushed, shoved, scratched, or restrained	
• Threatened with a knife, gun, or other weapon	
• Sexually assaulted, harmed, or hurt	
• Physically harmed in some other way (specify):	
Examples of Psychological Abuse	
• Yelled at, called names, insulted	
• Threatened with physical injury	
• Locked in a room	
• Stalked or followed around	
• Psychologically abused in some other way (specify):	
Examples of Neglect by Others or Self	
• Denied adequate care and supervision (especially in cases of physically or mentally impaired persons	
• Not treated for physical health problems	
• Isolated from others	
• Inappropriately dressed for weather or environmental conditions	
• Lacking adequate shelter	
• Neglected in some other way (specify):	
Examples of Exploitation	
• Money, property, or other assets used, taken, sold, or transferred without consent	
• Signature forged on checks or other financial and legal documents	
• Large sums of money withdrawn from bank accounts (without her/his knowledge)	
• Exploited in some other way (specify):	

FIGURE 25-1 Actual Abuse Tool. (From Anetzberger, G. J., Ejaz, F. K., Bass, D. M., & Nagpaul, K. (1999). *Abuse against older Ohioans in home and community based settings: Screening tools and referral protocol for service providers for stopping abuse against older Ohioans.* Cleveland: Benjamin Rose Institute. Reproduced with the permission of The Benjamin Rose Institute.)

Addressing Elder Abuse

Problem Complexity

Elder abuse situations are complex. They usually embody multiple abuse forms experienced over a period of time. For example, it is not uncommon to find represented the combination of physical abuse, psychological abuse, and financial abuse or self-neglect and financial abuse. Elder abuse situations often concern multiple parties. In addition to the victim and perpetrator, this might include alarmed neighbors, worried family members, involved service providers, and even public officials called to deal with a perceived community nuisance or crisis.

Elder abuse situations can transcend both civil and criminal codes. Such laws typically reflect three philosophical underpinnings upon which American society operates:

• Personal freedom: Various state adult protective service and nursing home bill of rights laws underscore each individual's constitutional right to liberty and privacy. As a result, most such laws emphasize decision making

Name of Client_____ Case Number_____

The Suspected Abuse Tool **is designed to help you recognize common signs or symptoms of abuse**. It does not contain all possible signs and is not intended to replace your own judgment. It is a supplement that assists in recognizing common signs of domestic violence, abuse, neglect, or exploitation. A single check indicates suspected abuse and requires an appropriate referral for further investigation.

Please check any signs reported to you or that your directly observe for this client.	(check)
Signs of Physical Abuse	
• Bruises, welts, cuts, or wounds, cigarette or rope burn marks, or blood on person/clothes	
• Internal injuries, including broken or fractured bones, sprains, or muscle injuries	
• Painful body movements, such as limping, trouble sitting/standing (not illness related)	
• Coded or vague or indirect references to sexual assault or unwanted sexual advances	
• Other signs of physical abuse (specify):	
Signs of Psychological Abuse	
• Sense of resignation and hopelessness with vague references to mistreatment	
• Behavior that is passive, helpless, withdrawn	
• Anxious, trembling, clinging, fearful, scared of someone/something	
• Self-blame for current situation and partner/caregiver behavior	
• Other signs of psychological abuse (specify):	
Signs of Neglect by Others or Self	
• Unclean physical appearance	
• Inadequate food or meal preparation supplies in household	
• Underweight, physically frail or weak, or dehydrated	
• Underuse or overuse of, or confusion about, prescription or over-the-counter medications	
• Inadequate utilities, including lack of heat, water, electricity, or toilet facilities	
• Unsafe or unclean environment, including insect infestation or uncared-for animals	
• Neglected household finances, including unpaid bills or rent	
• Other signs of neglect (specify):	
Signs of Exploitation	
• Overpayment for goods or services	
• Unexplained changes in power of attorney, wills, or other legal documents	
• Missing checks or money, or unexplained decreases in bank accounts	
• Missing personal belongings	
• Other signs of exploitation (specify):	

FIGURE 25-2 Suspected Abuse Tool. (From Anetzberger, G. J., Ejaz, F. K., Bass, D. M., & Nagpaul, K. (1999). *Abuse against older Ohioans in home and community based settings: Screening tools and referral protocol for service providers for stopping abuse against older Ohioans.* Cleveland: Benjamin Rose Institute. Reproduced with the permission of The Benjamin Rose Institute.)

and self-determination by older adults to the extent of their functional capabilities. They also provide for the notification of older adults regarding investigations and interventions taken on their behalf.

• Parens partriae: Laws regarding protective services, guardianship or conservatorship, and hospitalization of persons with mental disorders reflect the societal responsibility to promote the health and safety of vulnerable persons. Consequently, related laws define interventions to prevent, correct, or discontinue elder abuse or delineate circumstances under which surrogate decision making or involuntary intervention may be considered to promote the welfare of incapacitated older adults.

• Police powers: Criminal laws concerned with domestic violence, rape, theft, and other

Name of Client _____   Case Number _____

The Risk of Abuse Tool identifies common risk factors associated with cases of elder abuse and/or domestic violence. The Risk of Abuse Tool indicates whether the problem is likely to occur in a possible vicitm, a possible perpetrator, or both. A question intended for a possible vicitm is shaded in the column referring to the possible perpetrator, and vice versa. A question intended for both possible victim and possible perpetrator is identified by nonshaded columns next to the corresponding screening question. Service providers are encouraged to place a check mark in the appropriate row/question if they identify a particular problem/risk factor in either one or both columns.

RISK FACTOR SCREENING QUESTIONS	Possible victim (check)	Possible perpetrator (check)
Past neglect, Abuse, or Criminal Offenses		
• Is there a history of past abuse, violence (including use of guns/weapons, or neglect)?		
• Was the person convicted of abuse or another violent crime (including violation of a court order) in the past?	■	
• Is there current violence toward family members or pets, or access to guns?	■	
Relationship Problems Between Possible Victim and Perpetrator		
• Is there evidence of current or past relationship problems (including abuse/violence)?		
• Are there relationship problems specific to issues of power, control, dominance, coercion, and manipulation?	■	
• Is there evidence of extreme jealousy and possessiveness?		
• Do parties have unrealistic expectations of each other?		
Physical, Emotional, or Mental Health-Related Problems		
• Are there problems with anger and hostility?		
• Are there problems with use of alcohol or drugs or medications?		
• Are there mental health (including depression) or emotional problems?		
• Is the person a "blamer"?		
• Are there problems in physical health or functional activities (ADLs or IADLs)?		
• Is there evidence of cognitive or memory impairment?		
• Does the possible victim lack a regular doctor?		■
• Is the possible victim emotionally dependent?		■
• Is there evidence of behavior problems?		
• Is there a lack of understanding of the medical condition?		
• Does the possible perpetrator have problems with employment or work?	■	
Caregiving and Social Support		
• Is there evidence of a lack of social support?		
• Is there evidence of social isolation?		
• Is there difficulty with or reluctance performing care-related tasks?		
• Is there stress or strain or inexperience with caregiving?	■	
• Is the possible perpetrator caring for other dependent family members?	■	
• Is financial dependency a problem?		
Environmental and Household Characteristics		
• Do the possible victim and perpetrator share a household?		
• Does the house have hazardous environmental conditions?		■

FIGURE 25-3 Risk of Abuse Tool. (From Anetzberger, G. J., Ejaz, F. K., Bass, D. M., & Nagpaul, K. (1999). *Abuse against older Ohioans in home and community based settings: Screening tools and referral protocol for service providers for stopping abuse against older Ohioans.* Cleveland: Benjamin Rose Institute. Reproduced with the permission of The Benjamin Rose Institute.)

offenses acknowledge the role of society to remove dangerous or unhealthy situations and hold accountable those who commit socially reprehensible acts.

Finally, elder abuse situations tend to be ethically charged. They call upon adult protective service workers and others involved in problem prevention or resolution to thoughtfully and carefully balance often conflicting principles, like autonomy and beneficence or accountability and nonmalfeasance. For instance, how do you best serve a self-neglecting, cognitively intact older adult who refuses help? Does one report an elder abuse situation, as required by law and professional codes of ethics, when doing so may place the physically abused elder in grave danger? Is elder abuse a private matter, or by its very nature, is it subject to public scrutiny (Anetzberger, 1999)?

Service System Roles

The complexity of elder abuse situations means that no single service system or professional discipline can, or should, have the sole responsibility for addressing the problem. Rather, the responsibility falls across multiple systems and disciplines. The most important six systems are listed in Table 25-2. They are described with respect to their general purpose and usefulness to elder abuse victims. Three systems make up the foundation of elder abuse interventions: adult protective services, law enforcement, and domestic violence programs. They provide essential integrative service for victims as well as intervention during crisis or around the time of abuse occurrence. Three other systems build upon the services provided by the foundation systems. First-level help comes from health care and legal and victim assistance. Together these systems address the consequences of elder

TABLE 25-2 Key Service Systems for Elder Abuse Intervention

System	Purpose	Usefulness to Victims
Adult protective services	Adult protective services is authorized by law to receive reports of abuse, neglect, or exploitation targeting older adults; investigate the reports and determine the need for protective services to correct or discontinue the elder abuse; provide or arrange protective services; and sometimes facilitate court-ordered involuntary intervention under emergency and select other circumstances.	Adult protective services typically sees cases of self-neglect or neglect by a caregiver. However, the system usually has the primary responsibility for case handling all reported elder abuse situations. In so doing, it will work with other agencies and systems in coordinating needed assistance.
Law enforcement	Law enforcement acts to address violations of law and represents first responders in many crisis situations. A significant amount of law enforcement is directed at domestic disputes that frequently become violent and situations of financial fraud and abuse.	Law enforcement has the authority to arrest perpetrators of domestic violence in later life, enforce restraining orders, and signal to all involved that violence is not acceptable behavior. The system also responds to other elder abuse crimes perpetrated in community and institutional settings, and may accompany adult protective services in conducting investigations or carrying out involuntary interventions in situations deemed dangerous.
Domestic violence programs	Domestic violence programs work to insure safety for victims of domestic violence and to hold perpetrators accountable for their abusive behavior. Services typically include 24-hour crisis lines, emergency shelters, legal advocacy, support groups, counseling, education, and information	Although historically domestic violence programs were designed for non-elderly women and most still serve very few older victims, the services they provide can help older victims, particularly if they are organized to be sensitive to the special needs

System	Purpose	Usefulness to Victims
	and referral. Emphasis is placed on women as victims, insuring confidentiality, and empowering victims to voluntarily seek help. They are often closely associated with rape crisis centers, which offer crisis intervention, counseling, advocacy, and accompaniment to medical and court appointments for those who experience sexual abuse.	and circumstances of this population. Minimally this means having handicap accessible facilities, providing linkage to health care, and employing staff who, or training existing staff to understand aging-related issues and resources.
Health care	Health care represents the various hospitals, clinics, practitioner offices, mental health agencies, long-term care facilities, and other organizations established to diminish illness, disability, and suffering, including providing emergency and ongoing treatment for physical injuries and mental anguish caused by elder abuse.	Health care provides essential treatment for the effects of elder abuse. It is particularly important for older people, because they frequent the health care system more than younger people, and they have greater trust and confidence in physicians and other health care workers. The injuries experienced by older victims are more likely to heal slowly and cause permanent damage, thereby requiring the assistance of health care providers for a longer time period. Furthermore, health care providers are critical to abuse detection and service referral.
Legal and victim assistance	Legal services available through legal aid societies and other sources provide victims with representation and help in matters ranging from lawsuits to overturning guardianship appointments. Victim assistance programs, located in prosecutor's offices or police departments, provide legal advocacy, counseling, court accompaniment, and information about victim compensation.	The services of an attorney may be required for older victims in divorce proceedings and to protect their right to property and retirement income or benefits. Legal options can be confusing and the justice system daunting without the guidance, reassurance, and help of victim advocates found in victim assistance programs.
Aging network	The aging network represents various programs and services targeting older adults, including congregate and home-delivered meals, transportation and escort services, personal care and housekeeping, friendly visiting and socialization, and adult day care and home maintenance or repairs. The system is organized and funded under the Older Americans Act by the U.S. Administration on Aging. It is administered through state units on aging and more than 600 area agencies on aging as well as tribal organizations.	Aging network services can help victims manage at home without an abusive caregiver. They also can provide reassurance, support, and service access for those socially isolated and at risk.

abuse and provide victims with restoration or redress. Second-level help comes from the aging network, source of that vast collection of supportive, clinical, and life-enhancing services created out of the Older Americans Act and delivered through senior centers, offices on aging, congregate meals sites, and health or social service agencies. A key component of the aging network also has characteristics of the foundation systems: the long-term care ombudsman program.

The long-term care ombudsman program operates through federal and state law to advocate for residents in nursing home, board and care, and assisted-living settings. It does this by identifying, investigating, and resolving individual and system complaints that diminish the quality of life for residents because they compromise health, safety, and personal rights (Huber, Borders, Netting, & Nelson, 2001). Ombudsman staff and volunteers routinely deal with elder abuse. In FY 1998 they received about 20,000 complaints involving abuse, gross neglect, or exploitation and 10,000 related to financial abuse or property misappropriation (Administration on Aging, 2000). During a two-year period, ombudsman also handled 1700 complaints of sexual abuse (Burgess et al., 2000). Data from the National Ombudsman Reporting System show that physical abuse and resident-to-resident abuse were reported more than other abuse forms during the period 1997–2002 (Jogerst, Daly, & Hartz, 2005).

It is important to note that each service system has its own philosophy, strategies, and services, and, therefore, its own approach to addressing elder abuse. The complexity of the problem and uniqueness of each elder abuse situation mean that the same approach, or combination of approaches, will not fit every abuse occurrence. Therefore, particular approaches need to be thoughtfully selected, reflecting clear understanding of situation dynamics and the appropriateness of the varied service systems.

Intervention Strategies

Elder abuse situations demand the achievement of four goals:

1. Medical problems must be treated, including any injuries and emotional distress caused by the abuse.
2. Methods for securing victim safety must be identified, including plans for those victims who choose to remain in the abusive setting.
3. Help must be extended to victims to enable them to regain a sense of control and mastery, lost or compromised as a result of elder abuse. Information on available community resources is a first step in accomplishing this goal.
4. The cause of elder abuse must be determined and eliminated. This requires removing the risk factors for abuse occurrence (Anetzberger, 2005).

There is little evaluative research on elder abuse service systems and programs. Therefore, we simply do not know what works and what does not work in addressing elder abuse (Fulmer & Anetzberger, 1995; National Research Council, 2003; Wilber & Nielson, 2002). There is some evidence, however, that services and programs vary by targeted recipient.

Several studies suggest that most services target victims. Very little help is offered to perpetrators, although they are more likely to accept and benefit from it. Furthermore, few services are provided to either victims or perpetrators—just one or two typically, and they customarily reflect services extended to frail older people in general. Victims tend to accept and benefit most from concrete or empowerment services. The former is illustrated by medical care, home-delivered meals, and housekeeping; the latter by support groups, legal services, and advocacy. Perpetrators tend to accept and benefit from counseling, education, and training (Nahmiash & Reis, 2000; Sengstock, Hwalek, & Petrone, 1989; Vinton, 1991, 1992).

Multidisciplinary Teams

The effective involvement of several service systems and professional disciplines in addressing elder abuse is best realized through multidisciplinary teams (M-teams). These are groups of systems or professionals assembled for the purpose of identifying elder abuse and developing recommendations to treat it (Teaster & Nerenberg, 2004). Some M-teams are formed to serve the needs of a particular organization, like a hospital, and others work on behalf of entire communities or regions, like the San Francisco Consortium for the Prevention of Elder Abuse and the Consortium Against Adult Abuse, which covers the five counties of northeast Ohio. Some M-teams have a specific focus, such as the Fiduciary Abuse Specialist Teams that originated in California (Allen, 2000; Aziz, 2000) or those that do fatality review. However, most deal with all elder abuse forms and contexts, and sometimes other geriatric issues as well, such as Denver's Community Bioethics Committee (Otto, 2000).

M-teams usually provide case analysis, program planning, education, and advocacy (Bernotavicz, 1982; Mixson et al., 1991; Teaster & Nerenberg, 2004). Most begin small and informal. Many evolve into formal associations, with select membership and structured proceedings (Nerenberg, 1991). All M-teams work to improve elder abuse interventions in three ways (Anetzberger, Dayton, Miller, McGreevey, & Schimer, 2005):

• Offering a more holistic perspective on the problem than possible with a single system or discipline
• Sharing the responsibility for case handling
• Promoting professional relationships toward a community-wide approach to elder abuse

■ Summary

Elder abuse is neither a new phenomenon nor entirely a recently recognized health and social problem. Still, the path to collective awareness and action in the United States and elsewhere has been slow and remains incomplete. Unfortunately, time is running out for better understanding elder abuse through empirical study and identifying effective strategies to prevent and treat the problem through program evaluation. The "coming of [old] age" of the baby boomers assures greater occurrence of elder abuse in the future just by the sheer size of this generation. However, there are reasons to believe that baby boomers may experience elder abuse more than past generations of older adults. This is because baby boomers possess characteristics that increase their risk of abuse occurrence. For example, they are more likely to live alone, thereby increasing the likelihood of self-neglect and financial abuse. They have had more divorces and fewer children, leaving them with less available close family to provide care or social support and increasing the potential for neglect and psychological abuse or neglect. They have greater wealth and feeling of entitlement, leading to possible resentment over what may be seen as intergenerational inequity, thereby increasing the possibility of financial abuse and violation of rights.

Simply stated, it is critical that public attention be given to elder abuse and that policy and funding be directed at problem understanding and intervention. If we wait, the adage "too little, too late" may become the epitaph for elder abuse victims as it has for so many other vulnerable groups in the past.

Case Study

The occupational therapist visits Catherine at home as a follow-up to her recent discharge from a nursing facility for rehabilitative services. Catherine lives with her husband Hank in a two-story house with the only bathroom and bedrooms on the second floor. Catherine and Hank are in their mid-70s and have been married over 50 years. Catherine suffered a stroke several weeks ago, leaving her with right-sided paralysis and mild expressive aphasia. During the visit, the therapist learns that Catherine fell the evening before, injuring and bruising her right leg and arm. No medical attention was sought. Catherine seems frail and anxious. She also is unkempt, with uncombed hair and clothes smelling of urine. Hank is vague about the fall and becomes defensive when asked questions about Catherine's care. He is adamant that she could do more for herself, if she would only try. Hank seems intoxicated and angry with Catherine. However, he states that he can manage her by himself. He does not want to bother other people with his problems.

Questions

1. Are there indications of elder abuse in this situation? If so, what examples, signs, or risk factors are evident?
2. Should the occupational therapist report the situation to authorities? If uncertain about reporting, what additional information is needed to make that decision?

Review Questions

1. Why are there no universally accepted definitions and forms of elder abuse?
2. Discuss the evolution of elder abuse recognition as a health and social problem in the United States.
3. Distinguish between elder abuse prevalence, incidence, and reporting.
4. Why do professionals fail to report elder abuse to authorities despite the widespread existence of state mandatory reporting laws?
5. What theories have been proposed for explaining elder abuse?
6. What are the differences between examples, signs, and risk factors for elder abuse?
7. What are screening or assessment instruments used for in elder abuse detection and referral?
8. What are the most important service systems for addressing elder abuse?
9. Identify the benefits of multidisciplinary teams in elder abuse identification and intervention.

Web-Based Resources

For helpful information about the experience of elder abuse, visit:

www.inpea.net, **International Network for the Prevention of Elder Abuse,** date connected October 12, 2007. Provides epidemiologic data from around the world, as well as links to policy and prevention information.

http://www.ncea.aoa.gov/ncearoot/Main_Site/index.aspx, **National Center on Elder Abuse,** date connected April 10, 2008. Posted by the U.S. Administration on Aging, this site provides epidemiologic data, strategies for evaluating individuals to identify abuse, and an array of resources to assist in intervention. Links to many other sites are provided.

www.ncall.us, **National Clearinghouse on Abuse in Later Life,** date connected October 12, 2007. Material suitable both for professionals and lay individuals that describes elder abuse, provides resources, and offers suggestions for evaluation and intervention. Available in both Hmong and Spanish as well as English.

http://preventelderabuse.org, **National Committee for the Prevention of Elder Abuse,** date connected October 12, 2007. Links are provided to resources, networking opportunities, and information about the problem and potential policies to reduce elder abuse.

REFERENCES

Achenbaum, W. A. (1978). *Old age in the new land: American experience since 1790.* Baltimore: John Hopkins University Press.

Administration on Aging. (2000). *FY 1998 Long-term care ombudsman report with comparisons of national data for FY 1996–1998.* Washington, DC: Administration of Aging.

Allen, J. V. (2000). Financial abuse of elders and dependent adults: The FAST (Financial Abuse Specialist Team) approach. *Journal of Elder Abuse & Neglect. 12*(2), 85–91.

American Bar Association Commission on Law and Aging. (2005). *Information about laws related to elder abuse.* Unpublished manuscript.

American Public Welfare Association. (1962). *Guide statement on protective services for older adults.* Chicago: American Public Welfare Association.

Anetzberger, G. J. (1987). *The etiology of elder abuse by adult offspring.* Springfield, IL: Charles C Thomas.

Anetzberger, G. J. (1993). Elder abuse programming among geriatric education centers. *Journal of Elder Abuse & Neglect, 5*(3), 69–87.

Anetzberger, G. J. (1997). Elderly adult survivors of family violence: Implications for clinical practice. *Violence Against Women, 3*(5), 499–514.

Anetzberger, G. J. (1999). Ethical issues in personal safety. In T. F. Johnson (Ed.), *Handbook on ethical issues in aging* (pp. 187–219). Westport, CT: Greenwood.

Anetzberger, G. J. (2001a). Introduction. *Journal of Elder Abuse & Neglect, 13*(2), 1–2.

Anetzberger, G. J. (2001b). Elder abuse identification and referral: The importance of screening tools and referral protocols. *Journal of Elder Abuse & Neglect, 13*(2), 3–22.

Anetzberger, G. J. (2005). Clinical management of elder abuse: General considerations. In G. J. Anetzberger (Ed.), *The clinical management of elder abuse* (pp. 27–41). Binghamton, NY: Haworth Press.

Anetzberger, G. J., Dayton, C., Miller, C. A., McGreevey, J. F., Jr., & Schimer, M. (2005). Multidisciplinary teams in the clinical management of elder abuse. In G. J. Anetzberger (Ed.), *The clinical management of elder abuse* (pp. 157–171). Binghamton, NY: Haworth Press.

Anetzberger, G. J., Korbin, J. E., & Austin, C. (1994). Alcoholism and elder abuse. *Journal of Interpersonal Violence, 9*(2), 184–193.

Anetzberger, G. J., Korbin, J. E., & Tomita, S. K. (1996). Defining elder mistreatment in four groups across two generations. *Journal of Cross-Cultural Gerontology, 11,* 187–212.

Anonymous. (2002). Protecting older Americans: A history of federal action on elder abuse, neglect, and exploitation. *Journal of Elder Abuse & Neglect, 14*(2/3), 9–85.

Ansello, E. F. (1996). Causes and theories. In L. A. Baumhover & S. C. Beall (Eds.), *Abuse, neglect, and exploitation of older persons: Strategies for assessment and intervention* (pp. 9–29). Baltimore, MD: Health Professions Press.

Aziz, S. J. (2000). Los Angeles County Fiduciary Abuse Specialist Team: A model for collaboration. *Journal of Elder Abuse & Neglect, 12*(2), 79–83.

Baba, J., Colon, M., & Cruz, C. (1996). *Domestic violence and late adulthood.* Unpublished Masters Thesis, Graduate School of Social Work, University of Puerto Rico, San Juan.

Baker, A. A. (1975). Granny-battering. *Modern Geriatrics, 5*(8), 20–24.

Balaswamy, S. (1993). *Organizational barriers to implementing the adult protective services legislation.* Cleveland, OH: Adult Protective Service Consortium and Western Reserve Area Agency on Aging.

Barry, M. C. (1963, March). *Responsibilities of the social welfare profession in providing guardianship and protective services.* Paper presented at the Seminar on Protective Services for Older People, Harriman, NY.

Bass, D. M., Anetzberger, G. J., Ejaz, F. K., & Nagpaul, K. (2001). Screening tools and referral protocol for stopping abuse against older Ohioans: A guide for service providers. *Journal of Elder Abuse & Neglect, 13*(2), 23–38.

Bernotavicz, F. (1982). *Improving protective services for older Americans: A national guide series: Community role.* Portland, ME: University of Southern Maine, Human Services Development Institute.

Blenkner, M., Bloom, M., Nielson, M., & Weber, R. (1974). *Final report: Protective services for older people, findings from the Benjamin Rose Institute study.* Cleveland, OH: The Benjamin Rose Institute.

Block, M. R., & Sinnott, J. D. (Eds.). (1979). *The battered elder syndrome: An exploratory study.* College Park, MD: University of Maryland, Center of Aging.

Boldy, D., Horner, B., Crouchley, K., Davey, M., & Boylen, S. (2005). Addressing elder abuse: Western Australian case study. *Australasian Journal on Aging, 24*(1), 3–8.

Bristowe, E., & Collins, J. B. (1989). Family mediated abuse of non-institutionalized elder men and women living in British Columbia. *Journal of Elder Abuse & Neglect, 1*(1), 45–54.

Brown, A. J., Fernandez, R., & Griffith, T. M. (1990). *Service provider perceptions of elder abuse among the*

Navaho. Flagstaff, AZ: Northern Arizona University, Social Research Laboratory.

Buchwald, D., Tomita, S., Hartman, S., Furman, R., Dudden, M., & Manson, S. M. (2000). Physical abuse of urban Native Americans. *Journal of General Internal Medicine, 15,* 562–564.

Burgess, A. W., Dowdell, E., & Prentky, R. (2000). Sexual abuse of nursing home residents. *Journal of Psychosocial Nursing, 38,* 11–18.

Burr, J. J. (1982). *Protective services for adults: A guide to exemplary practice in states providing protective services to adults in the OHDS programs.* Washington, DC: Administration on Aging, U.S. Department of Health and Human Services.

Burston, G. R. (1975). Granny-battering. *British Medical Journal, 3*(5983), 592.

Butler, R. N. (1975). *Why survive: Being old in America.* New York: Harper & Row.

Callahan, J. J., Jr. (1988). Elder abuse: Some questions for policymakers. *The Gerontologist, 28*(4), 453–458.

Capezuti, E., Brush, B. L., & Lawson, W. T. (1997). Reporting elder mistreatment. *Journal of Gerontological Nursing, 23*(7), 24–32.

Carp, F. M. (2000). *Elder abuse in the family: An interdisciplinary model for research.* New York: Springer.

Chang, J., & Moon, A. (1997). Korean American elderly's knowledge and perceptions of elder abuse: A qualitative analysis of cultural factors. *Journal of Multicultural Social Work, 6*(1/2), 139–154.

Clark, A. N. G., Mankikar, G. D., & Gray, I. (1975). Diogenes syndrome: A clinical study of gross neglect in old age. *The Lancet I, 790,* 366–368.

Comijs, H. C., Penninx, B. W. J. H., Knipscheer, K. P. M., & VanTilburg, W. (1999). Psychological distress in victims of elder mistreatment: The effects of social support and coping. *Journals of Gerontology. Series B: Psychological Sciences and Social Sciences, 54*(4), 240–245.

Comijs, H. C., Pot, A. M., Smit, J. H., Bouter, L. M., & Jonker, C. (1998). Elder abuse in the community: Prevalence and consequences. *Journal of the American Geriatrics Society, 46,* 885–888.

Compton, S. A., Flanagan, P., & Gregg, W. (1997). Elder abuse in people with dementia in Northern Ireland: Prevalence and predictors in cases referred to a psychiatry of old age service. *International Journal of Geriatric Psychiatry, 12*(6), 632–635.

Cooney, C., & Mortimer, A. (1995). Elder abuse and dementia: A pilot study. *International Journal of Social Psychiatry, 41*(4), 276–283.

Coyne, A. C., Potenza, M., & Berbig, L. J. (1996). Abuse in families coping with dementia. *Aging, 367,* 93–95.

Coyne, A. C., Reichman, W. E., & Berbig, L. J. (1993). The relationship between dementia and elder abuse. *American Journal of Psychiatry, 150*(4), 643–646.

Daniels, R. S., Baumhover, L. A., & Clark-Daniels, C. L. (1989). Physicians' mandatory reporting of elder abuse. *The Gerontologist, 29*(3), 321–327.

Douglass, R. L., Hickey, T., & Noel, C. (1980). *A study of maltreatment of the elderly and other vulnerable adults.* Ann Arbor, MI: University of Michigan, Institute of Gerontology.

Dyer, C. B., Pavlik, V. N., Murphy, K. P., & Hyman, D. J. (2000). The high prevalence of depression and dementia in elder abuse or neglect. *Journal of the American Geriatrics Society, 48,* 205–208.

Faulkner, L. R. (1982). Mandating the reporting of suspected cases of elder abuse: An inappropriate, ineffective, and ageist response to the abuse of elder adults. *Family Law Quarterly, 16,* 69–91.

Federal Interagency Forum on Aging-Related Statistics. (2004, November). *Older Americans 2004: Key indicators of well-being.* Washington, DC: U.S. Government Printing Office.

Ferguson, D., & Beck, C. (1983). H.A.L.F.—A tool to assess elder abuse within the family. *Geriatric Nursing, 4,* 301–304.

Fischer, D. H. (1978). *Growing old in America.* Oxford: Oxford University Press.

Fisher, B. S., & Regan, S. L. (2006). The extent and frequency of abuse in the lives of older women and their relationship with health outcomes. *The Gerontologist, 46* (2), 200–209.

Fredrikson, K. I. (1989). Adult protective services: Changes with the introduction of mandatory reporting. *Journal of Elder Abuse & Neglect, 1*(2), 59–70.

Fulmer, T., & Anetzberger, G. J. (1995). *Knowledge about family violence interventions in the field of elder abuse.* Unpublished paper for the Committee on the Assessment of Family Violence Interventions of the National Research Council and Institute of Medicine.

Fulmer, T., Guadagno, L., Dyer, C. B., & Connolly, M. T. (2004). Progress in elder abuse screening and assessment instruments. *Journal of the American Geriatrics Society, 52,* 297–304.

Fulmer, T., & O'Malley, T. A. (1987). *Inadequate care of the elderly: A health care perspective on abuse and neglect.* New York: Springer.

Fulmer, T., Paveza, G., Abraham, I. I., & Fairchild, S. (2000). Elder neglect assessment in the emergency department. *Journal of Emergency Nursing, 26,* 436–443.

Gilbert, D. A. (1986). The ethics of mandatory elder abuse reporting statutes. *Advances in Nursing Science, 8*(2), 51–62.

Gioglio, G. R., & Blakemore, P. (1983). *Elder abuse in New Jersey: The knowledge and experience of abuse among older New Jerseyans.* Trenton, NJ: New Jersey Department of Human Resources and New Jersey Department of Community Affairs.

Greenberg, J. R., McKibben, M., & Raymond, J. A. (1990). *Journal of Elder Abuse & Neglect, 2,* 73–86.

Griffin, L. W., Williams, O. J., & Reed, J. G. (1998). Abuse of African American elders. In R. K. Bergen (Ed.), *Issues in intimate violence* (pp. 267–284). Thousand Oaks, CA: Sage.

Harris, S. B. (1996). For better or for worse: Spouse abuse grown old. *Journal of Elder Abuse & Neglect, 8*(1), 1–33.

Homer, A. C., & Gilleard, C. (1990). Abuse of elderly people by their caregivers. *British Medical Journal, 301*(6765), 1359–1362.

Horowitz, G., & Estes, C. (1971). *Protective services for the aged.* Washington DC: U.S. Department of Health, Education, and Welfare.

Huber, R., Borders, K., Netting, F. E., & Nelson, H. W. (2001). Data from long-term ombudsman programs in six states—The implications of collecting resident characteristics. *The Gerontologist, 41,* 61–68.

Hudson, M. F. (1991). Elder mistreatment: A taxonomy with definitions by Delphi. *Journal of Elder Abuse & Neglect, 3*(2), 1–20.

Hudson, M. F., Armachain, W. D., Beasley, C. M., & Carlson, J. R. (1998). Elder abuse: Two native American views. *The Gerontologist, 38*(5), 538–548.

Hudson, M. F., Beasley, C., Benedict, R. H., Carlson, J. R., Craig, B. F., Herman, C., & Mason, S. C. (2000). Elder abuse: Some Caucasian-American views, *Journal of Elder Abuse & Neglect, 12*(1), 89–114.

Hwalek, M., & Sengstock, M. (1986). Assessing the probability of abuse of the elderly: Towards the development of a clinical screening instrument. *Journal of Applied Gerontology, 5,* 153–173.

Jogerst, G., Daly, J., & Hartz, A. (2005). Ombudsman program characteristics related to nursing home abuse reporting. *Journal of Gerontological Social Work, 46*(1), 85–98.

Johnson, T. (1986). Critical issues in the definition of elder mistreatment. In K. A. Pillemer & R. S. Wolf (Eds.), *Elder abuse: Conflict in the family* (pp. 167–196). Dover, MA: Auburn House.

Jones, J. S. (1990). Geriatric abuse and neglect. In G. Bosker, G. R. Schwartz, J. S. Jones, & M. Sequeria (Eds.), *Geriatric emergency medicine* (pp. 533–542). St. Louis, MO: C.V. Mosby.

Kastenbaum, R., & Mishara, B. (1971). Premature death and self-injurious behavior in old age. *Geriatrics, 26,* 71–81.

Kivela, S., Kongas-Saviaro, P., Kesti, E., Pahkala, K., & Ijas, M. (1992). Abuse in old age—Epidemiological data from Finland. *Journal of Elder Abuse & Neglect, 4*(3), 1–18.

Kosberg, J. I. (1979). *Family conflict and abuse of the elderly: Theoretical and methodological issues.* Paper presented at the 32nd Annual Scientific Meeting of the Gerontological Society of America, Washington, DC.

Kosberg, J. I., & Garcia, J. L. (Eds.). (1995). Elder abuse: International and cross-cultural perspectives. *Journal of Elder Abuse & Neglect, 6*(3/4), 71–89..

Krassen Maxwell, E., & Maxwell, R. J. (1992). Insults to the body civil: Mistreatment of elderly in two Plain Indian tribes. *Journal of Cross-Cultural Gerontology, 7,* 3–23.

Lachs, M. S., Berkman, L., Fulmer, T., & Horowitz, R. (1994). A prospective community-based pilot study of risk factors for the investigation of elder mistreatment. *Journal of the American Geriatrics Society, 42*(2), 169–173.

Lachs, M. S., & Pillemer, K. (1995). Abuse and neglect of elderly persons. *The New England Journal of Medicine, 332*(7), 437–443.

Lachs, M. S., Williams, C., O'Brien, S., Hurst, L., & Horwitz, R. (1997). Risk factors for reported elder abuse and neglect: A nine-year observational cohort study. *The Gerontologist, 37*(4), 469–474.

Lachs, M. S., Williams, C. S., O'Brien, S., Pillemer, K. A., & Charlson, M. E. (1998). The mortality of elder mistreatment. *Journal of the American Medical Association, 280*(5), 428–432.

Lafata, M. J., & Helfrich, C. A. (2001). The occupational therapy elder abuse checklist. *Occupational Therapy in Mental Health, 16*(3/4), 141–161.

Lau, E. E., & Kosberg, J. I. (1979). Abuse of the elderly by informal care providers. *Aging, 299–300,* 10–15.

Le, Q. K. (1997). Mistreatment of Vietnamese elderly by their families in the United States. *Journal of Elder Abuse & Neglect, 9*(2), 51–62.

Longes, J. (1992). Race and type of maltreatment in an elder abuse system. *Journal of Elder Abuse & Neglect, 4*(3), 61–83.

Macolini, R. M. (1995). Elder abuse policy: Considerations in research and legislation. *Behavioral Sciences and the Law, 13,* 349–363.

Malley-Morrison, K., Nolido, N. E. -V., & Chawla, S. (2006). International perspectives on elder abuse: Five case studies. *Educational Gerontology, 32,* 1–11.

McLaughlin, J. S., Nickell, J. P., & Gill, L. (1980). An epidemiological investigation on elderly abuse in Southern Maine and New Hampshire. In U.S. Senate Special Committee on Aging & U.S. House Select Committee on Aging, *Elder abuse: Joint hearing* (pp. 111–147). Washington, DC: U.S. Government Printing Office.

Meagher, M. S. (1993). Legal and legislative dimensions. In B. Byers & J. E. Hendricks (Eds.), *Adult protective services: Research and practice.* (pp. 87–107). Springfield, IL: Charles C Thomas.

Mixson, P., Chelucci, K., Heisler, C., Overman, W., Sripada, P., & Yates, P. (1991). The case of Mrs. M—A multidisciplinary team staffing. *Journal of Elder Abuse & Neglect, 3*(4), 41–55.

Montoya, V. (1997). Understanding and combating elder abuse in Hispanic communities. *Journal of Elder Abuse & Neglect, 9*(2), 5–17.

Moon, A., & Williams, O. (1993). Perceptions of elder abuse and help-seeking patterns among African-American, Caucasian American, and Korean-American elderly women. *The Gerontologist, 33*(3), 386–395.

Moskowitz, S. (1998). Saving granny from the wolf: Elder abuse and neglect—The legal framework. *Connecticut Law Review, 31,* 77–204.

Mouton, C. P., Rodabough, R. J., Rovi, S. L. D., Hunt J. L., Talamantes, M. A., Brzyski, R. G., et al. (2004). Prevalence and 3-year incidence of abuse among post-menopausal women. *American Journal of Public Health, 94*(4), 605–612.

Nahmiash, D., & Reis, M. (2000). Most successful intervention strategies for abused older adults. *Journal of Elder Abuse & Neglect, 12*(3/4), 53–70.

Nerenberg, L. (1991). The San Francisco Consortium Multidisciplinary Team: Another perspective. *Journal of Elder Abuse & Neglect, 3*(3), 66–71.

National Association of State Units on Aging. (2005). *Nursing home abuse risk prevention profile and checklist.* Washington, DC: National Center on Elder Abuse.

National Center on Elder Abuse. (1998, September). *The national elder abuse incidence study.* Washington, DC: Author.

National Center on Elder Abuse. (2001, December). *The National Policy Summit on Elder Abuse: National action agenda, 2002.* Washington, DC: Author.

National Center on Elder Abuse. (2006). *The basics.* Retrieved April 10, 2008, from http://www.ncea.aoa.gov/ncearoot/Main_Site/index.aspx

National Research Council. (2003). *Elder mistreatment: Abuse, neglect, and exploitation in an aging America.* Washington, DC: The National Academies Press.

Ockleford, E., Barnes-Holmes, Y., Morichelli, R., Morjaria, A., Scocchera, F., Furniss, F., et al. (2003). Mistreatment of older women in three European countries. *Violence Against Women, 9*(12), 1458–1464.

Ogg, J., & Bennett, G. C. J. (1992). Elder abuse in Britain. *British Medical Journal, 305,* 998–999.

O'Malley, H., Segars, H., Perez, R., Mitchell, V., & Knuepfel, G. M. (1979). *Elder abuse in Massachusetts: A survey of professionals and para-professionals.* Boston: Legal Research and Services for the Elderly.

O'Neill, V. (1965). Protecting older people. *Public Welfare, 23*(2), 119–127.

Osgood, N. J., & Manetta, A. A. (2000–2001). Abuse and suicidal issues in older women. *OMEGA, 42*(1), 71–81.

Otto, J. M. (2000, March/April). Bioethics committee aids APS workers in making complex medical decisions for incapacitated adults. *Victimization of the Elderly and Disabled, 2*(6), 89, 94.

Paveza, G. J., Cohen, D., Eisdorfer, C., Freels, S., Semla, T., Ashford, W., et al. (1992). Severe family violence and Alzheimer's disease: Prevalence and risk factors. *The Gerontologist, 32,* 493–497.

Phillips, L. R. (1983). Abuse and neglect of the frail elderly at home: An exploration of theoretical relationships. *Journal of Advanced Nursing, 8,* 379–392.

Phillips, L. R. (1986). Theoretical explanations of elder abuse: Competing hypotheses and unresolved issues. In K. A. Pillemer & R. S. Wolf (Eds.), *Elder abuse: Conflict in the family* (pp. 197–217). Dover, MA: Auburn House.

Pillemer, K. A. (1986). Risk factors in elder abuse: Results from a case-control study. In K. A. Pillemer & R. S. Wolf (Eds.), *Elder abuse: Conflict in the family* (pp. 239–263). Dover, MA: Auburn House.

Pillemer, K., & Finkelhor, D. (1988). The prevalence of elder abuse: A random sample survey. *The Gerontologist, 28,* 51–57.

Pillemer, K. A., & Finkelhor, D. (1989). Causes of elder abuse: Caregiver stress versus problem relatives. *American Journal of Orthopsychiatry, 59,* 179–187.

Pillemer, K., & Prescott, D. (1989). Psychological effects of elder abuse: A research note. *Journal of Elder Abuse & Neglect, 1*(1), 65–74.

Pillemer, K., & Suitor, J. J. (1992). Violence and violent feelings: What causes them among family givers? *Journal of Gerontology, 47,* S165–S172.

Pitsiou-Darrough, E. N., & Spinellis, C. D. (1995). Mistreatment of the elderly in Greece. *Journal of Elder Abuse and Neglect, 6*(3/4), 45–64.

Podnieks, E. (1992). National survey on abuse of the elderly in Canada. *Journal of Elder Abuse & Neglect, 4*(1/2), 5–58.

Reay, A. M., & Browne, K. D. (2001). Risk factors for caregivers who physically abuse or neglect their elderly parents. *Aging and Mental Health, 5*(1), 56–62.

Regan, J. J. (1990). *The aged client and the law.* New York: Columbia University Press.

Reis, M., & Nahmiash, D. (1998). Validation of the Indicators of Abuse (IOA) screen. *The Gerontologist, 38,* 471–480.

Sanchez, Y. M. (1999). Elder mistreatment in Mexican American communities: The Nevada and Michigan experiences. In T. Tatara (Ed.), *Understanding elder abuse in minority populations* (pp. 67–77). Philadelphia: Brunner/Mazel.

Sengstock, M. C., Hwalek, M., & Petrone, S. (1989). Services for aged abuse victims: Service types and related factors. *Journal of Elder Abuse & Neglect, 1*(4), 37–56.

Stearns, P. J. (1986). Old age family conflict: The perspective of the past. In K. A. Pillemer & R. S. Wolf (Eds.), *Elder abuse: Conflict in the family* (pp. 3–24). Dover, MA: Auburn House.

Stein, K. F. (1991). A national agenda for elder abuse and neglect research: Issues and recommendations. *Journal of Elder Abuse & Neglect, 3*(3), 91–108.

Steinmetz, S. K. (1978, February). *Overlooked aspects of family violence: Battered husbands, battered siblings, and battered elderly.* Testimony presented to the U.S. House Committee on Science and Technology, Washington, DC.

Steinmetz, S. K. (1988). *Duty bound: Elder abuse and family care.* Newbury Park, CA: Sage.

Steinmetz, S. K., & Amsden, D. J. (1983). Dependent elders, family stress and abuse. In T. Brubaker (Ed.), *Family relationships in later life* (pp. 173–192). Beverly Hills, CA: Sage.

Straus, M. A. (1979). Measuring intrafamily conflict and violence: The Conflict Tactics (CT) Scale—Form A. *Journal of Marriage and the Family, 41,* 75–88.

Tatara, T. (1995, May). *An analysis of state laws addressing elder abuse, neglect, and exploitation.* Washington, DC: National Center on Elder Abuse.

Tatara, T. (1996, June). *Elder abuse: Questions and answers.* Washington, DC: National Center on Elder Abuse.

Tatara, T., & Kuzmeskus, L. (1997). *Summaries of statistical data on elder abuse in domestic settings for FY 95 and FY 96.* Washington, DC: National Center on Elder Abuse.

Tauriac, J. J., & Scruggs, N. (2006). Elder abuse among African Americans. *Educational Gerontology, 32,* 37–48.

Teaster, P. B. (2003). *A response to the abuse of vulnerable adults: The 2000 survey of state adult protective services.* Washington, DC: National Center on Elder Abuse.

Teaster, P. B., & Nerenberg, L. (2004). *A national look at elder abuse multidisciplinary teams.* Washington, DC: National Committee for the Prevention of Elder Abuse.

Teaster, P. B., & Roberto, K. A. (2004). Sexual abuse of older adults: APS cases and outcomes. *The Gerontologist, 44*(6), 788–796.

Teaster, P. B., Dugar, T. A., Meniondo, M. S., & Otto, J. M. (2005, May 12). *The 2004 survey of state adult protective services: Abuse of adults 60 years of age and older.* Washington, DC: National Center on Elder Abuse.

Thobaben, M. (1989). State elder/adult abuse and protection laws. In R. Filinson & S. R. Ingman (Eds.), *Elder abuse: Practice and policy* (pp. 138–152). New York: Human Services Press.

Tomita, S. (1994). The consideration of cultural factors in the research of elder mistreatment with an in-depth look at the Japanese. *Journal of Cross-Cultural Gerontology, 9,* 39–52.

Tornstam, L. (1989). Abuse of the elderly in Denmark and Sweden: Results from a population study. *Journal of Elder Abuse & Neglect, 1,* 35–44.

United Nations Economic and Social Council. (2002, February 25–March 1). *Abuse of older persons: Recognizing and responding to abuse of older persons in a global context.* Document of the Commission for Social Development presented at the Second World Assembly on Aging, New York.

U.S. Department of Health and Human Services. (1992). *Report from the Secretary's Task Force on Elder Abuse.* Washington, DC: Author.

U.S. General Accounting Office. (1991). *Elder abuse: Effectiveness of reporting laws and other factors.* Washington, DC: Author.

U.S. House Select Committee on Aging. (1981, April 3). *Elder abuse (An examination of a hidden problem).* Comm. Pub. No. 97-277. Washington, DC: U.S. Government Printing Office.

U.S. House Select Committee on Aging. (1990). *Elder abuse: A decade of shame and inaction.* Comm. Pub. No. 101-752. Washington, DC: U.S. Government Printing Office.

U.S. Senate Special Committee on Aging. (1977). *Protective services for the elderly: A working paper.* Washington, DC: U.S. Government Printing Office.

University of New Hampshire. (1986). *Elder abuse and neglect: Recommendations from the Research Conference on Elder Abuse and Neglect.* Durham, NH: University of New Hampshire.

Vinton, L. (1991). An exploratory study of self-neglectful elderly. *Journal of Gerontological Social Work, 18*(1/2), 55–67.

Vinton, L. (1992). Services planned in abusive elder care situations. *Journal of Elder Abuse & Neglect, 4*(3), 85–99.

Watson, M. M. (1995). *Silent suffering: Elder abuse in America: Conference summary and recommendations for the 1995 White House Conference on Aging.* Unpublished manuscript.

Wilber, K. H., & Nielsen, E. K. (2002). Elder abuse: New approaches to an age-old problem. *The Public Policy and Aging Report, 12*(2), 1, 24–27.

Wolf, R. S., Godkin, M. A., & Pillemer, K. A. (1984). *Elder abuse and neglect: Final report from Three Model Projects.* Worcester, MA: University of Massachusetts Medical Center, University Center on Aging.

Wolf, R. S., Godkin, M. A., & Pillemer, K. A. (1986). Maltreatment of the elderly: A comparative analysis. *Pride Institute Journal of Long Term Home Health Care, 5,* 10–17.

Wolf, R. S., & Li, D. (1999). Factors affecting the rate of elder abuse reporting to a state protective services program. *The Gerontologist, 39*(2), 222–228.

Wolf, R. S., & Pillemer, K. A. (1989). *Helping elderly victims: The reality of elder abuse.* New York: Columbia University Press.

Zborowsky, E. (1985). Developments in protective services: A challenge for social workers. *Journal of Gerontological Social Work, 8*(3/4), 71–83.

Zink, T., Regan, S., Jacobson, C. J., Jr., & Pabst, B. (2003). Cohort, period, and aging effects: A qualitative study of older women's reasons for remaining in abusive relationships. *Violence Against Women, 9,* 1429–1441.

CHAPTER 26

The End of Life

Rosalind A. Bye, PhD MAppSc(OT) • Gwynnyth M. Llewellyn, PhD, DipOT. MEd DipContEd • Karl E. Christl, BAppSc (Physiotherapy) LLB (Hons)

You can't experience being alive without one day realizing that you have to die . . . But it's just as impossible to realize you have to die without thinking how incredibly amazing it is to be alive.

J. Gaarder, *Sophie's World,* Phoenix House, London, 1995

OBJECTIVES

By the end of this chapter, readers will be able to:

1. Understand key theoretical principles of life span development as it relates to ageing and death.
2. Define palliative care and hospice philosophy.
3. Understand the unique palliative care needs of older people.
4. Understand international health policy related to palliative care services for older people.
5. Identify the role of occupational therapy in palliative care for older people.
6. Identify appropriate occupational therapy outcomes in palliative care for older people and their families.
7. Identify support strategies for occupational therapists working in this clinical area.

Working with people at the end of their lives is both a challenge and a privilege. The challenge for therapists is to find an approach to helping clients that meets the clients' and their families' needs and helps them manage the transition from life to death. The privilege is to witness this very special time of life and, in doing so, gain new understandings about the meaning of life and the inevitability of death for us all. Further, it is important to recognize that elders face an array of losses with which they must cope. Loss of friends, loss of function, and loss of socially sanctioned roles all require a period of mourning and adjustment. The discussion in this chapter reflects a process that can occur with any of these life changes.

This chapter aims to examine the role that occupational therapists play when working with older people who are terminally ill. Some therapists may choose to specialize in the care of people with terminal illness and assist many clients who are known to be dying. Others, such as those working in aged care settings, may encounter many clients who are near the end of life. Regardless of work setting or clinical specialty, it is likely that all therapists, over the course of their careers, will work with at least one older client who is dying. This is particularly so given the worldwide aging population and the growth in health services to this group internationally (Davies & Higginson, 2004). Therefore, it is important for all therapists to understand the issues people face at the end of their lives so that they are prepared to assist clients at this stage.

Older people are frequently devalued in the wider social context that values youth and productivity and measures people's worth by their social and economic status (Black, 2006; Giles & Reid, 2005). Such ageism has been shown to exist across many cultures (Giles & Reid, 2005). People who are terminally ill can also experience stigma. They can be viewed as a failure by a medical system that is primarily designed to cure and rehabilitate (Tigges & Marcil, 1988). Therefore, when an older person is dying, they can experience the double stigma of both their age and of having a terminal illness. Research has shown that these two issues have led to a situation where older people who are dying have had limited health services to meet their unique needs (Davies & Higginson, 2004). Lewis and Bottomley (1994) note the danger that older people may not receive optimum health care as a result of the perception that they would have died soon anyway. Funding of care for an older person at this stage of life is a hotly debated issue that raises many ethical and moral issues (Kaufman, 2000). As a result, funding and policy development for those with terminal illness has tended to focus on the provision of high-end care in inpatient **hospice** settings for people dying of illnesses such as cancer (Davies, 2004; Davies & Higginson, 2004). Such an approach has failed to address the unique needs of people "dying old" (Amella, 2003, p. 41), with complex comorbidity and other social and emotional needs related to their life stage or living situation (Davies, 2004; Davies & Higginson, 2004; Kristjanson, Toye, & Dawson, 2003).

There is now clear evidence that older people who are dying have experienced an underassessment of their pain, a lack of information and

involvement in decision making, a lack of home care, a lack of access to specialist services, and a lack of **palliative** care within nursing and residential homes (Davies & Higginson, 2004). To counteract this problem, the World Health Organization has prioritized the care of older people who are dying and released two evidence-based reports to guide policy and planning of health services: *What are the palliative care needs of older people and how might they be met?* (Davies, 2004) and *Better palliative care for older people* (Davies & Higginson, 2004). These two evidence-based reports are essential reading for all health professionals across the globe working with older people who are dying, as they establish clear needs of this group of clients, identify priority areas for care, and outline strategies for clinical practice and service development in this area. Key principles contained in these documents, along with other recent research on palliative care for older people will be further outlined in this chapter.

Occupational therapists play an important part in the care of people who are dying. However, working with people at the end of their lives can be a challenge for health professionals such as occupational therapists, who are predominantly trained to cure and rehabilitate (American Occupational Therapy Association [AOTA], 2005; Bye, 1998). The emphasis on rehabilitation and independence is a cornerstone of the occupational therapy profession. With this emphasis comes the expectation that clients will improve, be able to return to greater independence in daily life, and go on to live full, productive lives. In contrast, this plan does not happen when working with older clients who are dying. People at the end of their lives progressively deteriorate in terms of their functional independence, lose the ability to participate fully in life, and often require a significant amount of care from others leading up to death (S. A. Murray, Kendall, Boyd, & Sheikh, 2005).

And yet, it is possible for end-of-life to be a satisfying period, one that allows for a sense of fulfillment, and that provides both elders and their loved ones with a meaningful sense of closure. Occupational therapists can contribute greatly to ensuring that their clients have this experience of a "good death."

Therefore, this chapter will explore how working with older clients at the end of their lives requires therapists to reframe practice away from the traditional goals of rehabilitation and the emphasis on independence and improvement (Bye, 1998; Dawson & Barker, 1995). In doing so, therapists must modify their professional goal of helping clients to lead long, productive, balanced, independent lives—ideas that are not applicable to older clients who are dying. Instead, therapists need to help these clients live in the moment, have quality of life, and live out their last days participating in occupations they enjoy and that are meaningful to this stage of life (AOTA, 2005; Bye, 1998; Jacques & Hasselkus, 2004). Therapists also need to help clients make the transition from life to death by addressing their need for closure in life and facilitating the necessary care they will require when they are no longer able to participate fully in daily routines (AOTA, 2005; Bye, 1998). As such, therapists aim to affirm clients' remaining lives at the same time as they help them prepare for their death (Bye, 1998). When this occurs, therapists can feel that they have made an important contribution to clients' lives, even when the final outcome is death.

Normative Development: Ageing and The End of Life

The inevitability of death as the end point of our lives is still unchallenged despite modern-day advances in medicine and technology. For most of us, our lives will end sometime before the age of 90 years. Statistics from developed countries reveal that after reaching 65 years, people now live, on average, another 12 to 22 years, with France and Japan having the highest life expectancies (Davies & Higginson, 2004). If you are female, it is likely you will live longer than the men in your life, on average another 6 years (Davies & Higginson, 2004). If you are male and make it to 80, there will be twice as many women of your age (Davies & Higginson, 2004).

The awareness of our own mortality can encourage us to try and live a meaningful and rewarding life in the years we have here on earth. A sobering thought presented in Richard Carlson's popular book, *Don't sweat the small stuff... and it's all small stuff* (1997) is to remember that in 100 years from now (not that long really), there will be all new people on our planet. So unless there is a major breakthrough in medicine to extend our lives, most of us will be part of

history, hopefully having lived a long, healthy, meaningful life. Carlson (1997) suggests that understanding this fact can help us gain a more balanced perspective, encouraging us to focus on the big things in life rather than on our everyday minor worries.

Dying old is the expected norm in developed countries, where people live with access to modern health care, hygiene, and good diets (Chasteen & Madey, 2003). Living to a "ripe old age" is perhaps the goal of most of us. Chasteen and Madey (2003) found in their research study that death in old age was viewed by both younger and older participants as less tragic than the death of a younger person because an "older person has lived a full life, has had a 'turn at bat,' and is possibly waiting for death" (p. 314).

There is now a significant body of literature and research related to ageing and how people come to terms with the likelihood that death is closer with advancing age. As people live a long life, the experience of loss and grief may not be unfamiliar (Neimeyer, Wittkowski, & Moser, 2004). It is likely that they have experienced multiple losses throughout their lives: loss of health, mobility, productivity, or independence, as well as the death of spouses, family, and friends (K. M. Bennett, Smith, & Hughes, 2005; Lewis & Bottomley, 1994). This exposure to the loss and death of others can heighten the older person's awareness that these occurrences are a natural part of a long life.

Research reviewed by Neimeyer et al. (2004) reveals that acceptance of one's own death is associated with greater life satisfaction and a stronger religious belief. Nearing the end of life may trigger a search for the meaning of one's life and a renewed awareness or interest in spirituality (Dalby, 2006). For example, Moremen's (2005) interviews with older women about the meaning of life revealed they were engaged in a process of spiritual questioning, experiencing a need to feel connected with others, identified existential angst about life and death, had thoughts about death and dying, and had changes in their reliance on organized religion to a greater or lesser extent. Moremen (2005) concludes that spiritual questioning and the search for life meaning is a "natural part of the ageing process as one approaches the end of the lifespan" (p. 309). As death looms closer, people search for answers to questions about their place in the universe, their relationship to a higher power, and the relationship between themselves and their loved ones (Moremen, 2005).

Is death something that older people fear? In their review of research on death attitudes, Neimeyer et al. (2004) conclude that a substantial body of evidence reveals that anxiety and fear about death decrease from mid-life to old age, and this holds true in research including ethnically diverse samples. However, this does not mean that older people do not fear death at all or that they have no concerns about how their lives will end (Fry, 2003). Fry argues that the fear of death remains one of the most pervasive concerns for older people—in particular, fear of a lengthy dying process and fear of abandonment at the time of dying. Neimeyer et al.'s (2004) conclusions support Fry's (2003) conclusions, showing that older people are fearful about the loss of control leading up to death. Note that these are fears about the process of dying, not about death itself. In addition, elders are concerned about the possibility of an afterlife.

Fortner and Neimeyer's (1999) meta-analysis of research on death attitudes revealed that death anxiety was increased in a certain group of older people—namely, those who had more physical health problems; a reported history of psychological distress; weaker religious beliefs; and lower "ego integrity," life satisfaction, or resilience. In addition, this study found evidence that a person's place of residence also predicted death concerns, with older people living in nursing homes or other institutions being more fearful of death compared to those living independently. Fry's (2003) research adds to this picture by noting that an older person's sense of self-efficacy can reduce death fears, with a high sense of spiritual health efficacy being the most robust protector against death fears for both men and women.

Research shows that the wish of most older people is to die peacefully in their sleep in their own home (Neimeyer et al., 2004). However, whether or not this occurs will largely depend on the older person's health at the time of their death and their need for health care if their illness is considered terminal.

Older People and Terminal Illness

Despite an awareness of death's natural place at the end of life, the objective reality of a terminal diagnosis or life-limiting chronic illness brings with it a certainty that the end of life will occur sooner rather than at some unknown time in the future. Therefore, although an individual may be elderly, and at a time of life when death is considered "natural" or "expected," a terminal diagnosis may still bring with it shock and sadness as individuals grieve for experiences and goals that will never be realized as their health worsens and their lives draw to a close (Black, 2006).

Psychologically, impending death from a known terminal illness is confronting in the extreme. Stage theories of the psychological process of dying have been put forward. The most well known is that developed by Elizabeth Kubler-Ross (1969). Kubler-Ross identified five stages people pass through when they are aware they are dying: initial denial, anger, bargaining, depression, and final acceptance. These stages are now recognized as not being a linear process, but instead as possible reactions to the status of being terminally ill.

More recently, it has been argued that how one copes with the dying process mirrors lifelong coping strategies and behaviors, rather than being a universal set of behaviors and emotions for all people with terminal illness (Lindley-Davis, 1991; Neimeyer et al., 2004). Common emotions related to the experience of terminal illness have been identified. For example, fear and uncertainty are reported by many people with a terminal illness (Lloyd & Coggles, 1990; Pizzi, 1986; Reimer & Davies, 1991). Fear may not be of death itself but of the unknown, of potential pain and loss of self-image, of losing physical and cognitive functions, of the side effects of treatment, of people's reaction to their status as an individual who is dying, or of isolation and separation from others (Kellehear, 1984; Lloyd & Coggles, 1990; Werth, Gordon, & Johnson, 2002). Uncertainty may relate to the reason for the terminal disease, how to function in the short and long term, whether or not the disease is fatal, whether it is possible to live and die with dignity, and whether loved ones will cope after death (Lindley-Davis, 1991; Werth et al., 2002).

The first step toward working effectively with older clients at the end of their lives is to achieve a better understanding of the nature and course of terminal illness for older people (S. A. Murray et al., 2005). However, in doing so, it is very important to remember that clients are much more than their illness, the terminal diagnosis, or their age. The reductionist approach of the medical model of care and the increasingly advanced medical management of diseases such as cancer can at times seem to overshadow the individual identity of clients. There is a danger that health professionals may focus too intently on the illness and its effects and forget about the individual, his or her end-of-life needs, and his or her need to maintain dignity during this time (Pleschberger, 2007). Rather than focus on the illness, occupational therapists must view terminal illness in relation to how it influences older clients' daily lives and their ability to participate in desired occupations that are personally, socially, or culturally meaningful at the end of life (Jacques & Hasslekus, 2004).

Terminal illness takes many forms—for example, cancers, cardiac and respiratory illnesses, and liver disease (Amella, 2003; Mesler, 1995; S. A. Murray et al., 2005). As the worldwide population ages, the patterns of illness that cause death are also changing (Davies & Higginson, 2004). In 2020, it is predicted that the five leading causes of death will be ischemic heart disease; cerebrovascular disease; chronic obstructive pulmonary disease; lower respiratory infections; and lung, trachea, and bronchial cancer (J. L. Murray & Lopez, 1997).

The type of illness or disease will shape an older person's experience of death and dying and the care he or she will require at the end of life. In addition, older clients may have additional age-related conditions such as dementia (Sampson, Ritchie, Lai, Raven, & Blanchard, 2005) or other sensory or physical changes (Kristjanson et al., 2003) that influence their health and functioning. The challenge with older clients who have terminal illnesses concurrent with other health conditions is distinguishing between changes in health due to some other health complaint, and those caused by the advancement of the disease that will eventually cause their death.

Due to the complexity of older people's health problems, Amella (2003) notes that older people often present with a pattern of ill health leading up to their death that is different than that of a younger person dying from cancer:

> Because dying may be a more lingering process in older adults (eg, progression of heart failure vs. acute myocardial infarction), they actually may be dying for a much longer time, and thus may experience a plethora of

> symptoms. ...The older person experiences numerous trips to the hospital with miraculous recoveries, but each time, a small decrement in capacity occurs. Physiologic reserve, the capacity to bounce back from illness, wanes later in life. Loss of reserve culminates a final insult from which the individual can no longer recover, and death occurs. (p. 41)

This means that medical professionals can often not provide a clear prognosis for older clients, as rather than a predictable "downhill decline" of illnesses such as cancer, a "roller-coaster" trajectory is observed (Amella, 2003, p. 41).

It is important to understand how a terminal illness can affect a person's abilities, and in the older person, how that illness will interact with other health conditions (Davies & Higginson, 2004). Physically, serious illnesses can ravage a person's body. Loss of energy, muscle weakness, pain, nausea, sensory loss, and loss of appetite are common features (Davies, 2004). Illnesses have varying motor, sensory, and neurological effects on clients' bodies. For example, if a client has breast cancer, she may also develop metastases at two or more separate levels in the spine (Rashleigh, 1996). The metastases may cause neurological problems, such as paraparesis due to spinal cord compression (Gray, 1989). This same client may also have orthopedic difficulties such as pain and reduced range of movement in the shoulder following mastectomy. Removal of auxiliary lymph nodes during the mastectomy, followed by radiotherapy, may also cause **lymphedema** in the upper limb (Mason, 1993). Another client with a terminal brain tumor may experience cognitive and behavioral difficulties, and depending on the site of the tumor, various sensory and motor losses may occur. A client with heart failure or chronic obstructive pulmonary disease may experience shortness of breath on exertion and be severely restricted in the performance of daily activities (Davies, 2004).

S. A. Murray et al. (2005) have identified evidence-based **typical illness trajectories** to assist the complex clinical reasoning required by health professionals working with people who are dying. Three illness trajectories emerged from their review of research literature and analysis of their own research data from previous investigations. The first illness trajectory is represented by a *short period of decline leading up to death.* Such a trajectory is typical of the progression of certain cancers. The second trajectory is more representative of heart and lung or other organ failure and is characterized by *long-term limitations with intermittent serious episodes* across a 2- to 5-year period. Despite a prolonged period of illness, when death comes it seems "sudden" and is usually caused by the person being unable to fight off another exacerbation of their condition. The third trajectory is characterized by a *prolonged dwindling of health* due to illnesses such as dementia, generalized frailty, or multiple body system failure in old age. The person's death may be finally caused by an acute illness, such as pneumonia, or a traumatic event such as a fractured neck of the femur.

Understanding the course of an older client's illness, and how it interacts with other health complaints, allows the therapist to better understand the short-term and long-term impact of the older person's health on participation in daily occupations. In addition, therapists can use the concept of these trajectories to hypothesize how the person's illness will impact on the person's social supports and influence future planning related to the individual's living situation, potential need for environmental modifications, and coordination of care needs. This approach aims to ensure that a therapist working with this diverse group of clients does not take a "one-size-fits-all" approach to service provision for older clients who are dying (S. A. Murray et al., 2005). By tailoring therapy to meet the unique needs of older clients and their families, therapists can contribute to the achievement of what has been termed "a good death."

A Good Death

The concept of a **good death** has been proposed from research involving interviews with people who are terminally ill (Kellehear, 1984, 1990; Kellehear & Lewin, 1989; McNamara et al., 1995). The good death does not refer to a particular moment in time when the person actually dies but relates to the process or style of dying, leading up to and including death (Kaufman, 2000). It is a conceptualization of a series of social events between the dying person and others, such as family, friends, health professionals, clergy, and so on. The person who is dying directs these events and interactions. The pattern of dying will be a reflection of the person's particular sociocultural background and be "good" or "bad" relative to each individual's context (Kellehear, 1990).

Kellehear (1990) states that the good death includes five features:

1. An awareness of dying by the individual and others
2. Social adjustments and personal preparations for death, such as talking to friends and family, spending more time with loved ones, and delegating responsibility of personal affairs to another
3. Public preparations, including financial, funeral, or religious preparations
4. Work change, for example, relinquishing the work role if not already retired
5. Making last farewells to others, both formally and informally over time

Research has shown that preparing to die needs to go hand in hand with preparing to live out the remaining life with quality (Curtis et al., 2002; Kellehear, 1990; Patrick, Curtis, Engelberg, Nielsen, & McCown, 2003). This seemingly dual state of people living while imultaneously having the experience of terminal illness and being aware of imminent death has been termed *living until dying,* or living with death (DeSpelder & Strickland, 1992; Saunders, 1983). Making the best of each moment and each day is an important part of living with a terminal illness.

Patrick et al. (2003) sums up the challenge faced by older people who are dying:

> Older adults face what is perhaps the ultimate challenge for successful aging: dying and death. ...The challenge is to come to terms with dying and death so that death occurs without undue discomfort, according to one's goals and wishes, and within the context of one's beliefs and cultural traditions. (p. 410)

Occupational therapists can significantly influence quality of life by enhancing participation by the older client or their caregivers in daily occupations that work toward the achievement of a good death (AOTA, 2005). Adopting a palliative care approach to everyday practice is one way to ensure therapists fulfill this role in an effective manner.

The Palliative Care Approach

The care of clients who are dying is known as *palliative care.* Palliative care is now an established medical specialty that meets the needs of clients whose illnesses cannot be cured. There are many definitions of palliative care. However, what is common to all these definitions is that palliative care emphasizes symptom control, quality of life, and helping individuals live life to the fullest while still being able to prepare for death (Box 26-1) (Doyle et al., 1998; Saunders,

1998; World Health Organization, 2007; Woodruff, 1993).

People prepare for death and live their remaining lives in varied social settings: the home, hospital, hospice, or nursing home. Individuals may come and go from these settings during the course of their illness, thereby having contact with various health care professionals during this time. A palliative care approach can be applied to client care in any of these settings (e.g., Cooper & Littlechild, 2004; Glare et al., 2003; P. Hudson, 2003;

BOX 26-1 Definition, Aims, and Principles of Palliative Care

DEFINITION – WORLD HEALTH ORGANIZATION (2007)

Palliative care is an approach that improves the quality of life of patients and their families facing the problem associated with life-threatening illness, through the prevention and relief of suffering by means of early identification and impeccable assessment and treatment of pain and other problems, physical, psychosocial and spiritual. Palliative care:

- Provides relief from pain and other distressing symptoms;
- Affirms life and regards dying as a normal process;
- Intends neither to hasten or postpone death;
- Integrates the psychological and spiritual aspects of patient care;
- Offers a support system to help patients live as actively as possible until death;
- Offers a support system to help the family cope during the patients illness and in their own bereavement;
- Uses a team approach to address the needs of patients and their families, including bereavement counselling, if indicated;
- Enhances quality of life, and may also positively influence the course of illness;
- Is applicable early in the course of illness, in conjunction with other therapies that are intended to prolong life, such as chemotherapy or radiation therapy, and includes those investigations needed to better understand and manage distressing clinical complications.

AIM

"To enable the dying person to live until he dies, at his own maximum potential, performing to the limit of his physical activity and mental capacity with control and

independence wherever possible. If he is recognized as the unique person he is and helped to live as part of his family and in other relationships, he can still reach out to his hopes and expectations to what has deepest meaning for him and end his life with a sense of completion." (Saunders, 1998, p viii)

Dame Cicely Saunders,
one of the founders of the
hospice and palliative care movement

PRINCIPLES OF PALLIATIVE CARE (BENNAHUM, 1996; DAVIES & HIGGINSON, 2004; SAUNDERS, 1998)

- Knowledge and honesty about terminal illness and death
- Continuous, coordinated care managed by a skilled multidisciplinary team
- Honest, open communication between staff, patient, and family
- Control of common symptoms of disease, especially palliation of pain in all its elements—physical, psychological, social, and spiritual
- Treatment of patient and family as single unit of care
- Client- and family-centered care
- Active care programs for different settings—home care, respite care, day care, or inpatient care
- Care that permits the client to express preferences for place of care and death
- Flexible health care systems to permit seamless co-ordination of care across acute, community or institutional care settings
- Program of bereavement care for family after death of the patient
- Ongoing research and education by staff

Pleschberger, 2007). For example, a therapist may encounter an older client who is living in a residential setting such as a nursing home. When the client is known to be terminally ill, a palliative care approach can assist the therapist to work with this client and meet the client's needs leading up to death.

There is clear evidence to support the effectiveness of key palliative care strategies such as pain and symptom control, collaborative and honest communication processes, spiritual support, care coordination across different settings, the use of a multidisciplinary team, and support strategies for families and caregivers (Davies & Higginson, 2004). In addition, preliminary evidence is emerging that reveals the positive impact of using the palliative care approach with people experiencing a range of health conditions (Davies & Higginson, 2004).

Underpinning the palliative care approach is the hospice philosophy. Many people misunderstand the term *hospice* and believe that it merely refers to a place where people go to die. Instead, the term "hospice" refers to the philosophy of care that is a foundation for a palliative approach. Hospice philosophy was developed to guide medical and allied health staff working in palliative care to meet the unique needs of the client and family dealing with terminal illness (Biswas, 1993). This is in contrast to the aims of the modern hospital, which are predominantly devoted to highly specialized, acute, curative care for patients (DeSpelder & Strickland, 1992).

The hospice philosophy of palliative care is based on minimizing pain and controlling symptoms by meeting the physical, psychological, emotional, and spiritual needs of both people with terminal illness and their families (Tigges & Marcil, 1988). Hospice philosophy acknowledges that although cure is no longer an option in the treatment of clients, there is still a vital role for health professionals in the care of people with terminal illness.

The aims and principles applied in palliative care assist clients to live comfortably, as free of pain and symptoms as possible, and to have quality in their remaining lives (see Box 26-1). As Hockley and Mowatt (1996) note: "One cannot change the final destination of our patients . . . this would be impossible short of a miracle. However, what we can try and do is influence the quality of that journey" (p. 13).

To that end, a team of researchers has been working on measuring the quality of dying and death for terminally ill clients (Curtis et al., 2002; Patrick et al., 2003). They constructed a measure from a series of literature reviews and qualitative case studies in an effort to improve palliative care for clients and families. The Quality of Dying and Death Instrument consists of 31 items across three domains: (1) quality of end-of-life care; (2) quality of life at the end of life; and (3) quality of dying and death (Box 26-2). A client's loved one or surrogate caregiver is interviewed once the client has died. They rate each item in relation to the client's last 7 days, or if the client was unconscious or unresponsive, over the month prior to death. Items are rated from 0 (terrible experience) to 10 (almost perfect experience). The total is obtained by adding scores on all items and dividing this by the number of items answered. This mean is then multiplied by 10 to obtain a score out of 100. Higher scores reveal better quality overall.

This instrument has shown good preliminary construct and cross-sectional validity and internal consistency reliability (Curtis et al., 2002) and has promise as an outcome measure in palliative care—a clinical field where measuring outcomes can be methodologically difficult due to many factors. Research is ongoing on this instrument. However, the point to be made here is that this instrument is a useful guide to health professionals working in palliative care as it identifies evidence-based, quality indicators that are known to be important to people who are dying and their families. What is also evident from this list of items is that being able to engage in meaningful occupation and participate in daily life is seen as a key indicator of the quality of a person's dying and death. The occupational therapy role is therefore a critical one in the palliative care team.

This role is reflected in the recently commissioned White Paper on Palliative Care commissioned in the United States by the Bureau of Health Professions (2007). This document outlines the following aspects of care: physical; psychological and psychiatric; social; spiritual, religious, and existential; ethical and legal; and cultural. In each

---

BOX 26-2   Quality of Dying and Death Instrument: Domains and Concepts

QUALITY OF END-OF-LIFE
- Continuous healing relationships through death and after death for loved ones
- Focus on the dying patient's needs and respect for treatment and dying preferences
- The dying patient as a source of control wherever possible; loved ones involved at all times
- Shared knowledge and information about prognosis and all aspects of care up to death
- Shared decision making based on evidence
- Transparency in care and decision processes
- Anticipation of individual needs both inside and outside care settings
- Cooperation and communication among providers
- Coordination among caregivers, patients and families

QUALITY OF LIFE AT THE END OF LIFE
- Physical
  ○ Self care
  ○ Activities of daily living
  ○ Walking

  ○ Mobility
  ○ Eating
  ○ Sleeping
- Psychosocial
  ○ Interaction with loved ones
  ○ Receiving and giving help
  ○ Contribution to community
  ○ Recreation
  ○ Sexual life
  ○ Income
  ○ Respect
  ○ Variety in life
- Cognitive and Communication
  ○ Thinking and remembering; speaking
- Overall happiness

QUALITY OF DYING AND DEATH
- Symptoms and personal care
- Preparation for end of life
- Moment of death
- Family
- Treatment preferences
- Whole-person concerns, meaning and purpose

---

of these aspects, the occupational therapist plays an important role in ensuring that patient and family concerns are addressed.

Occupational Therapy—Our Role in Palliative Care

In the past, the occupational therapy literature on working in palliative care was contradictory about the part therapists should play in the lives of clients who are terminally ill. On the one hand, authors described the traditional, rehabilitative, problem-oriented process of therapy as applied to people with terminal illness (Dawson, 1982; A. E. Holland & Tigges, 1981; Oelrich, 1974; Romsas & Rosa, 1985). This rehabilitative approach focused on maximizing functional independence and helping patients return to lost roles, activities, and relationships. Little attention was paid to the reality of progressive deterioration, permanent functional loss, and preparations for death.

The American Occupational Therapy Association's Practice Framework (2002) has been discussed in every chapter in this book. Its description of elements of performance and of occupational profiles is every bit as relevant at the end of life as at earlier life stages. It is consistent with discussion by authors who, during the 1980s and early 1990s began to present a palliative approach to occupational therapy that considered the individual's unique experience of dying and discussed how the therapist could assist the individual through this final stage of life (S. Bennett, 1991; Flanigan, 1982; Pizzi, 1984, 1986; Tigges, 1983, 1986, 1998; Tigges & Marcil, 1988; Tigges & Sherman, 1983). Deterioration of functional performance, emotions of grief and loss, the need to facilitate client autonomy, and preparing for death were now important considerations.

These contrasting viewpoints presented therapists with conflicting ideas about working with clients who were terminally ill. In reality, clients are seen by occupational therapists at various stages of terminal illness. In the early stages, it may be possible to apply certain principles of slow-stream rehabilitation to maintain independence for as long as possible. For example, a client who has reduced mobility may be assisted to mobilize more often by the gradual upgrading of activity and exercise levels. At the same time, however, the therapist is aware that the terminal diagnosis may limit the amount of functional gain possible. The reality of the eventual decline is in the therapist's mind and ensures that realistic therapy goals are set with the client and family.

Further along in the course of the illness, a traditional rehabilitative approach may no longer be possible, and this client may require an approach that aims to compensate for increasing needs. At this time, it may be appropriate to acknowledge that maintenance of function is no longer possible without the use of compensatory strategies, such as walking aids, increased supervision during mobility, and strategies to conserve energy during activities of daily living.

With time, even these strategies may no longer succeed, as advancing terminal illness leads to the eventual decline of function. At this time, a palliative approach can be used to support caregivers in providing the necessary care for the client. The client can be assisted to stay involved in decision making related to his or her care. This ensures the client's continued control over daily life occupations and guarantees participation in planning even when physical control and physical independence are no longer possible.

In short, therapists need to modify their approach to practice over the course of clients' illnesses and as needs change (Figure 26-1). This process of adopting the right approach at the right time ensures that clients' occupational needs and goals are met as life draws to a close. Therapists must balance the focus and approach of care to be in line with the changing needs of clients. This will not always be a linear process of moving from one stage to the next. Instead, as clients' needs fluctuate and change, therapists can adopt the right approach at the right time to find a match between therapy goals and strategies and client needs and abilities.

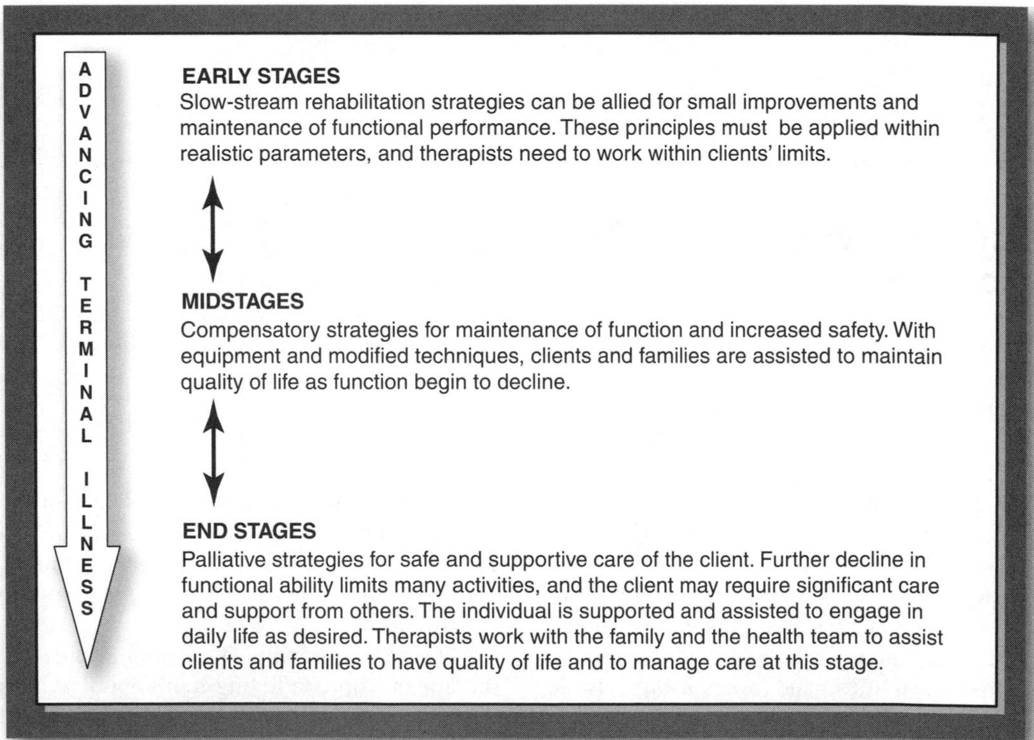

ADVANCING TERMINAL ILLNESS

EARLY STAGES
Slow-stream rehabilitation strategies can be allied for small improvements and maintenance of functional performance. These principles must be applied within realistic parameters, and therapists need to work within clients' limits.

MIDSTAGES
Compensatory strategies for maintenance of function and increased safety. With equipment and modified techniques, clients and families are assisted to maintain quality of life as function begin to decline.

END STAGES
Palliative strategies for safe and supportive care of the client. Further decline in functional ability limits many activities, and the client may require significant care and support from others. The individual is supported and assisted to engage in daily life as desired. Therapists work with the family and the health team to assist clients and families to have quality of life and to manage care at this stage.

FIGURE 26-1 As the client's illness advances, the therapist modifies the type of approach and the strategies used to best meet the client's needs. This process is not linear. A therapist may go back and forth between the approaches as the client's condition fluctuates and needs change.

Reframing Occupational Therapy for Palliative Care

Changing this balance as illness progresses may at times feel like therapy is achieving less and less with clients. Not only are clients old, potentially with other health difficulties related to aging, but they also are terminally ill. The continuation of the illness, the ongoing problems, and the increasing needs of clients can be overwhelming to an occupational therapist who is new to this area of practice. It is essential that therapists be clear about the important role they can play with such clients. Being unable to rehabilitate clients to solve underlying problems *permanently* should not discourage therapists from working with clients who are at the end of their lives.

Instead, therapists need to adopt a new approach to work effectively and gain a sense of achievement from their work (Bye, 1998). It must be remembered that many gains are made with clients throughout the course of therapy— for example, pain levels are reduced, mobility is improved and made safer, homes are modified so that clients can remain at home, clients are satisfied by being able to participate in everyday tasks and leisure activities, and caregivers are supported to care for their loved ones safely. Death still occurs, but the quality of the person's remaining life and his or her experience of dying have been enhanced by occupational therapy.

Therapy that Affirms Life and Helps Prepare for Death

Research has shown that occupational therapists working under a palliative approach reframe their practice to address the reality of clients' dual states of living and dying (Bye, 1998). Therapists aimed to meet the needs of clients at the end of life by adopting a client-centered approach to assessment, intervention, goal setting, and evaluation of outcomes. Furthermore, therapists identified a process of balancing the needs of clients who were in the dual state of living and dying. In doing so, therapists helped clients and their families both to affirm life and to prepare for death.

This approach is useful for understanding the complex needs of people with terminal illness. It recognizes that clients can be assisted to remain engaged in meaningful daily life occupations and, at the same time, be supported to come to terms with their mortality and prepare for death through participation in certain activities or planning for care needs. This process takes place by balancing the focus of client care to the engagement in occupations that will address remaining life goals *and* prepare the client and their family for death (Figure 26-2).

Recent research supports the occupational therapist's role in palliative care as being focused on occupations that continue to affirm life but also prepare for death. For example, Lyons, Orozovic, Davis, and Newman (2002) interviewed and observed day hospice participants to investigate the nature and purpose of their occupational engagement. They found that by *doing* occupational therapy, people were able to maintain a sense of well-being despite illness, which in turn reinforced a sense of *being* through engagement in pleasurable experiences and stimulating hospice day program activities. As a result, participants gained a sense of *becoming* through their occupational engagement and enjoyed the unexpected learning of new activities at the end of life and the opportunities to assist others also engaged in the program. Thus, Lyons et al. (2002) discovered that occupational engagement can be transformative even at the end of life.

Jacques and Hasselkus (2004) also investigated the meaning of occupation surrounding death and dying at a hospice facility. An ethnographic study over a 6-month period revealed four domains of occupation that were elements of the dying experience of participants. Clients wanted to "do things that matter" and therefore continue a meaningful engagement in life. They wanted to "get everything in order" as a means of preparing for death. Most felt it "takes so long to die" and engaged in waiting for death to come. Finally, the actual death and after-death experience also consisted of various occupations that hopefully helped to facilitate a "gentle good-bye" for the person who had died. These researchers concluded that

> ... occupation at the end of life may not be ordinary, familiar, or engaged in everyday. Rather, some occupations at the end of life seem to be unique to that point in time, unfamiliar, and engaged in only because of the expectation of a person's death. Further, some

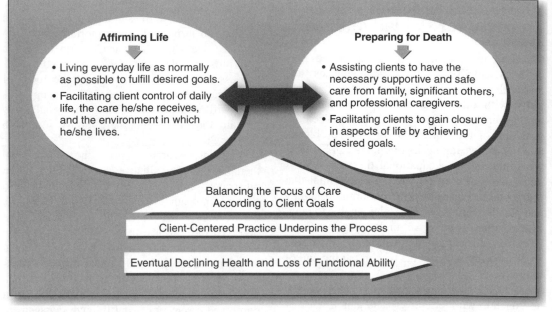

Affirming Life

- Living everyday life as normally as possible to fulfill desired goals.
- Facilitating client control of daily life, the care he/she receives, and the environment in which he/she lives.

Preparing for Death

- Assisting clients to have the necessary supportive and safe care from family, significant others, and professional caregivers.
- Facilitating clients to gain closure in aspects of life by achieving desired goals.

Balancing the Focus of Care According to Client Goals

Client-Centered Practice Underpins the Process

Eventual Declining Health and Loss of Functional Ability

FIGURE 26-2 Dual focus of therapy for clients with terminal illness: affirming life and preparing for death. Occupational therapy can help older people with terminal illness have a satisfactory quality of life by balancing care to encompass the dual reality of living with a terminal illness and dealing with impending death and decline in health.

occupations engaged in by people who are dying may be familiar, even ordinary in many ways, yet the nature of those occupational engagements seems changed in the presence of dying and impending death. (Jacques & Hasselkus, 2004, pp. 50–51)

Reframing the Processes of Therapy

By reframing certain ideas and understanding the altered nature and role of occupation at the end of life, occupational therapists can incorporate the principles and philosophy of hospice and palliative care into their daily work. Each stage of the problem-solving process of therapy can be adapted to suit the unique needs of an older client at the end of his or her life (Table 26-1) and to suit the illness trajectory the client is on, and the health care or community setting in which therapy takes place.

Reframing Referral

Referral to occupational therapy may come from clients' caregivers or other staff. In some situations, therapists may have access to all

clients where they work, and it is a matter of screening clients to determine whether there is a need for therapy services.

In palliative care, it is important to adopt a proactive approach to referral. Many times clients may not realize that they could benefit from occupational therapy. It may be difficult for clients to see how a therapist could help their situation when they have little knowledge of the role therapists play and feel that their options have been limited by a terminal diagnosis. Therapists can help clients achieve a sense of control again and participate more fully in daily life.

It is important for therapists to actively market their role to clients, caregivers, and other staff to ensure that appropriate referrals occur. Often, a quick talk with clients to discuss how they are managing from day to day can reveal needs. This short discussion can often open a range of possibilities that the client and caregiver had not considered. Educating clients, caregivers, and other staff about the options therapy can provide is essential to facilitating a sense of control over decisions related to daily life, activities, living environments, and caregiving. The use of posters and pamphlets for clients and caregivers is another way that therapists can "advertise" the availability of therapy on a

TABLE 26-1 **Reframing the Process of Occupational Therapy**

Stage	Key Issues in Palliative Care
Referral	Respond quickly because client's condition can change rapidly.
	Actively market therapy role to educate clients, caregivers, and the staff of available options.
Assessment	Use low-key approach—gentle, informal assessments that are not confronting or invasive to clients.
	Collect information from clients, caregivers, and other staff.
	Understand that assessment can be an emotional experience because it reveals to clients the extent of their problems and their loss of independence.
	Use empathy and listening skills to put clients at ease and build rapport and trust.
Goal Setting	Goals should be client- and family-centered.
	Help clients identify goals by providing them with options and possibilities. This will facilitate choice of desired goals.
	Keep goals short term to ensure that clients feel a sense of success, because they may have limited time in which to achieve them.
Intervention	Select and implement appropriate techniques related to client needs and goals.
	Modify techniques as necessary for a palliative approach; e.g., consider pain and fatigue levels during therapy, use temporary home modification rather than permanent methods, emphasize client control and quality of life rather than full functional independence.
Outcomes	Measure success of therapy by the achievement of client goals.
	Don't focus on permanency of outcomes because advancing illness and fluctuating client health are the reality.
	Examine whether therapy made a difference to the quality of clients' and caregivers' lives leading up to death.

hospital unit, hospice unit, day-care setting, or aged-care residential facility.

A terminal diagnosis puts the added pressure of response time onto therapists, as older clients' conditions can change rapidly. It is important to receive and attend to referrals as soon as possible because clients may have limited time to meet their desired goals. When someone is terminally ill, every moment counts. Speed of access to occupational therapy palliative care services has been shown to be a critical issue to clients and their caregivers (Kealy & McIntyre, 2005).

Referrals may relate to current problems or be aimed at preventing future difficulties and deterioration. Problems must be dealt with quickly to ensure comfort and quality of life, and to prevent further functional loss when possible. This is critical when working with older clients who may also have older caregivers. Problems with caregiving or environmental hazards can quickly develop into a need to relocate a client to a new care environment. Quick response to referral can diffuse problems, improve the situation for the client and caregivers, and increase quality of life. By responding quickly, therapists can prevent a crisis situation from occurring and alleviate the fears or concerns of older clients and their caregivers.

Reframing Assessment

Standard areas of occupational therapy assessment for older people are covered in the assessment process. Therapists may have their own particular methods, styles, and instruments they use for client assessment. This will depend on the theoretical framework guiding their clinical reasoning, clinical experience, and assessment and documentation techniques used at each work site.

Regardless of the particular format or focus of assessment, the assessment process in palliative care should be reframed so that assessments are "low key" (Bye, 1998). This avoids making the client feel as though he or she were being "tested." Rigorous, standardized assessments can be physically and emotionally taxing for older clients who are dying. Assessment usually reveals significant deterioration of functional ability and multiple complex care needs. This can be upsetting for clients as they realize the degree of their functional loss and dependence. Therapists need to balance their need to know and observe client function with how a client is feeling on that day and the possibility that a detailed physical or functional assessment may leave the client feeling exhausted and defeated. Gentle and informal methods can be used to focus on clients' current abilities and assess essential features of functional ability. A conversational style of interview can determine desired goals and build rapport with the client and significant others. Asking the client about what is of most concern to him or her can help prioritize multiple problems. Assessing the client over several shorter visits can ease them into the process of therapy and help build rapport and trust.

It is important to incorporate the views of others in the assessment process. Members of the family, other caregivers, and other professional team members can provide essential information to complete the assessment. For example, if a client is feeling unwell on the day of assessment, therapists can modify techniques of data collection. Instead of having the client take part in a self-care assessment, the occupational therapist can interview nursing staff or caregivers to provide information about such aspects as level of assistance required, major problems, and techniques used.

It is also critical to evaluate how the family is managing caregiving. Family members can feel anxious and worried about their ability to provide the necessary care (Baxandall & Reddy, 1993). It is standard practice in aged care and palliative care to include family members as part of the unit of care by therapists, and they therefore need to be included in the assessment process. An assessment should be conducted regarding caregivers' abilities and willingness to provide necessary end-of-life care. This assessment can then identify areas that need to be addressed in the later intervention related to supporting caregivers in their often difficult tasks.

The therapist should conduct an assessment of the client's environment with regard to safety, access, and comfort for both clients and caregivers. The therapist needs to keep in mind that clients' conditions are likely to progress and worsen with time. Eventually, many clients will spend prolonged periods in bed. Therefore, the bedroom, bed, and access to the toilet and shower need to be examined carefully to facilitate maximum care and comfort.

Reframing Goal Setting

Setting goals with older clients who are terminally ill is centered around their wishes and tailored to meet individual needs and solve problems. Goal setting guides the future intervention carried out by therapists in attempting to meet goals identified by clients. The goals identified by people who are dying relate to their final days of life and influence the quality of the remaining time. As a consequence, there is a precious quality to these goals (Bye, 1998). Goal setting must be client centered, and therapists should not make assumptions about the kinds of things that are important to older clients. Each client may have different goals to fulfill before his or her death. The achievement of these goals can assist clients to come to terms with their mortality and prepare for death. Therapists need to ask clients what they would like to do with their remaining time and then follow their lead.

Some clients find it difficult to identify goals beyond their medical care. Their life has revolved around medical treatment for so long that they can lose touch with the everyday things in life that they had previously enjoyed. A feeling of helplessness and hopelessness may result (Tigges, 1998). Spending time discussing likes and dislikes, interests, problems, and things they would like to do, can open up the range of possibilities available to clients. Clients often want to do basic, normal things (Bye, 1998; Jacques & Hasselkus, 2004). For example, clients may identify just wanting to wash or dry themselves when they are having a shower to achieve some privacy. Others may want to be pain free so they can sit and watch television with their families. Other examples might include being able to walk in the garden, sit at the table for meals, or listen to the radio. Being able to do everyday things is incredibly valuable to some clients because it gives them a sense of normality beyond their illness and the process of dying (Bye, 1998).

Other clients may have wishes related to family, friends, or leisure interests. Clients may wish to take part in a loved activity one more time with family or friends—for example, driving with the family to visit the local neighborhood, visiting the grave of a spouse a final time, or spending time with the family dog. Achieving these precious wishes helps clients prepare for death as they find closure to unfinished business and are able say goodbye to something or someone.

Clients may identify goals related to saying good-bye to their homes, pets, loved ones, and so on. Others may wish to write farewell letters or to make something to give to their families or friends to remember them by. Such activities help clients to find closure in aspects of life in preparation for death and become meaningful occupations at this time in life (Jacques & Hasselkus, 2004).

Going home to die is a common goal identified by clients. Some clients may not want to spend their last days in the hospital and just want to be in familiar surroundings with loved ones. Others may have a different view and prefer to spend their last days being cared for in a hospital or hospice. Some older clients may have limited caregivers in their life as their spouse may have already died, and their adult children live elsewhere. However, they may wish to return home for a short time and then be transferred into a hospital or hospice near the end of life. We cannot assume that all clients want to die in their homes or that all caregivers want this to happen. Both parties' goals are important to consider, and frequently clients are unable to achieve their goal unless caregivers are willing to accommodate them. This point illustrates that clients' goals exist within a wider context and, although "precious," also need to be feasible and realistic. The important role played by community or domiciliary palliative care therapists is vital to achieve a good death in the home environment (Kealey & McIntyre, 2005). Kealy and McIntyre's (2005) research into a community-based palliative care service revealed that clients and family were very satisfied with the role occupational therapists played in their overall care.

Because of the shortened life expectancy, therapists may believe that they are "working against the clock" to achieve clients' goals before they die (Bye, 1998). In addition, older clients usually experience rapid deterioration in the terminal stages, and there may be limited time to achieve activity-oriented goals before the client becomes too ill. The nature of terminal illness puts pressure on clients and therapists to achieve more active goals sooner rather than later as good days (for example, when the client is pain free or free of other symptoms) may be few and far between. Time should not be wasted by therapists and should be viewed with respect for each moment the client has remaining in his or her life.

Reframing Intervention

Clients with terminal illness lose a great deal—the ability to engage in daily activities due to physical losses, the ability to live independently at home, and the sense of themselves as competent people. Roles are lost, and self-esteem, body image, and confidence falter. Occupational therapists can work together to achieve goals with clients by addressing the functional performance problems blocking the achievement of occupational goals and thereby maximizing clients' abilities to participate in life. The processes of assessment and goal setting allow therapists to formulate intervention plans that will address identified problems and achieve desired goals (AOTA, 2005). The intervention strategies used to achieve these goals and manage problems include building up clients' internal resources, as well as facilitating external supports to compensate for the losses experienced and those expected (Bye, 1998).

Therapists can use education and functional retraining to develop clients' internal resources. As a result, clients gain knowledge and skills related to coping with the disease and its side effects, managing stress, conserving energy, and improving physical strength and endurance. These resources develop clients' abilities to deal with, compensate for, or adapt to losses they are experiencing to achieve their goals or solve identified problems.

To help clients manage problems and achieve goals even further, it is also crucial to build supports—both human and physical—that are external to the client. Human supports include professional caregivers, family, and friends. Strategies used to build external human supports include identifying, educating, and supporting caregivers to provide the necessary assistance. Physical supports include a variety of aids and environmental modifications that help clients manage loss of physical function. Kealy and McIntyre's (2005) research revealed that the provision of equipment and environmental modification were identified by clients and caregivers as some of the most helpful aspects of occupational therapy in palliative care.

Occupational therapists apply a wide variety of intervention strategies to achieve goals and solve problems for older people who are dying. Common intervention strategies, their aims, and their application in palliative care are summarized in Table 26-2. Therapists need to choose the appropriate strategies to apply to meet individual clients' goals and solve underlying problems. Traditional aged care therapy strategies may require modification when applied in palliative care. Occupational therapists may need to reconsider extensive home modification for older clients who are terminally ill; instead, short-term, temporary solutions may be found that solve problems quickly and inexpensively.

In sum, occupational therapists provide unique intervention strategies to help older clients who are dying manage problems and achieve goals at the end of their lives. Therapists need to keep in mind the central role of occupation in helping clients affirm life and prepare for death. Our unique role in the palliative care process must remain focused on

1. Maximizing occupational performance during an older person's final life stage
2. Understanding the meaning of engaging in occupation to an older person's sense of well-being
3. Recognizing the importance of participation in daily life to promote a positive sense of self
4. Being aware that particular occupations can help prepare people and their families for impending death (AOTA, 2005; Bye, 1998; Jacques & Hasselkus, 2004; Lyons et al., 2002)

Therapists have unique expertise to provide advice about the older person's continued engagement in life and to offer support as functional ability declines and care is needed in the

TABLE 26-2 Occupational-Therapy-Focused Assessment

Occupational Therapy Strategies	Aims and Application in Palliative Care
Activity modification	Aim
Energy conservation techniques Aids and equipment Caregiver assistance Safe methods and risk reduction	To facilitate continued engagement in life and participation in desired occupations. Techniques of activity analysis and task simplification and environmental modification allow clients to take part in meaningful occupations. This helps clients feel connected to normal life beyond medical aspects of care. Clients can be taught to save energy during some activities (e.g., showering) so they are able to have energy remaining to participate in desired activities (e.g., visiting family or friends).
Environmental modification	Aim
Home modification Aids and equipment Altered environmental layout Reduction of environmental hazards for safety	To reduce environmental demands as client function deteriorates, thereby promoting ongoing engagement in daily tasks, and facilitating ease and safety during caregiving tasks. Because of the client's shortened life expectancy, therapists and clients may choose to use temporary methods of environmental modification, which can solve problems quickly and are not too costly for clients. Environments should be altered in such a way that they remain familiar to clients and comfortable (e.g., avoid a medical or hospital atmosphere by creating homelike environments).
Therapeutic occupations	Aim
Facilitate engagement in normal, everyday activities Creative activities or gift making Leisure and recreation Day-care programs	To promote a sense of normality in life and develop an outlet for self-expression and creativity. Occupation creates a sense of mastery and engagement in life. Normal, everyday activities remind people of life before illness. Creative and leisure activities provide times for socialization, reminiscence, and expression of individuality. Gifts, letters, and life collages are examples of permanent end products of such activities that can be given to loved ones as keepsakes and expressions of farewell.

Occupational Therapy Strategies	Aims and Application in Palliative Care
Relaxation, stress management	**Aim**
Progressive muscle relaxation Meditation Active coping techniques Music and aromatherapy Relaxing environments	To promote a sense of peace, calm, and control during an otherwise difficult time. Specific relaxation and stress-management techniques can be taught to clients and caregivers to ease symptoms such as pain or nausea and to promote a sense of internal control and calm. This allows clients to take control of their bodies, which can otherwise seem controlled by illness.
Client education	**Aim**
Causes, effects, and treatment of client problems Education is essential in all aspects of occupational therapy.	To help clients understand the effects of illness on aspects of function. Education reduces anxiety by allowing open and honest dialogue about problems and treatment. Education promotes informed decision making about therapy.
Caregiver education and support	**Aim**
Safe caregiving techniques Manual handling and back care Client transfers Equipment use (e.g., hoists, wheel-chairs) Referral to support and services	To ensure safe caregiving techniques and protect the caregiver's physical status. Education on manual handling techniques and back care can prevent care-related injuries. Caregivers can be educated about the resources available to them to assist with caregiving tasks. From this knowledge base, they are able to make informed decisions about caregiving and the support they require. This can help caregivers feel better equipped to deal with the client's declining function and impending death.

time leading up to death. There is a need for ongoing research into the efficacy of occupational therapy interventions in palliative care so that future therapists have a stronger evidence base on which to plan interventions.

Reframing Outcomes

Therapists need to look differently at therapy outcomes in palliative care. In the rehabilitation unit, it is easy to objectively measure permanent gains that will help clients go on to lead fuller, more productive lives. Palliative care with older clients does not lead to the same type of therapy outcomes (Tigges, 1986). However, it is wrong to assume that there is only one outcome in palliative care—the death of the client. There are many outcomes of occupational therapy in palliative care. The achievement of these therapy outcomes is essential in determining whether a client is able to lead a meaningful and comfortable life before death.

First and foremost, therapists should examine whether client goals were achieved through therapy. This is one essential measure of the successful outcomes of therapy. For example,

did the client experience reduced pain? Was the caregiver able to manage more easily at home with the client? Was the client able to participate in family life for as long as possible? Did the client visit home for a final time to say goodbye to the pets? If these goals were achieved, then therapy was indeed a success.

Second, achievements in palliative care, particularly in the terminal phase of illness, need to be viewed on a day-to-day basis. Time often runs out in the palliative care environment, and although short-term goals were set, sometimes a client's condition worsens and he or she dies before goals were achieved. In this situation, the therapist needs to reflect on whether or not the *process* of therapy was successful. For example, did the client enjoy talking about and planning the visit home? Did the client gain a sense of control from the few short therapy sessions? Reflecting on the quality of the therapy process and the client–therapist relationship can reveal the success of therapy.

Research has pointed to four major outcomes identified by occupational therapists in palliative care (Bye, 1998):

1. Helping clients live as normally as possible within their otherwise changed reality
2. Helping clients achieve a sense of control in their lives
3. Helping clients and caregivers manage the care needed during the terminal stages so that they feel safe and supported
4. Facilitating a sense of closure in life by engaging in desired activities for a final time and making farewells to people, places, and things

These outcomes center on occupation and participation in daily life, and recognize clients' dual realities of living and dying. The first two outcomes are aimed at affirming clients' lives, and the latter two outcomes help clients and caregivers prepare for the impending death. The achievement of these outcomes helped therapists feel that they had made a difference in clients' lives and led to a sense of professional satisfaction (Bye, 1998).

Support Strategies for Therapists

Working with older clients reaching the end of their lives can be challenging and demanding, both professionally and personally. Prochnau, Liu, and Boman's (2003) qualitative study of occupational therapists working in palliative care found that therapists were satisfied with their work and viewed it as a source of personal and spiritual growth. However, therapists recognized the hardships and difficulties or dealing with death on a constant basis and identified the need for effective coping strategies such as ventilating feelings, self-nurturance, finding closure, and establishing clear professional boundaries. It is important for all therapists to build effective support strategies that deal proactively with the issues related to this area of work to help reduce burnout and stress and allow therapists to be more effective and find satisfaction in their work in the long term.

Education

Education is a critical strategy to support therapists entering into palliative care work with older people (Breaden, 1997). It is important to have a good grounding in aged care knowledge and skills, as well as a broad overview of different types of terminal illnesses and their courses, treatment, and outcomes. In addition, professional skills of communication, teamwork, and family-centered practice are essential skills for working effectively using a palliative care approach (Crawford & Price, 2003; Mattingly & Lawlor, 2003).

Education should also arm therapists with more than professional skills and knowledge. It should be an opportunity to examine some of the issues that staff members face when working with people who are dying (Rumbold, 2003). Education should provide opportunities for therapists to explore the meaning of life and death, personal values and beliefs surrounding death and dying, and the impact these have on working with clients. Examination of cultural and spiritual issues related to death and dying can allow therapists to gain awareness of clients' and families' needs during this time (Lickiss, 2003; Maddocks & Rayner, 2003). Even though most undergraduate or graduate health professional curricula contain some or all of these issues, the evidence suggests that in already crowded programs of study, palliative care receives only limited time and resources (Cairns & Yates, 2003).

With experience, therapists will learn a great deal from everyday work with clients. R. Hudson and Richmond (1997) note that each client's death teaches staff something new about the meaning of life and death. In addition, it can be useful to understand and learn about the experiences of clients by reading personal accounts written by people who are older and those who are terminally ill or their family and friends. For example, two honest and moving accounts written by daughters caring for elderly mothers are by the American occupational therapist, author, and academician Betty Hasselkus (1993) and by the French feminist philosopher Simone de Beauvoir (1969). These accounts allow readers to gain insight into the everyday world of people facing the issues of life and death. Therapists can learn a great deal from trying to see the situation from clients' and caregivers' perspectives. It is important to also read accounts that offer insight for therapists into cultural issues surrounding death and dying. This is particularly relevant when therapists are working with clients and families from cultural backgrounds other than their own or indigenous communities where the issues of loss and grief are prevalent due to historical political and social factors (Maddocks & Rayner, 2003). Integration of on-the-job learning, personal experience, and knowledge gained through formal education is essential for a well-rounded and skillful palliative care therapist.

Supportive Spiritual Rituals

Working with people who are dying has been shown to be particularly stressful, with health professionals at risk of burnout (J. M. Holland & Neimeyer, 2005). The symptoms of burnout include physical fatigue, cognitive weariness, and emotional exhaustion (J. M. Holland & Neimeyer, 2005). However, there are key strategies therapists can put into place to protect against the fatigue of being a caregiver constantly exposed to dying, death, and loss.

There is growing evidence that health care workers who attend to the spiritual aspect of their lives are more protected from burnout and stress when working with people who are dying. Spirituality is a broad term that may include how we find meaning in life, or a sense of coherence and wholeness (Rumbold, 2003). It may or may not pertain to religious expression or beliefs. Some gain a sense of spiritual wholeness by being with those they love, or in beautiful, natural surroundings, or through prayer or meditation (Rumbold, 2003).

J. M. Holland and Neimeyer's (2005) research investigated whether daily spiritual experiences protect health care workers from the unique stress of working with people who are dying. Daily spiritual experiences might include a sense of feeling blessed in daily life, or of being loved by a higher power. In a survey of 80 health professionals, results revealed that the frequency of daily spiritual experiences was negatively associated with workplace burnout. The researchers suggest the creation of workplace environments that encourage spiritual expression through everyday rituals.

There is a need for health care professionals to have a ritualized approach to protection against burnout, rather than casually doing something for yourself only once you are feeling down. Rituals add meaning and structure in our everyday lives (Breaden, 1997). We celebrate the passing of time with rituals such as birthdays and anniversaries. Dying is also surrounded by rituals to remember people's lives and acknowledge their passing. Funerals, remembrance services, prayer, and wakes are all examples of the way death is ritualized in society. Therapists working in palliative care can benefit from establishing their own spiritual rituals to remember clients and reflect on their work (Prochnau et al., 2003). It is common for palliative care or nursing home staff to attend the funerals of some clients to say goodbye to the client and to support the family during bereavement. Some hospice facilities hold regular remembrance services for clients who have died. Staff, hospice volunteers, and family can attend these sessions to remember clients and reflect on the care they provided (Rumbold, 2003). Therapists may also wish to talk about their experiences with other staff to debrief from sad or confronting experiences, visit the client for a final time to say goodbye, or visit the family after the death. Bye (1998) found that some occupational therapists visited the family home a couple of weeks after the death of the client to pick up loaned equipment such as wheelchairs and commodes. Therapists used this time to speak to the family, provide emotional support, and find closure in their work with that client.

Many palliative care settings have established support groups for staff to discuss how they are managing their work and dealing with issues of grief they may be experiencing related to clients' deaths. It is natural and normal for staff working in palliative care to feel these emotions. The important thing is to have effective support strategies in place to deal with these emotions as they arise, rather than allowing them to build up over time. Regular supportive rituals such as attending a support group promoting positive coping strategies and good work practices.

The type of supportive rituals adopted by therapists may be different for each client and will depend on factors such as the depth and length of the client–therapist relationship, the wishes of the family, and therapists' individual styles. "Rituals of remembering" (Breaden, 1997) provide opportunities for therapists to debrief, connect with their own spirituality, find closure, and reflect on the value and meaning of therapy with clients who are dying.

■ Summary

Occupational therapy is an essential component of comprehensive palliative care for older clients. Therapists working in this clinical area need to adopt a particular approach to their work. Adopting a palliative approach to practice means that therapists need to address clients' ongoing lives, as well as facilitate the preparations necessary for the impending death. Helping clients feel a sense of normality in everyday activities and facilitating their sense of control over daily life affirm clients' lives; organizing and providing supportive, safe care and offering opportunities for closure prepare clients for death. Achieving these outcomes assures therapists that they have made a difference in the lives of the clients (Hasselkus & Dickie, 1990, 1994).

Case Study

Marilyn is 70 years of age and lives with her husband Peter who is 74. They have been married for 4 years. Both had been married previously but had lost their spouses to cancer. They met at their local church and were married a year later. Recently Marilyn was diagnosed with liver cancer and is not expected to live more than 2 months. She is quite unwell and is unable to participate in daily activities for very long. She is now very thin and each day she becomes more frail and requires greater assistance from Peter to manage daily activities. She experiences pain and nausea, but some days manages better than others. Peter is now running the household and doing all the community tasks such as shopping and banking with the help of Marilyn's daughter who lives nearby. Marilyn's daughter also assists with Marilyn's personal care as the bathroom has a shower over the bath, and Marilyn finds this difficult to manage.

The couple is very sad as they feel their life together had just started and they had hoped to spend time traveling and spending time with their grandchildren. They were active in their church community and keen members of the volunteer committee helping isolated elderly people to remain in their own homes.

This year Marilyn and Peter had planned a party for their family and friends to celebrate their fifth wedding anniversary. The party is to occur in 4 weeks time but now they don't know whether to have it or not.

They hope that Marilyn can remain at home to die. However, they live close to an inpatient palliative care facility if needed. Marilyn's oncologist has referred her to the palliative care team at this center. The palliative care team will now take over Marilyn's care altogether. The occupational therapist from this team has received a referral to help this family and will be conducting a home visit tomorrow.

Questions

1. What are the issues being experienced by this couple and what goals might Marilyn and Peter have that are pertinent to you as an occupational therapist?
2. What might be some of the fears of Marilyn and Peter?
3. How will you approach this first meeting with Marilyn and Peter and what is your aim in this first visit? How will you explain your role?
4. Who else might you want to talk to in relation to their situation?
5. What types of intervention seem necessary and what is your time frame for intervention?
6. How will you monitor this family's progress?
7. What support services might the family require once Marilyn has died?

Review Questions

1. What personal experiences and beliefs do you have regarding old age and death and dying? How will these experiences and your beliefs influence your work in palliative care with older clients?
2. How does a person's life stage impact on their view of impending death and what factors may influence their acceptance or fear of this process?
3. How can occupational therapy enhance participation at the end stage of life despite a client's many health problems and activity limitations?
4. When working with an older client who is terminally ill, why do you need to take a "low key" approach to assessment of their occupational performance?
5. How will you ensure occupational therapy goals and intervention are client centered? Why is this an important approach for these clients?
6. Reflect on why you chose to become a therapist and what makes you satisfied in your work. Do you enjoy making a difference in clients' lives? What do you need to achieve to feel satisfied and successful as a palliative care therapist?

Web-Based Resources

For helpful information about the experience in the end of life, visit:

www.nethealthinc.com/cultural/, **Western Reserve Geriatric Education Center (2006),** date connected March 3, 2007. Online information about end of life. Units V and VI in particular deal with these issues.

www.growthhouse.org/palliat.html, **Growthhouse.org,** date connected October 12, 2007. Focuses primarily on medical aspects of palliative care and includes a variety of resources and links.

www.nhpco.org/templates/1/homepage.cfm, **National Hospice and Palliative Care Organization (n.d.),** date connected October 12, 2007. Focuses primarily on policy and advocacy to increase availability and quality of palliative care.

www.capc.org, **Center to Advance Palliative Care (2007),** date connected October 12, 2007. Provides information about educational opportunities, resources for practitioners, and links to other resources.

REFERENCES

Amella, E. J. (2003). Geriatrics and palliative care: Collaboration for quality of life until death. *Journal of Hospice and Palliative Care Nursing, 5*(1), 40–48.

American Occupational Therapy Association (AOTA). (2002). Occupational Therapy Practice Framework: Domain and process. *American Journal of Occupational Therapy, 56,* 609–639.

American Occupational Therapy Association (AOTA). (2005). Occupational therapy and hospice. *American Journal of Occupational Therapy, 59*(6), 671–675.

Baxandall, S., & Reddy, P. (1993). *The courage to care: The impact of cancer on the family.* Melbourne, Australia: David Lovell.

Bennahum, D. A. (1996). The historical development of hospice and palliative care. In D. C. Sheehan & W. B. Forman (Eds.), *Hospice and palliative care: Concepts and practice* (pp. 1–10). Sudbury, MA: Jones & Bartlett.

Bennett, K. M., Smith, P. T., & Hughes, G. M. (2005). Coping, depressive feelings and gender differences in late life widowhood. *Aging and Mental Health, 9*(4), 348–353.

Bennett, S. (1991). Issues confronting occupational therapists working with terminally ill patients. *British Journal of Occupational Therapy, 54,* 8–10.

Biswas, D. (1993). The medicalization of dying. In D. Clark (Ed.), *The future for palliative care* (pp. 132–139). Buckingham, England: Open University Press.

Black, H. K. (2006). The sacred self: Suffering narratives in old age. *Omega, 53*(1–2), 69–85.

Breaden, K. (1997). In the twilight: Alzheimer's disease and palliative care. In I. Maddocks (Ed.), *Palliative care: A study text* (pp. 281–291). South Australia: International Institute of Hospice Studies.

Bye, R. (1998). When clients are dying: Occupational therapists' perspectives. *Occupational Therapy Journal of Research, 18,* 3–24.

Cairns, W., & Yates, P. M. (2003). Education in palliative care. *Medical Journal of Australia, 179,* S26–S28.

Carlson, R. (1997). *Don't sweat the small stuff ... and it's all small stuff.* Sydney: Bantam Books.

Chasteen, A. L., & Madey, S. F. (2003). Belief in a just world and the perceived injustice of dying young or old. *Omega, 47*(4), 313–326.

Cooper, J., & Littlechild, B. (2004). A study of occupational therapy interventions in oncology and palliative care. *International Journal of Therapy and Rehabilitation, 11*(7), 329–333.

Crawford, G. B., & Price, S. D. (2003). Team working: Palliative care as a model of interdisciplinary practice. *Medical Journal of Australia, 179,* S32–S34.

Curtis, J. R., Patrick, D. L., Engelberg, R. A., Norris, K., Asp, C., & Byock, I. (2002). A measure of the quality of dying and death: Initial validation using after-death interviews with family members. *Journal of Pain and Symptom Management, 24*(1), 17–31.

Dalby, P. (2006). Is there a process of spiritual change or development associated with ageing? A critical review of research. *Aging and Mental Health, 10*(1), 4–12.

Davies, E. (2004). *What are the palliative care needs of older people and how might they be met?* Copenhagen: WHO Regional Office for Europe. Health Evidence Network Report: retrieved January 7, 2007, from www.euro.who.int/Document/E83747.pdf.

Davies, E., & Higginson, I. J. (2004). *Better palliative care for older people.* World Health Organization, Europe. Retrieved January 7, 2007, from www.euro.who.int.

Dawson, S. S. (1982). The role of occupational therapy in palliative care. *Australian Occupational Therapy Journal, 29,* 119–124.

Dawson, S., & Barker, J. (1995). Hospice and palliative care: A Delphi survey of occupational therapists' roles and training needs. *Australian Occupational Therapy Journal, 42,* 119–127.

de Beauvoir, S. (1969). *A very easy death.* England: Penguin, Harmondsworth.

DeSpelder, L. A., & Strickland, A. L. (1992) *The last dance. Encountering death and dying* (3rd ed.). Mountain View, CA: Mayfield.

Doyle, D., Hanks, G., Cherney, N. I., & Calman, K. (1998). Introduction. In D. Doyle, G. Hanks, N. I. Cherney, & K. Calman (Eds.), *Oxford textbook of palliative medicine* (2nd ed., pp. 3–8). England: Oxford University Press.

Flanigan, K. (1982). The art of the possible . . . occupational therapy in terminal care. *British Journal of Occupational Therapy, 45,* 274–276.

Fortner, B. V., & Neimeyer, R. A. (1999). Death anxiety in older adults: A quantitative review. *Death Studies, 23,* 387–411.

Fry, P. S. (2003). Perceived self-efficacy domains as predictors of fear of the unknown and fear of dying among older adults. *Psychology and Aging, 18*(3), 474–486.

Giles, H., & Reid, S. A. (2005). Ageism across the lifespan: Towards a self-categorization model of aging. *Journal of Social Issues, 61*(2), 389–404.

Glare, P. A., Auret, K. A., Aggarwal, G., Clark, K. J., Pickstock, S. E., & Lickiss, J. N. (2003). The interface between palliative medicine and specialists in acute-care hospitals: Boundaries, bridges and challenges. *Medical Journal of Australia, 179,* S29–S31.

Gray, R. (1989). The role of physiotherapy in hospice care. *Physiotherapy Practice, 5,* 9–16.

Hasselkus, B. R. (1993). Death in very old age: A personal journey of caregiving. *American Journal of Occupational Therapy, 47,* 717–723.

Hasselkus, B. R., & Dickie, V. A. (1990). Themes of meaning: Occupational therapists' perspectives on practice. *Occupational Therapy Journal of Research, 10,* 195–206.

Hasselkus, B. R., & Dickie, V. A. (1994). Doing occupational therapy: Dimensions of satisfaction and dissatisfaction. *American Journal of Occupational Therapy, 48,*145–154.

Hockley, J., & Mowatt, M. (1996). Rehabilitation. In R. A. Fisher & P. McDaid (Eds.), *Palliative day care* (pp. 13–21). London: Arnold.

Holland, A. E., & Tigges, K. N. (1981). The hospice movement. A time for professional action and commitment. *British Journal of Occupational Therapy, 44*(12), 373–376.

Holland, J. M., & Neimeyer, R. A. (2005). Reducing the risk of burnout in end-of-life-care setting: The role of daily spiritual experiences and training. *Palliative and Supportive Care, 3,* 173–181.

Hudson, P. (2003). Home-based support for palliative care families: Challenges and recommendations. *Medical Journal of Australia, 179,* S35–S37.

Hudson, R., & Richmond, J. (1997). The meaning of death in residential aged care. In I. Maddocks (Ed.), *Palliative care: A study text* (pp. 292–302). South Australia: International Institute of Hospice Studies.

Jacques, N. D., & Hasselkus, B. R. (2004). The nature of occupation surrounding dying and death. *Occupational Therapy Journal of Research, 24*(2), 44–53.

Kaufman, S. R. (2000). Senescence, decline, and the quest for a good death. *Journal of Aging Studies, 14*(1), 1–23.

Kealey, P., & McIntyre, I. (2005). An evaluation of the domiciliary occupational therapy service in palliative cancer care in a community trust: A patient and carers perspective. *European Journal of Cancer Care, 14,* 232–243.

Kellehear, A. (1984). Are we a "death-denying" society? A sociological review. *Social Science and Medicine, 18,* 713–723.

Kellehear, A. (1990) *Dying of cancer. The final year of life.* London: Harwood Academic.

Kellehear, A., & Lewin, T. (1989) Farewells by the dying: A sociological study. *Omega, Journal of Death and Dying, 19,* 275–292.

Kristjanson, L. J., Toye, C., & Dawson, S. (2003). New dimensions in palliative care: A palliative approach to neurodegenerative diseases and final illness in older people. *Medical Journal of Australia, 179,* S41–S43.

Kubler-Ross, E. (1969). *On death and dying.* New York: Macmillan.

Lewis, C. B., & Bottomley, J. M. (1994). *Geriatric physical therapy: A clinical approach.* Norwalk, CT: Appleton & Lange.

Lickiss, J. N. (2003). Approaching death in multicultural Australia. *Medical Journal of Australia, 179,* S14–S16.

Lindley-Davis, B. (1991). Process of dying: Defining characteristics. *Cancer Nursing, 14,* 328–333.

Lloyd, C., & Coggles, L. (1990). Psychosocial issues for people with cancer and their families. *Canadian Journal of Occupational Therapy, 57,* 211–215.

Lyons, M., Orozovic, N., Davis, J., & Newman, J. (2002). Doing-being-becoming: Occupational experiences of persons with life-threatening illnesses. *American Journal of Occupational Therapy, 56*(3), 285–295.

Maddocks, I., & Raynor, R. G. (2003). Issues in palliative care for indigenous communities. *Medical Journal of Australia, 179,* S17–S19.

Mason, M. (1993). The treatment of lymphoedema by complex physical therapy. *Australian Journal of Physiotherapy, 39,* 41–45.

Mattingly, C. F., & Lawlor, M. C. (2003). Disability experience from a family perspective. In E. B. Crepeau, E. S. Cohn, & B. A. Boyt-Schell (Eds.), *Willard and Spackman's occupational therapy* (10th ed., pp. 69–79). Philadelphia: Lippincott, Williams, & Wilkins.

McNamara, B., Waddell, C., & Colvin, M. (1995). Threats to the good death: The cultural context of stress and coping among hospice nurses. *Sociology of Health & Illness, 17,* 222–244.

Mesler, M. A. (1995). The philosophy and practice of patient control in hospice: The dynamics of autonomy versus paternalism. *Omega, Journal of Death and Dying, 30,* 173–189.

Moremen, R. D. (2005). What is the meaning of life? Women's spirituality at the end of the lifespan. *Omega, 50*(4), 309–330.

Murray, J. L., & Lopez, A. D. (1997). Alternative projections of mortality and disability by causes 1990–2020. Global burden of diseases study. *Lancet, 349,* 1498–1504.

Murray, S. A., Kendall, M., Boyd, K., & Sheikh, A. (2005). Illness trajectories and palliative care. *British Medical Journal, 330,* 1007–1011.

Neimeyer, R. A., Wittkowski, J., & Moser, R. P. (2004). Psychological research on death attitudes: An overview and evaluation. *Death Studies, 28,* 309–340.

Oelrich, M. (1974). The patient with a fatal illness. *American Journal of Occupational Therapy, 28,* 429–432.

Patrick, D. L., Curtis, J. R., Engelberg, R. A., Nielsen, E., & McCown, E. (2003). Measuring and improving the quality of dying and death. *Annals of Internal Medicine, 139*(5, part 2), 410–415.

Pizzi, M. (1984). Occupational therapy in hospice care. *American Journal of Occupational Therapy, 38,* 252–257.

Pizzi, M. (1986). Care of the terminally ill, part 1: General principles. In L. J. Davis & M. Kirkland (Eds.), *The role of occupational therapy with the elderly* (pp. 241–249). Rockville, MD: American Occupational Therapy Association.

Pleschberger, S. (2007). Dignity and the challenge of dying in nursing homes: The residents' view. *Age and Ageing, 36*(2), 197–202.

Prochnau, C., Liu, L., & Boman, J. (2003). Personal–professional connections in palliative care occupational therapy. *American Journal of Occupational Therapy, 57*(2), 196–204.

Rashleigh, L. (1996). Physiotherapy in palliative oncology. *Australian Journal of Physiotherapy, 42*(4), 307–312.

Reimer, J. C., & Davies, B. (1991). Palliative care: The nurse's role of helping families through the transition of "fading away." *Cancer Nursing, 14,* 321–327.

Romsas, E. P., & Rosa, S. A. (1985). Occupational therapy intervention for cancer patients with metastatic disease. *American Journal of Occupational Therapy, 39,* 79–83.

Rumbold, B. D. (2003). Caring for the spirit: Lessons from working with the dying. *Medical Journal of Australia, 179,* S11–S13.

Sampson, E. L., Ritchie, C. W., Lai, R., Raven, P. W., & Blanchard, M. R. (2005). A systematic review of the scientific evidence for the efficacy of a palliative care approach in advanced dementia. *International Psychogeriatrics, 17*(1), 31–40.

Saunders, C. M. (1983). The last stages of life. In C. A. Corr & D. M. Corr (Eds.), *Hospice care: Principles and practice* (pp. 5–11). London: Faber & Faber.

Saunders, C. (1998). Foreword. In D. Doyle et al. (Eds.), *Oxford textbook of palliative medicine* (2nd ed., pp. v–ix). England: Oxford University Press.

Tigges, K. N. (1983). Occupational therapy in hospice. In C. A. Corr & D. M. Corr (Eds.), *Hospice care. Principles and practice* (pp. 160–176). New York: Springer.

Tigges, K. N. (1986). Occupational therapy in hospice care. In L. Davis (Ed.), *Role of occupational therapy with the elderly* (pp. 261–264). Rockville, MD: American Occupational Therapy Association.

Tigges, K. N. (1998). Occupational therapy. In D. Doyle, G. Hanks, N. I. Cherney, & K. Calman (Eds.), *Oxford textbook of palliative medicine* (2nd ed., pp. 829–887). England: Oxford University Press.

Tigges, K. N., & Marcil, W. M. (1988). *Terminal and life threatening illness: An occupational behaviour perspective.* Thorofare, NJ: SLACK.

Tigges, K. N., & Sherman, L. M. (1983). The treatment of the hospice patient: From occupational history to occupational role. *American Journal of Occupational Therapy, 37,* 235–238.

Werth, J. L., Gordon, J. R., & Johnson, R. R. (2002). Psychosocial issues near the end of life. *Ageing and Mental Health, 6*(4), 402–412.

Woodruff, R. (1993). *Palliative medicine.* Melbourne, Australia: Asperula Pty Ltd.

World Health Organization (WHO). (2007). *WHO definition of palliative care.* Retrieved January 7, 2007, from www.who.int/cancer/palliative/definition/en/.

GLOSSARY

ABLEDATA: An Internet directory that provides a searchable database of assistive technology and rehabilitation devices.

Accommodation: The ability of the lens to adjust in order to keep objects focused on the retina.

Active life expectancy: The number of years of life that can be anticipated to be relatively free of disease and dysfunction that might limit participation in meaningful occupations.

Activity (ICF): The execution of a task or action by an individual; societal perspective of function.

Actual occupational performance: What an individual actually does.

Acute Care for the Elderly units (ACE): Specialized units providing acute care services for older adults, using a client-centered team approach.

Adaptable design: Involves making modifications to a standard design for the use of a particular individual with a disability, like adding large grips to kitchen utensils to help someone with rheumatoid arthritis (Story, 1998).

Adherence: The extent to which a client follows a health care professional's advice or recommendations.

ADL: Activities of daily living—an area of occupation that includes activities oriented toward taking care of one's own body. Also referred to as Basic Activities of Daily Living (BADL) and Personal Activities of Daily Living (PADL).

Agency: The ability of the individual to act on the environment.

Aging in place: Growing old in one's home and home community.

Age-related macular degeneration (AMD): An eye disease associated with aging that results in degeneration of the center of the retina (macula) and that gradually affects central vision.

Air conduction hearing test (audiometry): Hearing test in which tones of various frequencies are transmitted through binaural headphones.

Alternating attention: The capacity for mental flexibility that enables one to shift the focus of attention and move between tasks having different cognitive requirements (Parente & Anderson, 1991).

Amyloidosis: A histologic feature of aging characterized by the progressive deposition of amyloid protein.

Androgogy: The instructional process for adults.

Ankylosing spondylosis: A chronic inflammatory disease of the spine and sacroiliac.

Anorgasmia: The inability to reach orgasm.

Area agency on aging: A public or private non-profit agency designated by the state to address the needs and concerns of older adults as well as to implement the Older Americans Act at the local level.

Assessment: Refers to specific tools or instruments used during the evaluation process (AOTA, 1995).

Assistive Technology: A commercial, custom-fabricated, or homemade device.

Assistive technology device: Any item, piece of equipment, or product system, whether acquired commercially off the shelf, modified or customized, that is used to increase, maintain, or improve functional capabilities of individuals with disabilities (Technology Related Assistance for Individuals with Disabilities Act of 1988).

Astigmatism: A condition in which the cornea or lens has an abnormal curve, causing out-of-focus vision.

Atrial Fibrillation: An abnormal rhythm of the heart caused by irregular and rapid electrical discharges; as a result, the heart beats irregularly and, usually, rapidly.

Audiograms: Charts of hearing values.

Autotelic aspect: The individual experiences most or all of the various aspects of the activity as pleasurable, whether or not the activity was originally undertaken for its intrinsic value.

Baroreflex: Reflex sensitive to mechanical changes produced when pressure in the vessels in which it is located is altered.

Body function (ICF): The physiological or psychological function of a body system.

Body structure (ICF): The anatomical part of the body, such as an organ or limb and their components.

Bone mineral density: The amount of bone loss subtracted from the peak bone mass; measured in grams per unit area or volume.

Bone quality: Extent of architecture, mineralization, accumulated damage, and bone turnover.

Bone remodeling: The coordinated activity of **osteoblasts** and **osteoclasts.**

Cadence: Number of steps per unit of time.

Cardiac Output (CO): Stroke volume (amount of blood pumped by the heart in one contraction) × heart rate.

Caregiver: Person providing care to another. Informal caregivers are often spouse or partner, children, family members, and friends. Formal caregivers are various health professionals or paid support personnel.

Carotid sinus node disease: A condition of the sinus node (the heart's natural pacemaker) that causes insufficient or abnormal electrical impulses (arrhythmias).

Case Management: A system for assessing, planning treatment for, referring, and following up on clients in order to ensure the provision of continuous, comprehensive service and the coordination of payment and reimbursement for care.

Case Manager: An experienced health professional that works with clients, providers and insurers to coordinate all services deemed necessary to provide the client with a plan of medically necessary and appropriate health care.

Case mix adjustment: A Medicare term to describe the strategies used to adjust reimbursement for home health services based on the range of complexity of the needs of clients being seen.

Cataracts: A condition in which a cloudy or opaque area develops in the lens of the eye.

Catecholamine: Vasoactive neurotransmitter; also stimulates the sympathetic response in the fight-or-flight mechanism.

Choice reaction time: Time interval from the onset of a specific stimulus and paired specific response.

Chronic disease self-management: Individuals and families actively participating in the health care process, self-monitoring of symptoms or physiological processes, making informed decisions about their health, and managing the impact of the disease on their daily life.

Clinical utility: Usefulness of the particular assessment considering such aspects as the amount of time to complete, costs, ease of administration and interpretation, training requirements to administer the assessment, and availability of assessment manual and materials.

Cohort: A group of individuals of a particular age group who have shared historical events that have influenced their lives.

Cohort effect: The finding that a particular generation of individuals (a cohort) will have been influenced by historical and societal events that occurred during their lifetime.

Coitus: Sexual intercourse.

Colle's fracture: Fracture of the distal end of the radius.

Commission on Accreditation of Rehabilitation Facilities (CARF): An independent, not-for-profit organization that conducts an in-depth review of the quality of services offered by rehabilitation service providers and grants or denies accreditation dependent on whether the provider meets national standards of consumer-focused, state-of-the-art performance.

Comorbidity: Concurrent medical conditions that an individual exhibits in addition to the presenting medical problem.

Compliance (lung): The ratio of the change in lung volume to the change in transpulmonary pressure; an expression of the extensibility of the lung.

Comprehensive Geriatric Assessment (CGA): A multidimensional, interdisciplinary process that is used to determine an elderly person's medical, psychosocial, functional, and environmental needs, resources, and problems.

Comprehensive Outpatient Rehabilitation Facility (CORF): Term used to designate providers that offer a defined set of outpatient rehabilitation services that can be reimbursed.

Conductive hearing loss: Hearing loss associated with sound not being conducted efficiently through the outer ear or middle ear, or both.

Continuum of care: The system of services that support the well-being of older adults at every stage of functioning from independence to dependence.

Contrast sensitivity: The ability to see a target when there is limited contrast between the target and the background (Hyvarinen, 1996).

Convergence: The simultaneous inward movement of both eyes toward each other, typically in an effort to maintain single binocular vision.

Coping strategies: Strategies, either helpful or unhelpful, that are attempts to remedy problems.

Cornea: The eye's tough outer cover.

Crepitus: A grating, crunching, or popping sensation that occurs as a joint moves through range of motion.

Crystallized abilities: The accumulated practical skills and knowledge of the individual.

Culture: "The set of beliefs, rules of behavior, and customary behaviors maintained, practiced, and transmitted in a given society" (Hahn, 1995, p. 42).

Cultural competency: "Cultural and linguistic competence is a set of congruent behaviors, attitudes, and policies that come together in a system, agency, or among professionals that enables effective work in cross-cultural situations" (HHS Office of the Secretary, 2000, p. 80865).

Dark adaptation: The ability of the eye to recover its sensitivity in the dark, following exposure to a bright light.

Dead space: The volume of the lung that is not involved in gas exchange.

Declarative (explicit) memory: Refers to all memories that are consciously available, that is, information stored and retrieved explicitly from the external world. This information is about a specific event that has occurred at a specific time and place. Declarative memory also has two major subdivisions: **episodic memory** and **semantic memory.**

Decubitus ulcer: Ulcer caused by prolonged pressure over the affected area.

Deep venous thrombosis: Blood clot in a deep vein.

Dependency ratio: The ratio of individuals in paid employment (typically adults) to those ostensibly depending on them for financial support (usually children and elders who are not in the workforce).

Depth perception: A skill that allows one to judge distances away from the self (Zoltan, 1996).

Descriptive: Relative to the purpose of assessments, this includes the gathering of information to portray particular characteristics of individuals and enables the evaluator to differentiate or discriminate between people on the specific characteristic being measured (Law, 1987).

Diabetic retinopathy: The most common eye disease in people with diabetes, resulting from damage to the blood vessels in the retina.

Dichotic listening: Simultaneous presentation of different material to each ear.

Diffusing capacity: The ability of oxygen to diffuse from the alveolar airspaces into the pulmonary capillary.

Dihydroepiandosterone sulfate (DHEAS): Hormone produced primarily in the adrenal gland, where it reflects adrenal androgen production.

Disability: Limitation or inability to participate in roles and activities expected of an individual in a society because of impairments.

Disuse atrophy: Muscle atrophy that occurs with lack of physical activity.

Diuresis: Increased excretion of urine.

Divided attention: The allocation of attention to monitor stimuli simultaneously or to be able to perform multiple tasks at the same time.

Dose response: A relationship in which the change in amount, intensity, or duration of exposure is associated with a change in either an increase or decrease in risk of a specified outcome, such as body function or health response.

Double disability: A condition in which depression accompanies another physical or cognitive diagnosis, causing intensified functional loss because of the interaction of the two conditions.

Drusen: Yellow deposits of extracellular material in the macula.

Dynamic visual acuity: The ability to distinguish fine detail for objects moving relative to the observer (Keplinger, Schinar, & Scheiber, 1991).

Elder abuse: The infliction of injury or suffering on an older adult by her/himself or a trusted other person, usually a family member.

Elder abuse forms: Broad categories that incorporate examples of the problem with similar characteristics.

Encoding: The process by which information is moved from immediate memory to long-term memory.

Environment: Context within which one lives including the cultural, economic, institutional, physical, and social aspects or conditions.

Environmental press: The extent to which factors external to the individual affect the ease or difficulty of completing a task.

Episode of care: A Medicare term used to describe a single 60-day period for which service has been authorized.

Episodic memory: Relates to the types of memory that result from specific incidents in a life time.

Ethno-relativism: The belief that all cultures are equally valid and deserving of respect.

Evaluation: The gathering of information in order to assess and categorize, make appraisals, estimates, judgements; refers to "the process of obtaining and interpreting data necessary for intervention" (AOTA, 1995, p. 1072).

Everyday competence: Ability to accomplish normal daily tasks effectively and efficiently.

Everyday memory: A term used to describe the kind of memory needed to accomplish daily activities.

Extended Family: Blood relatives and in-laws beyond parents, children, and spouse. May include siblings, aunts, uncles, nieces, and nephews.

Family of origin: Family of one's youth, usually grandparents, parents, and siblings, although some definitions include aunts, uncles, and others.

Fictive kin: Individuals perceived as having family-like relationships, drawn together through voluntary choice.

Flow (synonyms): Involvement, serious leisure, committed leisure. The total engagement in an activity that characterizes leisure.

Fluid intelligence: The ability to adapt to and use new information in reasoning, solving, and integrating problems or novel information, corresponds to the subtests of the WAIS Performance scale.

Focused attention: The ability to focus on relevant stimuli.

Formal care network: Services and resources provided to older adults from agencies, institutions, and established housing options.

Frailty: An age-related pathological state of loss of physiologic reserve that leads to physical impairments, functional limitations, and disability.

Freezing: A sudden, unforeseen state of immobility. A clinical feature of Parkinson's disease and typically occurs during walking, attempts with turning, approaching a destination, or during the sequential execution of distinct movements.

Functional performance: The ability to engage in activities which are important to the individual within his or her environment

Functional Residual Capacity: The volume of air remaining in the lungs at the end of a normal expiration.

General Activities Programs: Events or tasks that satisfy interests and/or meet general activity needs which focus on enjoyment, stimulation, and repetition of present skills.

Geriatric Assessment Unit (GAU)/Geriatric Evaluation Unit (GEU): A distinct unit housed within a community hospital, a free-standing rehabilitation hospital, or a long-term care facility. Staffed by multi-disciplinary teams specializing in the management of the medical, social, physical, psychological, and economic well-being of older adults; rehabilitation goals are usually short-term.

Geriatric Evaluation and Management Unit (GEM): Typically a separate hospital ward that has been designed to facilitate care of the older adult client; provides interdisciplinary management of medical, rehabilitation, and psychosocial issues in an inpatient setting.

Geriatric Rehabilitation Unit (GAU): A distinct unit housed within a community hospital, a free-standing rehabilitation hospital, or a long-term care facility. Staffed by multi-disciplinary teams specializing in the management of the medical, social, physical, psychological, and economic well-being of older adults; rehabilitation goals are usually long-term.

Glaucoma: A condition in which fluid builds in the eyeball, resulting in increased intraocular pressure.

Global attention: Refers to all aspects of the ability to focus on stimuli in the environment and to process them.

Goal attainment scaling (GAS): An individualized measurement approach. It is a method of setting individualized client goals and measuring their attainment. GAS uses a 5-point rating scale (from $+2$ to -2) to reflect different levels of attainment with $+2$ being "much better than expected," $+1$ being "somewhat better than expected," 0 being the expected level of achievement, -1 being "somewhat less than expected" and -2 being much less than expected.

Good death: Conveys the idea that the emotional and physical challenges of dying can be addressed in such a way that death occurs in a comfortable and comforting environment.

Guanosine monophosphate (cGMP): Nucleotide that is found in RNA. It consists of the phosphate group, the pentose sugar ribose, and the nucleobase guanine.

Half-life: The time required to metabolize half of the amount of a substance taken in.

Happiness: A positive affect in the present moment.

Happy life expectancy: The number of years during which an individual can expect to live happily.

Health literacy: The capacity to obtain, process, and understand basic health information and services needed to make appropriate health decisions (USDHHS, 2000).

Health promotion: An approach to intervention focused on maintaining health and avoiding disease, rather than on treating disease once it has occurred.

Heart block: A condition in which conduction of the electrical impulses of the heart are faulty, causing a lack of coordination in the contraction of the atria and ventricles.

Heart rate reserve: Heart rate reserve = resting heart rate + (maximum heart rate − resting heart rate).

Hematoma: A confined swelling or mass of blood.

High-tech device: Typically involves microprocessors, and includes computer hardware and software.

Homebound status: Being unable to leave one's home unassisted.

Hospice: The hospice philosophy is based on minimizing pain and controlling symptoms by meeting the physical, psychological, emotional, and spiritual needs of both people with terminal illness and their families (Tigges & Marcil, 1988) once cure is no longer an option.

Hypokalemia: Extreme potassium depletion.

Hypostatic pneumonia: Pneumonia common in the elderly or debilitated patients who constantly remain in the same position.

Hypovolemia: Decreased blood volume.

Hypoxia: Deficiency of oxygen.

IADL: Instrumental activities of daily living—an area of occupation that included activities oriented toward interacting with the environment such as shopping or using the telephone.

Impairment: Abnormalities or losses of anatomical, physiological, emotional, or mental functions or structures; abnormalities or losses of the body structures or of a physiological or psychological function (WHO, 1998).

Incidence: Number of new cases of a phenomenon in a population over a period of time.

Informal care network: Services and resources provided to older adults from their families, friends, and neighbors.

Interdisciplinary team: A team in which members are involved in problem-solving beyond the scope of their own discipline, and then work toward goal attainment within their scope of practice.

Iris: Pigmented, circular structure of the eye (e.g., our iris color is our eye color).

Isokinetic strength: Muscle force generated against resistance at a constant rate of movement.

Isometric strength: Static muscle strength.

Isotonic contraction: Muscle activation in which there is a concentric or eccentric contraction of muscle fibers causing joint movement.

Isotonic strength: Dynamic muscle strength.

Kinematic gait analysis: Evaluation of the movement of the body as a whole and/or body segments in relation to each other during ambulation.

Kinesthesia: The sensation and awareness of movement.

Kinetic gait analysis: Evaluation of the forces involved in ambulation.

Kitwood's Model of Dementia: Conceptualized dementia as the manifestation of five factors interacting with one another: personality, biography, neurologic impairment, physical health, and social psychology.

Legally blind: Visual acuity of 20/200 or less in the least affected eye with the use of a correcting lens.

Leisure: An *experience*, that is, the perception that leisure "activities" are intrinsically motivated, freely chosen, and allow one to disengage from some of the concerns of real life.

Lens: Clear, circular structure of the eye that changes shape to bring objects at different distances into focus on the retina.

Lifelong education: An approach to learning that recognizes the ability of individuals to assimilate and apply information throughout their lives.

Life satisfaction: A subjective assessment of life as a whole, both past and present.

Linkage Services: Community resources, such as outreach or information and referral, which connect individuals with available services or service providers with each other.

Long-term (delayed) memory: That part of memory which stores a seemingly unlimited amount of information for an indefinite amount of time (as little as 30 seconds or as long as decades). Long-term memory is typically conceptualized as two types of memory: **declarative (explicit) memory** (which includes **semantic** and **episodic memory**) and **procedural memory.**

Low-tech device: Any device traditionally used by therapists, such as button hooks and reachers.

Low vision: Serious visual loss that is uncorrectable by medical or surgical intervention or with eyeglasses.

Lymphedema: A condition in which swelling occurs distal to a site where lymph nodes have been surgically removed. The lymph system is no longer available to drain fluids from the area.

Macula: Central area of the retina.

Macular degeneration: Deterioration of the central portion of the retina.

Meaningful: Identified by the individual as meeting a central psychological or emotional need, or conveying an important message to self or others.

Meissner's corpuscle: Encapsulated mechanoreceptor sensitive to light touch and vibration.

Metabolic equivalent (MET): One MET is equal to 3.5 mL/kg of body weight per minute.

Middle-old: Older adults between the ages of 76 and 84. This category was not originally identified by Neugarten (1976) when she categorized elders as young-old or old-old, but is sometimes seen in literature on aging.

Mild cognitive impairment: Minor changes in cognitive ability that are noticeable to the individual, but that do not impede normal daily function or rise to the level at which a diagnosis of dementia would be warranted.

Minimum Data Set (MDS): A core set of screening, clinical, and functional status elements, including common definitions and coding categories, that forms the foundation of the comprehensive assessment for all residents of long-term care facilities certified to participate in Medicare or Medicaid.

Monosynaptic connection: A single connection between the axon of one neuron and the dendrite of another.

Montessori-based activities: Activities utilizing Montessori educational principles, which are quite similar to principles used in occupational therapy.

Motivation: The reason one chooses to engage in an activity.

Motor unit: Functional unit of a muscle consisting of a single nerve cell and its axon, plus all muscle fibers innervated by the axon.

Multidisciplinary team: A discipline-oriented team, with each team member responsible for his or her own unique scope of practice.

Muscle power: The ability to generate force rapidly; calculated as the product of the muscle force generated by the velocity of movement.

Muscle synergy: The functional coupling of groups of muscles that act together as a unit.

Mutual cultural accommodation: A process by which all parties in the therapeutic process negotiate an agreement that respects their most central cultural values, but also provides a specific action plan (Bonder et al., 2002).

Myers-Menorah Park/Montessori-Based Assessment System (MMP/MAP): An activities-based assessment system for moderate to advanced dementia providing information to help develop activity programming for long-term care residents.

Myotonia: Tonic spasm or temporary rigidity of one or more muscles, often characteristic of various muscular disorders.

Needs assessment: Data gathering and analysis focused on determining the needs of an individual or a group of individuals, with emphasis on identifying appropriate goals for intervention.

Nuclear family: Most often defined as parents and their children. Sometimes grandparents are included in this network.

Obsolescence: When a worker can no longer do a job because the demands of the job become incongruent with a worker's knowledge, skills, and attitudes.

Occupation: Groups of functional tasks and activities in which a person engages over the life course including self-care, productivity, and leisure.

Occupation (as used in Occupational therapy): Occupation is everything people do to occupy themselves, including looking after themselves, enjoying life, and contributing to the social and economic fabric of their communities.

Occupational performance: The ability to do day-to-day activities to one's satisfaction; the outcome of the transaction that occurs among the person, environment, and occupation.

Occupational performance potential: What an individual is capable of doing.

Oculomotor skills: The coordinated use of extraocular eye muscles necessary for binocular vision and the efficient performance of conjugate eye movements (Warren, 2006).

Oldest-old: Older adults from age 85 on (Neugarten, 1976).

Olfaction: The sense of smell.

Orthostatic hypotension: A drop in blood pressure occurring with a change in position from lying to standing.

Orthostatic Intolerance: The development of symptoms during upright standing.

Orthostatism: The ability of the body to maintain normal cardiac output, in particular, cerebral perfusion, during assumption of the upright body position.

Osteoblasts: Bone cells responsible for bone formation.

Osteoclasts: Bone cells responsible for bone resorption.

Osteopenia: A decrease in bone mineral density.

Ototoxic drugs: Medications that cause damage to the ear, resulting in hearing loss.

Outcome: Change in functional performance over time; measures that are used to evaluate the change following intervention.

Pacinian corpuscle: Encapsulated mechanoreceptor sensitive to vibration and rapid changes in the tissue's mechanical state.

Palliative care: The active total care of patients whose disease is not responsive to curative treatment.

Parenchyma: The key elements of an organ essential to its functioning.

Participation: Ability of an individual to engage in roles and activities expected of an individual within a society; nature and extent of a person's involvement in life situations in relation to impairments, health conditions, activities, and contextual factors; it may be restricted in nature, duration, and quality (WHO, 1998).

Perceived control: Individuals who feel a sense of control over their circumstances.

Peripheral vision: The ability to perceive the presence or movement of stimuli in the periphery beyond the area of immediate focus that constitutes one's central vision (Warren, 2006).

Pernicious anemia: A chronic condition caused by impaired absorption of vitamin B12 due to decreased intrinsic factor secretion.

Phonemes: Speech sounds

Phosphodiesterase 5 (PDE5): An enzyme found in cytoplasm that catalyzes the transfer of a phosphate group to a fructose compound during the metabolism of glucose (Encarta ® World English Dictionary © & (P) 1998–2004 Microsoft Corporation. All rights reserved).

Polymyalgia rheumatica: A disorder characterized by proximal muscle pain and stiffness.

Pitch: Frequency of vibration that qualifies sound from low to high.

Post-prandial hypotension: Drop in blood pressure occurring after a meal.

Postural control: The ability to control the body's position in space for the purposes of **postural orientation** and **postural stability.**

Postural orientation: The ability to maintain an appropriate relationship between body segments, and between the body and the environment for a task (Horak & Macpherson, 1996).

Postural stability: Balance

Postural sway: Small oscillating movements of the body over the feet during bipedal standing.

Prediction: To foretell on the basis of observation, experience, or assessment; in the situation of assessments, to include items related to a specific characteristic in order to forecast another trait; see examples in text.

Premature ventricular contraction: A condition in which the ventricles electrically discharge and contract before the normal electrical discharges arrive from the SA node.

Premorbid: Prior to the development of the disease.

Presycusis: Age-related progressive loss of hearing.

Presbyopia: Age-related decline of accommodation for near vision.

Prevalence: Total number of cases of a phenomenon in a particular population at a specific time.

Prevention: Approaches in OT that focus on individuals at-risk for occupational performance problems; designed to promote healthy lifestyles.

Preventive occupation: The "application of occupational science in the prevention of disease and disability and the promotion of health and well-being of individuals and communities through meaningful engagement in occupations" (Scaffa, 2001).

Problem-solving: Systematic efforts to understand the characteristics of problems and identify potential strategies for remedying them.

Procedural (non-declarative or implicit) memory: Refers to memory that is expressed through performance rather than conscious recall, such as information acquired through skill learning (e.g., how to ride a bicycle), habit formation (e.g., knowing to put toothpaste on the toothbrush before brushing one's teeth), classical conditioning, emotional learning, and priming.

Product and technology: "Natural or human made products or systems of products, equipment, and technology in an individual's immediate environment, that are gathered, created, produced or manufactured" (WHO, p. 591).

Professional competence: Ability to function effectively in the tasks considered essential in a profession.

Program evaluation: A systematic process of examining the effectiveness of a program, to determine whether it is accomplishing its goals or needs modification.

Programmed (developmental-genetic) theories: Explain aging as the result of genetically pre-programmed changes in structure and function of cells and the organism.

Proprioception: The awareness of body segments in relationship to each other and in relationship to the environment.

Prospective memory: The ability to remember future intentions (Sohlberg & Mateer, 1989)

Prospective payment system: An insurance system in which the insurer identifies what it will pay prior to the delivery of care.

Pseudodementia: Depression that presents with symptoms similar to those of other dementias, but characterized by slowed response, poor attention, and psychomotor retardation.

Psychomotor retardation: Slowing of cognitive and motor processes subsyndromal depression: a pattern of depressive symptoms that are not severe or pervasive enough to meet the diagnostic criteria for a depressive disorder.

Pupil: The opening in the iris through which light enters the eye.

Purposeful Activity: Goal-directed behaviors that the individual considers meaningful.

Quality of life: A qualitative or subjective assessment of current circumstances.

Recumbency: Lying down

Rehabilitation efficiency: The amount of functional gains per day of service.

Reliability: Accuracy or precision of a measure; if we measure the same thing again and again, will we get the same or similar results?

Religion: "Consists of socially shared patterns of behavior and belief that seek to relate humans to the superhuman" (Howard & Howard, 1997 pp. 181–182).

Reporting: Referral of situations known or suspected to reflect a specific problem to agencies charged under law to investigate it.

Residual volume: The volume of air remaining in the lungs after a maximal expiration.

Retrospective payment: Payment based on the actual cost of care provided for a client.

Sarcopenia: Loss of muscle mass associated with aging.

Sclera: The tough, opaque eye tissue; the eye's protective outer coat—"the white of the eye."

Scotomas: Blind spots in the eye's field of vision.

Screening: Usually a short, easy to administer and accurate assessment of a particular function such as depression or mental status; often used to determine if more testing is needed.

Screening or assessment instruments: Various tools developed to improve and systematize the process of identifying persons experiencing specific problems, those at risk of the problems, or both.

Secondary (long-term) memory: Contains an unlimited amount of information for almost any length of time (Grady, 1998).

Selective attention: Ability to filter extraneous or distracting stimuli.

Self-efficacy: A belief that one can organize and execute courses of action needed to achieve a desired goal or succeed at a desired undertaking.

Semantic memory: The ability to store and recall meaning (Harrell, et al., 1992).

Senior centers: Organized environments that provide recreational, educational, and nutritional group activities and coordinate various social and health services for older adults.

Sensorineuronal hearing loss: Hearing loss secondary to problems with the cochlea and neural connections to the brain and auditory cortex.

Sensory modality: A communication channel associated with one of the senses; an input channel.

Service systems: Organized groups of programs and procedures that function interdependently to address particular problems or needs.

Short-term (immediate) memory (also sometimes referred to as "primary" or "active" memory): That part of memory which stores a limited amount of information for a limited amount of time (roughly 15–45 seconds). In order to overcome this, and retain information for longer, information must be periodically repeated, or *rehearsed*—either by articulating it out loud, or by mentally simulating such articulation. In this way, the information will re-enter the short-term store and be retained for a further period.

Simple reaction time: Time interval from the onset of a simple stimulus to the response.

Social participation: "Activities associated with organized patterns of behavior that are characteristic and expected for an individual interacting with others within a given social context" (AOTA, 2002).

Sociocusis: Hearing loss due to repeated noise exposure.

Somesthesia: Awareness of sensations, for example, light and deep touch, vibration, pain, and temperature.

Spaced Retrieval (SR): Giving persons practice successfully remembering information over increasing time intervals.

Spirituality: "Stresses the person's subjective perception and experience of something or someone greater than himself or herself" (Howard & Howard, p. 181).

Stigma: Prejudicial devaluing by a social group based on some characteristic or trait.

Standardized: In this case, an assessment that has been developed to be administered in a specific way which may include specific instructions, specific materials to be presented in a specified way, and so on; therapists may require training to use standardized assessments; and standardized assessments must be administered in a standard fashion to maintain the integrity of the instrument and the findings.

Stochastic theories: Explain aging as resulting from the accumulation of "insults" from the environment, which eventually reach a level incompatible with life.

Stria vascularis: The upper part of the spiral ligament of the scala media that contains numerous small blood vessels.

Stride length: The distance from the point of heel strike of one extremity to the point of heel strike of the same extremity.

Stroke volume: The amount of blood pumped by the heart in one contraction.

Sub-acute care: An alternative to prolonged hospitalization for the medically stable patient in need of intense therapies, close monitoring, and/or extensive nursing interventions.

Subjective well-being: A perception by the individual that he or she is currently experiencing a positive sense of life and circumstances with regard to both subjective and objective measures, including living environment, income, and other relevant factors.

Substance P: Major neurotransmitters of primary afferent nociceptive fibers.

Successful aging: A concept proposed by many gerontologists, and popularized by Rowe and Kahn (1998) that suggests that the aging process is a positive one for elders who are able to maintain meaningful engagement with activities, avoid disease and disability, and maintain health.

Sustained attention: Ability to maintain focus over time.

Syncope: Fainting due to inadequate blood flow to the brain.

Therapeutic environment: An environment, both at the level of the resident's proximal space and the institution in general, that's supportive of delivering quality activity programming.

Tinnitus: A perception of a ringing or tinkling sound (typically) in the ear, without the presence of an acoustic stimulus.

Transdisciplinary team: A team in which one member is chosen to be the primary leader who is responsible for care delivery regardless of her or his discipline; other team members contribute information and recommendations.

Transgenerational, or life-span, design: Considers the changes individuals experience as they age (Story, 1998).

Typical illness trajectories: An attempt to categorize patterns that emerge during the end-of-life period, so that interventions can be created to match identified needs (Descried, et al., 2005).

Universal design: Is defined as "the design of products and environments that can be used and experienced by people of all ages and abilities, to the greatest extent possible, without adaptation" (Story, 1998, p. 4).

Useful field of view (UFOV): The spatial area within which an individual can be quickly alerted to visual stimuli in a variety of situations (Keplinger, 1998).

Validity: The extent to which an instrument or procedure measures the construct that it purports to measure.

Vasocongestion: The increased amount of blood concentration in body tissues that occurs during sexual arousal.

Velocity: Distance divided by the time (speed). A measure of a body's motion in a given direction.

Visual Acuity: A measure of the clarity of one's vision which can be defined as the ability to distinguish the details of an object and resolve its spatial properties at various distances (Strano, 1989; Warren, 1993a; Warren, 1993b; Zoltan, 1996).

Visual attention: Ability required to shift the focus of vision efficiently from one stimulus to another (Warren, 1993a; Warren, 1993b; Warren, 2006).

Volunteerism: Provision of service in community settings without commensurate financial remuneration for the benefit of individuals, groups, or organizations.

Wellness: The individual's perception of physical and psychological well-being characterized by adequate physical capacity for accomplishment of desired activities, coupled with overall satisfaction with one's life situation (Gallup, 1999).

Working memory: Can be thought of as simultaneously holding information in mind (storage) and using that information to perform a task (processing).

Index